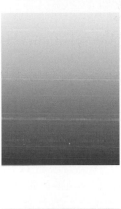

Basic Pathology

Basic Pathology

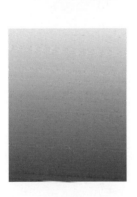

VINAY KUMAR, MD
Charles T. Ashworth Professor of Pathology
Southwestern Medical School
Southwestern Medical Center at Dallas
The University of Texas
Dallas, Texas

RAMZI S. COTRAN, MD
Frank Burr Mallory Professor of Pathology
Harvard Medical School
Chairman, Department of Pathology
Brigham and Women's Hospital
Boston, Massachusetts

STANLEY L. ROBBINS, MD
Visiting Professor of Pathology
Harvard Medical School
Senior Pathologist, Brigham and Women's Hospital
Boston, Massachusetts

fifth edition

W.B. SAUNDERS COMPANY
Harcourt Brace Jovanovich, Inc.
Philadelphia
London   Toronto   Montreal   Sydney   Tokyo

W. B. SAUNDERS COMPANY
Harcourt Brace Jovanovich, Inc.

The Curtis Center
Independence Square West
Philadelphia, Pennsylvania 19106

Library of Congress Cataloging-in-Publication Data

Kumar, Vinay.
    Basic pathology / Vinay Kumar, Ramzi S. Cotran, Stanley L. Robbins. 5th ed.
      p.   cm.
    Robbins' name appears first on earlier editions.
    Includes bibliographical references and index.

    ISBN 0-7216-3732-9

    1. Pathology.   I. Cotran, Ramzi S.   II. Robbins, Stanley L. (Stanley Leonard).
III. Title.
    [DNLM: 1. Pathology.   QZ 4 K955b]
RB111.K895   1992
616.07 — dc20
DNLM/DLC   92-3578

Editor: Jennifer Mitchell
Designer: Ellen Bodner-Zanolle
Production Manager: Peter Faber
Manuscript Editor: Lorraine Zawodny and Suzanne Enright
Illustration Specialist: Lisa Lambert

Listed here is the latest translated edition of this book together with the language of the translation and the publisher. 5/5/91, 4th edition, Spanish, Nueva Editorial Interamericana S.A., Mexico City, Mexico.

Listed here is the latest translated edition of this book together with the language of the translation and the publisher. 1/22/91, 4th edition, Vol II, Japanese, Hirokawa Publishing Company, Tokyo, Japan.

Listed here is the latest translated edition of this book together with the language of the translation and the publisher. 5/21/90, 4th edition, Volume 1, Japanese, Hirokawa Publishing Company, Tokyo, Japan.

Listed here is the latest translated edition of this book together with the language of the translation and the publisher. 3/20/91, 4th edition, Spanish, Nueva Editorial Interamericana S.A. de C.V., Mexico City, Mexico.

Listed here is the latest translated edition of this book together with the language of the translation and the publisher. 3/20/91, 4th edition, Turkish, Gunes Bookshops and Publishing Ltd. Co., Ankara, Turkey.

BASIC PATHOLOGY, Fifth Edition   ISBN 0-7216-3732-9

Last digit is the print number: 9   8   7   6   5   4   3   2

VINAY KUMAR AND RAMZI COTRAN
DEDICATE THIS BOOK TO
THEIR FRIEND AND COLLEAGUE,
STANLEY L. ROBBINS,
FOR A LIFETIME OF DEVOTION TO
THE TEACHING OF PATHOLOGY

Preface

How different is this edition from the previous one? Only the pages will prove, but we can say that extensive revision was dictated not by our compulsion to tamper but the need to incorporate the rapid advances in the understanding of diseases at the molecular level. Few areas of pathology have remained untouched by the new biology. Witness the advances that have been made into the molecular bases of cell injury, inflammation, carcinogenesis, and immune responses, to name a few. To introduce the new information without encroaching on the space devoted to basic concepts and classic morphologic descriptions was a challenge that necessitated several changes. Because regulation of cell growth and the interaction of cells with the extracellular matrix is central to the understanding of physiologic and neoplastic proliferations, we believed it was possible and desirable to draw together the biochemical and molecular events in cell proliferation into a single new chapter, Repair: Cell Growth, Regeneration, and Wound Healing (Chapter 3). The discussion in this chapter sets the stage for the subsequent discussion of oncogenes and cancer suppressor genes in Chapter 7, Neoplasia. To provide a more cohesive discussion of the basic and clinical aspects of tumors, the previous edition's two chapters on neoplasia have been combined into one. Another addition is Chapter 9, The Response to Infection. It highlights the host-parasite interactions so as to provide the student with a firm basis for the understanding of specific infectious diseases that are discussed throughout the text.

To accommodate these two new chapters without increasing the size of the book, we elected to consolidate environmental diseases and nutritional disorders into a single chapter and to delete the chapter on dental diseases. The latter change was motivated in part by the belief that dental students usually need greater details of dental pathology than can be reasonably accommodated in a general textbook. We have elected to provide shorter bibliographies on the grounds that *Basic Pathology* is not a reference text. The articles included in the reference lists are up-to-the-minute reviews or major papers on important subjects. For those interested, these readings should be helpful guides to more detailed listings of primary articles.

Encouraged by the positive response to the introduction of schematic illustrations and flow charts in the previous edition, we have expanded their use and have added a second color to enhance their clarity. Once again, to restrict the size of the text, care was taken to add only those figures that we believed would significantly enhance understanding. A major effort was also undertaken to replace old photographs with new, more crisp illustrations.

Despite the extensive changes and revisions, our goals remain substantially unaltered. We have strived to provide a balanced and accurate picture of the central body of knowledge of pathology. To the extent possible, we have attempted to correlate structural changes, be they subcellular or macroscopic, to clinical manifestations. And finally, we retain our conviction that a student text should not be merely an ornament on the bookshelf but should actually be read, and with pleasure. Judging by the reception accorded the previous editions, we are led to believe that our philosophy has been widely accepted, for which we are grateful; we only hope that the present edition will be a worthy successor to its forebears.

Acknowledgments

It is a great pleasure to acknowledge the help of many individuals without whose help this book could not have been written. First and foremost we are indebted to our personal editorial assistants: Ms. Beverly Shackelford, Ms. Debbie Watts, and Ms. Robyn Arndt (VK), Ms. Cathleen Curtin (RC), and Ms. Robin Lee (SR). For Beverly, this was not merely a project, but a special crusade to which she gave her ultimate effort and attention. There is no aspect of this book in which she was not involved, from researching the literature to the subtle art of choosing between "which" and "that" in a given sentence. Debbie (in Dallas) typed manuscript with single-minded devotion, and cheerfully accepted the fact that even the most "final" of the final drafts was not really final until it was in the hands of the editor in Philadelphia. Cathy and Robin (in Boston) were no less vital to this text. They conducted literature searches, typed and edited manuscript, and organized the seemingly endless "bits and pieces" that go into the preparation of a large manuscript. To all, our sincere thanks.

Special thanks are owed to Ms. Lynne Waltman, Ms. Marcia Williams, Mr. Jerry Tyson, and Mr. Robert Rubin. Lynne, whose art first appeared on the pages of *Robbins Pathologic Basis of Disease,* has continued to work with one of us (VK). Marcia created the new artwork for the Boston-based authors (RC and SR). Bob and Jerry are responsible for many of the excellent new photographs. We owe thanks to all of them for their many contributions.

Our contributors deserve special mention for their willingness to lend their expertise, time, and effort in revising some chapters. Dr. Mary Lipscomb (Professor of Pathology, Southwestern Medical School, Dallas) bore the major burden by rewriting the chapters Environmental Diseases, The Respiratory System, and The Liver and the Biliary Tract. Drs. John Samuelson (Assistant Professor, Department of Tropical Health, Harvard School of Public Health, Boston) and Arlene Sharpe (Assistant Professor of Pathology, Harvard Medical School, Boston) wrote the new chapter The Response to Infection. Dr. James Morris (Head of Neuropathology, The Radcliffe Infirmary, Oxford, England) revised his chapter The Nervous System. To each one we are deeply indebted.

Many colleagues helped by providing illustrative material and by offering helpful critiques. All those who gave us choice photographs have been acknowledged in the credits attached to their contribution(s). For any unintended omissions, our deepest apologies. Several of these benefactors deserve particular thanks (in alphabetical order): Dr. David Bloom (Brigham and Women's Hospital) for providing CT scans of pituitary adenomas; Dr. Dennis Burns (University of Texas, Southwestern Medical School) for providing several new illustrations and helpful comments for many chapters; Dr. Matthew Frosch (Brigham and Women's Hospital) for illustrations and expert critical analysis of CNS diseases; Dr. Jose Hernandez (University of Texas, Southwestern Medical School) for reviewing the sections relating to hematopoietic disorders; Dr. Eva Horvath for offering us gem-quality electron micrographs of pituitary lesions, Dr. Merle Legg (New England Deaconess Hospital) for the many illustrations of thyroid lesions; and Dr. Franz von Lichtenberg (Brigham and Women's Hospital) for the incorporation into the chapter The Responses to Infection of selected segments of text and illustrations from his chapter Infectious Disease in *Robbins Pathologic Basis of Disease,* 4th ed. We are grateful to Drs. Donald Ingber and Tucker Collins (Brigham and Women's Hospital) for critical review of the new chapter on cell growth, and to Dr. Merton Bernfield (Brigham and Women's Hospital) for use of syllabus material on the extracellular matrix. We also thank Drs. Christopher Crum and Helmut Rennke (at Brigham and Women's Hospital) and Drs. Charles Petty, Nancy Schneider, John Weissler, and Donald Wheeler (at the University of Texas, Southwestern Medical School) for helpful suggestions and critiques of the text in areas of their special expertise, and last but not least Dr. Mark Flomenbaum (Brigham and Women's Hospital) for graciously lending a hand whenever needed.

Many at W.B. Saunders deserve recognition for their unfailing support and encouragement, well beyond their professional obligations. Chief among them (in no particular order) are Ms. Jennifer Mitchell (editor), Ms. Lorraine Zawodny (copy editor), Mr. Peter Faber (production manager), Ms. Ellen Bodner-Zanolle (designer), Ms. Lisa Lambert (illustration coordinator), Mr. Richard Zorab (former editor), and Mr. Lew Reines, the president of W.B. Saunders. To all of these and to the undoubtedly numerous unsung heroes, our grateful thanks.

We would be remiss if we failed to acknowledge our families. For their tolerance of our absences, physically and emotionally, for their freely offered encouragement, and for their faith in us and our task, many, many thanks.

Finally, VK and SR wish to publicly acknowledge and welcome Dr. Ramzi Cotran, who came aboard as a coauthor with this edition. It was only natural that Dr. Cotran, senior author of *Robbins Pathologic Basis of Disease* ("big Robbins"), join the team for *Basic Pathology*. His well-known pursuit of excellence and dedication to the teaching of pathology will be readily apparent in this revision.

Contents

1

GENERAL PATHOLOGY

ONE
Cell Injury and Adaptation 3

TWO
Acute and Chronic Inflammation 25

THREE
Repair: Cell Growth, Regeneration, and Wound Healing ....[Repair].......... 47

FOUR
Disorders of Vascular Flow and Shock 61

FIVE
Genetic Diseases 83

SIX
Disorders of the Immune System 117

SEVEN
Neoplasia 171

EIGHT
Environmental Diseases 217
MARY F. LIPSCOMB, M.D.

NINE
The Response to Infection 261
JOHN C. SAMUELSON, M.D., Ph.D.
ARLENE SHARPE, M.D., Ph.D.

2 _____

DISEASES OF ORGAN SYSTEMS

TEN
Diseases of Blood Vessels.. 277

ELEVEN
The Heart 305

TWELVE
The Hematopoietic and Lymphoid Systems............................... 333

THIRTEEN
The Respiratory System.. 385
MARY F. LIPSCOMB, M.D.

FOURTEEN
The Kidney and Its Collecting System 437

FIFTEEN
The Gastrointestinal Tract 473

SIXTEEN
The Liver and the Biliary Tract 523
MARY F. LIPSCOMB, M.D.

SEVENTEEN
The Pancreas 569

EIGHTEEN
The Male Genital System 589

NINETEEN
The Female Genital System and the Breast............................. 607

TWENTY
Diseases of the Endocrine System 643

TWENTY-ONE
The Musculoskeletal System 681

TWENTY-TWO
The Nervous System 705
JAMES H. MORRIS, M.A., D.Phil., B.M., B.Ch.

Index.. 737

1

GENERAL
PATHOLOGY

ONE

Cell Injury and Adaptation

DEFINITIONS
CAUSES OF CELL INJURY
MECHANISMS OF CELL INJURY
    Ischemic and Hypoxic Injury
    Free Radical Mediation of Cell Injury
    Chemical Injury
    Other Examples of Free Radical Injury
    Cellular Aging
MORPHOLOGY OF CELL INJURY
    Patterns of Acute Cell Injury
        Reversible Injury
        Necrosis
        Apoptosis
SUBCELLULAR RESPONSES TO INJURY
LYSOSOMES: HETEROPHAGY AND
AUTOPHAGY
INDUCTION (HYPERTROPHY) OF SMOOTH
ENDOPLASMIC RETICULUM
MITOCHONDRIAL ALTERATIONS
CYTOSKELETAL LESIONS
INTRACELLULAR ACCUMULATIONS
    Lipids
        Fatty Change
        Cholesterol and Cholesterol Esters
    Other Intracellular Accumulations
        Proteins
        Glycogen
        Complex Lipids and Carbohydrates
        Pigments
CELLULAR ADAPTATIONS OF GROWTH
AND DIFFERENTIATION
    Atrophy
    Hypertrophy
    Hyperplasia
    Metaplasia
PATHOLOGIC CALCIFICATION
    Dystrophic Calcification
    Metastatic Calcification

DEFINITIONS

Modern pathology is both a science and a clinical practice. As a science it focuses on the mechanisms by which cells, tissues, and organs are injured and on the structural changes that underlie disease processes. The clinical practice of pathology involves the use of molecular, microbiological, immunologic and morphologic techniques on cells, tissues, and fluids to establish the diagnosis and guide therapy of disease.

All forms of tissue injury start with molecular or structural alterations in cells. It is necessary then to begin our consideration of pathology with an examination of disease at the cellular and subcellular levels.

The normal cell is a restless, pulsating microcosm, constantly modifying its structure and function in response to changing demands and stresses. Until these stresses become too severe, the cell tends to maintain a relatively narrow range of structure and function, so-called _normal homeostasis_. If the cell encounters excessive physiologic stresses or certain pathologic stimuli, it can undergo _adaptation,_ achieving an altered but steady state while preserving the health of the cell despite continued stress. The principal cellular adaptations are _atrophy, hypertrophy,_ and _hyperplasia,_ which are discussed later in this chapter. If no adaptive response is possible or the cell's adaptive capability is exceeded, _cell injury_ develops. Cell injury is _reversible_ up to a certain point, but with severe or persistent stress, the cell suffers _irreversible_ injury and is fated to die.

We can draw an analogy to a stately tree exposed to a wind storm. Up to a point, the tree bends and yields to the wind but rapidly resumes its erectness when the stresses abate. More severe wind may break branches and strip leaves, but such injury is compatible with recovery and survival. A hurricane, however, may be more than the tree can withstand and leaves the tree an uprooted victim of stresses too great for survival.

The relationships among normal, adapted, and reversibly and irreversibly injured cells as exemplified in heart muscle are shown in Figure 1–1. A myocardial fiber subjected to persistent increased load, such as occurs in hypertension, adapts by undergoing _hypertrophy_—an increase in size—sufficient to pump against an increased load. The same fiber, subjected to ischemia caused by coronary artery occlusion, may be either reversibly injured if the occlusion is incomplete and of brief duration or may undergo irreversible injury if the occlusion is complete and prolonged.

The most common morphologic pattern of cell death is _coagulative necrosis,_ manifested by denatura-

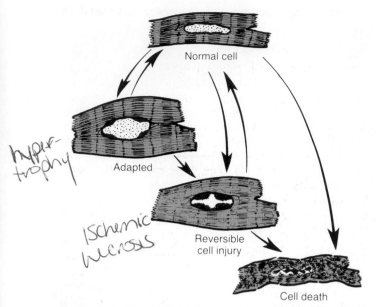

hyper-trophy

Ischemic necrosis

Figure 1–1. The relationships among normal, adapted, reversibly injured, and dead myocardial cells. The cellular adaptation depicted here is hypertrophy, and the type of cellular injury is ischemic necrosis.

tion of cytoplasmic protein and breakdown of cell organelles. A second and distinctive pattern, recently shown to underlie cell death in several important physiologic and pathologic processes, is called *apoptosis* (derived from the Greek for "dropping off"). Its chief morphologic features are chromatin condensation and fragmentation, and the mechanisms by which apoptosis is induced differ from those of necrosis, as we shall see (p. 14).

Whether a specific form of stress induces adaptation or causes reversible or irreversible injury and the morphologic pattern that results depends not only on the nature and severity of the stress but also on many variables relating to the cells themselves, such as particular vulnerability, differentiation, blood supply, nutrition, and previous state of the cell.

All stresses and noxious influences exert their effects first at the molecular level. The time lag required to produce the morphologic changes of cellular adaptation, injury, or death varies with the discriminatory ability of the methods used to detect these changes. With histochemical or ultrastructural techniques, changes can be seen in minutes or hours, but it may be much longer before they become evident with the light microscope or on gross examination of the tissue.

The following sections consider first the broad categories of stresses and noxious influences that induce reversible injury, cell death, and adaptation; then each of these three states is taken up individually.

CAUSES OF CELL INJURY GCHIPMAN!

The stresses that induce altered morphologic states in the cell range from the gross physical violence of a

crushing blow to the single gene defect that underlies many metabolic diseases. The broad categories of causes of cell injury and adaptations include (1) hypoxia, (2) chemicals and drugs, (3) physical agents, (4) microbiological agents, (5) immune mechanisms, (6) genetic defects, (7) nutritional imbalances, and (8) aging.

HYPOXIA. Hypoxia, an extremely important and common cause of cell injury and cell death, impinges on aerobic oxidative respiration. Hypoxia follows (1) loss of blood supply (ischemia) when the arterial flow or the venous drainage is impeded by vascular disease or thrombi; this is the most common cause of hypoxia; (2) inadequate oxygenation of the blood owing to cardiorespiratory failure; and (3) loss of the oxygen-carrying *capacity* of the blood, as in anemia or carbon monoxide poisoning (producing a stable carbon monoxyhemoglobin that blocks oxygen transport).

CHEMICALS AND DRUGS. Chemicals and drugs are important causes of cell adaptation, injury, and death. Virtually any chemical agent or drug may be implicated. Even an innocuous substance such as glucose, if sufficiently concentrated, may so derange the osmotic environment of the cell that it causes injury or cell death. Agents commonly known as poisons may cause severe cell damage and possibly death of the whole organism. Many of these chemicals and drugs effect their changes by acting on some vital function of the cell, such as membrane permeability, osmotic homeostasis, or the integrity of an enzyme or cofactor.

PHYSICAL AGENTS. Trauma, extremes of heat or cold, sudden changes in atmospheric pressure, radiant energy, and electrical energy all have wide-ranging effects on cells. These effects are discussed in Chapter 8 (Environmental Diseases).

MICROBIOLOGIC AGENTS. These agents range from the submicroscopic viruses to the large tapeworms. In between are the rickettsiae, bacteria, fungi, and higher forms of parasites. The ways by which biologic agents cause injury are diverse and are discussed in Chapter 9.

IMMUNOLOGIC REACTIONS. Although the immune system serves in the defense against biologic agents, immune reactions may, in fact, cause cell injury. The anaphylactic reaction to a foreign protein is a prime example, and reactions to endogenous self-antigens are thought to be responsible for autoimmune diseases (see Chapter 6).

GENETIC DEFECTS. Genetic injury may result in gross defects, such as the congenital malformations associated with Down's syndrome, or in subtle alterations in protein structure, such as the production of hemoglobin S in sickle cell anemia. The major genetic abnormalities are discussed in Chapter 5.

NUTRITIONAL IMBALANCES. It is sad to report that deficiencies in nutrition not only are important causes of cell injury today but threaten to become devastating problems in the future. Protein-calorie deficiencies among underprivileged populations are the most obvious examples. Avitaminoses are also rampant in deprived groups and are not uncommon even in industrialized nations having relatively high standards of living. Ironically, excesses in nutrition are also important causes of morbidity and mortality. Diets rich in animal _fats_ are strongly implicated in atherosclerosis and obesity and increase vulnerability to many disorders.

AGING. The mechanisms of cellular adaptations and injury in aging cells are discussed on page 10.

MECHANISMS OF CELL INJURY

The problem of unraveling the molecular sequence of events responsible for cell injury has proved to be immensely complex. Injury to cells may have many causes, and there is probably no common final pathway of cell death. The many macromolecules, enzymes, and organelles within the cell are so closely interdependent that it is difficult to differentiate the primary target of injury from the secondary ripple effects. The "point of no return," i.e., the point at which irreversible damage and cell death occur, is still largely undetermined.

With certain injurious agents, the mechanisms and loci of attack are well defined. Cyanide represents an intracellular asphyxiant in that it inactivates cytochrome oxidase. Certain anaerobic bacteria, such as _Clostridium perfringens_, elaborate phospholipases, which attack phospholipids in cell membranes. Other isolated examples exist, but the modes of action of many injurious agents are more complex. Oxygen, however, plays a central role in cell injury (Fig. 1–2). Lack of oxygen clearly underlies the pathogenesis of cell injury in ischemia, but in addition _partially reduced activated oxygen species are important mediators of cell death_ in many pathologic conditions. As we shall see, these free radical species cause lipid peroxidation and other deleterious effects on cell structure. In the following account we concentrate on hypoxic injury, injury induced by free radicals, and certain forms of chemical injury as model systems. Cell injury induced by bacteria and viruses is discussed in Chapter 9.

ISCHEMIC AND HYPOXIC INJURY

The sequence of events following acute hypoxic injury has been studied extensively in humans, experimental animals, and culture systems. Here we review the mechanisms underlying these events (Fig. 1–3) and the ultrastructural changes in reversible and irreversible injury (Fig. 1–4). The latter precede the alterations seen with the light microscope.

REVERSIBLE INJURY. _The first point of attack of hypoxia is the cell's aerobic respiration, i.e., oxidative phosphorylation by mitochondria._ The generation of adenosine triphosphate (ATP) thus slows down or stops. This loss of ATP has widespread effects on many systems within the cell. In particular, the activity of the ouabain-sensitive adenosinetriphosphatase (ATPase) of the cell membrane is decreased, causing failure of the active membrane "sodium pump," accumulation of sodium intracellularly, and diffusion of potassium out of the cell. The net gain of solute is accompanied by an iso-osmotic gain of water, producing _acute cellular swelling._

The decrease in cellular ATP and associated increase in adenosine monophosphate (AMP) also stimulate the enzyme phosphofructokinase, which results in an increased rate of anaerobic glycolysis to maintain the cell's energy sources by generating ATP from glycogen. Glycogen is thus rapidly depleted, a phenomenon that can be appreciated histologically if tissues are stained for glycogen (such as with the periodic acid–Schiff stain [PAS]). Glycolysis results in the accumulation of lactic acid and inorganic phosphates from the hydrolysis of phosphate esters. _This reduces the intracellular pH._

The next phenomenon to occur is _detachment of ribosomes from the granular endoplasmic reticulum and dissociation of polysomes into monosomes._ If hypoxia continues, other alterations take place and, again, are reflections of increased membrane permeability and diminished mitochondrial function. _Blebs may form at the cell surface._ "Myelin figures" (concentric laminations), derived from the plasma as well as organellar membranes, are seen within the cytoplasm or extracellularly. At this time the mitochondria appear normal, slightly swollen, or actually condensed; the endoplasmic reticulum is dilated; and the entire cell is markedly swollen.

All the above disturbances are reversible if oxygenation is restored. However, if ischemia persists, irreversible injury ensues.

IRREVERSIBLE INJURY. Irreversible injury is associated morphologically with severe vacuolization of the mitochondria, including their cristae; extensive damage to plasma membranes; swelling of lysosomes; and particularly if the ischemic zone is reperfused—massive _calcium influx_ into the cell. _Amorphous, calcium-rich densities develop in the mitochondrial matrix._ In the myocardium, these are early indications

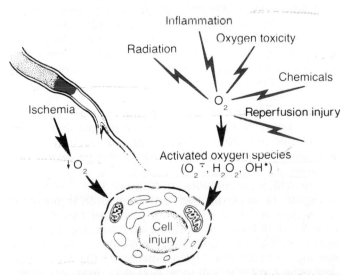

Inflammation
Oxygen toxicity
Radiation
Chemicals
O_2
Ischemia
Reperfusion injury
$\downarrow O_2$
Activated oxygen species
$(O_2^-, H_2O_2, OH^\bullet)$
Cell injury

Figure 1–2. The critical role of oxygen in cell injury. Ischemia causes cell injury by reducing cellular oxygen supplies, whereas other stimuli, such as radiation, induce damage via toxic activated oxygen species.

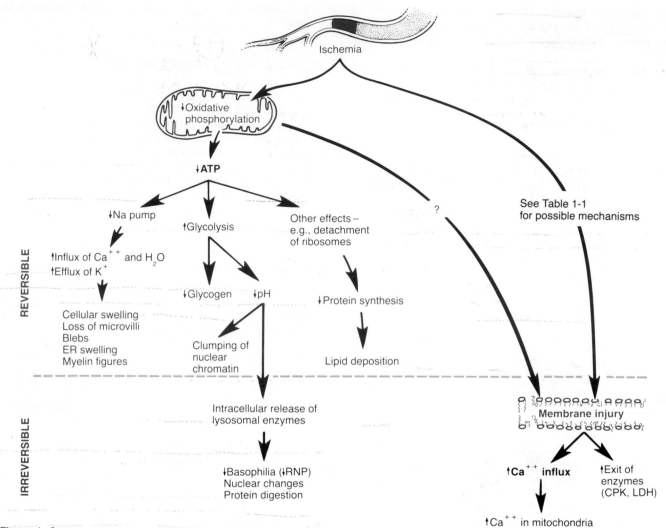

Figure 1-3. Postulated sequence of events in ischemic injury. Note that although reduced oxidative phosphorylation and ATP levels have a central role, ischemia causes direct membrane damage by mechanisms outlined in Table 1-1.

of irreversible injury and can be seen as soon as 30 to 40 minutes after ischemia. There is continued loss of proteins, essential coenzymes, and ribonucleic acids from the hyperpermeable membranes. The cells may also leak metabolites, which are vital for the reconstitution of ATP, thus further depleting net intracellular high-energy phosphates.

The falling pH leads to injury to the lysosomal membranes, followed by leakage of their enzymes into the cytoplasm, activation of acid hydrolases, and enzymatic digestion of cytoplasmic and nuclear components.

Following cell death, cell organelles are progressively degraded, and there is leakage of cellular enzymes into the extracellular space and, conversely, entry of extracellular macromolecules from the interstitial space into the dead cell. Finally, the dead cell may become replaced by large masses, composed of phospholipids, in the form of "myelin figures." These are then either phagocytosed by other cells or degraded further into fatty acids. _Calcification_ of such fatty acid residues may occur with the formation of calcium soaps.

Mechanisms of Irreversible Injury. The sequence of events for hypoxia was described as a continuum from its initiation to ultimate digestion of the lethally injured cell by lysosomal enzymes. But at what point did the cell actually die? _And what are the critical events in irreversible injury?_ Two phenomena consistently characterize irreversibility. The first is the _inability to reverse mitochondrial dysfunction_ (lack of oxidative phosphorylation and ATP generation) upon reperfusion or reoxygenation, and the second is the development of _profound disturbances in membrane function._

It would be reasonable to consider that progressive depletion of ATP in itself at some critical juncture constitutes a lethal event, but the evidence on this issue is conflicting. Although numerous alterations in mitochondrial structure and function are found in ischemic tissues, it has been possible experimentally to dissociate these changes as well as ATP depletion from the inevitability of cell death.

A great deal of evidence favors cell membrane damage as a central factor in the pathogenesis of irrevers-

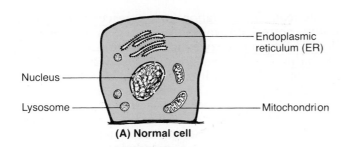

(A) Normal cell

Nucleus

Lysosome

Endoplasmic reticulum (ER)

Mitochondrion

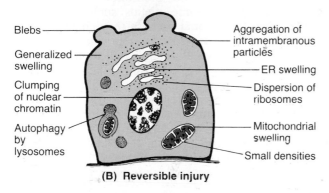

Blebs

Generalized swelling

Clumping of nuclear chromatin

Autophagy by lysosomes

Aggregation of intramembranous particles

ER swelling

Dispersion of ribosomes

Mitochondrial swelling

Small densities

(B) Reversible injury

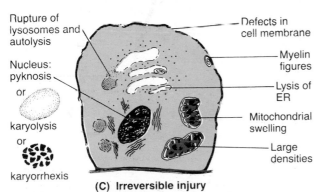

Rupture of lysosomes and autolysis

Nucleus: pyknosis

or

karyolysis

or

karyorrhexis

Defects in cell membrane

Myelin figures

Lysis of ER

Mitochondrial swelling

Large densities

(C) Irreversible injury

Figure 1–4. Schematic representation of the ultrastructural changes in reversible (*B*) and irreversible (*C*) cell injury (see text).

ible cell injury. Loss of volume regulation, increased permeability to extracellular molecules such as inulin, and demonstrable plasma membrane ultrastructural defects occur in the earliest stages of irreversible injury.

At least four potential causes have been implicated in the induction of membrane damage, and all may play a role (Table 1–1).

1. *Progressive loss of membrane phospholipids.* In ischemic liver, irreversible injury is associated with a marked decrease in the content of membrane phos-

pholipids. One explanation for phospholipid loss may be increased phospholipid degradation due to activation of endogenous phospholipases by the increased cytosolic calcium concentration induced by ischemia. Oxygen deprivation is known to release calcium sequestered in mitochondria and endoplasmic reticulum, thus raising cytosolic calcium. Progressive phospholipid loss can also presumably occur owing to decreased ATP-dependent reacylation or de novo synthesis of phospholipids.

2. *Cytoskeletal abnormalities.* In the presence of cell swelling, which occurs in ischemia, damage to the cytoskeleton may result in detachment of the cell membrane from the cytoskeleton, rendering the membrane susceptible to stretching and rupture. A potential mechanism in cytoskeletal protein degradation is the activation of intracellular *proteases*, possibly induced by increased cytosolic calcium.

3. *Toxic oxygen radicals.* As discussed later, partially reduced oxygen species are highly toxic molecules, which cause injury to cell membranes and other cell constituents. Such oxygen radicals are increased in ischemic tissues *upon restoration of blood flow* and may be the cause of the so-called *reperfusion injury. The toxic oxygen species are thought to be produced largely by polymorphonuclear leukocytes that infiltrate the site of ischemia during reperfusion.* If reperfusion does not occur, lethal ischemic cell injury will still eventually ensue, but toxic oxygen species are not involved.

4. *Lipid breakdown products.* These catabolic products accumulate in ischemic cells as a result of phospholipid degradation and have a detergent effect on membranes. *massive influx of Ca²⁺*

Whatever the mechanism(s) of membrane injury, the resultant loss of membrane integrity causes further influx of calcium from the extracellular space, where it is present in high concentrations ($>10^{-3}$ M), into the cells. When, in addition, the ischemic tissue is reperfused to some extent, as may occur in vivo, the scene is set for massive influx of calcium. The role of this calcium influx in determining irreversibility is controversial. However, calcium is taken up avidly by mitochondria after reoxygenation and permanently poisons them, inhibits cellular enzymes, denatures proteins, and causes the cytologic alterations characteristic of coagulative necrosis.

To summarize, *hypoxia affects the oxidative phosphorylation and hence the synthesis of vital ATP supplies; membrane damage is critical to the development of lethal cell injury; and calcium is a potential mediator of the morphologic alterations in cell death.*

FREE RADICAL MEDIATION OF CELL INJURY

One important mechanism of cell damage, already alluded to in the discussion of ischemic reperfusion, is injury induced by free radicals, particularly by acti-

TABLE 1–1. POTENTIAL MECHANISMS OF MEMBRANE INJURY

Loss of membrane phospholipids
   Increased degradation
   Decreased synthesis
Cytoskeletal alterations
Toxic oxygen radicals
Lipid breakdown products

vated oxygen species. Free radical injury is emerging as a final common pathway of tissue damage in such varied processes as chemical and radiation injury, oxygen and other gaseous toxicity, cellular aging, microbial killing by phagocytic cells, inflammatory damage, tumor destruction by macrophages, and others (see Fig. 1–2).

What is a free radical? In most atoms, the electron orbitals are filled with paired electrons spinning in opposite directions, thus canceling each other's physicochemical reactivity. A free radical is a chemical species that has a single unpaired electron in an outer orbital. In such a state the radical is extremely reactive and unstable and enters into reactions in cells with inorganic or organic chemicals—particularly with key molecules in membranes and nucleic acids. Moreover, free radicals initiate autocatalytic reactions whereby molecules with which they react are themselves converted into free radicals to thus propagate the chain of damage.

Radicals may be initiated within cells by the absorption of radiant energy (e.g., ultraviolet light, x-rays) or in the reduction-oxidation (redox) reactions that occur during normal physiologic processes, or they may be derived from the enzymatic metabolism of exogenous chemicals. Radiant energy may lyse water to release the radicals $OH\cdot$ (hydroxyl ion) and $H\cdot$. Another free radical is superoxide O_2^-, which is derived by reduction of molecular oxygen. Normally oxygen is reduced to water, but in some reactions involving oxidases (such as xanthine oxidase) in mitochondria, lysosomes, peroxisomes, and plasma membrane O_2^- may be formed (Fig. 1–5). Some metals such as iron and copper, called transitional because they change valency states, can accept or donate free electrons during transit and thereby catalyze free radical formation—the Fenton reaction ($Fe^{++} + H_2O_2 \rightarrow Fe^{+++} + OH\cdot + OH^-$). Iron is important in toxic oxygen injury, because the $OH\cdot$ generated is particularly toxic. However, most of the free iron is in the ferric (Fe^{+++}) form and has to be reduced to ferrous (Fe^{++}) form to be active in the Fenton reaction. This reduction is enhanced by superoxide ion, and thus *a source of iron and superoxide are required for maximal oxidative cell*

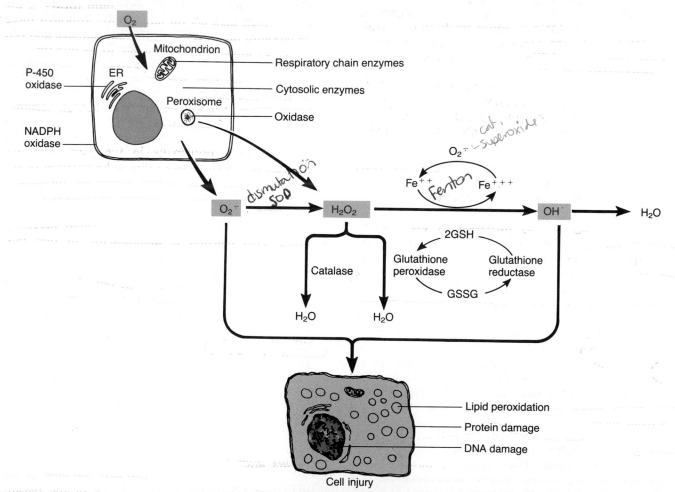

Figure 1–5. Formation of reactive oxygen species and anti-oxidant mechanisms in biologic systems. O_2 is converted to superoxide (O_2^-) by oxidative enzymes in the ER, mitochondria, plasma membrane, peroxisomes, and cytosol. O_2^- is converted to H_2O_2 by dismutation and thence to $OH\cdot$ by the Cu^{++}/Fe^{++} catalyzed Fenton reaction. H_2O_2 is also derived directly from oxidases in peroxisomes. Not shown is another potentially injurious radical, singlet oxygen. Resultant free radical damage to lipid (peroxidation), proteins, and DNA leads to various forms of cell injury. Note that superoxide catalyzes the reduction of Fe^{+++} to Fe^{++}, thus enhancing $OH\cdot$ generation by the Fenton reaction. The major antioxidant enzymes are SOD, catalase, and glutathione peroxidase.

injury. Certain exogenous chemicals such as CCl_4 can also be converted into free radicals, as will be discussed below.

The effects of these reactive species are wide-ranging, but four reactions are particularly relevant to cell injury.

1. *Lipid peroxidation of membranes.* Free radicals in the presence of oxygen may cause peroxidation of lipids within plasma and organellar membranes and damage endoplasmic reticulum, mitochondria, and other microsomal components. Polyunsaturated lipids, such as those in membranes, possess double bonds between some of the carbon atoms. Such bonds are vulnerable to attack by oxygen-derived free radicals. The lipid-radical interactions yield peroxides, which are themselves unstable and reactive, and an autocatalytic chain reaction ensues, resulting in extensive membrane, organellar, and cellular damage.

2. *Nonperoxidative mitochondrial damage.* This effect is not dependent on lipid peroxidation and results in loss of mitochondrial function, mimicking the effects of hypoxia on mitochondria.

3. *Lesions in deoxyribonucleic acid (DNA).* Reactions with thymine in DNA produce single-strand breaks in DNA, and such DNA damage has been implicated both in cell killing and in eventual malignant transformation of cells.

4. *Cross-linking of proteins.* Cross-linking of such labile amino acids as methionine, histidine, cystine, and lysine raises havoc throughout the cell, in particular inactivating enzymes, especially sulfhydryl enzymes.

Once free radicals are formed, how does the body get rid of them? They may spontaneously decay. Superoxide, for example, is unstable and decays automatically into oxygen and hydrogen peroxide. The rate of such decay is significantly increased by the catalytic action of *superoxide dismutases* (SOD) found in many cell types $(O_2^- + O_2^- + 2H \xrightarrow{+SOD} H_2O_2 + O_2)$. A number of other enzymes—*gluthatione peroxidase*, for example—also provide defense against free radicals $(2OH^{\cdot} + 2GHS \rightarrow 2H_2O + GSSG)$. *Catalase*, present in peroxisomes, decomposes H_2O_2 $(2H_2O_2 \rightarrow O_2 + 2H_2O)$ (see Fig. 1–5). From an evolutionary point of view such enzymes may have evolved to protect cells from free radical injury. Alternatively, endogenous or exogenous antioxidants—e.g., vitamin E; sulfhydryls such as cysteine or glutathione; and ceruloplasmin—may either block the initiation of free radicals or inactivate them.

In summary, the net potential for free radical injury flows from the balance between their initiation and their being scavenged. Thus cells are more or less vulnerable to free radical injury, depending on the presence and quantity of defensive enzymes and antioxidants that serve as protective mechanisms.

Although free radicals are discussed here mainly in the context of their damaging effects on tissues, it should be pointed out that free radicals are also utilized by phagocytic cells to kill ingested microbes (p.

32). This, then, is one of several examples whereby a given reaction can be beneficial or harmful to the integrity of the organism, depending on the context in which it occurs.

CHEMICAL INJURY

Chemicals induce cell injury by one of two mechanisms:

1. Some chemicals can act *directly* by combining with some critical molecular component or cellular organelle. For example, in *mercuric chloride poisoning,* mercury binds to the sulfhydryl groups of the cell membrane and other proteins, causing increased membrane permeability and inhibition of ATPase-dependent transport. Many antineoplastic chemotherapeutic agents and antibiotic drugs also induce cell damage by direct cytotoxic effects.

2. Most other toxic chemicals are not biologically active but must be converted to reactive toxic metabolites, usually by the P-450 mixed function oxidases in the smooth endoplasmic reticulum (SER) of the liver, which then act on target cells. Although these metabolites might cause membrane damage and cell injury by *direct covalent binding* to membrane protein and lipids, the most important mechanism of cell injury involves the formation of *reactive free radicals* and subsequent lipid peroxidation, as detailed earlier. Carbon tetrachloride (CCl_4), acetaminophen, and bromobenzene belong to this category. CCl_4, for example, is converted to the toxic free radical $CCl_3^{\cdot}$, principally in the liver. The free radicals produced locally cause autooxidation of the polyenoic fatty acids present within the membrane phospholipids. There, oxidative decomposition of the lipid is initiated, and organic peroxides are formed after reacting with oxygen (lipid peroxidation). This *reaction is autocatalytic* in that new radicals are formed from the peroxide radicals themselves. Thus, rapid breakdown of the structure and function of the endoplasmic reticulum is due to decomposition of the lipid. *It is no surprise, therefore, that CCl_4-induced liver cell injury is both severe and extremely rapid in onset.* Within less than 30 minutes there is a decline in hepatic protein synthesis of both plasma proteins and endogenous protein enzymes, and within 2 hours, swelling of SER and dissociation of ribosomes from the rough endoplasmic reticulum (RER) (Fig. 1–6). Accumulation of lipid then ensues, owing to the inability of cells to synthesize lipoprotein from triglycerides and "lipid acceptor protein." Mitochondrial injury occurs after injury to the endoplasmic reticulum, and this is followed by progressive swelling of the cells due to increased permeability of the plasma membrane. Plasma membrane damage is thought to be caused by relatively stable fatty aldehydes, which are produced by lipid peroxidation in the SER but are able to act at distant sites. This is followed by massive influx of calcium and cell death.

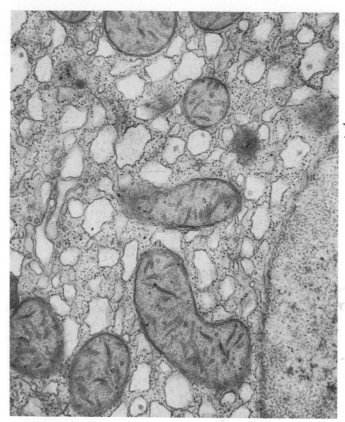

Figure 1-6. Rat liver cell after carbon tetrachloride intoxication, showing well-developed swelling of endoplasmic reticulum and shedding of ribosomes. Mitochondria at this stage are unaltered. (Courtesy of Dr. O. Iseri.)

OTHER EXAMPLES OF FREE RADICAL INJURY

RADIATION INJURY. This is an injury mediated by radiolysis of water, producing free radicals such as OH·, H·, and HOO·. These radicals may then interact with membranes, nucleic acids, or other key elements within the cell. Autocatalytic reactions are initiated that may ultimately result in the induction of mutations or the death of the cell.

OXYGEN TOXICITY. The lung is subject to injury when exposed to high concentrations of O_2. Free radical formation is believed to underlie the pulmonary changes of *oxygen toxicity* in patients requiring high-level oxygen inhalation therapy. Analogous changes may underlie the ocular injuries (retrolental fibroplasia) in newborns placed in incubators having high levels of oxygen.

INFLAMMATION AND ATHEROSCLEROSIS. Oxygen-derived reactive species, largely from leukocytes, are important mediators of cell injury in various types of inflammation (p. 38). Recent evidence also suggests that oxidized lipid products are important in the pathogenesis of atherosclerosis (p. 38).

AGING. The accumulation of injury caused by free radicals over the years may be responsible for certain aspects of *cellular aging.* Lipofuscin, a brownish-yellow granular intracellular pigment, accumulates in a variety of tissues (particularly the heart, liver and brain) as a function of age. The pigment represents complexes of lipid and protein that are derived from the peroxidation of polyunsaturated lipids of subcellular membranes.

CELLULAR AGING *Cont from p. 5*

Aging has many dimensions and can be characterized in many ways. Shakespeare probably did it best in his elegant description of the Seven Ages of Man. It begins at the moment of conception, involves the differentiation and maturation of the organism and its cells, at some variable point of time leads to the progressive loss of functional capacity characteristic of senescence, and ends in death. We discuss cellular aging here because it could represent the progressive accumulation over the years of alterations in structure and function that may lead to cell death or at the least diminished capacity of the cell to respond to injury.

A number of cell functions decline progressively with age. Oxidative phosphorylation by aged mitochondria is reduced, as is DNA and RNA synthesis of structural and enzymatic proteins and of cell receptors. Senescent cells have a decreased capacity for uptake of nutrients and for repair of chromosomal damage. The morphologic alterations in aging cells include irregular and abnormal lobed nuclei, pleomorphic vacuolated mitochondria, decreased endoplasmic reticulum, and distorted Golgi apparatus. Concomitantly, there is a steady accumulation of the pigment lipofuscin, which as described previously, represents a product of lipid peroxidation.

Several theories have been proposed to explain cellular aging (Fig. 1-7).

The *"wear and tear" group of theories* implies that the aging process in cells is the consequence of continual exposure throughout life to adverse exogenous influences leading to progressive encroachment on the cells' survivability. A favored scenario invokes the progressive effects of free radical damage throughout life. This damage can occur by repeated environmental exposure to such influences as ionizing radiation, to a progressive reduction of antioxidant defense mechanisms (e.g., vitamin E, glutathione peroxidase, etc.), or both. The accumulation of lipofuscin is consistent with free radical damage, but there is no evidence that the pigment itself is toxic to cells. A second wear and tear theory claims that posttranslational modifications of intracellular and extracellular proteins, which are known to occur with age, underlie the morphologic and functional changes in cell aging. One such modification is nonenzymatic glycosylation of proteins, leading to the formation of advanced glycosylation end products capable of cross-linking adjacent proteins. Such end products, as we shall see, play a role in the pathogenesis of diabetes. Age-related glycosylation of lens proteins underlies senile cataracts.

A second group of theories is the so-called genome-

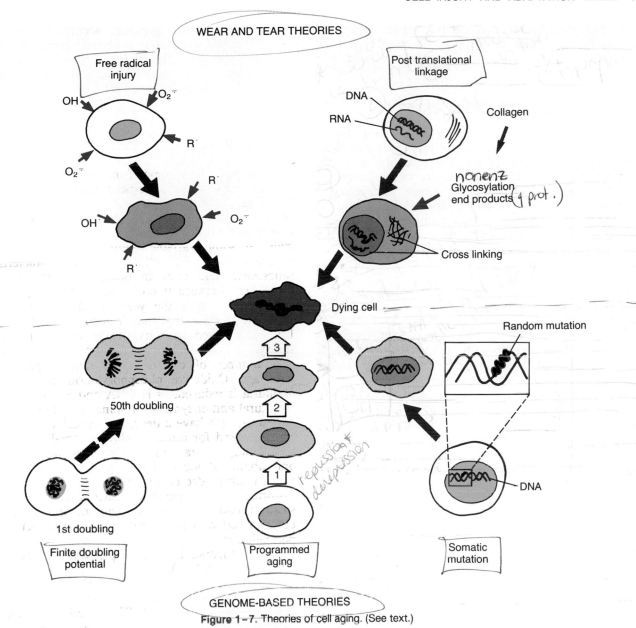

Figure 1-7. Theories of cell aging. (See text.)

based theories, which hold that progressive cellular damage occurs owing to intrinsic properties of cells determined by genetic factors.

- *The somatic mutation hypothesis* proposes that errors of DNA replication are not accurately repaired and will ultimately impinge on the viability and survivability of cells. Indeed, repair systems for DNA do slow in later life. However, although mutations are readily produced in cells by irradiation, these do not consistently affect lifespan.

- *The programmed aging hypothesis* assumes a predetermined sequence of events leading ultimately to senescence. Repression and derepression of genetic programs are presumably involved, explaining the orderly death of the anucleate squames that are shed from the epidermal surface of the skin and the programmed senescence terminating in the death of the Pacific salmon after spawning.

- *The finite cell replication hypothesis* proposes that cell aging is determined by a built-in genetic program of senescence that limits the doubling potential of cells. Normal cells in tissue culture undergo about fifty doublings, after which they stop dividing and become senescent. The significance of the limit to cell doublings, however, has been questioned, and it is not clear how this concept would apply to postmitotic cells, such as neurons or striated muscle cells.

Much more might be said about the mechanisms responsible for the cell alterations that occur in cell aging, but it suffices here to say that according to the present best evidence, some of these mechanisms are probably merely an extension of those involved in the maturation and differentiation of cells, and others are due to environmental influences that may interact with these mechanisms.

Against this background of the agents and their mediators that cause cell injury, we now turn to a description of the morphology of injured cells.

MORPHOLOGY OF CELL INJURY

The cellular morphologic changes induced by various stimuli can be divided into ① patterns of _acute cell injury_ discussed earlier—reversible and irreversible cell injury leading to _necrosis_ or _apoptosis,_ ② _subcellular alterations_ that occur largely as a response to more chronic or persistent injurious stimuli, and ③ _intracellular accumulations_ of a number of substances —lipids, carbohydrates, proteins—as a result of derangements in cell metabolism or excessive storage.

PATTERNS OF ACUTE CELL INJURY

Reversible Injury

In classic pathology, the morphologic changes resulting from nonlethal injury to cells were termed degenerations, but today they are more simply designated _reversible injuries._ Two patterns can be recognized under the light microscope: _cellular swelling_ and _fatty change._ Cellular swelling appears whenever cells are incapable of maintaining ionic and fluid homeostasis; its pathogenesis has been described earlier. _Fatty change,_ under some circumstances, may be another indicator of reversible cell injury. It is manifested by the appearance of small or large lipid vacuoles in the cytoplasm and occurs in hypoxic and various forms of toxic injury. It is a less universal reaction, principally encountered in cells involved in and dependent on fat metabolism, such as the hepatocyte and myocardial cell. Fatty change, particularly in the liver, can also be a manifestation of a number of metabolic derangements and is described further as a form of intracellular accumulation (p. 17).

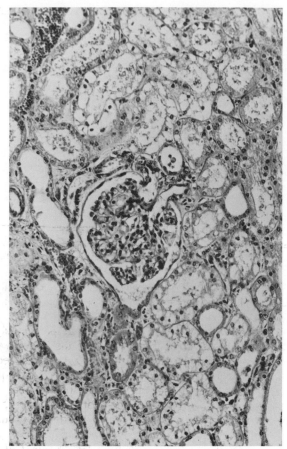

Figure 1–8. Swelling of renal tubular epithelial cells seen in the center field above and below the glomerulus. The cleared, vacuolated cells contain dark displaced nuclei, suggesting that the swelling has been followed by death of the cells.

pearance of phospholipid-rich amorphous densities; (3) **dilatation of the endoplasmic reticulum** with detachment and disaggregation of polysomes; and (4) **nucleolar** alterations, with disaggregation of granular and fibrillar elements.

Cellular swelling is the first manifestation of almost all forms of injury to cells. It is a difficult morphologic change to appreciate with the light microscope; it may be more apparent at the level of the whole organ. When if affects all cells in an organ, it causes some pallor, increased turgor, and increase in weight of the organ. Microscopically, small clear vacuoles may be seen within the cytoplasm. These vacuoles presumably represent distended and pinched-off or sequestered segments of the endoplasmic reticulum. This pattern of nonlethal injury is sometimes called **hydropic change** or **vacuolar degeneration** (Fig. 1–8).

The ultrastructural changes of reversible cell injury previously described (see Fig. 1–4B) include (1) **plasma membrane alterations** such as blebbing, blunting, and distortion of microvilli; creation of myelin figures; and loosening of intercellular attachments; (2) **mitochondrial changes,** including swelling, rarefaction, and the ap-

Necrosis

Cells can be recognized as dead with the light microscope only after they have undergone a sequence of morphologic changes. The most common (and until recently only) pattern of cell death recognized is _necrosis,_ caused by the _progressive degradative action of enzymes on the lethally injured cell._ Two essentially concurrent processes bring about the changes of necrosis: (1) enzymic digestion of the cell and (2) denaturation of proteins. The catalytic enzymes are derived either from the dying or dead cells themselves, in which case the enzymic digestion is referred to as _autolysis,_ or from the lysosomes of immigrant leukocytes, termed _heterolysis._ Depending on whether denaturation of proteins or enzymic digestion is ascendent, one of two quite distinctive patterns of cell necrosis develops. In the former instance, _coagulative necrosis_ develops. In the latter, progressive catalysis of cell structures leads to so-called *liquefactive necrosis.* Both of these processes require hours to develop and so there would be no detectable changes in cells if, for example, a myocardial infarct caused sudden death. The only telling evidence might be occlusion of a coronary artery.

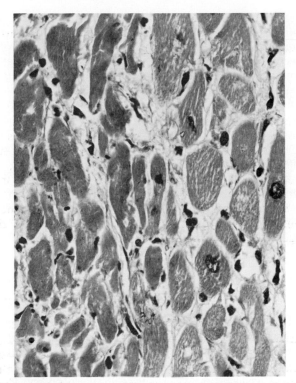

Figure 1–9. Myocardium, with preserved normal fibers on the right. The left half of the figure reveals coagulative necrosis of the fibers, with loss of nuclei and clumping of the cytoplasm but with preservation of basic outlines of the cells.

The necrotic cells show increased eosinophilia, attributable in part to the loss of normal basophilia imparted by the RNA in the cytoplasm and in part to the increased binding of eosin to denatured intracytoplasmic proteins. The cell may have a more glassy homogenous appearance than normal cells, due mainly to the loss of glycogen particles. When enzymes have digested the cytoplasmic organelles, the cytoplasm becomes vacuolated and appears moth-eaten. Finally, calcification of the dead cells may occur.

Nuclear changes also occur in sublethally and lethally injured cells. They appear in the form of one of three patterns (see Fig. 1–4C). The basophilia of the chromatin may fade **(karyolysis)**, a change that presumably reflects the activation of the DNAses as the pH of the cell drops. A second pattern is **pyknosis**, characterized by nuclear shrinkage and increased basophilia. Here the DNA apparently condenses into a solid, shrunken basophilic mass. In the third possible pattern, known as **karyorrhexis**, the pyknotic or partially pyknotic nucleus undergoes fragmentation. With the passage of time (a day or two), in one way or another the nucleus in the necrotic cell totally disappears.

Once the cell has died and has undergone the early alterations described above, one of three distinctive sequences ensues. The mass of necrotic cells may undergo **coagulative necrosis, liquefactive necrosis,** or, in special circumstances, **caseous necrosis.**

Coagulative necrosis implies preservation of the basic outline of the coagulated cell for a span of at least some days. Presumably the injury or the subsequent increasing intracellular acidosis denatures not only structural proteins but also enzymic proteins and so blocks the proteolysis of the cell. **The process of coagulative necrosis is characteristic of hypoxic death of cells in all tissues save the brain.** The myocardial infarct is a prime example. Here, acidophilic, coagulated, anucleate cells persist for weeks (Fig. 1–9). Ultimately the necrotic myocardial cells are removed by fragmentation and phagocytosis of the cellular debris by scavenger white cells and by the action of proteolytic lysosomal enzymes brought in by the immigrant white cells.

Liquefactive necrosis resulting from autolysis or heterolysis is mainly characteristic of focal bacterial infections, since bacteria constitute powerful stimuli to the accumulation of white cells (Fig. 1–10). For obscure reasons, hypoxic death of cells within the central nervous system evokes liquefactive necrosis, yet hypoxic death of heart muscle cells, liver cells, kidney cells, and in fact most other cells in the body is followed by coagulative necrosis. Whatever the pathogenesis, liquefaction essentially digests the dead carcasses of cells and often leaves a tissue defect filled with immigrant leukocytes, creating an abscess.

Caseous necrosis, a distinctive form of coagulative necrosis, is encountered most often in foci of tubercu-

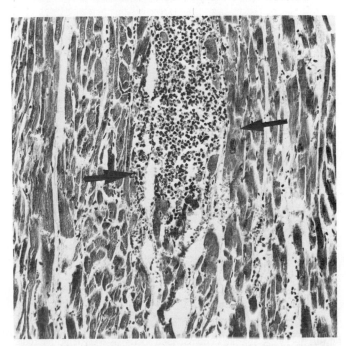

Figure 1–10. Liquefactive necrosis of a focus in the myocardium caused by bacterial seeding. The focus is filled with white cells, creating a myocardial abscess *(arrows).*

lous infection. The term "caseous" is derived from the gross appearance (white and cheesy) of the area of necrosis. Histologically the necrotic focus appears as amorphous granular debris seemingly composed of fragmented, coagulated cells enclosed within a distinctive inflammatory border known as a granulomatous reaction (p. 42). It is important to be able to recognize this morphologic pattern, because it is evoked by only a limited number of agents. Among these, tuberculosis is preeminent, as discussed in greater detail on page 416.

Enzymic fat necrosis is a term that is well fixed in medical parlance but does not in reality denote a specific pattern of necrosis. Rather, it is descriptive of **focal areas of destruction of fat resulting from abnormal release of activated pancreatic enzymes into the substance of the pancreas and the peritoneal cavity.** This occurs in the uncommon but calamitous abdominal emergency known as "acute pancreatic necrosis." In this condition, discussed more completely on page 581, activated pancreatic enzymes escape from acinar cells and ducts; the activated enzymes liquefy fat cell membranes, and the activated lipases split the triglyceride esters contained within fat cells. The released fatty acids combine with calcium to produce grossly visible chalky white areas, which enable the surgeon and the pathologist to identify this disease on inspection of involved fat depots. Histologically, the necrosis takes the form of foci of shadowy outlines of necrotic fat cells, the lipid content of which has been lipolyzed, surrounded by an inflammatory reaction (Fig. 1–11).

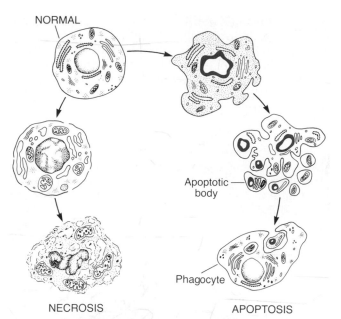

Figure 1–12. Cell necrosis and apoptosis. In apoptosis the initial changes consist of nuclear chromatin condensation and fragmentation, followed by phagocytosis of apoptotic bodies. There is also cellular blebbing. (Adapted from Walker, N. I., et al.: Patterns of cell death. Methods Achiev. Exp. Pathol. *13:*18–32, 1988.)

Ultimately, in the living patient, most necrotic cells and their debris disappear by a combined process of enzymic digestion and fragmentation, with phagocytosis of the particulate debris by leukocytes. If necrotic cells and cellular debris are not promptly destroyed and reabsorbed, they tend to attract calcium salts and other minerals and to become calcified. This phenomenon, so-called *dystrophic calcification,* is considered on page 23.

Apoptosis

This pattern of cell death has long been recognized by morphologists, but only recently has it been appreciated as a distinctive and important mode of cell injury, which should be differentiated from the common coagulative necrosis (Fig. 1–12). Its designation as apoptosis (pronounced by "Greekophiles" with a silent "p"—"apotosis") though unwieldy, appears to be established. It usually involves single cells or clusters of cells that appear on sections stained with hemotoxylin and eosin (H and E) as round or oval masses of intensely eosinophilic cytoplasm and dense nuclear chromatin fragments (Fig. 1–13). These chromatin fragments (apoptotic bodies) are taken up and degraded by adjacent phagocytic cells.

Three features characterize cells undergoing apoptosis: (1) chromatin condensation and formation of membrane blebs, (2) fragmentation of DNA into nucleosome-sized parts, and (3) a requirement for RNA and protein synthesis. The latter characteristic has led to the additional description of the process as "programmed cell death" or cell suicide, since it apparently involves active metabolism by the dying cell. The sequence of events leading to apoptosis is still unclear, but it is currently thought the process requires activa-

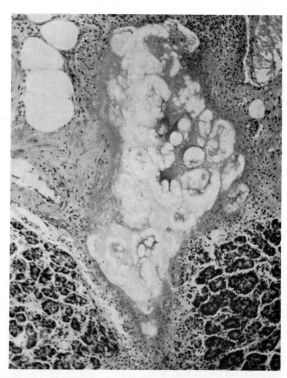

Figure 1–11. A sharply circumscribed focus of enzymatic necrosis of fat. Shadowy outlines of fat cells persist, surrounded by a zone of inflammation. The focus is surrounded by normal pancreatic substance.

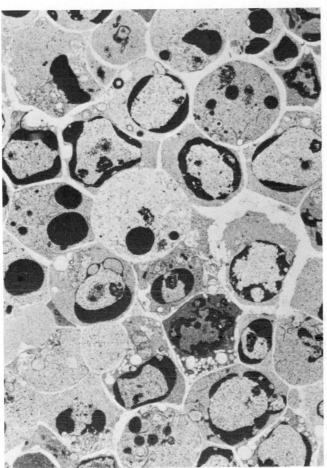

Figure 1-13. Apoptotic bodies in lymphoma cells. Some nuclear fragments show peripheral crescents of compacted chromatin, whereas others are uniformly dense. (From Kerr, J. F. R., and Harmon, B. V.: Definition and incidence of apoptosis: An historical perspective. *In* Tomei, L. D., and Cope, F. O. (eds.): Apoptosis: The Molecular Basis of Cell Death. Cold Spring Harbor, New York, Cold Spring Harbor Laboratory Press, pp. 5–29, 1991.)

tion of an endogenous endonuclease, perhaps via increases in cytosolic calcium, which results in the fragmentation of DNA and subsequent cellular changes.

Apoptosis is thought to be responsible for numerous physiologic events including the programmed destruction of cells during embryogenesis; for hormone-dependent involution, as occurs, for example, in the endometrium during the menstrual cycle; and for the death of immune cells after cytokine depletion. Indeed apoptosis may be the mechanism by which autoreactive T cells are deleted in the developing thymus, leading to the phenomenon of negative selection (p. 137). However, apoptosis may also be triggered by pathologic stimuli such as irradiation and virus infections. For example, apoptotic cell fragments are found in liver cells in viral hepatitis, where they are known as Councilman bodies.

SUBCELLULAR RESPONSES TO INJURY

To this point in the chapter, the focus has been on the cell as a unit. However, certain conditions are associated with rather distinctive alterations in cell organelles. Some of these alterations coexist with those described for acute lethal injury; others represent more chronic forms of cell injury, and others still are adaptive responses that involve specific cellular organelles. Here we shall touch on only some of the more common or interesting of these reactions.

LYSOSOMES: HETEROPHAGY AND AUTOPHAGY

Lysosomes are membrane-bound cytoplasmic bodies, 0.2 to 0.8 μm in diameter, that contain a variety of hydrolytic enzymes. They are involved in the breakdown of phagocytosed material in one of two ways (Fig. 1–14).

HETEROPHAGY. In this phenomenon materials from the external environment are taken up through the process of *endocytosis.* Uptake of particulate matter is known as *phagocytosis,* and that of soluble smaller macromolecules as *pinocytosis.* Heterophagy is most common in the "professional" phagocytes, such as neutrophils and macrophages, but also occurs in other cell types. Examples of heterophagocytosis include the uptake and digestion of bacteria by neutrophilic leukocytes and the removal of necrotic cells by macrophages. Fusion of the phagocytic vacuole with a lysosome then occurs with eventual digestion of the engulfed material.

AUTOPHAGY. In this process, intracellular organelles and portions of cytosol are first sequestered from the

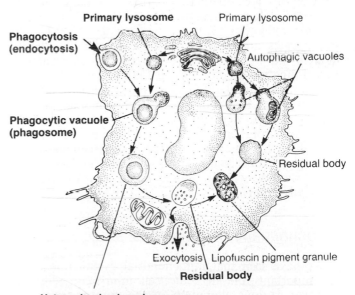

HETEROPHAGY   AUTOPHAGY

Primary lysosome   Primary lysosome

Phagocytosis
(endocytosis)   Autophagic vacuoles

Phagocytic vacuole
(phagosome)

Residual body

Exocytosis Lipofuscin pigment granule
Residual body

**Heterophagic phagolysosome
(secondary lysosome)**

Figure 1-14. Schematic representation of autophagy *(right)* and heterophagy *(left).* (Redrawn from Fawcett, D. W.: A Textbook of Histology, 11th ed. Philadelphia, W. B. Saunders Co., 1986, p. 17.)

cytoplasm in an *autophagic vacuole* formed from ribosome-free regions of the RER, which then fuses with preexisting primary lysosomes or Golgi elements to form an *autophagolysosome*. Autophagy is a common phenomenon involved in the removal of damaged organelles during cell injury and the cellular remodeling of differentiation and is particularly pronounced in cells undergoing atrophy induced by nutrient deprivation or hormonal involution.

The enzymes in the lysosomes are capable of breaking down most proteins and carbohydrates, but some lipids remain undigested. Lysosomes with undigested debris may persist within cells as *residual bodies* or may be extruded. *Lipofuscin pigment* granules, discussed earlier, represent undigested material that results from intracellular lipid peroxidation. Certain indigestible pigments, such as carbon particles inhaled from the atmosphere or inoculated pigment in tattoos, can persist in phagolysosomes of macrophages for decades.

Lysosomes are also wastebaskets in which cells sequester abnormal substances when these cannot be adequately metabolized. Hereditary *lysosomal storage disorders,* marked by deficiencies of enzymes that degrade various macromolecules, cause abnormal amounts of these compounds to be sequestered in the lysosomes of cells all over the body, particularly neurons, leading to severe abnormalities.

INDUCTION (HYPERTROPHY) OF SMOOTH ENDOPLASMIC RETICULUM

It is known that protracted human use of barbiturates leads to a state of increased tolerance, so that repeated doses lead to progressively shorter time spans of sleep. The patients have thus "adapted" to the medication. This adaptation is due to induction of an increased volume (hypertrophy) of the smooth endoplasmic reticulum (SER) of hepatocytes (Fig. 1–15). Barbiturates are detoxified in the liver by oxidative demethylation, which involves the P-450–centered mixed-function oxidase system found in the SER. The barbiturates stimulate *(induce)* the synthesis of more enzymes as well as more SER. In this manner the cell is better able to detoxify the drugs and so adapt to its altered environment. The mixed-function oxidase system of the SER is also involved in the metabolism of other exogenous compounds—carcinogenic hydrocarbons, steroids, carbon tetrachloride, alcohol, insecticides, and others.

MITOCHONDRIAL ALTERATIONS

We have seen that mitochondrial dysfunction plays an important role in acute cell injury. In addition, however, various alterations in the number, size, and shape of mitochondria occur in some pathologic conditions. For example, in cell hypertrophy and atrophy there is an increase and decrease, respectively, in the number of mitochondria in cells. Mitochondria may

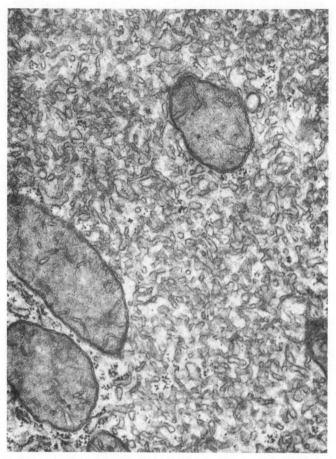

Figure 1–15. Electron micrograph of liver from phenobarbital-treated rat showing marked increase in smooth ER. (From Jones, A. L., and Fawcett, D. W.: Hypertrophy of the agranular endoplasmic reticulum in hamster liver induced by phenobarbital. J. Histochem. Cytochem., *14*:215, 1966. Courtesy of Dr. Fawcett.)

assume extremely large and abnormal shapes (megamitochondria). These can be seen in the liver in alcoholic liver disease and in certain nutritional deficiencies. In certain inherited metabolic diseases of skeletal muscle, the *mitochondrial myopathies,* defects in mitochondrial metabolism are associated with increased numbers of mitochondria that often are unusually large, have abnormal cristae, and contain crystalloids.

CYTOSKELETAL LESIONS

Abnormalities of the cytoskeleton underlie a variety of pathologic states. The *cytoskeleton* consists of microtubules (20 to 25 nm in diameter), thin actin filaments (6 to 8 nm), thick myosin filaments (15 nm), and various classes of intermediate filaments (10 nm). Several other nonpolymerized and nonfilamentous forms of contractile proteins also exist. Cytoskeletal abnormalities may be reflected by (1) defects in cell function, such as cell locomotion and intracellular organelle movements, or (2) in some instances by intracellular accumulations of fibrillar material. Only a few examples are cited.

Functioning myofilaments and microtubules are essential for various stages of leukocyte migration and phagocytosis, and functional deficiencies of the cytoskeleton appear to underlie certain defects in leukocyte movement toward an injurious stimulus (chemotaxis, p. 29) or the ability of such cells to perform phagocytosis adequately. For example, a defect of microtubule polymerization in the *Chédiak-Higashi syndrome* causes delayed or decreased fusion of lysosomes with phagosomes in leukocytes and thus impairs phagocytosis of bacteria. Some drugs, such as cytochalasin B, inhibit microfilament function and thus affect phagocytosis. Defects in the organization of microtubules can inhibit sperm motility to cause male sterility, and at the same time can immobilize the cilia of respiratory epithelium, causing interference with the ability of this epithelium to clear inhaled bacteria, leading to bronchiectasis (the *immotile cilia syndrome*).

Accumulations of intermediate filaments may be seen in certain types of cell injury. For example, the *Mallory body*, or "alcoholic hyalin," is an eosinophilic intracytoplasmic inclusion in liver cells that is highly characteristic of alcoholic liver disease. Such inclusions are now known to be composed largely of intermediate filaments of predominantly *prekeratin*. The *neurofibrillary tangle* found in the brain in Alzheimer's disease contains microtubule associated proteins and neurofilaments, a reflection of a disrupted neuronal cytoskeleton.

INTRACELLULAR ACCUMULATIONS ____

Under some circumstances, normal cells may accumulate abnormal amounts of various substances. These substances may accumulate either transiently or permanently and may be harmless to the cells, but on occasion they may also be severely injurious. The location of the substance may be in either the cytoplasm or the nucleus; in the former location *it is most frequently within lysosomes.*

The processes that may result in abnormal intracellular accumulations are many, but most can be divided into three general types.

- *A normal endogenous substance is produced at a normal or increased rate, but the rate of metabolism is inadequate to remove it.* An example of this type of process is *fatty change* in the liver.
- *A normal or abnormal endogenous substance accumulates because it cannot be metabolized.* The most common cause is *lack of an enzyme* that blocks a specific metabolic pathway, so that some particular metabolite cannot be used. When the enzyme lack is due to a genetically determined inborn error of metabolism, the disorders are referred to as *storage diseases* (p. 94).
- *An abnormal exogenous substance is deposited* and accumulates because the cell has neither the enzymic machinery to degrade the substance nor the ability to transport it to other sites. Accumulations of carbon particles and such nonmetabolizable chemicals as silica particles are examples of this type of alteration.

LIPIDS ____

Fatty Change ____

Fatty change refers to any abnormal accumulation of fat within parenchymal cells. *The appearance of fat vacuoles within cells, whether small or large, represents an absolute increase in intracellular lipids.* Although itself an indicator of nonlethal injury, fatty change is sometimes the harbinger of cell death and in many situations is encountered in cells adjacent to those that have died and undergone necrosis. Fatty change is most often seen in the liver, since it is the major organ involved in fat metabolism, but it may also occur in heart, muscle, kidney, and other organs.

Different mechanisms account for fatty change, dependent on the cause and cell involved. Fatty changes in the liver (fatty liver) in industrialized nations is most commonly caused by alcohol abuse. Alcohol is a hepatotoxin that alters mitochondrial and microsomal functions. Increased free fatty acid synthesis, diminished triglyceride utilization, decreased fatty acid oxidation, a block in lipoprotein excretion, and enhanced peripheral lipolysis—thus increasing delivery and hepatic uptake of free fatty acids—have all been implicated in alcohol-induced fatty liver (see p. 547). Other causes of fatty liver include protein malnutrition, diabetes mellitus, obesity, and hepatotoxins.

The significance of fatty change depends on the cause and severity of accumulation. It may have no effect on cellular function when mild. More severe fatty change may impair cellular function, but unless some vital intracellular process is irreversibly impaired (such as in carbon tetrachloride poisoning), fatty change per se is reversible. As a severe form of injury, therefore, fatty change may precede cell death, *but it should be emphasized that cells may die without undergoing fatty change.*

Fatty change is most often seen in the liver and heart, but it may occur in other organs.

LIVER. In the liver, mild fatty change may not affect the gross appearance. With progressive accumulation, the organ enlarges and becomes increasingly yellow until, in extreme instances, the liver may weigh 3 to 6 kg and may be transformed into a bright yellow, soft, greasy organ.

Fatty change is first manifested light microscopically by the appearance of small fat vacuoles in the cytoplasm around the nucleus. As the process progresses, the vacuoles coalesce to create cleared spaces that displace the nucleus to the periphery of the cell (Fig. 1–16). Occasionally, contiguous cells rupture, and the enclosed fat globules coalesce to produce so-called fatty cysts.

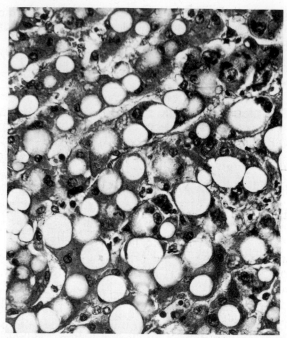

Figure 1–16. High-power detail of fatty change of liver. The variability in size of vacuoles is evident. In some cells, the well-preserved nucleus is squeezed into the displaced rim of cytoplasm about the fat vacuole.

HEART. Lipid, as a neutral fat, is sometimes found in heart muscle in the form of small droplets. It occurs in two patterns. In one, prolonged moderate hypoxia such as that produced by profound anemia causes intracellular deposits of fat, which create grossly apparent bands of yellowed myocardium alternating with bands of darker, red-brown, uninvolved myocardium (tigered effect). In the other pattern of fatty change produced by more profound hypoxia or some forms of myocarditis (e.g., diphtheritic), the myocardial cells are uniformly affected.

Cholesterol and Cholesterol Esters

As detailed previously, the overload of parenchymal liver cells by triglycerides is termed "fatty change." By quite different mechanisms, _phagocytic cells may become overloaded with lipid (triglycerides, cholesterol, and cholesteryl esters)._ Scavenger macrophages, wherever in contact with the lipid debris of necrotic cells or abnormal forms of plasma lipid, may become stuffed with lipid because of their phagocytic activities. They become filled with minute vacuoles of lipids so as to impart a foaminess to their cytoplasm _(foam cells)._ The pathogenesis of foam cell formation in atherosclerosis is discussed on p. 281.

OTHER INTRACELLULAR ACCUMULATIONS

Proteins

Protein accumulations may be encountered in cells either because excesses are presented to the cells or because the cells synthesize excessive amounts. Normally trace amounts of albumin, filtered through the glomerulus, are reabsorbed in the proximal convoluted tubules. Any disorder producing heavy proteinuria leads to pinocytotic reabsorption of the protein. When these pinocytotic vesicles in the epithelial cells fuse with lysosomes, hyaline cytoplasmic droplets, which appear pink in hematoxylin and eosin stains, are formed. If the proteinuria abates, the protein droplets are metabolized and disappear. Accumulations of immunoglobulins synthesized in the cisternae of the RER of plasma cells may create rounded, acidophilic _Russell bodies._

Glycogen

Excessive intracellular deposits of glycogen are seen in patients with an abnormality in either glucose or glycogen metabolism. Whatever the clinical setting, the glycogen masses appear as vacuoles within the cell. Diabetes mellitus is the prime example of a disorder of glucose metabolism. In this disease, glycogen is found in renal tubular epithelium, as well as within liver cells, beta-cells of the islets of Langerhans, and heart muscle cells.

Glycogen also accumulates within the cells in a group of closely related disorders, all genetic, collectively referred to as the _glycogen storage diseases, or glycogenoses_ (p. 94). In these diseases, some abnormal or normal forms of glycogen cannot be metabolized. These diseases represent instances in which massive stockpiling of substances within cells causes secondary injury and cell death.

Complex Lipids and Carbohydrates

In certain forms of storage diseases resulting from inborn errors of metabolism, abnormal complexes of carbohydrates and lipids accumulate that cannot be metabolized normally. These substances collect within cells throughout the body, principally those in the reticuloendothelial system, causing hepatomegaly and splenomegaly. Examples include the mucopolysaccharidoses and Gaucher's, Tay-Sachs, and Neimann-Pick diseases, in which the abnormal products are complex lipids. These intracellular deposits may become extreme and cause death not only of the cell but also of the patient.

Pigments

Pigments can either be exogenous, coming from outside the body, or endogenous, synthesized within the body itself.

The most common *exogenous pigment* is *carbon* or *coal dust*, which is a ubiquitous air pollutant of urban life. When inhaled, it is picked up by alveolar macrophages and transported through lymphatic channels to the regional tracheobronchial lymph nodes *(anthracosis)*. Aggregates of coal dust may induce a fibroblastic reaction or even emphysema and thus cause a serious lung disease known as *coal worker's pneumoconiosis.*

Endogenous pigments include lipofuscin, melanin, and certain derivatives of hemoglobin. *Lipofuscin* was described earlier (p. 10). In tissue sections it appears as a yellow-brown, finely granular intracytoplasmic pigment. It is seen in cells undergoing slow, regressive changes and is particularly prominent in the liver and heart.

Melanin (derived from the Greek work *melas,* meaning black) is an endogenous, non–hemoglobin-derived, brown-black pigment formed when the enzyme tyrosinase catalyzes the oxidation of tyrosine to dihydroxyphenylalanine in melanocytes.

Hemosiderin is a hemoglobin-derived, golden-yellow to brown granular or crystalline pigment in which form iron is stored in cells. Iron is normally stored in association with a protein, apoferritin, to form ferritin micelles. Hemosiderin pigment represents aggregates of ferritin micelles (Fig. 1–17). Under normal conditions small amounts of hemosiderin can be seen in the mononuclear phagocytes of the bone marrow, spleen, and liver, all actively engaged in red cell breakdown.

Excesses of iron cause hemosiderin to accumulate within cells, either as a localized process or as a systemic derangement.

Local excesses of iron and hemosiderin result from gross hemorrhages or the myriad minute hemorrhages that accompany severe vascular congestion. The best example of localized hemosiderosis is the common bruise. Following local hemorrhage, the area is at first red-blue. With lysis of the erythrocytes, the hemoglobin eventually undergoes transformation to hemosiderin. Macrophages take part in this process by phagocytizing the red cell debris, and then lysosomal enzymes eventually convert the hemoglobin, through a sequence of pigments, into hemosiderin. The play of colors through which the bruise passes reflects these transformations. The original red-blue color of hemoglobin is transformed to varying shades of green-blue, comprising the local formation of biliverdin (green bile), then bilirubin (red bile), and thereafter the iron moiety of hemoglobin is deposited as golden-yellow hemosiderin.

Whenever there are causes for *systemic overload of iron,* hemosiderin is deposited in many organs and tissues, a condition called *hemosiderosis.* It is seen with (1) increased absorption of dietary iron, (2) impaired utilization of iron, (3) hemolytic anemias, and (4) transfusions, as the transfused red cells constitute an exogenous load of iron. These conditions are discussed in Chapter 12.

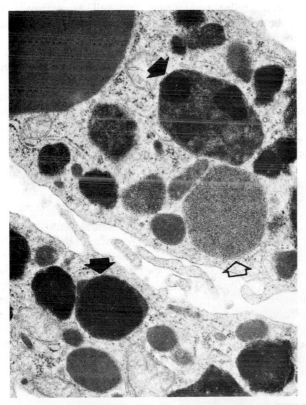

Figure 1–17. Hemosiderin granules in human splenic sinusoidal lining cells. Ferritin micelles *(open arrow)* are concentrated within phagosomes. The osmiophilic material *(arrows)* is probably lipid. A recently engulfed (undigested) red blood cell is present in the upper left hand corner.

Morphologically the pigment appears as a coarse, golden, granular pigment lying within the cell's cytoplasm. When the basic cause is the localized breakdown of red cells, the pigmentation is found at first in the reticuloendothelial cells in the area. In systemic hemosiderosis, it is found at first in the mononuclear phagocytes of the liver, bone marrow, spleen, and lymph nodes and in scattered macrophages throughout other organs such as the skin, pancreas, and kidneys. With progressive accumulation, parenchymal cells throughout the body (principally in the liver, pancreas, heart, and endocrine organs) become pigmented. Iron can be visualized in tissues by the Prussian blue histochemical reaction, in which colorless potassium ferrocyanide is converted by iron to blue-black ferric ferrocyanide.

In most instances of systemic hemosiderosis, the pigment does not damage the parenchymal cells or impair organ function. However, the more extreme accumulation of iron in a disease called *hemochromatosis* (p. 554) is associated with liver and pancreatic damage, resulting in liver fibrosis and diabetes mellitus.

CELLULAR ADAPTATIONS OF GROWTH AND DIFFERENTIATION

As explained earlier, cells must constantly adapt, even under normal conditions, to changes in their environment. These *physiologic adaptations* usually represent responses of cells to normal stimulation by hormones or endogenous chemical substances—for example, as in the enlargement of the breast and induction of lactation by pregnancy. *Pathologic adaptations* may share the same underlying mechanisms, but they provide the cells with the ability to modulate their environment and perhaps escape injury. Cellular adaptation, then, is a state that lies intermediate between the normal, unstressed cell and the injured, overstressed cell.

There are numerous types of cellular adaptations. Some involve *up- or down-regulation of specific cellular receptors* involved in metabolism of certain components—for example, in the regulation of cell surface receptors involved in the uptake and degradation of low-density lipoproteins (LDL) (p. 87). Others are associated with the *induction of new protein synthesis by the target cell.* These proteins, such as heat shock or stress shock proteins, may protect cells from certain forms of injury. Although the precise function of these proteins in higher organisms is still unclear, they have been conserved in structure through evolution, from *Escherichia coli* to man, and must have a survival role. Other adaptations involve a switch by cells from producing one type of a family of proteins to another or markedly overproducing one protein; such is the case in cells producing various types of collagens and extracellular matrix proteins in chronic inflammation and fibrosis (p. 55). Molecular techniques have increased our understanding of how such cellular responses occur—at the level of *receptor binding, signal transduction, transcription, translation,* or *regulation of protein packaging and release.*

In this section we consider the adaptive changes in cell growth and differentiation that are particularly important in pathologic conditions. These include atrophy (decrease in cell size), hypertrophy (increase in cell size), hyperplasia (increase in cell number), and metaplasia (change in cell type).

ATROPHY

Shrinkage in the size of the cell by loss of cell substance is known as atrophy. It represents a form of adaptive response. When a sufficient number of cells are involved, the entire tissue or organ diminishes in size, or becomes atrophic (Fig. 1–18).

The apparent causes of atrophy are (1) decreased workload, (2) loss of innervation, (3) diminished blood supply, (4) inadequate nutrition, (5) loss of endocrine stimulation, and (6) aging. Some of these stimuli are clearly physiologic, whereas others are clearly pathologic. However, the fundamental cellular change is identical in all, representing a retreat by the cell to a smaller size at which survival is still possible. The cell contains fewer mitochondria and myofilaments and less endoplasmic reticulum.

The biochemical mechanisms of atrophy are not very well understood. There is a finely regulated balance between protein synthesis and degradation in normal cells, and either decreased synthesis, increased catabolism, or both may cause atrophy. Hormones, particularly insulin, thyroid hormones, glucocorticoids, and prostaglandin, influence such protein turnover. For example, slight increases of protein degradation over a long period of time may result in atrophy, as seems to occur in some muscular dystrophies.

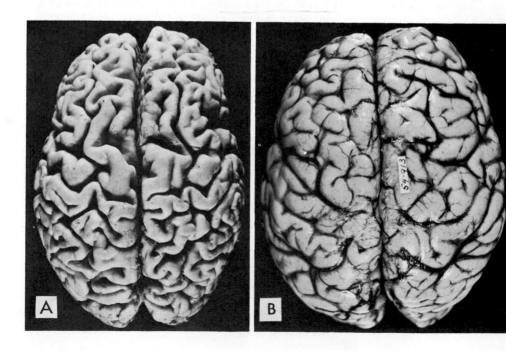

Figure 1–18. *A,* Physiologic atrophy of the brain in an 82-year-old male. The meninges have been stripped. *B,* Normal brain of a 35-year-old male.

In many situations atrophy is also accompanied by marked increases in the number of *autophagic vacuoles.* Some of the cell debris within the autophagic vacuole may resist digestion and persist as membrane-bound *residual bodies* that may remain as sarcophagi in the cytoplasm. An example of such residual bodies is the *lipofuscin granule,* discussed earlier. When present in sufficient amounts, they impart a *brown discoloration* to the tissue (brown atrophy).

HYPERTROPHY _____

Hypertrophy refers to an increase in the size of cells and, with such change, an increase in the size of the organ. Hypertrophy can be caused by increased functional demand or by specific hormonal stimulation and may occur *under both physiologic and pathologic conditions.* The physiologic growth of the uterus during pregnancy involves both hypertrophy and hyperplasia. The cellular hypertrophy is stimulated by estrogen through smooth muscle estrogen receptors, which allow for interactions of the hormones with nuclear DNA, eventually resulting in increased synthesis of smooth muscle proteins and increase in cell size. This, then, is physiologic hypertrophy effected by hormonal stimulation. Hypertrophy as an adaptive response is exemplified by muscular enlargement. The striated muscle cells in both the heart and skeletal muscle are most capable of hypertrophy, perhaps because they cannot adapt to increased metabolic demands by mitotic division and the formation of more cells to share the work (Fig. 1–19).

The environmental change that produces hypertrophy of striated muscle appears mainly to be increased workload. In the heart a stimulus is high blood pressure; in skeletal muscles, heavy work. Synthesis of more proteins and filaments occurs, achieving a balance between the demand and the cell's functional capacity. The greater number of myofilaments permits an increased workload with a level of metabolic activity per unit volume of cell not different from that borne by the normal cell. Thus the draft horse readily pulls the load that would break the back of a pony.

But what are the initial signals for increased protein synthesis? In the heart, there are at least two mechanisms: first, mechanical stretch per se, perhaps through a stretch receptor, triggers RNA synthesis and protein production; second, activation of α-adrenergic receptors on the surface of myocytes alters gene expression for certain contractile proteins.

Whatever the exact mechanism of hypertrophy, it eventually reaches a limit beyond which enlargement of muscle mass is no longer able to compensate for the increased burden, and cardiac failure, for example, ensues. At this stage a number of "degenerative" changes occur in the myocardial fibers, of which the most important are lysis and loss of myofibrillar contractile elements. The limiting factors for continued hypertrophy and the causes of regressive changes are incompletely understood; they may be due to limitation of the vascular supply to the enlarged fibers, to

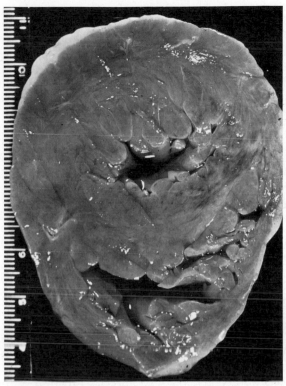

Figure 1–19. A cross section of a heart with marked left ventricular hypertrophy. The left ventricular wall is over 2 cm in thickness (normal, 1 to 1.5 cm). On the right side of the interventricular septum, the mottled, dark area is a focus of fresh ischemic necrosis (myocardial infarct).

diminished oxidative capabilities of mitochondria, or to alterations in protein synthesis and degradation.

HYPERPLASIA _____

Hyperplasia constitutes an increase in the number of cells in an organ or tissue. Hypertrophy and hyperplasia are closely related and often develop concurrently in tissues that are capable of cell division, such as the epidermis.

Cardiac and skeletal muscle cells have no capacity for hyperplastic growth and thus usually undergo only hypertrophy. (The determinants of cell growth are discussed more fully on page 47.)

Hyperplasia can be *physiologic* or *pathologic.*

Physiologic hyperplasia is divided into (1) *hormonal hyperplasia,* best exemplified by the proliferation of the epithelium of the female breast at puberty and during pregnancy; and (2) *compensatory hyperplasia,* i.e., hyperplasia that occurs when a portion of the tissue is removed or diseased. For example, when a portion of the liver is removed, mitotic activity in the remaining cells begins as early as 12 hours after hepatectomy, eventually restoring the liver to its normal weight—at which time mitoses cease. The stimuli for cell proliferation in this setting are polypeptide growth factors and hormones, which are produced by remnant hepatic cells. Such growth factors are discussed in greater detail in Chapter 3, but the specific factors that appear to be involved in liver regeneration are transforming growth factor–α (TGF-α), transforming growth factor–β (TGF-β), and a heparin-binding polypeptide called hepatopoietin.

Most forms of *pathologic hyperplasia* are instances of excessive hormonal stimulation or are the effects of growth factors on target cells. An example of hormonally induced abnormal hyperplasia sometimes develops in the endometrium. After a normal menstrual period there is a rapid burst of proliferative activity that might be viewed as reparative proliferation in the endometrium. This proliferation is potentiated by pituitary hormones and ovarian estrogen and abated by progesterone. If the normal balance between estrogen and progesterone is disturbed, resulting in absolute or relative increases in estrogen, hyperplasia results. Hyperplasia is a common cause of abnormal menstrual bleeding; the hyperplastic process remains controlled, nonetheless: if estrogenic stimulation abates, the hyperplasia disappears. This differentiates the process from cancer, in which, as we shall see on page 195, cells continue to grow. However, *pathologic hyperplasia constitutes a fertile soil in which cancerous proliferation may eventually arise.* Thus patients with hyperplasia of the endometrium are at increased risk of developing endometrial cancer.

Hyperplasia is also an important response of connective tissue cells in wound healing, in which proliferating fibroblasts and blood vessels, stimulated by growth factors (p. 51), aid in repair. Stimulation by growth factors is also involved in the hyperplasia that is associated with certain *virus infections* such as papilloma viruses causing skin warts.

Although hypertrophy and hyperplasia are two distinct processes, frequently both occur together, and may well be triggered by the same mechanism. Estrogen-induced growth in the uterus involves both increased DNA synthesis and enlargement of smooth muscle and epithelium. Both processes are initiated by binding of estrogen to a receptor complex in the cytoplasm of target cells. In certain instances, however, even potentially dividing cells, such as renal epithelial cells, undergo hypertrophy but not hyperplasia. Growth inhibitors, such as TGF-β, may be involved in this phenomenon. In *nondividing cells* (such as myocardial fibers), only hypertrophy occurs. Nuclei in such cells have a much higher DNA content than normal myocardial cells, probably because the cells arrest in the G$_2$ phase of the cell cycle without undergoing mitosis.

METAPLASIA

Metaplasia is a reversible change in which one adult cell type (epithelial or mesenchymal) is replaced by another adult cell type. It, too, represents an adaptive substitution for cells more sensitive to stress by other cell types better able to withstand the adverse environment. Metaplasia is best seen in the form of squamous change that occurs in the respiratory tract in the habitual cigarette smoker. The normal columnar ciliated epithelial cells of the trachea and bronchi are replaced focally or widely by stratified squamous epithelial cells. Stones in the excretory ducts of the salivary glands, pancreas, or bile ducts may cause replacement of the normal secretory columnar epithelium by nonfunctioning stratified squamous epithelium (Fig. 1–20). A deficiency of vitamin A induces squamous metaplasia in the respiratory epithelium. In all these instances, the more rugged stratified squamous epithelium is able to survive under circumstances in which the more fragile specialized epithelium most likely would have succumbed.

Metaplasia may also occur in mesenchymal cells but less clearly as an adaptive response. Fibroblasts may become transformed to osteoblasts or chondroblasts to produce bone or cartilage where it is normally not encountered. For example, bone is occasionally formed in soft tissues, particularly in foci of injury. This process represents a form of "divergent differentiation."

PATHOLOGIC CALCIFICATION

Pathologic calcification is a common process that implies the abnormal deposition of calcium salts, together with smaller amounts of iron, magnesium, and other mineral salts. When the deposition occurs in dead or dying tissues, it is known as *dystrophic calcification: it may occur despite normal serum levels of calcium and in the absence of derangements in calcium metabolism.* In contrast, the deposition of calcium salts in normal tissues is known as *metastatic calcification, and it almost always reflects some derangement in calcium metabolism, leading to hypercalcemia.*

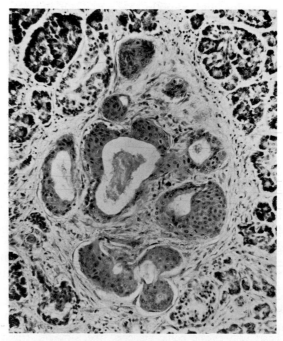

Figure 1–20. Metaplastic transformation of adult columnar epithelial cells to adult stratified squamous cells in pancreatic ducts.

DYSTROPHIC CALCIFICATION _____

This alteration is encountered in areas of coagulation, in caseous and liquefactive necrosis, and in foci of enzymic necrosis of fat whenever the necrotic tissue persists for a long period of time. It commonly develops in damaged heart valves, hampering their function (Fig. 1–21). Calcification is almost inevitable in the atheromas of advanced atherosclerosis, which, as will be seen, are focal intimal injuries in the aorta and larger arteries that are characterized by the accumulation of lipids (p. 283).

> Whatever the site of deposition, the calcium salts appear macroscopically as fine, white granules or clumps, often felt as gritty deposits. Sometimes, a tuberculous lymph node is virtually converted to stone. Histologically calcification appears as **intracellular** or **extracellular** basophilic deposits or **both**. In time **heterotopic bone** may be formed in the focus of calcification.

The pathogenesis of dystrophic calcification involves *initiation* and *propagation* leading ultimately to the formation of crystalline calcium phosphate. Initiation in *extracellular* sites occurs in membrane-bound *vesicles* about 200 nm in diameter; in normal cartilage and bone they are known as *matrix vesicles,* whereas in pathologic calcification they seem to be derived from degenerating or aging cells. It is thought that calcium is concentrated in these vesicles by its affinity for acidic phospholipids, and the phosphates accumulate as a result of the action of membrane-bound

phosphatases. Initiation of *intracellular* calcification occurs in the *mitochondria* of dead or dying cells that accumulate calcium, as described earlier. Propagation and crystal formation then occur, dependent on the concentration of Ca^{++} and PO_4 in the extracellular spaces, the presence of mineral inhibitors, and the degree of collagenization. Collagen appears to increase the rate of crystal proliferation.

Although dystrophic calcification may be simply a "tell-tale" sign of previous cell injury, it is often a cause of organ dysfunction. Such is the case in calcific valvular disease and atherosclerosis, as becomes clear in the further discussion of these diseases.

METASTATIC CALCIFICATION _____

This alteration may occur in normal tissues whenever there is hypercalcemia. Hypercalcemia also accentuates dystrophic calcification. The causes of hypercalcemia include [1] hyperparathyroidism; [2] vitamin D intoxication; [3] systemic sarcoidosis; [4] milk-alkali syndrome; [5] hyperthyroidism; [6] idiopathic hypercalcemia of infancy; [6] Addison's disease (adrenocortical insufficiency); increased bone catabolism associated with multiple myeloma, metastatic cancer, and leukemia; and decreased bone formation, as occurs in immobilization. Hypercalcemia also arises in some instances of advanced renal failure. The resulting phosphate retention leads to secondary hyperparathyroidism.

> Metastatic calcification may occur widely throughout the body but principally affects the interstitial tissues of the blood vessels, kidneys, lungs, and gastric mucosa. In all these sites, the calcium salts morphologically resemble those described in dystrophic calcification. On occasion extensive involvement of the lungs produces remarkable changes in x-ray films and respiratory deficits. Massive deposits in the kidney (nephrocalcinosis) may in time cause renal damage.

The cellular and subcellular alterations described in this chapter are not merely of anatomic interest; they are fundamental to all the diseases discussed in this book as well as those that have escaped our tender ministrations.

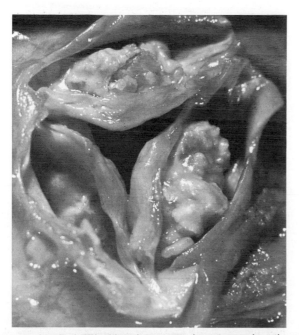

Figure 1–21. A view looking down onto the unopened aortic valve in a heart with calcific aortic stenosis. The semilunar cusps are thickened and fibrotic. Behind each leaflet are seen irregular masses of piled-up dystrophic calcification.

Bibliography _____

Chipman, J. K.: Mechanisms of cell toxicity. Curr. Opin. Cell Biol. *1:*231–234, 1989. (Summary of recent work on biochemical mechanisms of cell injury.)

Dunn, W. A.: Studies on the mechanisms of autophagy. J. Cell Biol. *110:*1923–1945, 1990.

Fairweather, D. S., and Evans, J. G.: Aging. *In* Cohen, R. D., Lewis, B., Alberti, K. G. M. M., and Denman, A. M. (eds.). The Metabolic and Molecular Basis of Acquired Disease. London, Bailliére Tindall, 1990, pp. 213–236.

Farber, J. L., Kyle, M. E., and Coleman, J. B.: Mechanisms of cell injury by activated oxygen species. Lab. Invest. *62:*670–679, 1990. (Review of role of free radicals and lipid peroxidation in cell injury.)

Fausto, N., and Mead, J. E.: Regulation of liver growth: Proto-oncogenes and transforming growth factors. Lab. Invest. *60:4*, 1989. (Review of studies on the mechanisms of hyperplasia in the liver.)

Jones, A. L., and Fawcett, D. W.: Hypertrophy of the agranular endoplasmic reticulum in hamster liver induced by phenobarbital. J. Histochem. Cytochem. *14:*215, 1966. (A classic description of organelle hypertrophy induced by drugs.)

Majno, G., et al.: Cellular death and necrosis: Chemical, physical, and morphologic changes in rat liver. Virchows Arch. *333:*421, 1960. (A classic description of the biochemistry and morphology of cell death.)

Mergner, W. J., Jones, R. T., and Trump, B. F. (eds.): Cell Death. Mechanisms of Acute and Lethal Cell Injury, Vol. 1. New York, Field and Wood Medical Publishers, 1990. (A compendium of articles dealing with biochemical mechanisms of cell injury.)

Michaelopoulos, G. K.: Liver regeneration: molecular mechanisms of growth control. FASEB J. *4:*176–187, 1990.

Schoen, F. J., et al.: Calcification: pathology, mechanisms and strategies of prevention. J. Biomed. Mater. Res. *22:*A1, 1988. (A summary of the mechanisms of calcification.)

Tomei, L. D., and Cope, F. O. (eds.): Apoptosis: The Molecular Basis of Cell Death. New York, Cold Spring Harbor Laboratory Press, 1991.

Walker, N. I., et al.: Patterns of cell death. Methods Achiev. Exp. Pathol. *13:*18–32, 1988. (A good review of differences between necrosis and apoptosis.)

Weinberg, J. M.: The cell biology of ischemic injury. Kidney Int. *39:*476–500, 1991. (A discussion of the role of alterations in purine nucleotide metabolism, calcium, phospholipids, and oxidants in ischemic injury in the kidney.)

Wolf, G., and Nielson, E. G.: Molecular mechanisms of renal hypertrophy and hyperplasia. Kidney Int. *39:*401–420, 1991. (A review of growth factors and signal mechanisms associated with hypertrophy and hyperplasia.)

Wyllie, A. H.: Glucocorticoid-induced thymocyte apoptosis is associated with endogenous endonuclease activation. Nature *282:*555–556, 1980. (Landmark paper on the pathogenesis of apoptosis.)

TWO

Acute and Chronic Inflammation

ACUTE INFLAMMATION
VASCULAR CHANGES
  Changes in Vascular Flow and Caliber
  Increased Vascular Permeability (Vascular
  Leakage)
CELLULAR EVENTS: LEUKOCYTE EXUDATION
AND PHAGOCYTOSIS
  Margination and Adhesion
  Emigration and Chemotaxis
  Phagocytosis and Degranulation
  Leukocyte Activation and Tissue Injury
  Defects in Leukocyte Function
SUMMARY OF THE ACUTE INFLAMMATORY
RESPONSE
CHEMICAL MEDIATORS OF INFLAMMATION
  Vasoactive Amines
  Plasma Proteases
  Arachidonic Acid Metabolites — Prostaglandins
    and Leukotrienes
  Platelet-Activating Factor
  Cytokines
  Leukocyte Products
  Other Mediators

CHRONIC INFLAMMATION
DEFINITION AND CAUSES
  Chronic Inflammatory Cells
  Granulomatous Inflammation
ROLE OF LYMPHATICS AND LYMPHOID TISSUE
MORPHOLOGIC PATTERNS IN ACUTE AND
CHRONIC INFLAMMATION
SYSTEMIC MANIFESTATIONS OF
INFLAMMATION

In Chapter 1 we saw how various exogenous and endogenous stimuli can cause cell injury. These same stimuli also provoke, in the vascularized connective tissues, a complex reaction called inflammation. Inflammation is fundamentally a protective response whose ultimate goal is to rid the organism of both the initial cause of cell injury (e.g., microbes or toxins) and the consequences of such injury, the necrotic cells and tissues. Humans could not long survive injury without the protective responses of inflammation. Infections would run amok, burns would not heal, and wounds would remain festering, open sores.

The inflammatory response involves the connective tissue, including plasma, circulating cells, blood vessels, and cellular and extracellular constituents of connective tissue (Fig. 2–1). Two types of inflammation are recognized. *Acute inflammation* is of relatively short duration, lasting for a few minutes, several hours, or a few days, and its main characteristics are the exudation of fluid and plasma proteins and the emigration of leukocytes, predominantly neutrophils. *Chronic inflammation*, on the other hand, is of longer duration and is associated histologically with the presence of lymphocytes and macrophages and with the proliferation of blood vessels and connective tissue.

The vascular and cellular responses of inflammation are mediated by chemical factors derived from plasma or cells and triggered by the inflammatory stimulus. Such chemical mediators, acting together or in sequence, then influence the evolution of the inflammatory response. But necrotic cells or tissues themselves, whatever the cause of cell death can also trigger the elaboration of inflammatory mediators. Such is the case with the acute inflammation following myocardial infarction.

Inflammation is closely interwoven with the process of *repair*. Inflammation serves to destroy, dilute, or wall off the injurious agent, but in turn it sets into motion a series of events that tend to heal the damaged tissue. During repair, the injured tissue is replaced by *regeneration* of native parenchymal cells, or by filling of the defect with fibroblastic scar tissue *(scarring),* or most commonly by a combination of these two processes.

Although inflammation and repair are basically defense mechanisms, they are *potentially harmful.* Indeed, an overreactive inflammatory response (hypersensitivity) to a bee sting can cause death. Similarly, scarring, such as sometimes follows bacteria-induced inflammatory reactions in the pericardial sac, may so encase the heart in dense fibrous tissue that it permanently impairs cardiac function. Notwithstanding such possible untoward consequences, the inflammatory and reparative responses are fundamental to the survival of the organism, as we shall see.

25

CONNECTIVE TISSUE   VESSELS   CONNECTIVE TISSUE
MATRIX   CELLS

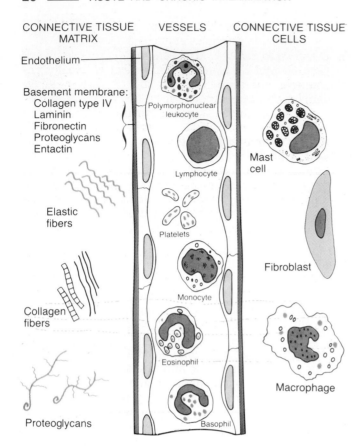

Endothelium

Basement membrane:
Collagen type IV
Laminin
Fibronectin
Proteoglycans
Entactin

Polymorphonuclear
leukocyte

Mast
cell

Lymphocyte

Elastic
fibers

Platelets

Fibroblast

Collagen
fibers

Monocyte

Eosinophil

Macrophage

Proteoglycans

Basophil

Figure 2–1. Intravascular cells, connective tissue cells and extracellular matrix involved in the inflammatory response.

Acute Inflammation

Acute inflammation is the immediate and early response to an injurious agent. Since the two major defensive components against microbes—antibodies and leukocytes—are normally carried in the bloodstream, it is not surprising that vascular phenomena play a major role in acute inflammation. Therefore, acute inflammation has three major components: *(1) alterations in vascular caliber that lead to an increase in blood flow, (2) structural changes in the microvasculature that permit the plasma proteins and leukocytes to leave the circulation, and (3) emigration of the leukocytes from the microcirculation and their accumulation in the focus of injury.* These components account for the classical local signs of acute inflammation, immortalized by Celsus (first century A.D.): heat *(calor),* redness *(rubor),* swelling *(tumor),* and pain *(dolor).* A fifth clinical sign, loss of function *(functio laesa),* was later added by Virchow.

VASCULAR CHANGES

CHANGES IN VASCULAR FLOW AND CALIBER

Changes in vascular flow and caliber begin very early after injury and develop at varying rates, depend-

ing on the severity of the injury. The changes occur in the following order:

1. Following an inconstant and transient vasoconstriction of arterioles, lasting a few seconds, *vasodilatation* occurs. This first involves the arterioles and then results in opening of new microvascular beds in the area. Thus comes about *increased blood flow,* the hallmark of the early hemodynamic changes in acute inflammation and the cause of the heat and the redness (Fig. 2–2). How long vasodilatation lasts depends on the stimulus; it is followed by the next event:

2. *Slowing of the circulation.* This is brought about by *increased permeability of the microvasculature,* with the outpouring of protein-rich fluid into the extravascular tissues. The latter results in concentration of red cells in small vessels and increased viscosity of the blood, reflected by the presence of <u>dilated small vessels packed with red cells</u>—termed *stasis.* As stasis develops one begins to see peripheral orientation of leukocytes, principally neutrophils, along the vascular endothelium, a process called *leukocytic margination.* Leukocytes stick to the endothelium, at first transiently then more avidly, and soon afterward they migrate through the vascular wall into the interstitial tissue, in a process called *emigration.*

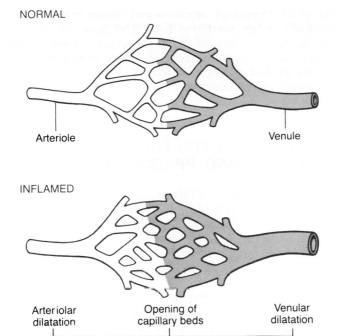

NORMAL

Arteriole   Venule

INFLAMED

Arteriolar   Opening of   Venular
dilatation   capillary beds   dilatation

Increased blood flow

Figure 2–2. Alterations in blood flow associated with inflammation.

fects <u>only venules</u> 20 to 60 μm in diameter, leaving capillaries and arterioles unaffected.

2. *Direct endothelial injury, resulting in endothelial cell necrosis and detachment.* This effect is usually encountered in severe injuries and is due to direct damage to the endothelium by the injurious stimulus, as for example by severe burns or lytic bacterial infections. In most instances leakage starts immediately after injury and is sustained at a high level for several hours or days until the damaged vessels are thrombosed or repaired. The reaction is known as the *immediate sustained response. All levels of the microcirculation are affected, including venules, capillaries, and arterioles.* Endothelial cell detachment is often associated with platelet adhesion and thrombosis.

Delayed prolonged leakage is a curious type of direct injury that *begins after a delay of 2 to 12 hours, lasts for several hours or even days, and involves venules and capillaries.* Such leakage is caused, for example, by mild-to-moderate thermal injury, x- or ultraviolet irradiation, and certain bacterial toxins. The late-appearing sunburn is a good example of a delayed reaction.

INCREASED VASCULAR PERMEABILITY (VASCULAR LEAKAGE) _____

In the earliest phase of inflammation, vasodilatation and increased blood flow increase intravascular hydrostatic pressure, resulting in increased filtration of fluid from the capillaries. This fluid contains little protein, being essentially an ultrafiltrate of blood plasma; it is called a *transudate.* Transudation is soon overshadowed by an increase in permeability of the vessel wall, which leads to the escape into the interstitium of protein-rich fluid, termed *exudate. The loss of protein-rich fluid from the plasma reduces the intravascular osmotic pressure and increases the osmotic pressure of the interstitial fluid;* together they lead to a marked *outflow* of fluid and its accumulation in the interstitial tissue (Fig. 2–3). This net increase of extravascular fluid is called *edema.*

Normal fluid exchange and microvascular permeability are critically dependent on an intact endothelium. How then does the endothelium become leaky in inflammation? At least four mechanisms are known (Fig. 2–4).

1. *Endothelial cell contraction, leading to the formation of widened intercellular junctions, or intercellular gaps.* This is by far the most common mechanism of vascular leakage and is elicited by histamine, bradykinin, and virtually all other chemical mediators of inflammation. This type of vascular leakage occurs rapidly after exposure to the mediator and its binding to receptors on endothelial cells and is usually short lived (15 to 30 minutes); it is thus known as the *immediate transient response.* It af-

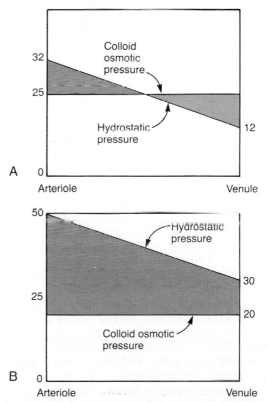

Figure 2–3. Blood pressure and plasma colloid osmotic forces in normal and inflamed microcirculation. *A,* Normal hydrostatic pressure of about 32 mm Hg at arterial end of capillary and 12 mm Hg at venous end. Mean capillary pressure equals colloid osmotic pressure (horizontal line). *B,* Acute inflammation. Mean capillary pressure is increased because of arteriolar dilatation, while osmotic pressure is reduced because of protein leakage across venule. Result is net excess of extravasated fluid. (Redrawn from Wright, G. P.: An Introduction to Pathology. 3rd ed. London, Longmans, Green and Co., 1958.)

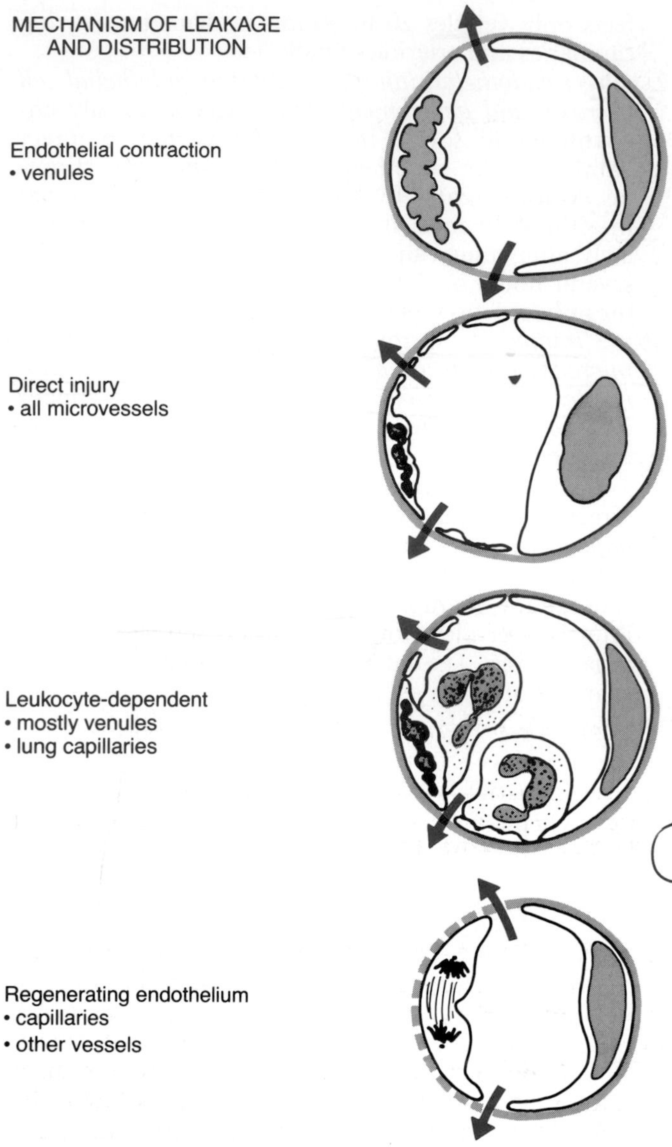

MECHANISM OF LEAKAGE
AND DISTRIBUTION

Endothelial contraction
• venules

Direct injury
• all microvessels

Leukocyte-dependent
• mostly venules
• lung capillaries

Regenerating endothelium
• capillaries
• other vessels

Figure 2-4. Diagrammatic representation of the four mechanisms of increased vascular permeability in inflammation.

3. *Leukocyte-dependent endothelial injury.* Leukocytes aggregate and adhere to endothelium relatively early in inflammation. As we shall see (p. 38), such leukocytes may be activated in the process, releasing toxic oxygen species and proteolytic enzymes, which then cause endothelial injury or detachment— resulting in increased permeability.

4. *Leakage from regenerating capillaries.* During repair, endothelial cells proliferate and form new blood vessels (granulation tissue p. 52). These capillary sprouts remain leaky until the endothelial cells differentiate and form intercellular junctions, accounting for the edema characteristic of healing inflammation.

It should be noted that although these four mechanisms are separable all may play a role in response to one stimulus. For example, in various stages of a thermal burn, leakage results from chemically mediated endothelial contraction as well as direct and

leukocyte-dependent injury—and from regenerating capillaries when the burns heal. This accounts for the life-threatening loss of fluid in severely burned patients. In addition, different chemical mediators may be activated in consecutive phases of the inflammatory response and account for sustained and prolonged responses.

CELLULAR EVENTS: LEUKOCYTE EXUDATION AND PHAGOCYTOSIS ————

A critical function of inflammation is the delivery of leukocytes to the site of injury. Leukocytes kill bacteria and other microbes and degrade necrotic tissue and foreign antigens. Unfortunately, leukocytes may also prolong inflammation and induce tissue damage by releasing enzymes, chemical mediators, and toxic oxygen radicals.

The sequence of events in the leukocyte journey can be divided into (1) margination, rolling, and adhesion; (2) emigration toward a chemotactic stimulus; (3) phagocytosis and intracellular degradation; and (4) leukocyte activation, with extracellular release of leukocyte products (Fig. 2-5).

MARGINATION, ROLLING, AND ADHESION ————

In normally flowing blood, erythrocytes and leukocytes are confined to a central axial column, leaving a cell-poor layer of plasma in contact with endothelium. As blood flow slows early in inflammation (as a result of the increased vascular permeability), white cells fall out of the central column, tumble slowly and roll along the endothelium of venules, and finally rest at some point where they adhere. The initial process is called *margination,* and in time the endothelium appears to be virtually lined by white cells, a phenomenon called *pavementing.* When the leukocytes adhere, they resemble "pebbles or marbles over which a stream runs without disturbing them." This process of leukocyte-endothelial adhesion is a necessary prelude to all the subsequent leukocytic events.

Although several factors influence adhesion (for example, calcium ions and surface charge) it is now clear that leukocyte adhesion is principally determined by the binding of complementary adhesion molecules on the leukocyte and endothelial surfaces, like a key and lock. A number of such adhesion molecules have been identified (Table 2-1). Stimulation of adhesion in inflammation is caused by induction of the surface expression of new adhesion molecules, or by increasing their number, or by altering their affinity to each other. Some agents act on the leukocytes, others on endothelial cells, and still others on both cell types.

Two examples of these important interactions are shown in Figure 2-6. In the first, the chemical mediator C5a (page 36) induces in the leukocyte increased surface expression of a family of three integrin glycoproteins called LFA-1, Mac-1, and P150-95 (the

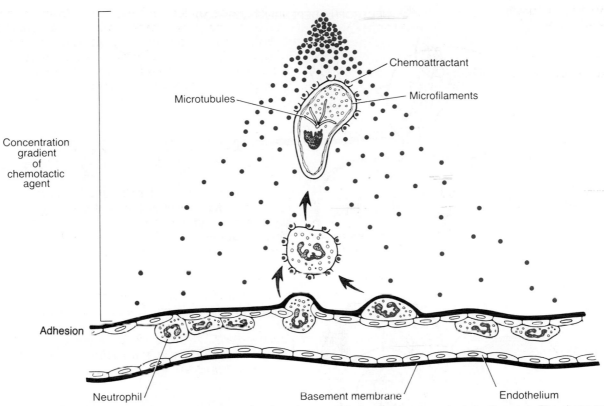

Figure 2-5. Schematic diagram depicting adhesion and emigration of neutrophils in response to a chemotactic agent. The chemoattractant binds to cell surface receptors on neutrophils. For simplicity the leukocytes within blood vessels are shown without the receptors.

CD11/CD18 complex). These integrins have identical beta subunits and different alpha subunits. In addition to increasing the numbers of such molecules, C5a also induces a conformational change in their structure, such that their binding affinity to their endothelial ligands is enhanced, causing increased leukocyte adhesion. The ligand on endothelial cells for LFA-1 and Mac-1 is another adhesion glycoprotein called intercellular adhesion molecule 1 (ICAM-1). In contrast to the effects of C5a, other chemical mediators such as interleukin 1 (IL-1) stimulate leukocyte adhesion by inducing synthesis or increased surface expression of adhesive proteins *on endothelial cells,* which then bind with receptors on leukocytes, *an endothelium-dependent effect.* Three such endothelial adhesion molecules are

endothelial leukocyte adhesion molecule 1 (ELAM-1), involved in neutrophil adhesion; ICAM-1, involved in neutrophil and lymphocyte adhesion; and VCAM-1 (vascular cell adhesion molecule), involved in lymphocyte and monocyte adhesion. Certain mediators, such as tumor necrosis factor (TNF), increase adhesion by affecting the expression of both leukocyte and endothelial molecules.

EMIGRATION AND CHEMOTAXIS

Following adhesion—and almost certainly stimulated by this adhesive interaction—leukocytes move along the endothelial surface, insert pseudopods into the junctions between the endothelial cells, squeeze through interendothelial junctions, and assume a position between the endothelial cell and the basement membrane. Eventually they traverse the basement membrane and escape into the extravascular space (see Fig. 2-5). Neutrophils, monocytes, lymphocytes, eosinophils, and basophils all use the same pathway.

In most types of acute inflammation, neutrophils emigrate first and monocytes later. Since there are also many more neutrophils than monocytes in the blood, in the first 24 to 48 hours most acute inflammatory infiltrates are predominantly neutrophilic (Fig. 2-7). By 48 hours, however, monocytes take over, owing to three factors: (1) Short-lived neutrophils disintegrate and disappear after 24 to 48 hours, whereas monocytes

TABLE 2-1. ENDOTHELIUM-LEUKOCYTE ADHESION MOLECULES

Endothelial Adhesion Molecule	Receptor on Leukocyte	Function
ELAM-1	Sialyl Lewis X	Neutrophil adhesion
ICAM-1	Integrins LFA-1, Mac-1 (CD11a,b/CD18)	Neutrophil, lymphocyte adhesion
VCAM-1	Integrin VLA-4	Lymphocyte, monocyte adhesion

NEUTROPHIL-DEPENDENT ADHESION

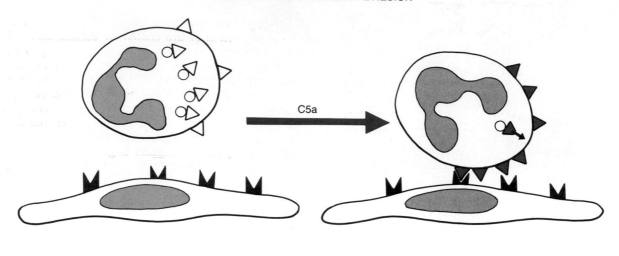

ENDOTHELIUM-DEPENDENT ADHESION

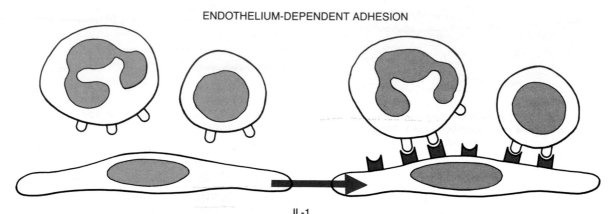

IL-1

Figure 2–6. Two mechanisms of induction of leukocyte-endothelium adhesion in inflammation. C5a causes an increase in the number and avidity of leukocyte adhesion molecules (neutrophil-dependent adhesion), whereas cytokines (e.g., IL-1) induce the surface expression of adhesion molecules on the endothelium (an endothelium-dependent effect). Certain mediators (e.g., TNF) trigger both effects.

survive longer. (2) Monocyte emigration is sustained long after neutrophil emigration ceases. (3) Chemotactic factors for neutrophils and monocytes are activated at different phases of the response.

Leukocytes are thought to emigrate in tissues toward the site of injury, along a chemical gradient, in a process called *chemotaxis* (see Fig. 2–5). Both exogenous and endogenous substances can act as chemotactic agents for leukocytes, among them (1) *soluble bacterial products;* (2) *components of the complement system,* particularly C5a (p. 36); and (3) *products of the lipoxygenase pathway of arachidonic acid (AA) metabolism,* particularly leukotriene B4 (discussed in the section on chemical mediators).

But how does the headless leukocyte "see" (or "smell") the chemotactic agents, and how do these diverse substances actually induce directed cell movement? Although not all the answers are known, several important steps and second messengers are recognized (Fig. 2–8). Binding of chemotactic agents to specific receptors on the cell membranes of leukocytes results in activation of phospholipase C (mediated by a unique G protein), leading to the hydrolysis of phosphatidylinositol-4,5-biphosphate (PIP_2), to inositol-1,4,5-triphosphate (IP_3) and diacylglycerol (DAG), and the release of calcium, first from intracellular stores and subsequently from the influx of extracellular calcium. It is the increased cytosolic calcium that triggers the assembly of contractile elements responsible for cell movement. It also activates phospholipase A_2, which as we shall see (p. 38) converts membrane phospholipids to arachidonic acid. In addition, DAG, through its activation of protein kinase C, is involved in various phases of leukocyte activation, degranulation, and secretion, which occur when there is a very strong chemotactic stimulus or during phagocytosis.

PHAGOCYTOSIS AND DEGRANULATION

Phagocytosis consists of recognition and attachment of the particle to be ingested by the leukocyte; its engulfment, with subsequent formation of a phagocytic

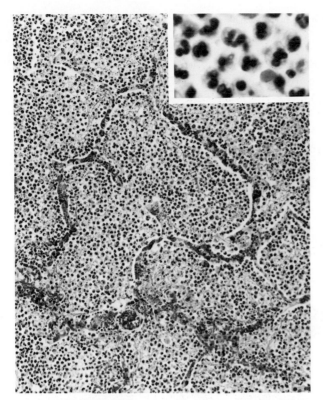

Figure 2–7. Photomicrograph of an acutely inflamed lung (pneumonia) showing emigration of inflammatory cells into the alveoli. Most of the cells in the exudate are neutrophils *(inset)*. (Courtesy of Dr. Charles L. White III, Department of Pathology, Southwestern Medical School, Dallas, TX.)

vacuole, and killing or degradation of the ingested material (Fig. 2–9).

Recognition and attachment of bacteria is accomplished when they are coated by certain serum factors called *opsonins,* which bind to specific receptors on the leukocytes. The two major serum opsonins and their leukocyte receptors are (1) the Fc fragment of the immunoglobulin G (IgG) molecule and its receptor, called FcR, and (2) the C3b fragment of complement, generated by immune or nonimmune mechanisms, and the C3b receptor (C3bi or Mac-1). Binding of the opsonized particles triggers engulfment. Extensions of the cytoplasm (pseudopods) flow around the object to be engulfed, eventually forming a phagocytic vacuole (see Fig. 2–9). The vacuole then fuses with the limiting membrane of a lysosomal granule, resulting in discharge of the granule's contents into the phagolysosome and *degranulation* of the leukocyte. The process is associated with phospholipase C activation, diacylglycerol and IP₂ production, protein kinase C activation, and increased concentration of cytosolic calcium, the latter two acting as second messengers to initiate cellular motile events.

The ultimate step in phagocytosis of bacteria is *killing and degradation. Bacterial killing is accomplished largely by reactive oxygen species.* Phagocytosis

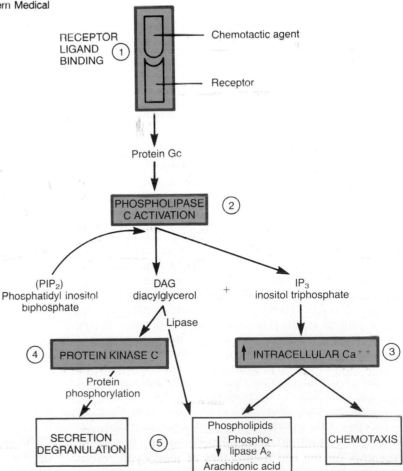

Figure 2–8. Biochemical events in leukocyte activation. The key events are (1) receptor-ligand binding, (2) phospholipase-C activation, (3) increased intracellular calcium, and (4) activation of protein kinase C. The biologic activities (5) resulting from leukocyte activation include chemotaxis, elaboration of arachidonic acid metabolites, secretion, and degranulation.

process is assoc w/:
PLC activation
DAG + IP₂ prod.
PKC activation
↑ [ ] cytosolic Ca²⁺)
   2nd mess-
initiate cell
motile events

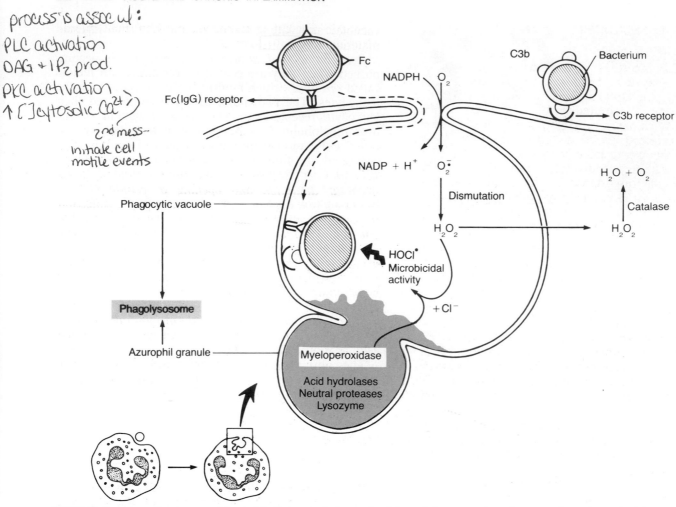

Figure 2–9. Schematic diagram of bacterial phagocytosis by neutrophils and the generation of oxygen-dependent microbicidal mechanisms within the phagolysosome.

stimulates *a burst in oxygen consumption by the leukocytes and the activation of a leukocyte oxidase* (NADPH oxidase), which oxidizes NADPH (reduced nicotinamide adenine dinucleotide) and in the process reduces oxygen to superoxide ion (O_2^-).

$$2O_2 + NADPH \xrightarrow{oxidase} 2O_2^- + NADP^+ + H^+$$

Superoxide is converted into hydrogen peroxide, mostly by spontaneous dismutation ($O_2^- + 2H^+ \rightarrow H_2O_2$). Hydrogen peroxide is then reduced by the enzyme *myeloperoxidase* (present in the azurophil granules of neutrophils) in the presence of a halide such as chloride, to HOCl· ($H_2O_2 + Cl^- \xrightarrow{MPO}$ HOCl· + H_2O). HOCl· is a powerful oxidant and antimicrobial agent. Hydroxyl ions, also formed during oxidative metabolism, are additional antimicrobial agents. Failure of oxidative metabolism during phagocytosis, as occurs in *chronic granulomatous disease of childhood* (CGD), makes these patients unusually susceptible to recurrent infections (p. 33). Microbes can also be killed by non–oxygen-dependent substances in the leukocyte granules, including *bacterial permeability–increasing (BPI) protein, lysozyme, lactoferrin, and a group of newly discovered arginine-rich cationic peptides called defen-*

sins. The pH of the phagolysosome drops to between 4 and 5 after phagocytosis, allowing acid hydrolases to degrade the dead microorganisms.

④ LEUKOCYTE ACTIVATION AND TISSUE INJURY

Under certain circumstances, leukocyte activation during chemotaxis and phagocytosis results in the release of products not only within the phagolysosome but also potentially into the extracellular space. The most important of these substances are (1) *lysosomal enzymes;* (2) *oxygen-derived active metabolites,* described earlier; and (3) *products of AA metabolism,* including prostaglandins and leukotrienes. These products are in themselves powerful mediators that cause endothelial injury and tissue damage and amplify the effects of the initial inflammatory stimulus. Thus, if persistent and unchecked, the leukocytic infiltrate itself becomes the offender, and indeed leukocyte-dependent tissue injury underlies many human diseases, such as rheumatoid arthritis and certain forms of chronic lung disease. This will become evident in the discussion of chronic inflammation.

DEFECTS IN LEUKOCYTE FUNCTION _____

From the preceding discussion it is obvious that leukocytes play a cardinal role in host defense. Not surprisingly, therefore, defects in leukocyte function, both genetic and acquired, lead to increased vulnerability to infections. Impairments of virtually every phase of leukocyte function—from adherence to vascular endothelium/to microbicidal activity—have been described. Although individually rare, these disorders underscore the importance of the complex series of events that must occur in vivo following invasion by microorganisms. Only the most important of the leukocyte defects are briefly noted here.

1. *Defects in adhesion.* The classic example is *leukocyte adhesion deficiency,* an autosomal recessive disorder caused by a deficiency in the biosynthesis of the B chain of the leukocyte integrins described earlier (LFA-1, Mac-1), which mediate leukocyte-endothelial adhesion (p. 29).
2. *Defects in chemotaxis.* These can be classified into two major categories, intrinsic and extrinsic: Intrinsic cellular defects include, for example, Chédiak-Higashi syndrome and diabetes mellitus. In Chédiak-Higashi syndrome, an autosomal recessive disorder, there are multiple abnormalities, including disordered assembly of microtubules, which impair locomotion. Extrinsic defects include defective generation of chemotactic factors, as occurs, for example, in complement deficiency states.
3. *Defects in phagocytosis.* These may also be intrinsic cellular defects (e.g., neutrophil "actin dysfunction," or diabetes mellitus), or extrinsic (deficiencies of immunoglobulins or complement, and the resultant failure of opsonization of the leukocytes).
4. *Defects in microbicidal activity.* This is illustrated by the childhood disease chronic granulomatous disease (CGD), a genetic abnormality in which there is a deficiency of NADPH oxidase. As a result, engulfment of bacteria is not followed by activation of oxygen-dependent killing mechanisms. The defective killing of bacteria by CGD neutrophils is somewhat selective. Many bacteria produce hydrogen peroxide, which can be utilized by neutrophils to form bactericidal compounds, since the myeloperoxidase-halide system is normal; however, certain bacteria such as *Staphylococcus aureus* possess catalase, which inactivates hydrogen peroxide and thus prevents its utilization by the neutrophils. Against such bacteria the CGD neutrophils are defenseless. In contrast, a measure of resistance is present against catalase-negative bacteria such as pneumococci.
5. *Mixed defects.* In some diseases, exemplified by diabetes mellitus and Chédiak-Higashi syndrome, several defects are present. The latter is characterized by neutropenia, decreased chemotaxis, defective degranulation, and delayed microbial killing. The neutrophils and other leukocytes present have giant granules that can be readily appreciated in peripheral blood smears. The molecular basis of this genetic disorder is unknown, but abnormal microtubule function is suspected.

SUMMARY OF THE ACUTE INFLAMMATORY RESPONSE _____

At this point it would be profitable to review the events in acute inflammation discussed so far. The vascular phenomena are characterized by increased blood flow to the injured area, resulting mainly from arteriolar dilatation and opening of capillary beds. Increased vascular permeability results in the collection of protein-rich extravascular fluid, which forms the exudate. Plasma proteins leave the vessels, either through widened interendothelial cell junctions of the venules or by direct endothelial cell injury. The leukocytes, predominantly neutrophils, first adhere to the endothelium via adhesion molecules, then leave the microvasculature and migrate to the site of injury under the influence of chemotactic agents. Phagocytosis of the offending agent follows, which may lead to the death of the microorganism. During chemotaxis and phagocytosis activated leukocytes may release toxic metabolites and proteases extracellularly, potentially causing endothelial and tissue damage.

CHEMICAL MEDIATORS OF INFLAMMATION _____

Having described the events in acute inflammation, we can now turn to a discussion of the chemical mediators that account for the events. So many mediators have been identified that we are confronted with an embarrassment of riches. While the multitude may have survival value for the organism (and also for investigators searching for mediators), they are most difficult for students to learn and remember. Here we review only general principles and highlight some of the more important mediators.

1. Mediators originate either from *plasma* or from *cells* (Fig. 2–10). Plasma-derived mediators (for example, complement) are present in plasma in *precursor forms* that *must be activated,* usually by a series of proteolytic changes, to acquire their biologic properties. Cell-derived mediators are normally *sequestered in intracellular granules* (for example, histamine in mast cells) which need to be secreted or *are synthesized de novo* (for example, prostaglandins) in response to a stimulus.
2. Once activated and released from the cell, most of these mediators quickly decay (for example, AA metabolites) or are inactivated by enzymes (for example, kininase inactivates bradykinin), or otherwise scavenged (antioxidants scavenge toxic oxygen metabolites). There is thus a system of checks and balances in the regulation of mediator actions.
3. Almost all mediators perform their biologic activity by initially *binding to specific receptors on target cells.*

CHEMICAL MEDIATORS

Figure 2–10. Chemical mediators of inflammation.

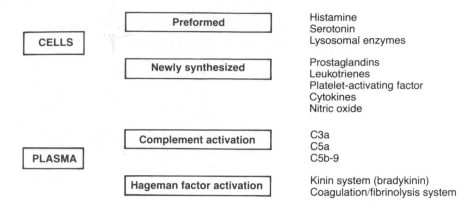

4. A chemical mediator can stimulate the release of mediators by target cells themselves. These secondary mediators may be identical or similar to the initial mediators but may also have opposing activities. They provide mechanisms for amplifying—or in certain instances counteracting—the initial mediator action.

We will now discuss the specific mediators.

VASOACTIVE AMINES

HISTAMINE. *Histamine* is widely distributed in tissues, the richest source being the mast cells that are normally present in the connective tissue adjacent to blood vessels. It is also found in blood basophils and platelets. Preformed histamine is present in mast cell granules and is released by mast cell degranulation in response to a variety of stimuli: (1) physical injury such as trauma or heat, (2) immune reactions involving binding of antibodies to mast cells (p. 122), (3) fragments of complement called anaphylatoxins, (4) cationic lysosomal proteins derived from neutrophils, and (5) certain neuropeptides. In humans, histamine causes dilatation of the arterioles and increases vascular permeability of the venules. It is considered to be the principle mediator of the immediate phase of increased vascular permeability, causing venular endothelial contraction and widening of the interendothelial cell junctions, as we have seen. Soon after being released from mast cells, histamine is inactivated by histaminase. In addition to its role in vascular phenomena, histamine has been reported to be chemotactic for eosinophils.

SEROTONIN. *Serotonin* (5-hydroxytryptamine) is a second vasoactive mediator. Release of serotonin from platelets (the platelet release reaction) is stimulated when platelets aggregate after contact with collagen and antigen-antibody complexes. Although serotonin induces effects similar to those of histamine in rodents, its role as an inflammatory mediator in humans is not established.

PLASMA PROTEASES

A variety of phenomena in the inflammatory response are mediated by three interrelated plasma-derived factors—kinins, complement, and the clotting system (Fig. 2–11).

THE KININ SYSTEM. Activation of the kinin system leads to the formation of bradykinin. Like histamine, bradykinin causes arteriolar dilatation, increased permeability of venules due to contraction of endothelial cells, and extravascular smooth muscle contraction. It is rapidly inactivated by kininases present in plasma and tissues, and its role is limited to the early phase of increased vascular permeability.

Bradykinin is a polypeptide derived from plasma, where it is present in a precursor form called *high–molecular weight kininogen (HMWK)*. This precursor glycoprotein is cleaved by a proteolytic enzyme, *kallikrein,* which must be activated from its own precursor, prekallikrein, by activated factor XII of the clotting system (Hageman factor), which results from contact of factor XII with the injured tissues, especially collagen and vascular basement membrane. Figure 2–11 illustrates the close interaction between the clotting and the kinin-generating system and also the amplifying effect of kallikrein on the activation of Hageman factor.

THE COMPLEMENT SYSTEM. The complement system consists of a series of plasma proteins that play an important role in both immunity and inflammation. Complement components present as inactive forms in plasma are numbered C1 through C9. Although it is not our intention to go into the detailed sequence of the activation of the "complement cascade," a brief review of the salient features will be helpful to our discussion. The most critical step in the elaboration of the biologic functions of complement is the activation of the third component, C3 (Fig. 2–12). All other complement components can be grouped into functional units in relation to their interaction with C3. Cleavage of C3 can occur by the so-called *classical pathway,* which is triggered by fixation of C1 to antibody (IgM or IgG) combined with antigen. Activation

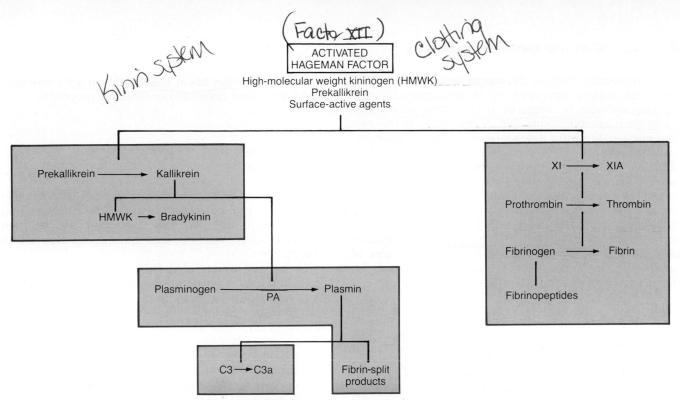

Figure 2–11. Plasma mediator systems triggered by activation of Hageman factor. PA = plasminogen activator.

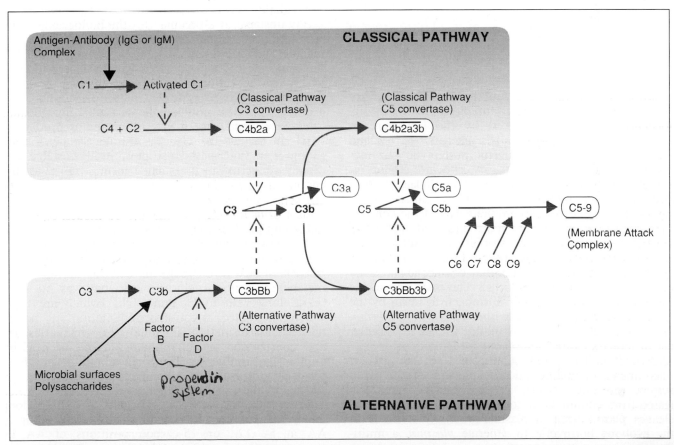

Figure 2–12. Overview of complement activation pathways. The classical pathway is initiated by C1 binding to antigen-antibody complexes, and the alternative pathway is initiated by C3b binding to various activating surfaces, such as microbial cell walls. The C3b involved in alternative pathway initiation may be generated in several ways, including spontaneously, by the classical pathway, or by the alternative pathway itself (see text). Both pathways converge and lead to the formation of inflammatory complement mediators (C3a and C5a) and the membrane attack complex. In this figure, bars over the letter designations of complement components indicate enzymatically active forms and dashed lines indicate proteolytic activities of various components. (Modified from Abbas, A. K., et al.: Cellular and Molecular Immunology. Philadelphia, W. B. Saunders Co., 1991, p. 261.)

can also occur through the *alternate* pathway, which does not require activation by antigen-antibody complexes, and can be triggered by bacterial polysaccharides such as endotoxins and human IgA. It involves the participation of a distinct set of serum components called the properdin system (properdin [P], factors B and D). Whichever pathway is involved in the cleavage of C3, there is a single amplification mechanism composed of the alternate pathway proteins, which promote further conversion of C3 to C3b. Once C3b is generated, it utilizes a common final *effector* sequence involving C5 through C9, which leads to the generation of several biologically active factors and lysis of antibody-coated cells. Complement-derived factors affect a variety of phenomena in acute inflammation:

1. *Vascular phenomena.* C3a and C5a (also called anaphylatoxins), which are the split products of the corresponding complement components (see Fig. 2–12), increase vascular permeability and cause vasodilatation by releasing histamine from mast cells. C5a also activates the lipoxygenase pathway of AA metabolism in neutrophils and monocytes, causing further release of inflammatory mediators.
2. *Chemotaxis.* As mentioned previously, C5a, a split product of C5, causes adhesion of neutrophils to the endothelium and is chemotactic for monocytes and neutrophils.
3. *Phagocytosis.* C3b, when fixed to the bacterial cell wall, acts as an opsonin and favors phagocytosis by neutrophils and macrophages, which bear cell surface receptors for C3b.

Among the complement components, C3 and C5 are undoubtedly the most important mediators. Their significance is further enhanced by the fact that, in addition to the mechanisms discussed above, C3 and C5 can be activated by several proteolytic enzymes present within the inflammatory exudate. These include plasmin and lysosomal enzymes released from neutrophils (see discussion later in this chapter). Thus, the chemotactic effect of complement and the complement-activating effects of neutrophils can set up a self-perpetuating cycle of neutrophil emigration.

THE CLOTTING SYSTEM. The clotting system (p. 67) is a series of plasma proteins that can be activated by Hageman factor (see Fig. 2–11). The final step of the cascade is the conversion of fibrinogen to fibrin by the action of thrombin. During this conversion, *fibrinopeptides* are formed, which induce increased vascular permeability and are chemotactic for leukocytes.

The *fibrinolytic system* contributes to the vascular phenomena of inflammation by means of the kinin system (see Fig. 2–11). Plasminogen activator (released from endothelium, leukocytes, and other tissues) cleaves plasminogen, a plasma protein that binds to the evolving fibrin clot to generate *plasmin,* a multifunctional protease. Plasmin is important in lysing fibrin clots, but in the context of inflammation it has the following actions: (1) it activates Hageman factor (XII), releasing factor XIIA, which initiates the cascade to generate bradykinin; (2) it cleaves C3, the third component of complement, to produce C3 fragments;

and (3) it degrades fibrin to form fibrin split products, which may have permeability-inducing properties.

ARACHIDONIC ACID METABOLITES: PROSTAGLANDINS AND LEUKOTRIENES _____

Products derived from the metabolism of AA affect a variety of biologic processes including inflammation and hemostasis and play important physiologic roles in the renal, cardiovascular, and pulmonary systems, to name a few.

AA is a polyunsaturated fatty acid that is present in large amounts in phospholipids of the cell membrane. It is released from membrane phospholipids due to activation of cellular phospholipases by inflammatory stimuli or by other chemical mediators such as C5a. During inflammation, lysosomes of neutrophils are believed to be an important source of phospholipases. AA metabolism proceeds along one of two major pathways (Fig. 2–13), which are named after the enzymes that initiate the reactions:

THE CYCLOOXYGENASE PATHWAY. This leads initially to the formation of a cyclic endoperoxide, prostaglandin G_2 (PGG_2), which in turn is converted into prostaglandin H_2 (PGH_2) by a peroxidase. PGH_2, itself highly unstable, is a precursor of the biologically active end products of the cyclooxygenase pathway. These include PGE_2, PGD_2, $PGF_{2\alpha}$, PGI_2 (prostacyclin), and thromboxane (TXA_2), each of which is derived from PGH_2 by the action of a specific enzyme. Some of these enzymes have restricted tissue distribution. For example, platelets contain the enzyme thromboxane synthetase, and hence TXA_2 is the major product of PGH_2 in these cells. TXA_2 is a potent platelet-aggregating agent and vasoconstrictor, itself unstable and rapidly converted to its inactive form TXB_2. Vascular endothelium, on the other hand, lacks thromboxane synthetase but posseses prostacyclin synthetase, which leads to the formation of prostacyclin (PGI_2) and its stable end product $PGF_{1\alpha}$. Prostacyclin is a vasodilator and a potent inhibitor of platelet aggregation. The opposing roles of TXA_2 and PGI_2 in hemostasis are further discussed on page 67. PGD_2 is the major metabolite of the cyclooxygenase pathway in mast cells; along with PGE_2 and PGF_2 (which are more widely distributed) it causes vasodilatation and potentiates edema formation. It should be noted that aspirin and nonsteroidal antiinflammatory agents such as indomethacin inhibit cyclooxygenase and thus inhibit prostaglandin synthesis. Lipoxygenase, however, is not affected by these antiinflammatory agents.

LIPOXYGENASE PATHWAY. The initial reaction along this pathway is the addition of a hydroperoxy group to AA at 5-, 12-, or 15-carbon positions of AA by enzymes called 5-, 12-, or 15- lipoxygenases, respectively. 5-Lipoxygenase is the predominant enzyme in neutrophils, and the metabolites derived by its actions are the best-characterized. The 5-hydroperoxy derivative of AA, 5-HPETE, is quite unstable and is either reduced to 5-HETE (which is chemotactic for neutro-

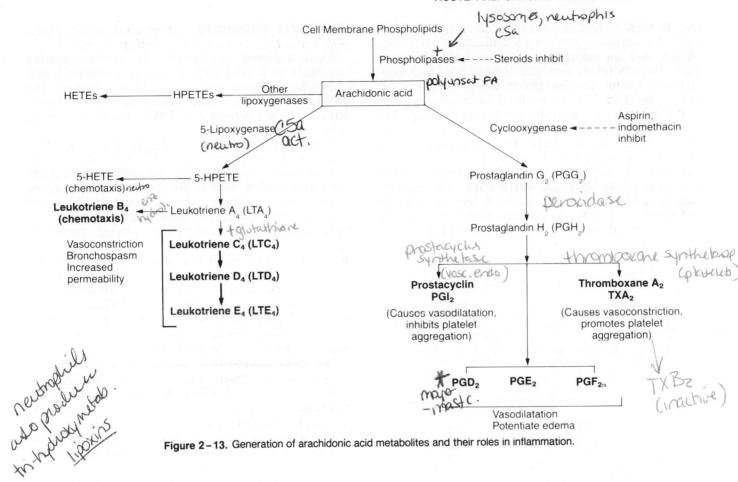

Figure 2-13. Generation of arachidonic acid metabolites and their roles in inflammation.

phils) or converted into a family of compounds collectively called *leukotrienes*. The first leukotriene generated from 5-HPETE is called leukotriene A_4 (LTA_4), which in turn gives rise to leukotriene B_4 (LTB_4) by enzymatic hydrolysis or to leukotriene C_4 (LTC_4) by addition of glutathione. LTC_4 is converted to leukotriene D_4 (LTD_4) and finally to leukotriene E_4 (LTE_4). LTB_4 is a potent chemotactic agent and causes aggregation of neutrophils. LTC_4, LTD_4, and LTE_4 cause vasoconstriction, bronchospasm, and increased vascular permeability. Neutrophils also produce trihydroxy-metabolites of AA called *lipoxins*. These metabolites have powerful pro-inflammatory effects but their role in vivo is still unclear.

In summary, prostaglandins and leukotrienes can mediate virtually every step of acute inflammation. Although the effects of the AA metabolites have been investigated most extensively in vitro, there is mounting evidence for their role in vivo. Prostaglandins and leukotrienes can be found in inflammatory exudates, and agents that suppress cyclooxygenase (aspirin, indomethacin) also suppress inflammation in vivo. Glucocorticoids, which are powerful antiinflammatory agents, may act at least in part by inducing the synthesis of a protein that inhibits phospholipase A_2. Recall that phospholipases are required for the generation of AA from the phospholipids of the cell. Thus, glucocorticoids, by blocking the synthesis of AA, may effectively prevent the subsequent generation of prostaglandins and leukotrienes. Finally, variations in

arachidonic acid metabolism may account for some of the beneficial effects of *fish oil*. Diets rich in fish oil contain essential fatty acids of the $\omega 3$ variety (e.g., *linolenic acid*) rather than $\omega 2$ linoleic acid found in most animal or vegetable fat. The $\omega 3$ fatty acids serve as poor substrates for conversion to active metabolites of the cyclooxygenase, and particularly the lipoxygenase, series. Such diets inhibit platelet aggregation to inhibit thrombosis and prevent certain inflammatory processes.

PLATELET-ACTIVATING FACTOR

Platelet-activating factor (PAF) is another phospholipid-derived mediator. It has long been known as a factor, derived from antigen-stimulated IgE-sensitized basophils, which causes platelets to aggregate and release their contents. Its chemical structure is acetyl glycerol ether phosphocholine (AGEPC). In addition to platelet stimulation, PAF causes increased vascular permeability, leukocyte aggregation and adhesion, chemotaxis, and a number of systemic hemodynamic changes. A variety of cell types, including basophils, neutrophils, monocytes, and endothelium, can elaborate PAF. It appears to act directly on target cells, but it also stimulates the synthesis of other mediators, particularly prostaglandins and leukotrienes, by leukocytes and other cells.

CYTOKINES

Cytokines are polypeptides produced by many cell types (but principally activated lymphocytes and macrophages) that modulate the function of other cell types. Long known to be involved in cellular immune responses, these products have additional effects that play important roles in the inflammatory response. Cytokines that appear to be important mediators of inflammation are IL-1, TNF, and IL-8.

IL-1 and TNF share many biologic properties. Both are produced by activated macrophages and IL-1 by many other cell types as well. Their secretion can be stimulated by endotoxin, immune complexes, toxins, physical injury, and a variety of inflammatory processes. They induce their effects in three ways: they can act on the same cell that produces them (an *autocrine* effect); on cells in the immediate vicinity (as in lymph nodes and joint spaces; a *paracrine* effect); or systemically, as with any other hormone (*endocrine* effect). Their most important actions in inflammation are the local effects on endothelium, the systemic acute-phase reactions, and the effect on fibroblasts (Fig. 2–14). In particular they induce the synthesis and surface expression of the endothelial adhesion molecules that mediate leukocyte sticking and increase surface thrombogenicity of the endothelium. They are largely responsible for the fever seen in acute inflammation. TNF also causes aggregation and activation of neutrophils and the release of proteolytic enzymes from mesenchymal cells, thus contributing to tissue damage. IL-8 is a small (8000 Kd) polypeptide, produced by activated macrophages and other cell types, that is a powerful chemoattractant and activator of neutrophils.

LEUKOCYTE PRODUCTS

When activated by chemotactic agents, immune complexes, or a phagocytic challenge, neutrophils and macrophages release oxygen-derived free radicals and lysosomal enzymes, which may contribute to inflammation. *Oxygen-derived metabolites* are implicated in three responses:

- *Endothelial cell damage with resultant increased vascular permeability.*
- *Inactivation of antiproteases,* such as α_1-antitrypsin, discussed earlier. Potentially this may lead to unopposed protease activity with increased destruction of structural components of tissue, such as elastin.
- *Injury to other cell types* (tumor cells, red cells, parenchymal cells).

As discussed in Chapter 1, serum, tissue fluids, and target cells possess antioxidant protective mechanisms that detoxify these potentially harmful oxygen-derived radicals. *Thus, the influence of oxygen-derived free radicals in any given inflammatory reaction depends on the balance between the production and inactivation of these metabolites by cells and tissues.*

Lysosomal contents of neutrophils, when released, provide several mediators of acute inflammation. These are released from neutrophils by several mechanisms: following death of neutrophils, by leakage during the formation of the phagocytic vacuole, and by reverse endocytosis. In the latter process, attempted phagocytosis of immune complexes attached to flat surfaces leads to exocytosis (expulsion) of lysosomal enzymes into the medium. The effects of many of these substances were discussed earlier in this section and will be mentioned briefly here. *Neutral proteases* including enzymes such as elastase, collagenase, and cathepsin can mediate tissue injury by degrading elastin, collagen, and other tissue proteins. Proteases may cleave C3 and C5 directly to generate anaphylatoxins. Kallikrein released from the lysosomes promotes the generation of bradykinin. Cationic proteins include several biologically active factors that (1) increase vascular permeability by causing mast cell degranulation, (2) possess chemotactic activity for monocytes, and (3) immobilize neutrophils at the site of inflammation.

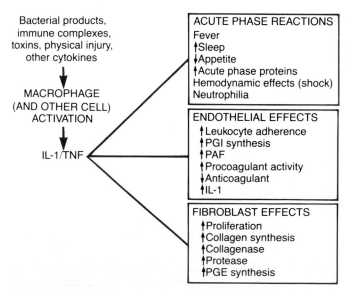

Figure 2–14. Major effects of interleukin 1 (IL-1) and tumor necrosis factor (TNF) in inflammation.

TABLE 2–2. SUMMARY OF MEDIATORS IN INFLAMMATION

Event	Mediator or Mechanism
Vasodilatation	Histamine, bradykinin, prostaglandins-I_2, E_2, D_2, $F_{2\alpha}$
Increased vascular permeability	Histamine, bradykinin, C3a and C5a (anaphylatoxins), leukotriene C_4, D_4, E_4, PAF, oxygen metabolites
Chemotaxis	LTB_4, C5a, bacterial products, neutrophil cationic proteins, cytokines (TNF, IL-8)
Fever	IL-1, TNF
Pain	PGE_2, bradykinin
Tissue damage	Oxygen free *radicals*, lysosomal enzymes

Other Mediators

Neuropeptides, such as substance P, cause vasodilatation and increased vascular permeability both directly and by stimulating mast cell degranulation. They are probably involved in neurogenic inflammation. *Nitric oxide* produced by endothelium, macrophages, and other cells causes vasodilation and is potentially cytotoxic. It is currently receiving close scrutiny as a possible mediator in physiologic and pathologic processes in which vasodilatation and tissue damage occur.

A summary of the mediators in inflammation is presented in Table 2–2.

Chronic Inflammation

DEFINITION AND CAUSES

Acute inflammation may have one of four outcomes:

1. *Complete resolution.* In a perfect world, all inflammatory reactions, once they have succeeded in neutralizing the injurious stimulus, should end with restoration of the site of acute inflammation to normal. This is called resolution and is the usual outcome when the injury is limited or short lived or when there has been little tissue destruction. Resolution involves neutralization of the chemical mediators, with subsequent return of normal vascular permeability, cessation of leukocytic infiltration, and finally removal of edema fluid, leukocytes, foreign agents, and necrotic debris from the battleground (Fig. 2–15). Lymphatics and phagocytes play a role in these events, as we shall see.
2. *Healing by scarring* occurs after substantial tissue destruction, or when the inflammation occurs in tissues that do not regenerate, or when there is abundant fibrin exudation. Scarring is detailed in Chapter 3.
3. *Abscess formation,* which occurs particularly in infections with pyogenic organisms, and
4. Progression to *chronic inflammation.* Chronic inflammation may arise in one of two ways. It may follow acute inflammation, or the response may be chronic almost from the onset. Acute to chronic transition occurs when the acute inflammatory response cannot be resolved, owing either to the persistence of the injurious agent or to some interference in the normal process of healing. For example, bacterial infection of the lung may begin as a focus of acute inflammation (pneumonia), but its failure to resolve may lead to extensive tissue destruction and formation of a cavity in which the inflammation continues to smolder, leading eventually to a chronic lung abscess. Another example of chronic inflammation with a persisting stimulus is peptic ulcer of the duodenum or stomach. Peptic ulcers may persist for years and as we shall see (p. 487) are manifested by both acute and chronic inflammatory tissues.

In most settings chronic inflammation is initiated as a primary process. Often the injurious agents are less toxic than those that lead to acute inflammation. Three major groups can be identified:

1. *Persistent infections* by certain intracellular microorganisms, such as tubercle bacilli, *Treponema pallidum* (causative organism of syphilis), and certain fungi. These organisms are of low toxicity and evoke an immune reaction called delayed hypersen-

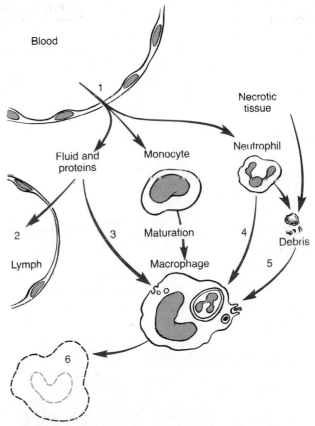

Figure 2–15. Events in the resolution of inflammation: (1) return to normal vascular permeability; (2) drainage of edema fluid and proteins into lymphatics or (3) by pinocytosis into macrophages; (4) phagocytosis of neutrophils; and (5) necrotic debris by macrophages; and (6) disposal of macrophages. Note the central role of macrophages in resolution. (Modified from Haslett, C., Henson, P. M.: *In* Clark, R., Henson, P. M. (eds.): The Molecular and Cellular Biology of Wound Repair. New York, Plenum Press, Inc., plc, 1988.)

sitivity (p. 130). The inflammatory response often takes a specific pattern called a granulomatous reaction, which is discussed later in this chapter.

2. *Prolonged exposure to nondegradable inanimate material;* an example is silica particles, which after being inhaled for a prolonged period set up a chronic inflammatory response in the lungs called *silicosis* (p. 223). Silica may act as both a chemical and a mechanical irritant.

3. Under certain conditions, immune reactions are set up against the individual's own tissues, leading to *autoimmune diseases* (see p. 138). In these diseases, autoantigens evoke a self-perpetuating immune reaction that results in several important chronic inflammatory diseases, such as rheumatoid arthritis.

CHRONIC INFLAMMATORY CELLS _____

In contrast to acute inflammation, which is manifested by vascular changes, edema, and leukocytic infiltration, chronic inflammation is characterized by infiltration with mononuclear cells, which include macrophages, lymphocytes, and plasma cells (Fig. 2–16), tissue destruction, and fibrosis. Macrophages play a central role in these processes, and we will begin our discussion with a brief review of the biology of macrophages.

Macrophages are but one component of the *mononuclear phagocyte system (MPS)*, previously known as the reticuloendothelial system (RES) (Fig. 2–17A). The MPS consists of closely related cells of bone marrow origin, including blood monocytes, and tissue macrophages. The latter are diffusely scattered in the

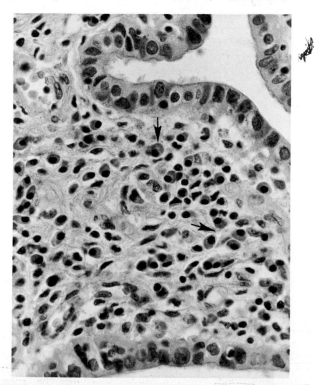

Figure 2–16. Chronic inflammation of the fallopian tube. The subepithelial connective tissue is infiltrated with mononuclear white cells, principally plasma cells marked by eccentric nuclei *(see arrows).*

connective tissues or clustered in organs such as the liver (Kupffer cells), spleen and lymph nodes (sinus histiocytes), and lungs (alveolar macrophages). All arise from a common precursor in the bone marrow, which gives rise to blood monocytes. From the blood, monocytes migrate into various tissues and transform into macrophages. The half-life of blood monocytes is about one day, whereas the life span of tissue macrophages is several months.

In addition to phagocytosis, already discussed, macrophages possess several other features that are important in their role as inflammatory cells. *They have the potential of being "activated,"* a process that results in an increase in cell size, increased levels of lysosomal enzymes, more active metabolism, and greater ability to phagocytose and kill ingested microbes. Macrophage activation is a complex multistep process occurring in response to external stimuli that must be presented in an orderly sequence. Activation signals include lymphokines (such as γ-interferon) secreted by sensitized T lymphocytes, bacterial endotoxins, and contact with fibronectin-coated surfaces and a variety of chemicals, some of which are generated during acute inflammation. Following activation, the *macrophages secrete a wide variety of biologically active products* that are important mediators of the tissue destruction and fibrosis characteristic of chronic inflammation (Fig. 2–17B). These can be grouped into the following major categories (Table 2–3):

1. *Enzymes:* both neutral and acid proteases. Several neutral proteases such as elastase and collagenase were previously mentioned as mediators of tissue damage in inflammation. Others, such as plasminogen activator, trigger the production of plasmin and greatly amplify the generation of pro-inflammatory substances.

2. *Plasma proteins:* These include complement proteins and coagulation proteins such as tissue factor and factors V, VII, IX, and X.

3. *Reactive metabolites of oxygen.*

4. *Lipid mediators* including products of AA metabolism and PAF.

5. *Cytokines,* such as IL-1 and TNF.

6. *Growth factors,* which influence the proliferation of a variety of cell types.

It should be noted that although this impressive arsenal of mediators, enzymes, and factors makes macrophages powerful allies in the body's defense against unwanted invaders, the very same weaponry can also induce considerable tissue damage when macrophages are inappropriately activated, as may occur in autoimmune diseases. Thus, *tissue destruction is one of the hallmarks of chronic inflammation.*

Returning to the presence of macrophages at sites of chronic inflammation, it must be obvious that they are derived from blood monocytes that emigrate from the blood vessels under the influence of chemotactic factors. The steady release of lymphocyte-derived factors (p. 38) is an important mechanism by which macrophages continue to accumulate at the site of chronic inflammation. Once in the tissues, macrophages have

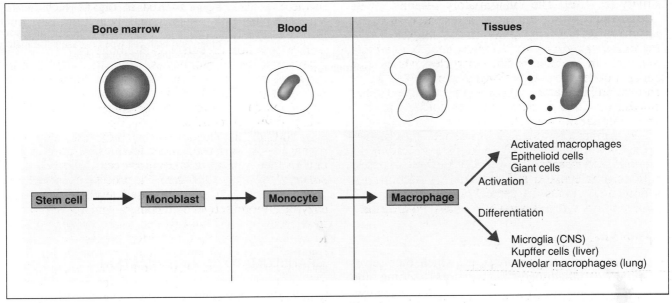

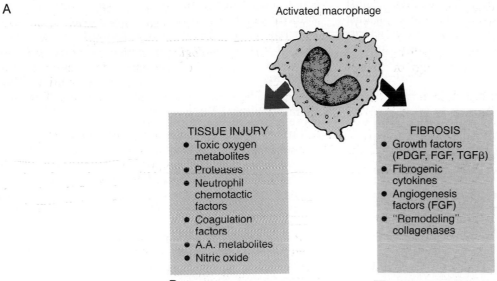

Figure 2–17. A, Maturation of mononuclear phagocytes. B, Macrophage products involved in tissue destruction and fibrosis. (A from Abbas, A. K., et al.: Cellular and Molecular Immunology. Philadelphia, W. B. Saunders Co., 1991, p. 21.)

TABLE 2–3. PRODUCTS RELEASED
BY MACROPHAGES

1. Enzymes
   Neutral proteases
      Elastase
      Collagenase
      Plasminogen activator
   Acid hydrolases
      Phosphatases
      Lipases
2. Plasma proteins
   Complement components (e.g., C1 to C5, properdin)
   Coagulation factors (e.g., factors V, VII, tissue factor)
3. Reactive metabolites of oxygen
4. Arachidonic acid metabolites
5. Cytokines (IL-1, TNF, IL-8)
6. Growth factors (PDGF, EGF, FGF)

the ability to survive for long periods, outliving neutrophils, which may have been the earliest cells to arrive. Macrophages also have a limited capacity to divide. Fusion of macrophages can lead to formation of large cells having multiple nuclei, called giant cells (p. 131).

Other types of cells present in chronic inflammation are lymphocytes, plasma cells, and eosinophils. *Lymphocytes* are mobilized in both antibody- and cell-mediated immune reactions, but also, for reasons unknown, in non–immune-mediated inflammation. They have a reciprocal relationship to macrophages in chronic inflammation (Fig. 2–18). Lymphocytes can be activated by contact with antigen. Activated lymphocytes produce *lymphokines*, and one of these, γ-interferon, is a major stimulator of monocytes and macrophages. Products of activated macrophages (mono-

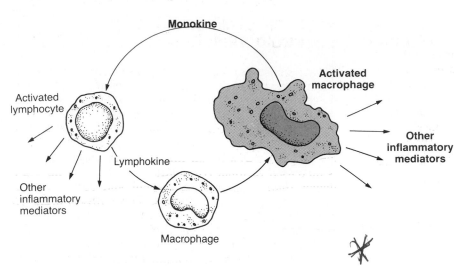

Figure 2–18. Macrophage-lymphocyte interactions in chronic inflammation. Activated lymphocytes and macrophages influence each other, and both cell types release inflammatory mediators that affect other cells.

kines) in turn activate lymphocytes, which themselves also produce inflammatory mediators—setting the stage for persistence of the inflammatory response. *Plasma cells* produce antibody, directed either against persistent antigen in the inflammatory site or against altered tissue components. *Eosinophils* are characteristic of immune reactions mediated by IgE and of parasitic infections. Their granules contain *major basic protein* (MBP), a highly cationic 14,000-Kd protein that is toxic to parasites but also causes lysis of mammalian epithelial cells.

Finally, fibrosis—the proliferation of fibroblasts and accumulation of excess extracellular matrix—is a common feature of many chronic inflammatory diseases and is an important cause of loss of organ function. The mechanisms of inflammatory fibrosis are similar to those that obtain during repair and are discussed in Chapter 3.

GRANULOMATOUS INFLAMMATION _____

This distinctive pattern of chronic inflammatory reaction encountered in relatively few diseases is described in more detail on page 130. Tuberculosis is the archetype of the granulomatous diseases, but sarcoidosis, cat-scratch disease, lymphogranuloma inguinale, leprosy, brucellosis, syphilis, and some of the mycotic infections, berylliosis, and reactions to irritant lipids are also included (Table 2–4). Recognition of the granulomatous pattern in a biopsy is important because of the limited number of possible conditions that cause it, some of which are extremely threatening.

A granuloma consists of a microscopic aggregation of macrophages that may be transformed into epithelium-like cells (and are therefore designated epithelioid cells) surrounded by a collar of mononuclear leukocytes, principally lymphocytes and occasionally plasma cells

TABLE 2–4. EXAMPLES OF GRANULOMATOUS INFLAMMATIONS

Disease	Cause	Tissue Reaction
Bacterial		
Tuberculosis	*Mycobacterium tuberculosis*	Noncaseating tubercle (granuloma prototype): a focus of epithelioid cells, rimmed by fibroblasts, lymphocytes, histiocytes, occasional Langhans' giant cell; caseating tubercle: central amorphous granular debris, loss of all cellular detail; acid-fast bacilli
Leprosy	*Mycobacterium leprae*	Acid-fast bacilli in macrophages; granulomas and epithelioid types
Syphilis	*Treponema pallidum*	Gumma: Microscopic to grossly visible lesion, enclosing wall of histiocytes; plasma cell infiltrate; center cells are necrotic without loss of cellular outline
Cat-scratch disease	Gram-negative bacillus	Rounded or stellate granuloma containing central granular debris and recognizable neutrophils; giant cells uncommon
Parasitic		
Schistosomiasis	*Schistosoma mansoni, S. haematobium, S. japonicum*	Egg emboli; eosinophils
Fungal		
	Cryptococcus neoformans	Organism is yeast-like, sometimes budding; 5 to 10 μm; large, clear capsule
	Coccidioides immitis	Organism appears as spherical (30–80 μm) cyst containing endospores of 3–5 μm each
Inorganic Metals and Dusts		
Silicosis, berylliosis		Lung involvement; fibrosis
Unknown		
Sarcoidosis		Noncaseating granuloma: giant cells (Langhans' and foreign-body types); asteroids in giant cells; occasional Schaumann's body (concentric calcific concretion); no organisms

(Fig. 2–19). In the usual hematoxylin and eosin preparations the epithelioid cells have a pale pink granular cytoplasm with indistinct cell boundaries, often appearing to merge into one another. The nucleus is less dense than that of a lymphocyte (vesicular), is oval or elongate, and may show folding of the nuclear membrane. Older granulomas develop an enclosing rim of fibroblasts and connective tissue. Frequently, but not invariably, *large giant cells* are found in the periphery or sometimes in the center of granulomas. These giant cells may attain diameters of 40 to 50 μm. They comprise a large mass of cytoplasm containing 20 or more small nuclei.

There are two types of granulomas:

- *Foreign body granulomas,* incited by relatively inert foreign bodies.
- *Immune granulomas.* Two factors determine the formation of immune granulomas: the presence of indigestible particles or organisms (such as the tubercle bacillus) and T cell–mediated immunity to the inciting agent. Products of activated T lymphocytes, principally γ-interferon, are important in transforming macrophages into epithelioid cells and multinucleate giant cells.

To summarize, granulomatous inflammation is a specific type of chronic reaction characterized by accumulations of modified macrophages (epithelioid cells) and initiated by a variety of infectious and noninfectious agents. The presence of *poorly digestible irritants or T cell–mediated immunity to the irritant, or both,* appears to be necessary for granuloma formation.

ROLE OF LYMPHATICS AND LYMPHOID TISSUE

Lymphatics are almost as pervasive as capillaries. In tissues terminal lymphatics are blind-ended, thin-walled tubes. All are lined with continuous endothelium having loose cell junctions. One function of lymphatics is to drain the small amount of low-protein tissue fluid that is normally formed by ultrafiltration of the blood (p. 27). In an inflammatory response, there is increased regional lymphatic flow of a fluid having a higher than usual protein content and containing increased numbers of leukocytes. These vessels drain off the fluid and cells from the area of reaction and are important in the resolution of inflammation (see Fig. 2–15). Regrettably, lymphatic drainage also provides channels for the dissemination of the injurious agent. Inflammatory involvement of lymphatic channels *(lymphangitis)* and the regional filtering lymph nodes *(reactive lymphadenitis)* may develop. Reactive lymphadenitis is associated with a variety of changes, prominent among which are enlargements of the lymphoid follicles and increases in the number of histiocytes lining the sinuses. Often there is phagocytosis of cell debris by the phagocytic cells of the sinuses and follicles. Occasionally polymorphonuclear cells and particulate debris can be identified in the sinuses. If significant numbers of viable bacteria drain to the node, they may set up secondary sites of necrosis, which leads to the destruction of the lymph node and accumulation of exudate in these sites.

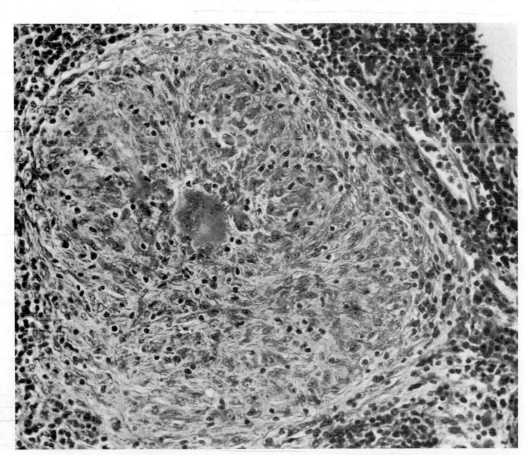

Figure 2–19. A granuloma with a central Langhans'-type giant cell surrounded by epithelioid cells (large pale cells) and lymphocytes.

Nevertheless, the regional lymph nodes constitute important secondary lines of defense, which, in general, tend to screen off the infection from the remainder of the body. As would be expected, if these secondary lines of defense are overwhelmed, the inflammatory reaction may extend throughout the body. This dissemination is encountered only in severe inflammatory reactions and usually implies drainage of the infection through the entire lymphatic system and then into the blood as well. With microbiologic infections that involve the bloodstream, cells of the MPS, particularly Kupffer cells of the liver and splenic macrophages, constitute the main line of defense. When infections become generalized, tender lymphadenopathy appears, accompanied by hepatomegaly and splenomegaly. For this reason, the astute clinician always palpates for enlargement of the lymph nodes, liver, and spleen in febrile patients suspected of having a disseminated microbiologic infection.

MORPHOLOGIC PATTERNS IN ACUTE AND CHRONIC INFLAMMATION _____

The severity of the reaction, its specific cause, and the particular tissue and site involved all introduce morphologic variations in the basic patterns of acute and chronic inflammation.

SEROUS INFLAMMATION. Serous inflammation is marked by the outpouring of a thin fluid that, depending on the site of injury, is derived from either the blood serum or the secretions of mesothelial cells lining the peritoneal, pleural, and pericardial cavities. The skin blister resulting from a burn represents a large accumulation of fluid, either within or immediately beneath the epidermis of the skin.

FIBRINOUS INFLAMMATION. With more severe injuries and the resulting greater vascular permeability, larger molecules pass the vascular barrier. A fibrinous inflammatory exudate develops when the vascular leaks are large enough to permit the passage of fibrinogen molecules. A fibrinous exudate is characteristic of inflammation in body cavities, such as the pericardium and pleura. Histologically, fibrin appears as an eosinophilic meshwork of threads, or sometimes as an amorphous coagulum (Fig. 2–20). Fibrinous exudates may be removed by fibrinolysis, and other debris by macrophages. This process, called *resolution,* may restore normal tissue structure, but when the fibrin is not removed it may stimulate the ingrowth of fibroblasts and blood vessels and thus lead to scarring. Conversion of the fibrinous exudate to scar tissue *(organization)* within the pericardial sac will lead either to opaque fibrous thickening of the pericardium and epicardium in the area of exudation or, more often, to the development of fibrous strands that bridge the pericardial space. It is evident, then, that fibrinous exudation may have more serious consequences than serous exudation.

SUPPURATIVE OR PURULENT INFLAMMATION. This form of inflammation is characterized by the production of large amounts of pus or purulent exudate.

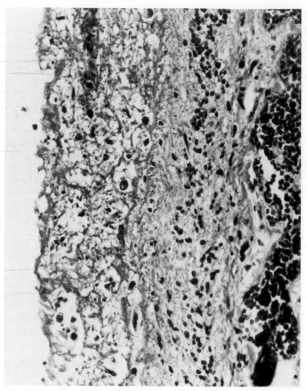

Figure 2–20. Fibrinous inflammation of the pleura. A meshwork of fibrin strands on the left is seen overlying the congested and inflamed pleura. (Courtesy of Dr. Charles L. White III, Department of Pathology, University of Texas, Southwestern Medical School, Dallas, TX.)

Certain organisms (e.g., staphylococci) produce this localized suppuration and are therefore referred to as pyogenic (pus-producing) bacteria. A common example of an acute suppurative inflammation is acute appendicitis. *Abscesses are localized collections of pus caused by suppuration buried in a tissue, organ, or confined space.* They are produced by deep seeding of pyogenic bacteria into a tissue. Abscesses have a central region that appears as a mass of necrotic white cells and tissue cells. There is usually a zone of preserved neutrophils about this necrotic focus, and outside this region vascular dilatation and parenchymal and fibroblastic proliferation occur, indicating the beginning of repair. In time, the abscess may become walled off by connective tissue that limits further spread. Pyogenic infections of the skin range from the simple hair follicle infection *(folliculitis)* to the *furuncle* (also called a "boil"), which involves suppuration of subcutaneous tissue, to multiple deep-seated abscesses called *carbuncles.* Certain organisms such as *streptococci* cause an acute edematous and purulent inflammation (called *cellulitis*) that tends to trek rapidly through large areas of tissue such as an entire arm, the face, or the abdominal wall.

ULCERS. *An ulcer is a local defect, or excavation, of the surface of an organ or tissue that is produced by the sloughing (shedding) of inflammatory necrotic tissue.* Ulceration can occur only when an inflammatory necrotic area exists on or near the surface. It is most

Figure 2–21. A low-power cross section of duodenal ulcer crater with a dark inflammatory exudate in the base.

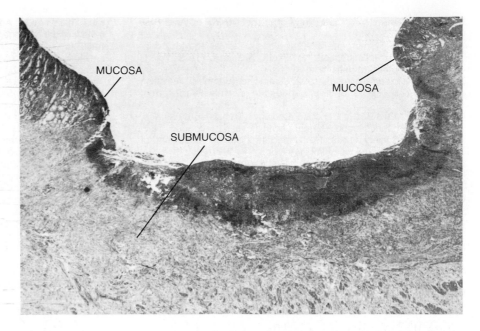

MUCOSA

MUCOSA

SUBMUCOSA

commonly encountered in ① inflammatory necrosis of the mucosa of the mouth, stomach, intestines, or genitourinary tract, and ② subcutaneous inflammations of the lower extremities in older persons who have circulatory disturbances that predispose to extensive necrosis. Such lesions are best exemplified by the peptic ulcer of the stomach or duodenum (Fig. 2–21). During the acute stage, there is intense polymorphonuclear infiltration and vascular dilatation in the margins of the defect. With chronicity, the margins and base of the ulcer develop fibroblastic proliferation, scarring, and the accumulation of lymphocytes, macrophages, and plasma cells.

SYSTEMIC MANIFESTATIONS OF INFLAMMATION

Systemic manifestations of inflammation are all too familiar to anyone who has suffered a severe sore throat or a respiratory tract infection. *Fever* is one of the most prominent systemic manifestations, particularly in inflammatory states associated with spread of organisms into the bloodstream. It is now thought that cytokines, principally IL-1 and TNF, are involved in the origin of fever (p. 38). These cytokines are produced by leukocytes (and other cell types) in response to infectious agents or to immune and toxic reactions. They reach the brain and interact with *vascular* receptors in the thermoregulatory center of the hypothalamus. *Either by direct action of the cytokines or, more likely, through local prostaglandin (PGE) production,* there eventually is sympathetic nerve stimulation, vasoconstriction of skin vessels, decrease in heat dissipation, and fever.

Leukocytosis is a common feature of inflammatory reactions, especially those induced by bacterial infection. The leukocyte count usually climbs to 15,000 or 20,000 cells per mm³, but sometimes it may reach extraordinarily high levels of 40,000 to 100,000 cells. These extreme elevations are referred to as *leukemoid reactions* because they are similar to the white cell counts of leukemia. The leukocytosis occurs initially because of *accelerated release* of cells from the bone marrow postmitotic reserve pool (caused by IL-1 and TNF) and is associated with an increase in the number of more immature neutrophils in the blood ("shift to the left"). However, prolonged infection also induces proliferation of precursors in the bone marrow, caused by increased production of cytokines (*colony-stimulating factors*). This stimulation of CSF production is also mediated by IL-1 and TNF.

Certain infections (typhoid fever and infections caused by viruses, rickettsiae, and certain protozoa) are associated with a decreased number of circulating white cells (*leukopenia*). Leukopenia is also encountered in infections that overwhelm patients debilitated by disseminated cancer or rampant tuberculosis.

This concludes our discussion of the cellular and molecular events in acute and chronic inflammation. But we have not told the whole story, because an important component has, to this point, been omitted — the changes induced by the body's attempts to heal the damage, the process of *repair.* The repair of injury begins almost as soon as the inflammatory changes have begun. It involves fundamental processes of cell proliferation and differentiation, and connective tissue formation. These are reviewed next.

Bibliography

Bevilacqua, M. P., et al.: Identification of an inducible endothelial-leukocyte adhesion molecule, ELAM-1. Proc. Natl. Acad. Sci. USA *84*:9238, 1987. (Description of the first endothelial adhesion molecule.)

Beutler, B., Cerami, A.: The biology of cachectin/TNF-α. Ann. Rev. Immunol. *7*:625, 1989.

Cochrane, C. G., Gimbrone, M. A., Jr. (eds.): Cellular and Molecular Mechanisms of Inflammation. New York, Academic Press. Vol. 1, 1990: Receptors of Inflammatory Cells; Vol. 2, 1991: Vascular Adhesion Molecules. Vol. 3, 1992: Leukocyte-Endothelial Adhesion Molecules. (A series of brief, up-to-date summaries of current work.)

Cohnheim, J.: Lectures in General Pathology. (Translated by McKee, A. D., from the second German edition, vol. 1.) London, New Sydenham Society, 1889. (An important historical document of Cohnheim's descriptions of inflammation.)

Dinarello, C. A., et al.: New concepts of the pathogenesis of fever. Rev. Infect. Dis. *10*:168, 1989. (A summary of the mechanisms of fever production, particularly the role of cytokines.)

Gallin, J. I., et al. (eds.): Inflammation: Basic Principles and Clinical Correlates. New York, Raven Press, 1989. (A multiauthor book covering all aspects of acute and chronic inflammation. A new edition is expected in 1993.)

Kelley, W. N., et al. (eds.): Textbook of Rheumatology. 4th ed. Philadelphia, W. B. Saunders, 1992. (The first part of this book contains up-to-date chapters on the cellular components of inflammation.)

Kunkel, S. L., et al.: Cellular and molecular aspects of granuloma-tous inflammation. Am. J. Resp. Cell. Mol. Biol. *1*:439, 1989. (A review of the pathogenesis of granuloma formation.)

Lehrer, R. J., Gans, T., Selsted, M. E.: Defensins: Endogenous antibiotic peptides of animal cells. Cell *64*:229, 1991. (A summary of the most recent nonoxidative mechanism of bacterial killing.)

Lewis, R. A., Austen, K. F., Soberman, R. J.: Leukotrienes and other products of the 5-lipoxygenase pathway. N. Engl. J. Med. *323*:645, 1990. (A review of arachidonic acid metabolites important in inflammation.)

Majno, G., Palade, G. E.: Studies on inflammation. I. The effect of histamine and serotonin on vascular permeability: An electron microscopic study. J. Biophys. Biochem. Cytol. *11*:571, 1961; and Majno, G., et al.: Studies on inflammation. II. Effects of histamine and serotonin along the vascular tree: A topographic study. J. Biophys. Biochem. Cytol. *11*:607, 1961. (The first classic descriptions of the ultrastructural basis of inflammation.)

Osborn, L.: Endothelial adhesion molecules in inflammation. Cell *62*:3, 1990. (A brief review of adhesion molecules.)

Pober, J. S., Cotran, R. S.: Overview: the role of endothelial cells in inflammation. Transplantation 50:537–544, 1990.

Ward, P. A., Varani, J.: Mechanisms of neutrophil-mediated killing of endothelial cells. J. Leuk. Biol. *48*:97, 1990.

Weiss, S. J.: Tissue destruction by neutrophils. N. Engl. J. Med. *320*:365, 1989.

THREE

Repair: Cell Growth, Regeneration, and Wound Healing

REGENERATION
THE CELL CYCLE AND TYPES OF CELLS
    Control of Cell Growth
        Molecular Events in Cell Growth
        Growth Inhibition
        Growth Factors
REPAIR BY CONNECTIVE TISSUE
    Description of Healing Wounds
    Mechanisms of Wound Healing
        Extracellular Matrix and Cell-Matrix
            Interactions
        Collagen Synthesis, Degradation, and
            Wound Strength
PATHOLOGIC ASPECTS OF REPAIR
OVERVIEW OF THE INFLAMMATORY-
REPARATIVE RESPONSE

The body's ability to replace dead cells and repair damage induced by local injury are critical to survival. Repair begins very early in the process of inflammation and involves two distinct processes: (1) *regeneration of injured tissue by parenchymal cells of the same type*, sometimes leaving no residual trace of the previous injury; and (2) *replacement by connective tissue*, or *fibroplasia*, which in its permanent state constitutes a scar. In most instances, both processes contribute to repair. In addition, both regeneration and fibroplasia are determined by essentially similar mechanisms involving cell growth and differentiation, as well as cell-matrix interactions. The latter are particularly important. Orderly renewal of the epithelial tissues of skin and viscera requires the continued presence of the *basement membrane* (BM). This specialized extracellular matrix (ECM) functions as an extracellular scaffold for accurate regeneration of preexisting structures. Maintenance of BM integrity provides for specificity of cell type and polarity and, as we shall see, influences cell migration, growth, and morphogenesis during repair.

In this chapter we review some of the general features of regeneration, cell growth, and connective tissue repair, describe the healing of skin wounds as a specific prototype of the repair process, and briefly discuss pathologic aspects of repair.

Regeneration

THE CELL CYCLE AND TYPES OF CELLS

The cell growth cycle, as should be familiar to you (Fig. 3–1), consists of G_1 (presynthetic), S (DNA synthesis), G_2 (premitotic), and M (mitotic) phases. Quiescent cells are in a physiologic state called G_0. The cells of the body are divided into three groups on the basis of their regenerative capacity and their relationship to the cell cycle.

1. *Continuously dividing cells* (also called *labile cells*) follow the cell cycle from one mitosis to the next and continue to proliferate throughout life, replacing cells that are continuously being destroyed. Tissues that contain labile cells include surface epithelia such as stratified squamous surfaces of the skin, oral cavity, vagina, and cervix; the lining mucosa of all the excretory ducts of the glands of the body (e.g., salivary glands, pancreas, biliary tract); the columnar epithelium of the gastrointestinal tract, uterus, and fallopian tubes; the transitional epithelium of the urinary tract and cells of the splenic, lymphoid, and hematopoietic tissues.

2. *Quiescent (or stable) cells* usually demonstrate a

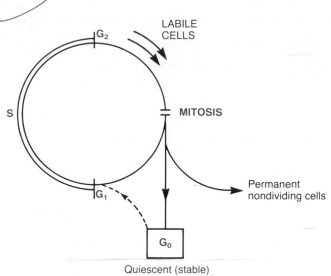

Figure 3–1. Cell populations and the phases of the cell cycle. Continuously dividing cells (labile cells) go around the cell cycle from one mitosis to the next. Nondividing cells have left the cycle and are destined to die without dividing again. Quiescent G_0 cells are neither cycling nor dying and can be induced to reenter the cycle by an appropriate stimulus. (Modified from Baserga, R.: The cell cycle. N. Engl. J. Med. *304*:453, 1981.)

low normal level of replication; however, these cells can undergo rapid division in response to a variety of stimuli and are thus capable of reconstituting the tissue of origin. They are considered to be in G_0, but can be stimulated into G_1 by an appropriate stimulus. In this category are the parenchymal cells of virtually all the glandular organs of the body, such as liver, kidney, and pancreas; mesenchymal cells such as fibroblasts and smooth muscle; and vascular endothelial cells. The regenerative capacity of stable cells is best exemplified by the ability of the liver to regenerate after hepatectomy and following toxic, viral, or chemical injury (p. 50).

3.) *Nondividing (permanent) cells* have left the cell cycle and cannot undergo mitotic division in postnatal life. To this group belong the nerve cells and the skeletal and cardiac muscles cells, the regenerative attempts of which (at least in mammals) are of no practical importance.

Except for tissues composed solely (or largely) of nondividing cells most tissues of adults consist of a mixture of cells that includes continuously dividing cells, quiescent cells that occasionally go back to the cell cycle, and nondividing cells.

CONTROL OF CELL GROWTH

Injury, cell death, and mechanical deformation of tissues can all stimulate cell proliferation; however, it is now clear that cell growth is controlled largely by chemical factors in the environment, which either stimulate or inhibit cell proliferation. An excess of

stimulators or a deficiency of inhibitors will lead to net growth, and in the case of cancer, uncontrolled growth, as we shall see (p. 185). Although growth can be accomplished by shortening the cell cycle or decreasing the rate of cell loss (as occurs in tumors) *the most important factors are those that recruit G_0 cells into the cell cycle.*

Although many chemical substances can affect cell growth, the most important are *polypeptide growth factors* present in serum or produced by cells. Some of these substances are *competence factors,* which do not stimulate DNA synthesis but render cells in G_0 or G_1 competent to do so; others are *progression factors,* which stimulate DNA synthesis in competent cells. Certain growth factors also initiate cell migration, differentiation, and tissue remodeling and may be involved in various stages of wound healing.

MOLECULAR EVENTS IN CELL GROWTH

Recently there has been an explosion in our understanding of the molecular events that lead to cell proliferation induced by growth factors, stemming largely from the discovery in the early 1980s that oncogenes (genes that are involved in cancer formation) are highly homologous to cellular genes involved in normal growth control pathways (protooncogenes). Protooncogenes and oncogenes are discussed in detail in the chapter on neoplasia (Chapter 7). Here we shall review the chain of molecular events that leads to cell division and the proteins that participate in the control of cell growth, as these are critical to understanding repair and neoplasia (Fig. 3–2).

- *Ligand-receptor binding.* Cell growth is initiated by the binding of a putative growth factor (ligand) to specific receptors either at the cell surface or inside the cell. Most of the growth factors have receptors on the plasma membrane, but steroid receptors are intracellular, interacting with lipophilic ligands that cross the cell membrane to interact with the receptor in the nucleus or cytoplasm.

- *Growth factor receptor activation.* Most growth factor receptors (such as epidermal growth factor [EGF] and platelet-derived growth factor [PDGF] receptors, p. 51) are equipped with intrinsic protein tyrosine kinase activity, which is activated after ligand binding. Such receptor protein kinases have a large glycosylated extracellular ligand–binding domain, a single hydrophobic transmembrane region, and a cytoplasmic domain that contains the tyrosine kinase activity (Fig. 3–3). Ligand binding induces a conformational alteration of the extracellular domain, which in turn induces dimerization of receptors. It is thought that this dimerization, by allowing interactions between adjacent cytoplasmic domains, leads to activation of the kinase.

Other transmembrane growth factor receptors which do not possess endogenous kinase activity recruit intracellular protein kinases to the cell periphery. The net result in either case is activation of

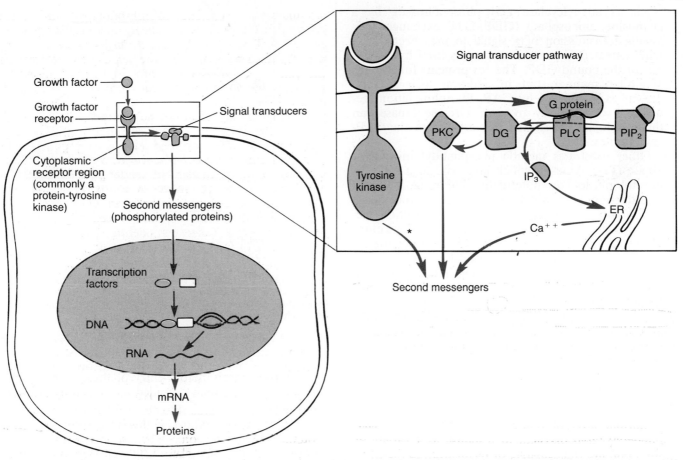

Figure 3-2. Cellular events initiated by growth factors shown here for PDGF (see text). The inset on the right illustrates some of the events in signal transduction. Certain growth factor receptors do not possess tyrosine kinase activity, as shown here, but recruit protein kinases (PKC) to the cell periphery. See Figure 3-3.

a protein phosphorylation cascade, which stimulates quiescent cells to enter the growth cycle.

- *Signal transduction and second messengers.* Tyrosine kinases are essential for signal transduction and thus *phosphorylation of tyrosine residues on one or more target proteins must be a critical event in the transfer of signals for cell proliferation.* Several substrates for tyrosine kinases have been identified (Fig. 3-3). The first one, phospholipase C-γ, catalyzes the degradation of phosphatidyl-4,5 biphosphate, resulting in the generation of two second messengers: inositol 1,4,5-triphosphate, which releases intracellular calcium stores, and diacylglycerol (DG). DG in turn activates protein kinase C (PKC), a member of a family of serine threonine kinases that are partially bound to the plasma membrane and are thus in the same perimembrane region as the kinases of the receptors.

The second enzyme that is phosphorylated by receptor (and cytoplasmic) tyrosine kinases is the guanosine triphosphatase (GTPase)-activating protein (GAP). This protein stimulates the activity of the *ras* p21 protein, which is one of the two GTPases implicated in the regulation of cell proliferation—the other being the well-known G proteins. Both of these proteins function by coupling extracellular signals (such as growth factors) to cellular effectors

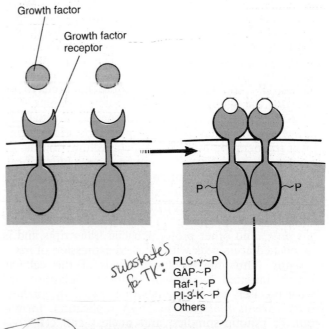

Figure 3-3. A possible mechanism for receptor tyrosine kinase activation. Engagement of PDGF receptor by PDGF causes a conformational alteration in its extracellular domain, in turn inducing dimerization of receptors, activation of the kinase, and subsequent phosphorylation of substrate proteins (see text).

(such as adenylcyclase and phospholipase), by a guanosine diphosphate (GDP)-GTP exchange. Following transmission of a signal to the effector protein, activated G protein inactivates itself by hydrolysis of the bound GDP. The *ras* proteins function in a similar manner, but in addition their GTPase activity is stimulated by GAP. Phosphorylation (activation) of GAP by receptor tyrosine kinase can thus modulate the signals that arise from the GAP-*ras* complex.

Other substrates include phosphatidyl inositol 3^1 kinase (PI-3^1 kinase), which gives rise to a series of inositol phosphates potentially important in signal transduction; and Raf-1, a serine threonine kinase that phosphorylates a number of transcription factors. Protein phosphorylation is counteracted by a number of *cellular phosphatases,* which are receiving increased attention as regulators of cell growth. Activation or inactivation of such phosphatases has been shown to correlate respectively with inhibition or stimulation of cell growth.

- *Transcription factors.* The precise method by which the signals for mitosis are transferred across the cytoplasm is unknown. It is known, however, that when quiescent cells are exposed to growth factors, a large number of cellular genes are induced. These have been divided into *early growth-regulated genes,* whose mRNAs increase well before mid-G_1 of the cell cycle and which are induced *in the absence of protein synthesis;* and *late growth-regulated genes* whose mRNAs start to increase in mid-G_1, or even at the G_1-G_s boundary, and which are dependent on protein synthesis. The functions of many of these genes are unknown and most are probably not directly involved in the regulation of cell proliferation. However, among the growth-regulated genes are a number of proteooncogenes in which mutations may be associated with malignant transformation (p. 185). Some, such as *myc, fos, jun,* code for transcription factors and are involved in the regulation of DNA synthesis, and possibly cell division. The *jun* protooncogene, for example, encodes part of the transcription factor AP-1 and *fos* encodes a protein that binds to *jun* forming the whole of the AP-1 protein complex. The importance of these protooncogenes in normal cell growth is well exemplified by their expression during liver regeneration after partial hepatectomy in rats. As you recall, partial hepatectomy induces a burst of cell proliferation in the remnant hepatic cells, so that the liver size returns to normal within two weeks of the surgical operation. As seen in Figure 3–4, DNA synthesis in these cells is preceded by increased expression of *fos, myc,* and other protooncogene transcripts and is associated at its peak with marked expression of *ras.*

- *Cyclins.* Thus far we have discussed the cellular events initiated by growth factor stimulation, but what precisely are the signals that trigger the orchestrated events that lead to DNA replication, formation of mitotic spindles, and nuclear and cell division? The evidence is now clear that these processes are controlled in part by changes in the intracellular concentration of a group of proteins called *cyclins,* which are induced during the cell cycle. G_1 cyclins

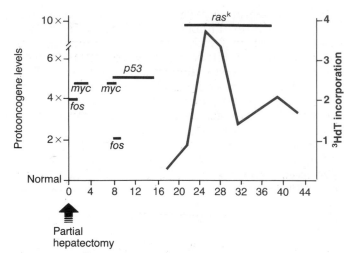

Figure 3–4. Expression of protooncogenes after partial hepatectomy and its relation to DNA synthesis by hepatocytes, shown here by the level of 3H-thymidine incorporation. Note that there is induction of fos, myc, and p53 prior to the onset of DNA synthesis. Ras^k peaks during the S phase. (Courtesy of Dr. Nelson Fausto, Brown University, Providence, RI.)

levels rise sharply before entry of the cell into the S phase. They are then degraded and reach basal levels at the end of the S phase. During the G_2 phase, genes for a second set of cyclins called G_2 or *B cyclins* are induced. Following cell division the G_2 cyclins are degraded and in the presence of a stimulus, the daughter cells start a new cell cycle again. Both cyclins associate with a constitutive enzyme p34^{cdc} kinase and the cyclin-kinase complex phosphorylates, proteins involved in the formation of the mitotic spindle and DNA replication.

To summarize, polypeptide growth factors bind to and activate their receptors, many of which possess kinase activity. Their activation phosphorylates several substrates that are involved in the generation of second messengers. These in turn transmit the signals to the nucleus where activation of transcription factors leads to the initiation of DNA synthesis, and ultimately, cell division. This process of cycling is tuned by a family of proteins, appropriately called *cyclins.*

Growth Inhibition

The other side of the coin in cellular growth control is growth inhibition. The existence of growth inhibitory signals that maintain the integrity of a tissue has been suspected for decades from observations that populations of cells in culture or in vivo can limit one another's growth. *Contact inhibition* of growth in confluent cultures is one such manifestation of growth inhibition. There is also in vivo evidence for growth suppression. In the model of partial hepatectomy discussed earlier the liver cells stop multiplying when the liver has attained its normal preoperative size and configuration, suggesting the action of an inhibitory signal. The recent discovery that loss of tumor suppressor genes (or antioncogenes) occurs in certain cancers suggests that such genes encode components of some cellular inhibitory pathway (p. 191). Growth inhibition, like growth stimulation, apparently utilizes polypeptide factors and signal transducers, including cell surface receptors, cytoplasmic second messengers, and transcription regulators. Few of these mechanisms have been well described, although work with tumor suppressor genes give some clues. One polypeptide factor that acts as a growth inhibitor of many cell types is transforming growth factor-β (TGF-β). Insoluble extracellular matrix molecules may also serve to suppress cell responsiveness to soluble mitogens in the local tissue microenvironment. Both of these factors are described later.

Finally, it should be mentioned that these two pathways—growth inhibition and growth stimulation—almost certainly intertwine along their intracellular routes. One example is the interaction of the tumor suppressor gene of neurofibromatosis (NF-1) with the normal *ras* p21 protein, serving to inactivate the p21 protein. You will recall that the *ras* protein is involved in signal transduction after stimulation by growth factors.

Growth Factors

Having reviewed the molecular events in cell growth, we can now turn to a description of some of the polypeptide growth factors, particularly those that are involved in inflammatory repair.

1. *Epidermal growth factor* is a 6045-dalton polypeptide that is purified from submaxillary glands of mice or from human urine (urogastrone) and was first discovered by its ability to cause precocious separation of the eyelids of newborn mice. EGF is mitogenic for a variety of epithelial cells and fibroblasts in vitro and causes hepatic cell division in vivo. It is a progression factor that stimulates cell division by binding to specific tyrosine kinase receptors on the cell membrane, followed by the events described earlier. The EGF receptor is c-*erb* β-1 (p. 186).

2. *Platelet-derived growth factor*. This is a highly cationic protein (of approximately 30,000 daltons) composed of two chains (A and B). PDGF is stored in the platelet α granules and released upon platelet activation. It can also be produced by activated macrophages, endothelial and smooth muscle cells, and a variety of tumor cells. PDGF causes both migration and proliferation of fibroblasts, smooth muscle cells, and monocytes, but has other pro-inflammatory properties as well. It binds to two types of specific receptors (α and β) that have protein kinase activity, but unlike EGF, it triggers the cell cycle by acting as a competence factor, so it requires a progression factor for mitogenesis (e.g., EGF, plasma, insulin). PDGF is active in vivo: when applied directly to surgical incisions, there is enhancement of monocyte influx, collagen synthesis, and tensile strength in the wounds.

3. *Fibroblast growth factors*. First described as fibroblast mitogens extracted from bovine brain and pituitary, fibroblast growth factors (FGFs) represent a family of polypeptide growth factors that have many other activities, including, in particular, *the ability to induce all the steps necessary for new blood vessel formation (angiogenesis),* both in vivo and in vitro (p. 194). FGFs have a strong affinity for heparin (heparin-binding growth factors) and consist of basic groups and acidic forms. Basic FGF is present in the extracts of many organs and is elaborated by activated macrophages, whereas acidic FGF is confined to neural tissue.

4. *Transforming growth factors α and β.* These factors were initially extracted from sarcoma virus–transformed cells and were thought to be involved in transformation of normal cells to cancer. TGF-α has homology to EGF, binds to the EGF receptor, and produces most of the biologic activities of EGF.

TGF-β, on the other hand, has more varied and often conflicting effects. TGF-β is a *growth inhibitor* to most epithelial cell types in culture and is implicated in cessation of cell growth after partial hepatectomy. Its effect appears to be mediated by the inhibition of c-*myc* transcription, possibly by activating the product of the retinoblastoma suppressor gene (see p. 189). Its effects on fibroblasts and smooth muscle proliferation are variable. In low concentrations it induces the synthesis and secretion of PDGF and is thus indirectly mitogenic. In high concentrations it is growth inhibitory, owing to its ability to inhibit the expression of PDGF receptors. TGF-β also stimulates fibroblast chemotaxis and the production of collagen and fibronectin by cells, at the same time inhibiting collagen degradation, *all effects favoring fibrogenesis.* TGF-β is produced by different cell types, including platelets, endothelium, T cells, and macrophages.

5. Many *cytokines* are growth factors, and indeed there is so much overlap between these two groups of mediators as to make distinctions between them tenuous. *IL-1* and *TNF*, for example, are mitogenic and chemotactic for fibroblasts, and they stimulate the synthesis of both collagen and collagenase by fibroblasts. They are known as the *fibrogenic cytokines.* TNF is also angiogenic in vivo.

Before we leave the topic of growth factors, several points should be made.

- First, *a number of growth inhibitors are known to be produced in inflammation.* One of these, TGF-β, was already considered. Others include interferon-α, prostaglandin E_2, and heparin; all three inhibit fibroblast and smooth muscle proliferation in vitro.

- Second, growth factors also have effects on cell locomotion, contractility, and differentiation—effects that may be as important to inflammatory repair and wound healing as the growth-promoting effects. Many of these effects may be mediated in part through growth factor–induced alterations of the extracellular matrix, as we shall see (p. 55).

- Third, *macrophages,* which may be abundant in healing wounds, may play a central role in these processes because they can be induced to secrete growth factors (PDGF, FGF), fibrogenic cytokines (IL-1, TNF), growth inhibitors (TGF-β, prostaglandins), and enzymes involved in tissue degradation and organization (see Fig. 2–17B, p. 41).

- Fourth, growth factors act by endocrine, paracrine, or autocrine signaling. Paracrine stimulation is most common in connective tissue repair by healing wounds, in which a factor produced by one cell type has its growth effect on adjacent cells, usually of a different cell type (for example, macrophage-derived growth factors acting on fibroblasts). Many cells, however, have receptors to their endogenously produced growth factors (autocrine stimulation), a process that plays a role in compensatory epithelial hyperplasia (such as hepatic regeneration) and particularly in tumors (p. 186).
- Finally, as we shall see later, the genes that encode for some of these growth factors or their receptors show extensive sequence homology with oncogenes (for example, PDGF with c-sis and the EGF receptor with c-erb b), suggesting involvement of these growth factors in cancer formation.

REPAIR BY CONNECTIVE TISSUE _____

Cell growth and differentiation are central to the second important process in the repair of tissue damage — replacement of nonregenerated parenchymal cells by connective tissue, which in time produces a scar. There are four components to this process:

- Migration and proliferation of fibroblasts
- Deposition of extracellular matrix
- Formation of new blood vessels (angiogenesis)
- Maturation and organization of the scar, also known as remodeling.

The process of repair begins early in inflammation. Sometimes as early as 24 hours after injury, fibroblasts and vascular endothelial cells begin proliferating to form (by three to five days) the specialized type of tissue (granulation tissue) that is the hallmark of healing. The term granulation tissue derives from its pink, soft, granular appearance on the surface of wounds, but it is the histologic features that are characteristic: the proliferation of new small blood vessels and fibroblasts (Fig. 3–5). Migration of fibroblasts to the site of injury and their subsequent proliferation are undoubtedly triggered by growth factors such as PDGF, EGF, FGF, and TGF-β and the fibrogenic cytokines derived in part from inflammatory macrophages. Some of these growth factors also stimulate synthesis of collagen and other connective tissue molecules. In early stages more proteoglycans are formed; later collagen predominates.

New vessels originate by budding or sprouting of preexisting vessels, a process called angiogenesis or neovascularization. Angiogenesis is an important biologic process, which, as we shall see (p. 194), is also involved in the progressive growth of tumors. At least four steps are needed in the development of a new

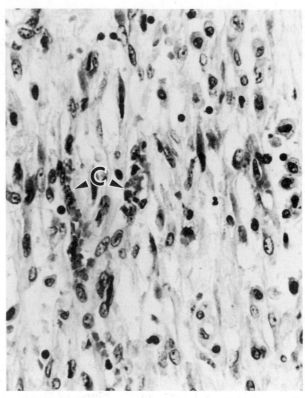

Figure 3–5. Granulation tissue containing spindle-shaped fibroblasts, mononuclear inflammatory cells, and capillaries (C) embedded in loose ground substance. (Courtesy of Dr. Charles L. White III, Department of Pathology, Southwestern Medical School, Dallas, TX.)

capillary vessel (Fig. 3–6): (1) proteolytic degradation of the basement membrane of the parent vessel to allow formation of a capillary sprout and subsequent cell migration; (2) migration of endothelial cells toward the angiogenic stimulus; (3) proliferation of endothelial cells, just behind the leading front of migrating cells; and (4) maturation of endothelial cells and organization into capillary tubes. These new vessels have leaky interendothelial junctions, allowing the passage of proteins and red cells into the extravascular space. *Thus new granulation tissue is often edematous.* Indeed, this leakiness accounts for much of the edema that persists in healing wounds long after the acute inflammatory response has subsided (Fig. 2–4, p. 28).

Several factors can induce angiogenesis in vivo and in vitro, including basic FGF and a newly described vascular endothelial growth factor (VEGF). Basic FGF is an excellent candidate for mediating angiogenesis: it induces proteinase secretion by endothelial cells, which is necessary for the initial basement membrane degradation; it triggers endothelial cell migration and proliferation required to form new vessels; and in the presence of appropriate matrix components it causes tube formation in the migrating proliferating cells. Basic FGF also binds to heparin in basement membranes and can presumably be released from such damaged membranes.

Figure 3–6. Four steps in angiogenesis. Parent mature vessel is on the left. 1. Basement membrane and ECM matrix degradation. 2. Endothelial migration. 3. Endothelial proliferation (mitosis). 4. Organization and maturation. (Adapted from Ausprunk, D. H.: *In* Houck, J. C. [ed.]: Chemical Messengers of the Inflammatory Process. Amsterdam, Elsevier/North Holland, 1979.)

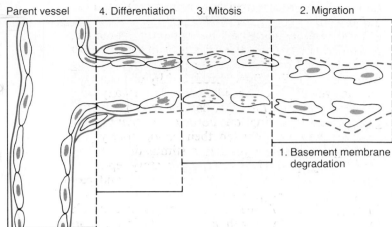

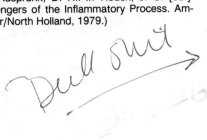

Macrophages are almost always present in granulation tissue, busily ridding the area of extracellular debris, fibrin, and other foreign matter; and, if the appropriate chemotactic stimuli persist, neutrophils, eosinophils, and lymphocytes are also seen. Mast cells are also present in great numbers. With further healing, there is an increase in extracellular constituents, mostly collagen, and a decrease in the number of active fibroblasts and new vessels. Many of the blood vessels characteristic of the early stages undergo thrombosis and dissolution, and their various cells are reabsorbed and digested by macrophages. The end result of granulation tissue is a scar composed of inactive-looking, spindle-shaped fibroblasts, dense collagen, fragments of elastic tissue, extracellular matrix (ECM), and relatively few vessels.

With this background we can now turn to a discussion of the healing of skin wounds, a process that involves both epithelial growth and formation of connective tissue discussed above.

DESCRIPTION OF HEALING WOUNDS

The least complicated example of wound repair is the healing of a clean, uninfected surgical incision approximated by surgical sutures (Fig. 3–7). Such healing is referred to as *primary union or healing by first intention.* The incision causes death of a limited number of epithelial cells and connective tissue cells as well as disruption of epithelial basement membrane continuity. The narrow incisional space immediately fills with clotted blood containing fibrin and blood cells; dehydration of the surface clot forms the well-known scab that covers the wound.

Within 24 hours, neutrophils appear at the margins of the incision, moving toward the fibrin clot. The epidermis at its cut edges thickens *as a result of mitotic activity of basal cells,* and within 24 to 48 hours spurs of epithelial cells from the edges both migrate and grow along the cut margins of the dermis, depositing

basement membrane components as they move. They fuse in the midline beneath the surface scab, thus producing a continuous but thin epithelial layer.

By day 3, the neutrophils have been largely replaced by macrophages. *Granulation tissue* progressively invades the incision space. Collagen fibers are now present in the margins of the incision, but at first these are vertically oriented and do not bridge the incision. Epithelial cell proliferation continues, thickening the epidermal covering layer.

By day 5, the incisional space is filled with granulation tissue. Neovascularization is maximal. Collagen fibrils become more abundant and begin to bridge the incision. The epidermis recovers its normal thickness, and differentiation of surface cells yields a mature epidermal architecture with surface keratinization.

During the second week, there is continued accumulation of collagen and proliferation of fibroblasts. The leukocytic infiltrate, edema, and increased vascularity have largely disappeared. At this time, the long process of blanching begins, accomplished by the increased accumulation of collagen within the incisional scar, accompanied by regression of vascular channels.

By the end of the first month, the scar comprises a cellular connective tissue devoid of inflammatory infiltrate, covered now by intact epidermis. The dermal appendages that have been destroyed in the line of the incision are permanently lost. Tensile strength of the wound increases thereafter, but it may take months for the wounded area to obtain its maximal strength.

When there is more extensive loss of cells and tissue, as occurs in infarction, inflammatory ulceration, abscess formation, and surface wounds that create large defects, the reparative process is more complicated. *The common denominator in all these situations is a large tissue defect that must be filled.* Regeneration of parenchymal cells cannot completely reconstitute the original architecture. Abundant granulation tissue grows in from the margin to complete the repair. This form of healing is referred to as *secondary union or healing by second intention.*

Secondary healing differs from primary healing in several respects:

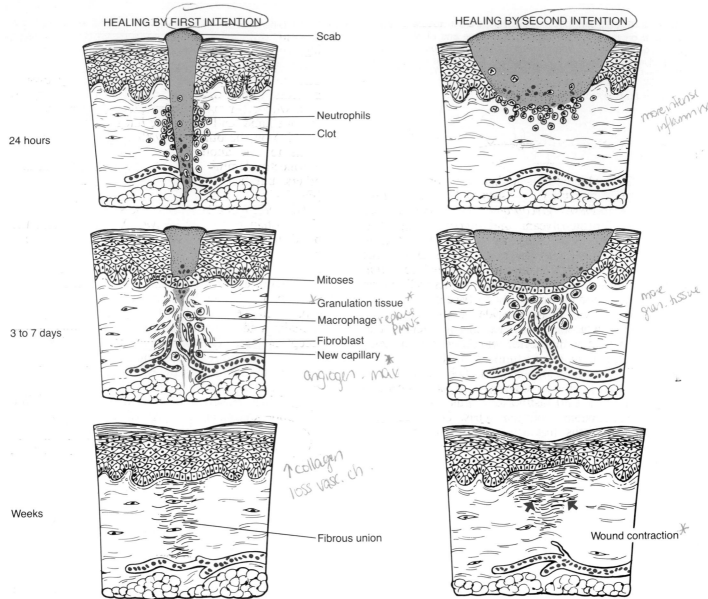

HEALING BY FIRST INTENTION

HEALING BY SECOND INTENTION

24 hours

— Scab
— Neutrophils
— Clot

more intense inflamm rxn

3 to 7 days

— Mitoses
— Granulation tissue *
— Macrophage *replace PMNs*
— Fibroblast
— New capillary *

angiogen. mark

more gran. tissue

Weeks

↑ collagen loss vasc. ch

— Fibrous union

Wound contraction *

Figure 3–7. Steps in wound healing by first intention *(left)* and second intention *(right)*. In the latter, the resultant scar is much smaller than the original wound, owing to wound contraction.

1. Inevitably, large tissue defects initially have more fibrin and more necrotic debris and exudate that must be removed. Consequently, the *inflammatory reaction is more intense.*

2. *Much larger amounts of granulation tissue are formed.* When a large defect occurs in deeper tissues, such as in a viscus, granulation tissue with its numerous *scavenger white cells* bears the full responsibility for its closure, because drainage to the surface cannot occur.

3. Perhaps the feature that most clearly differentiates primary from secondary healing is the phenomenon of *wound contraction,* which occurs in large surface wounds. Large defects in the skin of a rabbit are reduced in approximately six weeks to 5 to 10% of their original size, largely by contraction. Contraction has been ascribed, at least in part, to the presence of *myofibroblasts*—altered fibroblasts that

have many of the ultrastructural and functional features of contractile smooth muscle cells.

MECHANISMS OF WOUND HEALING

Wound healing, as we have seen, is a complex (but orderly) phenomenon involving a number of well-orchestrated processes, including regeneration of parenchymal cells, migration and proliferation of both parenchymal and connective tissue cells, synthesis of ECM proteins, remodeling of connective tissue and parenchymal components, and collagenization and acquisition of wound strength. The mechanisms underlying many of these events are similar to those that occur during embryogenesis and are also relevant to the abnormal growth in cancer. We have already discussed, for example, the role of growth factors in causing migration, proliferation, and differentiation of epithelial cells, in connective tissue formation, and in the growth of new vessels. Equally important in wound healing are the influences of interactions between cells and the extracellular matrix on the same processes—migration, proliferation, and differentiation.

Extracellular Matrix and Cell-Matrix Interactions

The ECM, which forms a significant proportion of the volume of any tissue, consists of *fibrous structural proteins* and *adhesive glycoproteins* embedded in a gel composed of proteoglycans and glycosaminoglycans. ECM occurs in two forms: as interstitial matrix in connective tissues, and as a basement membrane around epithelial and certain mesenchymal cells (endothelium and smooth muscle). Besides its well-known function of providing turgor to soft tissues and rigidity to skeletal tissues, ECM provides a substratum to which cells can adhere, migrate, and proliferate, and directly influences the form and function of cells. There are three components in most ECMs:

- *The collagens* are composed of a triple helix of three polypeptide α chains, having a gly-x-y repeating sequence. About 30 distinct α chains form approximately 15 distinct collagen types. Some collagen types form fibrils (e.g., the interstitial or fibrillar collagens, types I, III, and V), whereas others (e.g., type IV) are nonfibrillar and are components of basement membranes. The interstitial collagens form a major proportion of the connective tissue in healing wounds, and particularly in scars, and will be discussed further separately.

- The *adhesive glycoproteins* are structurally diverse proteins whose major property is their ability to bind with other extracellular matrix components, on the one hand, and to specific integral cell membrane proteins on the other. They thus link ECM components to one another and to cells. They include fibronectin, laminin, thrombospondin, tenascin, and others, but here we will discuss only the first two (Fig. 3–8).

  Fibronectin is a large (400,000 kd) multifunctional glycoprotein consisting of two chains held together by disulfide bonds. Associated with cell surfaces, basement membranes, and pericellular matrices, fibronectin is produced by fibroblasts, monocytes, endothelial cells, and other cells. Fibronectin binds to a number of other ECM components (including collagen, fibrin, heparin, and proteoglycans) via specific domains and to cells via *integrin* receptors. These receptors are transmembrane glycoproteins, and their intracellular domains interact with elements of the cytoskeleton to signal cell locomotion or differentiation. Many integrins bind to matrix proteins by recognizing the specific amino acid sequence of the tripeptide arginine-glycine-aspartic acid (RGD), a sequence that is thought to play a key role in cell adhesion. For these reasons, fibronectin is directly involved in attachment, spreading, and migration of

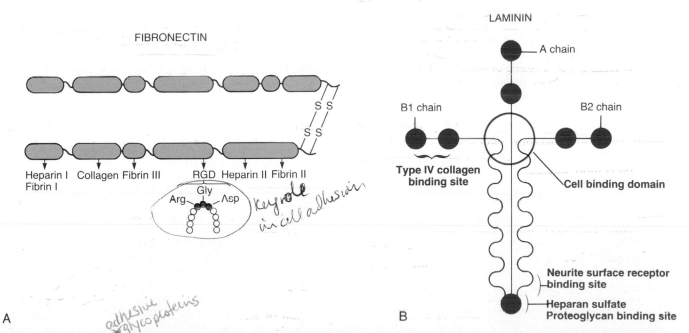

Figure 3–8. The fibronectin molecule (A) consists of a dimer held by S—S bonds. Note the various domains that bind to extracellular matrices and the cell-binding domain containing an Arg/Gly/Asp sequence. The cross-shaped lamina (B) molecule spans basement membranes and has ECM and cell-binding domains. (B reproduced, with permission, from The Annual Review of Cell Biology, Vol. 3, © 1987 by Annual Reviews Inc.)

cells. In addition, it serves to enhance the sensitivity of certain cells, such as capillary endothelial cells, to the proliferative effects of growth factors such as FGF. This has been ascribed to the ability of fibronectin to activate intracellular chemical signaling pathways and to modulate cell shape. In healing skin wounds a large quantity of fibronectin, mostly plasma-derived, appears in the extracellular matrix in the first two days after wound healing. Thereafter, fibronectin is actively synthesized by proliferating endothelial cells.

Laminin, another glycoprotein that is important in wound healing, is the most abundant glycoprotein in basement membranes. It is a large (800 to 1,000 kd) cross-shaped structure, which spans the basement membrane and binds on the one hand with specific receptors on the surface of cells and on the other with matrix components such as collagen type IV and heparan sulfate. Laminin is also believed to mediate cell attachment to connective tissue substrates; in culture, it alters the growth, survival, morphology, differentiation, and motility of various cell types. In endothelial cell cultures exposed to FGF, laminin causes alignment of endothelial cells and subsequent capillary tube formation, a most critical event in angiogenesis. Other ECMs can also induce capillary tube formation; however, the molecular pathways that link ECM composition to the control of cell form and function are much less clear than those that are involved in cell growth, described earlier. It is likely, however, that receptors for growth factors and different ECM molecules may share common intracellular signaling mechanisms.

- _Proteoglycans_ comprise the third component of the ECM. Proteoglycans consist of glycosaminoglycans (e.g., dermatan sulfate and heparan sulfate) linked covalently to a protein core. Glycosaminoglycans without a protein core such as hyaluronic acid can also be found in tissues. They have diverse roles in regulating connective tissue structure and permeability. Proteoglycans can also be integral membrane proteins and are thus modulators of cell growth and differentiation. For example, _syndecan_, an integral membrane glycoprotein, binds collagen, fibronectin, thrombospondin, and certain growth factors such as

basic fibroblast growth factor. It associates with actin cytoskeleton and has been shown to maintain the morphology of epithelial sheets.

To summarize, wound healing involves at least two signals, one soluble and the other insoluble. Soluble molecules are largely polypeptide growth factors and growth inhibitors. Insoluble factors are the extracellular matrices such as laminin, fibronectin, and collagens, and these usually act in concert as regulators of cell growth and differentiation. Table 3–1 summarizes the growth factors that seem to be important in mediating angiogenesis, fibroblast migration, proliferation, and collagen deposition in wound healing. Figure 3–9 is a model of the interactions between growth factors, extracellular matrix, and cell responses.

Collagen Synthesis, Degradation, and Wound Strength

The development of wound strength and scarring is related primarily to the deposition of collagen in healing wounds. As previously described, collagen synthesis by fibroblasts begins early in wound healing, by day 3 or 5, and continues for several weeks, depending on wound size. Collagen synthesis is stimulated by several factors, including growth factors (PDGF, FGF) and cytokines (IL-1, TNF), which are secreted by leukocytes in healing wounds. Net collagen accumulation, however, depends not only on synthesis but also on collagen degradation.

Collagen degradation is achieved by a family of zinc metalloproteinases of which the most studied is _collagenase_. These metalloproteinases are important in the tissue remodeling that occurs not only during wound healing but also in normal embryonic development. (These are also important in initiating angiogenesis, as we have seen, and in cancer metastases, p. 197.) Collagenase, which is produced by a variety of cell types (fibroblasts, macrophages, neutrophils, synovial cells, and some epithelial cells), can cleave collagen under physiologic conditions, cutting the triple helix into two unequal fragments, which are then susceptible to digestion by other proteases. This is potentially harmful to the organism, but the enzyme is elaborated

TABLE 3–1. MAJOR GROWTH FACTORS IN WOUND HEALING

	PDGF	B FGF	TGF-β	TGF-α/EGF	IL-1 or TNF
Angiogenesis in vivo	O	+	+*	+*	+*
Chemotaxis					
Monocytes	+	+	+	?	+
Fibroblasts	+	+	+	O	+
Endothelium	O	+	−	+	?
Mitogenesis					
Fibroblasts	+	+	±	+	+
Endothelium	O	+	−	+	O or −
Collagen synthesis	+	?	+	?	+
Collagenase secretion	+	+	+	+	+

Key: +, stimulates; −, inhibits; O, no effect; *, effect may be indirect.

Figure 3–9. Scheme of possible mechanisms by which extracellular matrix (ECM) and growth factors influence cell shape, motility, and growth. Receptors for ECM, such as the integrins—which recognize the RGD sequence—interact with the cytoskeleton and initiate the production of diffusible second messengers, which act on both nucleus and cytoplasm to cause the cell responses, as illustrated. Cell surface receptors to growth factors also initiate second messengers, which modulate cell growth, locomotion, and differentiation. (Adapted from Madri, J., et al.: *In* Simionescu, N., and Simionescu, M. [eds.]: Endothelial Cell Biology. New York, Plenum Publishing Co., 1988.)

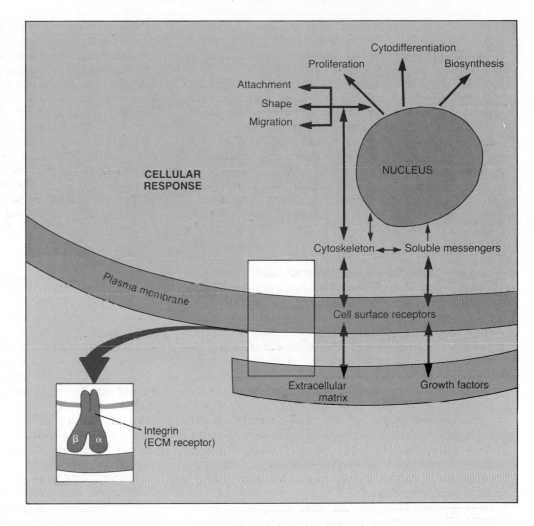

in a latent (zymogen) form that can be activated by certain chemicals (HOCl·) and enzymes (plasmin, proteases). In addition, activated collagenases can be rapidly inhibited by specific tissue inhibitors of metalloproteinase (TIMP). There are thus multiple checks against the uncontrolled action of these proteinases. Nevertheless, it is thought that the collagenases of neutrophils, macrophages, and fibroblasts play a role in degrading collagen in inflammation and wound healing. Degradation aids in the débridement of injured sites and also in the remodeling of connective tissue necessary to repair the defect.

We now turn to the questions of how long it takes for a skin wound to achieve its maximal strength and which substances contribute to this strength. Carefully sutured wounds have approximately 70% of the strength of unwounded skin immediately after surgery, largely owing to the placement of the sutures. When sutures are removed, usually at the end of the first week, wound strength is approximately 10%, but it increases rapidly over the next four weeks. This rate of increase then slows and virtually reaches a plateau at approximately the third month after the original incision. This plateau is reached at about 70 to 80% of the tensile strength of unwounded skin, which indeed may persist for life.

The recovery of tensile strength can therefore be represented by a sigmoid curve terminating in a plateau below the original level of the unwounded skin. The structural or biochemical explanation of this curve still eludes us. It is not merely a function of collagen synthesis, because the curve of tensile strength does not parallel that of collagen increase in the wound, but it may be related to the type of collagen produced. Thus, although adult skin collagen is type I, collagen deposited early in granulation tissue is type III, characteristic of embryonic skin. During maturation of the scar, type III is replaced by adult type I collagen.

We can conclude this discussion of wound healing and collagenization by emphasizing that the healing wound, as a prototype of many other processes of tissue repair, is a dynamic and changing environment. The early phase is one of inflammation, followed by a stage of fibroplasia, followed by tissue remodeling and scarring. Different mechanisms occurring at different times trigger the release of chemical signals that modulate the orderly migration, proliferation, and differentiation of cells and the synthesis and degradation of extracellular matrix proteins. These proteins, in turn, directly affect cellular events and modulate cell responsiveness to soluble growth factors. Many of the molecular details in this scenario are unknown, but it is remarkable that despite the many seemingly disjointed activities, the process of wound healing is so well coordinated.

PATHOLOGIC ASPECTS OF REPAIR _____

Cell growth and fibroplasia were discussed in this chapter as salutary phenomena in repair, and we reviewed only the orderly healing of wounds in normal persons. But these processes are modified by a number of known influences and some unknown ones, sometimes impairing the quality and adequacy of the reparative process.

- *Many systemic and local host factors influence the adequacy of the inflammatory-reparative response.* Nutrition has profound effects on wound healing. Protein deficiency, for example, and particularly vitamin C deficiency, inhibit collagen synthesis and retard healing. *Glucocorticoids* have well-documented antiinflammatory effects, which influence various components of inflammation and fibroplasia. Of the local factors, *infection* is the single most important cause of delay in healing. *Mechanical factors* such as increased abdominal pressure may cause rupture of abdominal wounds, called *wound dehiscence. Inadequate blood supply* usually caused by arteriosclerosis or venous abnormalities that retard venous drainage also impair healing. Finally, *foreign bodies* such as unnecessary sutures or fragments of steel, glass, or even bone constitute impediments to healing.

- *The tissue in which the injury has occurred* is also a factor to be considered. Perfect repair can occur only in tissues made up of stable and labile cells, whereas all injuries to tissues composed of permanent cells must inevitably give rise to scarring and, at the most, very slight restoration of specialized elements. Such is the case with healing of a myocardial infarction. The location of the injury, or the character of the tissue in which the injury occurs, likewise is of considerable importance from yet another standpoint. There are many situations in the body in which inflammations arising within tissues or tissue spaces (pleural, peritoneal, synovial cavities) develop extensive exudates. Under these circumstances, repair may occur by digestion of the exudate, initiated by the proteolytic enzymes of leukocytes, and resorption of the dissolved exudate. This mechanism of dealing with an exudative inflammation is called *resolution*. If no necrosis of fixed tissue cells has occurred, perfect restitution of the preexisting architecture is attained. Conversely, in the presence of substantial necrosis, granulation tissue grows into the exudate and converts it into masses of fibrous tissue, a process referred to as organization.

- Aberrations of growth may occur even in what may begin initially as normal wound healing. The accumulation of excessive amounts of collagen may give rise to a raised tumorous scar known as a *keloid*.

Keloid formation appears to be an individual predisposition, and for reasons unknown this aberration is somewhat more common in blacks. We still do not know the mechanisms of keloid formation. Another deviation in wound healing is the formation of excessive amounts of granulation tissue, which protrudes above the level of the surrounding skin and in fact blocks reepithelialization. This has been called *exuberant granulation* or, with more literary fervor, *proud flesh*. Excessive granulations must be removed by cautery or surgical excision to permit restoration of the continuity of the epithelium. Finally (fortunately rarely), incisional scars or traumatic injuries may be followed by exuberant proliferations of fibroblasts and other connective tissue elements that may, in fact, recur after excision. Called *desmoids,* or *aggressive fibromatoses,* these lie in the interface between benign proliferations and malignant (though low-grade) tumors. Indeed, the line between the benign hyperplasias characteristic of repair and neoplasia is frequently finely drawn, as we shall see.

- The mechanisms underlying the fibroplasia of wound repair—cell proliferation, cell-cell interactions, cell-matrix interactions, and ECM deposition—are similar to those that occur in the chronic inflammatory fibrosis of such diseases as rheumatoid arthritis, lung fibrosis, and hepatic cirrhosis. The same growth factors (e.g., PDGF, TGF-β) are involved, and there is an important role for fibronectin and other ECM components. Unlike orderly wound healing, however, the diseases are associated with persistence of initial stimuli for fibroplasia or the development of immune and autoimmune reactions in which lymphocyte-monocyte interactions sustain the synthesis and secretion of growth factors and fibrogenic cytokines (p. 51); or the unchecked actions of enzymes and other biologically active molecules. Collagen degradation by collagenases, for example, which is important in the normal remodeling of healing wounds, causes much of the joint destruction in rheumatoid arthritis (p. 145). The molecular mechanisms that regulate orderly fibroplasia, and that may become aberrant in chronic inflammatory fibrosis, are obviously of utmost importance and currently are subjects of much interest.

do not get orderly fibrosis

OVERVIEW OF THE INFLAMMATORY-REPARATIVE RESPONSE _____

At this point, a backward look may help to relate the multitude of changes that occur simultaneously or sequentially in the inflammatory-reparative response. Figure 3–10 offers an overview of the possible pathways. This schema reemphasizes certain important concepts. Not all injuries result in permanent damage; some are resolved with almost perfect repair. More often, the injury and inflammatory response result in residual scarring. Although it is functionally imperfect, the scarring provides a permanent patch that permits

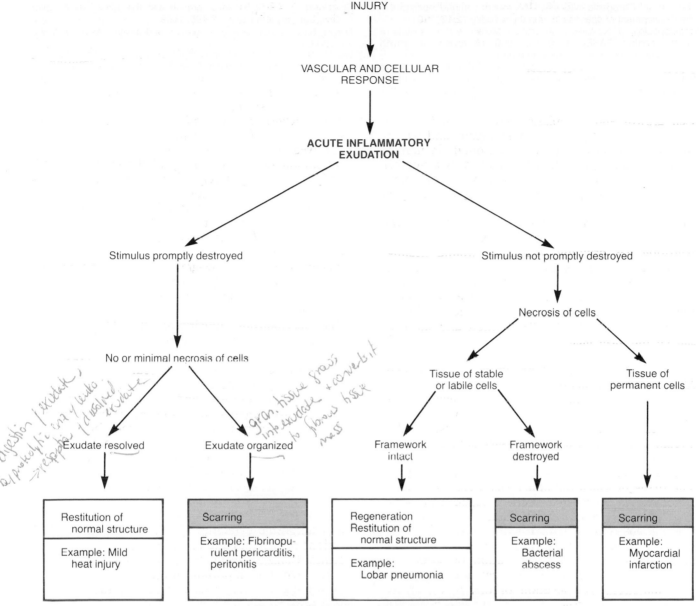

Figure 3–10. Pathways of reparative response.

the residual parenchyma more or less to continue functioning. Sometimes, however, the scar itself is so large or so situated that it may cause permanent dysfunction, as for example in a healed myocardial infarct. In this case, the fibrous tissue not only represents a loss of preexisting contractile muscle but also constitutes a permanent burden to the overworked residual muscle.

Bibliography

Baserga, R.: The Biology of Cell Reproduction. Cambridge, MA, Harvard University Press, 1985. (A highly readable, concise text on cell cycle and cell growth.)

Clark, R. A. F., Henson, P. M. (eds.): The Molecular and Cell Biology of Wound Repair. New York, Plenum Press, 1988. (A multiauthored, comprehensive work dealing with mechanisms of cell proliferation, migration and differentiation, and fibroplasia in wound healing; a second edition is in preparation.)

Damsky, C. H., Bernfield, M.: Cell-cell contact and extracellular matrix. Curr. Opinion Cell Biol. 2:813, 1990. (A review of several aspects of ECM biology.)

Gabbiani, G., Ryan, G. B., Majno, G.: Presence of modified fibroblasts in granulation tissue and their possible role in wound contraction. Experientia 27:549, 1971. (The first classic description of the myofibroblast.)

Gross, M., Dexter, M.: Growth factors in development, transformation and tumorigenesis. Cell 64:271, 1991. (A brief review of growth factors and the relationship between growth and differentiation.)

Hay, E. D. (ed.): The Cell Biology of the Extracellular Matrix. 2nd ed. New York, Plenum Press, 1992. (A comprehensive text of ECM.)

Heldin, C. H., Westermark, B.: Platelet-derived growth factor and autocrine mechanisms of oncogenic processes. Crit. Rev. Oncogenesis 2:109, 1991. (A review of PDGF, its receptor, signal transduction pathways, and autocrine growth.)

Ingber, D. E., Folkman, J.: How does extracellular matrix control capillary morphogenesis? Cell 58:803, 1989.

Kovacs, E. J.: Fibrogenic cytokines: The role of immune mediators in the development of scar tissue. Immunol. Today 12:17, 1991.

Michaelopoulos, G. K.: Liver regeneration: Molecular mechanisms of growth control. FASEB J. 4:176, 1990. (A review of growth factors and inhibitors in liver regeneration.)

Moses, H. L., Young, E. J., Piekenpol, J. A.: TGF-β stimulation and inhibition of cell proliferation. Cell 63:245, 1990. (A short essay summarizing how TGF-β can both inhibit and stimulate cell growth.)

Studzinski, G. P.: Oncogenes, growth and the cell cycle: An overview. Cell Tissue Kinetics 22:405, 1989.

Travali, S., et al.: Oncogenes in growth and development. FASEB J. 4:3209, 1990.

Woessner, J. F. Jr.: Matrix metalloproteinases and their inhibitors in connective tissue remodeling. FASEB J. 5:2145, 1991.

FOUR

Disorders of Vascular Flow and Shock

EDEMA
HYPEREMIA OR CONGESTION
HEMORRHAGE
THROMBOSIS
    Microcirculatory Thrombosis — Disseminated
      Intravascular Coagulation
EMBOLISM
    Fat Embolism
    Caisson Disease
    Amniotic Fluid Embolism (Amniotic Fluid
      Infusion)
INFARCTION
SHOCK

Survival of cells and tissues is exquisitely dependent on the oxygen provided in a normal blood supply. What may be less apparent is their dependence on a normal fluid balance. Approximately 60% of a person's lean body weight is water. This is divided between the intracellular compartment (40%) and the extracellular compartment (interstitial fluid, 15%; plasma water, 5%). Derangements in either blood supply or fluid balance cause some of the most commonly encountered disorders in medical practice: edema, congestion, hemorrhage, shock, and the three interrelated conditions — thrombosis, embolism, and infarction. Not only are these disorders common, they are major causes of mortality. Pulmonary edema is often the terminal event in most forms of heart disease. Hemorrhage and shock are virtually daily problems in the emergency room of any large hospital. Thrombosis, embolism, and infarction underlie three of the most important disorders in industrialized nations: myocardial infarction, pulmonary embolism, and cerebrovascular accidents (strokes). This chapter, then, deals with the predominating mechanisms of morbidity and mortality.

EDEMA

The term *edema* refers to the accumulation of abnormal amounts of fluid in the intercellular tissue spaces or body cavities. It may occur as a generalized or localized disorder. The term *anasarca* is used when the edema is severe and generalized, producing marked swelling of the subcutaneous tissues. Edematous collections in the various serous cavities of the body are given the special designations *hydrothorax, hydropericardium,* and *hydroperitoneum* (more commonly called *ascites).* The fluid of noninflammatory edema, such as develops in hydrodynamic derangements, is a transudate, low in protein and other colloids, with a specific gravity usually below 1.012. Inflammatory collections of fluid are rich in proteins (see p. 27) and therefore have a higher specific gravity — usually over 1.020.

Edema is the result of an increase in the forces that tend to move fluids from the intravascular compartment into the interstitial fluid. The normal interchange of fluid, as proposed by Starling, is regulated by the hydrostatic and osmotic pressures within and without the vascular compartment (Fig. 4–1). *The opposing effects of intravascular hydrostatic pressure and plasma colloid osmotic pressure are the major factors to be considered in the pathogenesis of edema.* At the arteriolar end of the capillary bed, the hydrostatic pressure is about 35 mm Hg. At the venular end it falls to 12 to 15 mm Hg. The colloid osmotic pressure of the plasma is 20 to 25 mm Hg, rising slightly at the venular end as fluid escapes (Fig. 4–2). Thus fluid leaves at the arteriolar end of the capillary bed and returns at the venular end. Not all of the fluid in the interstitial spaces returns to the venules; some is drained off through the lymphatics, to be returned to the bloodstream only indirectly.

From this brief review of the formation and drainage of interstitial fluid we can deduce that edema will occur when there is:
- *an increase in intravascular hydrostatic pressure*
- *a fall in colloid osmotic pressure of the plasma*
- *an impairment in the flow of lymph.*

These constitute the important *primary causes* of noninflammatory edema. To this list must be added *renal retention of salt and water,* which may be a primary disturbance when there is kidney disease or may be a secondary event contributing to edema of other causes. Table 4–1 lists the primary causes of edema and the associated clinical conditions. Not included in this table is inflammatory edema, which, as already discussed (p. 27), results from an increase in

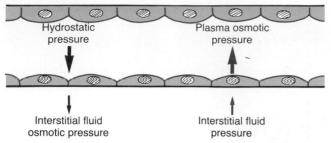

Figure 4–1. Factors affecting the flow of fluid across capillary walls. Intravascular hydrostatic pressure and interstitial fluid osmotic pressure tend to move fluid outward. Conversely, interstitial fluid pressure and plasma osmotic pressure draw fluid inward.

vascular permeability brought about by the action of chemical mediators.

Increased hydrostatic pressure may result from an impaired venous outflow, most frequently encountered in the lower extremities, secondary to the development of obstructive thromboses. The resulting edema is localized to the legs. A generalized increase in venous pressure and systemic edema occurs when there is congestive heart failure (p. 305) affecting right ventricular function. Although increased venous hydrostatic pressure is an important factor, the pathogenesis of cardiac edema is far more complex (Fig. 4–3). Congestive heart failure is associated with reduced cardiac output and reduced renal blood flow. Through a series of complex regulatory mechanisms, a reduction in renal perfusion or perfusion pressure triggers the renin-angiotensin-aldosterone axis, resulting in renal retention of sodium and water _(secondary aldosteronism)_. Expansion of the intravascular volume resulting from this sequence of events does not improve renal perfusion, since the failing heart is unable to increase cardiac output. With the extra fluid load (which the heart is unable to handle) there is further increase in venous pressure and edema formation. Thus a vicious circle of fluid retention and worsening edema sets in. Not surprisingly, therefore, restriction of salt intake and administration of diuretics and aldosterone antagonists reduce the edema of congestive heart failure.

Reduced osmotic pressure of the plasma results from

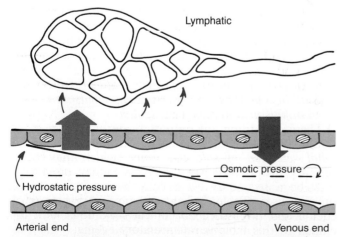

Figure 4–2. Normal formation and drainage of interstitial fluid.

TABLE 4–1. CAUSES OF EDEMA

Primary Cause	Clinical Examples	
	Localized Edema	Generalized Edema
Increased hydrostatic pressure	Venous obstruction Thrombosis External compression (e.g., tumors)	Congestive heart failure
Reduced colloid osmotic pressure of plasma— hypoalbuminemia	None	(a) Excessive loss of albumin (e.g., renal disease) (b) Decreased synthesis of albumin (e.g., diffuse liver disease)
Lymphatic obstruction	Neoplastic or inflammatory obstruction	None
Sodium retention	None	Renal disease with salt retention

excessive loss or reduced synthesis of serum albumin. The most important cause of increased loss of albumin is certain diseases of the kidney in which the glomerular basement membrane becomes abnormally permeable to albumin. The resulting _nephrotic syndrome_ (p. 444) is characterized by generalized edema. Reduced synthesis of serum proteins occurs with diffuse diseases of the liver, such as cirrhosis (p. 545), or in association with malnutrition (p. 243). In all these instances, movement of fluid from the intravascular to the interstitial compartment leads to a contraction of plasma volume. Predictably, a reduction in renal perfusion follows, and secondary aldosteronism sets in. However, the retained salt and water cannot correct the deficit in plasma volume, because the primary defect of too little serum proteins persists. Once again, we see that the edema initiated by one mechanism gets complicated by secondary salt and fluid retention.

Lymphatic obstruction is another primary cause of edema. Impaired lymphatic drainage and consequent lymphedema is usually localized and may result from inflammatory or neoplastic obstruction. Filariasis, a parasitic infection, often causes massive fibrosis of the lymph nodes and lymph channels in the inguinal region. The resulting edema of the external genitalia and the lower limbs is so extreme it is called _elephantiasis_. Cancer of the breast is sometimes treated by removal or irradiation of the entire breast along with all or most of the lymph nodes in the axilla. Consequently, postoperative edema of the arm often follows such therapy and can be a troublesome clinical problem.

Sodium retention, along with obligate water retention, has already been mentioned as a contributing factor in several forms of edema. Salt retention may be a primary cause of edema when there is acute reduc-

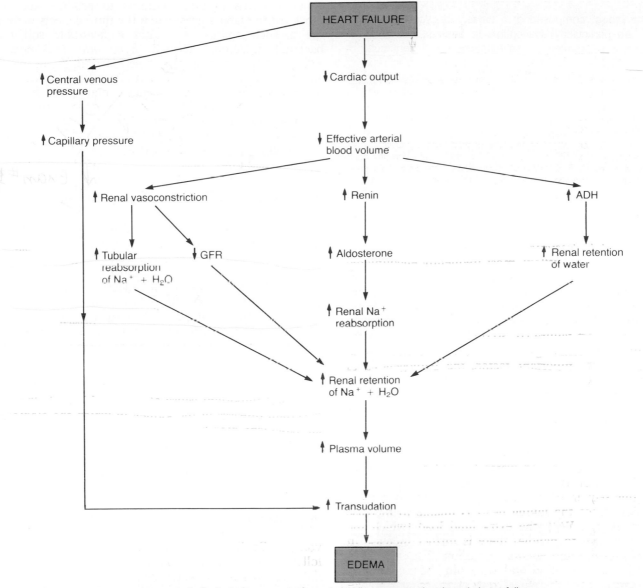

Figure 4–3. Projected sequence of events leading to systemic edema in heart failure.

tion in renal function, as may be encountered in poststreptococcal glomerulonephritis (p. 449) or in acute renal failure (p. 457). The retained salt and water cause expansion of intravascular fluid volume and lead secondarily to increased hydrostatic pressure and, consequently, edema.

MORPHOLOGY. The morphologic changes of edema are much more evident grossly than microscopically. Although any organ or tissue in the body may be involved, edema is encountered most often in three sites: the subcutaneous tissues, usually in the lower extremities; the lungs; and the brain.

Subcutaneous edema of the lower parts of the body is a prominent manifestation of cardiac failure, particularly failure of the right ventricle. Although right ventricular failure obviously affects the entire systemic venous return to the heart, edema is most prominent in the lower extremities because they are subject to the highest hydrostatic pressures. If the patient is confined to bed, sacral edema may become evident. **Since the distribution of the edema is influenced by gravity, it is termed "dependent."**

Edema produced by **renal dysfunction** results from proteinuria and sodium retention. It tends to be generalized and more severe than cardiac edema, affecting all parts of the body equally. However, it may manifest itself initially in tissues that have a loose connective tissue matrix, such as the eyelids **(periorbital edema).** Such generalized edema merits the designation "anasarca." Finger pressure over edematous subcutaneous tissue will squeeze out the fluid and produce pitted depressions, hence the common clinical term **pitting edema.** Incision of edematous subcutaneous tissues discloses increased oozing of interstitial fluid, but it is usually slight and difficult to appreciate.

The **lungs**, composed of a loose, honeycombed tissue, are particularly susceptible to edema. <u>Pulmonary edema is a prominent manifestation of left ventricular failure</u> (Fig. 4–4). It may also be encountered in renal failure, in the so-called adult respiratory distress syndrome, in infections of the lung, and in hypersensitivity reactions. The changes are described more fully in the consideration of congestive heart failure on page 305.

Edema of the **brain** is encountered in a variety of clinical circumstances, such as brain trauma, meningitis, encephalitis, hypertensive crises, and any form of obstruction to the venous outflow of the brain. This condition is described on page 707.

CLINICAL CORRELATION. Edema may give rise to minor clinical problems, or it can be lethal. Edema of the subcutaneous tissues in cardiac or renal failure is important chiefly because it indicates underlying disease, but it sometimes impairs healing of wounds or infections. Because edema of the lungs (pulmonary edema) impairs normal ventilatory function, it may be lethal. The <u>fluid first collects within the alveolar walls around the capillaries, producing an "alveolocapillary block" in oxygen diffusion</u>. The impact on ventilatory function may seem disproportionate to the relatively

small amounts of fluid required to produce such a block. In the later stages, when the fluid collects within the alveolar spaces, it creates a favorable soil for bacterial infection, termed *hypostatic pneumonia*. Edema of the brain can be a serious clinical problem and may cause death if it is sufficiently marked. The increased mass of brain substance may cause herniation of the cerebellar tonsils into the foramen magnum or may cause shearing stresses on the blood supply to the brain stem. Both conditions secondarily impinge on medullary centers to cause death.

↓ Exam #4

HYPEREMIA OR CONGESTION

These synonyms refer to a local increased volume of blood caused by dilatation of the small vessels. *Active hyperemia* results from an augmented arterial inflow, such as occurs in the muscles during exercise, at sites of inflammation, and in the pleasing neurovascular dilatation termed blushing. *Passive congestion* results from diminished venous outflow such as follows cardiac failure or obstructive venous disease. Thus, in cardiac failure the appearance of edema is almost always accompanied by passive congestion, giving rise to the more appropriate designation *congestion and edema*. *Chronic passive congestion of the lungs is one of the most reliable postmortem indicators of left ventricular cardiac failure.* When congestion is encountered in the lower extremities, the legs are abnormally cool and either pale, owing to the predominance of edema, or dusky blue-gray, owing to the venous congestion accompanying the edema.

HEMORRHAGE

Hemorrhage obviously implies rupture of a blood vessel. Rupture of a large artery or vein is almost always caused by some form of injury, such as trauma, atherosclerosis, or inflammatory or neoplastic erosion of the vessel wall. Rupture of a large artery in the brain is a frequent cause of death in hypertensive patients (Fig. 4–5). An increased tendency to hemorrhage is encountered in a wide variety of clinical disorders known collectively as the *hemorrhagic diatheses*. These are discussed in Chapter 12.

to deprive "body" 161

Hemorrhages may be external and exsanguinating. When the blood is trapped within the tissues of the body, the accumulation is referred to as a *hematoma*. Rupture of the aorta, for example in a dissecting or atherosclerotic aneurysm, may cause a massive retroperitoneal hematoma with sufficient loss of blood to cause death. When the blood accumulates in one of the body cavities it is referred to as *hemothorax, hemopericardium, hemoperitoneum,* or *hemarthrosis.* *bleeding into a joint* Minute hemorrhages into the skin, mucous membranes, or serosal surfaces are known as *petechiae.* Slightly larger hemorrhages are designated *purpura.* A large (over 1 to 2 cm in diameter) subcutaneous hematoma, an example of which is the common bruise, is called an *ecchymosis.* The released hemoglo-

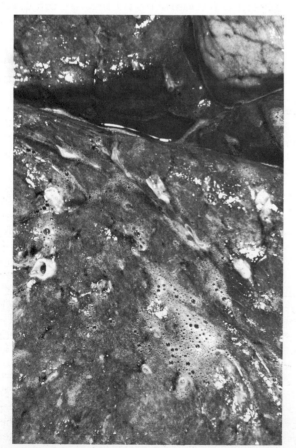

Figure 4–4. Pulmonary edema. A close-up view of the transected surface of a very wet lung, from which frothy edema fluid exudes.

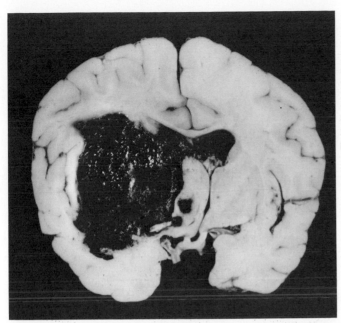

Figure 4–5. A fatal intracerebral hemorrhage. (Courtesy of Dr. Dennis Burns, Department of Pathology, Southwestern Medical School, Dallas, TX.)

bin is converted into bilirubin and eventually into hemosiderin. Patients who sustain a large hemorrhage, such as massive gastrointestinal bleeding, a pulmonary hemorrhage or infarct (p. 74), or a hematoma, sometimes become jaundiced owing to the breakdown of red cells and subsequent release of bilirubin.

The significance of hemorrhage depends on the volume of blood loss, the rate of loss, and the site of hemorrhage. Sudden losses of up to 20% of the blood volume or slow losses of even larger amounts may have little clinical significance. Larger or more acute losses may induce hemorrhagic (hypovolemic) shock (p. 78). The site of the hemorrhage is, of course, important; a hemorrhage that would be trivial in the subcutaneous tissues may cause death when located in the brain stem. Repeated external hemorrhages (i.e., those in which the blood is shed—as from the skin, gastrointestinal tract, or female genital tract) represent losses of not only blood volume but also of valuable iron. Usually the small but repeated volume losses are rapidly corrected by movement of water from the interstitial spaces into the vascular compartment, but the chronic loss of iron may lead to an iron deficiency anemia. In contrast, when the red cells are retained, as occurs with hemorrhages into the body cavities, joints, or tissues, the iron can be recaptured for synthesis of hemoglobin.

THROMBOSIS _____

The formation of a clotted mass of blood in the noninterrupted cardiovascular system is known as *thrombosis*, and the mass itself is termed a *thrombus*. Blood clotting, when it plugs a severed vessel, may be life saving; when it occludes a functioning vessel sup-

plying a vital structure, it may be life threatening. In addition, some part or all of the thrombus may break loose to create an *embolus* that flows downstream to lodge at a distant site. Thrombosis and embolism are, then, closely interrelated, as is indicated by the commonly used term *thromboembolism.* The potential consequence of both thrombosis and embolism is ischemic necrosis of cells and tissue, known as *infarction.* Thromboembolic infarctions of the heart, lungs, and brain are dominating causes of morbidity and mortality in industrialized nations and account collectively for more deaths than those caused by all forms of cancer and infectious disease together. Here we consider the subject of thrombosis, and in later sections, embolism and infarction.

PATHOGENESIS. The development of a thrombus is best viewed as the consequence of inappropriate activation of the process of normal hemostasis. We should briefly review, then, normal hemostasis.

Normal Hemostasis. When a vessel is severed it almost immediately contracts, owing to reflex neurogenic mechanisms, possibly augmented by such humoral factors as *endothelin,* a potent endothelium-derived vasoconstrictor. Such vascular contraction is most evident in vessels that have well-defined muscular walls, but it also occurs in the sphincteric mechanisms situated at the junction of metaarterioles and capillaries, thereby shutting off capillary beds. Soon, however, the vascular spasm abates and bleeding would resume were it not for activation of the platelet and coagulation systems. We can dissect the ensuing process of hemostasis by considering the three major contributors to it: (1) *endothelial cell injury,* (2) *platelets,* and (3) *the coagulation system.*

Endothelial cells modulate several aspects of the hemostasis-coagulation sequence. On the one hand they possess antiplatelet, anticoagulant, and fibrinolytic properties; on the other hand they exert procoagulant functions (Fig. 4–6). Only some properties of the "schizophrenic" endothelial cells are summarized here. Consider first those aspects of the endothelium that oppose clotting.

1. Antiplatelet properties. *Intact endothelium insulates the blood platelets and coagulation proteins from the highly thrombogenic subendothelial components, principally collagen.* Platelets flowing in the bloodstream do not adhere to the endothelium. This antiplatelet function seems intrinsic to the plasma membrane of endothelium and is not dependent upon the production of prostacyclin (PGI_2). On the other hand, once platelets are "activated" (following focal endothelial injury), they are inhibited from adhering to the surrounding uninjured endothelial cells by the action of PGI_2 and nitric oxide, which are powerful inhibitors of platelet aggregation and potent vasodilators. PGI_2 is a well-known arachidonic acid derivative whereas nitric oxide, an endothelium-derived relaxing factor, is generated by enzymatic transformation of L-arginine. Their synthesis in endothelial cells is stimulated by adenosine diphosphate (ADP), thrombin, and other undefined serum factors produced during coagulation.

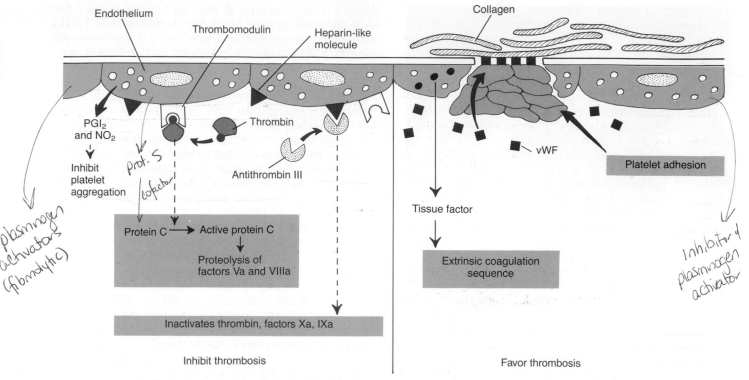

Figure 4–6. A schematic illustration of the procoagulant and anticoagulant activities of endothelial cells.

2. **Anticoagulant Properties.** These are mediated by membrane-associated heparin-like molecules and thrombomodulin, a specific thrombin receptor (see Fig. 4–6). The *heparin-like molecules* act indirectly; they catalyze the actions of naturally occurring anticoagulant protein antithrombin III, which inactivates thrombin and several other coagulation factors, including factor Xa. *Thrombomodulin* also acts indirectly. It binds thrombin and in so doing converts thrombin from a procoagulant to an anticoagulant. Thrombin that is bound to thrombomodulin activates protein C, a powerful naturally occurring anticoagulant. Activated protein C inhibits clotting by proteolytic cleavage of factors Va and VIIIa. Protein S, synthesized by endothelial cells, serves as a cofactor for the anticoagulant activity of protein C.
3. **Fibrinolytic Properties.** Endothelial cells react against blood clots by synthesizing plasminogen activators that promote fibrinolytic activity in the blood and help to clear fibrin deposits from endothelial surfaces.

While on the one hand endothelial cells oppose blood clotting and thrombosis, on the other hand they are prohemostatic, affecting both platelets and coagulation proteins. As mentioned earlier, endothelial injury leads to the first step in hemostasis: adhesion of platelets to subendothelial collagen. Endothelial cells synthesize and secrete von Willebrand's factor (vWF), which is essential for the adhesion of platelets to collagen and other surfaces. Tissue factor released from endothelial cells that have been injured or perturbed (for example, by exposure to tumor necrosis factor [TNF] or interleukin 1 [IL-1]) activates the extrinsic clotting pathway. Endothelial cells are also known to express binding sites for activated forms of factors IX and X, and cell-bound factors seem to be more active than their counterparts in solution. Another prothrombotic effect of endothelial cells is mediated through the secretion of an inhibitor of plasminogen activator, which depresses fibrinolysis.

In summary, intact endothelial cells, although multifunctional, predominantly serve to inhibit platelet adherence and initiation of blood clotting. Conversely, injury to endothelial cells represents a loss of anticlotting mechanisms and thus contributes to hemostasis and, as will be seen, to thrombosis.

Platelets, as must already be evident, play a key role in normal hemostasis. In their circulating form, they appear as relatively smooth discs enclosed within a typical plasma membrane, itself coated by a glycocalyx. Within the platelets are two specific types of granules. *Alpha granules* contain fibrinogen, fibronectin, factors V and VIII, platelet factor 4 (a heparin-neutralizing polypeptide), and platelet-derived growth factor (PDGF). The other form of granules are *electron-dense bodies* that are the storage sites for a nonmetabolic pool of adenine nucleotides (adenosine diphosphate [ADP], adenosine triphosphate [ATP]), ionized calcium, histamine, serotonin (5-HT), and epinephrine.

With injury to a vessel, platelets are exposed to a number of elements in the vascular wall—subendothelial collagen, capillary basal lamina, fibroblasts, and smooth muscle cells. Although all are capable of causing platelet adhesion, collagen is the most powerful stimulus. On contact with collagen, for example, plate-

hemostasis
= "arrest of bleeding"

lets undergo a number of changes, which can be listed as *adhesion, release reaction (or secretion), and aggregation.* Together these phenomena are referred to as "platelet activation" (Fig. 4–7).

Platelet adhesion to collagen is mediated in large part by interactions with von Willebrand's factor (vWF). This large molecule acts as a bridge between platelet surface receptors (mostly glycoprotein Ib) and the exposed collagen. In patients with an inherited deficiency of vWF (von Willebrand's disease, p. 382) platelet adhesion to collagen and other surfaces is impaired. Adhesion of platelets to subendothelial collagen is followed soon by *secretion*—or the so-called *release reaction*—during which ADP, serotonin, and various other platelet contents are released. Secretion of ADP is a particularly important event since ADP causes platelet aggregation (platelets adhering to other platelets) and it also augments the release of ADP from other platelets. Thus an autocatalytic reaction is set into motion that leads to the build-up of an enlarging platelet aggregate. Initially, platelet aggregation is reversible, so the breach in the vessel wall is sealed by a "temporary hemostatic plug." Soon, however, under the influence of thrombin, thromboxane A_2 (TXA_2, discussed below), and increasing amounts of ADP, platelets contract, and a mass of irreversibly aggregated platelets ("viscous metamorphosis") is produced. It will be recalled (p. 36) that TXA_2 is a prostaglandin that is synthesized by the platelets and, like prostacyclin, is a product of the cyclooxygenase pathway of arachidonic acid metabolism (p. 36). However, prostacyclin (PGI_2) and TXA_2 have opposing actions: prostacyclin inhibits platelet aggregation and is a vasodilator, whereas TXA_2 is a powerful aggregator and vasoconstrictor. *The interplay of PGI_2 and TXA_2 constitutes a finely balanced mechanism for modulation of human platelet function, which, in the normal state, prevents intravascular platelet aggregation and clotting but following endothelial injury favors the formation of hemostatic plugs.*

The build-up of a platelet mass at a site of vascular injury serves many functions. It alone may suffice as a hemostatic plug to control bleeding in small vessels. The aggregated platelets make available platelet factor 3 for the coagulation sequence. *Platelet factor 3 (unlike most other platelet constituents) is not a secreted product but rather a phospholipid complex that is activated or in some manner exposed on the platelet surface.* This phenomenon is of singular importance, since virtually every step in the coagulation sequence discussed below requires a phospholipid surface (see Fig. 4–9). The platelet surface therefore serves as a haven for the accumulation of thrombin, which itself is a potent inducer of platelet aggregation. Thus a feedback loop is built into the platelet system, augmenting the build-up of a hemostatic plug while contributing to the clotting sequence. Fibrin, the end product of coagulation, serves to cement the aggregated platelets. The events described thus far are summarized in Figure 4–7.

3. The *coagulation system,* the third component of the hemostatic process, is a major contributor to thrombus formation. It is not our intention to delve into the details of the clotting sequence but to highlight certain general principles and concepts with relevance to hemostasis and thrombogenesis.

- The coagulation sequence comprises, in essence, a series of transformations of proenzymes to activated enzymes (serine proteases), culminating in the formation of thrombin, which converts the soluble plasma protein fibrinogen to the insoluble fibrous protein fibrin (Fig. 4–8).

- Each reaction in the coagulation pathway results from the assembly of a reaction complex composed of an *enzyme* (activated coagulation factor), a *substrate* (proenzyme form of coagulation factor), and a *cofactor* (reaction accelerator). These components are assembled on a *phospholipid surface* and held together by *calcium ions.* Thus clotting tends to remain localized to sites where such an assembly can occur, e.g., on the surface of activated platelets. One of the key reactions in blood clotting, conversion of factor X to Xa, is illustrated in Figure 4–9. It has been customary to divide the blood coagulation scheme into an *extrinsic* and *intrinsic* pathway, both of which converge at the point where factor X is activated (see Fig. 4–8). However, it is now clear that such a division is probably an artifact of testing methods in vitro and that there are several interconnections between the so-called intrinsic and extrinsic pathways. An important example of such "crosstalk" between pathways is the demonstration that

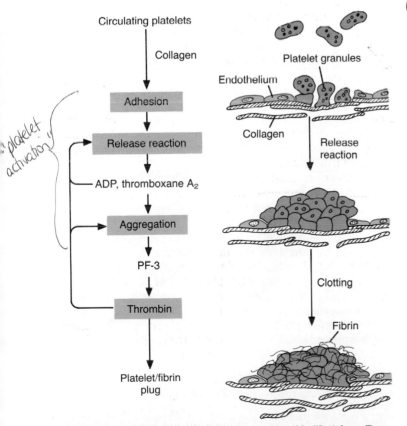

platelet activation

Figure 4–7. Platelet functions in hemostasis. (Modified from Taussig, M. J.: Processes in Pathology. 2nd ed. Oxford, Blackwell Scientific, 1984, p. 627.)

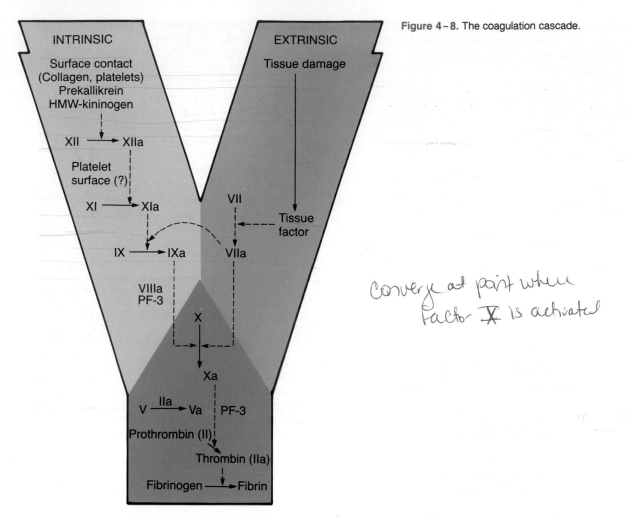

Figure 4–8. The coagulation cascade.

Converge at point where factor X is activated

the conversion of factor IX to IXa is brought about not only by the "contact-activated" factors of the intrinsic pathway but also by factor VII, the initiator of the extrinsic pathway (see Fig. 4–8).

Once the coagulation cascade has been activated, it must be contained to the local site of vascular injury lest clotting involve the entire vascular tree. The naturally occurring anticoagulants fall into three basic groups:

1. *Antithrombins*, exemplified by antithrombin III, are characterized by their ability to inhibit the activity of thrombin and other serine proteases—factors IXa, Xa, XIa, and XIIa. Antithrombin is activated by binding to heparin-like molecules on endothelial cells and by the therapeutic administration of heparin.

2. *Proteins C and S* are two vitamin K–dependent proteins characterized by their ability to inactivate cofactors Va and VIIIa. These two, it will be recalled, serve as reaction accelerators in the coagulation cascade. The activation of protein C by endothelium-associated thrombomodulin has already been described.

3. The *plasminogen-plasmin* system serves to break down fibrin and check fibrin polymerization. The proteolytic conversion of plasminogen to its active form, plasmin, is accomplished either by a factor

XII–dependent pathway or by plasminogen activators (PA). There are two groups of PAs: (1) *urokinase-like* PA (uPA) is present in plasma and various

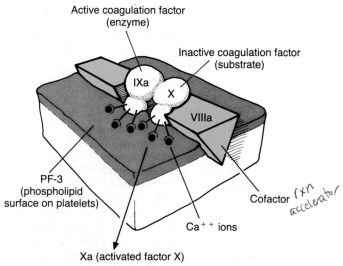

Figure 4–9. A schematic illustration of the conversion of factor X to factor Xa. The reaction complex consisting of an enzyme (factor IXa), a substrate (factor X), and a reaction accelerator (factor VIIIa) are assembled on the surface of platelets. Ca⁺⁺ ions hold the assembled components together and are essential for reaction. (Modified from Mann, K. G.: Clin. Lab. Med. 4:217, 1984.)

tissues and activates plasminogen in the fluid phase; (2) *tissue type PA (tPA)*, synthesized principally by endothelial cells, is active when attached to fibrin. The affinity for fibrin makes tPA a much more useful therapeutic reagent. The fibrin split products, once released, serve as potent anticoagulants. Plasminogen is also activated by a bacterial product, streptokinase. With this overview of normal hemostasis, attention can be turned to its participation in the formation of thrombi.

Thrombogenesis. The influences that predispose to thrombus formation are endothelial injury, stasis or turbulence of blood flow, and hypercoagulability of the blood.

(1) *Endothelial injury* is the dominant influence in thrombogenesis and the only one which by and of itself may lead to thrombus formation. This is amply documented by the frequency with which thrombi appear on ulcerated plaques in severely atherosclerotic arteries, particularly in the aorta; at sites of traumatic or inflammatory injury to vessels; and within the cardiac chambers when there has been injury to the endocardium, as may occur with myocardial infarction or in any form of myocarditis. The injury may be subtler in nature—hemodynamic stresses of hypertension, bacterial toxins, or endotoxins—and such adverse influences as homocystinuria, hypercholesterolemia, and products absorbed from cigarette smoke may also represent potential causes of endothelial injury. Overt in many of these situations and perhaps covert in others is endothelial damage and exposure of subendothelial collagen (as well as other platelet activators), adherence of platelets (Fig. 4–10), release of tissue factor, and local depletion of prostacyclin and plasminogen activator. However, it should be stressed that the endothelial injury may be subtle and not detectable even under the electron microscope.

(2) *Stasis and turbulence* (with its pockets of stasis) constitute major thrombogenic influences. In normal laminar blood flow, all of the formed elements are separated from the endothelial surface by a clear plasmatic zone. Stasis and turbulence (1) disrupt laminar flow and permit platelets to come into contact with the endothelium; (2) prevent dilution of activated clotting factors to subcritical concentrations; (3) retard the inflow of clotting factor inhibitors; (4) permit the build-up of platelet aggregates and nascent fibrin either in the sluggish stream or in the pockets of stasis; (5) promote endothelial cell hypoxia and injury, predisposing to platelet and fibrin deposition as well as reducing release of TPA; additionally, (6) the turbulence is a mechanism for endothelial injury. *Stasis plays a dominant role in venous flow because of the low velocity of blood flow in veins.* Several investigators have documented the origin of venous thrombi in the sinuses behind the valve cusps in the deep veins of the lower leg. A similar phenomenon probably occurs in the auricular appendages of the heart when there is atrial fibrillation or massive dilatation of the atria, as for example with mitral stenosis. Stasis and turbulence undoubtedly contribute to the development of thrombi

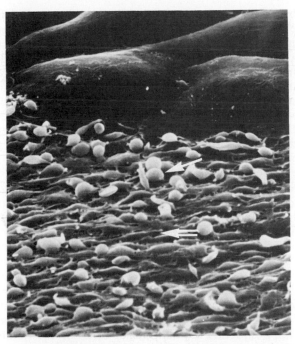

Figure 4–10. Scanning electron micrograph of an area of experimental endothelial denudation with only a few intact endothelial cells seen above. Numerous platelets are adherent to the subendothelium. Discoid and rounded platelets *(arrow)* are seen on top of an earlier layer of tightly adherent, elongated, flattened platelets *(double arrow)*. (Courtesy of Dr. C. Haudenschild, Mallory Institute of Pathology, Boston, MA.)

within aneurysmal dilatations, which are already favored sites for thrombosis because of the underlying vascular disease and endothelial injury (e.g., atherosclerosis leading to aneurysm formation).

(3) *Hypercoagulability* can be defined as an alteration of the blood or, specifically, the clotting mechanism that in some way predisposes to thrombosis. This is not a common cause of thrombogenesis. The best-understood and prototypic hypercoagulable states are associated with an inherited lack of the natural anticoagulants antithrombin III, protein C, or protein S. Affected patients present with venous thrombosis and recurrent thromboembolism in adolescence or early adult life. Although these hereditary disorders are quite uncommon, it is easy to understand the basis of thrombotic tendencies in these patients. It is much more difficult to unravel the pathogenesis of the thrombotic diathesis in several more common clinical settings such as nephrotic syndrome, following severe trauma or burns, in later pregnancy, with cardiac failure, and in disseminated cancer. In some of these settings, for example with cardiac failure or following trauma, other influences such as stasis or vascular injury may be the most important mechanism. But the frequency of thrombosis in patients having disseminated cancer and in late pregnancy (discussed more completely on p. 72), and the increased frequency of both venous and arterial thromboses in females who have used oral contraceptives, point to hypercoagulability as the predisposing mechanism. Unfortunately in

most of these instances it has been difficult to define the precise basis for hypercoagulability. In users of oral contraceptives an increase in concentrations of plasma fibrinogen, prothrombin, and factors VII, VIII, and X can be demonstrated, as can a decrease in fibrinolytic activity; yet it has not been possible to prove a cause-and-effect relationship between the abnormalities in laboratory tests and increased thromboses. In patients with disseminated cancer, secretion of thrombogenic factors or release of procoagulant products from necrotic tumor cells has been proposed as the basis for the tendency toward thrombosis.

Some patients with high titers of *autoantibodies directed against anionic phospholipids* (so-called lupus anticoagulant) have a high frequency of arterial and venous thrombosis. Some of them have manifestations of a well-defined autoimmune disease such as systemic lupus erythematosus (p. 139), but in others thrombosis is the major or only clinical manifestation. The mechanism by which antiphospholipid antibodies promote thrombosis in vivo are unknown. Possibilities include induction of platelet aggregation, inhibition of prostacyclin production by endothelial cells, or interference in the generation of protein C. In summary, despite suggestive clinical and some laboratory evidence, the role of a hypercoagulable state in thrombogenesis is difficult to document. The only exceptions to this generalization are the inherited deficiencies of antithrombin III or proteins C and S, already mentioned.

slower-moving blood of the veins, the coagulation simulates that in a test tube. Thus, these thrombi have a much richer admixture of erythrocytes and are therefore known as **red, coagulative, or stasis thrombi.** On transection laminations are not well developed, but tangled strands of fibrin can usually be seen. **Phlebothrombosis most commonly affects the veins of the lower extremities (90%) in approximately the following order of frequency: deep calf, femoral, popliteal, and iliac veins.** Less commonly, venous thrombi may develop in the periprostatic plexus, or the ovarian and periuterine veins. Sometimes they occur in the portal vein or its radicles or in the dural sinuses.

Venous thrombi can be readily confused with postmortem clots at autopsy. The postmortem clot forms a cast of the vessel, but it is rubbery and gelatinous. The dependent portions of the clot where the red cells have settled by gravity tend to resemble dark red currant jelly. The supernatant, free of red cells, has a yellow "chicken fat" appearance. Characteristically the postmortem clot is not attached to the underlying wall. In contrast, coagulation thrombi are more firm, almost always have a point of attachment, and on transection disclose barely visible tangled strands of pale gray fibrin.

Arterial and venous thrombi vary enormously in size. They range from small, irregular, roughly spherical masses to enormously elongated, snake-like structures

MORPHOLOGY OF THROMBI. Thrombi may develop anywhere in the cardiovascular system: in chambers of the heart, or in arteries, veins, or capillaries. Those arising in the arterial side of the circulation (including the heart) differ somewhat from those arising in the venous side. Arterial or cardiac thrombi usually begin at a site of endothelial injury or turbulence, either from some lesion or because a vessel bifurcates or branches. Classically the arterial thrombus is a dry, friable, tangled gray mass that on transection usually discloses darker gray lines of aggregated platelets interspersed between paler layers of coagulated fibrin. These lamellae are known as the **lines of Zahn.** When arterial thrombi arise in the capacious chambers of the heart or in the aorta, they are usually applied to one wall of the underlying structure and thus are termed **mural thrombi** (Fig. 4–11). Mural thrombi also develop in abnormal dilatations of arteries (aneurysms). In arteries smaller than the aorta the thrombus usually builds up rapidly until it completely obstructs the lumen, producing a so-called **occlusive thrombus.** Any artery may be affected, but the most common and most important sites of involvement in order of frequency are as follows: coronary, cerebral, femoral, iliac, popliteal, and mesenteric arteries. **The term "thrombus," unless otherwise designated, implies the occlusive type.**

Venous thrombosis, also known as **phlebothrombosis**, is almost invariably occlusive. In fact, the thrombus often creates a long cast of the lumen of the vein. In the

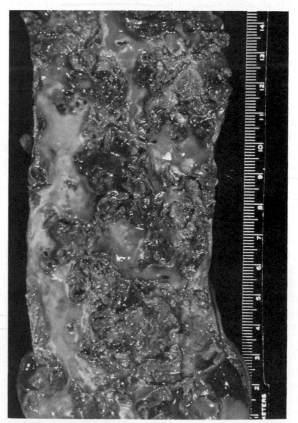

Figure 4–11. Numerous friable mural thrombi superimposed on advanced atherosclerotic lesions of the aorta.

that are formed when a long tail builds up behind the occluding head. In the arterial circulation the tail builds up retrograde to the direction of flow. On the venous side the tail extends in the direction of the blood flow, that is, toward the heart. Often such propagations extend to the next major vascular branch.

A small or large area of attachment to the underlying vessel or heart wall is characteristic of all thromboses. Frequently the attachment is most firm at the point of origin, and the propagating tail may or may not be attached. It is this loosely attached tail which, in veins, is most likely to fragment to create an embolus. On the arterial side of the circulation, embolization usually implies detachment of the entire or almost the entire thrombus.

In special circumstances thrombi may be deposited on the heart valves. Blood-borne infections may attack heart valves (**bacterial** or **infective endocarditis),** creating ideal sites for the development of thrombotic masses. These masses, laden with microorganisms, are referred to as vegetations. Less commonly, noninfective, **verrucous endocarditis** may appear in patients who have systemic lupus erythematosus (p. 139). Vegetations may also develop on uninfected valves— **nonbacterial (thrombotic) endocarditis** in older patients with terminal cancers or other chronic ailments, and sometimes in young patients with nonfatal disorders. In these conditions hypercoagulability of the blood, subtle endothelial injuries, or both are invoked as the causative mechanisms.

If a patient survives the immediate effects of vascular obstruction, what happens to the thrombus over the course of days and weeks? One of the following sequences evolves: (1) the thrombus may propagate and eventually cause obstruction of some critical vessel, (2) it may embolize, (3) it may be removed by fibrinolytic activity, or (4) it may undergo organization and become recanalized—that is, incorporated within the vessel wall. The first two eventualities need no further comment here. There is evidence that fibrinolytic removal may occur. By angiography, pulmonary thromboemboli have been observed to shrink rapidly and even be totally lysed soon after they develop. Such a happy outcome is most likely within the first day or two, presumably because as the thrombus ages and the fibrin undergoes continued polymerization, it is more resistant to proteolysis. It is relevant in this connection to note that infusion of fibrinolytic agents such as recombinant TPA and streptokinase within hours of the acute event is currently employed in the management of massive pulmonary thromboemboli and coronary thrombosis.

When a thrombus persists in situ for a few days, it is likely to become **organized.** This term refers to the ingrowth of granulation tissue, subendothelial smooth muscle cells, and mesenchymal cells into the fibrinous thrombus. In time the thrombus becomes populated with these spindle cells, and capillary channels are formed. Simultaneously the surface of the thrombus becomes covered with a layer of endothelial cells. The capillary channels may anastomose to create thoroughfares from one end of the thrombus to the other through which blood may flow, reestablishing to some extent the continuity of the lumen of the original vessel. This process is known as **recanalization** of the thrombus (Fig. 4–12).

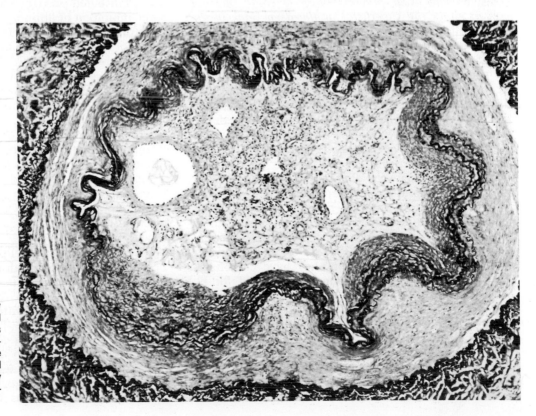

Figure 4–12. A low-power view of a thrombosed artery stained for elastic tissue. The lumen is delineated by the partially degenerated internal elastic membrane and is totally filled with organized clot, now traversed by many newly formed recanalized channels.

In this manner the thrombus is converted into a vascularized subendothelial mass of connective tissue and eventually incorporated into the wall of the vessel. With the passage of time and the contraction of the mesenchymal cells, only a fibrous lump or thickening may remain to mark the site. Occasionally, instead of becoming organized, the center of the thrombus undergoes enzymic digestion and softens. This action presumably reflects the release of lysosomal enzymes derived from the trapped leukocytes and platelets. This sequence is particularly likely in large thrombi within aneurysmal dilatations or within mural thrombi in the cardiac chambers. If a bacteremia occurs, such softened debris is an ideal culture medium for conversion of the thrombus into a septic mass of pus.

CLINICAL CORRELATION. Thrombi are critically important for two reasons: (1) *they cause obstruction of arteries and veins* and (2) *they provide possible sources of emboli.* Venous thrombi may cause congestion and edema in dependent parts, but a far graver consequence is that thrombi, most frequently those arising in the deep veins of the legs, are responsible for one of the major causes of death in the United States—namely, pulmonary embolization and infarction (p. 406). In contrast, although arterial thrombi may of course embolize, much more important is their obstructive role in myocardial infarction, when the coronary arteries are involved, and in cerebral infarction, when the arteries in the brain are involved.

As pointed out earlier, most venous thrombi are occlusive. *The great preponderance of these thrombi arise in either the superficial or the deep veins of the leg.* Superficial thrombi usually occur in the saphenous system, particularly when there are varicosities. Such thrombi may cause local congestion and swelling, pain, and tenderness along the course of the involved vein, but only rarely do they embolize. However, the local edema and impaired venous drainage predispose the skin to infections from slight trauma and to the development of *varicose ulcers.* It is the *deep thrombi in the larger outflow veins of the legs (e.g., popliteal, femoral, and iliac veins) that are the most serious because they may embolize.* They may also cause edema of the foot and ankle and produce pain and tenderness on compression of the calf muscles (by either squeezing the calf muscles or forced dorsiflexion of the foot), known as Homans' sign. However, in *approximately half of the patients such thrombi are entirely asymptomatic* and are recognized only when they have embolized. The venous obstruction is soon compensated for by the opening of collateral bypass channels of drainage. The most serious aspect of venous thrombosis in the deep veins of the leg, as mentioned, is its potential for causing pulmonary embolization and infarction.

It is necessary to digress for a moment to clarify the commonly used clinical term *"thrombophlebitis."* This *designation is often applied to phlebothrombosis because* the pain, tenderness, and erythema sometimes encountered at the local site are vaguely ascribed to a chronic inflammatory reaction in the wall of the involved vein, hence the term thrombophlebitis. Morphologic studies, however, rarely disclose significant inflammatory changes in such vessels, and the pain, tenderness, and erythema are more reasonably attributed to local vascular stasis, edema, and distention of the affected vessel. Thus, *there is no valid distinction between phlebothrombosis and thrombophlebitis.*

Specific clinical settings in which venous thrombosis is most likely to occur have already been mentioned in the discussion of thrombogenesis but for emphasis are repeated here. *They include cardiac failure, severe trauma or burns, postoperative and postpartum states, the nephrotic syndrome, disseminated cancer* (and in fact, all serious illnesses), and the use of oral contraceptives. Cardiac failure is an obvious cause of sluggish venous circulation. Trauma, surgery, and burns usually imply reduced physical activity, injury to vessels, release of procoagulant substances from tissues, and reduced tPA activity. The incidence of postoperative deep vein thrombosis is estimated to be 15 to 30% after general surgery and 45 to 70% after orthopedic procedures. Many factors act in concert to predispose to thrombosis in the puerperal and postpartum states. During delivery there is trauma to vessels and the potential for the entrance of amniotic fluid, bearing platelet-aggregating and possibly procoagulant factors into the pelvic veins (p. 75). But, in addition, there is a distinct hazard of venous thrombosis in the third trimester of pregnancy, as well as in the postdelivery period, giving rise to the designation "milk leg" or "phlegmasia alba dolens" (painful white leg). The basis for such predisposition is not entirely clear but has been attributed to hypercoagulability as well as to some inhibition of fibrinolysis.

Predisposition to venous thrombosis in any of the veins of the body in patients with visceral cancer, particularly with abdominal neoplasms (such as carcinoma of the pancreas), was first noted by Trousseau and so is referred to as *Trousseau's sign.* Frequently the thrombi develop at one site only to disappear and reappear elsewhere, giving rise to the pattern known as *migratory thrombophlebitis.* The basis for such a thrombotic diathesis probably involves a number of influences, including age, surgical procedures, confinement to bed, and, in addition, development of hypercoagulability due to release of procoagulant material from tumor cells. Thus there are many possible mechanisms leading to a thrombotic diathesis in cancer.

Regardless of specific clinical setting, advanced age, bed rest, and immobilization increase the hazard. The reduced physical activity in older age lessens the milking action of muscles in the lower leg and so slows venous return. Immobilization and bed rest carry the same implications.

Despite some persisting controversies, *it is generally accepted that women who use oral contraceptives containing at least 50 µg of estrogen are at an increased risk of developing thrombosis and its attendant complications such as embolism.* This subject is discussed in

DISORDERS OF VASCULAR FLOW AND SHOCK _____ **73**

greater detail on page 229; suffice it to say that the risk is highest in women between 35 and 45 years of age, and concurrent cigarette smoking compounds the hazards of thrombotic disease considerably.

Arterial thrombi are particularly likely to develop in patients with myocardial infarction, rheumatic heart disease, florid atherosclerosis, and aneurysmal dilatations of the aorta or other major arteries. Myocardial infarction usually is associated with damage to the adjacent endocardium, providing a site for the origin of a mural thrombus, usually within the left ventricle (Fig. 4–13). Stasis and turbulence within the affected cardiac chamber are usually also present because of dyskinetic contraction of the myocardium or the development of cardiac irregularities. Advanced age, bed rest, and impaired circulation compound the problem. Rheumatic heart disease often leads to marked stenosis of the mitral valve and, along with it, stasis within the markedly dilated left atrium and atrial appendage. Concurrently, cardiac arrhythmias may augment the stasis. Florid atherosclerosis underlying the dominant causes of mortality in industrialized nations—myocardial infarction and stroke—is a prime initiator of thromboses for what must now be obvious reasons. But, in addition to all of the serious obstructive consequences, thrombi in the aorta and in the cardiac chambers often yield fragments that embolize to such sites as the brain, the kidney, the legs, and the spleen. Other tissues or organs may also be affected, but the brain, kidneys, and spleen constitute prime targets because of their large blood flow volume. The iliac, femoral, and more distal arteries of the lower legs represent the "ends of the line" of the aortic flow.

Although many high-risk clinical disorders have been cited, it should be emphasized that thrombosis may occur in any clinical setting and sometimes arises in otherwise healthy, active young persons, particularly those whose work involves long periods of standing or sitting. Therefore, no individual is immune, and ultimately thrombosis is an unpredictable, puzzling disorder of quixotic nature.

MICROCIRCULATORY THROMBOSIS— DISSEMINATED INTRAVASCULAR COAGULATION

In many disease states, minute thrombi form in widely dispersed sites within the microcirculation, principally in capillaries and venules. The thrombi are largely made up of aggregated platelets admixed with some fibrin. They are rarely visible on gross inspection but in the aggregate can cause circulatory insufficiency, principally in the lungs, brain, heart, and kidneys. Disseminated intravascular coagulation (DIC) is not a primary disorder; rather, it is a complication of some underlying disease which, in some manner, activates the processes involved in blood clotting. Paradoxically, the innumerable small thrombi may lead to a hemorrhagic diathesis. The bleeding tendency is probably attributable to the rapid consumption of platelets and clotting factors; hence DIC is sometimes also referred to as *defibrination syndrome* or *consumption coagulopathy*. The clinical settings in which DIC is encountered are extremely diverse and are discussed in greater detail on page 378. It suffices here that this complex clotting disorder may, on the one hand, cause clinical manifestations by occlusion of the microcirculation in one or more organs or, on the other hand, lead to a serious hemorrhagic diathesis.

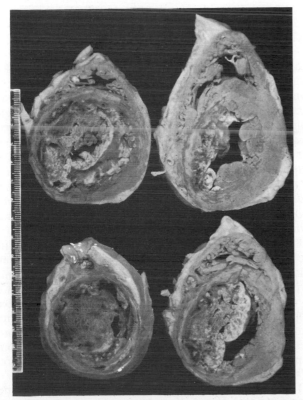

Figure 4–13. Multiple transections of the ventricles of a heart with a recent myocardial infarction. The left ventricle is virtually filled with thrombus, particularly toward the apex of the heart.

EMBOLISM

Embolism refers to occlusion of some part of the cardiovascular system by the impaction of some mass (embolus) *transported to the site through the bloodstream.* The great majority of emboli represent some part or the whole of a dislodged thrombus, hence the commonly used term *thromboembolism.* Much less commonly, embolization is produced by droplets of fat, undissolved air or gas bubbles, atherosclerotic debris (cholesterol emboli), tumor fragments, bits of bone marrow, or any other substance that gains entry to the bloodstream (such as a bullet). Collectively, the unusual forms account for less than 1% of all embolisms, and so, unless otherwise indicated, embolism is considered to be thrombotic in origin.

Embolism may occur within either the venous or the arterial system. **In approximately 95% of instances, venous emboli arise from thrombi** within the veins of the leg in the locations previously mentioned (p. 70). Much more rarely they arise in pelvic veins, inferior vena cava, or elsewhere. They drain through progressively larger channels, usually pass through the right heart, and become lodged in the pulmonary circulation (Fig. 4–14). Regrettably, not one but many emboli may become dislodged, often at recurrent intervals. Thus, **the patient who has had one pulmonary embolus is at high risk of having more.** Indeed, at times the pulmonary circulation is peppered by a shower of small fragments. Rarely, a large, snake-like mass may become coiled upon itself and lodge in one of the valvular orifices of the right side of the heart. Alternatively, it may impinge on the bifurcation of the main pulmonary artery and sit astride the two major subdivisions, thus creating a **saddle embolus.** The size of the vessel occluded obviously depends on the size of the mass. As discussed in greater detail on p. 407, the morphologic consequences of pulmonary embolism (e.g., infarction, hemorrhage) depend on the size of the embolus and the state of pulmonary circulation.

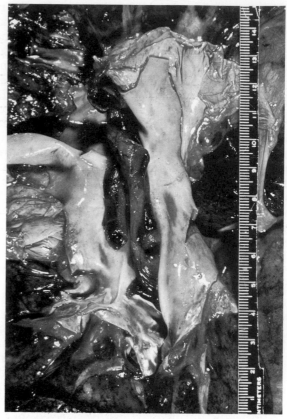

Figure 4–14. The opened major pulmonary arteries in the root of the lung. A large, coiled embolus having the diameter of one of the large veins in the leg was the cause of the sudden death of this patient.

Pulmonary embolism, the most serious form of thromboembolic disease, is an extremely important and common clinical problem. Meticulous dissection of the lungs reveals evidence of pulmonary embolism in as many as 64% of autopsies. Many of these emboli are small, produce no clinical symptoms, and are of little significance. Nonetheless, surveys have disclosed that pulmonary embolism is the prime or contributing cause of death in about 15% of hospitalized patients and one of the most common causes of death among hospitalized patients in the United States. The clinical course of pulmonary thromboembolism is discussed on page 407.

Arterial emboli most commonly arise from intracardiac mural thrombi. Less often they take origin from mural thrombi in an aortic aneurysm or from those overlying atherosclerotic plaques in the aorta or some other large artery. Infrequently arterial emboli arise from fragmentation of a vegetation on a heart valve (discussed in more detail on p. 323). Occlusive thrombi in arteries of medium to small size rarely embolize because they are usually firmly lodged at their sites of origin. In contrast to venous emboli, arterial masses usually follow a shorter pathway because they travel through vessels of progressively diminishing caliber. The site of lodgement depends to a considerable extent on the point of origin of the thromboembolus and the volume of blood flow through an organ or tissue. The consequences of such emboli are somewhat dependent on the richness of the vascular supply of the affected tissue, its vulnerability to ischemia, and the caliber of the vessel occluded. These considerations are dealt with on page 77.

FAT EMBOLISM

Minute globules of fat can often be demonstrated in the circulation following fractures of the shafts of long bones (which have fatty marrows) and, rarely, with soft tissue trauma and burns. Presumably the microglobules are released by injury to marrow or adipose tissue and gain access to the circulation by rupture of the marrow vascular sinusoids or venules. It should be emphasized that whereas *traumatic fat embolism can be demonstrated anatomically in approximately 90% of individuals who sustain severe skeletal injuries, only about 1% of these individuals manifest clinical signs or symptoms known as fat embolism syndrome.* It is characterized by pulmonary insufficiency (resembling the acute respiratory distress syndrome, p. 399), neurologic symptoms, anemia, and thrombocytopenia. Typically the symptoms appear after a latent period of 24 to 72 hours after injury. There is sudden onset of tachypnea, dyspnea, and tachycardia. Neurologic symptoms include irritability and restlessness, which progress to delirium or coma. Petechial skin rash is common. The fat embolism syndrome is fatal in about 10% of cases.

The pathogenesis of this symptom complex is not entirely clear but is believed to involve both mechanical obstruction and chemical injury. It is proposed that microaggregates of neutral fat cause occlusion of pulmonary or cerebral microvasculature, and the free fatty acids released from fat globules result in toxic injury to the vascular endothelium. The petechial skin rash is related to rapid onset of thrombocytopenia. Presumably myriad fat globules become coated with platelets, thus depleting circulating platelets.

The microscopic demonstration of fat microglobules in tissues or organs requires special techniques using frozen sections and fat stains because the emboli are dissolved out of the blood by the usual solvents employed in paraffin embedding of tissues. Sometimes the microemboli can be identified in the gross specimen by gentle pressure on fresh tissue slices immersed in saline, which releases the droplets and permits them to float to the surface.

CAISSON DISEASE

A particular form of gas embolism, known as *caisson disease* or *decompression sickness,* may appear in deep sea and scuba divers, in underwater construction workers, and in individuals in unpressurized aircraft that ascend rapidly to high altitudes. As deep sea divers descend to greater depths, air pressure is increased within the diving suit and helmet to compensate for the water pressure. The gases within the pressurized air are dissolved in the blood, tissue fluid, and fat. If the diver then ascends to the surface too rapidly, the dissolved oxygen, carbon dioxide, and nitrogen may come out of solution in the form of minute bubbles. Although the first two gases are rapidly solubilized, the nitrogen is of low solubility and persists as minute bubbles. Essentially the same sequence transpires with ascent from normal atmospheric pressures to the rarefied atmosphere of high altitudes.

The formation of minute gas bubbles within the skeletal muscles and supporting tissues in and about joints creates what is known as *the bends.* Emboli may induce foci of necrosis in the brain, highly vascularized bones, the heart, or other tissues or organs. In the lungs, edema, hemorrhages, and focal atelectasis or emphysema may appear, sometimes leading to sudden respiratory distress, called *the chokes.* Treatment of gas embolism consists of placing the individual in a compression chamber where the barometric pressure may be raised. This speeds the solution of the gas bubbles and permits slow decompression of the individual. However, when this condition is unrecognized, or when such therapy is not available, serious medical consequences may occur, as is still evident among native sponge and pearl divers in many locales around the world.

AMNIOTIC FLUID EMBOLISM (AMNIOTIC FLUID INFUSION)

This disorder of mysterious origin occurs in about one in 50,000 to 80,000 deliveries. As the other major causes of maternal mortality—pulmonary thrombo-

embolism, hemorrhage, and toxemia—decrease in incidence, amniotic embolism is assuming increased importance because it can be fatal, totally unpredictable, and largely unpreventable. Typically it appears in older, multiparous patients who have a tumultuous labor, and it is characterized by sudden dyspnea, cyanosis, collapse, hemorrhage, and often convulsions followed by coma. The classic findings in the pulmonary arterioles and capillaries at autopsy are epithelial squames from fetal skin; lanugo hairs; fat from vernix caseosa; and mucin, presumed to be from the fetal gastrointestinal tract. Extensive fibrin thrombi, indicative of DIC (p. 378), are found in the small vessels of uterus, lung, kidney, thyroid, and myocardium.

The pathogenesis of amniotic fluid embolism is still unclear. There is little doubt that the symptom complex is triggered by infusions of amniotic fluid into the blood. Such entry may occur through endocervical veins, the uteroplacental site, or lacerations of the uterus or cervix. At one time it was thought that particulate matter within the amniotic fluid (e.g., epithelial squames, vernix caseosa) was responsible for the pulmonary vascular obstruction. It is now suspected that vasoactive substances within the amniotic fluid such as prostaglandins may be the cause of pulmonary vasoconstriction. Additionally, one or more thrombogenic factors within the amniotic fluid induce intravascular coagulation, leading in effect to DIC and its attendant complications such as hemorrhages and acute renal failure. Present therapy is directed toward countering shock and hypoxemia, and controlling DIC.

INFARCTION

An infarct is an area of ischemic necrosis within a tissue or an organ, produced by occlusion of either its arterial supply or its venous drainage. Nearly all infarcts result from thrombotic or embolic occlusion, but sometimes infarction may be caused by other mechanisms, such as ballooning of an atheroma secondary to hemorrhage within a plaque. Other uncommon causes include twisting of the vessels to the ovary or a loop of bowel, compression of the blood supply of a loop of bowel in a hernial sac, or trapping of a viscus under a peritoneal adhesion. In these last-mentioned situations the veins alone or both the veins and arteries may be blocked, but often the final occlusive episode is thrombotic closure of the already narrowed vessel. However, vascular occlusion does not always produce infarction, as will become clear later.

Nearly 99% of infarcts are caused by thromboembolic events and almost all are the result of arterial occlusions. Emboli arising in the heart or major arteries must impact in arteries. Similarly, venous thromboemboli lodge in the pulmonary arterial system and so cause arterial infarcts. Although venous thrombosis may cause infarction of some tissue or organ, more often it merely induces venous obstruction. Usually bypass channels develop, providing some outflow from the area, which in turn permits some improvement in the arterial inflow. Infarcts caused by venous thrombosis are more likely in organs having a single venous outflow channel, such as the testis and ovary.

Infarcts are crudely divided into two types — white (anemic) and red (hemorrhagic). This distinction is quite arbitrary and is based merely upon the amount of hemorrhage that occurs in the area of infarction at the moment of vascular occlusion. This in turn depends on the solidity of the tissue involved and on the type of vascular compromise (venous or arterial). Most infarcts in solid organs result from arterial occlusion and are white or pale. The solidity of the tissue limits the amount of hemorrhage into the area of ischemic necrosis. **The heart, spleen, and kidneys exemplify solid, compact organs that develop white or pale infarcts. In contrast, the lung usually suffers hemorrhagic or red infarction** (Fig. 4–15). This loose, spongy organ permits blood to collect in the infarct from the anastomotic capillary circulation in the margins of the necrotic area. Hemorrhagic infarction is also encountered in those organs in which the venous outflow is limited to the obstructed vessel and in which bypass channels cannot develop. The ovary and the testis are the best examples of such. The entire ovarian blood supply and outflow pass through the mesovarium, and the testicular venous drainage traverses the spermatic cord. A twist in either of these organs may occlude only the thin-walled

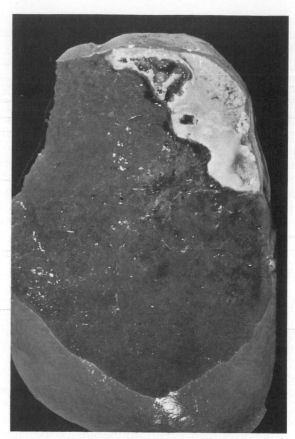

Figure 4–16. The transected surface of a spleen with a 1-week-old, pale, sharply demarcated infarct.

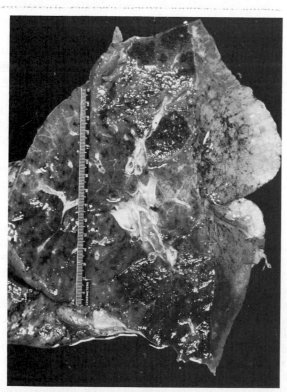

Figure 4–15. The transected surface of a lung shows several dark hemorrhagic infarcts, most evident at the apex and lower right. The infarction is recent and poorly demarcated from the adjacent, preserved lung substance.

venous outflow tract. Similarly, hemorrhagic venous infarction may be encountered in loops of the intestine or in the brain (from bilateral occlusion of the jugular vein). Another uncommon mechanism for hemorrhagic infarction of the brain deserves passing mention. An arterial embolus may impact in a large artery such as the middle cerebral and induce a large area of nonhemorrhagic infarction. Subsequently, the embolus may shatter and the small fragments may move onward into smaller vessels, permitting "reflow" and hemorrhage into the primary area of ischemia.

All infarcts, red and white, tend to be wedge shaped, with the occluded vessel at the apex and the periphery of the organ forming the base. Sometimes the margins are quite irregular, reflecting the pattern of vascular supply from adjacent vessels. When the base is a serosal surface, there is often a covering fibrinous exudate. At the outset, all infarcts are poorly defined and slightly hemorrhagic. In solid organs in which the lesions have relatively little hemorrhage, the contained red cells are laked and the released hemoglobin either diffuses out or is transformed to hemosiderin. **Thus, in the course of approximately 48 hours, infarcts in solid organs become progressively more pale and more sharply delimited** (Fig. 4–16). In spongy organs, such as the lungs, too many red cells are present to permit the lesion ever to become pale. The infarct is at first spongy and cyanotic (red-blue). Over the course of a few days, it becomes more firm and brown, reflecting the development of hemosiderin pigment. The margins of both types of infarcts, in the course of a few days, become progressively better defined. The delimitation is produced by the hyperemia accompanying the acute inflammatory response from the surrounding vital substance.

The dominant histologic characteristic of infarction is ischemic coagulative necrosis of affected cells (p. 12). It should be noted, however, that if the patient dies immediately after having sustained the infarction, insufficient time may have elapsed to permit the enzymic alteration in cells that follows cell death. Thus, for example, in sudden death after myocardial infarction both light and electron microscopy may disclose no demonstrable cytologic or histologic changes in the heart. The dynamic sequence and time required for the appearance of changes following cell death have been described in Chapter 1, to which reference should be made for an understanding of this important consideration. In hemorrhagic or red infarcts, the suffusion of red cells often seems to obliterate the native underlying architecture. In this connection, the pulmonary hemorrhage is distinguished from an infarct by preservation of the native structure. Only the alveolar spaces are filled with red cells; the alveolar walls, blood vessels, and stroma are preserved.

Most infarcts are ultimately replaced by scar tissue, which often contains hemosiderin granules as residues of the broken down red cells.

When an infarct is produced by an infected embolus **(septic embolus)**, as may occur with a fragment of a bacterial vegetation from a heart valve, or when organisms of bacteremic origin seed the area of devitalized tissue, the infarct virtually is converted to an abscess.

FACTORS THAT CONDITION THE DEVELOPMENT OF AN INFARCT. Occlusion of an artery or vein may have little or no effect on the involved tissue or it may cause death of the tissue, and indeed of the individual. *The major determinants include (1) the nature of the vascular supply, (2) the rate of development of the occlusion, (3) the vulnerability of the tissue to hypoxia, and (4) the oxygen-carrying capacity of the blood.*

Nature of Vascular Supply. The availability of an *alternative or newly acquired source of blood supply* is perhaps the most important factor in determining whether occlusion of a vessel will cause damage.

As is well known, the lungs have a dual blood supply from pulmonary and bronchial arteries. Hence blockage of a small radicle of the pulmonary arterial tree may be without effect in a young person who has normal bronchial circulation. The same applies to the liver, with its double blood supply of hepatic artery and portal vein. In the young, healthy individual, occlusion of one point in the circle of Willis may be without effect if the patient's vessels are not narrowed by preexisting disease. Infarction or gangrene of the hand or forearm is almost never encountered, because

of the double arterial supply through the radial and ulnar arteries, with their numerous interconnections. Such sequelae could occur only if both major arteries were simultaneously occluded.

Newly acquired *collateral circulation* may be equally effective in preventing infarction. The coronary arterial supply to the myocardium is an excellent case in point. Small anastomoses normally exist between the three major coronary trunks—that is, the left anterior descending, the left circumflex, and the right coronary arteries. If one of these trunks is slowly narrowed, as by an atheroma, these anastomoses may enlarge sufficiently to prevent infarction, even though the major coronary artery is eventually occluded.

Rate of Development of Occlusion. Slowly developing occlusions are less likely to cause infarction since they provide an opportunity for alternative pathways of flow and anastomotic bypass channels to develop.

Vulnerability of Tissue to Hypoxia. The susceptibility of the tissue to hypoxia influences the likelihood of infarction. Neurons of the nervous system undergo irreversible damage when deprived of their blood supply for 3 to 4 minutes. Myocardial cells, although hardier than neurons, are also quite sensitive to anoxia. In contrast, the fibroblasts within the myocardium are unaffected and are quite resistant to hypoxia. The epithelial cells of the proximal renal tubules are much more vulnerable to hypoxia than are the other segments of the nephron.

Oxygen-Carrying Capacity of Blood. *The oxygen level of the blood* will obviously be of significance in determining the effect of vascular occlusion or narrowing. The anemic or cyanotic patient tolerates arterial insufficiency less well than does the normal patient. Occlusion of a small vessel might lead to an infarction in those so handicapped, whereas it would be without effect at normal levels of oxygen transport. In this way, cardiac decompensation with its circulatory stasis and possibly reduced levels of oxygen saturation of the blood contribute to, and indeed may be critical in, determining whether the patient with a pulmonary arterial occlusion will develop only a pulmonary hemorrhage or an infarction.

CLINICAL CORRELATION. Infarction of tissues underlies some of the most frequent as well as most serious clinical disorders. The two most common forms of infarction are myocardial and pulmonary. The primary cause of death today in the United States and in other industrialized nations is coronary heart disease, and the great preponderance of these deaths results from myocardial infarction. Less awesome, but still gravely significant, is pulmonary infarction. Infarction of the brain (p. 714) is another very common killer infarct. Infarction of the small or large intestine happily is not a common disease, but when it does occur, it is frequently fatal. Less grave, but nonetheless productive of clinical signs and symptoms and possibly of serious disease, are renal and splenic infarcts.

Infarctions tend to have a special gravity because they are most common in patients least able to withstand them. Thus infarcts tend to occur in aged individuals with advanced atherosclerosis or cardiac decompensation. The postoperative and postdelivery periods are also times of increased vulnerability. The anemic or cyanotic patient is often fragile and poorly prepared for further insult. The triad of thrombosis, embolism, and infarction therefore resembles the proverbial vultures always hovering over the heads of those least able to withstand the attack.

↑ #1

SHOCK   *from p. 65

Shock, often loosely called "vascular collapse," may develop following any serious assault on the body's homeostasis. In the final analysis *shock constitutes widespread hypoperfusion of cells and tissues due to reduction in the blood volume or cardiac output, or redistribution of blood resulting in a decrease of effective circulating volume.* The reduced perfusion of cells and tissues if unchecked leads to irreversible injury and death of the cells, and eventually of the patient.

Shock may be precipitated by any massive insult to the body, such as profuse hemorrhage, severe trauma or burns, extensive myocardial infarction, massive pulmonary embolism, or uncontrolled bacterial sepsis. All these causes of shock can be grouped into mechanistic categories presented in Table 4–2. A review of this table will indicate that the mechanisms underlying cardiogenic and hypovolemic shock are fairly obvious. As might be expected, they are *associated with low cardiac output, hypotension, impaired tissue perfusion, and cellular hypoxia.* The basis of septic shock is much more complex and still imperfectly understood. The majority of cases of septic shock are caused by endotoxin-producing gram-negative bacilli—*Escherichia coli, Klebsiella pneumoniae, Proteus* species,

Pseudomonas aeruginosa, Serratia, and *Bacteroides*—hence the term *endotoxic shock.* However, gram-positive cocci such as pneumococci and streptococci may produce a similar syndrome. In contrast to hypovolemic and cardiogenic shock, the *cardiac output in septic shock is not low at the outset;* however, the total peripheral resistance is inappropriately low, owing to arteriolar vasodilatation. This results principally from release of vasoactive mediators such as complement components (Fig. 4–17; see also Chapter 2), but direct toxic injury to the vessels may also be involved. As a consequence, veins (the so-called capacitance vessels) become engorged with blood, producing peripheral pooling. *The disproportion between the circulating blood volume and the expanded volume of the circulatory bed thus induces a state of relative hypovolemia, and impaired perfusion results.* Sequestration of large volumes of blood in the capacitance vessels impairs venous return and leads eventually to low cardiac output. Endotoxins or other bacterial toxins play havoc on many other fronts: *Endothelial injury* leads to activation of both the intrinsic and extrinsic clotting pathways, leading to *disseminated intravascular coagulation,* which further aggravates tissue hypoxia. Activation of *complement* generates many factors, including those that increase vascular permeability and attract neutrophils. Accumulation of neutrophils in tissues, particularly the lung, followed by release of their enzymes and production of toxic free radicals, damages the pulmonary epithelium and initiates the acute respiratory distress syndrome (ARDS) (p. 399). Recent studies suggest that endotoxin-mediated activation of the mononuclear phagocyte system and the consequent release of TNF-α is a key event in the pathogenesis of septic shock (Fig. 4–17). This cytokine signals the synthesis and release of a whole array of secondary mediators, including prostaglandins and platelet-activating factors. TNF-α also promotes intravascular coagulation and capillary thrombosis. Indeed, most of the metabolic and hemodynamic effects of endotoxins can be mimicked by the infusion of TNF-α in laboratory animals. Conversely, antibodies directed against this cytokine can reverse experimentally induced septic shock. In addition to causing the release of biologically active mediators, bacterial toxins also cause direct injury to cells and tissues. Thus, even the cells that are well perfused fail to extract adequate oxygen from the blood. This results in a subnormal arteriovenous oxygen difference often noted in septic shock. *To summarize, septic shock is associated with distributive defects (peripheral pooling), endotoxin-mediated activation of the inflammatory-immune response, and direct toxic injury to cells and tissues. All of these acting in concert lead to failure of multiple organ systems and in many cases death.*

STAGES OF SHOCK. Shock is a progressive disorder that, if uncorrected, may lead to death. Unless the insult is massive and rapidly lethal (e.g., a massive hemorrhage from a ruptured aortic aneurysm or an extensive infarct affecting the left ventricle), shock tends to evolve through three stages (Fig. 4–18): (I) an

TABLE 4–2. CLASSIFICATION OF SHOCK

Type of Shock	Clinical Examples	Principal Mechanisms
Cardiogenic	Myocardial infarction, rupture of heart, arrhythmias, cardiac tamponade, pulmonary embolism	Failure of myocardial pump due to intrinsic myocardial damage or extrinsic pressure or obstruction to outflow
Hypovolemic	Hemorrhage, fluid loss (e.g., vomiting, diarrhea, burns)	Inadequate blood or plasma volume
Septic	Overwhelming bacterial infections: gram-negative septicemia ("endotoxic shock") or gram-positive septicemia	Peripheral vasodilatation and pooling of blood; cell membrane injury, endothelial cell injury with DIC
Neurogenic	Anesthesia, spinal cord injury	Peripheral vasodilatation with pooling of blood

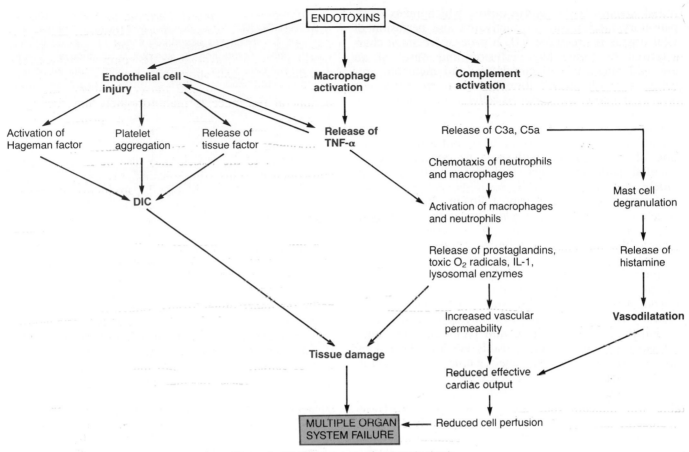

Figure 4–17. Pathogenesis of endotoxic shock.

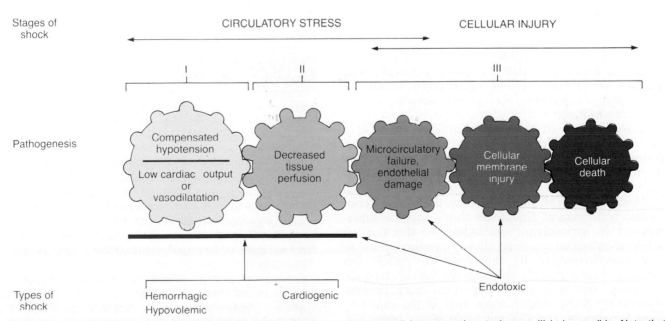

Figure 4–18. Pathogenesis and stages of shock. Stage I is nonprogressive, stage II is progressive, and stage III is irreversible. Note that endotoxic shock is multifactorial; it is associated with vasodilatation, decreased tissue perfusion, endothelial damage, and direct cellular injury. (Modified from Wyngaarden, J. B., Smith, L. H., Jr.: Cecil Textbook of Medicine. 17th ed. Philadelphia, W. B. Saunders, 1985, p. 212.)

(I) initial *nonprogressive phase* during which reflex compensatory mechanisms are activated and perfusion of vital organs is preserved; (II) a *progressive stage* characterized by tissue hypoperfusion and onset of an ever-widening circle of circulatory and metabolic imbalances; and finally (III) an *irreversible stage* that sets in after the body has incurred cellular and tissue injury so severe that even if therapy corrects the hemodynamic defects survival is not possible. Admittedly, these stages are somewhat arbitrary, but a brief discussion of this sequence will serve to integrate the sequential pathophysiologic and clinical alterations in shock.

During "early shock" (say, following blood loss), a *variety of neurohumoral mechanisms come into play to maintain cardiac output and blood pressure.* These include the baroreceptor reflexes, release of catecholamines, activation of the renin-angiotensin axis, antidiuretic hormone release, and generalized sympathetic stimulation. The effect of all these is to produce *tachycardia, peripheral vasoconstriction, and conservation of fluid by the kidney.* The vasoconstrictor response is responsible for the coolness and pallor of skin. Since the coronary and cerebral vessels are less affected by the sympathetic response, their caliber is not significantly affected and thus oxygen continues to be delivered to these vital organs. Obviously, therapeutic maneuvers have the best chance of success at this stage. Uncorrected, shock passes imperceptibly to the progressive phase, during which the vital organs begin to experience significant hypoxia. With persistent oxygen deficit there is impairment of intracellular aerobic respiration, followed by anaerobic glycolysis and excessive production of lactate, which often induces metabolic *lactic acidosis.* The lowering of pH in the tissues obtunds the vasomotor response; arterioles dilate and blood begins to pool in the microcirculation. Peripheral pooling not only worsens the cardiac output, it also favors anoxic injury to endothelial cells, thereby setting the stage for DIC. Release of TXA_2, a potent platelet aggregator, has also been implicated in the occlusion of microvasculature. With widespread tissue hypoxia, the function of vital organs begins to deteriorate; often *the patient is confused and the urinary output begins to fall.*

At some point in the downward spiral there is a transition from the reversible to the irreversible stage. Widespread cell injury allows leakage of lysosomal enzymes that further aggravate the shock state. *The ischemic pancreas is believed to liberate a myocardial depressant factor (MDF),* worsening the already poor cardiac performance. Endotoxic shock may be superimposed on hypovolemic or cardiogenic shock if the ischemic intestinal mucosa allows intestinal flora to enter the circulation. By this stage *the patient has complete renal shutdown due to acute tubular necrosis.* In closing, one may ask, When does shock become irreversible? Some would argue that if the initiating cause is removed, shock is reversible at any stage. The issue is moot, but one fact is not: death from shock, despite the heroic measures afforded by modern intensive care units, is still an everyday happening.

MORPHOLOGY. The cellular and tissue changes induced by shock are essentially those of hypoxic injury; only their distribution is somewhat distinctive. These were detailed earlier, in Chapter 1. Late stages of shock are characterized by **failure of multiple organ systems** and hence the cellular changes may appear in any tissue. They are particularly evident in the brain, heart, lungs, kidneys, adrenals, and gastrointestinal tract.

The **brain** may develop so-called ischemic encephalopathy, discussed on page 713.

The **heart** may undergo a variety of changes. Extensive lesions such as myocardial infarction or myocardial disease may, of course, be present. In addition, subendocardial hemorrhages and necrosis, or "zonal lesions," sometimes appear in all forms of shock. The term zonal lesions refers to apparent hypercontraction of a myocyte, inducing shortening and scalloping of the sarcomere, fragmentation of the Z band, distortion of the myofilaments, and displacement of the mitochondria away from the intercalated disc. Subendocardial hemorrhages and zonal lesions are not diagnostic of shock and may be seen following administration of catecholamines or after prolonged use of the heart-lung bypass pump in cardiac surgery.

The **kidneys** may be severely affected in shock, and so oliguria, anuria, and electrolyte disturbances constitute major clinical problems. The renal changes are referred to as **acute tubular necrosis**, but because similar changes may be encountered in other settings, they are described in detail on page 458.

The **lungs** are seldom affected in pure hypovolemic shock because they are resistant to hypoxic injury, but when the vascular collapse is caused by bacterial sepsis or trauma, changes may appear that are referred to as "shock lung." The pulmonary lesions result from diffuse alveolar damage and give rise to ARDS. Because these anatomic changes may be caused by a variety of clinical derangements, they are described on page 399.

The **adrenal** alterations encountered in shock comprise in essence those common to all forms of stress and so might be referred to as **"the stress response."** Early there is focal depletion of lipids in the cortical cells beginning in the zona reticularis and then spreading progressively outward into the zona fasciculata. This loss of corticolipids implies not adrenal exhaustion but rather reversion of the relatively inactive vacuolated cells to metabolically active cells that utilize stored lipids for the synthesis of steroids.

The **gastrointestinal tract** may suffer patchy mucosal hemorrhages and necroses, referred to as "hemorrhagic enteropathy" (p. 497; Fig. 4–19).

The **liver** may sometimes develop fatty change and, with severe perfusion deficits, central necrosis.

Virtually all of these organ changes may revert to normal if the patient survives. However, loss of neurons from the brain and of myocytes from the heart is, of course, irreversible. Moreover, persistent pulmonary septal edema may be converted into septal fibrosis, which is irreversible. However, most patients who suffer shock so severe as to produce irreversible changes succumb before these alterations become well developed.

Figure 4–19. Hemorrhagic enteropathy in the colon. The superficial mucosa is entirely obscured by the extensive hemorrhage; only the bases of the colonic glands are visible. The submucosa is unaffected.

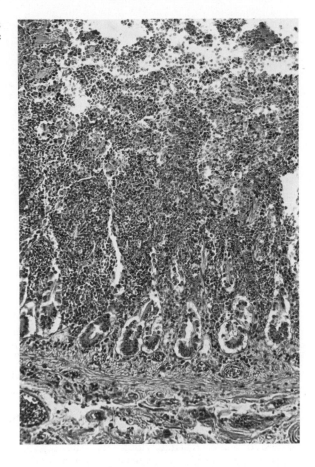

CLINICAL COURSE. The clinical manifestations depend on the precipitating insult. In hypovolemic and cardiogenic shock, *the patient presents with hypotension; an ashen gray pallor; cool, clammy skin; weak, thready pulse; and rapid cardiac and respiratory rates. With uncontrolled sepsis, however, the skin may be warm and indeed flushed owing to peripheral vasodilation.* The course of the patient in shock is beset with a sequence of hazards and pitfalls. The initial threat to life stems from the underlying catastrophe that precipitated the shock, such as the myocardial infarct, severe hemorrhage, or uncontrolled bacterial infection. However, the cardiac, cerebral, and pulmonary changes secondary to the shock state materially worsen the problem. Soon electrolyte disturbances and metabolic acidosis make their unwanted contributions. If all of these grave problems are survived, *the patient enters a second phase dominated by renal insufficiency* as is detailed on page 457. This may appear any time from the second to the sixth day and is marked by a progressive fall in urine output. Without going into detail, serious fluid and electrolyte imbalances now appear. If these can be managed with appropriate therapy, return of renal function is heralded by a "urinary flood tide." During this diuretic phase there is an increased vulnerability to microbiologic infections.

It is evident that the postshock course of the patient does not lack for threats to life. The prognosis varies with the origin of shock and its duration. For example, 80% of young, otherwise healthy patients with hypovolemic shock survive with appropriate management, whereas cardiogenic shock associated with extensive myocardial infarction, and gram-negative shock carry a mortality rate of 70 to 80%, even with the best care currently available.

Bibliography

Hawiger, J.: Formation and regulation of platelet and fibrin hemostatic plug. Hum. Pathol. *18*:111, 1987. (An excellent account of the mechanism of hemostasis with emphasis on platelet functions.)

High, K. A.: Antithrombin III, protein C, and protein S. Naturally occurring anticoagulant proteins. Arch. Pathol. Lab Med. *112*:28, 1988. (A succinct review of the basic and clinical aspects relating to these three proteins.)

Hirsh, J., Buchanan, M. R., Ofosu, F. A., et al.: Evolution of thrombosis. Ann. NY Acad. Sci. *516*:586, 1987. (An overview of the mechanisms involved in venous thrombosis.)

Moser, K. M.: Venous thromboembolism. Am Rev Resp Dis *141*:235, 1990. (A state of the art review of the pathogenesis and complications of venous thrombosis.)

Parillo, J. E. (moderator): NIH Conference. Septic shock in humans. Ann. Int. Med. *113*:227, 1990. (A detailed review of the pathogenesis of cardiovascular dynamics and management of septic shock.)

Pearson, J. D.: Endothelial cell biology. Radiology *179*:9, 1991. (A concise overview of the many roles played by endothelial cells in hemostasis.)

Tracey, K. J., Vlassara, H., Cerami, A.: Cachectin/tumor necrosis factor. Lancet *i*:1122, 1989. (A short summary of the biochemistry of TNF and its role in diseases including septic shock.)

Van Besouw, J. P., Hinds, C. J.: Fat embolism syndrome. Br. J. Hosp. Med. *42*:304, 1989. (A brief review of the pathogenesis and effects of fat embolism.)

Vane, J. R., Anggard, E. E., Botting, R. M.: Regulatory functions of the vascular endothelium. N. Engl. J. Med. *323*:27, 1990. (A very good overview of the biology of prostacyclin, EDRF, and endothelins.)

FIVE

Genetic Diseases

MENDELIAN DISORDERS (DISEASES CAUSED BY SINGLE-GENE DEFECTS)
   Autosomal Dominant Conditions
      Marfan's Syndrome
      Familial Hypercholesterolemia
      Neurofibromatosis
   Autosomal Recessive Disorders
      Cystic Fibrosis
      Phenylketonuria
      Galactosemia
      Albinism
      Glycogen Storage Disorders
         (Glycogenoses)
      Lysosomal Storage Diseases
      Mucopolysaccharidoses
   X-Linked Disorders
DISORDERS WITH MULTIFACTORIAL
POLYGENIC) INHERITANCE
   Gout
DISORDERS WITH VARIABLE MODES
OF TRANSMISSION
      Hereditary Malformation
      Ehlers-Danlos Syndromes
CYTOGENETIC DISORDERS
   Autosomal Disorders
      Down's Syndrome (Trisomy 21)
   Sex Chromosome Disorders
      Klinefelter's Syndrome
      XYY Males
      Turner's Syndrome
      Fragile X Syndrome
MOLECULAR DIAGNOSIS OF GENETIC
DISEASES
OTHER DIAGNOSTIC APPLICATIONS OF
RECOMBINANT DNA TECHNIQUES

Medical genetics, not too long ago considered an obscure subject, has by now permeated virtually every branch of medicine. While classical genetics was often viewed as a mere catalog of rare syndromes and disorders, the "new genetics" has provided penetrating insights into common disorders such as cancer and diabetes. Indeed, Victor McKusick, an eminent geneticist, recently said, "Genetics is to biology what the atomic theory is to physical sciences." Much of the recent progress in medical genetics has resulted from application of recombinant DNA techniques. It is possible, for example, to excise human genes and insert them into appropriate "cloning vectors." The human gene when recombined with the DNA of the cloning vector can be replicated, transcribed, and translated. This technique has opened up new possibilities of piece-by-piece analysis of human genetic material. Indeed, an international effort to map and sequence the entire human genome is now under way. Some examples of the impact of recombinant DNA technology on medicine follow:

- *Molecular basis of human diseases.* Recombinant DNA technology has been applied most extensively to the study of genetic diseases. Two general strategies, illustrated in Figure 5–1, have been utilized. The classic approach is useful for diseases such as phenylketonuria (PKU), hemoglobinopathies, and several inborn errors of metabolism. In these disorders the identity of the affected protein and its functions are known. A variety of methods permit researchers to isolate the relevant normal gene, clone it, and determine the molecular changes that affect the gene in patients with the disorder. For example, cloning of the hemoglobin gene led to the discovery that a single base substitution changes hemoglobin A to sickle hemoglobin and produces the concomitant changes in the physicochemical properties of hemoglobin, giving rise to sickle cell anemia.

- Much more exciting and widely applicable is the so-called reverse genetics, or new genetics. This approach does not depend on a knowledge of the biochemical abnormality or the nature of the defective gene product. Indeed, in many genetic disorders the identity of the mutant protein is not known. Reverse genetics therefore relies on the chromosomal localization of the affected gene. Once the region in which the gene maps has been localized within reasonably narrow limits (by techniques called chromosome walking or chromosome jumping), the next step is to clone several pieces of DNA from the relevant segment of the genome. Among several candidate genes thus isolated, the "culprit" can be

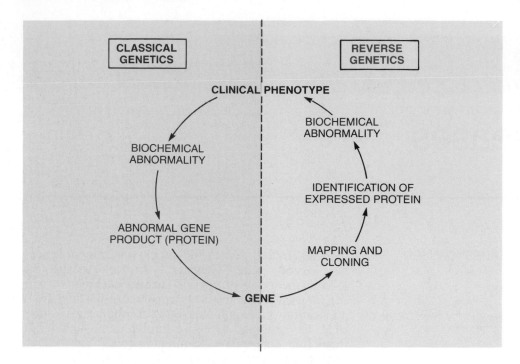

CLASSICAL GENETICS

REVERSE GENETICS

CLINICAL PHENOTYPE

BIOCHEMICAL ABNORMALITY

ABNORMAL GENE PRODUCT (PROTEIN)

GENE

BIOCHEMICAL ABNORMALITY

IDENTIFICATION OF EXPRESSED PROTEIN

MAPPING AND CLONING

Figure 5–1. A schematic illustration of the strategies employed in classic and reverse genetics. The classic approach begins with relating the clinical phenotype to biochemical-protein abnormalities, followed by isolating the mutant gene. The reverse genetic strategy begins by mapping and cloning the disease gene without any knowledge of the gene product. Identification of the gene product and the mechanism by which it produces the disease follows the isolation of the mutant gene.

identified by noting differences (mutations) between corresponding isolates from affected and unaffected individuals. Expression in vitro of the cloned DNA, followed by identification of the protein products, can then be utilized to pinpoint the aberrant protein encoded by the mutant gene. This approach has been used successfully with many diseases, including most recently the identification of the genes for cystic fibrosis (on chromosome 7) and neurofibromatosis (on chromosome 17).

Another powerful tool for studying the molecular pathogenesis of human diseases—both genetic and acquired—was created when it became possible to insert molecularly cloned human DNA into the germ line of mice. The technique of producing such *transgenic mice* involves microinjection of a cloned gene into the pronucleus of the fertilized mouse egg, followed by implantation of the zygotes into the oviducts of pseudopregnant female mice. Using appropriate gene constructs it is possible to target the expression of the introduced gene in specific tissues such as the beta cells of the pancreatic islets. Transgenic mice are proving to be extremely useful in the study of diseases as diverse as viral hepatitis, diabetes mellitus, and neoplasia.

- *Production of human biologically active agents.* An array of ultrapure biologically active agents can now be produced in virtually unlimited quantities by inserting the requisite gene into bacteria or other suitable cells in tissue culture. Some examples of genetically engineered products already in clinical use include tissue plasminogen activator (tPA) for the treatment of thrombotic states, growth hormone for the treatment of deficiency states, erythropoietin to reverse the anemia of renal disease, and myeloid growth and differentiation factors (GM-CSF, G-CSF) to enhance production of monocytes and neutrophils in states of poor marrow function.

- *Gene therapy.* The goal of treating genetic diseases by transfer of somatic cells transfected with the normal gene, although not yet attained, is tantalizingly close. Most interest is focused on transplantation of patients' hematopoietic stem cells that have been transfected with the cloned normal gene. The first attempts at human gene therapy have been undertaken in patients with immunodeficiency resulting from a lack of the enzyme adenosine deaminase (ADA). It is expected that the expression of the transferred ADA gene in the marrow cells will restore enzyme levels in vivo, thereby reversing the state of immunoincompetence that characterizes ADA-deficient patients.

- *Disease diagnosis.* Molecular probes are proving to be extremely useful in the diagnosis of both genetic and nongenetic (e.g., infectious) diseases. The diagnostic applications of recombinant DNA technology are detailed at the end of this chapter.

With this background of new genetics we can turn to the traditional classification of human diseases into three categories: (1) those that are genetically determined, (2) those that are almost entirely environmentally determined, and (3) those to which both nature and nurture contribute. Advances in knowledge, however, have tended to blur these distinctions. At one time microbial infections were cited as examples of disorders arising wholly from environmental influences, but it is now clear that to some extent heredity conditions the immune response and the susceptibility to microbiologic infections. Despite these uncertainties, there is a large and ever-growing list of disorders referred to as genetic diseases, whose prevalence is not generally appreciated.

Surveys indicate that as many as 20% of the pediatric inpatients in university hospital populations suffer from disorders of genetic origin. These data describe only the tip of the iceberg. Chromosome aberrations have been identified in up to 50% of spontaneous abortuses during the first trimester. Only those mutations compatible with independent existence constitute the reservoir of genetic disease in the population at large. Many more abortuses must have had gene mutations.

It is beyond the scope of this book to review normal human genetics. It is necessary, however, to clarify several commonly used terms—*hereditary, familial,* and *congenital.* Hereditary disorders, by definition, are derived from one's parents, are transmitted in the gametes through the generations, and therefore are familial. The term congenital simply implies "present at birth." It should be noted that some congenital diseases are not genetic, as for example congenital syphilis. On the other hand, not all genetic diseases are congenital; patients with hereditary Huntington's chorea, for example, begin to express their condition only after the third or fourth decade of life.

Genetic disorders fall into three major categories: (1) *those related to mutant genes of large effect,* (2) *diseases with multifactorial (polygenic) inheritance,* and (3) *those arising from chromosomal aberrations.* The first category, sometimes referred to as "mendelian disorders," includes many relatively rare conditions such as the storage diseases and inborn errors of metabolism, all resulting from single-gene mutations of large effect. Most of these conditions are hereditary and familial. The second category includes some of the most common disorders of humans, such as hypertension and diabetes mellitus. Multifactorial or polygenic inheritance implies that both genetic and environmental influences condition the expression of a phenotypic characteristic or disease. The third category includes disorders that have been shown to be the consequence of numerical or structural abnormalities in the chromosomes.

Each of these three categories will now be discussed separately.

MENDELIAN DISORDERS (DISEASES CAUSED BY SINGLE-GENE DEFECTS)

Single-gene defects (mutations) follow the well-known mendelian patterns of inheritance. Thus, the conditions they produce are often called mendelian disorders. The number of known mendelian disorders has grown rapidly to more than 4000. Although individually each is rare, together they account for approximately 1% of all adult admissions to hospitals and about 6 to 8% of all pediatric hospital admissions. Table 5–1 lists some of the more common mendelian disorders and their prevalence. Many of these are discussed in this chapter; most of the remaining ones are described elsewhere in the text. First, however, we

TABLE 5–1. PREVALENCE OF SELECTED MONOGENIC DISORDERS AMONG LIVEBORN INFANTS*

Disorder	Estimated Prevalence
Autosomal Dominant	
Familial hypercholesterolemia	1 in 500
Polycystic kidney disease	1 in 1250
Huntington's disease	1 in 2500
Hereditary spherocytosis	1 in 5000
Marfan's syndrome	1 in 20,000
Autosomal Recessive	
Sickle cell anemia	1 in 625 (US blacks)
Cystic fibrosis	1 in 2000 (Caucasians)
Tay-Sachs disease	1 in 3000 (US Jews)
Phenylketonuria	1 in 12,000
Mucopolysaccharidoses (all types)	1 in 25,000
Glycogen storage diseases (all types)	1 in 50,000
Galactosemia	1 in 57,000
X-Linked	
Duchenne muscular dystrophy	1 in 7000
Hemophilia	1 in 10,000

* From Wyngaarden, J. B., and Smith, L. H., Jr.: Cecil Textbook of Medicine. 18th ed. Philadelphia, W. B. Saunders, 1988, p. 147.

will briefly review some general concepts of medical genetics.

Mutations involving single genes follow one of three patterns of inheritance: autosomal dominant, autosomal recessive, and X-linked. Although gene expression is usually described as dominant or recessive, it should be remembered that in some cases both alleles of a gene pair may be fully expressed in the heterozygote—a condition called *codominance.* Histocompatibility and blood group antigens are good examples of codominant inheritance as well as *polymorphism* (multiple allelic forms of a single gene).

A single-gene mutation may lead to many phenotypic effects *(pleiotropy)* and, conversely, mutations at several genetic loci may produce the same trait *(genetic heterogeneity).* For example, Marfan's syndrome, which results from a basic defect in connective tissue, is associated with widespread effects involving the skeleton, eye, and cardiovascular system, all of which stem from a common abnormality in connective tissues. On the other hand, profound childhood deafness, an apparently homogeneous clinical entity, can result from any of 16 different types of autosomal recessive mutations. Recognition of genetic heterogeneity not only is important in genetic counseling but also facilitates the understanding of the pathogenesis of common disorders such as diabetes mellitus (p. 569).

AUTOSOMAL DOMINANT CONDITIONS

Autosomal dominant disorders are manifested in the heterozygous state, so at least one parent of an index case is usually affected; both males and females are affected and both can transmit the condition. When an affected person marries an unaffected one, every child has one chance in two of having the disease. The following features also pertain to autosomal dominant diseases:

- With every autosomal dominant disorder, some patients do not have affected parents. Such patients owe their disorder to new mutations involving either the egg or the sperm from which they were derived. Their siblings are neither affected nor at increased risk of developing the disease. The proportion of patients who develop the disease as a result of a new mutation is related to the effect of the disease on reproductive capability. If a disease markedly reduces reproductive fitness, most cases would be expected to result from new mutations. Many new mutations seem to occur in germ cells of relatively older fathers. For example, in sporadic cases of Marfan's syndrome fathers of affected children are about seven years older than the average.

- Clinical features can be modified by reduced penetrance and variable expressivity. Some individuals inherit the mutant gene but are phenotypically normal. This is referred to as *reduced penetrance.* The factors that affect penetrance are not clearly understood, but this phenomenon is clearly important for genetic counseling because such phenotypically normal persons can transmit the disease and so belong to a skipped generation. In contrast to penetrance, if a trait is seen in all individuals carrying the mutant gene but is expressed differently among individuals, the phenomenon is called *variable expressivity.* For example, polydactyly may be expressed in toes or in fingers as one or more extra digits.

- In autosomal dominant disorders a 50% reduction in the normal gene product is associated with clinical symptoms. Since a 50% loss of enzyme activity can usually be compensated for, involved genes usually do not encode for enzyme proteins. Two major categories of nonenzyme proteins are usually affected in autosomal dominant disorders: (1) those involved in regulation of complex metabolic pathways, often subject to feedback control (examples are membrane receptors and transport proteins) and (2) key structural proteins such as collagen and cytoskeletal components of the red cell membrane (e.g., spectrin). The biochemical mechanisms by which a 50% reduction in the levels of such proteins results in an abnormal phenotype are not fully understood. In some cases, the product of the mutant gene may interfere with the function of residual normal protein. In transgenic mice, for example, even a 10% expression of a mutant collagen gene adversely affects the function of normal collagen.

- In many conditions the age of onset is delayed: symptoms and signs do not appear until adulthood (as in Huntington's disease).

Marfan's Syndrome

In this autosomal dominant disorder of connective tissues the basic biochemical abnormality remained mysterious for years. It was logical to suspect some defect in collagen or elastin, the two major structural elements of connective tissue; however, molecular studies failed to define either regulatory or structural defects involving the major fibrillar collagens. Although *fragmentation of elastic tissue is a common finding in Marfan's syndrome,* no primary abnormality of elastin molecules could be documented. In view of these disappointing results, attention focused on another component of the connective tissue: microfibrillar fibers. These serve as scaffolding for the deposition of elastin and are considered integral components of elastic elements. Both qualitative and quantitative defects in *fibrillin,* a glycoprotein component of the microfibrillar fibers, have been noted in Marfan's patients. Recent molecular studies firmly implicate fibrillin proteins as the primary culprit in Marfan's syndrome. One of the fibrillin genes (FBN1) and Marfan's locus have both been mapped to chromosome 15q21.1. Furthermore, mutations in the FBN1 gene have been found in patients with Marfan's syndrome.

Although connective tissue throughout the body is affected, the principal clinical manifestations relate to three systems—skeleton, eyes, and cardiovascular system.

Skeletal abnormalities are the most obvious feature of Marfan's syndrome. Patients have a slender, elongated habitus with abnormally long legs and arms; a high, arched palate; and hyperextensibility of joints. A variety of spinal deformities such as severe kyphoscoliosis may appear. The chest is classically deformed, presenting either pectus excavatum (deeply depressed sternum) or a pigeon-breast deformity. President Lincoln is thought to have had features suggestive of Marfan's syndrome. The most characteristic **ocular change** is bilateral dislocation or subluxation of the lens due to weakness of its suspensory ligaments. It should be noted that the ciliary zonules that support the lens are devoid of elastin and made up exclusively of microfibrillary fibers. Most serious, however, is the involvement of the **cardiovascular system.** Fragmentation of the elastic fibers in the tunica media of the aorta predisposes to aneurysmal dilatation and aortic dissection (p. 296). The cardiac valves, especially the mitral and tricuspid, may be excessively distensible and regurgitant **(floppy valve syndrome),** giving rise to congestive cardiac failure (p. 305). Death from aortic rupture may occur at any age. Although some patients with this disorder survive into the seventh and eighth decades, the average age at death is 30 to 40 years.

Familial Hypercholesterolemia

Familial hypercholesterolemia is perhaps the most common of all mendelian disorders; the frequency of heterozygotes is one in 500 in the general population. *It is caused by a mutation in the gene that specifies the receptor for low-density lipoprotein (LDL),* the form in which 70% of total plasma cholesterol is transported. As you know, cholesterol may be derived from the diet or from endogenous synthesis. Dietary triglycerides and cholesterol are incorporated into chylomicrons (containing apoproteins C-11, B-48, E) in the intestinal mucosa, which drain via the gut lymphatics into the blood. These chylomicrons are hydrolyzed by an endothelial lipoprotein lipase in the capillaries of muscle and fat. The chylomicron remnants, rich in cholesterol, are then delivered to the liver. Some of the cholesterol enters the metabolic pool (to be described), and some is excreted as free cholesterol or bile acids into the biliary tract. The endogenous synthesis of cholesterol and LDL begins in the liver (Fig. 5–2). The first step in the synthesis of LDL is the secretion of triglyceride-rich, very low-density lipoproteins (VLDL) by the liver into the blood. In the capillaries of adipose tissue and muscle the VLDL particle undergoes lipolysis and is converted to intermediate-density lipoprotein (IDL). As compared to VLDL, the triglyceride content of IDL is reduced and that of cholesteryl esters enriched, but it retains on its surface two of the three VLDL-associated apoproteins, B-100 and E. Further metabolism of IDL occurs along two pathways: most of the IDL particles are taken up by the liver through the LDL receptor described below; others are converted to cholesterol-rich LDL by a further loss of triglycerides and apoprotein E. Two thirds of the resultant LDL is metabolized by the LDL receptor pathway and the rest by an LDL receptor–independent pathway, to be described later. The LDL receptor binds to apoproteins B-100 and E and hence is involved in the transport of both LDL and IDL. Although the LDL receptors are widely distributed, approximately 75% are located on hepatocytes, so liver plays an extremely important role in LDL metabolism.

The first step in the receptor-mediated transport of LDL involves binding to the cell surface receptor, followed by endocytotic internalization (Fig. 5–3). Within the cell the endocytic vesicles fuse with the lysosomes, and the LDL molecule is enzymically degraded, resulting ultimately in the release of free cholesterol into the cytoplasm. The cholesterol not only is utilized by the cell for membrane synthesis but also takes part in intracellular cholesterol homeostasis by a sophisticated system of feedback control.

- It suppresses cholesterol synthesis by inhibiting the activity of the enzyme 3-hydroxy-3-methylglutaryl (3HMG) coenzyme A reductase, which is the rate-limiting enzyme in the synthetic pathway.
- It activates the enzyme cholesterol acyltransferase, which favors esterification and storage of excess cholesterol.
- It down-regulates the synthesis of cell surface LDL receptors, thus protecting cells from excessive accumulation of cholesterol.

The transport of LDL that does not involve LDL receptors, alluded to earlier, appears to take place in cells of the mononuclear-phagocyte system, and possibly in other cells as well. Monocytes and macrophages have receptors for chemically modified (e.g., acetylated or oxidized) LDL. The amount catabolized by this "scavenger receptor" pathway is directly related to the plasma cholesterol level.

In familial hypercholesterolemia mutations in the LDL receptor gene impair the synthesis of critical membrane-related receptors and so impair intracellular transport and catabolism of the LDL, resulting in the accumulation of LDL cholesterol in the plasma. In addition, the absence of LDL receptors on the liver cells also impairs the transport of IDL into the liver, and hence a greater proportion of plasma IDL is converted into LDL. Thus patients with familial hypercholesterolemia develop excessive levels of serum cholesterol owing to the combined effects of reduced catabolism and excessive biosynthesis (see Fig. 5–2).

Familial hypercholesterolemia is an autosomal dominant disease. Heterozygotes have a two- to threefold elevation of plasma cholesterol levels, whereas homozygotes may have in excess of a fivefold elevation. Although their cholesterol levels are elevated from birth, heterozygotes remain asymptomatic until adult life, when they develop cholesterol deposits (xanthomas) along tendon sheaths and premature atherosclerosis resulting in coronary artery disease. Homozygous persons are much more severely affected, developing cutaneous xanthomas in childhood and often dying of myocardial infarction by age 15 years.

Analysis of the cloned LDL receptor gene has revealed that at least 16 different mutations can give rise to familial hypercholesterolemia. These can be grouped

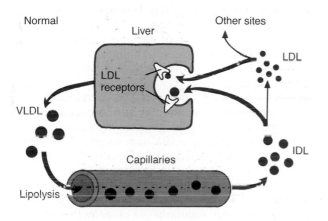

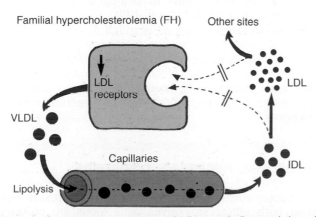

Figure 5–2. Schematic illustration of LDL metabolism and the role of the liver in its synthesis and catabolism, in normal persons and those with familial hypercholesterolemia (FH). (VLDL, very–low density lipoprotein; IDL, intermediate-density lipoprotein.)

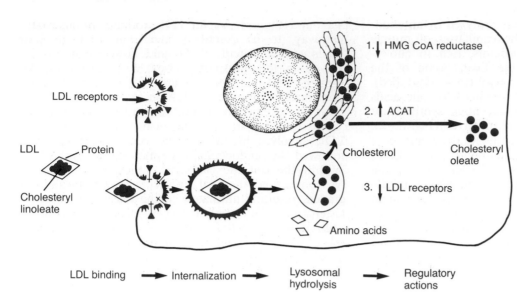

Figure 5-3. Sequential steps in the LDL pathway in cultured mammalian cells. (LDL, low-density lipoprotein; HMG CoA reductase, 3-hydroxy-3-methylglutaryl coenzyme A reductase; ACAT, acyl-CoA:cholesterol acyltransferase.) (From Goldstein, J. L., Brown, M. S.: The LDL receptor defect in familial hypercholesterolemia. Implications for pathogenesis and therapy. Med. Clin. North Am. *66*:335, 1982.)

in four categories. Class I mutations, the most prevalent form, are associated with loss of receptor synthesis; with class II mutations, the receptor protein is synthesized but its transport from endoplasmic reticulum to Golgi is impaired; class III mutations produce receptors that are transported to the cell surface but fail to bind LDL normally; class IV mutations, the rarest of all, give rise to receptors that fail to internalize after binding to LDL.

It should be emphasized that familial hypercholesterolemia is only one of several forms of hyperlipoproteinemia, most of which are not genetically determined (p. 279).

Neurofibromatosis

Neurofibromatoses comprise at least two autosomal dominant disorders, affecting approximately 100,000 persons in the United States. They are referred to as neurofibromatosis-1 (previously known as *von Recklinghausen's disease*) and neurofibromatosis-2 (previously called bilateral *acoustic neurofibromatosis*). Although the occurrence of neurogenic tumors is common to both, the two entities are clinically and genetically distinct. *Neurofibromatosis-1,* which accounts for more than 90% of cases, has three major features. (1) *Multiple neurofibromas* develop, usually in the form of pedunculated nodules protruding from the skin. The neurofibromas are discrete, generally unencapsulated, soft nodules. In some cases, the tumors form large, multilobar, pendulous masses (plexiform neurofibromas). Although derived from Schwann cells, they contain a tangled array of all the elements found in peripheral nerves (i.e., Schwann cells, neurites, and fibroblasts). Similar tumors ranging from microscopic to monstrous masses may occur in every conceivable site (along nerve trunks, the cauda equina, cranial nerves, in the retroperitoneum, orbit, tongue, and gastrointestinal tract, for example). (2) Pigmented skin lesions known as *café au lait spots* sometimes overlie a

neurofibroma. Infrequently, patients with von Recklinghausen's disease have only the café au lait spots, an example of variable expressivity of a genetic defect. (3) Pigmented iris hamartomas, called *Lisch nodules,* do not present any clinical problem but are helpful in establishing the diagnosis.

In addition to being a disfiguring condition, neurofibromatosis may be extremely serious, either by virtue of the location of a lesion (e.g., within the spinal canal) or because one or more of the benign neurofibromas becomes transformed into a malignant neoplasm (in approximately 3% of patients). Usually the neurogenic sarcomas arise in the plexiform tumors attached to large nerve trunks of the neck or extremities. These patients also are at greater risk of developing other tumors, particularly optic gliomas, meningiomas, and pheochromocytomas. Skeletal lesions are also common and may manifest as scoliosis and erosive bone defects.

The genetic basis of neurofibromatosis is beginning to be unraveled. The affected gene has been mapped to chromosome 17, and it seems to encode a protein that acts as a negative regulator of a growth-stimulating pathway and thus seems to belong to the family of tumor suppressor genes (see p. 189).

Type 2 neurofibromatosis is much rarer than type 1. Although most patients have peripheral neurofibromas and café au lait spots, *the defining feature of this variant is the presence of bilateral acoustic neuromas.* The gene for type 2 neurofibromatosis has been mapped to chromosome 22, but its function remains unknown.

AUTOSOMAL RECESSIVE DISORDERS _____

Because autosomal recessive disorders result only when both alleles at a given gene locus are mutants, such disorders are characterized by the following features: (1) the trait does not usually affect the parents, but siblings may show the disease; (2) siblings have one chance in four of being affected (i.e., the recurrence risk is 25% for each birth); (3) if the mutant gene occurs with a low frequency in the population, there is a strong likelihood that the proband is the product of a consanguineous marriage. In contrast to those of autosomal dominant diseases, the following features generally apply to most autosomal recessive disorders.

- The expression of the defect tends to be more uniform than in autosomal dominant disorders.
- Complete penetrance is common.
- Onset is frequently early in life.
- Although new mutations for recessive disorders do occur, they are rarely detected clinically. Since the affected individual is an asymptomatic heterozygote, several generations may pass before the descendants of such a person mate with heterozygotes and produce affected offspring.
- In many cases enzyme proteins are affected by the mutation. In heterozygotes equal amounts of normal and defective enzyme are synthesized. Usually the natural "margin of safety" ensures that cells with half their usual complement of the enzyme function normally.

To illustrate possible mechanisms by which an enzyme deficiency may give rise to an autosomal recessive disorder, Figure 5–4 provides an example of an enzyme reaction in which the substrate is converted by intracellular enzymes through intermediates into an end product. In this example the final product exerts feedback control on enzyme 1. A minor pathway producing small quantities of M1 and M2 also exists. The biochemical consequences of an enzyme defect in such a reaction have two major implications: (1) Depending on the site of the block, *accumulation of the substrate* may be accompanied by build-up of one or both intermediates. Moreover, an increased concentration of intermediate 2 may stimulate the minor pathway and thus lead to an excess of M1 and M2. Under these conditions tissue injury may result if the precur-

sor, the intermediates, or the products of alternate minor pathways are toxic in high concentrations. For example, in galactosemia, the deficiency of galactose-1-phosphate uridyltransferase leads to accumulation of galactose and to consequent tissue damage. A deficiency of phenylalanine hydroxylase results in the accumulation of phenylalanine. Excessive accumulation of complex substrates within the lysosomes due to deficiency of degradative enzymes is responsible for a group of diseases generally referred to as *lysosomal storage diseases* (p. 94). (2) *The enzyme defect can lead to a metabolic block and a decreased amount of an end product* that may be necessary for normal function. For example, a deficiency of melanin may result from lack of tyrosinase, which is necessary for the biosynthesis of melanin from its precursor tyrosine. This results in the clinical condition called albinism, to be discussed later. If the end product is a feedback inhibitor of the enzymes involved in the early reactions (in Fig. 5–4 it is shown that P inhibits E1), the deficiency of the end product may permit overproduction of intermediates and their catabolic products, some of which may be injurious at high concentrations. A prime example of a disease with such an underlying mechanism is the Lesch-Nyhan syndrome (p. 100).

Enzyme deficiencies may act in other ways as well. For example, α-1-antitrypsin is a protease inhibitor whose chief function is to inactivate neutrophil elastase. In patients with α_1-antitrypsin deficiency, the elastic tissue in the walls of pulmonary alveoli falls prey to the unopposed destructive activity of neutrophil elastase, leading eventually to emphysema (p. 392).

With this background, we will discuss some of the more common autosomal recessive diseases. Many others in this category, including sickle cell disease and other hemoglobinopathies, thalassemias, and α_1-antitrypsin deficiency, are discussed elsewhere in this book.

Cystic Fibrosis

With an incidence of 1 in 2000 live births, cystic fibrosis (CF) is the most common lethal genetic disease that affects Caucasian populations. It is distinctly uncommon among Orientals and blacks. CF is associated with a widespread defect in the secretory process of all exocrine glands. Indeed, abnormally viscid mucus secretions that block the airways and the pancreatic ducts are responsible for the two most important clinical manifestations: *recurrent and chronic pulmonary infections,* and *pancreatic insufficiency.* In addition, although the exocrine sweat glands are structurally normal (and remain so throughout the course of this disease) *high levels of sweat sodium chloride is a consistent and characteristic biochemical abnormality in CF.*

Until recently, there was no unifying hypothesis that could explain both the production of abnormal mucus and the increased level of sweat sodium chloride in CF. However, recent electrophysiologic studies on sweat ducts and airway epithelium point conclusively to a fundamental defect in the transport of chloride

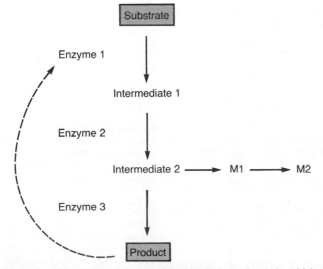

Figure 5–4. A scheme of a possible metabolic pathway in which a substrate is converted to an end product by a series of enzyme reactions. (M1, M2, products of a minor pathway.)

(Cl⁻) ions, and possibly other anions, across epithelia. The changes in mucus are now considered to be secondary to the disturbance in fluid and electrolyte transport.

Relative *impermeability* of epithelial cell membranes to Cl⁻ ions seems to be the primary defect in CF; however, the impact of this defect on transport functions is tissue specific. In the sweat ducts, for example, inability to reabsorb Cl⁻ (and concomitantly sodium [Na⁺]) leads to salty sweat. In the respiratory tract, on the other hand, the impaired transport of Cl⁻ ions across the epithelial cell membrane causes a series of secondary effects that lead to *increased* movement of sodium and water from the air space to blood, thereby lowering the water content of airway secretions. It remains unclear, however, whether the primary defect in the respiratory epithelium is a failure of Cl⁻ secretion into the airways or whether, as indicated in Figure 5-5, impaired reabsorption of Cl⁻ from the airways is paramount.

The molecular basis of the defect in Cl⁻ transport is not yet understood. The CF gene, mapped to chromosome 7, has been cloned, and its product is a membrane-associated protein that serves as a Cl⁻ channel. Approximately 70% of patients have a single mutation involving the deletion of three nucleotides that encode phenylalanine. Precisely how this change affects ion transport is under active investigation.

MORPHOLOGY. The anatomic changes in cystic fibrosis are highly variable and depend on the age at onset and severity of expression of this genetic disorder. **Pancre-** **atic abnormalities** are present in approximately 80% of patients. These may consist only of accumulations of mucus, leading to dilatation of ducts; in more advanced cases the ducts may become totally plugged, causing atrophy of the exocrine glands (Fig. 5-6); the islets of Langerhans are spared. The ducts may be converted into cysts separated only by islets of Langerhans and an abundant fibrous stroma, a picture that gives rise to the designation "fibrocystic disease of the pancreas." Loss of pancreatic secretion may lead to severe malabsorption, particularly of fats. A resultant lack of vitamin A, a fat-soluble vitamin, may then contribute to squamous metaplasia of the linings of the ducts. Changes similar to those in the pancreas may develop in the salivary glands. **Pulmonary lesions** are seen in almost every case and they are the most serious aspect of this disease. Retention of abnormally viscid mucin within the small airways leads to dilatation of bronchioles and bronchi with secondary infection, so that severe chronic bronchitis (p. 396), bronchiectasis (p. 397), and lung abscesses (p. 424) are frequent sequelae. *Staphylococcus aureus* and *Pseudomonas aeruginosa* are the two pathogens most commonly isolated in CF patients. For reasons not clear, the mucoid form of *P. aeruginosa*, rarely found in persons who do not have CF, is found in more than 50% of those who have the disease. The subtended pulmonary parenchyma may undergo emphysema (p. 392) or atelectasis (p. 386). Obstruction of the small bowel secondary to impacted viscid mucin (**meconium ileus**) is not an uncommon complication in newborns. In approximately 25% of patients, inspissation of mucin within the bile ducts impairs excretion of bile,

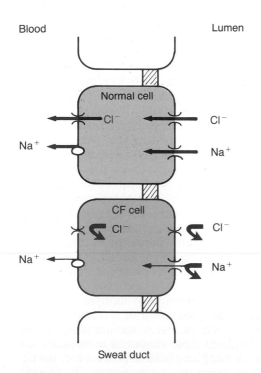

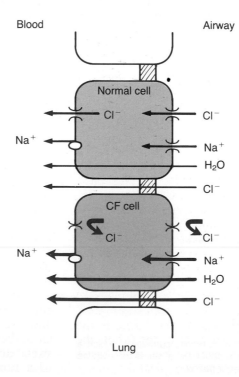

Figure 5-5. A schematic illustration of the transport of Cl⁻ and other electrolytes in normal cells and in cells of patients with cystic fibrosis. A fundamental defect in the transport of Cl⁻ ions leads to multiple effects. In the sweat duct there is decreased reabsorption of NaCl (*left*). In the airways, according to the one model (*right*), despite a decrease in Cl⁻ reabsorption across the apical membrane of CF cells, a net increase in NaCl (and water) absorption gives rise to dehydrated mucus. Note that the increased movement of Cl⁻ across the airway epithelium is not transcellular but paracellular. (Modified from Quinton, P. M.: Cystic fibrosis: A decrease in electrolyte transport. FASEB J. 4:2709, 1990.)

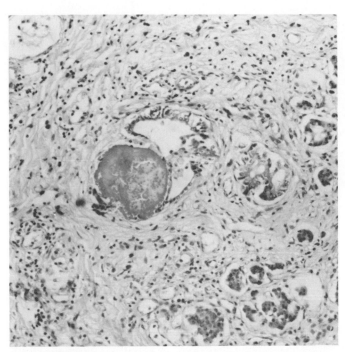

Figure 5–6. Cystic fibrosis of the pancreas. A dilated duct plugged with inspissated mucin is seen in center field. The atrophic acini are completely replaced by fibrous tissue that contains several surviving islets of Langerhans. (Courtesy of Dr. Dennis Burns, Department of Pathology, Southwestern Medical School, Dallas, TX.)

adding to the malabsorption problems. In time, **biliary cirrhosis** (p. 552) may develop, but in only about 2% of patients. The exocrine glands of the male reproductive tract are affected and in adults this often leads to sterility.

The clinical manifestations of this condition are extremely varied and range from mild to severe, from onset at birth to onset years later. Approximately 5 to 10% of the cases come to clinical attention at birth or soon after because of an attack of meconium ileus. More commonly, manifestations of malabsorption (e.g., large, foul stools, abdominal distention, and poor weight gain) appear during the first year of life. The faulty fat absorption may induce deficiency states of the fat-soluble vitamins, resulting in manifestations of avitaminosis A, D, or K. If the child survives these hazards, pulmonary problems such as chronic cough, persistent lung infections, obstructive pulmonary disease, and cor pulmonale may make their appearance. Persistent pulmonary infections are responsible for 80 to 90% of the deaths. With improved control of infections, more patients are now surviving to adulthood; median life expectancy is approximately 26 years.

The diagnosis of CF is based on clinical findings and the biochemical abnormalities in sweat. A properly administered and interpreted sweat test is crucial to the diagnosis. An increase in sweat electrolytes (often the mother makes the diagnosis because her baby tastes salty) along with one or more major clinical features is necessary for diagnosis. Until recently there has been no reliable test for detection of heterozygotes or for antenatal diagnosis; however, since the CF gene has been cloned and more than two thirds of the patients owe their disease to a single mutation, the detection of carriers with the most common mutation is now possible.

Phenylketonuria

There are several variants of this inborn error of metabolism. The most common form, referred to as classic PKU, is quite common in persons of Scandinavian descent and is distinctly uncommon in blacks and Jews.

Homozygotes with this autosomal recessive disorder classically have a severe lack of phenylalanine hydroxylase, leading to hyperphenylalaninemia and PKU. Affected babies are normal at birth but within a few weeks develop a rising plasma phenylalanine level, which in some way impairs brain development. Usually by six months of life severe mental retardation becomes all too evident; fewer than 4% of untreated phenylketonuric children have IQ values greater than 50 or 60. About one third of these unfortunate children are never able to walk, and two thirds cannot talk. Seizures, other neurologic abnormalities, decreased pigmentation of hair and skin, and eczema often accompany the mental retardation in untreated children. Hyperphenylalaninemia and the resultant mental retardation can be avoided by restriction of phenylalanine intake early in life. Hence a number of screening procedures are routinely used for detection of PKU in the immediate postnatal period.

Many clinically normal female PKU patients who were treated with diet early in life have now reached childbearing age. Most of them have discontinued dietary treatment and have marked hyperphenylalaninemia. Children born to such women are profoundly mentally retarded and have multiple congenital anomalies, even though the infants themselves are heterozygotes. This syndrome, termed *maternal PKU*, results from the teratogenic effects of phenylalanine that crosses the placenta and affects the developing fetus. Hence, *it is imperative that maternal phenylalanine levels be lowered by dietary means prior to conception.*

The biochemical abnormality in PKU is an inability to convert phenylalanine into tyrosine. In normal children, less than 50% of the dietary intake of phenylalanine is necessary for protein synthesis. The rest is converted to tyrosine by the phenylalanine hydroxylase system, which has several components in addition to the enzyme phenylalanine hydroxylase (Fig. 5–7). With a block in phenylalanine metabolism due to lack of phenylalanine hydroxylase, minor shunt pathways come into play, yielding phenylpyruvic acid, phenyllactic acid, phenylacetic acid, and o-hydroxyphenylacetic acid, which are excreted in large amounts in the urine in PKU. Some of these abnormal metabolites are excreted in the sweat, and phenylacetic acid in particular imparts a strong musty or mousy odor to affected

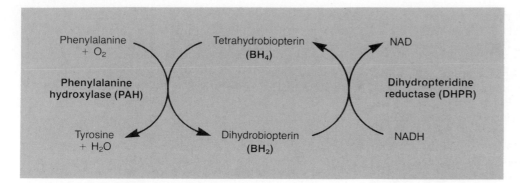

Figure 5-7. The phenylalanine hydroxylase system.

infants. It is believed that excess phenylalanine or its metabolites contribute to the brain damage in PKU.

At the molecular level, several mutant alleles of the phenylalanine hydroxylase gene have been identified. It seems that only those mutations that result in severe deficiency of the enzyme result in classic PKU. In those with a partial deficiency of phenylalanine hydroxylase, only modest elevations of phenylalanine levels occur without any neurologic damage. This condition, referred to as *benign hyperphenylalaninemia,* is important to recognize because the affected individuals may well test "positive" in the widely utilized Guthrie screening test but will not develop the stigmata of classic PKU. Measurement of serum phenylalanine levels is necessary to differentiate benign hyperphenylalaninemia and PKU.

As alluded to earlier, a number of variant forms of PKU have been identified. They account for 3 to 10% of all cases of PKU and result from deficiencies of enzymes other than phenylalanine hydroxylase. For instance, some patients lack dihydropteridine reductase (DHPR, Fig. 5-7). Like those with classic PKU, they are also unable to metabolize phenylalanine, but in addition they have associated abnormalities of tyrosine and tryptophan metabolism, since DHPR is required for hydroxylation of these two amino acids. The concomitant impairment of tyrosine and tryptophan hydroxylation leads to disturbance in the synthesis of

neurotransmitters, and neurologic damage is not arrested despite normalization of phenylalanine levels. *It is clinically important to recognize these variant forms of PKU because they cannot be treated by dietary control of phenylalanine levels.*

Galactosemia

Galactosemia is an autosomal recessive disorder of galactose metabolism. Normally, lactose, the major carbohydrate of mammalian milk, is split into glucose and galactose in the intestinal microvilli by lactase. Galactose is then converted to glucose in three steps (Fig. 5-8). *Two variants of galactosemia have been identified. In the more common variant there is a total lack of galactose-1-phosphate uridyl transferase, involved in reaction 2. The rare variant arises from a deficiency of galactokinase, involved in reaction 1.* Because galactokinase deficiency leads to a milder form of the disease not associated with mental retardation, it is not considered in our discussion. As a result of the transferase lack, galactose-1-phosphate accumulates in many locations, including liver, spleen, lens of the eye, kidney, heart muscle, cerebral cortex, and erythrocytes. Alternative metabolic pathways are activated, leading to the production of galactitol, which also accumulates in the tissues. Heterozygotes may have a mild defi-

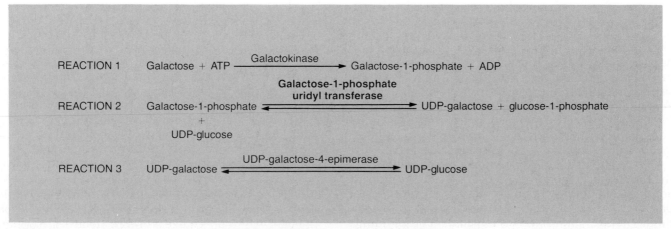

Figure 5-8. Pathways of galactose metabolism.

ciency but are spared the clinicomorphologic consequences of the homozygous state.

The liver, eyes, and brain bear the brunt of the damage. The early-to-develop *hepatomegaly* is due largely to fatty change, but in time widespread scarring that closely resembles the cirrhosis of alcohol abuse may supervene (p. 546). *Opacification of the lens (cataracts)* develops, probably because the lens absorbs water and swells as galactitol, produced by alternate metabolic pathways, accumulates and increases its tonicity. *Nonspecific alterations appear in the central nervous system,* including loss of nerve cells, gliosis, and edema, particularly in the dentate nuclei of the cerebellum and the olivary nuclei of the medulla. Similar changes may occur in the cerebral cortex and white matter.

There is still no clear understanding of the mechanism of injury to the liver and brain. Toxicity has been imputed to galactose-1-phosphate. Alternatively, galactitol has been indicted as the toxic product. It is also possible that the abnormal galactose metabolism interferes with the formation of galactose-containing cerebral lipids.

Almost from birth these infants *fail to thrive. Vomiting* and *diarrhea* appear within a few days of milk ingestion. *Jaundice and hepatomegaly* usually become evident during the first week of life and may seem to be a continuation of the physiologic jaundice of the newborn. The *cataracts* develop within a few weeks, and within the first 6 to 12 months of life, mental retardation may be detected. Even in untreated infants the mental deficit is usually not as severe as that of PKU. Accumulation of galactose and galactose-1-phosphate in the kidney impairs amino acid transport, resulting in aminoaciduria. There is an increased frequency of fulminant *Escherichia coli* septicemia.

Most of the clinical and morphologic changes can be prevented by early removal of galactose from the diet for at least the first two years of life. Control instituted soon after birth prevents the cataracts and liver damage and permits almost normal mental development. When galactosemia is recognized later, the changes in the lens and liver (if cirrhosis has not occurred) may be reversible, but the mental retardation is irreversible. The diagnosis can be suspected by the demonstration in the urine of a reducing sugar other than glucose, but tests that directly identify the deficiency of the transferase in leukocytes and erythrocytes are more reliable. Antenatal diagnosis is possible in cultured fibroblasts from amniotic fluid.

Albinism

Albinism need be mentioned only briefly, since, happily, it is not a serious clinical disorder. It is not a single entity, but rather a heterogeneous group of inherited disorders characterized by an inability to synthesize melanin. The major clinical manifestation is hypopigmentation of the skin, hair, and eyes *(oculocutaneous albinism)* or just the eyes *(ocular albinism).* Most variants of albinism are transmitted as autosomal recessive traits, but certain pedigrees suggest dominant transfer and others, X-linked transmission. In some genetic variants the absence of pigmentation results from a deficiency of tyrosinase. In others the precise defect is not known. Tyrosinase, you may recall, is involved in the conversion of tyrosine to 3,4-dopa, necessary for the synthesis of melanin. The lack of pigmentation of skin, hair, sclera, and iris is of consequence only insofar as it permits light to pour through the unpigmented iris and sclera, thus causing retinal injury, and the absence of melanin pigmentation of the skin makes these patients vulnerable to skin cancer (including malignant melanoma).

Glycogen Storage Disorders (Glycogenoses)

An inherited deficiency of any one of the enzymes involved in glycogen synthesis or degradation can result in excessive accumulation of glycogen or some abnormal form of glycogen in various tissues. The type of glycogen stored, its intracellular location, and the tissue distribution of the affected cells vary, depending on the specific enzyme deficiency. Regardless of the tissue or cells affected, the glycogen is most often stored within the cytoplasm, or sometimes within nuclei. One variant, Pompe's disease, is a form of *lysosomal storage disease* because the missing enzyme is localized to lysosomes. Most glycogenoses are inherited as autosomal recessive diseases, as is common with "missing enzyme" syndromes.

The biochemical consequences of individual enzyme deficiencies can best be appreciated in the context of normal glycogen metabolism. Hence a few comments on glycogen metabolism that are of particular relevance to the understanding of glycogen storage diseases are in order. Glycogen is a very large branched polysaccharide of glucose (molecular weight 250 to 100,000 Kd). A specific enzyme (amylo-1,4:1,6-transglucosidase) is necessary to initiate branching during synthesis. Conversely, during degradation the phosphorylases split glucose-1-phosphate from the branches until about four glucose residues remain on each branch, leaving a branched oligosaccharide called limit dextrin. This can be further degraded only by the debranching enzyme (amylo-1,6-glucosidase). In addition to traveling these major metabolic pathways, glycogen is also broken down in the lysosomes by acid maltase; if the lysosomes are deficient in this enzyme, the membrane-enclosed glycogen is not accessible to degradation by the cytoplasmic enzymes such as phosphorylases. Approximately a dozen forms of glycogenoses have been described on the basis of specific enzyme deficiencies. On the basis of pathophysiology they can be grouped into three categories:

- *Hepatic forms.* Liver contains several enzymes that synthesize glycogen for storage and also break it down into free glucose. Hence a deficiency of the hepatic enzymes involved in glycogen metabolism is associated with two major clinical effects: *enlargement of the liver due to storage of glycogen and hypoglycemia due to a failure of glucose production* (Fig. 5–9). Von Gierke's disease (type I glycogenosis), resulting from a lack of glucose-6-phosphatase,

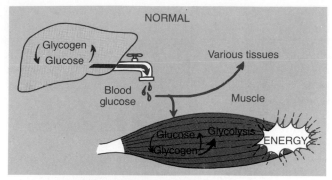

NORMAL

Glycogen
Glucose

Blood
glucose

Various tissues

Muscle

Glucose
Glycogen

Glycolysis

ENERGY

GLYCOGEN STORAGE DISEASE—HEPATIC TYPE

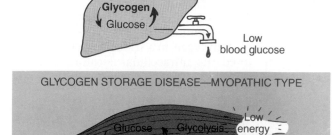

Glycogen
Glucose

Low
blood glucose

GLYCOGEN STORAGE DISEASE—MYOPATHIC TYPE

Glucose
Glycogen

Glycolysis

Low
energy
output

Figure 5–9. *Top,* A simplified scheme of normal glycogen metabolism in the liver and skeletal muscles. *Middle,* The effects of an inherited deficiency of hepatic enzymes involved in glycogen metabolism. *Bottom,* The consequences of a genetic deficiency in the enzymes that metabolize glycogen in skeletal muscles.

is the most important example of the hepatic form of glycogenoses (Table 5–2).

- *Myopathic forms.* In striated muscle, glycogen, derived by the glycolytic pathway, is an important source of energy. When enzymes that are involved in glycolysis are deficient, glycogen storage occurs in muscles and there is an associated muscle weakness due to impaired energy production. Typically, *the myopathic forms of glycogen storage diseases are marked by muscle cramps following exercise and failure of exercise to induce an elevation in blood lactate* levels owing to a block in glycolysis. McArdle's disease (type V glycogenosis), resulting from a deficiency of muscle phosphorylase, is the prototype of myopathic glycogenoses.

- Two other forms of glycogenosis do not fit into either of the two categories described above. Type II glycogenosis (Pompe's disease) is caused by a deficiency of lysosomal acid maltase, and so is associated with deposition of glycogen in virtually every organ, but cardiomegaly is most prominent. Brancher glycogenosis (type IV) is caused by deposition of an abnormal form of glycogen, with detrimental effects on the liver, heart, and muscles.

The principal subgroups of glycogen storage diseases are summarized in Table 5–2.

Lysosomal Storage Diseases

Lysosomes, as is well known, contain a variety of hydrolytic enzymes that are involved in the breakdown of complex substrates, such as sphingolipids and mu-

TABLE 5–2. PRINCIPAL SUBGROUPS OF GLYCOGENOSES

Clinicopathologic Category	Specific Type	Enzyme Deficiency	Morphologic Changes	Clinical Features
Hepatic type	Hepatorenal—von Gierke's disease (type I)	Glucose-6-phosphatase	Hepatomegaly—intracytoplasmic accumulations of glycogen and small amounts of lipid; intranuclear glycogen Renomegaly—intracytoplasmic accumulations of glycogen in cortical tubular epithelial cells	Failure to thrive, stunted growth, hepatomegaly, and renomegaly. Hypoglycemia due to failure of glucose mobilization, often leading to convulsions. Hyperlipidemia and hyperuricemia resulting from deranged glucose metabolism; many patients develop gout and skin xanthomas. Bleeding tendency due to platelet dysfunction. Mortality approximately 50%
Myopathic type	McArdle's syndrome (type V)	Muscle phosphorylase	Skeletal muscle only—accumulations of glycogen predominant in subsarcolemmal location	Painful cramps associated with strenuous exercise. Myoglobinuria occurs in 50% of cases. Onset in adulthood (>20 years). Muscular exercise fails to raise lactate level in venous blood. Compatible with normal longevity
Miscellaneous types	Generalized glycogenosis—Pompe's disease (type II)	Lysosomal glucosidase (acid maltase)	Mild hepatomegaly—ballooning of lysosomes with glycogen creating lacy cytoplasmic pattern Cardiomegaly—glycogen within sarcoplasm as well as membrane-bound Skeletal muscle—similar to heart (see Cardiomegaly)	Massive cardiomegaly, muscle hypotonia, and cardiorespiratory failure within two years. A milder adult form with only skeletal muscle involvement presents with chronic myopathy

copolysaccharides, into soluble end products. These large molecules may be derived from the turnover of intracellular organelles that enter the lysosomes by autophagocytosis, or they may be acquired from outside the cells by phagocytosis. With an inherited lack of a lysosomal enzyme, catabolism of its substrate remains incomplete, leading to the accumulation of the partially degraded insoluble metabolite within the lysosomes (Fig. 5–10). As might be expected, these missing-enzyme syndromes are inherited as autosomal recessive disorders, and the storage of insoluble intermediates occurs mainly in cells of the mononuclear phagocyte system, since they ingest and degrade senescent red cells, leukocytes, and other tissue breakdown products.

The numerous lysosomal storage diseases can be divided into broad categories based on the biochemical nature of the substrates and the accumulated metabolites (Table 5–3). Within each group are several entities, each resulting from the deficiency of a specific enzyme. Fortunately for both medical students and the potential victims of the diseases, most of these conditions are very rare, and their detailed description is better relegated to specialized texts and reviews. Only a few of the more common mucopolysaccharidoses (see Table 5–3) are considered here. Type 2 glycogen storage disease (Pompe's disease), also a lysosomal disorder, was discussed earlier.

GAUCHER'S DISEASE. There are three autosomal recessive variants of Gaucher's disease. Common to all three is variably *deficient activity of a glucocerebrosidase* that normally cleaves the glucose residue from ceramide. This leads to an accumulation of glucocerebrosides in the reticuloendothelial cells and the formation of so-called *Gaucher cells.* Normally, the glycolipids derived from the breakdown of blood cells, particularly erythrocytes, are sequentially degraded. In Gaucher's disease the degradation stops at the level of glucocerebrosides, which, in transit through the blood as macromolecules, are engulfed by the phagocytic

TABLE 5–3.
LYSOSOMAL STORAGE DISORDERS

Disease	Enzyme Deficiency	Major Accumulating Metabolite
Glycogenoses		
Type 2—Pompe's disease	Lysosomal glucosidase	Glycogen
Sphingolipidoses		
G_{M1}—gangliosidoses	G_{M1} ganglioside β-galactosidase	G_{M1} ganglioside, galactose-containing oligosaccharides
G_{M2}—gangliosidoses:		
Tay-Sachs disease	Hexosaminidase A	G_{M2} ganglioside
Gaucher's disease	Glucocerebrosidase	Glucocerebroside
Neimann-Pick disease	Sphingomyelinase	Sphingomyelin
Mucopolysaccharidoses		
MPS 1 H (Hurler)	α-L-iduronidase	Heparan sulfate Dermatan sulfate
MPS II (Hunter) (X-linked recessive)	L-iduronosulfate sulfatase	Heparan sulfate Dermatan sulfate
Glycoproteinoses	Enzymes involved in degradation of oligosaccharide side chains of glycoproteins (several)	Several, depending on specific enzyme

cells of the body, especially those in the liver, spleen, and bone marrow. *These phagocytes (Gaucher cells) become enlarged, sometimes up to 100 μm, because of the accumulation of distended lysosomes, and develop a pathognomonic cytoplasmic appearance characterized as "wrinkled tissue paper"* (Fig. 5–11). No distinct vacuolation is present.

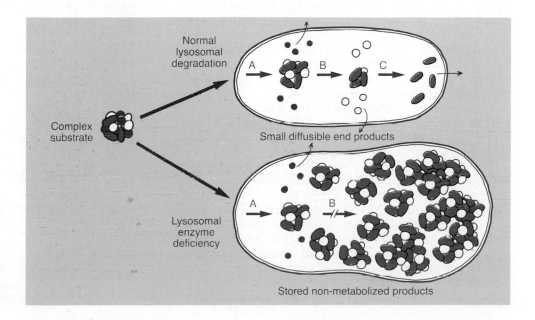

Figure 5–10. A schematic diagram illustrates the pathogenesis of lysosomal storage diseases. In the example illustrated, a complex substrate is normally degraded by a series of lysosomal enzymes (A, B, and C) into soluble end products. If there is a deficiency or malfunction of one of the enzymes (e.g., B), catabolism is incomplete and insoluble intermediates accumulate in the lysosomes.

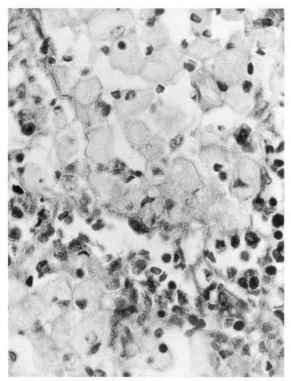

Figure 5–11. The spleen in Gaucher's disease. The large vacuo-lated cells have a ground-glass appearance and contain some faint wavy lines, creating some resemblance to wrinkled tissue paper.

One variant, *type I, also called the chronic nonneu-ronopathic form, accounts for 99% of cases of Gaucher's disease.* It is characterized by hepatospleno-megaly and the absence of central nervous system involvement. The spleen often enlarges massively, fill-ing the entire abdomen. Gaucher cells are found in the liver, spleen, lymph nodes, and bone marrow. Marrow replacement and cortical erosion may produce radio-graphically visible skeletal lesions as well as a reduc-tion in the formed elements of blood. Hypersplenism (p. 383) also contributes to the anemia and leuko-penia. Type I has a predilection for Ashkenazi Jews and, unlike other variants, is compatible with long life. The type II variant is highly lethal, affects children by six months of age, and is characterized by severe central nervous system involvement. Although liver and spleen are also involved, the clinical features are dominated by neurologic disturbances.

The type III (juvenile) variant involves the brain as well as viscera, but the course is intermediate between type I and II. The three variants result from distinct mutations that affect the glucocerebrosidase gene.

The level of glucocerebrosidase in leukocytes or cultured fibroblasts is helpful in diagnosis and in the detection of heterozygotes. Current therapy is aimed at enzyme replacement by infusion of purified glucocere-brosidase. On the horizon is somatic gene therapy involving infusion of autologous hematopoietic stem cells transfected with the normal glucocerebrosidase gene in vitro.

NIEMANN-PICK DISEASE. This designation refers to a group of disorders that are clinically, biochemically,

and genetically heterogeneous. The unifying feature of the Niemann-Pick group of diseases is the lysosomal accumulation of sphingomyelin and cholesterol. Bio-chemically, *two major groups can be distinguished:* patients with a deficiency of the sphingomyelin cleav-ing enzyme sphingomyelinase (types A and B), and others in which this enzyme activity is normal or nearly so (types C and D). In the latter types there is a primary defect in intracellular cholesterol esterification and transport, but the defective gene product has yet to be identified. All types are rare, so our remarks will be confined to the sphingomyelinase-deficient, type A variant, which accounts for 75 to 80% of all cases. With a deficiency of sphingomyelinase, the breakdown of sphingomyelin into ceramide and phosphorylcholine is impaired and excess sphingomyelin accumulates in all phagocytic cells and in the neurons. The phagocytic cells become stuffed with droplets or particles of the complex lipid, imparting a fine vacuolation or foami-ness to the cytoplasm (Fig. 5–12). Because of their high content of phagocytic cells, the organs most se-verely affected are the spleen, liver, bone marrow, lymph nodes, and lungs. As in Gaucher's disease, splenic enlargement may be striking. In addition, the entire central nervous system, including spinal cord and ganglia, is involved in this tragic, inexorable pro-cess. The affected neurons are enlarged and vacuolated owing to the storage of lipids. This variant manifests itself in infancy with massive visceromegaly and severe neurologic deterioration. Death usually occurs within the first five years of life. Estimation of sphingomye-

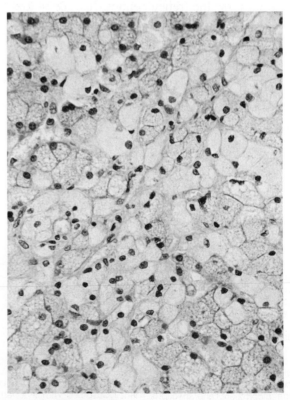

Figure 5–12. Niemann-Pick disease. The foamy vacuolation of the cells in the spleen results from accumulations of sphingomyelin.

linase activity in the leukocytes or cultured fibroblasts can be used for diagnosis of suspected cases as well as for detection of carriers. Antenatal diagnosis is possible by the use of cultured fibroblasts obtained by amniocentesis.

TAY-SACHS DISEASE OR G_{M2} GANGLIOSIDOSIS TYPE 1. Gangliosidoses are characterized by accumulation of gangliosides, principally in the brain, due to a deficiency of a catabolic lysosomal enzyme. Depending on the ganglioside involved, these disorders are subclassified into G_{M1} and G_{M2} categories. Tay-Sachs disease, by far the commonest of all gangliosidoses, is characterized by deficiency of the enzyme hexosaminidase A, which is necessary for the degradation of G_{M2}. The brain is principally affected, since it is most involved in ganglioside metabolism. *The storage of G_{M2} occurs within neurons, axon cylinders of nerves, and glial cells throughout the central nervous system.* Affected cells appear swollen, possibly foamy, and not dissimilar from those in Niemann-Pick disease. Electron microscopy reveals a whorled configuration within lysosomes (Fig. 5–13). These anatomic changes are found throughout the central nervous system (including the spinal cord), peripheral nerves, and autonomic nervous system. The retina is usually involved as well.

Like the other lipidoses, Tay-Sachs disease is most common among Ashkenazi Jews, among whom the frequency of heterozygous carriers is estimated to be one in 30. Heterozygotes can be reliably detected by estimating the level of hexosaminidase A in the serum. Antenatal diagnosis is possible, and the detection of Tay-Sachs disease in the fetus is generally viewed as an indication for therapeutic abortion. Infants who are born suffer from mental retardation, blindness, and severe neurologic dysfunctions, which lead to certain death within two or three years.

Mucopolysaccharidoses

Mucopolysaccharidoses (MPS) are characterized by defective degradation—and therefore storage—of mucopolysaccharides in various tissues. You may recall that mucopolysaccharides form a part of ground substance and are synthesized in the connective tissues by fibroblasts (p. 56). Most of the mucopolysaccharide is secreted into the ground substance, but a certain fraction is degraded within lysosomes. Several enzymes are involved in this catabolic pathway; it is the lack of these enzymes that leads to accumulation of mucopolysaccharides within the lysosomes. Several clinical variants of MPS, classified numerically from MPS I to MPS VII, have been described, each resulting from the deficiency of one specific enzyme. Within a given group (e.g., MPS I, characterized by a deficiency of α-L-iduronidase) subgroups exist that result from *different* mutant alleles at the same gene locus. Thus, the severity of enzyme deficiency and the clinical picture are often different, even within subgroups. *The mucopolysaccharides that accumulate within the tissues include dermatan sulfate, heparan sulfate, keratan sulfate, and, in some cases, chondroitin sulfate.*

In general, the MPSs are progressive disorders characterized by involvement of multiple organs, including liver, spleen, heart, and blood vessels. Most are associated with coarse facial features, clouding of the cornea, joint stiffness, and mental retardation. Urinary excretion of the accumulated mucopolysaccharides is often increased. All except one are inherited as autosomal recessive conditions; one variant, Hunter's syndrome, is an X-linked recessive disease. Of the seven recognized variants, only two well-characterized syndromes are discussed briefly here.

Hurler's syndrome, also called MPS I H, results from a deficiency of α-L-iduronidase. Affected children have a life expectancy of six to ten years. Like patients with most other forms of MPS, they develop coarse facial features associated with skeletal deformities, which creates an appearance referred to as gargoylism. Death is often due to cardiac complications resulting from the formation of raised endothelial and endocardial lesions by the deposition of mucopolysaccharides in the coronary arteries and heart valves. Accumulation of dermatan sulfate and heparan sulfate is seen in cells of the mononuclear phagocyte system, in fibroblasts, and within endothelium and smooth muscle cells of the vascular wall. The affected cells are swollen and have clear cytoplasm, resulting from the accumulation of PAS-positive material within engorged, vacuolated lysosomes. Lysosomal inclusions are also found in neurons, accounting for the mental retardation. Although most of the clinical features can be explained

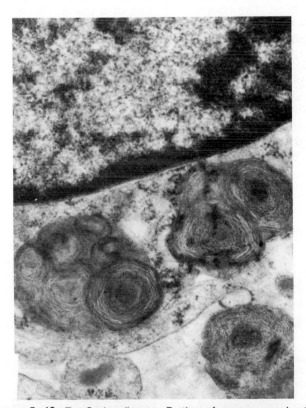

Figure 5–13. Tay-Sachs disease. Portion of a neuron under the electron microscope shows prominent lysosomes with whorled configurations. Part of the nucleus is shown above. (Courtesy of Dr. Joe Rutledge, Southwestern Medical School, Dallas, TX.)

on the basis of excessive storage of mucopolysaccharides, joint stiffness, for example, probably results from disturbances in collagen synthesis, which occur secondary to the derangement in the ground substance.

The other variant of MPS, called *Hunter's syndrome,* differs from Hurler's syndrome in its mode of inheritance (X-linked), the absence of corneal clouding, and often its milder clinical course. As in Hurler's syndrome, *the accumulated mucopolysaccharides in Hunter's syndrome are heparan- and dermatan sulfate, but this results from a deficiency of L-iduronate sulfatase.* Despite the difference in enzyme deficiency, an accumulation of identical substrates occurs because breakdown of heparan- and dermatan sulfate requires both L-iduronidase and the sulfatase; if either one is missing, further degradation is blocked.

X-LINKED DISORDERS

Sex-linked (better known as X-linked) disorders are transmitted by heterozygous female carriers virtually only to sons, who of course are *hemizygous* for the X chromosome. Heterozygous females rarely express the full phenotypic change, owing to the presence of the paired normal allele; however, because of the inactivation of one of the X chromosomes in females (discussed later) it is remotely possible for the normal allele to be inactivated in the vast majority of cells, permitting full expression of the disease in heterozygous females. An affected male does not transmit the disorder to sons, but all daughters are carriers. Sons of heterozygous women have, of course, one chance in two of receiving the mutant gene. To date, no Y-linked diseases are known. Save for determinants that dictate male differentiation, the only characteristic that may be located on the Y chromosome is the not altogether devastating attribute of hairy ears.

There are a very few X-linked dominant diseases. Their inheritance pattern is characterized by transmission of the disease to 50% of the sons and daughters of an affected heterozygous female. An affected male cannot transmit the disease to his sons, but all daughters are affected. One example of such a disease is vitamin D–resistant rickets.

X-linked recessive disorders are much less common than those arising from autosomal mutations. Some of the more important conditions having this mode of transmission are presented elsewhere: glucose-6-phosphate dehydrogenase deficiency (p. 341), hemophilia A and hemophilia B (p. 382), and agammaglobulinemia (p. 154). Some variants of inborn errors of metabolism have already been cited as being X-linked—for example, one form of MPS (Hunter's syndrome). Other X-linked disorders—such as Fabry's disease, Duchenne's and Becker's muscular dystrophies (p. 697), and nephrogenic diabetes insipidus—are too rare for inclusion here. Without regrets we can proceed, then, to the next category of genetic disease.

DISORDERS WITH MULTIFACTORIAL (POLYGENIC) INHERITANCE

Multifactorial (also called polygenic) inheritance is involved in many of the physiologic characteristics of humans (e.g., height, weight, blood pressure, hair color). *A multifactorial physiologic or pathologic trait may be defined as one governed by the additive effect of two or more genes of small effect but conditioned by environmental, nongenetic influences.* Even monozygous twins reared separately may achieve different heights because of nutritional or other environmental influences. When surveyed in a large population, phenotypic attributes governed by multifactorial inheritance fall on a continuous, Gaussian distribution (Fig. 5–14). Presumably there is some threshold effect, so that a disorder becomes manifest only when a certain number of effector genes as well as conditioning environmental influences are involved. The threshold effect also explains why parents of a child with a polygenic disorder may themselves be normal. Once the threshold value is exceeded, the severity of the disease is directly proportional to the number and the degree of influence of the pathologic genes.

Multifactorial disorders run in families because family members share many of their genes as well as environmental influences. The risk of a disorder's being expressed depends to a large extent on the relationship of the family member to the proband. However, all multifactorial disorders involve environmental influences, so risk factors are, at best, approximations. The concordance rate of a disease in monozygous twins is significantly less than 100% when multifactorial inheritance is involved. However, the chance of concordance in monozygous twins is much higher than that between first-degree relatives (siblings, parents, and offspring). For most multifactorial disorders, the first-degree relatives of the affected individual have a 5 to 10% risk of developing the disease. Since second-degree relatives (uncles, aunts) share only one fourth of their genes with the proband, their risk of developing the disease is only in the range of 0.5 to 1%.

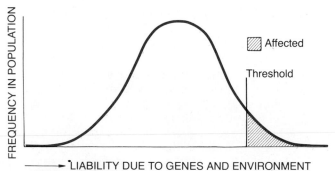

Figure 5–14. Multifactorial inheritance. The continuous distribution of the liability to develop a multifactorial disease is determined by many genes and the environment. A threshold of liability indicates the limit beyond which disease is expressed (From Elsas, L. J., Priest, J. H.: Medical genetics. *In* Sodeman, W. A., Sodeman, T. M. [eds.]: Pathologic Physiology: Mechanisms of Disease. 7th ed. Philadelphia, W. B. Saunders, 1985, p. 61.)

This form of inheritance is believed to underlie such common diseases as diabetes mellitus, hypertension, gout, schizophrenia, manic depression, and certain forms of congenital heart disease, as well as some skeletal abnormalities. Hypertension provides an excellent example of multifactorial inheritance. There is good evidence that the level of blood pressure of an individual, at least in some part, is under genetic control, apparently governed by multiple genes of small effect. The pressure levels of the population at large fall along a continuous Gaussian curve of distribution. At some arbitrary level of blood pressure, hypertension is said to exist, since pressures above this level are associated with a significant disadvantage to the individual. (Hypertension is described in Chapter 14.) Here we will discuss gout as a prototypic multifactorial metabolic disorder.

GOUT

Gout is a genetic or acquired disorder of uric acid metabolism that leads to hyperuricemia and consequent acute and chronic arthritis. The recurrent but transient attacks of acute arthritis are triggered by the precipitation into the joints of monosodium urate (MSU) crystals from supersaturated body fluids. Over a span of years, the progressive accumulation of urates and recurrent attacks of inflammation lead to chronic destructive arthritis. MSU crystals are deposited in and around the joints as well as other tissues, creating inflammatory foci known as *tophi*, the morphologic hallmark of gout. Whatever its pathophysiology, *the essential biochemical requirement for the development of clinical gout is hyperuricemia,* but a clear distinction should be made between hyperuricemia and gout. A plasma urate value above 7 mg/100 ml is considered elevated, since this exceeds the saturation value for urate in plasma. By this definition, 2 to 18% of the Western hemisphere's population have hyperuricemia, but the prevalence of gout ranges from 0.13 to 0.37%. Obviously, other factors that remain poorly understood must be involved in the transition of hyperuricemia into gout.

CLASSIFICATION AND PATHOPHYSIOLOGY. Gout is traditionally classified (Table 5–4) as *primary* when the basic metabolic defect is unknown or when the main manifestation of a known defect is hyperuricemia and gout. Because approximately 90% of all cases of gout fall into this category it will be the major focus of our discussion. *Secondary* gout refers to cases in which the hyperuricemia is secondary to some other acquired or genetic disorder. In these patients gout is not the main clinical disorder.

Elevation of the level of serum uric acid can be due to its overproduction or reduced excretion, or both. To understand the mechanisms underlying disturbances in uric acid production or excretion in gout a brief review of normal uric acid synthesis and excretion is warranted.

As is well known, uric acid is the end product of

TABLE 5–4. CLASSIFICATION OF GOUT

Clinical Category	Metabolic Defect
Primary Gout (90% of cases)	
Enzyme defects unknown (85 to 90% of primary gout)	1. Overproduction of uric acid a. Normal excretion (majority) b. Increased excretion (minority) 2. Underexcretion of uric acid with normal production
Known enzyme defects— e.g., partial HGPRT deficiency (rare)	Overproduction of uric acid
Secondary Gout (10% of cases)	
1. Associated with increased nucleic acid turnover —e.g., leukemias	Overproduction of uric acid with increased urinary excretion
2. Chronic renal disease	Reduced excretion of uric acid with normal production
3. Inborn errors of metabolism—e.g., complete HGPRT deficiency (Lesch-Nyhan syndrome)	Overproduction of uric acid with increased urinary excretion

purine metabolism. Increased synthesis of uric acid, a common feature of primary gout, results from some abnormality in the production of purine nucleotides. The synthesis of purine nucleotides occurs along two pathways, referred to as the de novo and salvage pathways (Fig. 5–15).

- The de novo pathway involves synthesis of purines and then uric acid from nonpurine precursors. The starting substrate for this pathway is ribose-5-phosphate, which is converted through a series of intermediates into purine nucleotides (inosinic acid, guanylic acid, and adenylic acid). This pathway is controlled by a complex array of regulatory mechanisms. Particularly important for our discussion are (1) the negative (feedback) regulation of the enzyme amidophosphoribosyl transferase (amido PRT) and PRPP synthetase by purine nucleotides, and (2) the allosteric activation of amido PRT by its substrate 5-phosphoribosyl-1-pyrophosphate (PRPP).

- The salvage pathway represents a mechanism by which free purine bases derived from catabolism of purine nucleotides, breakdown of nucleic acids, and dietary intake are utilized for the synthesis of purine nucleotides. This occurs in a single-step reaction whereby free purine bases (hypoxanthine, guanine, and adenine) condense with PRPP to form the purine nucleotide precursors of uric acid (inosinic acid, guanylic acid, and adenylic acid, respectively). These reactions are catalyzed by two transferases: hypoxanthine guanine phosphoribosyl transferase (HGPRT) and adenine phosphoribosyl transferase (APRT).

Excretion of uric acid occurs principally through the kidney. Uric acid is freely filtered across the glomeru-

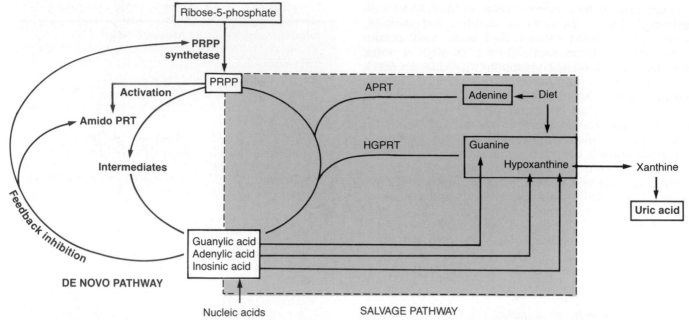

Figure 5–15. Purine biosynthesis and catabolism. The shaded area on the right represents the salvage pathway of purine synthesis. On the left is the de novo pathway.

lus, but 98 to 100% is reabsorbed in the early part of the proximal convoluted tubules. A proportion (~10%) is then secreted back into the tubule lumen by a more distal region of the tubule.

On the basis of uric acid synthesis and excretion, patients with primary gout can be divided into three subsets: (1) *a majority with overproduction and no increased urinary excretion,* (2) *a minority with overproduction and increased urinary excretion, and* (3) *a significant minority (30%) with no overproduction but a primary renal abnormality associated with underexcretion.* Although excessive purine biosynthesis occurs in over two thirds of those with gout, the precise metabolic defect that leads to excessive production can be identified in only a minority of cases. Nevertheless, these rare patients with known enzyme defects have provided valuable information on the regulation of purine biosynthesis and potential mechanisms of hyperuricemia. This is illustrated by patients with an inborn genetic deficiency of the enzyme HGPRT.

Complete lack of HGPRT gives rise to *Lesch-Nyhan syndrome.* This X-linked genetic condition, seen only in males, is characterized by the excretion of excessive amounts of uric acid, severe neurologic disease with mental retardation, and self-mutilation. Because there is an almost complete lack of HGPRT, the synthesis of purine nucleotides by the salvage pathway is blocked. This has two effects: an accumulation of PRPP, a key substrate for the de novo pathway, and increased activity of the enzyme amido PRT due to the dual effect of allosteric activation brought about by PRPP and reduced feedback inhibition due to reduction in purine nucleotides. Both of these conditions have the effect of augmenting purine biosynthesis (by the de novo pathway), resulting eventually in excess production of the end product, uric acid. It should be noted

that typical gouty arthritis is neither common nor a prominent clinical feature, and hence the Lesch-Nyhan syndrome is considered an example of secondary gout.

Less severe deficiencies of this enzyme ("partial" HGPRT deficiency, see Table 5–4) may occur, and these patients present clinically with severe gouty arthritis, beginning in adolescence, that is associated in some cases with mild neurologic disease.

Informative as these genetic disorders may be to the understanding of the pathways of purine metabolism, collectively they account for fewer than 15% of cases of overproduction of uric acid. In the vast majority of patients with primary gout, the cause of excessive uric acid synthesis is not known.

As in the case of primary gout, the hyperuricemia of *secondary gout* can result from overproduction or underexcretion of uric acid (see Table 5–4). Most cases of secondary gout associated with excessive production result from the increased breakdown of cells and nucleic acid turnover, such as occurs in myeloid metaplasia, chronic myeloid leukemia, polycythemia vera, and acute myelogenous and lymphocytic leukemias.

Reduced excretion of uric acid, such as occurs with chronic renal disease or following administration of drugs, may produce secondary gout. Particularly implicated among the drugs are thiazide diuretics, presumably owing to their effect on tubule transport of uric acid. In all cases of secondary gout, the metabolic pool of uric acid is increased and this condition may lead to disease that is indistinguishable from the primary idiopathic form.

INHERITANCE. It should be obvious from our discussion that primary gout is merely a common end point of a heterogeneous group of biochemical disorders. Given this, more than one mode of genetic transmission may be expected. The most common form of primary gout, which affects males predominantly, is believed to have a polygenic or multifactorial mode of inheritance. Environmental factors such as drugs, dietary levels of purines, and alcohol often act in concert with genetic factors. The male preponderance has been attributed to the fact that before menopause women normally have lower serum concentrations of urate. An autosomal dominant pattern of inheritance has also been reported in some families. In gout associated with HGPRT deficiency, transmission is X linked, as already described.

MORPHOLOGY. The distinctive morphologic as well as clinical features of gout are (1) acute arthritis, (2) chronic tophaceous arthritis, and (3) tophi in soft tissues.

The **acute arthritis** takes the form of an acute inflammatory synovitis made distinctive by the microcrystals of urates in the joint effusion. Although ultimately any joint in the body may be affected, in order of frequency, the following joints are involved: great toe (90% of patients), instep, ankle, heel, knee, and wrist.

The inflammatory response in the joints is initiated by the formation of MSU crystals within the synovial fluid, and possibly within the synovial membrane. MSU crystals directly or indirectly activate a remarkable number of cellular and humoral inflammatory mediators (Fig. 5–16). A partial listing follows:

- Neutrophils play an important role in acute gouty arthritis. Crystals themselves and other chemotactic influences (see Fig. 5–16) cause accumulation of neutrophils in the joint. Phagocytosis of crystals has consequences, including release of toxic free radicals, prostaglandins, and leukotrienes (LTB4), and, ultimately, lysosomal enzymes, brought about by the lysis of neutrophils.
- Interleukin 1 and tumor necrosis factor α produced by monocytes or synovial living cells are responsible for several local and systemic effects. They stimulate synovial cells and chondrocytes to release collagenases, cause fever, and are chemotactic to neutrophils.
- Hageman factor, activated by MSU crystals, leads to production of mediators such as kinins and complement fractions.

As a result of the inflammatory process, the synovial membranes are congested, swollen, and heavily infiltrated with neutrophils, macrophages, lymphocytes, and some plasma cells. When the episode of crystallization abates and the formed crystals are resolubilized, the acute attack remits.

Although the sequence of events as outlined is generally accepted, several questions remain unanswered. What initiates crystallization of urates in joint spaces? Why are certain peripheral joints preferentially involved? Why is there no correlation between the serum level of

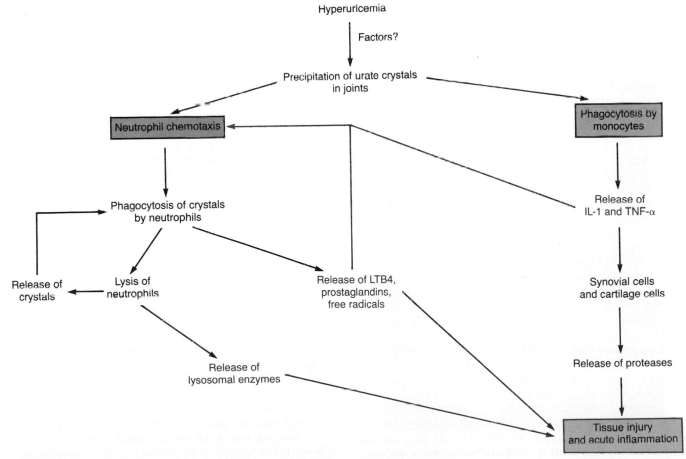

Figure 5–16. Pathogenesis of acute gouty arthritis.

uric acid and occurrence of gouty arthritis? The marked predilection of acute gout for peripheral joints may relate to their lower temperature, since solubility of urates is significantly reduced as the temperature is lowered. The normal temperature of the ankle joint is 29°C, whereas in the knee joint it is 33°C. Solubility of the urate crystals in the joint fluid is also affected by its content of proteoglycans, hyaluronic acid, and chondroitin sulfate. Alterations in the normal structure or concentration of various proteoglycans may therefore be an important factor in the pathogenesis of acute gouty arthritis. Such alterations may be genetic or acquired (for example, by repeated joint trauma).

Chronic arthritis evolves from the continued precipitation of urates in the recurrent attacks of acute arthritis. The urates produce heavy encrustations on the articular surface, and some deposits penetrate deep (Fig. 5–17). Large aggregations of urates are now formed within the subarticular bone or in the soft tissues about the joint. These deposits create the pathognomonic tissue lesion of gout, **the tophus. The tophus is a mass of crystalline or amorphous urates surrounded by an intense inflammatory reaction of macrophages, lymphocytes, and fibroblasts. Large foreign body–type giant cells, which are often wrapped around masses of precipitated salts, are very prominent** (Fig. 5–18). As tophi develop in joints, the articular cartilage and the underlying bone are eroded, and progressive destruction of the joint ensues, simulating the changes of advanced osteoarthritis. In-

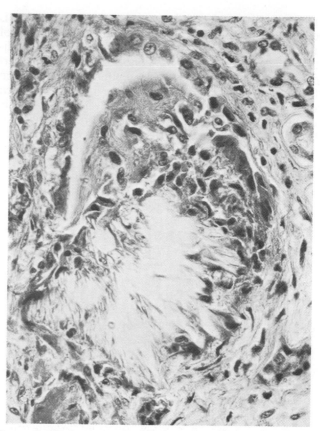

Figure 5–18. A tophus of gout. The deposit of urate crystals is surrounded by an inflammatory reaction of fibroblasts, occasional lymphocytes, and giant cells.

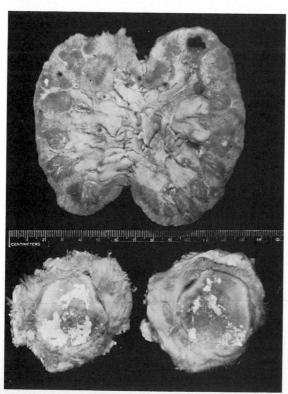

Figure 5–17. Urate deposits in gout. Several white urate deposits are seen within the pyramids of the opened kidney. Below, the white encrustations are seen on the articular surfaces of the patellae.

deed, secondary osteoarthritis often supervenes in gouty arthritis.

Tophi are also likely to develop in the periarticular ligaments, tendons, connective tissues, olecranon and patellar bursas, and the ear lobes. Less frequently they appear in the kidneys; skin of the fingertips, palms, or soles; nasal cartilages; aorta; myocardium; and aortic or mitral valves. Very rarely, tophi develop in the central nervous system, eyes, tongue, larynx, penis, and testes.

Urate crystals are water soluble, and nonaqueous fixatives such as absolute alcohol are necessary to preserve them in histologic sections. When preserved, they are demonstrable with routine or, more effectively, with silver staining techniques. The crystals are brilliantly anisotropic with polarized light microscopy.

Although the formation of tophi can be reasonably related to hyperuricemia, there exists a poorly understood association between cardiovascular disease, obesity, and gout. Without going into the perplexing plethora of details, we can state that (1) gouty and hyperuricemic patients tend to be at increased risk of hypertension and atherosclerosis and their attendant complications; (2) hyperuricemic patients tend to be heavier than controls; and (3) the association between hypertension and gout cannot be explained on the basis of coexisting obesity or impaired renal function. Hypertension and obesity thus appear to be independently associated with gout. Undoubtedly, hypertension contributes to the increased frequency of coronary artery disease seen in patients with gout.

Other than the joints, the **kidney** is the organ most commonly involved in gout. Three types of lesions directly related to gout may be seen. The most common is **urate nephropathy** resulting from the deposition of MSU crystals in the medullary interstitium, the pyramids, and papillae (see Fig. 5–17). In time, distinctive microtophi with a typical foreign body giant cell reaction are formed. Tophus formation in the cortex is rare. (2) Acute obstructive renal failure resulting from **intratubular deposition of free uric acid crystals** is a well-known complication in patients with myeloproliferative disorders. These cases of secondary gout are associated with severe hyperuricaciduria, especially at initiation of chemotherapy, when massive nucleic acid breakdown occurs. (3) **Uric acid stones** are formed, particularly in subjects who excrete more than 1100 mg of uric acid per day. In such cases the incidence of stones approaches 50%, and secondary complications of obstructive uropathy such as pyelonephritis are also increased. In addition to these lesions, nephrosclerosis due to the increased prevalence of hypertension may also appear. It should be pointed out that urate nephropathy, which is the commonest renal lesion, does not result in renal functional impairment per se. Rather, when functional impairment appears it is most closely correlated with hypertension (and nephrosclerosis), urinary obstruction, and aging.

CLINICAL CORRELATION. From the clinical standpoint, gout has many faces. It may disclose its presence by a severe attack of arthritis early in its course, but equally often it smolders as a subclinical disease. Three stages have been delineated. *Stage 1 is designated as hyperuricemic asymptomatic gout.* Silent hyperuricemia is present in 25 to 33% of relatives of patients with the overt disease. *Stage 2 is acute gouty arthritis,* characterized by flare-ups that may last a few days to weeks but are followed by complete remissions (intercritical periods) that last months to years. *Stage 3, chronic tophaceous gout,* is the likely sequel to years of recurrent acute arthritis. Persistent disabling joint disease may develop within a few years or only after many decades of acute attacks. Involvement of the kidney by one or more of the mechanisms cited above gives rise to proteinuria, passage of gravel, and azotemia. Indeed, about 20% of those with chronic gout die of renal failure.

Gout can be a satisfying disease to the physician because the correct diagnosis and appropriate therapy have much to offer the patient.

DISORDERS WITH VARIABLE MODES OF TRANSMISSION

Hereditary Malformations

Congenital malformations may be familial and genetic or may be acquired by exposure to teratogenic agents in utero. Hereditary malformations are associated with several modes of transmission. Certain common congenital malformations are multifactorial disorders, whereas others are transmitted by single mutant genes; still others are caused by chromosomal aberrations. Some of the multifactorial defects that have a frequency of one or more per 1000 births are listed in Table 5–5. These disorders run in families and present significant risks to blood relatives. As already discussed, the more genes an individual shares with the affected family member (proband), the greater is the probability that the individual will develop the malformation. Thus, first-degree relatives of an individual with a hereditary harelip have a 35 to 40 times greater chance of being similarly affected than do control populations; the risk for second-degree relatives is sevenfold, and for third-degree relatives, threefold. In some malformations of multifactorial origin, environmental influences that contribute to the expression of the disease can be identified. For example, in the infant with a genetic vulnerability to congenital hip dislocation, premature weight bearing or trauma may unmask the problem. The importance of recognizing these multifactorial traits lies, then, in the possibility of controlling environmental factors that contribute to the expression of the disorder. Other hereditary malformations are transmitted by single mutant genes. For the most part, these monogenic errors of morphogenesis take the form of localized lesions affecting a single organ or system (e.g., the fingers, eyes, or small intestine). Alterations associated with several abnormal karyotypes almost invariably are widespread malformations; the best examples are the autosomal trisomies (e.g., Down's syndrome), presented later in this chapter.

Detecting the underlying cause of congenital malformations is obviously necessary for genetic counseling, especially because some syndromes that closely resemble each other have different modes of transmission. It is also important to exclude nongenetic causes of congenital malformation, such as fetal exposure to teratogenic drugs and viruses.

Ehlers-Danlos Syndromes

Ehlers-Danlos syndromes (EDS) are characterized by defects in collagen synthesis and structure. As such they belong to the same general category as Marfan's

TABLE 5–5. MALFORMATIONS THAT OCCUR IN AT LEAST 1 IN 1000 BIRTHS*

Diagnosis	Incidence/1000 Births
Cleft lip (with or without cleft palate)	1.0
Congenital heart defects	6.0
Pyloric stenosis	3.0
Anencephaly	2.0
Spina bifida cystica	2.5
Congenital dislocation of the hip	1.0

* Modified from Carter, C. O.: Genetics of common single malformations. Br. Med. Bull. *32:*21, 1976.

syndrome but are discussed here because of variable modes of transmission of the different types. All of them are single-gene disorders, but the mode of inheritance encompasses all three of the mendelian patterns. This should not be surprising, since biosynthesis of collagen is a complex process that may be disturbed by genetic errors that affect the structural genes or the genes that code for the enzymes necessary for post-transcriptional events such as cross-linking of collagen fibers. Since abnormalities of collagen biosynthesis underlie all the variants of EDS, it is advisable to review collagen synthesis. It suffices to recall here that on the basis of chemical analyses, several distinct types of collagen have been found in humans. They have characteristic tissue distributions and are the products of different genes. To some extent the clinical heterogeneity of EDS can be explained on the basis of mutations in different collagen genes.

Ten clinical and genetic variants of EDS are recognized. Since defective collagen is present in all of the variants, certain clinical features are common to all.

As might be expected, tissues rich in collagen, such as skin, ligaments, and joints, are frequently involved in most variants of EDS. Because the abnormal collagen fibers lack adequate tensile strength, *skin is hyperextensible and joints are hypermobile.* These features permit grotesque contortions, such as bending the thumb backward to touch the forearm and bending the knee forward to create almost a right angle. Indeed, it is believed that most contortionists have one of the EDS; however, a predisposition to joint dislocation is one of the prices paid for this virtuosity. *The skin is extraordinarily stretchable, extremely fragile, and vulnerable to trauma.* Minor injuries produce gaping defects, and surgical repair or any surgical intervention is accomplished with great difficulty because of the lack of normal tensile strength. *The basic defect in connective tissue may lead to serious internal complications:* rupture of the colon and large arteries (EDS type IV), ocular fragility with rupture of cornea and retinal detachment (EDS type VI), and diaphragmatic herniae (EDS type I) among others.

The molecular bases of EDS are varied. They include the following:

- Deficiency of the enzyme lysyl hydroxylase. Decreased hydroxylation of lysyl residues in type I collagen interferes with the normal cross-links among collagen molecules.
- Deficient synthesis of type III collagen due to mutations in the pro-α_1 (III) gene.
- Defective conversion of procollagen type I to collagen, resulting from a mutation in the type I collagen gene.

CYTOGENETIC DISORDERS _____

Before we embark on the discussion of chromosomal aberrations it should be recalled that karyotyping is the basic tool of the cytogeneticist. A karyotype is the photographic representation of a stained metaphase spread in which the chromosomes are arranged in order of decreasing length. A variety of techniques for staining of chromosomes have been developed. With the widely used Giemsa stain (G-banding) technique, each chromosome set can be seen to possess a distinctive pattern of alternating light and dark bands of variable widths (Fig. 5–19). With recent improvements (high-resolution banding), as many as 2000 bands per karyotype can be recognized. The use of banding techniques allows certain identification of each chromosome, as well as precise localization of structural changes in the chromosomes, to be described later.

Chromosomal abnormalities are much more frequent than is generally appreciated. It is estimated that approximately 1 of 200 newborn infants has some form of chromosomal abnormality. The figure is much higher in fetuses that do not survive to term. It is estimated that in 50% of first-trimester abortions the fetus has a chromosomal abnormality. Cytogenetic disorders may result from alterations in the number or structure of chromosomes and may affect autosomes or sex chromosomes.

NUMERICAL ABNORMALITIES

In humans the normal chromosome count is 46 (i.e., $2n = 46$). Any exact multiple of the haploid number *(n)* is called euploid. Chromosome numbers such as $3n$ and $4n$ are called *polyploid.* Polyploidy generally results in a spontaneous abortion. Any number that is not an exact multiple of *n* is called *aneuploid.* The chief cause of aneuploidy is nondisjunction of a homologous pair of chromosomes at the first meiotic division or a failure of sister chromatids to separate during the second meiotic division. The latter may also occur during somatic cell division, leading to the production of two aneuploid cells. Failure of pairing of homologous chromosomes followed by random assortment (anaphase lag) can also lead to aneuploidy. When nondisjunction occurs at the time of meiosis, the gametes formed have either an extra chromosome $(n + 1)$ or one less chromosome $(n - 1)$. Fertilization of such gametes by normal gametes would result in two types of zygotes: trisomic, with an extra chromosome $(2n + 1)$, or monosomic $(2n - 1)$. *Monosomy involving an autosome is incompatible with life, whereas trisomies of certain autosomes and monosomy involving sex chromosomes are compatible with life.* These, as we shall see, are usually associated with variable degrees of phenotypic abnormalities. *Mosaicism* is a term used to describe the presence of two or more populations of cells in the same individual. In the context of chromosome numbers, postzygotic mitotic nondisjunction would result in the production of a trisomic and a monosomic daughter cell; the descendants of these cells would then produce a mosaic. As we shall discuss later, mosaicism affecting sex chromosomes is common, whereas autosomal mosaicism is not.

STRUCTURAL ABNORMALITIES

Structural changes in the chromosomes usually result from chromosome breakage followed by loss or rearrangement of material. Such changes are usually designated using a cytogenetic shorthand in which "p"

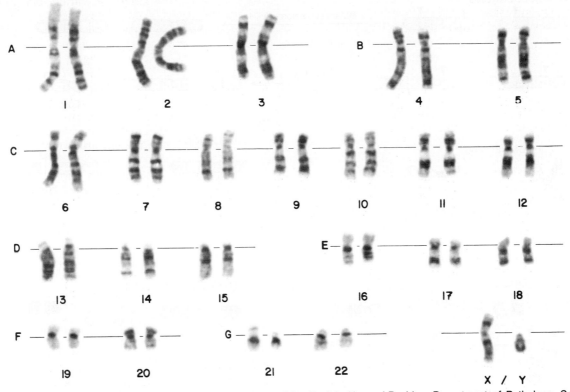

Figure 5-19. A normal male karyotype with G banding. (Courtesy of Dr. Patricia Howard-Peebles, Department of Pathology, Southwestern Medical School, Dallas, TX.)

(petit) denotes the short arm of a chromosome and "q" the long arm. Each arm is then divided into numbered regions (1, 2, 3, and so on) from centromere outward, and within each region the bands are numerically ordered (Fig. 5-20). Thus 2q34 indicates chromosome 2, long arm, region 3, band 4. Loss and gain of material is denoted by minus and plus sign, respec-

tively. The patterns of chromosomal rearrangement following breakage (diagrammed in Fig. 5-21) are as follows:

Translocation implies transfer of a part of one chromosome to another chromosome. The process is usually reciprocal (i.e., fragments are exchanged between two chromosomes). In genetic shorthand, transloca-

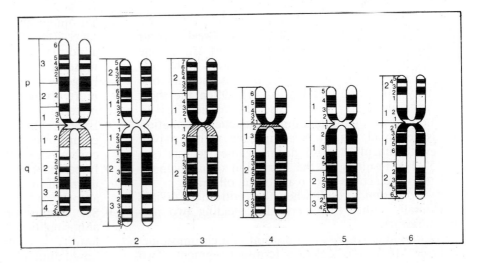

Figure 5-20. Diagrammatic representation of mid-metaphase chromosome bands to indicate nomenclature of arms, regions, and bands. (After Yunis, J. J., Chandler, M. S.: The chromosomes of man—Clinical and biologic significance. A review. Am. J. Pathol. *8*:466, 1977.)

☐ Negative or pale-staining G bands

■ Positive G bands

▨ Variable bands

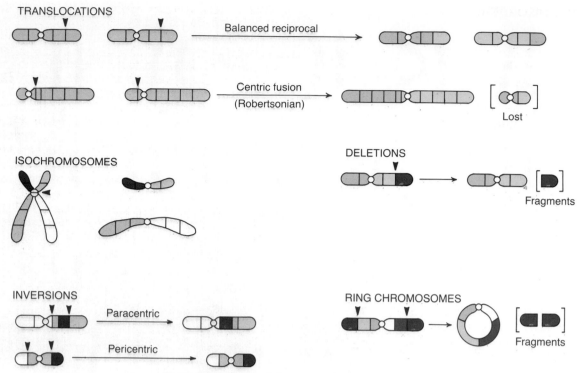

Figure 5–21. Types of chromosomal rearrangements.

tions are indicated by "t" followed by the involved chromosomes in numeric order, for example, t(14q;21q). When the entire broken fragments are exchanged, the resulting balanced reciprocal translocation (see Fig. 5–21) is not harmful to the carrier, who has the normal number of chromosomes and the full complement of genetic material. However, during gametogenesis, abnormal (unbalanced) gametes will be formed, resulting in abnormal zygotes. A special pattern of reciprocal translocation involving two acrocentric chromosomes is called *centric fusion type* or *Robertsonian translocation.* Typically the breaks occur close to the centromere, affecting the short arm in one and the long arm in the other. Transfer of the segments leads to one very large chromosome and one extremely small one (see Fig. 5–21). Often the short fragments are lost. In this case the carrier has 45 chromosomes, but the amount of genetic information lost is so small that it is compatible with survival. However, difficulties arise during gametogenesis (see Fig. 5–23), resulting in the formation of unbalanced gametes, which could lead to abnormal offspring.

Isochromosomes result when the centromere divides horizontally rather than vertically, yielding two new chromosomes.

Deletion involves loss of a portion of a chromosome. A single break may delete a terminal segment. Two interstitial breaks, with reunion of the proximal and distal segments, may result in loss of an intermediate segment. The isolated fragment, which lacks a centromere, almost never survives and thus many genes are lost.

Inversions occur when there are two interstitial breaks in a chromosome and the segment reunites after a complete turnaround.

A *ring chromosome* is a variant of a deletion. Following the loss of segments from each end of the chromosome, the arms unite to form a ring.

Against this background, we can turn first to some general features of chromosomal disorders, followed by some specific examples of diseases involving changes in the karyotype.

- Chromosomal disorders may be associated with absence (deletion, monosomy), excess (trisomy), or abnormal rearrangements (translocations) of chromosomes.
- In general, loss of chromosomal material produces more severe defects than does gain of chromosomal material.
- Excess chromosomal material may result from a complete chromosome (trisomy) or part of an extra chromosome (Robertsonian translocation).
- Imbalances of sex chromosomes (excess or loss) are tolerated much better than similar imbalances of autosomes.
- Sex chromosomal disorders often produce subtle abnormalities, sometimes not detected at birth. Infertility, a common manifestation, cannot be diagnosed until adolescence.
- In most cases chromosomal disorders result from de novo changes—i.e., parents are normal and risk of recurrence in siblings is low. An uncommon but important exception to this principle is exhibited by the translocation form of Down's syndrome.

AUTOSOMAL DISORDERS _____

Three autosomal trisomies (21, 18, and 13) and one deletion syndrome (cri du chat), which results from partial deletion of the short arm of chromosome 5, were the first chromosomal abnormalities identified. Within the past few years, several additional trisomies and deletion syndromes have been described. Most of these disorders are quite uncommon, and all are characterized by clinical features that should permit ready recognition. Some of the features of the three most common entities are presented in Figure 5–22.

Only trisomy 21 occurs with sufficient frequency to merit further consideration.

Down's Syndrome (Trisomy 21) _____

Down's syndrome is the most common of the chromosomal disorders. About 92 to 95% of affected persons have trisomy 21, so their chromosome count is 47. As mentioned earlier, the most common cause of trisomy, and therefore of Down's syndrome, is meiotic nondisjunction. The parents of such children have a normal karyotype and are normal in all respects. *Maternal age has a strong influence on the incidence of Down's syndrome.* It occurs once in 1550 live births in women younger than 20 years, in contrast to 1 in 25 live births for mothers older than 45 years. The correlation with maternal age suggests that in most cases the meiotic nondisjunction of chromosome 21 occurs in the ovum. Indeed in 80% of cases the extra chromosome is of maternal origin. The reason for the increased susceptibility of the ovum to nondisjunction may lie in the fact that all ova are present from birth and as such are vulnerable to potentially harmful environmental influences. The increasing incidence of nondisjunction with age may be related to cumulative exposure to such environmental influences. No effect of paternal age has been found in those cases where the extra chromosome is derived from the father.

In about 4% of all patients with Down's syndrome, the extra chromosomal material is present not as an extra chromosome but as a translocation of the long arm of chromosome 21 to chromosome 22 or 14. Such cases are usually familial, and the translocated chromosome is inherited from one of the parents, who is most frequently a carrier of a Robertsonian translocation. The consequences of the mating of a 14-21 translocation carrier (who may be phenotypically normal, with a chromosome count of 45) and a normal individual are depicted in Figure 5–23. Although theoretically the carrier has one chance in three of bearing a *live* child with Down's syndrome, the observed frequency of affected children in such cases is much lower. The reasons for this discrepancy are not well understood. Approximately 2% of Down's patients are mosaics, usually having a mixture of 46- and 47-chromosome cells. These result from mitotic nondisjunction of chromosome 21 during an early stage of embryogenesis. Symptoms in such cases are variable and milder, depending on the proportion of abnormal cells.

The clinical features of Down's syndrome are illustrated in Figure 5–23. The combination of epicanthic folds and flat facial profile accounted for the unfortunate earlier designation "Mongolian idiocy." Down's syndrome is a leading cause of mental retardation. The degree of mental retardation is severe: IQs vary from 25 to 80. Congenital malformations are common and quite disabling. Approximately 40 to 60% of patients with trisomy 21 are afflicted with cardiac malformations, which are responsible for most of the deaths in early childhood. Serious infections are another important cause of morbidity and mortality. As with most other clinical features, the basis of increased susceptibility to infection is not clearly understood. The chromosomal imbalance in some undefined manner also increases the risk of developing acute leukemias.

The overall prognosis for individuals with Down's syndrome has improved remarkably in the recent past, owing to better control of infections. Currently, it is estimated that approximately 80% of those without congenital heart disease can expect to survive 30 years. The outlook is less favorable for those with cardiac malformations. The majority of those who survive into middle age develop histologic, metabolic, and neurochemical changes of Alzheimer's disease (p. 726). Many develop frank dementia. The basis of this association is being actively investigated with the hope of finding clues to the pathogenesis of Alzheimer's disease.

SEX CHROMOSOME DISORDERS _____

A number of abnormal karyotypes involving the sex chromosomes, ranging from 45,X to 49,XXXXY, are compatible with life. Indeed, males who are phenotypically normal have been identified who have two and even three Y chromosomes. Such extreme karyotypic deviations are not encountered with the autosomes. In large part this latitude relates to two facts: (1) lyonization of X chromosomes and (2) the scant amount of genetic information carried by the Y chromosome. The consideration of lyonization must begin with the *Barr body,* or *sex chromatin,* a prominent clump of chromatin attached to the nuclear membrane in the interphase nuclei of all somatic cells of females. In 1962, Lyon proposed that *the X, or Barr, body represents one genetically inactivated X chromosome.* This inactivation occurs early in fetal life, about 16 days after conception, and randomly inactivates either the paternal or the maternal X chromosome in each of the primitive cells representing the developing zygote. Once inactivated, the same X chromosome remains genetically neutralized in all of the progeny of these cells. Moreover, it is now established that *all but one X chromosome is inactivated and so a 48,XXXX female has only one active X chromosome and three Barr bodies.* This phenomenon explains why normal females do not have a double dose (as compared with the male) of phenotypic attributes coded by the X chromosome. Lyon's hypothesis also explains why normal females are in reality mosaics, containing two cell populations—one with an active maternal X, the

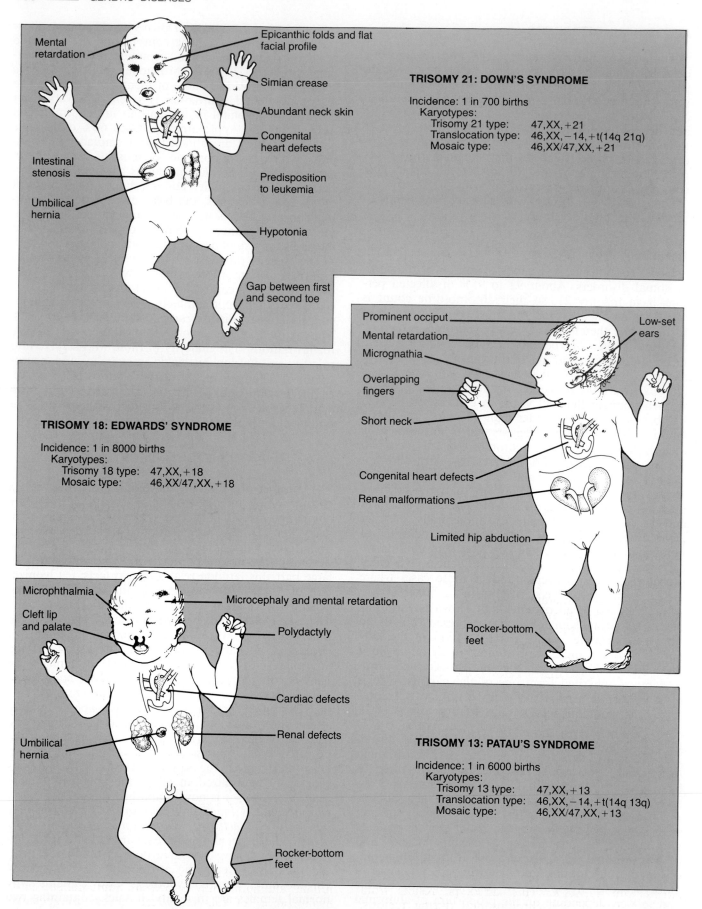

Mental retardation

Epicanthic folds and flat facial profile

Simian crease

Abundant neck skin

Congenital heart defects

Intestinal stenosis

Umbilical hernia

Predisposition to leukemia

Hypotonia

Gap between first and second toe

TRISOMY 21: DOWN'S SYNDROME

Incidence: 1 in 700 births
Karyotypes:
Trisomy 21 type: 47,XX,+21
Translocation type: 46,XX,−14,+t(14q 21q)
Mosaic type: 46,XX/47,XX,+21

Prominent occiput

Mental retardation

Micrognathia

Overlapping fingers

Short neck

Congenital heart defects

Renal malformations

Limited hip abduction

Low-set ears

Rocker-bottom feet

TRISOMY 18: EDWARDS' SYNDROME

Incidence: 1 in 8000 births
Karyotypes:
Trisomy 18 type: 47,XX,+18
Mosaic type: 46,XX/47,XX,+18

Microphthalmia

Cleft lip and palate

Umbilical hernia

Microcephaly and mental retardation

Polydactyly

Cardiac defects

Renal defects

Rocker-bottom feet

TRISOMY 13: PATAU'S SYNDROME

Incidence: 1 in 6000 births
Karyotypes:
Trisomy 13 type: 47,XX,+13
Translocation type: 46,XX,−14,+t(14q 13q)
Mosaic type: 46,XX/47,XX,+13

Figure 5–22. Clinical features and karyotypes of selected autosomal trisomies.

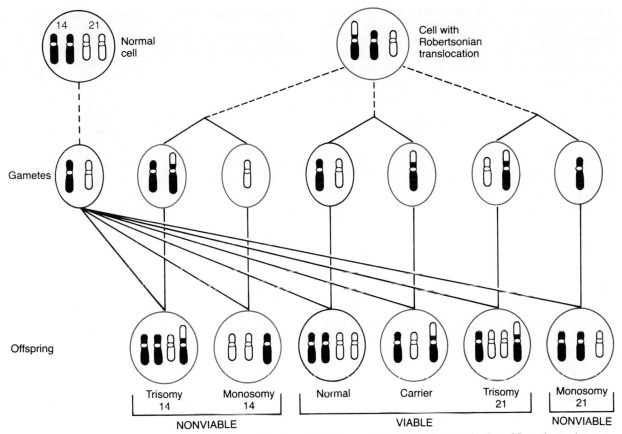

Figure 5-23. Consequences of Robertsonian translocation (14–21) on gametogenesis and production of Down's syndrome.

other with an active paternal X. This can be easily demonstrated if a female is heterozygous for an X-linked gene. For example, there are many alleles for the glucose-6-phosphate dehydrogenase (G6PD) gene, which code for G6PD isoenzymes. If a number of fibroblasts from such a woman are cloned, two different populations containing two distinctive forms of G6PD can be demonstrated.

Extra Y chromosomes are readily tolerated because the only information known to be carried on the Y chromosome appears to relate to male differentiation. It should be noted that whatever the number of X chromosomes, the presence of a Y invariably dictates the male phenotype. The Y body appears as a small, brightly fluorescent spot in interphase nuclei stained with fluorescent dyes and examined with the ultraviolet microscope. The genes for male differentiation are located on the short arm of the Y.

Three disorders arising in aberrations of sex chromosomes are described briefly.

Klinefelter's Syndrome

This syndrome is best defined as male hypogonadism that develops when there are at least two X chromosomes and one or more Y chromosomes. Most patients are 47,XXY. This karyotype results from nondisjunction of sex chromosomes during meiosis. The extra X chromosome may be of maternal or paternal origin. Advanced maternal age and a history of irradiation of either parent may contribute to the meiotic error resulting in this condition. Approximately 15% of patients show mosaic patterns, including 46,XY/47,XXY, 47,XXY/48,XXXY, and variations on this theme. The presence of a 46,XY line in mosaics is usually associated with a milder clinical condition.

Although the following description applies to most of the patients, it should be noted that Klinefelter's syndrome is associated with a wide range of clinical manifestations. In some it may be expressed only as *hypogonadism,* but most patients have a distinctive body habitus with *an increase in length between the soles and the pubic bone,* which creates the appearance of an elongated body. *Reduced facial and body hair* and *gynecomastia* are also frequently noted. The testes are markedly reduced in size, sometimes to only 2 cm in greatest dimension. Along with the *testicular atrophy,* the serum testosterone levels are lower than normal, and urinary gonadotropin levels are elevated.

The principal clinical effect of this syndrome is sterility. Only rare patients, presumably mosaics with a large proportion of 46,XY cells, are fertile. The sterility is due to impaired spermatogenesis, sometimes to the extent of total azoospermia. A variety of testicular tubular alterations may be present. Some patients have hyalinization of tubules, which appear as ghostlike structures in tissue section. Others have rare, apparently normal testicular tubules mixed with atrophic tubules that have virtually no spermatogenic germ cells, the so-called *tubule dysgenesis* pattern. Still others have very embryonic-looking tubules, as though development had been arrested in early fetal life. In all forms, Leydig cells are prominent, owing to either hyperplasia or an apparent increase related to loss of tubules. Although Klinefelter's syndrome may be associated with mental retardation, *the degree of intellectual impairment is typically mild, and in some cases undetectable.* The reduction in intelligence is correlated with the number of extra X chromosomes. Thus, in patients with the most common variant (XXY), intelligence is nearly normal, but in those with rare variant forms involving additional X chromosomes, significantly subnormal levels of intelligence as well as more severe physical abnormalities are found.

XYY Males

XYY karyotype results from nondisjunction at the second meiotic division during spermatogenesis. Most of these individuals are phenotypically normal, although they may be somewhat taller than usual, but they have been reported to display antisocial behavior. This remains a controversial issue and requires long-term prospective studies for resolution.

Turner's Syndrome

Turner's syndrome, characterized by primary hypogonadism in phenotypic females, results from partial or complete monosomy of the short arm of the X chromosome. In approximately 55% of the patients, the entire X chromosome is missing, resulting in a 45,X karyotype. These patients are the most severely affected, and the diagnosis can often be made at birth or early in childhood. Typical clinical features associated with 45,X Turner's syndrome include significant growth retardation leading to abnormally short stature (below third percentile); webbing of the neck; low posterior hairline; cubitus valgus (an increase in the carrying angle of the arms); shield-like chest with widely spaced nipples; high, arched palate; lymphedema of hands and feet; and a variety of congenital malformations such as horseshoe kidney and coarctation of the aorta (Fig. 5–24). Affected girls fail to develop normal secondary sex characteristics, the genitalia remain infantile, breast development is inadequate, and little pubic hair appears. Most have primary amenorrhea, and morphologic examination reveals transformation of the ovaries into white streaks of fibrous stroma devoid of follicles. Ovarian estrogen levels are low, and the loss of feedback inhibition leads to elevated levels of pituitary gonadotropin. In adult patients a combination of short stature and primary

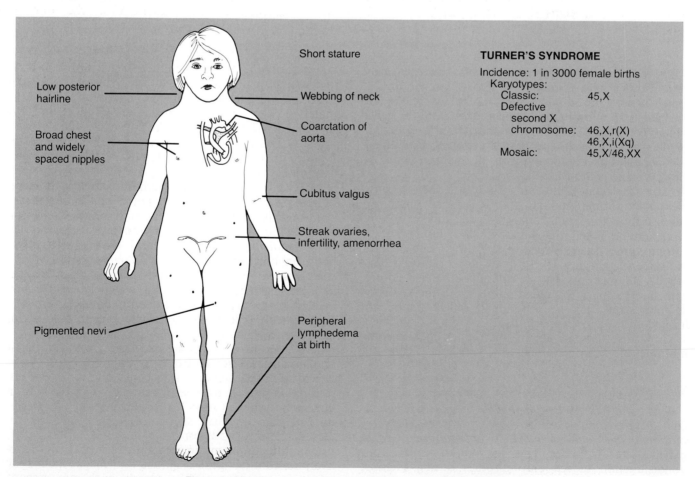

Figure 5–24. Clinical features and karyotypes of Turner's syndrome.

amenorrhea should prompt strong suspicion of Turner's syndrome. The diagnosis is established by karyotyping.

Approximately 45% of patients with Turner's syndrome are either mosaics (one of the cell lines being 45,X) or have deletions of the small arm of one X chromosome. Combinations of deletions and mosaicism are reported. It is important to appreciate the karyotypic heterogeneity associated with Turner's syndrome because it is responsible for significant variations in the phenotype. In contrast to the patients with monosomy X described above, those that are mosaics or deletion variants may have an almost normal appearance and may present only with primary amenorrhea.

It is pertinent to recall the Lyon' hypothesis in the context of Turner's syndrome. If only one active X chromosome were necessary for the development of normal females (as proposed in the Lyon hypothesis), patients with partial or complete loss of one X chromosome would not be expected to display the stigmata of Turner's syndrome. In view of this inconsistency and other observations, the Lyon hypothesis has recently been modified. It is now believed that although one X chromosome is inactivated in all cells during embryogenesis, it is selectively reactivated in germ cells prior to first meiotic division. Furthermore, it seems that certain X-chromosome genes remain active on both X chromosomes in many somatic cells of normal females. Thus it seems that two copies of some X-linked genes are essential for normal gametogenesis and female development.

Fragile X Syndrome

This syndrome is characterized by mental retardation and an inducible cytogenetic abnormality in the X chromosome (Fig. 5–25). The cytogenetic alteration is induced by certain culture conditions and is *seen as a*

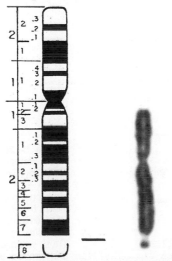

Figure 5–25. Fragile X, seen as discontinuity of staining. (Courtesy of Dr. Patricia Howard-Peebles, Southwestern Medical School, Dallas, TX.)

discontinuity of staining or constriction in the long arm of the X chromosome. Fragile X syndrome is one of the most common causes of familial mental retardation. It was originally believed to follow an X-linked pattern of inheritance; however several recent observations, such as the presence of mental retardation in 30% of carrier females and the absence of clinical features in approximately 20% of carrier males, suggest a much more complex mode of inheritance. Clinically affected males have moderate to severe mental retardation. Although a variety of physical abnormalities have been reported, they are inconstant and not readily apparent. *The only distinctive physical abnormality that can be detected in postpubertal males is macroorchidism* (enlargement of testes). Demonstration of the fragile X by karyotypic studies is essential for diagnosis.

MOLECULAR DIAGNOSIS OF GENETIC DISEASES

Traditionally the diagnosis of mendelian disorders has depended on the identification of abnormal gene products (e.g., mutant hemoglobin or enzymes) or their clinical effects such as anemia or mental retardation (e.g., PKU). Now it is possible to identify mutations at the level of DNA and offer gene diagnosis for several mendelian disorders. The use of recombinant DNA technology for the diagnosis of inherited diseases has several distinct advantages over other techniques:

- *It is remarkably sensitive.* The amount of DNA required for diagnosis by molecular hybridization techniques can be readily obtained from 100,000 cells. Furthermore, the use of the polymerase chain reaction (PCR) allows greater than 200,000-fold amplification of DNA or RNA, making it possible to utilize as few as 10 or 100 cells for analysis. Tiny amounts of whole blood or even dried blood can supply sufficient DNA for PCR amplification.
- *DNA-based tests are not dependent on a gene product* that may be produced only in certain specialized cells (e.g., brain) or expression of a gene that may occur late in life. Because all normal cells of the body contain the same DNA, each postzygotic cell carries the mutant gene in inherited genetic disorders.

These two features have profound implications for the prenatal diagnosis of genetic diseases because a sufficient number of cells can be obtained from a few milliliters of amniotic fluid or from a biopsy of chorionic villus that can be performed as early as the first trimester.

There are two distinct approaches to the diagnosis of single gene diseases by recombinant DNA technology: (1) direct detection of mutations and (2) indirect detection based on linkage of the disease gene with a harmless "marker gene." These two methods are described below.

DIRECT GENE DIAGNOSIS

Victor McKusick, an eminent geneticist, has appropriately called direct gene diagnosis the "diagnostic biopsy of the human genome." It depends on the detection of an important qualitative change in the DNA. There are two variations of the direct gene diagnosis.

One technique relies on the fact that some mutations alter or destroy certain restriction sites on the normal DNA. For example, in the normal β-globin gene (HbA) there are three sites that are specifically recognized by the restriction enzyme Mst II (Fig. 5–26). The sickle mutation responsible for sickle cell anemia (p. 336) involves a single base pair change (A → T) in the sixth codon of the β-globin chain. The enzyme Mst II recognizes and cleaves the normal sequence but not the altered sequence, hence the mutant (hemoglobin S) gene loses one of the three Mst II–cutting sites. When DNA from a normal individual is digested with Mst II and hybridized with the radioactive cDNA probe specific for the 5' end of the β-globin gene, a single 1.15-kb band that reacts with the probe is detected on Southern blot analysis (such a band results from the formation of identical 1.15-kb fragments from each of the two normal chromosomes). On the other hand, a similar analysis of DNA from the cells of a patient homozygous for the HbS gene leads to the formation of a single, larger (1.35-kb) fragment, owing to the loss of the Mst II sites from both chromosomes. In persons heterozygous for the sickle mutation, the normal chromosome yields a 1.15-kb band, whereas the chromosome carrying the mutation gives rise to the 1.35-kb band. Thus Southern blot analysis reveals two different-sized bands, allowing detection of a heterozygote carrier.

If the mutation does not alter any known restriction site, an alternative approach based on the use of *allele-specific oligonucleotides* can be utilized (Fig. 5–27). For example, many cases of α_1-antitrypsin (α_1-AT) deficiency are due to a single G → A change in the α_1-AT gene, producing the so-called Z allele (p. 394). Two oligonucleotides, having at their center the single base by which the normal and mutant gene differ, are synthesized. Such allele-specific oligonucleotides can then be used as radiolabeled probes in a Southern blot analysis. The oligonucleotide containing the sequence of the normal gene hybridizes with both the normal and the mutant DNA, but hybridization to the mutant DNA is unstable, owing to the single base pair mismatch. Thus, under stringent conditions of hybridization, the labeled normal probe produces a strong autoradiographic signal with DNA from a normal individual, no signal in the DNA extracted from a patient homozygous for the mutant gene, and a faint signal with DNA from a heterozygote. With the probe containing the mutant sequence the pattern of hybridization is reversed. Of course heterozygotes react with

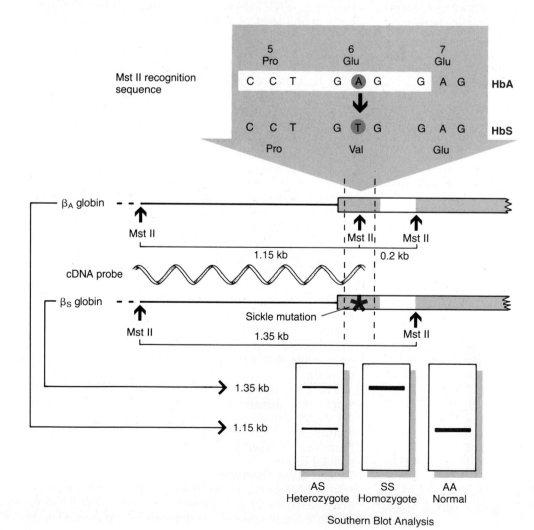

Figure 5–26. Direct gene diagnosis: detection of the sickle mutation by Southern blot analysis. An A → T substitution in the sixth codon of the β_A globin gene yields the β_S allele. This substitution eliminates an Mst II recognition site in the β globin DNA. Thus, when digested with Mst II and probed with an appropriate cDNA, the β_S allele generates a 1.35-kb fragment rather than the normal 1.15-kb fragment.

Figure 5–27. Direct gene diagnosis by using an oligonucleotide probe, and Southern blot analysis. *A,* A G→A change converts a normal α_1-antitrypsin allele (allele M) to a mutant Z allele. This change involves exon V of the α_1-antitrypsin gene, which lies between restriction sites for the enzymes Xba I and Hind III. *B,* The principle of oligonucleotide probe analysis. Two synthetic oligonucleotide probes, one corresponding in sequence to the normal allele (M allele probe) and the other corresponding to the mutant allele (Z allele probe), are lined up against normal and mutant genes, and the expected pattern of hybridization with different combinations is indicated on the right. *C,* The results of Southern blot analysis when DNA from normal individuals or those heterozygous or homozygous for the mutant Z allele is digested (with Xba I and Hind III) and probed with the normal (M) or Z oligonucleotide probe.

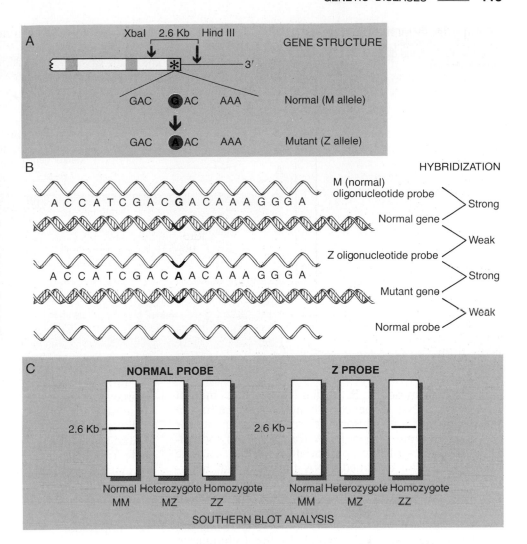

both probes because they carry one normal and one mutant gene.

LINKAGE ANALYSIS

Direct gene diagnosis is possible only if the mutant gene and its normal counterpart have been identified and cloned, and if their nucleotide sequences are known. In a large number of genetic diseases, including some that are relatively common, information about the gene sequence is lacking. Therefore, alternative strategies must be employed to track the mutant gene on the basis of its linkage to detectable genetic markers. In essence one has to determine whether a given fetus or family member has inherited the same relevant chromosomal region(s) as a previously affected family member. It follows, therefore, that the success of such a strategy depends on the ability to distinguish the chromosome that carries the mutation from its normal homologous counterpart. This is accomplished by exploiting naturally occurring variations in DNA sequences that give rise to the so-called *restriction fragment length polymorphisms* (RFLPs). Because RFLPs form the backbone of indirect DNA diagnosis, they will be discussed briefly.

Examination of DNA from any two persons will reveal variations in the DNA sequences involving approximately one nucleotide in every 200- to 500-base pair stretch. Most of these variations occur in noncoding regions of the DNA and are hence phenotypically silent; however, these single–base pair changes may abolish or create recognition sites for restriction enzymes, thereby altering the length of DNA fragments produced after digestion with certain restriction enzymes. Using appropriate DNA probes that hybridize with sequences in the vicinity of the polymorphic sites, it is possible to detect the DNA fragments of different lengths by Southern blot analysis. *To summarize, the term restriction fragment length polymorphism (RFLP) refers to variation in fragment length between individuals that results from DNA sequence polymorphisms.*

With this background we can discuss how RFLPs can be used in gene tracking. Figure 5–28 illustrates the principle of RFLP analysis. In this example of an autosomal recessive disease, both parents are heterozygote carriers and the children are normal, are carriers, or are affected. In the illustrated example, the normal chromosome (A) has two restriction sites (7.6-kb apart)

Figure 5-28. Schematic illustration of the principles underlying RFLP analysis in the diagnosis of genetic diseases.

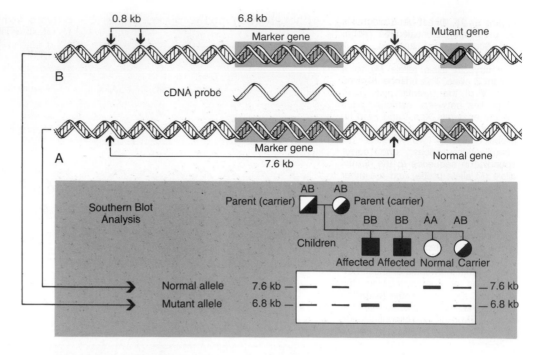

whereas chromosome B, which carries the mutant gene, has a DNA sequence polymorphism resulting in the creation of an additional (third) restriction site for the same enzyme. When DNA from such an individual is digested with the appropriate restriction enzyme and probed with a cloned DNA fragment that hybridizes with a stretch of sequences between the restriction sites, the normal chromosome yields a 7.6-kb band whereas the other chromosome produces a smaller, 6.8-kb, band. Thus, on Southern blot analysis two bands are noted. It is possible by this technique to distinguish family members who have inherited both normal chromosomes from those who are heterozygous or homozygous for the mutant gene.

To summarize, RFLP analysis makes it possible to track the transmission of a single chromosome region through a family and to see if a particular single-gene disease is co-inherited with a polymorphic site. It is therefore possible to utilize this method for antenatal diagnosis by examining fetal DNA. However, because the probe does not identify the disease gene itself, certain limitations become apparent:

- First, for prenatal diagnosis several relevant family members must be available for testing. A DNA sample from a previously affected child is necessary to determine the RFLP pattern that is associated with the homozygous genotype.
- Second, key family members must be heterozygous for an RFLP (i.e., the two homologous chromosomes must be distinguishable). This may require the use of multiple restriction enzymes and several different probes for closely linked genes.
- Third, normal exchange of chromosomal material between homologous chromosomes (recombination) during gametogenesis may lead to "separation" of the mutant gene from the polymorphism pattern with which it had been previously co-inherited. This

may lead to an erroneous genetic prediction in a subsequent pregnancy. Obviously, the closer the linkage, the smaller the likelihood of recombination and thus of a false result.

RFLPs have been useful in the antenatal diagnosis of cystic fibrosis, Huntington's disease, and adult polycystic kidney disease, among others. It is obvious that when a disease gene is identified and cloned (e.g., cystic fibrosis) direct gene diagnosis becomes the preferred method.

OTHER DIAGNOSTIC APPLICATIONS OF RECOMBINANT DNA TECHNIQUES _____

In principle, recombinant DNA techniques can be applied to any situation where detection of a genetic sequence is of diagnostic value. Consequently, DNA-based diagnosis is finding wide applications in many areas of medicine. Three are worthy of mention:

- *Diagnosis of infectious diseases:* Since every microbe has unique DNA or RNA sequences, molecular hybridization provides a powerful tool in the diagnosis of infectious diseases. Nucleic acid hybridization offers several advantages over other methods of diagnosis: (1) Unlike serologic techniques, hybridization is not dependent upon a host immune response, (2) organisms that grow slowly or poorly in culture can be readily detected, and (3) with PCR techniques, the size of sample needed is extremely small.
- *Diagnosis of neoplasms:* As will be discussed in Chapter 7, malignant transformation is associated with somatic mutations. In many instances, these mutations affect dominant oncogenes or recessive antioncogenes that can be readily detected by re-

combinant DNA technology. Although such methods are not widely utilized in the diagnosis of tumors, they are of significant supplemental value in the prognostication of certain tumors (e.g., neuroblastomas) and the diagnosis of some hematopoietic malignancies (e.g., chronic myeloid leukemia).

- *Determination of identity:* Since each human has a unique set of genes and associated DNA polymorphisms, it is possible to detect a distinctive pattern of expressed or silent genes in each person. Such genetic identification has obvious implications for forensic pathology. Specimens of hair, semen, and blood are being utilized to provide "molecular fingerprints" of considerable value in cases of rape, violent crime, and disputed paternity.

Bibliography

Abadi, R., Pascal, E.: The recognition and management of albinism. Opthalmol. Physiol. Opt. 9:3, 1989. (A detailed discussion of the several variants of albinism.)

Antonarakis, S. E.: Diagnosis of genetic disorders at the DNA level. N. Engl. J. Med. 320:153, 1989. (A very good overview of the clinical applications of recombinant DNA technology in the diagnosis of genetic diseases.)

Becker, M. A.: Clinical aspects of monosodium urate monohydrate crystal deposition disease (gout). Rheum. Dis. Clin. North Am. 14:377, 1988. (Discussion focuses primarily on the metabolic abnormalities in purine synthesis and excretion in gout.)

Bentler, E.: Gaucher's disease. N. Engl. J. Med. 325:1354, 1991. (A brief state-of-the-art overview of this rare condition.)

Cohen, P. R., Schneiderman, P.: Clinical manifestations of the Marfan syndrome. Int. J. Dermatol. 28:291, 1989. (A very good overview of Marfan's syndrome.)

Davis, P. B.: Cystic fibrosis from bench to bedside. New Engl. J. Med. 325:575, 1991. (A summary of the pathophysiology of cystic fibrosis and new therapeutic approaches.)

Eisenstein, B. I.: The polymerase chain reaction. A new method of using molecular genetics for medical diagnosis. N. Engl. J. Med. 322:178, 1990. (A brief and simple guide to PCR technology and its application.)

Elleder, M.: Niemann-Pick disease. Pathol. Res. Pract. 185:293, 1989. (A scholarly review that includes discussion of clinical features, histologic picture, and genetic variants.)

Grundy, S. M., Vega, G. L.: Causes of high blood cholesterol. Circulation 81:412, 1990. (A scholarly review of the metabolic aspects of familial and other forms of hypercholesterolemia.)

Martin, B. M., Sidransky, E., Ginns, E. I.: Gaucher's disease: Advances and challenges. Adv. Pediatr. 36:277, 1989. (An account of the clinical and molecular features of Gaucher's disease.)

McKusick, V. A.: The defect in Marfan syndrome. Nature 352:279, 1991. (An editorial summarizing data relating to the identification of Marfan gene product.)

Mulvihill, J. J. (moderator): NIH Conference Neurofibromatosis 1 (Recklinghausen's disease) and neurofibromatosis 2 (Bilateral acoustic neurofibromatosis). An update. Ann. Intern. Med. 113:39, 1990. (A detailed review of the genetics and clinical features of neurofibromatoses.)

Russell, D. W., Esser, V., Hobbs, H.: Molecular basis of familial hypercholesterolemia. Atherosclerosis 9(suppl.1):I-8, 1989. (A brief and up-to-date summary of the molecular pathology of FH.)

Scriver, C. R., Beaudet, A. L., Sly, W. S., Valle, D. (eds.): The Metabolic Basis of Inherited Disease. 6th ed. New York, McGraw Hill Information Services, 1989. (This two-volume text is a classic. It provides comprehensive accounts of the vast majority of genetic disorders.)

Terkeltaub, R. A., Ginsburg, M. H.: The inflammatory reaction to crystals. Rheum. Dis. Clin. North Am. 14:353, 1988. (A succinct discussion of the mechanisms and mediators of acute gouty arthritis.)

Woo, S. L. C.: Molecular basis and population genetics of phenylketonuria. Biochemistry 28:1, 1989. (A detailed account of the molecular defects in PKU.)

SIX

Disorders of the Immune System

CELLS OF THE IMMUNE SYSTEM
  T Lymphocytes
  B Lymphocytes
  Macrophages
  Dendritic and Langerhans' Cells
  Natural Killer Cells
CYTOKINES: MESSENGER MOLECULES OF THE IMMUNE SYSTEM
HISTOCOMPATIBILITY GENES (ANTIGENS)
  Significance of HLA Complex
IMMUNE MECHANISMS OF TISSUE INJURY
  Type I Hypersensitivity (Anaphylactic Type)
  Type II Antibody-Dependent Hypersensitivity
  Type III (Immune Complex–Mediated) Hypersensitivity
  Type IV (Cell-Mediated) Hypersensitivity
  Transplant Rejection
AUTOIMMUNE DISEASES
  Self-Tolerance
  Mechanisms of Autoimmune Disease
    Loss of Self-Tolerance
    Genetic Factors in Autoimmunity
    Microbial Agents in Autoimmunity
  Systemic Lupus Erythematosus
  Rheumatoid Arthritis
    Variants of Rheumatoid Arthritis
  Spondyloarthropathies
  Sjögren's Syndrome
  Systemic Sclerosis
  Polymyositis (Dermatomyositis)
IMMUNODEFICIENCY DISEASES
  Primary Immunodeficiency States
    X-Linked (Congenital) Agammaglobulinemia — Bruton's Disease
    Thymic Hypoplasia (DiGeorge's Syndrome)
    Severe Combined Immunodeficiency (Swiss-Type Agammaglobulinemia)
    Isolated Deficiency of IgA
    Common Variable Immunodeficiency

    Immunodeficiency with Thrombocytopenia and Eczema (Wiskott-Aldrich Syndrome)
  Secondary Immunodeficiencies
    Acquired Immunodeficiency Syndrome
AMYLOIDOSIS

The immune system is like the proverbial two-edged sword. On the one hand humans are dependent on the immune system for survival, and on the other hand they are vulnerable to disorders in its function ranging from immunodeficiency states to hypersensitivity disorders. Put more succinctly, the disorders range from those caused by "too little" to those caused by "too much or inappropriate" immunoreactivity. To encompass this spectrum, the various disorders of immune function are considered under the following headings:

- Immune mechanisms of tissue injury
- Autoimmune diseases
- Immunodeficiency diseases

We will also consider amyloidosis, a disease characterized by deposition of an abnormal protein (amyloid) in the tissues. Although not an immunologic disease in the traditional sense, it is clear that amyloidosis is associated with derangements of the immune apparatus.

Because abnormalities of lymphocyte functions are fundamental to immunologic disease, some recent advances in the understanding of lymphocyte biology are reviewed first and are followed by a brief description of the histocompatibility genes, because their products are relevant to both normal and abnormal immune responses.

CELLS OF THE IMMUNE SYSTEM

T LYMPHOCYTES

As is well known, T lymphocytes are the mediators of cellular immunity. T cells circulate in blood, where they comprise 60 to 70% of peripheral lymphocytes. *T lymphocytes are also found in the paracortical areas of lymph nodes and periarteriolar sheaths of the spleen.* Each T cell is genetically programmed to recognize a specific cell-bound antigen by means of an antigen-specific T-cell receptor (TCR). In approximately 95% of T cells, the TCR consists of a disulfide-linked heterodimer made up of an α and a β polypeptide chain (Fig. 6–1), each having a variable (antigen-binding) and a constant region. In a minority of peripheral blood T cells another type of TCR, composed of γ and δ polypeptide chains, is found. The TCRγ/δ cells tend to aggregate at epithelial interfaces such as the mucosa of the respiratory and gastrointestinal tracts. Both the α/β and γ/δ TCR are noncovalently linked to a cluster of five polypeptide chains referred to as the CD3 molecular complex. The CD3 proteins are nonvariable. They do not bind antigen but are involved in transduction of signals into the T cell after it has bound the antigen. T cell–receptor diversity is generated by somatic rearrangement of the genes that encode the α, β, γ, and δ TCR chains. As might be expected, every somatic cell has TCR genes from the germ line. During ontogeny, somatic rearrangements of these genes occur only in T cells; hence the *demonstration of TCR gene rearrangements by Southern blot analysis is a molecular marker of T-lineage cells.* Such analyses are utilized in classification of lymphoid malignancies (p. 361). Furthermore, because each T cell has a unique DNA rearrangement (and hence a unique TCR) it is possible to distinguish polyclonal (non-neoplastic) T-cell proliferations from monoclonal (neoplastic) T-cell proliferations.

In addition to CD3 proteins, T cells express a variety of other nonpolymorphic function–associated molecules, including CD4, CD8, and many so-called adhesion molecules such as CD2 and LFA-1 (CD11a). Of these, CD4 and CD8 are particularly important. They are expressed on two mutually exclusive subsets of T cells. CD4 is expressed on approximately 60% of mature CD3+ T cells, whereas CD8 is expressed on about 30% of T cells. Thus in normal healthy persons the CD4-CD8 ratio is about 2:1. Although initially discovered as markers of T-cell subsets, these T-cell membrane–associated glycoproteins are now known to play important roles in T-cell activation. During antigen presentation CD4 molecules on T cells bind to the nonpolymorphic portions of class II major histocompatability complex (MHC) molecules (p. 121) expressed on antigen-presenting cells. In contrast, CD8 molecules bind to class I MHC molecules during antigen presentation. Because of these properties, CD4+ helper/inducer T cells can recognize antigen only in the context of class II MHC antigens, whereas the CD8+ cytotoxic/suppressor T cells recognize cell bound antigens only in association with class I MHC antigens.

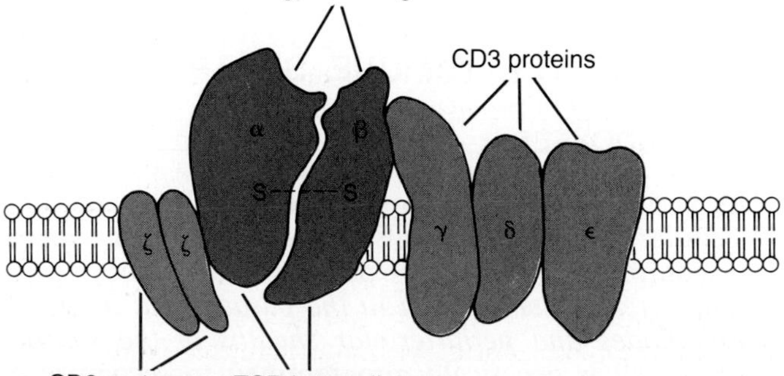

B LYMPHOCYTES

B lymphocytes constitute 10 to 20% of the circulating peripheral lymphocyte population. They are also present in bone marrow, peripheral lymphoid tissues such as lymph nodes, spleen, or tonsils, and in extra-lymphatic organs such as the gastrointestinal tract. In lymph nodes they are found in the superficial cortex. In the spleen they are found in the white pulp. At both sites they are aggregated in the form of lymphoid follicles, which upon activation develop pale-staining germinal centers.

Upon antigenic stimulation B cells form plasma cells that secrete immunoglobulins, which in turn are the mediators of humoral immunity. Of the five immunoglobulin isotypes, IgG, IgM, and IgA constitute 95% of serum immunoglobulins; IgE occurs in traces; and IgD occurs predominantly in a cell-bound form on the B-cell membrane. As is well known, monomeric IgM, present on the surface of all B cells, constitutes the antigen receptor on B cells. As with T cells, each B-cell receptor has a unique antigen specificity, derived in part from somatic rearrangements of immunoglobulin genes. *Thus the presence of rearranged immunoglobulin genes in a lymphoid cell is used as a molecular marker of B-lineage cells.* As with T cells, several nonpolymorphic molecules are expressed on B cells. These include CD19 and CD20, which are restricted to B cells and hence are of practical value in classification of lymphoid malignancies. The functions of these B cell–associated molecules are not yet clear.

MACROPHAGES

Macrophages are a part of the mononuclear phagocyte system and as such their role in inflammation was discussed in Chapter 2. Here we need only to emphasize that macrophages play several roles in the immune response.

- First, they are required to process and present antigen to immunocompetent T cells. The presence of class II MHC antigens (p. 121) on macrophages is considered critical for their antigen-presenting function. Since T cells (unlike B cells) cannot be triggered by free antigen, presentation of antigens by macrophages or other antigen-presenting cells (e.g., Langerhans' cells, discussed below) is obligatory for induction of cell-mediated immunity.
- They produce interleukin 1 (IL-1) and a whole array of soluble factors (monokines). Some of these, like IL-1, promote T- and B-cell differentiation; others

Figure 6–1. The T-cell receptor (TCR) complex. A schematic illustration of TCRα and TCRβ polypeptide chains linked to the CD3 molecular complex.

are proinflammatory (e.g., tumor necrosis factor-α [TNF α]). The functions of these soluble factors are discussed later.

- Macrophages lyse tumor cells by secreting toxic metabolites and proteolytic enzymes and as such may play a role in immunosurveillance.
- Macrophages are important effector cells in certain forms of cell-mediated immunity, such as the delayed hypersensitivity reaction.

DENDRITIC AND LANGERHANS' CELLS _____

Dendritic and Langerhans' cells comprise a population of cells that have dendritic cytoplasmic processes and large amounts of class II molecules on their cell surfaces. Dendritic cells are found in lymphoid tissues and Langerhans' cells occur in the epidermis. Both these cell types are extremely efficient in antigen presentation, and according to some they are the most important antigen-presenting (accessory) cells in the body. Unlike macrophages, they are poorly phagocytic, and hence they do not exhibit antimicrobial or scavenger cell activities.

NATURAL KILLER CELLS _____

Approximately 10 to 15% of the peripheral blood lymphocytes do not bear T-cell receptors or cell surface immunoglobulins. In the past these non-T, non-B cells were called "null cells." It is now recognized that these lymphocytes are endowed with an innate ability to lyse a variety of tumor cells, virally infected cells, and some normal cells, *without prior sensitization.* Hence they are called natural killer (NK) cells (Fig. 6-2). NK cells are believed to be a part of the "natural" (as opposed to adaptive) immune system that may be the first line of defense against neoplastic or virus-infected cells. Although they share some surface markers with T cells (e.g., CD2), NK cells do not rearrange T-cell receptor genes and are CD3⁻. Two cell surface molecules, CD16 and CD56, are widely utilized to identify NK cells. Of these, CD16 is of func-

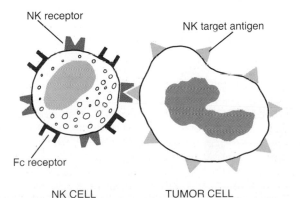

Figure 6-2. A schematic representation of the direct tumor cell killing by NK cells. Note that the Fc receptor of NK cells is not involved.

tional significance. It represents the Fc receptor for IgG and hence endows NK cells with another function — the ability to lyse IgG-coated target cells. This phenomenon, known as antibody-dependent cytotoxicity (ADCC), is described in greater detail later in this chapter (p. 126).

Morphologically, NK cells are somewhat larger than T and B lymphocytes, and unlike these two cell types, contain azurophilic cytoplasmic granules. Hence NK cells are sometimes referred to as large granular lymphocytes (LGLs).

CYTOKINES: MESSENGER MOLECULES OF THE IMMUNE SYSTEM _____

It is well known that the induction and regulation of the immune responses involve multiple interactions among lymphocytes, monocytes, inflammatory cells (e.g., neutrophils), and endothelial cells. Many such interactions are cognitive and so are dependent on cell-to-cell contact; however, in several instances cell interactions and effector functions are mediated by short-acting soluble mediators. Depending on the source, mediators are called *lymphokines* (lymphocyte-derived, such as the T cell–derived factor IL-2) or *monokines* (monocyte-derived, such as TNF-α). Because of an increasing awareness that many such factors have a wide spectrum of effects and that a given factor may be produced by several cell types, it is now customary to group these polypeptide mediators under the single rubric of *cytokines.*

We will not attempt to list the presently well-characterized and molecularly cloned cytokines, since any such list would soon be dwarfed by the torrent of new cytokines being isolated and reported every day by armies of toiling immunologists and cell biologists. Instead we will classify the presently known cytokines into four categories and then list some of their general properties.

- Cytokines that mediate natural immunity. Included in this group are IL-1, TNF-α, IL-6, type 1 interferons, and the IL-8 family. Certain of these cytokines (e.g., interferons) protect against viral infections, while others (e.g., IL-1, TNF-α, IL-8) initiate nonspecific inflammatory responses.
- Cytokines that regulate lymphocyte growth, activation, and differentiation. Within this category are IL-2, IL-4, and transforming growth factor–β (TGF-β). While IL-2 and IL-4 usually favor lymphocyte growth and differentiation, TGF-β is a powerful down-regulator of immune responses.
- Cytokines that activate inflammatory cells. In this category are γ interferon (IFN-γ), TNF-α, lymphotoxin (TNF-β), migration inhibitory factor, and IL-5. Most of these cytokines derived from T cells serve to activate the functions of nonspecific effector cells.
- Cytokines that stimulate hematopoiesis. Many cytokines generated during immune responses stimulate the growth and production of new blood cells by acting on hemopoietic progenitor cells. Several members of this family are called colony-stimulating

factors (CSFs) because they were initially detected by their ability to promote the growth of hemopoietic cell colonies from the bone marrow. Examples include granulocyte-macrophage (GM) CSF and granulocyte (G) CSF. IL-3 and IL-7, two other cytokines in this group, affect growth of lymphocyte progenitor cells.

It should be noted that this subdivision of cytokines into functional groups, although convenient, is somewhat arbitrary because, as will be noted below, cytokines such as IL-1 and TNF-α are pleotropic in their effects.

GENERAL PROPERTIES OF CYTOKINES

- Many individual cytokines are produced by several different cell types. For example IL-1 and TNF-α can be produced by virtually any cell.
- The effects of cytokines are pleiotropic: they act on many cell types. For example IL-2, initially discovered as a T-cell growth factor, is known to affect the growth and differentiation of B cells and of NK cells as well.
- Cytokines induce their effects in three ways: (1) they act on the same cell that produces them (*autocrine* effect), such as occurs when IL-2 produced by activated T cells promotes T-cell growth, (2) they affect other cells in their vicinity (*paracrine* effect), as occurs when IL-1 produced by antigen-presenting cells affects T cells during the induction of an immune response (p. 132), and (3) they affect many cells systemically (*endocrine* effect), the best examples in this category being IL-1 and TNF-α, which produce the acute-phase response during inflammation.
- Cytokines mediate their effects by binding to specific high-affinity receptors on their target cells. For example, IL-2 activates T cells by binding to high-affinity IL-2 receptors (IL-2R). Blockade of the IL-2R by monoclonal antibodies directed against the receptor prevents T-cell activation. This observation provides a means by which T-cell activation, when undesirable (as in transplant rejection), may be controlled.

The knowledge gained about cytokines is not merely of academic interest; it has practical therapeutic rami-

fications as well. First, by regulating cytokine production or action it may be possible to control the harmful effects of inflammation or tissue-damaging immune reactions. Second, cytokines produced by recombinant DNA technology can be administered to enhance immunity against cancer or microbial infections (immunotherapy). Both these avenues are currently being pursued on an experimental basis in humans.

HISTOCOMPATIBILITY GENES (ANTIGENS)

Although originally identified as antigens that evoke rejection of transplanted organs, histocompatibility molecules are now considered important in the regulation of the immune response as well as in resistance or susceptibility to a growing list of diseases. *The principal physiologic function of the cell surface histocompatibility molecules is to bind peptide fragments of foreign proteins for presentation to appropriate antigen-specific T cells.* Recall that T cells (unlike B cells) can recognize only membrane-bound antigens. The histocompatibility molecules and the corresponding genes are complex in structure and organization and are still incompletely understood. Here we summarize only the salient features of human histocompatibility antigens, primarily to facilitate understanding of their role in rejection of organ transplants and in disease susceptibility. Several genes code for histocompatibility antigens, but those that code for the most important transplantation antigens are clustered on a small segment of chromosome 6. This cluster constitutes the human major histocompatibility complex and is also known as the HLA complex (Fig. 6–3). It is equivalent to the murine H-2 complex. The initials HLA stand for human leukocyte antigens, as MHC-encoded antigens were initially detected on the white cells. The HLA system is highly polymorphic; that is, there are several alternative forms (alleles) of a gene at each locus. This, as we shall see, constitutes a formidable barrier in organ transplantation.

Based on their chemical structure, tissue distribution, and function, the MHC gene products are classified into three categories.

- *Class I antigens* are coded by three closely linked

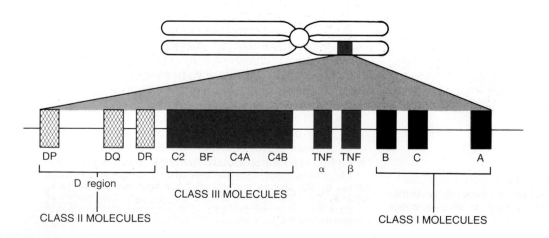

Figure 6–3. A schematic representation of the HLA complex and its subregions on human chromosome 6. The class III genes are not shown individually; they map within the region shown as a solid red rectangle. The relative distances between various genes and regions are not drawn to scale, and in some cases are unknown.

loci designated HLA-A, HLA-B, and HLA-C (see Fig. 6–3). Each of these molecules is a heterodimer, consisting of a polymorphic glycoprotein of 45,000 daltons (heavy chain or α chain) linked noncovalently to a smaller nonpolymorphic peptide called β_2-microglobulin. The latter is encoded by a gene on chromosome 15. *The extracellular portion of the α chain contains a cleft where foreign peptides bind to MHC molecules for presentation to T cells.* Class I antigens are present on virtually all nucleated cells and platelets.

- *Class II antigens* are coded for in a region known as HLA-D. There are at least three subregions, DP, DQ, and DR, within the originally defined HLA-D region. Class II antigens differ from class I antigens in several respects. Chemically, they exist as bimolecular complexes, but both of their constituent polypeptide chains are polymorphic. Unlike class I antigens, their tissue distribution is quite restricted; they are found mainly on antigen-presenting cells (monocytes and macrophages, dendritic cells), B cells, and some activated T cells. However, several other cell types, such as vascular endothelial cells, fibroblasts, and renal tubular epithelial cells, can be induced to express class II antigens by γ interferon, a lymphokine produced by activated T cells.

- *Class III proteins* are those components of the complement system (C2, C3, and Bf) that are coded within the MHC. Genes for the cytokines TNF-α and TNF-β are also encoded within the MHC. Although genetically linked to class I and II antigens, class III molecules and the cytokine genes do not act as histocompatibility (transplantation) antigens and will not be discussed further.

As already mentioned, a feature shared by class I and class II genes is the high degree of polymorphism. Each of the several alleles at these loci is designated by a number, such as HLA-A1, HLA-B5, and so forth. *All class I determinants and most (but not all) of the class II determinants evoke the formation of humoral antibodies in genetically nonidentical individuals.* This makes it possible to type these antigens by conventional serologic techniques such as antibody and complement-mediated lysis.

Because HLA antigens form an allelic series, an individual inherits only one determinant from each parent and can have no more than two different antigens for every locus. Thus, cells of a heterozygous individual express six different class I HLA antigens, three of maternal origin and three of paternal origin. Owing to the polymorphism at the major HLA loci, innumerable combinations of antigens can exist and therefore each individual in a noninbred population is likely to have a more or less unique antigenic profile, like a fingerprint on the cell surface.

Significance of HLA Complex

Organ Transplantation. HLA antigens were discovered in the course of transplantation studies, and they continue to present formidable barriers to the success of clinical organ transplantation. HLA antigens of the graft evoke both humoral and cell-mediated responses, which lead eventually to graft destruction, as discussed on page 132. Because the severity of the rejection reaction is related to the degree of HLA disparity between donor and recipient, HLA typing is of clinical significance in the selection of donor-recipient combinations.

Induction and Regulation of Immune Responses. As mentioned in the introduction to this section, the major physiologic function of the HLA molecules is to present antigens to T cells. Thus histocompatibility molecules play an important role in the induction of cellular as well as humoral immunity.

Class I MHC molecules bind to intracellularly synthesized peptides (e.g., viral antigens) and present them to CD8+ cytotoxic T lymphocytes. In this interaction, the T cell receptor recognizes the MHC-peptide complex and the CD8 molecule binds to the nonpolymorphic portion of the class I molecule (Fig. 6–4). It is important to note that *CD8+ cytotoxic T cells can recognize viral (or other) peptides only if presented as a complex with self class I antigens. This phenomenon is referred to as HLA restriction.* Since one of the important functions of CD8+ cytotoxic T cells is to eliminate virus-infected cells, and viral antigens can be recognized only when complexed to class I MHC molecules, it makes "good sense" to have widespread expression of class I HLA antigens.

In contrast to class I MHC molecules, the class II molecules are important for the presentation of anti-

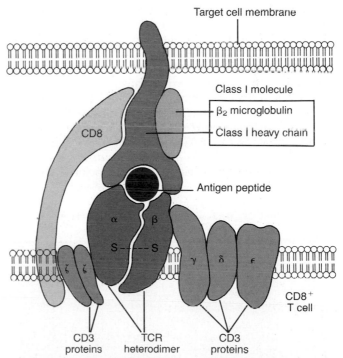

Figure 6–4. A schematic illustration of antigen recognition by CD8+ T cells. Note that the TCR (TCR heterodimer) recognizes a complex formed by the peptide fragment of the antigen and class I MHC molecule. The CD8 molecule binds to the nonpolymorphic portion of the class I molecule and thus acts as an accessory structure during antigen recognition.

gens to CD4+ helper T cells. The nature of antigens presented in association with class II molecules also differs. In general class II molecules present exogenous antigens that are first internalized and processed by antigen-presenting cells and then the class II–peptide complex is transported to the cell surface. Because CD4+ T cells can recognize foreign antigens only in the context of self class II molecules, they are referred to as being "class II restricted."

The role of class II antigens in the induction of helper T cells has an important bearing on the genetic regulation of the immune response. It is well known that the magnitude of immune responses is controlled by immune response (Ir) genes that map within the HLA-D region. Indeed, it is now believed that class II genes function as Ir genes. How class II antigens influence the magnitude of the immune response is not fully understood. It is conceivable that certain class II alleles code for cell surface (class II) molecules that form highly immunogenic complexes with a given antigen. This in turn would translate into a vigorous activation of helper T cells and a strong immune response. The consequence of inheriting such a class II gene would depend on the nature of the antigen and the type of immune response generated. For example, if the antigen were ragweed pollen and the response were production of IgE antibody, the individual would be genetically prone to type I hypersensitivity disease. On the other hand, good responsiveness to a viral antigen may be beneficial for the host.

HLA and Disease Association. A variety of diseases have been found to be associated with certain HLA types (Table 6–1). The best-known is the association between ankylosing spondylitis and HLA-B27; individuals who possess this antigen have a 90-fold greater chance (relative risk) of developing the disease than those who are negative for HLA-B27. The diseases that show association with HLA can be broadly grouped into the following categories: (1) *inflammatory diseases,* including ankylosing spondylitis and several postinfectious arthropathies, all associated with HLA-B27; (2) *inherited errors of metabolism,* such as hemochromatosis (HLA-A3) and 21-hydroxylase deficiency (HLA-BW47); (3) *autoimmune diseases,* including autoimmune endocrinopathies, associated with al-

leles at the DR locus. The mechanisms underlying these associations are not understood at present. In view of the physiologic role of the HLA complex in regulation of the immune response, it is somewhat easier to speculate on the possible mechanisms that may underlie the associations with immunologically mediated diseases. As was discussed above, HLA class II genes can regulate immune responsiveness. Accordingly, an association between certain autoimmune diseases and HLA-DR antigens may result from an exaggerated immune response to autoantigens.

IMMUNE MECHANISMS OF TISSUE INJURY

Immune responses (humoral or cell-mediated) to antigens of either endogenous or exogenous sources can cause tissue-damaging reactions. Classically these are called *hypersensitivity reactions* and the resultant tissue lesions *hypersensitivity disease.* The term hypersensitivity, however, is somewhat misleading as it implies abnormal or excessive sensitivity to an antigen. Hypersensitivity disease may result from perfectly usual or normal immune responses to an antigen (e.g., the rejection of tissue grafts from antigenically dissimilar donors). A better designation for hypersensitivity disease might be "diseases resulting from immune mediated tissue-damaging reactions," but, alas, this is too cumbersome a designation.

Hypersensitivity diseases (Table 6–2) are best classified on the basis of the immunologic mechanism mediating the disease. This approach is of great value, since it clarifies the manner in which the immune response ultimately causes tissue injury and disease. *In type I disease* the immune response releases vasoactive amines and other mediators derived from mast cells or basophils that affect vascular permeability and smooth muscle in various organs. In the *type II* disorder humoral antibodies participate directly in injuring cells by predisposing them to phagocytosis or to lysis. *Type III disorders* are best remembered as "immune complex diseases"; here humoral antibodies bind antigens and activate complement. The fractions of complement then attract neutrophils. Ultimately it is the activated complement and the release of neutrophilic enzymes and other toxic moieties (e.g., oxygen metabolites) that produce the tissue damage. *Type IV disorders* are examples of tissue injury in which cell-mediated immune responses with sensitized lymphocytes are the ultimate cause of the cellular and tissue injury. Each of these immune mechanisms is presented in the succeeding sections.

Type I Hypersensitivity (Anaphylactic Type)

Type I hypersensitivity is a rapidly occurring reaction that follows the combination of an antigen with antibody previously bound to the surface of mast cells and basophils. It is now recognized that many type I reactions have two well-defined phases: the initial response, characterized by vasodilatation, vascular leak-

TABLE 6–1. ASSOCIATION OF HLA
WITH DISEASE

Disease	HLA Allele	Relative Risk
Ankylosing spondylitis	B27	87.4
Postgonococcal arthritis	B27	14.0
Acute anterior uveitis	B27	14.6
Rheumatoid arthritis	DR4	5.8
Chronic active hepatitis	DR3	13.9
Primary Sjögren's syndrome	DR3	9.7
Insulin-dependent diabetes	DR3	5.0
	DR4	6.8
	DR3/DR4	14.3
Hemochromatosis	A3	8.2
21-Hydroxylase deficiency	BW47	15.0

TABLE 6-2. MECHANISMS OF IMMUNOLOGICALLY MEDIATED DISORDERS

Type	Prototype Disorder	Immune Mechanism
I Anaphylactic type	Anaphylaxis, some forms of bronchial asthma	Formation of IgE (cytotropic) antibody → release of vasoactive amines and other mediators from basophils and mast cells
II Cytotoxic type	Autoimmune hemolytic anemia, erythroblastosis fetalis, Goodpasture's disease	Formation of IgG, IgM → binds to antigen on target cell surface → phagocytosis of target cell or lysis of target cell by C8,9 fraction of activated complement or ADCC
III Immune complex disease	Arthus reaction, serum sickness, SLE, certain forms of acute glomerulonephritis	Antigen-antibody complexes → activated complement → attracted neutrophils → release of lysosomal enzymes and other toxic moieties
IV Cell-mediated (delayed) hypersensitivity	Tuberculosis, contact dermatitis, transplant rejection	Sensitized thymus-derived T lymphocytes → release of lymphokines and T cell-mediated cytotoxicity

age, and smooth muscle spasm, usually becomes evident within 5 to 30 minutes after exposure to an allergen and tends to subside in 60 minutes. In many individuals a second, "late-phase" reaction sets in 2 to 8 hours later without additional exposure to antigen and lasts for several days. This late phase reaction is characterized by more intense infiltration of tissues, with eosinophils, neutrophils, basophils, and monocytes as well as tissue destruction in the form of mucosal epithelial cell damage.

Because mast cells and basophils are central to the development of type I hypersensitivity, we will first review some of their salient characteristics and then discuss the immune mechanisms that underlie this form of hypersensitivity. Mast cells are bone marrow–derived cells that are widely distributed in the tissues. They are found predominantly near blood vessels and nerves and in subepithelial sites. As is well known, mast cell cytoplasm contains membrane-bound granules that possess a variety of biologically active mediators. In addition, mast cell granules contain acidic proteoglycans that bind basic dyes such as toluidine blue. Since the stained granules often acquire a color that is different from that of the native dye, they are referred to as "metachromatic" granules. As is detailed below, mast cells and basophils are activated by crosslinking of high-affinity IgE Fc receptors; in addition, mast cells may also be triggered by several other stimuli, such as complement components C5a and C3a (anaphylatoxins), both of which act by binding to their receptors on mast cell membrane. Other mast cell secretagogues include macrophage-derived cytokines (e.g., IL-8), some drugs such as codeine and morphine, mellitin (present in bee venom), and physical stimuli (e.g., heat, cold, sunlight). Basophils are similar to mast cells in many respects, including the presence of cell surface IgE Fc receptors as well as cytoplasmic granules. Unlike mast cells, however, basophils are not normally present in tissues but rather circulate in the blood in extremely small numbers. Like other granulocytes, they can be recruited to inflammatory sites.

In humans, type I reactions are mediated by IgE antibodies (also called reaginic antibodies); in other species, IgG antibodies can mediate anaphylactic reactions. The basic sequence of events in the pathogenesis of this form of hypersensitivity begins with the initial exposure to certain antigens (often called allergens). The allergen stimulates IgE production by B cells, a process that requires the assistance of helper T cells and is under the regulatory influence of suppressor-T cells. The IgE is strongly cytophilic for mast cells and basophils, which possess high-affinity receptors for the Fc portion of IgE. Once IgE is bound to the surface of mast cells, the individual is primed to develop type I hypersensitivity. Reexposure to the same antigen results in fixing of the antigen to cell-bound IgE, initiating a series of reactions that lead to the release of several powerful mediators that are responsible for the clinical features of type I hypersensitivity (Fig. 6-5). The mediator release requires that adjacent IgE molecules on the surface of mast cells and basophils be cross-linked by binding to a multivalent antigen. The cross-linking of cell-bound IgE induces a membrane signal that initiates several parallel and independent processes (Fig. 6-6)—one leading to mast cell degranulation with discharge of preformed or *primary mediators* and the other involving de novo synthesis and release of *secondary mediators* such as arachidonic acid metabolites.

PRIMARY MEDIATORS. Primary mediators are contained within mast cell granules and are of two types: (1) those that are rapidly released and act early in the course of a hypersensitivity reaction and (2) those that make up the granule matrix and are released slowly. Histamine is the most important mediator in the first category. It is known to cause increased vascular permeability, vasodilatation, bronchospasm, and increased secretion of mucus. Other rapidly released mediators include factors that are chemotactic for neutrophils and eosinophils. Accumulation of eosinophils is often prominent in these allergic reactions. The mediators that make up the granule matrix include heparin, neutral proteases (e.g., tryptase), and inflammatory factor of anaphylaxis. These factors are believed to participate in the late phase reaction of type I hypersensitivity. The neutral proteases can cleave comple-

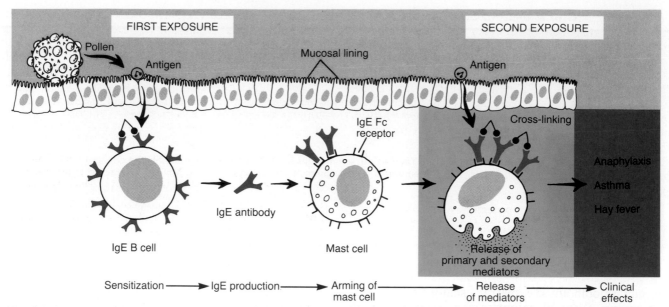

Figure 6–5. Sequence of events leading to type I hypersensitivity. (Modified from Roitt, I., et al.: Immunology. New York, Gower Medical Publishing, 1985, p. 19.2.)

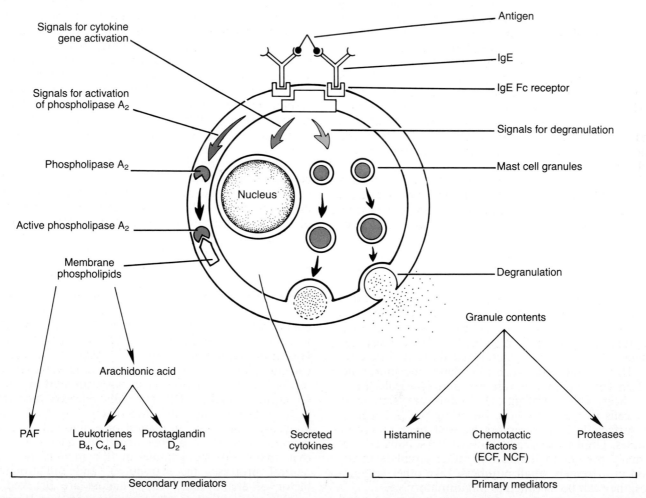

Figure 6–6. Activation of mast cells in type I hypersensitivity and release of their mediators. ECF = eosinophil chemotactic factor; NCF = neutrophil chemotactic factor.

ment components to generate additional chemotactic and inflammatory factors. C3a, for example, can cause further mast cell degranulation.

SECONDARY MEDIATORS. These include two classes of compounds: (1) lipid mediators and (2) cytokines. The lipid mediators are generated by sequential reactions in the mast cell membranes that lead to activation of phospholipase A_2, an enzyme that acts on membrane phospholipids to yield *arachidonic acid*. This, you may recall, is the parent compound from which leukotrienes and prostaglandins are derived by the 5-lipoxygenase and cyclooxygenase pathways, respectively (p. 36).

- *Leukotrienes* are extremely important in the pathogenesis of type I hypersensitivity. *Leukotrienes C_4 and D_4* are the most potent vasoactive and spasmogenic agents known. On a molar basis they are several thousand times more active than histamine in increasing vascular permeability and causing bronchial smooth muscle contraction. *Leukotriene B_4* is highly chemotactic for neutrophils, eosinophils, and monocytes.
- *Prostaglandin D_2* is the most abundant mediator derived by the cyclooxygenase pathway in mast cells. It causes intense bronchospasm as well as increased mucus secretion.
- *Platelet-activating factor* (PAF, p. 37) is another secondary mediator that causes platelet aggregation, release of histamine, and bronchospasm. Although its production is also initiated by the activation of phospholipase A_2, it is not a product of arachidonic acid metabolism.
- *Cytokines.* There is increasing evidence that mast cells can produce a variety of cytokines, including TNF-α, IL-1, IL-5, and IL-6. Some of these, in particular TNF-α, may contribute to the accumulation of inflammatory cells that occurs in the late phase.

In summary, a variety of chemotactic, vasoactive, and spasmogenic compounds (listed in Table 6–3) mediate type I hypersensitivity reactions. Some of these compounds are released rapidly from sensitized mast cells and are believed to be responsible for the intense immediate reactions associated with conditions such as systemic anaphylaxis. Others, such as granule matrix–associated factors and cytokines are probably responsible for the late-phase reactions. It is important to note that since histamine does not play an important role in late-phase reaction, antihistaminics are of little value after the initial phase. Control of the late phases usually requires broad-spectrum antiinflammatory drugs such as glucocorticosteroids.

CLINICAL MANIFESTATIONS. A type I reaction may occur as a systemic disorder or as a local reaction. Often this is determined by the route of antigen exposure. Systemic (parenteral) administration of protein antigens (such as antisera) and drugs (such as penicillin) results in *systemic anaphylaxis.* It should be remembered that once the individual is primed, the challenge dose of antigen may be extremely small (as for example, the tiny amounts used in skin testing for various forms of allergies). Within minutes after exposure, itching, hives, and skin erythema appear, followed shortly thereafter by striking respiratory difficulty, resulting presumably from constriction of respiratory bronchioles. Thus the principal organ affected is the lung, more specifically the smooth musculature of the pulmonary blood vessels and the respiratory passages. Pulmonary obstruction is accentuated by hypersecretion of mucus. Laryngeal edema may cause obstruction of the upper airway. In addition, the musculature of the entire gastrointestinal tract may be affected, with resultant vomiting, abdominal cramps, and diarrhea. The patient may go into shock and even die within the hour. At autopsy the findings may be surprisingly few, consisting principally of pulmonary edema and hemorrhages, sometimes accompanied by hyperdistention of the lungs and right-sided cardiac dilatation.

Systemic anaphylaxis is an important condition to bear in mind, because it is capable of causing death within minutes. It has been estimated, for example, that as many as 20% of persons treated with penicillin develop varying degrees of sensitivity to the drug, each

TABLE 6–3. SUMMARY OF THE ACTION OF MAST CELL MEDIATORS
IN TYPE I HYPERSENSITIVITY*

Action	Mediator	Source
Cellular infiltration	Leukotriene B_4	Membrane phospholipids
	Eosinophil chemotactic factor of anaphylaxis	Mast cell granules
	Neutrophil chemotactic factor of anaphylaxis	Mast cell granules
	* Inflammatory factors of anaphylaxis	Mast cell granule matrix
	* Cytokines	Mast cell granules
Vasoactive (vasodilatation, increased vascular permeability)	Histamine	Mast cell granules
	Platelet-activating factor (PAF)	Membrane lipids
	Leukotrienes C_4, D_4, E_4	Membrane lipids
	* Neutral proteases that activate complement	Mast cell granule matrix
	Prostaglandin D_2	Membrane lipids
Smooth muscle spasm	Leukotrienes C_4, D_4, E_4	Membrane lipids
	Histamine	Mast cell granules
	Prostaglandins	Membrane lipids
	PAF	Membrane lipids

* Important for late-phase reactions.

of whom is a potential candidate for an anaphylactic attack.

Local reactions generally occur on the skin or mucosal surfaces when they are the sites of antigenic exposure. The common forms of skin and food allergies, hay fever, and certain forms of asthma are examples of localized anaphylactic reactions. Presumably the synthesis of IgE occurs in the regional lymphoid tissues and local fixation to mast cells occurs. Susceptibility to localized type I reactions appears to be genetically controlled, and the term *atopy* is used to imply familial predisposition to such localized reactions. Patients who suffer from nasobronchial allergy (including hay fever and some forms of asthma) often have a family history of similar conditions; however, neither the number of genes involved nor the mode of inheritance is clear.

Before we close the discussion of type I hypersensitivity, it should be noted that the IgE antibodies are not merely "villains" that cause much human discomfort and diseases. They also play an important protective role in several parasitic infections. IgE antibodies are regularly produced in response to many helminthic infections. Figure 6–7 provides a schematic illustration of the process by which IgE antibodies serve to inflict damage on the schistosome larvae. The following points are worthy of note in this schema:

- IgE-sensitized mast cells do not cause direct damage to the parasites. Instead, they attract other leukocytes such as eosinophils by release of chemotactic factors.
- In addition to mast cells, eosinophils, platelets, and some macrophages possess Fc receptors for IgE.
- IgE-armed leukocytes attach to the surface of parasites and inflict damage by a variety of mechanisms. For example, eosinophils are capable of mediating antibody-dependent cellular cytotoxicity (described later); macrophages, on the other hand, release toxic oxygen metabolites and lysosomal enzymes.

Type II (Antibody-Dependent) Hypersensitivity _____

In type II hypersensitivity, antibodies are formed against target antigens that are either normal or altered cell membrane components. Unlike type III hypersensitivity reactions, discussed later, the antigens in this type of reaction are intrinsic to the cell or tissue that is damaged. Three different antibody-dependent mechanisms are involved in this type of hypersensitivity (Fig. 6–8).

COMPLEMENT-MEDIATED CYTOTOXICITY. In complement-mediated cytotoxicity, antibody reacts with a cell surface antigen, leading to fixation of complement and cell lysis. In addition, cells coated with antibodies become susceptible to phagocytosis, a process also favored by fixation of complement (p. 31). Blood cells are most commonly damaged by this mechanism, but antibodies can be directed against other tissue elements, such as glomerular basement membrane in Goodpasture's syndrome (p. 441). Clinically, antibody-mediated reactions occur in the following situations: (1) *Transfusion reactions,* in which red cells from an

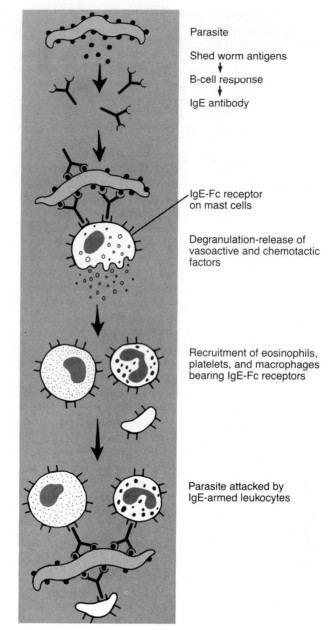

Parasite

Shed worm antigens

B-cell response

IgE antibody

IgE-Fc receptor on mast cells

Degranulation-release of vasoactive and chemotactic factors

Recruitment of eosinophils, platelets, and macrophages bearing IgE-Fc receptors

Parasite attacked by IgE-armed leukocytes

Figure 6–7. IgE-mediated destruction of parasites.

incompatible donor are destroyed after being coated with antibodies normally present in the recipient. Such antibodies are directed against blood group antigens. (2) *Rhesus incompatibility,* in which an Rh-negative mother is sensitized by red cells from an Rh-positive baby. The maternal Rh antibodies can cross the placenta and cause destruction of the Rh-positive fetal red cells. The resulting syndrome is called *erythroblastosis fetalis* (p. 343). (3) Some persons develop antibodies against their own blood elements, resulting in autoimmune hemolytic anemia, agranulocytosis, or thrombocytopenia. The possible reasons for such autoantibody formation are discussed in a later section (p. 138).

ANTIBODY-DEPENDENT CELL-MEDIATED CYTOTOXICITY (ADCC). This is the second possible mechanism involved in type II reactions. Many cell types that bear

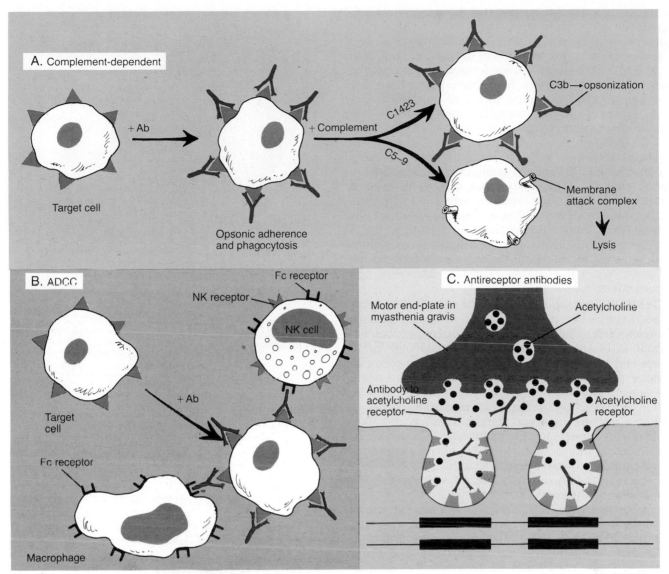

Figure 6–8. A schematic illustration of three different mechanisms of antibody-mediated injury in type II hypersensitivity. *A*, Complement-dependent reactions that lead to lysis of cells or render them susceptible to phagocytosis. *B*, Antibody-dependent cellular cytotoxicity (ADCC). IgG-coated target cells are killed by cells that bear Fc receptors for IgG (e.g., NK cells, macrophages). *C*, Antireceptor antibodies disturb the normal function of receptors. In this example, acetylcholine receptor antibodies impair neuromuscular transmission in myasthenia gravis.

receptors for the Fc portion of IgG cause the lysis of target cells coated with IgG antibody. Presumably this interaction involves the Fc receptors of the killer cells, which engage the Fc portion of the antibody coating the target cell (Fig. 6–8). *Lysis of the target cell requires contact but does not involve phagocytosis or fixation of complement.* ADCC can be mediated by a variety of cell types that bear Fc-IgG receptors. These include neutrophils, eosinophils, macrophages, and NK cells. Although in most cases IgG antibodies are involved in ADCC, in certain instances (for example, eosinophil-mediated ADCC against parasites, discussed above) IgE antibodies are utilized.

ANTIBODY-MEDIATED CELLULAR DYSFUNCTION. In some cases antibodies directed against cell surface receptors impair or dysregulate function without causing cell injury or inflammation. For example, in myasthenia gravis antibodies reactive with acetylcholine recep-

tors in the motor end plates of skeletal muscles impair neuromuscular transmission and therefore cause muscle weakness. The converse, i.e., antibody-mediated stimulation of cell function, is noted in Graves' disease. In this disorder, antibodies against the thyroid-stimulating hormone (TSH) receptor on thyroid epithelial cells stimulate the cells, resulting in hyperthyroidism.

Type III (Immune Complex–Mediated) Hypersensitivity

Type III hypersensitivity is mediated by antigen-antibody (immune) complexes that initiate an acute inflammatory reaction in the tissues. *Activation of complement and accumulation of polymorphonuclear leukocytes are important components of immune complex–mediated tissue injury.* The formation of immune complexes can be initiated by exogenous antigens such as bacteria and viruses or by endogenous antigens such as DNA. Pathogenetic immune complexes are either formed in the circulation and then deposited in the tissues or are formed at extravascular sites where antigen may have been planted (in situ immune complexes). Some forms of glomerular diseases in which immune complexes are formed in situ on the glomerular basement membrane are discussed in Chapter 14.

There are two patterns of immune complex-mediated injury. In one the complexes are deposited in various tissues of the body, thus causing a systemic pattern of injury. In the other the injury is localized to the site of formation, within a tissue or organ, of the complexes. Although the mechanism of tissue injury is the same, the sequence of events and the conditions leading to the formation of the immune complexes are different. We will, therefore, consider these two patterns separately.

SYSTEMIC IMMUNE COMPLEX DISEASE (SERUM SICKNESS TYPE). The pathogenesis of systemic immune complex disease can be resolved into three phases: (1) formation of antigen-antibody complexes in the circulation and (2) deposition of the immune complexes in various tissues, thus initiating (3) an inflammatory reaction in various sites throughout the body (Fig. 6–9). *Acute serum sickness* is the prototype of a systemic immune complex disease; it was at one time a frequent sequel to the administration of large amounts of foreign serum (e.g., horse antitetanus serum) used for passive immunization. It is now seen infrequently and in different clinical settings. For example, in one report 11 of 12 patients who were injected with horse antithymocyte globulin for treatment of aplastic anemia developed serum sickness. Approximately five days after the serum injection, antibodies directed against the serum components are produced; these react with the antigen still present in the circulation to form antigen-antibody complexes (the first phase). More is involved than the mere formation of immune complexes in the circulation; indeed, immune complexes are often formed during many immune responses, and they are removed from the circulation by the mononuclear phagocyte system. The factors that determine whether immune complex formation will lead to tissue deposition and disease are not fully understood, but two possible influences are as follows:

- Size of the complexes seems to be important. Very large complexes formed in great antibody excess are rapidly removed from the circulation by the mononuclear phagocytic cells and are therefore relatively harmless. The most pathogenic complexes are of small or intermediate size, circulate longer, and bind less avidly to phagocytic cells.
- Since the mononuclear phagocyte system normally serves to filter out the circulating immune complexes, its overload or intrinsic dysfunction increases the probability of persistence of immune complexes in the circulation and tissue deposition.

Tissue injury does not occur unless the circulating

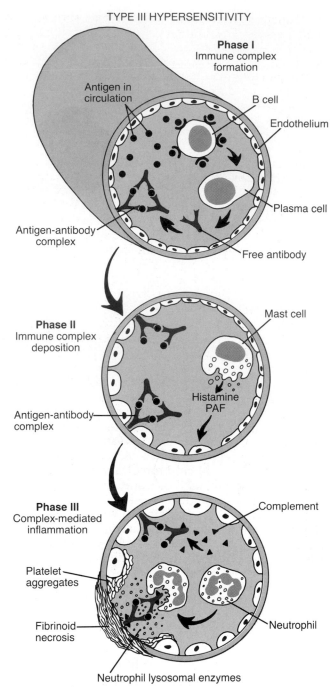

TYPE III HYPERSENSITIVITY

Phase I
Immune complex formation

Antigen in circulation

B cell

Endothelium

Plasma cell

Antigen-antibody complex

Free antibody

Phase II
Immune complex deposition

Mast cell

Histamine PAF

Antigen-antibody complex

Phase III
Complex-mediated inflammation

Complement

Platelet aggregates

Fibrinoid necrosis

Neutrophil

Neutrophil lysosomal enzymes

Figure 6–9. Schematic illustration of the three sequential phases in the induction of systemic type III (immune complex) hypersensitivity.

immune complexes are extravasated into various tissues (second phase). For complexes to leave the microcirculation there must be an increase in vascular permeability, mediated by small amounts of IgE induced shortly after administration of the antigen. Thus, a miniature type I (anaphylactic) reaction ensues, resulting in the release of histamine and platelet-activating factor, which are known to increase vascular permeability. Although this mechanism explains the vascular localization of the complexes, it fails to account for other tissue distributions. For reasons not entirely clear, the favored sites of immune complex deposition are kidneys, joints, skin, heart, serosal surface, and small vessels. Localization in the kidney could be explained in part by the filtration function of the glomerulus, with trapping of the circulating complexes in the glomeruli. Other factors that influence renal disposition are discussed later, in the context of glomerular diseases (p. 442). There is at present no satisfactory explanation for the peculiar localization of immune complexes in the other sites of predilection.

Once complexes are deposited in the tissues they initiate an acute inflammatory reaction (phase three). It is during this phase (approximately 10 days after antigen administration) that clinical features such as fever, urticaria, arthralgias, lymph node enlargement, and proteinuria appear. Central to the pathogenesis of tissue injury is the fixation of complement by the complexes, activation of the complement cascade, and release of biologically active fragments (p. 36), notably the anaphylatoxins (C3a and C5a), which increase vascular permeability and yield chemotactic factors for polymorphonuclear leukocytes. Phagocytosis of immune complexes by the accumulated neutrophils results in the release of lysosomal enzymes, such as neutral proteases, which can digest basement membranes, collagen, elastin, and cartilage. Tissue damage may also be mediated by free oxygen radicals produced by activated neutrophils. The released lysosomal enzymes serve to perpetuate the inflammatory process (p. 38). Immune complexes lead to other effects as well: aggregation of platelets and activation of Hageman factor, both of which augment the inflammatory process (Fig. 6–10). Microthrombi formed by platelet aggregation and initiation of clotting also contribute to the tissue injury by producing local ischemia.

It should be clear from the discussion above that only complement-fixing antibodies (i.e., IgG and IgM) are involved in type III hypersensitivity. The important role of complement in the pathogenesis of the tissue injury is supported by the observation that experimental manipulations that deplete serum complement levels greatly reduce the severity of the lesions, as does depletion of neutrophils. During the active phase of the disease, consumption of complement induces low serum levels.

The morphologic consequences of immune complex injury are dominated by acute necrotizing vasculitis, microthrombi, and superimposed ischemic necrosis accompanied by acute inflammation of the affected organs. The necrotic vessel wall takes on a smudgy eosinophilic appearance called "fibrinoid necrosis" (Fig. 6–11). Immune complexes can be visualized in the tissues, usually in the vascular wall, by both electron microscopy and immunofluorescence. In due course the lesions tend to resolve, especially when they were brought about by a single large exposure to antigen (e.g., acute serum sickness and acute poststreptococcal glomerulonephritis, p. 449); however, chronic immune complex disease develops when there is persistent antigenemia or repeated exposure to the antigen. This occurs in several human diseases, such as systemic lupus erythematosus (SLE), which is associated with persistent exposure to autoantigens. Often, however, despite the fact that the morphologic changes and other findings suggest immune complex disease, the inciting antigens are unknown. Included in this category are rheumatoid arthritis, polyarteritis nodosa, membranous glomerulonephritis, and several vasculitides.

LOCAL IMMUNE COMPLEX DISEASE (ARTHUS REACTION). *The Arthus reaction may be defined as a localized area of tissue necrosis resulting from acute immune complex vasculitis.* The reaction can be produced experimentally by injecting an antigen into the skin of a previously immunized animal. Antibodies against the antigen are therefore already present in the circulation. *Because of the large excess of antibodies,*

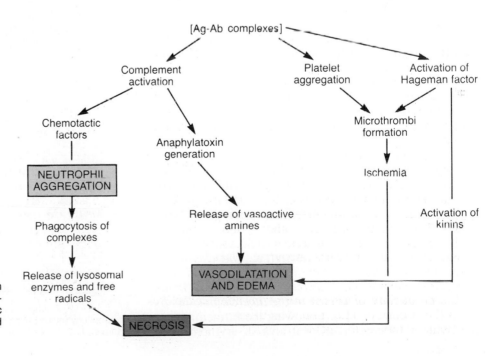

Figure 6–10. Schematic representation of the pathogenesis of immune complex–mediated tissue injury. The morphologic consequences are depicted as boxed areas.

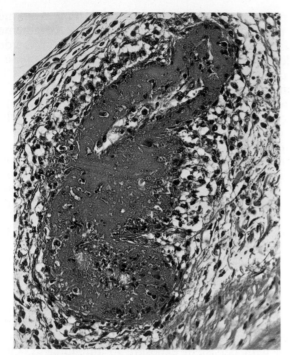

Figure 6-11. Immune complex vasculitis—acute fibrinoid necrosis of walls of small vessels.

immune complexes are formed; these are precipitated at the site of injection, especially within vessel walls, where the injected antigen is immediately bound to the circulating antibodies. Once the complexes are formed, the subsequent events are very similar to those described in the systemic pattern. Histologically, there is a severe necrotizing vasculitis and intense accumulation of neutrophils. Intrapulmonary Arthus-type reactions seem to be responsible for a number of diseases in humans, including farmer's lung, a hypersensitivity reaction to molds that grow on hay.

Type IV (Cell-Mediated) Hypersensitivity

Type IV hypersensitivity is mediated by T cells rather than antibodies. *Two types of reactions mediated by different T cell subsets are involved in type IV hypersensitivity:* (1) delayed type hypersensitivity, initiated by CD4+ T cells and (2) cellular cytotoxicity, mediated by CD8+ T cells. In both cases, the reaction is initiated by the exposure of sensitized T cells to specific antigens complexed to self MHC molecules, but the subsequent events are different. In delayed hypersensitivity CD4+ T cells secrete cytokines, leading to recruitment of other cells, especially macrophages, which are the major effector cells. In cell-mediated cytotoxicity, on the other hand, cytotoxic CD8+ T cells themselves assume the effector function.

DELAYED TYPE HYPERSENSITIVITY. *The classic example of a delayed hypersensitivity reaction is a positive Mantoux reaction (tuberculin test) elicited in an individual already sensitized to the tubercle bacillus by a prior infection* (p. 417). Following the intracutaneous injection of tuberculin, a local area of erythema and induration begins to appear at 8 to 12 hours, reaches a peak (approximately 1 to 2 cm in diameter) in 2 to 7 days, and thereafter slowly subsides. Histologically, cutaneous delayed hypersensitivity in humans is characterized by emigration of lymphocytes and monocytes from dermal venules, producing perivascular "cuffing" (Fig. 6-12). There is an associated increased microvascular permeability resulting from the formation of interendothelial gaps. Not unexpectedly, there is an escape of plasma proteins, giving rise to dermal edema and deposition of fibrin. In fully developed lesions, the lymphocyte-cuffed venules show marked endothelial hypertrophy and, in some cases, hyperplasia. With certain persistent or nondegradable antigens, the initial perivascular mononuclear cell infiltrate is replaced by macrophages over a period of two to three weeks. The accumulated macrophages often undergo a morphologic transformation into epithelial-like cells and are then referred to as epithelioid cells. *A microscopic aggregation of epithelioid cells, usually surrounded by a collar of lymphocytes, is referred to as a granuloma.* This pattern of inflammation that is characteristic of type IV hypersensitivity is called granulomatous inflammation. Recognition of a granuloma is of great importance because of the limited number of possible conditions that can cause it. In the usual hematoxylin and eosin preparations, the epithelioid cells have a pale pink granular cytoplasm with indistinct cell boundaries, often appearing to merge into one another. The nucleus is less dense (vesicular) than that of a lymphocyte, is oval or elongated, and may show folding of the

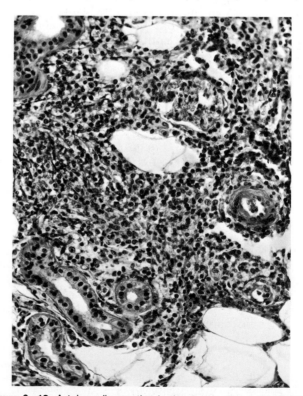

Figure 6-12. A tuberculin reaction in the dermis. There is infiltration of lymphocytes and macrophages about the small vessels and skin adnexa.

nuclear membrane. Older granulomas develop an enclosing rim of fibroblasts and connective tissue. Frequently, but not invariably, *large giant cells* are found in the periphery or sometimes in the center of granulomas. These giant cells may achieve diameters of 40 to 50 μm. They comprise a large mass of cytoplasm containing numerous (20 or more) small nuclei. Two types of giant cells are encountered. The *Langhans type* is said to be characteristic of tuberculosis but in reality may be found in any of the granulomatous reactions. The nuclei in this form tend to be arranged about the periphery of the cell, sometimes encircling the cytoplasm and at other times producing horseshoe patterns. The individual nuclei are quite small and have a diameter that is only a very small fraction of the diameter of the entire cell. *The foreign body–type giant cell* differs in that the numerous nuclei are scattered throughout the cytoplasm in no distinctive pattern. Both forms of giant cells are believed to arise from fusion of macrophages. Although some observers rely heavily on the finding of giant cells, *the identification of a granulomatous reaction actually rests on the recognition of epithelioid cells.*

The sequence of events in delayed hypersensitivity, as exemplified by the tuberculin reaction, begins with the first exposure of the individual to tubercle bacilli. CD4+ lymphocytes recognize antigens of tubercle bacilli in association with class II antigens on the surface of monocytes or other antigen-presenting cells that have processed mycobacterial antigens. This sensitization leads to the formation of "memory" T cells that remain in the circulation for long periods, sometimes years. Upon intracutaneous injection of tuberculin in such an individual, the sensitized T cells interact with the antigen on the surface of antigen-presenting cells and are activated (i.e., they undergo blast transformation and proliferation). These changes are accompanied by the secretion of a number of cytokines, which are responsible for the expression of delayed type hypersensitivity (Fig. 6–13). Cytokines most relevant to this reaction and their actions are as follows:

- IFN-γ is the most important mediator of delayed type hypersensitivity. It is an extremely potent activator of macrophages. Activated macrophages are altered in several ways: their ability to phagocytose and kill microorganisms is markedly augmented; they express more class II molecules on the surface, thus facilitating further antigen presentation; their capacity to kill tumor cells is enhanced; and they secrete several polypeptide growth factors, such as platelet-derived growth factor and TGF-β, that stimulate fibroblast proliferation and augment collagen synthesis. Thus activated, macrophages serve to eliminate the offending antigen, and if the activation is sustained fibrosis results.
- IL-2 causes autocrine and paracrine proliferation of T cells, which accumulate at sites of delayed hypersensitivity; included in this infiltrate are some antigen-specific CD4+ T cells and many more bystander T cells activated by IL-2.
- TNF-α and lymphotoxin are two cytokines that exert important effects on endothelial cells: (1) in-

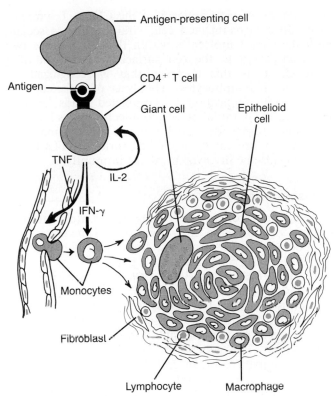

Figure 6–13. A schematic illustration of the events that give rise to the formation of granuloma in type IV hypersensitivity reactions. Note the role played by T cell–derived cytokines.

creased secretion of prostacyclin, which in turn favors increased blood flow by causing local vasodilatation, (2) increased expression of ELAM-1 (see p. 29), an adhesion molecule that promotes attachment of the passing lymphocytes and monocytes, and (3) induction and secretion of low–molecular weight chemotactic factors such as IL-8. Together all these changes in the endothelium facilitate the extravasation of lymphocytes and monocytes at the site of the delayed hypersensitivity reaction.

It is important to point out that although the generation of lymphokines is the result of a very specific interaction between the antigen and the sensitized T cells, the effects of lymphokines are not antigen specific. For example, macrophages activated by tuberculoprotein develop increased activity not only against tubercle bacilli but also against several unrelated bacteria. This type of hypersensitivity is a major mechanism of defense against a variety of intracellular pathogens, including mycobacteria, fungi, and certain parasites, and may also be involved in transplant rejection and tumor immunity.

T CELL–MEDIATED CYTOTOXICITY. In this variant of type IV hypersensitivity, sensitized CD8+ T cells kill antigen-bearing target cells. Such effector cells are called cytotoxic T lymphocytes (CTLs). CTLs, directed against cell surface histocompatibility antigens, play an important role in graft rejection, to be discussed next in this chapter. They also play a role in resistance to virus infections. As discussed earlier, class I MHC molecules play an extremely important role in the presentation of viral antigens to the CD8+ T lymphocytes. In a virus-infected cell, viral peptides associate with the class I molecules within the cell and the two are transported to the cell surface in the form of a complex. It is this complex that is recognized by cytotoxic T lymphocytes. The lysis of infected cells before viral replication is completed leads in due course to the elimination of the infection. It is believed that many tumor-associated antigens (p. 204) may also be similarly presented on the cell surface. CTLs therefore may also be involved in tumor immunity.

Transplant Rejection

Rejection of organ transplants is a complex immunologic phenomenon that involves cell-mediated and antibody-mediated responses, both of which are targeted on the HLA antigens in the graft.

T CELL–MEDIATED REJECTION. The classic acute rejection, which occurs within 10 to 14 days in non-immunosuppressed recipients, is largely the result of cell-mediated immunity. As already mentioned, this involves delayed hypersensitivity and T cell–mediated cytotoxicity. The generation of CTL in response to HLA-incompatible organ grafts starts when the recipient's lymphocytes encounter foreign HLA antigens on the surface of cells in the graft. It is believed that the donor lymphoid cells ("passenger lymphocytes"), especially dendritic cells contained within the grafts, are the most important immunogens, since they are rich in both class I and class II antigens. The CD4+ helper T-cell subset is triggered into proliferation by recognition of the class II specificities. At the same time, precursors of CD8+ CTL ("pre-killer T cells"), bearing receptors for class I HLA antigens, differentiate into mature CTLs. This process of differentiation is complex and incompletely understood. Involved are interactions of antigen-presenting cells, T-cell subsets, and soluble factors such as IL-1, IL-2, and IL-4 (see Fig. 6–14). Once mature CTLs are generated, they lyse the grafted tissue. In addition to the specific cytotoxic T cells, lymphokine-secreting CD4+ T cells are also generated as in the delayed hypersensitivity reaction. This leads to increased vascular permeability and local accumulation of mononuclear cells (lymphocytes and macrophages), as previously described. According to some investigators, the delayed hypersensitivity with its attendant microvascular injury produces tissue ischemia, which along with destruction mediated by accumulated macrophages is an important mechanism of graft destruction. The molecular basis of allorecognition by T cells is incompletely understood. According to one widely held view an alloantigen may be considered a modified self-antigen. According to this hypothesis a nonself-HLA molecule is recognized by a T cell that normally interacts with a complex of self-HLA molecules and a foreign peptide.

ANTIBODY-MEDIATED REJECTION. There is little doubt that T cells are of paramount importance in the rejection of organ transplants. This is supported by the inability of T cell–deprived animals to reject allografts. However, antibodies can also mediate rejection, and this process can take two forms. (1) *Hyperacute rejection occurs when preformed antidonor antibodies are present in the circulation of the recipient.* Such antibodies may be present in a recipient who has already rejected a kidney transplant. Multiparous women who develop anti-HLA antibodies against paternal antigens shed from the fetus may also have preformed antibodies to grafts taken from their husbands or children. Prior blood transfusions from HLA-nonidentical donors can also lead to presensitization, since platelets and white cells are particularly rich in HLA antigens. In such circumstances rejection occurs immediately after transplantation, because the circulating antibodies react with and deposit rapidly on the vascular endothelium of the grafted organ. Complement fixation occurs and an Arthus-type reaction follows. (2) Even in nonsensitized individuals, anti-HLA humoral antibodies develop concurrently with T cell–mediated rejection.

These antibodies are particularly important in mediating acute vascular rejection in recipients who have been treated with immunosuppressive drugs following transplantation. The immunosuppressive drugs suppress T-cell responses, but some formation of antibodies continues, causing damage by ADCC and complement fixation with the formation of immune complexes. In most cases, the major target of antibody-mediated damage is the vascular endothelium. Superimposed on the immunologically mediated vascular damage are platelet aggregation and coagulation, adding ischemic insult to the injury.

MORPHOLOGY OF REJECTION REACTIONS. Based on morphology and the mechanisms involved, rejection reactions have been classified as hyperacute, acute, and chronic.

The morphologic changes in these patterns are described as they relate to renal transplants. Similar changes would be encountered in any other vascularized visceral organ transplant.

Hyperacute Rejection. Hyperacute rejection may occur within minutes or a few hours in presensitized persons. **Basically, it is characterized by widespread acute arteritis and arteriolitis, thrombosis of vessels, and ischemic necrosis.** As indicated earlier, this pattern of rejection is mediated largely by humoral antibodies, which evoke an Arthus-like reaction. As a consequence of the arterial lesions, the graft never becomes vascularized and it undergoes ischemic necrosis. Virtually all arterioles and arteries exhibit characteristic acute fibrinoid necrosis of their walls, with narrowing or complete occlusion of the lumens by precipitated fibrin and cellular debris. Deposits of IgG, IgM, complement, and fibrin can be demonstrated within the vessel walls. It should be noted that with the current practice of cross-matching (i.e., testing recipients for the presence of antibodies directed against donor's lymphocytes) hyperacute rejection is no longer a significant clinical problem.

Acute Rejection. Acute rejection may occur within days of transplantation in the untreated recipient or may

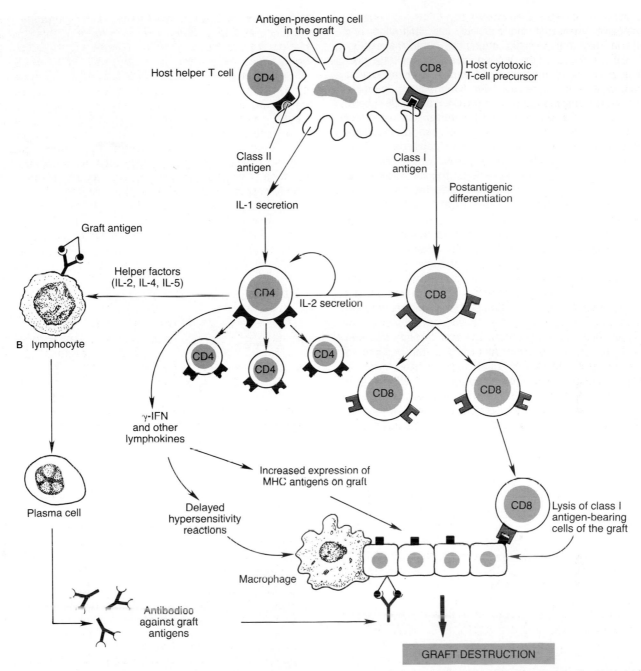

Figure 6–14. Schematic representation of events that lead to the destruction of histoincompatible grafts. Class I and class II antigens of the graft donor are recognized by CD8+ cytotoxic T cells and CD4+ helper cells, respectively, of the host. The interaction of the CD4+ cells with class II antigens leads to release of interleukin 1 (IL-1) and other co-stimulators from the antigen-presenting cells. IL-1 promotes the proliferation of CD4+ cells and the release of interleukin 2 (IL-2) from the cells. IL-2 further augments the proliferation of CD4+ cells and also provides helper signals for the differentiation of class I–specific CD8+ cytotoxic cells. In addition to IL-2, a variety of other soluble mediators (lymphokines) that promote B-cell differentiation and participate in the induction of a local delayed hypersensitivity reaction are produced by CD4+ helper cells. Eventually, several mechanisms converge to destroy the graft: (1) lysis of cells that bear class I antigens by CD8+ cytotoxic T cells, (2) antigraft antibodies produced by sensitized B cells, and (3) nonspecific damage inflicted by macrophages and other cells that accumulate as a result of the delayed hypersensitivity reaction.

appear suddenly months or even years later, when immunosuppression has been employed and terminated. As suggested earlier, acute graft rejection is a combined process in which both cellular and humoral tissue injury play parts. In any one patient, one or the other mechanism may predominate. Histologically, humoral rejection is associated with vasculitis, whereas cellular rejection is marked by an interstitial mononuclear cell infiltrate.

Acute cellular rejection is most commonly seen within the initial months after transplantation and is often accompanied by abrupt onset of clinical signs of failure of renal function. Histologically, there may be extensive interstitial mononuclear cell infiltration and edema, as well as mild interstitial hemorrhage (Fig. 6–15). In humans, the mononuclear cell infiltrate consists primarily of medium-sized and small lymphocytes along with some large blast-like lymphocytes. Immunoperoxidase staining reveals both CD4+ and CD8+ cells, as might be expected from the earlier discussion of graft rejection. Plasma cells are also seen in longstanding cases. Glomerular and peritubular capillaries contain large numbers of mononuclear cells, which may also invade the tubules and cause focal tubular necrosis. In the absence of an accompanying arteritis, these cellular rejections respond promptly to immunosuppressive therapy.

Acute rejection vasculitis (humoral rejection) may also be present in the acute reaction after transplantation or when immunosuppressive therapy is discontinued. The histologic lesions consist of necrotizing arteritis with endothelial necrosis; neutrophilic infiltration; deposition of immunoglobulins, complement, and fibrin; and thrombosis. The process may evolve to extensive glomerular necrosis and cortical arteriolar thrombosis, with resulting cortical infarction. Almost all of the patients so affected also have evidence of acute cellular rejection. More common than this acute type of vasculitis is so-called subacute vasculitis, which is characterized by marked thickening of the intima by a cushion of proliferating fibroblasts, myocytes, and foamy macrophages,

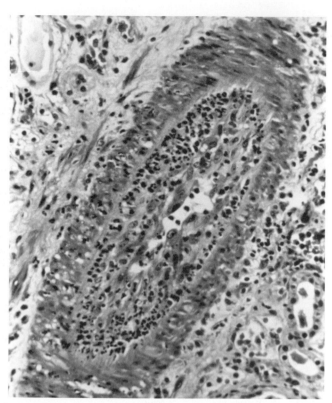

Figure 6–16. Acute humoral rejection of a renal allograft manifested by subacute vasculitis. The vascular intima is markedly thickened and inflamed. (Courtesy of Dr. Helmut Renké, Department of Pathology, Brigham and Women's Hospital, Boston, MA.)

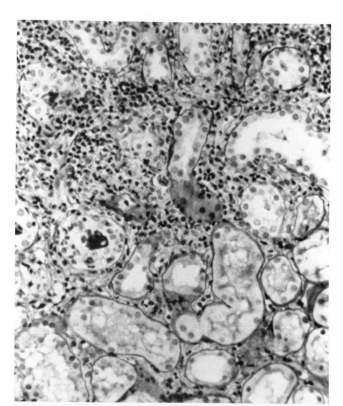

Figure 6–15. Acute cellular rejection of renal allograft manifested by a diffuse mononuclear cell infiltrate and interstitial edema. (Courtesy of Dr. Helmut Renké, Department of Pathology, Brigham and Women's Hospital, Boston, MA.)

often leading to luminal narrowing or obliteration. The thickened intima may be infiltrated by scattered neutrophils and mononuclear cells, and the walls of most of these arteries have deposits of immunoglobulin and complement (Fig. 6–16).

Chronic Rejection. Since most instances of acute graft rejection are more or less controlled by immunosuppressive therapy, chronic changes are commonly seen in the renal allograft. Patients with chronic rejections present clinically with a progressive rise in serum creatinine level (an index of renal dysfunction) over a period of four to six months. The vascular changes consist of dense intimal fibrosis, principally in the cortical arteries; the lesion probably is the end stage of the patterns of arteritis described in acute and subacute stages. These vascular lesions result in renal ischemia manifested by glomerular obsolescence, interstitial fibrosis, and tubular atrophy and shrinkage of the renal parenchyma. Together with the vascular lesions, the kidneys usually have interstitial mononuclear cell infiltrates containing large numbers of plasma cells and numerous eosinophils. This is taken as an indication of chronic cell-mediated rejection, but in truth it must be said that identification of the pathogenetic mechanisms in chronic graft rejection is much more difficult than it is in acute forms; it is further complicated by the contribution of ischemic damage to progressive renal dysfunction.

METHODS OF INCREASING GRAFT SURVIVAL. We are still far from the utopia in which diseased organs can be replaced as easily as worn-out automobile parts. Intensive efforts have been made to devise strategies that will prevent graft rejection. These include reduction in histocompatibility barriers, immunosuppression, or both.

Since HLA antigens are the major targets in transplant rejection, better matching of the donor and the recipient would, of course, improve graft survival. Obviously, monozygotic twins are the most perfectly matched and are ideal donors for each other. The benefits of HLA matching are most dramatic in intrafamilial (living, related donor) kidney transplants. For example, transplants from HLA-identical siblings have a survival rate of 90% at one year, compared with 56% if donor and recipient do not share either haplotype. However, the effects of HLA matching on graft survival (summarized below) in renal transplants from cadavers are less dramatic and depend on several variables, including the number and class of HLA antigens matched, ethnic composition of the population under study (relatively homogeneous versus heterogeneous), and concurrent immunosuppressive therapy.

- Three loci, HLA-A, -B, and -DR, are considered most relevant for matching. In general the more alleles that are matched the better is the graft survival.
- Of these three loci, matches at HLA-DR are most important. A DR mismatch largely negates the beneficial effect of A and B matches.
- Matching is more predictive of graft survival in relatively homogeneous populations (e.g., in Europeans) than in extensively outbred populations, as that of the United States.
- Effective immunosuppression, discussed below, often masks any beneficial effects of HLA matching.

Immunosuppression of the recipient is a practical necessity in all organ transplantation except in the case of identical twins. Even in transplants from HLA-identical siblings, there are minor non-HLA antigenic differences that can evoke a rejection reaction, albeit a mild one. Drugs and anti–T cell antibodies are the two common modes of immunosuppression employed. Among drugs, cyclosporin has emerged as a powerful and effective tool in preventing organ transplant rejection. It suppresses T cell–mediated immunity by inhibiting the transcription of cytokine genes, in particular the gene for IL-2. As alluded to above, HLA-mismatched renal grafts often fare as well as HLA-matched grafts when cyclosporin is employed for immunosuppression; however, the use of cyclosporin is limited by its significant renal toxicity. For this reason there is an ongoing search for less toxic immunosuppressive drugs. One such candidate, called FK506, has generated much excitement because in early trials it appears to be far more potent than cyclosporin and may be less toxic. Another avenue for immunosuppression is the administration of monoclonal anti-CD3 antibodies that react with all T cells. To make the anti–T cell therapy more selective, recent attempts are directed toward eliminating only those T cells that are activated by the grafted organ. Since activated T cells express receptors for IL-2, administration of anti–IL-2 receptor antibodies provides one such approach that is currently under investigation. Immunosuppression definitely improves graft survival, but it renders the individual vulnerable to opportunistic infections and high-grade lymphoid tumors. Often an immunosuppressed patient dies of disseminated and refractory infections rather than organ failure.

TRANSPLANTATION OF LIVER. Although kidney is the most frequently transplanted solid organ, transplantation of liver, heart, lungs, and pancreas is rapidly increasing. Liver transplantation is now performed at most large medical centers in the United States. The major indications are: extrahepatic biliary atresia, certain forms of cirrhosis, and inborn errors of metabolism such as α-1 antitrypsin deficiency. Unlike the case with kidney transplantation, no effort is made to match the histocompatibility antigens of the donor and host. This peculiarity may be related to the fact that HLA antigens are poorly expressed on liver cells. Furthermore, any possible detrimental effect of HLA mismatching is largely overcome by the use of potent immunosuppressive drugs such as cyclosporin. For those who survive the initial postoperative stage, a three-year survival rate of 70 to 90% can be expected.

TRANSPLANTATION OF HEMATOPOIETIC CELLS. Transplantation of bone marrow is a form of therapy increasingly employed for hematopoietic malignancies, aplastic anemias, and certain immune deficiency states. The recipient is given large doses of irradiation either to destroy the malignant cells (e.g., leukemias) or to create a graft bed (aplastic anemias), and the destroyed bone marrow is restored by marrow transplantation. Two major problems complicate this form of transplantation: graft-versus-host disease (GVH) and rejection of the transplant. *GVH disease* occurs when immunologically competent cells or their precursors are transplanted into recipients who are immunologically crippled because of the primary disease or from prior treatment with drugs or irradiation. When such recipients receive normal bone marrow cells from allogeneic donors, the immunocompetent T cells derived from the donor marrow recognize the recipient's tissue as "foreign" and react against them. This results in the generation of cytotoxic lymphocytes and lymphokine-secreting T cells, which are detrimental to the recipient's tissues. The resulting GVH syndrome causes *epithelial cell necrosis in three principal target organs —liver, skin, and gut mucosa—resulting in jaundice, skin rashes, and diarrhea.* GVH disease is a potential lethal complication that can be minimized but not eliminated by HLA matching. As a possible solution to this problem, T cells are depleted from the donor marrow. This protocol has proved to be the proverbial two-edged sword: the risk of GVH disease is reduced, but the incidence of graft failures and recurrence of leukemia increases. It seems that the schizophrenic T cells not only mediate GVH but are also required for the engraftment of the transplanted bone marrow stem cells and elimination of leukemia cells.

AUTOIMMUNE DISEASES _____

An immune reaction against "self antigens"—autoimmunity—is now a well-established cause of disease. In recent years a growing list of diseases has been attributed to autoimmunity. However, caution must be exercised in assigning an autoimmune cause to every disease in which autoantibodies can be demonstrated. It should be remembered that autoantibodies can be formed in response to injured, antigenically altered tissues. Moreover, autoantibodies can be demonstrated in a surprisingly large number of persons, particularly older ones, who are apparently entirely free of autoimmune disease. The designation of a condition as an autoimmune disease should therefore be based on (1) evidence of an autoimmune reaction, (2) the judgment that the immunologic findings are not merely secondary, and (3) the lack of any other identified cause for the disorder.

Despite uncertainties, a number of conditions have been designated autoimmune diseases (Table 6–4). They range from *single organ* (or *single cell*) *type disorders,* which involve specific immune reactions directed against one particular organ or cell type, to *multisystem diseases,* characterized by lesions in many organs, associated usually with a multiplicity of autoantibodies or cell-mediated reactions, or both. In most of the latter diseases the pathologic changes are found principally within the connective tissue and blood vessels of the various organs involved. Thus, these diseases were once called "collagen-vascular diseases" or "connective tissue diseases." As will be seen, the autoimmune reactions in these systemic diseases are not specifically directed against the constituents of connective tissue or blood vessels, but these older designations remain useful because they connote widespread lesions affecting many organs and systems.

The immunologic evidence that the diseases listed in Table 6–4 are indeed the result of autoimmune reactions is more compelling for some than for others. With SLE, the presence of a multiplicity of autoantibodies logically explains many of the observed changes. Moreover, the autoantibodies can be identified within the lesions by immunofluorescent and electron microscopic techniques. Few would dispute the assumption that SLE is an autoimmune disease. In many others, such as polyarteritis nodosa, an immune-mediated basis of tissue injury is suspected, but the nature of the antigen is not established. Indeed, in some cases an exogenous antigen may initiate the autoimmune attack.

Only the systemic autoimmune diseases are considered in this chapter. The single-target involvements are more appropriately discussed in the chapters that deal with specific organs. Before describing individual disorders we will consider the general nature of self-tolerance and theories about its loss.

SELF-TOLERANCE _____

Immune tolerance is defined as a state in which the individual is incapable of developing an immune re-

TABLE 6–4. AUTOIMMUNE DISEASES

Single Organ or Cell Type	Systemic
Probable	*Probable*
Hashimoto's thyroiditis	SLE
Autoimmune hemolytic anemia	RA
Autoimmune atrophic gastritis of pernicious anemia	Sjögren's syndrome
Autoimmune encephalomyelitis	Reiter's syndrome
Autoimmune orchitis	*Possible*
Goodpasture's syndrome*	Polymyositis-dermatomyositis
Autoimmune thrombocytopenia	Systemic sclerosis (scleroderma)
Insulin-dependent diabetes mellitus	Polyarteritis nodosa
Myasthenia gravis	
Graves' disease	
Possible	
Primary biliary cirrhosis	
Chronic active hepatitis	
Ulcerative colitis	
Membranous glomerulonephritis	

* Target is basement membrane of glomeruli and alveolar walls.

sponse against a specific antigen. *Self-tolerance refers to lack of immune responsiveness to the individual's own tissue antigens.* Obviously, self-tolerance is necessary for our tissues to live harmoniously with an army of lymphocytes. Before we consider the mechanisms underlying self-tolerance certain general features of tolerance are worthy of note:

- Tolerance obeys the same laws of antigen specificity that apply to other immune responses; thus it is restricted to the antigens used to induce tolerance. It follows that tolerance must result from physical or functional inactivation of antigen-specific T or B lymphocytes, or both.
- Self-tolerance is an acquired, or learned, characteristic. Genes that encode lymphocyte receptors that bind to self antigens are inherited by all individuals. Hence mechanisms that prevent the function of potentially auto reactive lymphocytes must exist in normal persons.
- Functionally immature lymphocytes are rendered tolerant more readily than fully mature cells. Thus it is postulated that self-tolerance is induced early in life when the developing lymphocytes come in contact with self antigens. However, because lymphocytes are produced continuously during life, mechanisms to render newly formed immature lymphocytes tolerant must operate throughout the life span of each individual.

Three major mechanisms are believed to prevent antiself reactivity in healthy individuals: clonal deletion, clonal anergy, and peripheral suppression (mediated for example, by suppressor T cells). These pathways of self-tolerance are illustrated in Figure 6–17 and briefly described next.

- *Clonal Deletion.* Clonal deletion is loss or deletion of self-reactive clones of either T lymphocytes or B

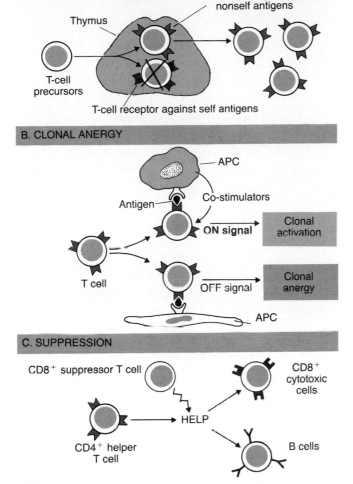

A. CLONAL DELETION

Thymus

T-cell receptor against
nonself antigens

T-cell
precursors

T-cell receptor against self antigens

B. CLONAL ANERGY

APC

Antigen — Co-stimulators

ON signal → Clonal activation

T cell

OFF signal → Clonal anergy

APC

C. SUPPRESSION

CD8+ suppressor T cell

CD8+ cytotoxic cells

HELP

CD4+ helper T cell

B cells

Figure 6–17. A schematic illustration of the three possible mechanisms of self-tolerance.

lymphocytes or both during their maturation. Indeed there is abundant evidence that *T lymphocytes that bear receptors for self antigens are deleted within the thymus during the process of T cell maturation.* It is proposed that many autologous protein antigens are expressed in the thymus in association with self MHC molecules. The developing T cells that express high-affinity receptors for such self antigens are "negatively selected," or deleted, and therefore the peripheral T-cell pool lacks potentially self-reactive cells. Whereas clonal deletion may also affect self-reactive B cells, this mechanism plays a less important role in B-cell tolerance. B cells that bear receptors for a variety of self antigens, including thyroglobulin, collagen, DNA, and myelin, can be readily demonstrated in normal humans. Hence B-cell tolerance must be maintained by other mechanisms.

- *Clonal Anergy.* This refers to prolonged or irreversible functional inactivation of lymphocytes, induced by encounter with antigens under certain conditions.

For example, it is well established that activation of antigen-specific CD4+ cells requires two signals: recognition of peptide antigen in association with class II MHC molecules on the surface of antigen-presenting cells (APCs) and a set of second signals delivered in the form of soluble "co-stimulatory factors" produced by APCs. If the antigen is presented by cells that cannot produce the necessary costimulators, a negative signal is delivered and the cell becomes anergic. Such a cell then fails to be activated even if the relevant antigen is presented by competent APCs (e.g., macrophages, dendritic cells) that can produce co-stimulators. Clonal anergy of T cells may occur during development in the thymus, if the thymic APCs fail to deliver the second signal. Thus the thymus plays a critical role in self-tolerance: during ontogeny self-reactive T cells may either be deleted or rendered functionally incompetent within the thymus. Clonal anergy affects B cells as well and is probably the major mechanism for B-cell tolerance to self antigens. The mechanisms of B-cell anergy are somewhat different from those that operate on T cells. It is believed that if B cells encounter antigen before they are fully mature, the antigen-receptor complex is endocytosed but, unlike mature B cells, such cells never reexpress their immunoglobulin receptors. Understandably, such cells are unable to respond to subsequent antigenic stimulation. In addition to antigen-induced loss of surface immunoglobulin receptors, other mechanisms of B-cell anergy are also postulated to exist.

- *Peripheral Suppression by T Cells.* Although clonal deletion and anergy are the primary mechanisms of self-tolerance, it is believed that additional failsafe mechanisms must also exist. Many factors, both cellular and humoral, that can actively suppress autoreactive lymphocytes have been described. However, most interest has focused on suppressor T cells. These cells, like cytotoxic T cells, are CD8+, but are believed to comprise a distinct subset. In experimental models it is possible to demonstrate inactivation of both helper T cells and B cells by suppressor T cells. Unfortunately, despite intensive efforts, the molecular mechanisms by which suppressor T cells recognize antigens and exert their suppressive effects have remained elusive.

In summary, prevention of autoimmunity is so vital to survival that several mechanisms have evolved to protect us from our "protectors." Deletion of autoreactive clones appears to be the major mechanism of self-tolerance in T cells. Because helper T cells are critical control elements for both cellular and humoral immunity, *tolerance of self-reactive T cells is extremely important for prevention of autoimmune diseases.* In contrast to T-cell tolerance, B-cell tolerance is maintained largely by clonal anergy. Because most self antigens are T dependent, autoantibody formation may be prevented by tolerance of either hapten-specific B cells or the relevant helper T cells or both. Lymphocytes (both T and B cells) that "leak" through the barriers of clonal deletion or anergy are restrained by suppressor mechanisms.

MECHANISMS OF AUTOIMMUNE DISEASE _____

Breakdown of one or more of the mechanisms of self-tolerance can unleash an immunologic attack on tissues that leads to the development of autoimmune diseases. Although immunocompetent cells are undoubtedly involved in mediating the tissue injury, we do not know the precise influences that initiate their reactions against self, but genetic factors and infectious agents are thought to be important. First the mechanisms involved in the breakdown of self-tolerance will be discussed, followed by the genetic and microbial factors.

Loss of Self-Tolerance _____

This can be best understood in the context of the mechanisms invoked in the maintenance of self-tolerance.

BYPASS OF HELPER T CELL TOLERANCE. It should be recalled that antibody responses against most self antigens require collaboration between hapten-specific B cells and carrier-specific helper T-cells. Tolerance to self antigens is often associated with clonal deletion of carrier-specific helper T cells in the presence of fully competent hapten-specific B cells. Therefore, this form of tolerance may be overcome, if the need for tolerant helper T cells is bypassed or substituted. This can be accomplished in one of several ways:

1. Modification of the Molecule. If the carrier determinant of a self antigen is modified, it may acquire new antigenic specificities, which will be recognized as foreign by clones of helper T cells that were not deleted (Fig. 6–18). These could then cooperate with the hapten-specific B cells, leading to formation of autoantibodies. Modification of the carrier may result from complexing of self antigens with drugs or microorganisms. For example, autoimmune hemolytic anemia, which occurs after the administration of certain drugs, may result from drug-induced alterations in the red cell surface (p. 342). Partial degradation of an autoantigen such as collagen could expose new carrier determinants; such degradation may be brought about by lysosomal enzymes (e.g., in rheumatoid arthritis).

2. Cross Reactions. These may occur between some human antigens and certain microbes if they share haptenic specificities. Normally, no autoantibody against the self hapten is formed, owing to T helper cell tolerance. However, infecting microorganisms may trigger an antibody response by presenting the cross-reacting hapten in association with their own carrier, which would be recognized by nontolerant helper T cells. Antibody capable of reacting with the infecting organisms and normal tissues would thus be formed. Such may be the case in rheumatic heart disease, which follows infection with certain streptococci. Streptococcal M protein appears to be a hapten that cross-reacts with sarcolemmal antigens of heart muscle.

3. Polyclonal Lymphocyte Activation. It was mentioned earlier that in some instances self-tolerance may be

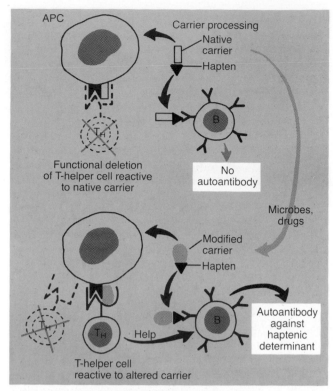

Figure 6–18. Tolerance of self-antigen (native carrier–hapten complex) owing to lack of T-cell help, and the loss of self-tolerance by modification of carrier.

maintained by anergy of autoreactive lymphocytes that were not deleted during development. Autoimmunity may occur if such self-reactive but anergic clones are stimulated and reactivated by antigen-independent mechanisms. In the case of B cells, several microbial products, especially endotoxins, can act as powerful polyclonal stimulants. Mice injected with endotoxins produce antibodies of many specificities, including autoantibodies. In humans such an event could follow infection with gram-negative bacteria. Infection of B cells with Epstein-Barr virus (EBV) could also achieve the same effects since all human B cells are activated by EBV.

IMBALANCE OF SUPPRESSOR-HELPER T-CELL FUNCTION. It may be expected from our discussion of suppressor T cells that any loss of their function will contribute to autoimmunity and, conversely, excessive T-cell help may drive B cells to extremely high levels of autoantibody production. Experimental evidence indeed suggests that this is true. There is an age-associated loss of suppressor T cells in the NZB × NZW (F1) mice, which develop an autoimmune disease similar to SLE as they age. Defects in suppressor T cell function or numbers (or both) have also been reported in human SLE, but this subject remains controversial. Enhanced helper T cell function manifested in the form of chronic hypersecretion of cytokines is seen in the SLE–prone MRL-1pr/1pr mice, and a somewhat similar increase in helper cell activity is also noted in certain patients with lupus.

Genetic Factors in Autoimmunity _____

There is little doubt that genetic factors play a significant role in the predisposition to autoimmune diseases. This conclusion is derived from three lines of evidence:

● Familial clustering of several human autoimmune diseases such as systemic lupus erythematosus, autoimmune hemolytic anemia, and autoimmune thyroiditis.
● Linkage of several autoimmune diseases with HLA, especially class II antigens.
● Induction of autoimmune diseases in transgenic rats. In humans, HLA-B27 is strongly associated with occurrence of certain autoimmune diseases such as ankylosing spondylitis. When cloned human HLA-B27 gene is introduced into the germ line of rats, some transgenic rats develop ankylosing spondylitis. This model provides direct evidence for genetic regulation of autoimmunity.

The precise role of MHC genes in autoimmunity is not entirely clear. Much attention has been focused on the mechanisms by which certain class II molecules predispose to autoimmunity. It is postulated that MHC antigens influence the clonal deletion of potentially autoreactive T cells within the thymus. Because clonal deletion in the thymus is based on high-affinity binding of the T-cell receptors with self antigens presented by class II molecules, it follows that if a given MHC allele presents an autoantigen poorly, the relevant autoreactive T-cell clone may not be deleted. Individuals who inherit such class II molecules may therefore be at increased risk of developing autoimmunity. A striking example, in this context, is presented by the association of type I (autoimmune) diabetes mellitus with certain HLA-DQ molecules (p. 57).

Microbial Agents in Autoimmunity _____

A variety of microbes, including bacteria, mycoplasmas, and viruses, have been implicated in triggering autoimmunity at one time or another.

Microbes may trigger autoimmune reactions in several ways. First, microbial antigens and autoantigens may become associated to form immunogenic units and bypass T-cell tolerance, as described earlier (p. 138). Second, some viruses (such as EBV) and bacterial products are nonspecific polyclonal B-cell mitogens and may thus induce formation of autoantibodies. Third, infection may result in loss of suppressor T-cell function by mechanisms that at present are not entirely clear. Viruses and other microbes, particularly certain bacteria such as streptococci and *Klebsiella* organisms, may share cross-reacting epitopes with self antigens, as discussed earlier. It must be obvious that there is no dearth of possible, and some plausible, mechanisms by which infectious agents may participate in the pathogenesis of autoimmunity. However, at present there is no clear evidence to implicate any microbe in the causation of human autoimmune disease.

Against this general background we turn to the individual systemic autoimmune diseases. Although each disease is discussed separately, it will be apparent that there is considerable overlap in their clinical, serologic, and morphologic features. Indeed, in some instances the term "overlap syndrome" best describes the patient's condition.

SYSTEMIC LUPUS ERYTHEMATOSUS _____

SLE is a febrile, inflammatory, multisystem disease of protean manifestations and variable behavior. It is best characterized by the following features: (1) *Clinically,* it is an unpredictable, remitting, relapsing disease of acute or insidious onset that may involve virtually any organ in the body; however, it principally affects the skin, kidneys, serosal membranes, joints, and heart. (2) *Anatomically,* all sites of involvement have in common vascular lesions with fibrinoid deposits. (3) *Immunologically,* the disease involves a bewildering array of antibodies of presumed autoimmune origin, especially antinuclear antibodies. The clinical presentation of SLE is so variable and bears so many similarities to other autoimmune connective tissue diseases (rheumatoid arthritis, polymyositis-dermatomyositis, and others) that it has been necessary to develop diagnostic criteria (Table 6–5). If a patient demonstrates four or more of the criteria during any interval of observation, the diagnosis of SLE is established.

SLE is a fairly common disease; its incidence may be as high as one case per 2500 persons in certain populations. There is a strong female preponderance —about 10 to 1. It usually arises in the second or third decade of life but may become manifest at any age, even in early childhood. The disease is more common and severe in black Americans.

ETIOLOGY AND PATHOGENESIS. A mountain of evidence points toward an autoimmune pathogenesis for SLE, but the cause or causes of the bewildering array of autoimmune reactions in these patients still elude us. First we shall present some of the immunologic findings, followed by the theories that attempt to explain their origins.

A host of autoantibodies, some of which may react with several targets, have been identified against both nuclear and cytoplasmic components of cells. *Antinuclear antibodies (ANA)* are directed against several nuclear antigens and can be grouped into four categories: (1) antibodies to DNA, (2) antibodies to histones, (3) antibodies to nonhistone proteins bound to RNA, (4) antibodies to nucleolar antigens. Several techniques are employed to detect ANAs. Clinically, the most commonly utilized method is indirect immunofluorescence, which detects a variety of nuclear antigens including DNA, RNA, and proteins *(generic ANA).* The pattern of nuclear fluorescence suggests the type of antibody present in the patient's serum. Four basic patterns are recognized:

● *Homogeneous or diffuse staining* usually reflects antibodies to deoxyribonucleoprotein and histones.
● *Rim or peripheral staining* patterns are most com-

TABLE 6–5. THE 1982 REVISED CRITERIA FOR THE CLASSIFICATION OF SLE*

1. Butterfly rash
2. Discoid lupus
3. Photosensitivity
4. Oral ulcers
5. Arthritis
6. Serositis
   a. Pleuritis: rub heard by a physician or pleural effusion, or
   b. Pericarditis: documented by EKG or rub, or evidence of pericardial effusion
7. Renal disorder
   a. Persistent proteinuria > 0.5 gm/dl/day
   b. Cellular casts: may be red cell, hemoglobin, granular, tubular, or mixed
8. Neurologic disorder
   a. Seizures: in the absence of offending drugs or known metabolic derangements
   b. Psychosis in the absence of offending drugs
9. Hematopoetic disorder
   a. Hemolytic anemia: with reticulocytosis or
   b. Leukopenia: 4000 cells/μl on two or more occasions or
   c. Lymphopenia: 1500 cells/μl on two or more occasions or
   d. Thrombocytopenia: 100,000/μl in the absence of offending drugs
10. Immunologic disorder
    a. Positive LE cell preparation or
    b. Anti-DNA: presence of antibody to untreated DNA in abnormal titer or
    c. Anti-Sm: presence of antibody to Sm nuclear antigen or
    d. False-positive STS known to be positive for at least six months and confirmed by TPI or FTA tests
11. Antinuclear antibody. An abnormal titer of antinuclear antibody by immunofluorescence or an equivalent assay at any point in time and in the absence of drugs known to be associated with "drug-induced lupus" syndrome

Key: STS, Serologic test for syphilis; TPI, treponemal inhibition; FTA, fluorescent treponemal antibody.

* The proposed classification is based on 11 criteria. For the purpose of identifying patients in clinical studies, a person shall be said to have SLE if any four or more of the 11 criteria are present serially or simultaneously, during any interval of observation.

Modified from Tan, E. M., et al.: The 1982 revised criteria for the classification of systemic lupus erythematosus. Arthritis Rheum. *25*:1271, 1982. Reprinted from Arthritis and Rheumatism Journal, copyright 1982. Used by permission of the American Rheumatism Association.

monly indicative of antibodies to double-stranded DNA.
- *Speckled pattern* refers to the presence of uniform or variable-sized speckles. It reflects the presence of antibodies to non-DNA nuclear constituents such as antibodies to histones and ribonucleoproteins. These components are easily extracted with salt solutions, and hence are sometimes called extractable nuclear antigens (ENAs). Examples include Sm antigen and SS-A and SS-B antigens (Table 6–6).
- *Nucleolar pattern* refers to the presence of a few discrete spots of fluorescence within the nucleus that represent antibodies to nucleolar RNA. This pattern is reported most often in patients with systemic sclerosis.

It must be emphasized, however, that the patterns are not absolutely specific for the type of antibody. The immunofluorescence test for ANA is quite *sensitive* for the detection of SLE, but it is not *specific*.

Table 6–6 shows that the ANAs detected by this technique are present not only in SLE but also in several other related autoimmune diseases. Furthermore, approximately 10% of normal persons have low titers of these antibodies. Some clinically useful ANAs are listed in Table 6–6. It will be noted that *antibodies to double-stranded DNA and the so-called Smith (Sm) antigen are virtually diagnostic of SLE.*

In addition to antinuclear antibodies, lupus patients have a host of other autoantibodies. Some are directed against elements of the blood such as red cells, platelets, and lymphocytes; others are directed against phospholipids. In recent years there has been much interest in antiphospholipid antibodies. They are present in 30 to 40% of lupus patients and react with a wide variety of anionic phospholipids. Some bind to cardiolipin antigen, used in syphilis serology, and therefore lupus patients may have a false positive test result for syphilis. Because phospholipids are required for blood clotting, patients with antiphospholipid antibodies may display abnormalities of in vitro clotting tests such as partial thromboplastin time. Therefore these antibodies are sometimes referred to as "lupus anticoagulant." Despite having a circulating anticoagulant that delays clotting in vitro, these patients have complications associated with a *pro*coagulant state. They have venous and arterial thromboses, which may be associated with recurrent spontaneous miscarriages and focal cerebral or ocular ischemia. The pathogenesis of thrombosis in patients with antiphospholipid antibodies is unknown. Proposed mechanisms include direct endothelial cell injury, antibody-mediated platelet activation, and inhibition of endogenous anticoagulants such as protein C.

Genetic Factors. The evidence that supports a genetic predisposition for SLE takes many forms.
- There is a high rate of concordance (30%) in monozygotic twins.
- Family members have an increased risk of developing SLE and clinically unaffected first-degree relatives may reveal autoantibodies.
- In North American Caucasian populations there is a positive association between SLE and the DR-2, DR-3, genes of the HLA complex.
- Some lupus patients (~6%) have inherited deficiencies of complement components. Lack of complement presumably impairs removal of immune complexes from the circulation and favors tissue deposition, giving rise to tissue injury (p. 129).

Nongenetic Factors. The impact of nongenetic factors in initiating autoimmunity is best exemplified by the occurrence of an SLE-like syndrome in patients receiving several *drugs,* such as procainamide and hydralazine. Most patients treated with procainamide for more than six months develop ANAs, and clinical features of SLE appear in 15 to 20%. *Sex hormones* seem to exert an important influence on the occurrence of SLE. Androgens appear to protect, whereas estrogens seem to favor the development of SLE. Witness the overwhelming female preponderance of the disease. Exposure to ultraviolet light is another environmental factor that exacerbates the disease in many individuals. Ultraviolet light may alter the anti-

TABLE 6-6. PREVALENCE OF ANTINUCLEAR
ANTIBODIES IN VARIOUS AUTOIMMUNE DISEASES*

Nature of Antigen	Antibody System	Disease				
		SLE (%)	Systemic Sclerosis —Diffuse (%)	Limited Scleroderma (%)	Sjögren's Syndrome (%)	Polymyositis (%)
Many nuclear antigens (DNA, RNA, proteins)	Generic ANA (indirect IF)	>95	70–90	70–90	50–80	40–60
Native DNA	Anti–double stranded DNA	40–60	<5	<5	<5	<5
Ribonucleoprotein (Smith antigen)	Anti-SM	20–30	<5	<5	<5	<5
Ribonucleoprotein	SS-A(Ro)	30–40	<5	<5	70–95	10
Ribonucleoprotein	SS-B(La)	15	<5	<5	60–90	<5
DNA topoisomerase I	Scl-70	<5	40–70	10	<5	<5
Centromeric proteins	Anticentromere	<5	<10	90	<5	<5
Histidyl-tRNA synthetase	Jo-1	<5	<5	<5	<5	25

Boxed entries indicate high correlation.
* Modified from Tan, E. M., et al.: Antinuclear antibodies (ANAs): Diagnostically specific immune markers and clues towards understanding systemic autoimmunity. Clin. Immunol. Immunopathol. 47: 121, 1988; McCarty, G. A.: Autoantibodies and their relation to rheumatic diseases. Med. Clin. North Am. 70:237, 1986; and Bernstein, R. M., and Matthews, M. B.: Autoantibodies to intracellular antigens, with particular reference to t-RNA and related proteins in myositis. J. Rheumatol. 14(Suppl 13):83, 1987.

genicity of tissues or possibly modulate immune responses.

Immunologic Factors. With the host of autoantibodies that have been described, it will come as no surprise that *B-cell hyperactivity is fundamental to the pathogenesis of SLE.* There is overwhelming evidence that B cells are "turned on" in these patients. The activation of B cells is polyclonal, and as such there is *increased production of antibodies to both self and nonself antigens.* What is the basis of this B-cell hyperactivity? In theory, excessive B-cell activation could result from an intrinsic defect in B cells, excessive stimulation by helper T cells, or a defect in suppressor T cells that fail to dampen the B-cell response. Studies with several murine models of SLE and analyses of immune cell populations in patients with SLE reveal that B-cell hyperactivity arises by diverse mechanisms, and evidence implicating each of the three pathways cited above has been uncovered. Thus it appears that SLE is a syndrome that can result from several different forms of immunologic derangements.

Mechanisms of Tissue Injury. Regardless of the exact sequence by which autoantibodies are formed, they are clearly the mediators of tissue injury. Most of the visceral lesions are mediated by immune complexes (type III hypersensitivity). DNA–anti-DNA complexes can be detected in the glomeruli. It is believed that free DNA binds first to the basement membrane, followed by the formation of DNA–anti-DNA complexes in situ. Low levels of serum complement and granular deposits of complement and immunoglobulins in the glomeruli further support the immune complex nature of the disease. On the other hand, autoantibodies against red cells, white cells, and platelets mediate their effects via type II hypersensitivity. There is no evidence that ANAs, which are involved in immune complex formation, can permeate intact cells. However, if cell nuclei are exposed, the ANAs can bind to them. In tissues, nuclei of damaged cells react with ANAs, lose their chromatin pattern, and become homogeneous, to produce so-called *LE bodies* or *hematoxylin bodies.* Related to this phenomenon is the *LE cell, which is seen only in vitro. Basically, the LE cell is any phagocytic leukocyte (neutrophil or macrophage) that has engulfed the denatured nucleus of an injured cell.* When blood is withdrawn and agitated, a sufficient number of leukocytes can be damaged to thus expose their nuclei to ANAs. The LE cell test is positive in up to 70% of patients with SLE. However, with newer techniques for detection of ANA, this test is now largely of historical interest.

To summarize, SLE appears to be a multifactorial disease involving complex interactions among genetic, hormonal, and environmental factors, all of which presumably act in concert to produce pronounced B-cell activation, resulting in the production of several autoantibodies. Each factor may be necessary but not enough per se for the expression of disease, and the relative importance of various factors may vary in different individuals.

MORPHOLOGY. The morphologic changes in SLE result largely from the formation of immune complexes in a variety of tissues. SLE is therefore a systemic disease with protean manifestations. Although many organs may be involved, some are affected more than others (Table 6–7). We will first discuss changes in small blood vessels that are common to all the affected tissues and then the specific anatomic lesions in the organs most frequently involved.

An **acute necrotizing vasculitis** affecting small arteries and arterioles classically is present in most affected tissues and organs (Fig. 6–19). The arteritis is characterized by necrosis and fibrinoid deposits within the vessel walls. Immunoglobulins, DNA, the third component of complement (C3), and fibrinogen have been found in the fibrinoid deposits within the arterial and arteriolar lesions. At a later stage, the involved vessels undergo fibrous thickening with luminal narrowing. Frequently, a perivascular lymphocytic infiltrate is present.

Skin lesions are prominent clinical findings in these patients. Classically, the lesion is an erythematous or maculopapular eruption over the malar eminences and bridge of the nose, creating a butterfly pattern. It is usually exacerbated by exposure to sunlight or to ultraviolet light in tanning parlors. Microscopically the areas of involvement show liquefactive degeneration of the basal layer of the epidermis, edema at the dermoepidermal junction, and swelling and apparent fusion of collagen fibers (Fig. 6–20). In an occasional patient the rash may occur on the neck, chest, back, or abdomen and may even be purpuric, bullous, or vesicular.

Deposits of immunoglobulin and complement can be seen along the dermoepidermal junction, in both the involved and the **uninvolved skin.** The granular immunoglobulin deposits in the uninvolved skin are considered highly specific for SLE and help differentiate it from other immunologic diseases with skin involvement. Twenty to thirty per cent of patients develop so-called **discoid lupus.** This takes the form of coin-shaped or

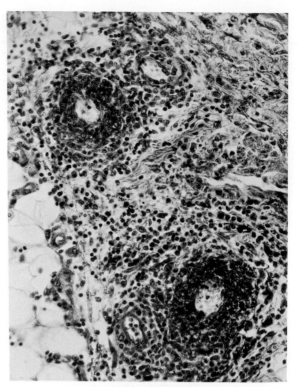

Figure 6–19. SLE. Two small arteries exhibit an acute necrotizing angiitis that has virtually destroyed the vessel walls. There is an extensive perivascular inflammatory infiltrate.

disc-like erythematous raised patches with adherent keratotic scaling, which may progress to atrophic scarring. These lesions may be present anywhere on the body. Discoid lesions may be present without the characteristic systemic involvement of SLE but approximately 5 to 10% of such cases eventually progress to SLE.

Serosal membranes, particularly the pericardium and pleura, may exhibit a variety of changes ranging from serous effusions or fibrinous exudation in acute cases to fibrous opacification in chronic cases. During the acute stages of serositis there is microscopic evidence of edema, focal vasculitis with perivascular lymphocytic infiltration, and foci of fibrinoid necrosis.

Cardiovascular system involvement is manifested primarily in the form of pericarditis. Symptomatic or asymptomatic pericardial involvement is present in the vast majority of patients. Myocarditis, manifested as nonspecific mononuclear cell infiltration, may also be present, but is less common. It may cause resting tachycardia and electrocardiographic abnormalities. Valvular endocarditis may occur, but it is clinically insignificant. In the era before the widespread use of steroids, the so-called Libman-Sacks endocarditis was more common. This **nonbacterial verrucous endocarditis** takes the form of single or multiple irregular 1 to 3 mm warty deposits on any valve in the heart, distinctively on **either surface of the leaflets** (i.e., on the surface exposed to the forward flow of the blood or on the underside of the

TABLE 6–7. DISTRIBUTION OF LESIONS IN SLE

Site of Lesion	Approximate Percentage of Cases
Joints*	95
Kidneys*	60
Heart*	50
Serous membranes*	40
Skin	80
Lymph node enlargement	60
Gastrointestinal tract	30
Central nervous system	30
Liver	25
Spleen	20
Eyes	20
Lungs	15
Peripheral nervous system	10

* Lesions cause major clinical findings.

Figure 6–20. Systemic lupus erythematosus involving the skin. *(A)* A hematoxylin and eosin–stained section shows liquefactive degeneration of the basal layer of epidermis and edema at the dermoepidermal junction. *(B)* Immunofluorescence micrograph stained for IgG reveals deposits of immunoglobulin along the dermoepidermal junction. (Courtesy of Dr. Candace Kasper, Department of Pathology, Southwestern Medical School, Dallas, TX.)

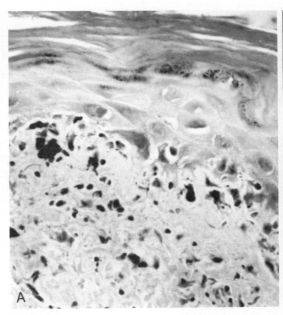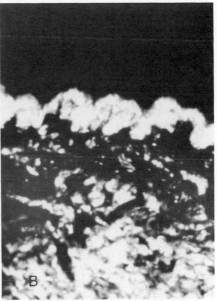

leaflet) (Fig. 6–21). Histologic examination of these lesions reveals deposits of fibrinoid associated with a surrounding mononuclear inflammatory reaction followed later by collagenization of the areas of inflammation.

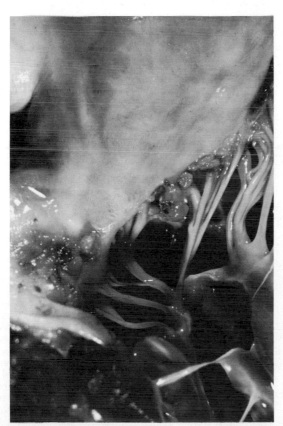

Figure 6–21. Libman-Sacks endocarditis of the mitral valve in lupus erythematosus. The small vegetations attached to the margin of the valve leaflet are easily seen.

Kidney involvement is one of the most important anatomic features of SLE, and renal failure is an important cause of death. Although the kidney appears normal by light microscopy in 30 to 40% of cases, almost all cases of SLE show some renal abnormality if examined by immunofluorescence and electron microscopy. According to the World Health Organization morphologic classification, five patterns are recognized: (1) normal by light-, electron-, and immunofluorescent microscopy (class I), which is quite rare; (2) mesangial lupus glomerulonephritis (class II); (3) focal glomerulonephritis (class III); (4) diffuse proliferative glomerulonephritis (class IV); and (5) membranous glomerulonephritis (class V)

Mesangial lupus nephritis is associated with mild clinical symptoms. There is a slight increase in the mesangial matrix and cellularity. However, granular mesangial deposits of IgG and C3 are almost invariably present, even in minimally affected glomeruli. Such deposits presumably represent the earliest change, since filtered immune complexes aggregate primarily in the mesangium, where they may be catabolized. Not infrequently, therefore, other alterations (to be described) are superimposed on the mesangial changes.

Focal glomerulonephritis implies involvement of only portions of fewer than 50% of glomeruli. Typically, one or several glomerular lobules within an otherwise normal glomerulus exhibit swelling and proliferation of endothelial and mesangial cells, foci of acute capillary necrosis infiltrated with neutrophils, and sometimes fibrinoid deposits and intracapillary thrombi. Focal lesions are usually associated with mild clinical manifestations such as microscopic hematuria and some proteinuria. Transitions to more serious forms of renal involvement may occur in some patients.

Diffuse proliferative glomerulonephritis is the most common form of renal lesion, affecting 45 to 50% of patients. The anatomic changes are dominated by proliferation of endothelial, mesangial, and, sometimes, epithelial cells. Thus there is hypercellularity of the glomeruli. Sometimes macrophages and proliferated epithelial cells fill Bowman's space to create crescent-shaped masses of cells, not surprisingly referred to as "crescents." In time these changes lead to sclerosis of the glomeruli. Most or all glomeruli are involved in both kidneys, and almost always entire glomeruli are affected. These patients are overtly symptomatic. Most have hematuria with moderate to severe proteinuria, hypertension, and renal insufficiency.

Membranous glomerulonephritis is the designation given to glomerular disease in which the principal histologic change consists of widespread thickening of the capillary wall. Membranous glomerulonephritis associated with SLE is very similar if not identical to that encountered in idiopathic membranous glomerulopathy and is described more fully on page 445. Thickening of glomerular capillary walls is the consequence of both the increased deposition of basement membrane–like material and the presence of irregular clumps of immune complexes deposited on the basement membrane. In advanced cases glomerular sclerosis may supervene. This form of glomerular lesion is almost always associated with severe proteinuria or the overt nephrotic syndrome (p. 444).

The pathogenesis of all forms of glomerulonephritis involves the deposition of DNA–anti-DNA complexes within the glomeruli. The immune deposits are seen within the mesangium as well as in subendothelial, intramembranous, and subepithelial locations. Subendothelial deposits are common in the diffuse proliferative variety but may occur in the membranous type as well (Fig. 6–22). When extensive, these deposits create a peculiar thickening of the capillary wall, which appears to resemble rigid "wire loops" on routine light microscopy (Fig. 6–23). Subepithelial deposits are relatively common in the membranous form of lupus nephritis.

Grossly, kidneys in lupus may be normal in size and color during the acute stages but sometimes are enlarged, pale, and dotted with punctate cortical hemorrhages. When glomerular sclerosis supervenes, contraction and a diffuse, fine cortical granularity appear.

Interstitial and tubular lesions are also seen in SLE. In approximately 50% of patients, granular deposits composed of immunoglobulin and complement are present around the tubules. Immune complex–mediated tubule injury leads to diffuse interstitial fibrosis.

Joint involvement, although very common clinically, **usually is not associated with striking anatomic changes nor with joint deformity.** When present it consists of swelling and a nonspecific mononuclear cell infiltration in the synovial membranes, occasionally accompanied by some increase in ground substance and focal areas of fibrinoid necrosis in the subepithelial connective tissue. Erosion of the membranes and destruction of articular cartilage such as occurs with rheumatoid arthritis is exceedingly rare. For this reason, even in advanced cases, permanent disabling joint disease is very uncommon in SLE.

Despite frequent clinical involvement, the morphologic basis of **central nervous system** symptoms is not clear. Proposed mechanisms include acute vasculitis with focal neurologic symptoms, and damage caused by neuron-reactive antibodies. Neuropsychiatric manifestations are seen more commonly in patients with antiphospholipid antibodies, but the basis of this association remains unclear.

The **spleen** may be of normal size or moderately enlarged. Capsular fibrous thickening is common, as is

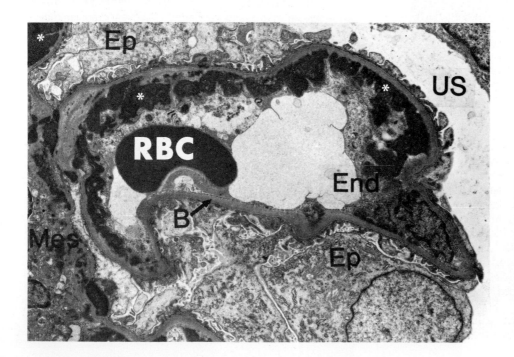

Figure 6–22. Electron micrograph of renal glomerular capillary loop from patient with systemic lupus erythematosus nephritis. Subendothelial dense deposits correspond to "wire loops" seen by light microscopy. (End, endothelium; Mes, mesangium; Ep, epithelial cell with foot processes; RBC, red blood cell in capillary lumen; B, basement membrane; US, urinary space; *, electron-dense deposits in subendothelial location. (Courtesy of Dr. Edwin Eigenbrodt. Department of Pathology, Southwestern Medical School, Dallas, TX.)

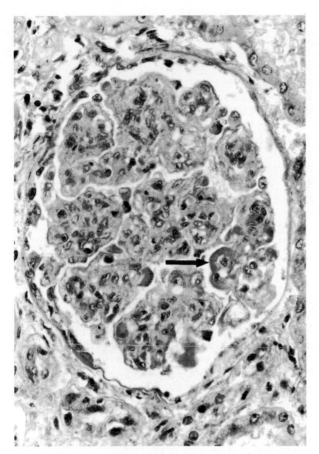

Figure 6-23. Lupus nephritis. A glomerulus with "wire loop" thickening of the basement membrane. (Courtesy of Dr. Fred Silva, Department of Pathology, Southwestern Medical School, Dallas, TX.)

follicular hyperplasia. One of the most constant alterations in spleens of both normal and abnormal size is a marked perivascular fibrosis, producing so-called **onion-skin lesions** around the central penicilliary arteries.

Many **other organs and tissues** may be involved. The changes consist essentially of acute vasculitis of the small vessels, foci of mononuclear infiltrations, and fibrinoid deposits. In addition, lungs may reveal interstitial fibrosis, along with pleural inflammation; liver reveals nonspecific inflammation of the portal tracts.

CLINICAL MANIFESTATIONS. The diagnosis of SLE may be obvious in a young female with a classic butterfly rash over the face, fever, pain but no deformity in one or more peripheral joints (feet, ankles, knees, hips, fingers, wrists, elbows, shoulders), pleuritic chest pain, and photosensitivity. However, in many patients the presentation of SLE is subtle and puzzling, taking forms such as a febrile illness of unknown origin, abnormal urinary findings, or joint disease masquerading as rheumatoid arthritis or rheumatic fever. ANAs can be found in virtually 100% of patients, but they can also be found in 50 to 80% of those with Sjögren's syndrome, in 80% with systemic sclerosis, and in 15 to 25% with adult rheumatoid arthritis, as well as in patients with other autoimmune

disorders. As mentioned earlier, anti–double-stranded DNA antibodies are considered highly diagnostic of SLE, and their titer seems to be correlated with the severity of renal disease. A variety of clinical findings may point toward renal involvement, including hematuria, red cell casts, proteinuria, and, in some cases, the classic nephrotic syndrome (p. 445). Varying levels of azotemia and renal failure are encountered in those with diffuse proliferative or membranous glomerulonephritis, or both. In most patients focal glomerulonephritis produces recurrent hematuria and mild proteinuria, but approximately 30% of patients with focal lesions develop renal failure. The hematologic derangements mentioned (Table 6-5) may in some cases be the presenting manifestation as well as the dominant clinical problem. In still others, mental aberrations, including psychosis or convulsions, may constitute prominent clinical problems. In addition, patients with SLE often have small retinal exudates (cytoid bodies) and such nonspecific complaints as malaise, anorexia, vomiting, and weakness.

The course of SLE is extremely variable and virtually unpredictable. Some unfortunate individuals have an acute onset and follow a progressively downhill course to death within months. More often the disease is characterized by flare-ups and remissions spanning a period of years and even decades. Acute attacks are usually treated by adrenocortical steroids or immunosuppressive drugs, and these drugs often control the acute manifestations. With cessation of therapy the disease usually recurs and is exacerbated. The prognosis appears to have improved significantly in the recent past; approximately 76% are alive 10 years after the onset of illness. In some part this apparent improvement derives from the earlier diagnosis and the recognition of milder forms of the disease. In addition to renal failure, other important causes of death are diffuse central nervous system involvement, intercurrent infections, and uncontrolled acute febrile illness.

RHEUMATOID ARTHRITIS

Rheumatoid arthritis (RA) is a systemic, chronic inflammatory disease that affects principally the joints and sometimes many other organs and tissues throughout the body as well. More specifically, *the disease is characterized by a nonsuppurative proliferative synovitis, which in time leads to the destruction of articular cartilage and progressive disabling arthritis.* When extraarticular involvement develops—for example, of the skin, heart, blood vessels, muscles, and lungs—RA assumes more than a passing resemblance to SLE, scleroderma, and polymyositis-dermatomyositis, and, along with these entities, is sometimes referred to as a connective tissue disease.

RA is a very common condition with a prevalence of approximately 1%. It usually has its onset in the third or fourth decade but may begin at any age. It is three to five times more common in women than in men. Since the pathogenesis of this condition will be facilitated by a knowledge of the morphologic changes, these will be reviewed first.

MORPHOLOGY. RA is a systemic disease that can cause significant damage to many organs. Its most destructive effects are seen in the joints. It produces symmetric arthritis, which affects principally the small joints of the hands and feet, ankles, knees, wrists, elbows, and shoulders. Typically, the proximal interphalangeal and metacarpophalangeal joints are affected, but distal interphalangeal joints are spared. Axial involvement, when it occurs, is limited to upper cervical spine; similarly hip joint involvement is extremely uncommon. The process begins as a nonspecific inflammatory synovitis characterized by swelling and hypertrophy of the synoviocytes and the underlying connective tissues. More advanced chronic synovitis shows (1) proliferation of synovial lining cells as well as subjacent cells, often with palisading of the synoviocytes; (2) marked hypertrophy of the synovium, with the formation of villi (finger-like projections); (3) lymphocytic and plasma cell infiltration (with perivascular predilection), sometimes with formation of lymphocytic nodules; (4) focal deposits of fibrinoid; and (5) foci of cellular necrosis (Fig. 6–24). The highly vascularized, inflammatory, reduplicated synovium that covers the articular cartilaginous surfaces is known as a **pannus** (mantle). With full-blown inflammatory joint involvement, periarticular soft tissue edema usually develops, which is classically manifested first by fusiform swelling of the proximal interphalangeal joints. Later, swelling of other affected joints may appear. With progression of the disease, the articular cartilage subja-

cent to the pannus is eroded and in time virtually destroyed. The subarticular bone may also be attacked and eroded. Eventually the pannus fills the joint space, and subsequent fibrosis and calcification may cause permanent ankylosis. A number of additional changes occur simultaneously.

Early in the disease the synovial fluid is increased in volume, becomes turbid because of an inflammatory infiltrate, and loses some of its mucin content (thus forming a poor mucin clot when mixed with dilute acetic acid). Although the synovial membrane is infiltrated by chronic inflammatory cells, the synovial fluid contains acute inflammatory cells. The contained neutrophils exhibit granular inclusions of phagocytized immune complexes. Joint motion may cause erosion of the exuberant pannus, leading to bleeding and fibrin clots. The eroded, devascularized cartilage may undergo calcification and fragmentation, adding foreign bodies to the inflammatory process. Osteoarthritis may supervene and compound the articular disability. The periarticular inflammatory response may lead to local myositis, followed by muscle atrophy, and is sometimes accompanied by more remote focal myositis in the form of collections of lymphocytes, plasma cells, and occasional epithelioid cells. Collectively, then, the musculoskeletal lesions in progressive disease cause marked motor disability and even permanent crippling disease.

Rheumatoid subcutaneous nodules eventually appear in about a quarter of patients; the nodules usually occur along the extensor surface of the forearm or other areas subjected to mechanical pressure. They are firm, nontender, oval or rounded masses up to 2 cm in

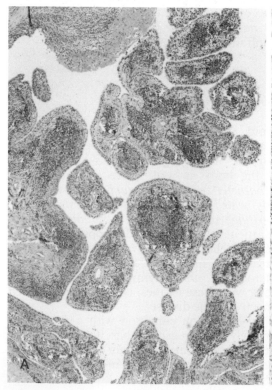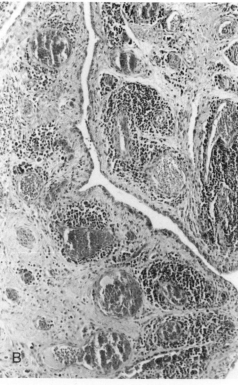

Figure 6–24. Rheumatoid arthritis. *(A)* Low magnification reveals marked synovial hypertrophy with formation of villi. *(B)* At higher magnification, highly vascular subsynovial tissue containing dense lymphoid aggregates is seen. (Courtesy of Dr. Sara Milchgrub and Mr. Rich Pucci, Department of Pathology, Southwestern Medical School, Dallas, TX.)

diameter. Less commonly these nodules appear in the Achilles tendons, on the back of the skull, overlying the ischial tuberosities, or along the tibia. They are characterized by a central focus of fibrinoid necrosis surrounded by a palisade of macrophages, which in turn is rimmed by granulation tissue. Rheumatoid nodules may also involve the viscera, including lung, spleen, pericardium, aorta, and the heart valves.

As it is a systemic disease, a number of other structures may be affected in RA. Acute necrotizing vasculitis may involve small or large arteries. Serosal involvement may manifest itself as fibrinous pleuritis or pericarditis, or both. Lung parenchyma may be damaged by progressive interstitial fibrosis. Ocular changes such as uveitis and keratoconjunctivitis (similar to those seen in Sjögren's syndrome) may be prominent in some cases.

ETIOLOGY AND PATHOGENESIS. There is little doubt that there is a genetic predisposition to RA and that the joint inflammation is immunologically mediated; however, the initiating agent(s) and the precise interplay between genetic and environmental factors remain to be clarified.

In all likelihood the disease is initiated by activation of helper T cells responding to some arthritogenic agent (microbe). Activated CD4+ cells produce a number of cytokines that have two principal effects: (1) activation of macrophages and other cells in the joint space, which release tissue-destructive enzymes and other factors that perpetuate inflammation, and (2) activation of the B-cell system, resulting in the production of antibodies, some of which are directed against self constituents; the resultant autoimmune reactions damage the joints and are believed to play an important role in disease progression. In the context of this general scheme we can now discuss the roles of genetic factors, T cells, cytokines, B cells, and infectious agents (Fig. 6–25).

Immunogenetics. The importance of genetic factors in the pathogenesis of RA is supported by the increased frequency of this disease among first-degree relatives and a high concordance rate in monozygotic twins. The role of genetic factors is further strengthened by the association of RA with certain class II MHC genes. A majority of patients with RA carry HLA-DR4 or HLA-DR1, or both. Recent molecular studies have revealed that the susceptibility-associated DR alleles share a common stretch of four amino acids located in the antigen-binding cleft of the DR molecule. Thus it seems that the *association between certain DR molecules and RA may be explained by the capacity of individuals carrying these DR determinants to bind an arthritogenic antigen, which in turn activates helper T cells and initiates disease.* Since HLA-DR molecules are critical for presentation of antigens to T cells, these molecular studies also support the primacy of T-cell immunity in the pathogenesis of RA.

T Cells. As mentioned earlier, rheumatoid synovium is heavily infiltrated with lymphocytes. The vast majority of these are CD4+ helper T-cells, which are often clustered in perivascular nodules in close contact with HLA-DR+ antigen-presenting cells. This cellular arrangement suggests in situ antigen presentation and activation of T cells. The role for T lymphocytes in initiating or perpetuating the disease is also supported by the observed improvement in symptoms when T cells are depleted by either thoracic duct drainage or total lymphoid irradiation.

Cytokines. Activated CD4+ cells are a well known source of cytokines, which activate other immune cells (e.g., B cells, other T cells) as well as macrophages. The latter in turn themselves secrete a variety of proinflammatory and tissue-degrading factors. The rheumatoid synovium is embarrassingly rich in both lymphocyte- and monocyte-derived cytokines. Included in this list are IL-1, IL-2, IL-6, GM-CSF, IFN-γ, and TNF-α and TGF-β. The activity of these cytokines can account for many features of rheumatoid synovitis. IL-1, TNF-α, IL-6, and IL-2, for example, promote T- and B-cell differentiation; IFN-γ, GM-CSF, and IL-2 activate macrophages. Local proliferation of synoviocytes and fibroblasts is stimulated by IL-1 and TGF-β. Finally, IL-1 stimulates synovial cells and chondrocytes to secrete proteolytic and matrix-degrading enzymes. Because of the multiple effects of IL-1 in initiating joint inflammation, it is not surprising that inhibitors of IL-1 are receiving serious consideration as therapeutic tools in RA and other inflammatory joint diseases.

B cells. Until recently, humoral autoimmunity was considered to be the primary abnormality in RA. This view was based on finding rheumatoid factors (RFs), which are autoantibodies in serum and synovial fluids directed against the Fc portion of IgG. Such autoantibodies exist among all immunoglobulin classes. The significance of circulating RFs in the pathogenesis is uncertain, but their presence in the joints is believed to contribute to the inflammatory reaction. Synovial fluid IgG rheumatoid factors self-associate (IgG–anti-IgG) to form immune complexes that fix complement, attract polymorphonuclear leukocytes, and lead to tissue injury by the classical type III hypersensitivity reaction (p. 127). Although there is general agreement that rheumatoid factors amplify joint inflammation, most investigators believe that their formation is secondary to helper T cell–induced B-cell hyperactivity. Why antibodies against autologous IgG are formed when B cells are stimulated remains unclear.

Role of infectious agents. Finally we come to the elusive infectious agent(s) whose antigens activate T cells. Many candidates have been considered, but none chosen. Included in the category of suspects are EBV, mycoplasmas, parvoviruses, and mycobacteria. Circumstantial evidence implicating each of these exists but in no case has a causal relationship been established. However, similarities of RA to known infectious arthritides such as Lyme disease continue to intrigue investigators and so the search goes on. So we must leave it that, although *joint damage in RA is of immune origin and appears to occur in genetically*

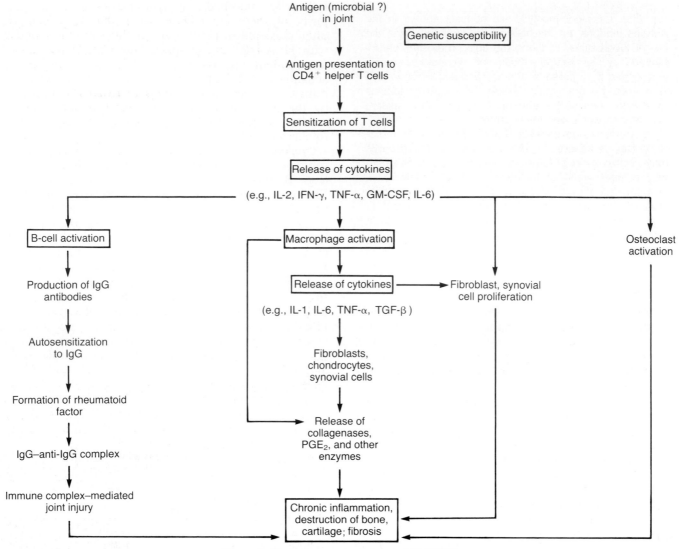

Figure 6–25. Pathogenesis of rheumatoid arthritis.

predisposed individuals, the precise trigger that initiates these reactions is still unknown.

CLINICAL COURSE. Although rheumatoid arthritis is basically a symmetric polyarticular arthritis, the joint involvement may be associated with constitutional symptoms such as weakness, malaise, and low-grade fever. Many of these systemic manifestations result from the same mediators that cause joint inflammation (e.g., IL-1 and TNF-α). The arthritis first appears insidiously, with aching and stiffness of the joints, particularly in the morning. As the disease advances the joints become enlarged, motion is limited, and in time complete ankylosis may appear. The fingers may become virtually immobilized in a claw-like position with ulnar deviation. At this stage of the disease, anemia is common. The vasculitis may give rise to Raynaud's phenomenon (p. 153), chronic leg ulcers, and gastrointestinal mucosal erosions, and indeed may cause infarction in the brain, heart, or intestines. It is obvious that with such multisystem involvement rheumatoid arthritis must be differentiated from systemic

lupus erythematosus, scleroderma, polymyositis-dermatomyositis, and Lyme disease, as well as other forms of arthritis. Helpful in differential diagnosis are (1) characteristic radiographic findings; (2) sterile, turbid synovial fluid with decreased viscosity, poor mucin clot formation, and inclusion-bearing leukocytes; and (3) rheumatoid factor (85 to 95% of patients). It must be appreciated, however, that rheumatoid factor may also be present with SLE, sarcoidosis, leprosy, syphilis, tuberculosis, bacterial endocarditis, and other diseases associated with persistent antigenemia.

The clinical course of RA is highly variable. In a minority of patients the disease may become stabilized or may even regress. Most of the remainder pursue a chronic, remitting, relapsing course. After 15 to 20 years, the majority of patients become permanently and severely crippled. RA is an important cause of reactive amyloidosis. This complication develops in 5 to 10% of these patients, particularly those with long-standing severe disease.

Variants of Rheumatoid Arthritis

Two variants of rheumatoid arthritis merit brief characterization. *Juvenile RA* refers to chronic idiopathic arthritis that occurs in children. It is not a single disease but a heterogeneous group of disorders that differ significantly from the adult form of RA. In general, the juvenile forms tend to involve large joints such as knees, wrists, and ankles rather than small joints. Rheumatoid factor and subcutaneous nodules are present only infrequently. One variant, previously called *Still's disease,* has an acute febrile onset and systemic manifestations including leukocytosis (15,000 to 25,000 cells per microliter), hepatosplenomegaly, lymphadenopathy, and skin rash. In about one third of patients the disease is monoarticular. Unlike those who have the classic form of RA, most patients with juvenile RA experience complete remission. *Felty's syndrome* comprises the triad of polyarthritis, splenomegaly, and leukopenia. In these patients the hematologic problems often dominate the clinical picture.

SPONDYLOARTHROPATHIES

For years, several entities in this group of disorders were considered variants of rheumatoid arthritis; however, careful clinical, morphologic, and genetic studies have revealed fundamental differences that distinguish these disorders from rheumatoid arthritis and hence they are segregated from it. The spondyloarthropathies are characterized by the following features:
- Pathologic changes that affect primarily the ligamentous attachments to bone rather than synovium.
- Frequent involvement of the sacroiliac joints along with peripheral inflammatory arthropathy.
- Absence of rheumatoid factor (hence the name seronegative spondyloarthropathies).
- Association with HLA-B27.

This group of disorders includes several clinical subsets, of which ankylosing spondylitis is the prototype. Others in this category are Reiter's syndrome, psoriatic arthropathy, spondylitis associated with inflammatory bowel diseases, and reactive arthropathies (that follow infections by *Yersinia, Shigella,* and *Salmonella* organisms). There is a considerable overlap in these conditions, and they are distinguished from each other according to the particular peripheral joint involved and associated extraskeletal manifestations (urethritis, conjunctivitis, uveitis; Table 6–8). It will be noted that sacroiliitis is common to all. Although these seronegative spondyloarthropathies are believed to be caused by immune mechanisms their pathogenesis remains obscure. As mentioned earlier (p. 139), clinical features of most of the spondyloarthropathies have been reproduced in HLA-B27 transgenic rats, clearly implicating the B27 gene in the pathogenesis of these conditions.

SJÖGREN'S SYNDROME

Sjögren's syndrome is a clinicopathologic entity characterized by dry eyes (keratoconjunctivitis sicca) and dry mouth (xerostomia) resulting from immune-mediated destruction of the lacrimal and salivary glands. It occurs as an isolated disorder (primary form), also known as the *sicca syndrome,* or more often in association with another autoimmune disease (secondary form). Among the associated disorders, RA is the most common, but some patients have SLE, polymyositis, systemic sclerosis, vasculitis, or thyroiditis.

ETIOLOGY AND PATHOGENESIS. Several lines of evidence support a role for *B-cell dysfunction* in the pathogenesis of Sjögren's syndrome, which is second only to SLE in its multiplicity of serum autoantibodies. Hypergammaglobulinemia is virtually always present, and most patients have rheumatoid factor in their sera, even in the absence of demonstrable RA. Approximately 50 to 80% of patients have antinuclear antibodies, and about 25% show positive results in the LE cell test. A majority of patients (~70%) with primary Sjögren's syndrome possess autoantibodies to two nuclear antigens, designated SS-A and SS-B. Those with anti SS-A antibodies are more likely to have systemic (extraglandular) manifestations. In view of the B-cell activation and formation of autoantibodies, it is not surprising that most patients have circulating immune complexes. The initial polyclonal B-cell activation gradually becomes oligoclonal, and in some patients eventually monoclonal, with the development of

TABLE 6–8. SOME FEATURES OF SPONDYLOARTHROPATHIES*

Feature	Ankylosing Spondylitis	Reiter's Syndrome	Psoriatic Arthropathy	Spondylitis with Inflammatory Bowel Disease	Reactive Arthropathy
HLA-B27	95%	80%	50%	50%	80%
Sacroiliitis	Always	Often	Often	Often	Often
Peripheral joints	Lower > upper (Often)	Lower usually	Upper > lower	Lower > upper	Lower > upper
Uveitis	++	++	+	+	+
Conjunctivitis	–	+	–	–	–
Urethritis	–	+	–	–	–
Skin involvement	–	+	++	–	–
Mucosal involvement	–	+	–	+	+

* Modified from Wyngaarden, J., Smith, L. H. (ed.): Cecil Textbook of Medicine. 18th ed. Philadelphia, W.B. Saunders, 1988, p. 2008.

a non-Hodgkin's lymphoma. The basis for all of these humoral immune reactions is still unclear; as with SLE, primary B-cell hyperactivity has been implicated. A role for T cells in the pathogenesis of Sjögren's syndrome is indicated by immunohistochemical studies of the inflammatory cells within the salivary and lacrimal glands. The infiltrate contains predominantly T cells of the helper phenotype, but some cytotoxic T cells are also found. It is tempting to speculate that the helper T cells aid both local formation of antibodies and activation of cytotoxic T cells, but firm evidence is lacking.

Genetic factors also play a role in the pathogenesis of Sjögren's syndrome. Patients with the primary form of the disease have an increased frequency of HLA-DR3, whereas those with associated rheumatoid arthritis are more likely to have HLA-DR4. These genetic studies suggest that despite several clinical similarities, patients with primary and secondary forms of Sjögren's syndrome constitute distinct subsets.

Morphology. The keratoconjunctivitis and xerostomia are the consequence of extensive damage to the lacrimal and salivary glands. Other secretory glands, including those in the nose, pharynx, larynx, trachea, bronchi, and vagina, may also be involved. When they are, all reveal an intense lymphocytic and plasma cell infiltration and destruction of the native architecture, similar to the changes encountered in Hashimoto's thyroiditis (p. 656; Fig. 6–26). Sometimes the lymphoid infiltrates create germinal follicles. These changes may be confused with lymphomatous invasion and, as noted above, in some instances true neoplastic transformation occurs.

The lack of tears in the eyes, resulting from the secretory lesions, leads to drying of the corneal epithelium, which becomes inflamed, eroded, and ulcerated. The oral mucosa may atrophy, with inflammatory fissuring and ulceration. Dryness and crusting of the nose may lead to ulcerations and even perforation of the nasal septum. When the respiratory passages are involved, secondary laryngitis, bronchitis, and pneumonitis may appear. Approximately 25% of the patients (especially those with anti-SS-A antibodies) develop extraglandular disease affecting the central nervous system, skin, kidneys, and muscles. Renal lesions take the form of mild interstitial nephritis associated with tubular transport defects. Unlike in SLE, glomerulonephritis is rare. Skin involvement is manifested by widespread vasculitis.

CLINICAL COURSE. Sjögren's syndrome predominantly affects females over 40 years of age. In approximately 60% of patients it is associated with other "connective tissue diseases." The diagnosis of primary Sjögren's syndrome can be made readily by the lack of moisture and by the secondary changes in the eyes and oral cavity. Some patients have mild arthritis, neuropathy, and Raynaud's phenomenon. Functional renal tubular defects, when present, include renal tubular acidosis, uricosuria, phosphaturia, and generalized

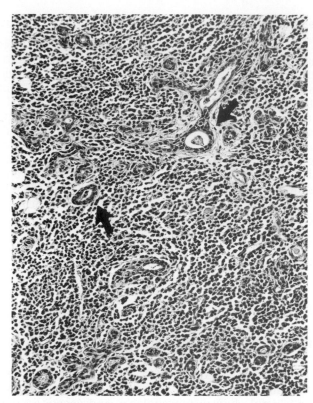

Figure 6–26. Sjögren's syndrome—submandibular gland. The intense lymphocytic and plasma cell infiltration virtually obscures the native architecture. Only a few residual ducts *(arrows)* can be identified.

aminoaciduria, characteristic of Fanconi's syndrome. Of particular interest is the development of B-cell lymphomas in approximately 1% of patients. In addition, about 10% of patients have had lesions designated as "pseudolymphomas." These comprise marked inflammatory hyperplastic changes within the salivary glands, bordering on the appearance of lymphoid cancer. It would therefore appear that in this disorder of probable immune origin, lymphoid hyperactivity may in time give rise to abnormal pseudolymphomatous proliferations and in some cases to true malignant lymphoid tumors.

SYSTEMIC SCLEROSIS

Although the designation *"scleroderma"* is time honored, this disorder is better called systemic sclerosis (SS) because it is characterized by inflammatory and fibrotic changes throughout the interstitium of many organs in the body. *Although skin involvement is the usual presenting symptom and eventually appears in approximately 95% of cases, it is the visceral involvement—of the gastrointestinal tract, lungs, kidneys, heart, and striated muscles—that produces the major disabilities and threatens life.* The disease may begin at any age, from infancy to the advanced years, but most often commences in the third to fifth decade.

Women are affected about three times more often than men.

In recent years, systemic sclerosis has been subclassified into two groups on the basis of its clinical course:

- *Diffuse scleroderma,* characterized by widespread skin involvement at onset, with rapid progression and early visceral involvement.
- *Limited scleroderma,* with relatively limited skin involvement, often confined to fingers and face. Involvement of the viscera occurs late, and hence in general the disease in these patients has a relatively benign course. This is also called the CREST syndrome (p. 153).

ETIOLOGY AND PATHOGENESIS. SS is a disease of unknown cause. Two major hypotheses have been offered: one favors a primary *immunologic* abnormality and the other affords primacy to *vascular injury* (Fig. 6–27). Regardless of the initiating event, it is obvious that activation of fibroblasts must be a part of the final common pathway in the pathogenesis of SS. Abnormal stimulation of SS fibroblasts is attested by their ability to synthesize and secrete excessive amounts of collagen when explanted in vitro. While increased biosynthesis of collagen is established, what triggers the fibroblasts to choke the tissue with collagen remains unknown.

According to the *immunologic hypothesis,* fibrosis is secondary to abnormal activation of the immune system. It is proposed that T cells responding to an as yet unidentified antigen accumulate in the skin and release cytokines that activate macrophages. Several monocyte-derived cytokines, such as IL-1, TNF-α, PDGF, and TGF-β can enhance fibroblast growth and up-regulate collagen synthesis. In support of this hypothesis, activated CD4+ helper T cells can be found in the skin of many patients with SS. Monocyte activation has also been documented. The possibility that the immune system may be playing a role in the pathogenesis of SS is further supported by the finding that several features of this disease (including the cutaneous sclerosis) are found in human GVH disease, a disorder that results from activation of T cells (p. 135). The presence of nonspecific serologic abnormalities such as hypergammaglobulinemia (50% of the cases), antinuclear antibodies (70 to 90% of cases), and rheumatoid factor (25% of cases) points to a possible role for disordered humoral immunity as well. Recently two antinuclear antibodies more or less unique to systemic sclerosis have been described. One of these, directed against DNA topoisomerase I, is highly specific; it is present in 28 to 70% of patients with diffuse scleroderma and in less than 1% of patients with other connective tissue diseases. The other, an anti-centromere antibody, is found in 80 to 90% of the patients with limited scleroderma (i.e., the CREST syndrome).

The *vascular hypothesis* rests on the consistent presence of microvascular disease early in the course of SS. Intimal fibrosis is evident in 100% of digital arteries of patients with SS. According to this view, recurrent endothelial injury affecting the microvasculature is the primary event. Telltale signs of endothelial injury (increased levels of factor VIII-von Willebrand factor) and increased platelet activation (increased percentage of circulating platelet aggregates) have been noted. It is proposed that repeated cycles of endothelial injury followed by platelet aggregation lead to release of platelet factors (e.g., PDGF, TGF-β) that trigger peri-adventitial fibrosis and eventual ischemic injury caused by widespread narrowing of the microvasculature. However, this simple and otherwise attractive hypothesis fails to explain the host of immunologic abnormalities noted in SS, so the mystery surrounding the pathogenesis of SS persists.

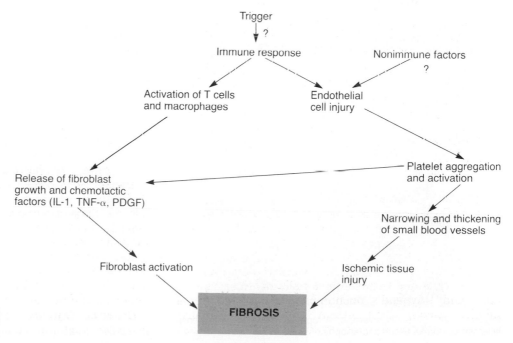

Figure 6–27. A schematic illustration of the possible mechanisms leading to systemic sclerosis.

MORPHOLOGY. Virtually any organ may be affected in SS, but the most prominent changes are found in the skin, musculoskeletal system, gastrointestinal tract, lungs, kidneys, and heart.

The changes in the **skin** almost always begin in the fingers and distal regions of the upper extremities and extend proximally to involve the upper arm, shoulders, neck, and face. In advanced cases the entire back and abdomen as well as the lower extremities may be affected. The earliest changes consist only of some dermal edema and possibly some increased ground substance, but as the disease advances, there is considerable increase in dermal collagen, with epidermal atrophy and loss of skin adnexa (Fig. 6–28). The walls of dermal capillaries and arterioles are markedly thickened and hyalinized. The fingers may take on a tapered, claw-like appearance, and the dermal fibrosis may limit motion in the joints. The sclerotic atrophy of the tips of the fingers often causes resorption of the terminal phalanges of the fingers. Focal and sometimes diffuse subcutaneous calcifications may develop, especially in patients with limited scleroderma (CREST syndrome). Recurrent traumatic ulcerations associated with chronic ischemia due to vascular occlusion may progress to autoamputation of the fingers. The face may take on the appearance of a drawn mask. A variety of superimposed changes may appear, including vitiligo and hyperpigmentation.

The **gastrointestinal tract** is affected in over half the patients. The most common manifestation consists of progressive atrophy and fibrosis of the esophageal wall, involving principally the submucosa and muscularis. This may be accompanied by atrophy and ulceration of the overlying mucosa. Almost invariably the small vessels in these areas show progressive thickening of their walls, accompanied by a perivascular infiltrate of lymphocytes. Similar atrophy and fibrosis may occur in the stomach, small bowel, and colon.

In the **musculoskeletal system** both joints and muscles are affected. Early in the disease a nonspecific inflammatory synovitis may appear, resembling the early stages of rheumatoid arthritis. With progression, the synovium undergoes collagenous sclerosis, followed in some cases by some bony resorption of the subjacent bone. At the same time sclerosis in the periarticular connective tissues limits joint motion. Destruction of joints, such as occurs with RA, is quite rare. Focal inflammatory infiltrates followed by fibrosis may appear in the skeletal muscles, and many of these patients develop muscle atrophy.

The **lungs** often develop diffuse interstitial fibrosis of the alveolar septa, accompanied by progressive thickening of the walls of the smaller pulmonary vessels. The fibrosis may lead to the production of microcysts. Thus patients with SS may develop lesions indistinguishable from those of idiopathic pulmonary fibrosis (honeycomb lung, p. 402).

The **kidneys** frequently (66% of cases) are damaged by a variety of lesions, but it is difficult to interpret the nature of the renal lesions, since many patients with SS and renal involvement have severe hypertension, known to induce renal injury. The principal changes are found in small arteries, which show concentric intimal proliferation, deposition of acid mucopolysaccharides, reduplication of the internal elastic lamina, and hyalinization. Although these vascular changes resemble those found in malignant hypertension, it should be noted that in SS they are restricted to vessels that are 150 to 500 μm in diameter, and, moreover, they are not always associated with hypertension. Indeed, hypertension is seen in only 30% of the cases; in 7 to 10% it takes the form of malignant hypertension. In those with hypertension the lesions in the kidney are more severe and often include fibrinoid necrosis of arterioles, focal necrosis of glomeruli, and microinfarcts. Other glomerular changes are nonspecific, such as localized basement membrane thickening and an increase in the mesangium. About half of the patients die of renal failure.

The **heart** may have focal interstitial fibrosis, principally in the perivascular areas, and occasionally there are perivascular infiltrates of lymphocytes and macrophages. Small intramyocardial arteries and arterioles may show vascular thickening. Because of the changes in the lungs, right-sided cardiac hypertrophy (cor pulmonale, p. 315) is often present.

Other sites may be affected, particularly nerve trunks, possibly related to microvascular lesions with ischemic and fibrotic alterations in the perineurium.

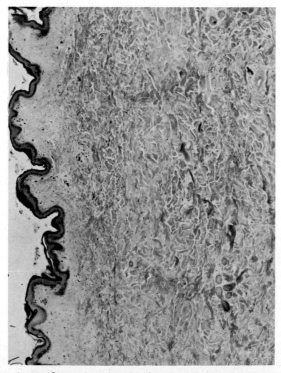

Figure 6–28. Systemic sclerosis. Atrophy of the skin, with dense sclerosis of dermal tissue and atrophy of skin adnexa.

CLINICAL COURSE. It must be apparent from the described anatomic changes that SS has many of the features of RA, SLE, and, as will be described, dermatomyositis. It is, however, *distinctive because of the striking cutaneous changes.* Almost all patients develop *Raynaud's phenomenon,* a vascular disorder characterized by reversible vasospasm of the arteries. Typically the hands turn white on exposure to cold, reflecting vasospasm, followed by a blue color as capillaries and venules dilate and blood stagnates. Finally, the color changes to red as reactive vasodilatation occurs. It should be noted that Raynaud's phenomenon may be noted prior to any organic changes in the skin. The progressive collagenization of the skin leads to atrophy of the hands, with increasing stiffness and eventually complete immobilization of the joints. The disability becomes more generalized as the trunk and extremities are affected. Difficulty in swallowing and gastrointestinal symptoms are inevitable consequences of the changes in the esophagus and lower gut. Malabsorption may appear if the submucosal and muscular atrophy and fibrosis involve the small intestine. Dyspnea and chronic cough reflect the pulmonary changes, and often these patients develop the so-called *stiff lung syndrome.* With advanced pulmonary involvement, secondary pulmonary hypertension may develop, leading in turn to right-sided cardiac dysfunction. Renal functional impairment secondary to both the advance of SS and the concomitant malignant hypertension frequently is marked.

Limited scleroderma, or the so-called CREST syndrome, is characterized by *c*alcinosis, *R*aynaud's phenomenon, *e*sophageal dysmotility, *s*clerodactyly, and *t*elangiectasia. Raynaud's phenomenon is frequently the presenting feature and is associated with limited skin involvement confined to the fingers and face. These two features may be present for decades before the appearance of distinctive visceral lesions.

The course of diffuse SS is difficult to predict. In most patients the disease pursues a steady, slow, downhill course over the span of many years, with gradual evolution of the cutaneous lesions and progressive deformity. Many develop crippling limitation of motion of various joints. In the absence of renal involvement, the life span may be normal. The overall 10-year survival rate ranges from 35 to 70%. The chances of survival are significantly better for patients with localized scleroderma than for those with the usual diffuse progressive disease.

POLYMYOSITIS (DERMATOMYOSITIS) _____

Polymyositis is a chronic inflammatory myopathy of uncertain cause. When a skin rash is also present it is called dermatomyositis. Clinically, the disease is characterized by symmetric proximal muscle weakness with varying degrees of pain, often accompanied by a rash about the eyes, face, and extensor surfaces of the limbs. The disease may occur at any age from infancy to late life; there are bimodal peaks in the age groups of five to 15 and 50 to 60 years.

The clinical expression of inflammatory myopathies is extremely varied. Muscle involvement may or may not be accompanied by cutaneous manifestations. In approximately 20% of patients, there is an associated connective tissue disorder such as SLE, systemic sclerosis, or Sjögren's syndrome. Dermatomyositis in children (juvenile dermatomyositis) seems to represent a distinct clinicopathologic entity. In this group of patients there is widespread vasculitis involving the skin and the gastrointestinal tract. As a result, bowel infarction with perforation and skin ulceration are prominent clinical features in addition to the myositis.

ETIOLOGY AND PATHOGENESIS. The belief that polymyositis-dermatomyositis is of immune origin is based in part on "guilt by association," because the clinical and anatomic features in some cases overlap with those of other connective tissue diseases with better-established immunopathogeneses (i.e., Sjögren's syndrome, RA, and SLE). Autoantibodies such as rheumatoid factor and ANAs have been found in some cases. Recent studies suggest that antibodies to the Jo-1 antigen, which is a subunit of histidyl-tRNA synthetase, are found principally in patients with polymyositis. Whether antibodies play any role in pathogenesis is unknown, except possibly in childhood dermatomyositis. The widespread vasculitis seen in this condition seems to be mediated by immune complexes that can be identified in the affected blood vessels. Cell-mediated immunity has also been implicated in the pathogenesis of polymyositis-dermatomyositis. Supporting this view is the presence of helper and cytotoxic T lymphocytes in the inflammatory infiltrate. These lymphocytes may damage the muscle fibers by cell-mediated cytotoxicity. What initiates the autosensitization is as obscure as it is in other autoimmune diseases. As usual, microbial agents are prime suspects because of sporadic reports of elevated antibody titers to viruses (coxsackie B) and *Toxoplasma gondii.* However, firm evidence linking any infectious agent to the causation of polymyositis is lacking.

MORPHOLOGY. The major anatomic features of polymyositis-dermatomyositis are muscle involvement and skin rash. Histologically, the following features are present: necrosis of foci or single muscle cells, phagocytosis of muscle cell fragments, and a prominent perivascular, endomysial, and perimysial inflammatory infiltrate (Fig. 6–29). In addition several nonspecific changes indicative of muscle fiber regeneration may also be noted. In chronic cases focal areas of fibrosis and/or replacement of muscle by fat may occur. Immunocytochemical studies reveal that in polymyositis most of the infiltrating cells are T lymphocytes that bear activation markers such as IL-2 receptors. Both CD4+ and CD8+ cells are found. In dermatomyositis a greater percentage of B cells suggests activation of humoral immunity.

The **skin rash** seen in approximately 40% of patients may be quite variable or it may be virtually diagnostic. The classic rash takes the form of a **lilac or heliotrope discoloration of the upper eyelids, with periorbital edema.** It is often accompanied by a scaling erythematous eruption or dusky red patches over the knuckles,

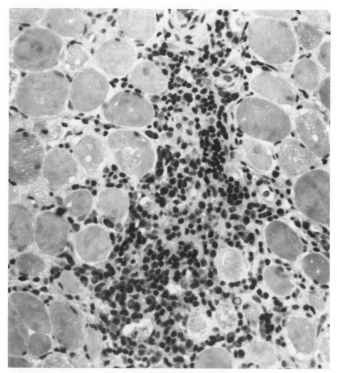

Figure 6-29. Polymyositis. A focus in skeletal muscle showing necrosis of muscle cells and infiltration by mononuclear cells. (Courtesy of Dr. Dennis Burns, Department of Pathology, Southwestern Medical School, Dallas, TX.)

elbows, and knees (Gottron's lesions). Histologically, dermal edema is seen in the early stages, with mononuclear infiltrates surrounding the dermal vessels.

In children, and in some acute involvements in adults, widespread necrotizing vasculitis may be present, involving the lungs, kidneys, heart, and other organs. This vasculitis is reminiscent of that encountered in polyarteritis. Diffuse interstitial pulmonary fibrosis is frequently present in adults with anti-Jo-1 antibodies.

CLINICAL COURSE. Polymyositis-dermatomyositis has, as its principal clinical finding, symmetric muscular weakness that is insidious but sometimes acute in onset. *The diagnosis cannot be entertained in the absence of muscle involvement.* It usually begins proximally in the shoulders and pelvic girdles and may then extend to the neck and eventually to the distal extremities. This pattern is not invariable. Frequently, weakness of the striated muscles of the pharynx leads to difficulty in swallowing. The skin rash may or may not be diagnostic. Occasionally, patients exhibit Raynaud's phenomenon or rheumatoid manifestations. As mentioned, there is considerable overlap of symptoms with SLE, systemic sclerosis, and rheumatoid arthritis, and, indeed, sometimes these diseases coexist. Moreover, it is hardly necessary to point out that many other muscle disorders (e.g., myasthenia gravis and the muscular dystrophies) must also be considered in the differential diagnosis. Electromyography allows distinc-

tion between inflammatory muscle disease and those caused by diseases of neurons and receptors. As might be expected, muscle injury is associated with elevations in enzymes such as creatine kinase and aldolases. Biopsy is required for diagnosis.

The course is characterized by remissions and exacerbations. Most patients experience remission with immunosuppressive therapy; overall the 5-year survival rate is 75% for adults and better for children.

Many, but not all, investigators believe that polymyositis, especially when accompanied by dermatomyositis, is associated with a 13 to 20% risk for malignancy. A wide variety of visceral malignancies including those affecting lung, ovary, and stomach have been linked with these disorders.

IMMUNODEFICIENCY DISEASES _____

The more we learn about the immune system, the more complex it appears. No less complex is the classification of immunodeficiency states. At one time, in blissful ignorance, these were simply categorized as a lack of B cells or T cells or sometimes of both forms of cells; but alas, many new subtleties have emerged. For example, it is now appreciated that ineffective immune responses may be caused not merely by lack of lymphocytes but also by disorders of immunoregulatory circuits. Despite many complexities, the immunodeficiencies can be broadly subdivided into primary diseases of genetic origin and those secondary to some underlying disorder. Our discussion will begin with a brief account of the primary immunodeficiencies, to be followed by more detailed description of the acquired immunodeficiency syndrome, better known as AIDS, the most devastating example of secondary immunodeficiency.

PRIMARY IMMUNODEFICIENCY STATES _____

Primary immunodeficiency states are experiments of nature that have greatly helped our understanding of the ontogeny and regulation of the immune system (Fig. 6-30). They usually come to attention early in life because of the vulnerability of the child to recurrent infections. Although these immune disorders are relatively uncommon, they are often devastating, and the infections are often fatal. A few of the more common syndromes will be characterized.

X-Linked (Congenital) Agammaglobulinemia — Bruton's Disease _____

The basic defect in this disorder is a failure of pre-B cells to differentiate into mature B cells. At the molecular level, the defect seems to reside in an inability to effect orderly and productive rearrangement of immunoglobulin heavy chain genes. It is one of the more common forms of primary immunodeficiency. As an X-linked disease, it is seen almost entirely in males, but sporadic cases have been described in females. It usually does not become apparent until about six

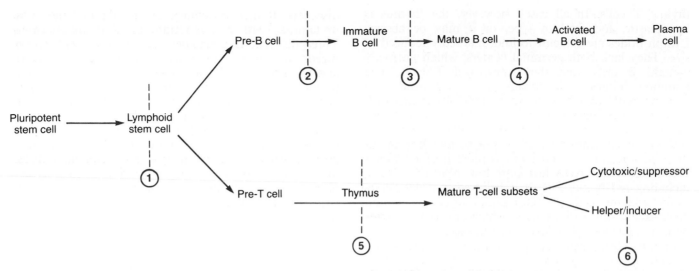

Figure 6–30. A simplified scheme of lymphocyte development. Numbers indicate cells or steps affected in various immunodeficiency states: 1, severe combined immunodeficiency; 2, Bruton's agammaglobulinemia; 3, isolated IgA deficiency, affects only immature IgA positive B cells; 4, one form of common variable immunodeficiency; 5, DiGeorge's syndrome; 6, AIDS.

months of age, when maternal immunoglobulins are depleted. In most cases, recurrent bacterial infections such as acute and chronic pharyngitis, sinusitis, otitis media, bronchitis, and pneumonia call attention to the underlying immune defect. Almost always the causative organisms are *Haemophilus influenzae, Streptococcus pyogenes, Staphylococcus aureus,* or the pneumococci. Most viral, fungal, and protozoal infections are handled normally by cell-mediated mechanisms, but there are some important exceptions to this generalization. These patients seem to be very susceptible to echovirus and enterovirus infections. They are also at increased risk for development of *Pneumocystis carinii* pneumonia. Persistent intestinal infections with *Giardia lamblia* may give rise to malabsorption. These observations indicate a role for antibodies in resistance against certain agents that are traditionally considered to be eliminated only by cell-mediated immunity. The classic form of this disease has the following characteristics:

- B cells are absent or remarkably decreased in the circulation, and the serum levels of all classes of immunoglobulins are depressed. Pre-B cells are found in normal numbers in bone marrow.
- Germinal centers of lymph nodes, Peyer's patches, the appendix, and tonsils are underdeveloped or rudimentary.
- There is remarkable absence of plasma cells throughout the body.
- T cell–system and cell-mediated reactions are entirely normal.

Autoimmune diseases occur with increased frequency in patients with Bruton's disease. Nearly half of these children develop a condition similar to rheumatoid arthritis that clears remarkably with restitutive immunoglobulin therapy. Similarly, lupus erythematosus (p. 139), dermatomyositis (p. 153), and other autoimmune disorders are more common in these patients. The basis of these peculiar associations is not known.

Thymic Hypoplasia (DiGeorge's Syndrome) ____

This disorder results from a lack of thymic influence on the immune system. *The thymus is usually rudimentary and T cells are deficient or absent in the circulation. They are similarly depleted in the thymus-dependent areas of the lymph nodes and spleen* (p. 117). Thus infants with this defect are extremely vulnerable to viral, fungal, and protozoal infections. Susceptibility to intracellular bacteria is also increased, because phagocytic cells that eliminate them require T cell–derived signals for activation. The B-cell system and serum immunoglobulins are entirely unaffected.

DiGeorge's syndrome results from a congenital malformation affecting the third and fourth pharyngeal pouches. These structures give rise to the thymus, parathyroid glands, and portions of lips, ears, and the aortic arch. Hence, in addition to thymic hypoplasia the parathyroid glands are also either hypoplastic or totally absent, often leading to tetany from hypocalcemia. Most of these infants have additional developmental defects affecting the face, ears, heart, and great vessels. Transplantation of thymus tissue has been successful in some of these infants. In others (with partial defects) immunity may improve spontaneously with age.

Severe Combined Immunodeficiency (Swiss-Type Agammaglobulinemia) ____

Severe combined immunodeficiency represents a constellation of syndromes all having in common variable defects in both humoral and cell-mediated immune responses. Several variants have been identified, all quite rare. Most affected persons have marked lymphopenia with a deficiency of both T and B cells. Others have normal numbers of B cells, which are nonfunctional owing to lack of T-cell help. Still others have normal numbers of circulating lymphocytes that bear the cell surface markers of very immature intrathymic T cells. In all cases, however, the thymus is hypoplastic and fetal in type, or it may be absent. Lymph nodes are difficult to find, markedly reduced in size. They lack both germinal centers, which normally contain B cells, and the paracortical T cells. The lymphoid tissues of the tonsils, gut, and appendix are also markedly hypoplastic. About 50% of patients with an autosomal recessive type of severe combined immunodeficiency have a lack of adenosine deaminase (ADA), an enzyme involved in purine metabolism. In these patients, T-cell deficiency is more profound than B-cell deficiency. ADA levels are low in all the tissues, including red blood cells. It is believed that deficiency of this enzyme leads to accumulation of adenosine and deoxy-adenosine triphosphate, which are toxic to lymphocytes, particularly of the T-cell lineage.

Infants with these severe immune handicaps are vulnerable to all forms of viral, fungal, and bacterial infections, and most die during the first year of life. A number of patients with severe combined immunodeficiency with or without ADA deficiency have been successfully treated by transplantation of normal histocompatible bone marrow cells, suggesting that these patients have normal thymus and bursa-equivalent tissues and that the basis of their T- and B-cell deficiency is defective lymphoid stem cells. ADA-deficient patients are prime candidates for somatic gene therapy. The ADA gene has been cloned and can be transfected into autologous bone marrow cells, which can then be reinfused into the patient. Results of initial attempts to correct ADA deficiency by this procedure should be available in the near future.

Isolated Deficiency of Immunoglobulin A

The commonest of all the primary immunodeficiency diseases, IgA deficiency affects about one in 700 individuals. Both serum and secretory IgA are deficient. Although most persons with this condition are asymptomatic, some present with a variety of symptoms, including respiratory infections, chronic diarrhea, and atopic disorders such as asthma. There is also a significant association with autoimmune diseases, the basis of which is not entirely clear. Some individuals with IgA deficiency are also deficient in IgG2 and IgG4 subclasses of immunoglobulin G. This subgroup of patients is particularly prone to develop infections. IgA deficiency may be familial or acquired in association with toxoplasmosis, measles, or some other virus infection. The pathogenesis of IgA deficiency seems to involve a block in the terminal differentiation of IgA-secreting B cells. Serum IgE antibodies to IgA are found in approximately 44% of the patients. Whether this observation is of any etiologic significance is unknown, but it has important clinical implications. When transfused with blood containing normal levels of IgA, some of these patients develop severe, sometimes fatal, anaphylactic reactions.

Common Variable Immunodeficiency

This relatively common but poorly defined derangement probably represents a heterogeneous group of disorders. It may be congenital or acquired, sporadic or familial (with an inconstant mode of inheritance). Three different immunologic causes have been recognized: intrinsic B cell defects, autoantibodies to B cells, and regulatory T-cell imbalances. The feature common to all patients is hypogammaglobulinemia, generally affecting all the antibody classes but sometimes only IgG. About two thirds of patients have *normal levels of circulating B cells,* which can recognize antigens and proliferate but fail to differentiate into plasma cells. Histologically the B-cell areas—the lymphoid follicles in the nodes, spleen, and gut—are markedly hyperplastic. The histologic findings support the notion that B cells can proliferate in response to antigen recognition. The symptoms resemble those of X-linked agammaglobulinemia, i.e., recurrent bacterial infections, but they start at a later age (15 to 20 years). Infestation with the intestinal parasite *Giardia lamblia* is also quite common and may lead to a spruelike syndrome. These patients also have a high rate of autoimmune diseases.

Immunodeficiency with Thrombocytopenia and Eczema (Wiskott-Aldrich Syndrome)

Wiskott-Aldrich syndrome is selected for presentation because it demonstrates the complexity of the immune system findings in some patients with primary immune deficiency syndromes. The Wiskott-Aldrich syndrome is an X-linked recessive disease characterized by eczema, thrombocytopenia, and recurrent infections. Classically, these patients show a poor antibody response to polysaccharide antigens (for example, those derived from pneumococcus types I and II) and as such they are vulnerable to recurrent infections by encapsulated bacteria (e.g., pneumococcus and *H. influenzae*). T- and B-cell numbers are normal initially, but by 6 years of age there is a profound loss of T cells and a progressive loss of cell-mediated immunity develops. The pathogenesis of this form of immunodeficiency is obscure. Patients have a defect in glycosylation of membrane proteins, including some that are expressed on T and B cells; however, the relationship of the impaired glycosylation to the immune deficiency is not clear.

SECONDARY IMMUNODEFICIENCIES

Secondary immune deficiencies are sometimes encountered in patients with malnutrition, infection, cancer, renal diseases, Hodgkin's disease, and sarcoidosis. They may also occur secondary to the use of immunosuppressive drugs such as corticosteroids and cancer therapeutic agents. Many of these secondary states can be accounted for by loss of immunoglobulins (as in proteinuric renal diseases), inadequate synthesis of immunoglobulins (as in malnutrition), or loss of lymphocytes (as may occur with drugs and systemic infections), but other mechanisms may also be operative. As a group, the secondary immunodeficiencies are more common than the disorders of genetic origin.

Here we will discuss only AIDS, which has assumed epidemic proportions in the last five years and has terrorized the entire world.

Acquired Immunodeficiency Syndrome (AIDS) _____

In June 1981, the Centers for Disease Control (CDC) of the United States reported that five young homosexual males in the Los Angeles area had contracted *Pneumocystis carinii* pneumonia. Two of the patients had died. This report signaled the beginning of an epidemic of a *retroviral disease characterized by profound immunosuppression associated with opportunistic infections, secondary neoplasms, and neurologic manifestations, which has come to be known as AIDS.* As of late 1991, approximately 200,000 patients with AIDS had been reported in the United States, and, based on serologic data, it is estimated that 1.5 to 2 million individuals have been infected with human immunodeficiency virus (HIV), the agent that causes AIDS. In central Africa the number of infected individuals is even larger. No less impressive is the explosion of new knowledge relating to HIV and its remarkable ability to cause this modern plague. So rapid is the pace of research on the molecular biology of HIV and its effects that any textbook that covers this topic is doomed to be out of date by the time it is published. It is with this sobering realization that an attempt will be made to summarize the currently available data on the epidemiology, cause, pathogenesis, and clinical features of HIV infection.

EPIDEMIOLOGY. Although AIDS was first described in the United States and this country has the majority of the reported cases, AIDS has now been reported from over 100 countries around the world, and the pool of HIV-infected persons in central Africa is quite large. Epidemiologic studies in the United States have identified five groups of adults at risk for developing AIDS. The case distribution in these groups is as follows:

Homosexual or bisexual males constitute by far the largest group, accounting for 70% of the reported cases. This includes 7% who were intravenous drug abusers as well.

Intravenous drug abusers with no previous history of homosexuality compose the next largest group, representing about 18% of all patients. They represent 60% of all cases among heterosexuals.

Hemophiliacs, especially those who received large amounts of factor VIII concentrates prior to 1985, make up 1% of all cases.

Recipients of blood and blood components who are not hemophiliacs but who received transfusions of HIV-infected whole blood or components (e.g., platelets, plasma) account for 2.5% of patients.

Heterosexual contacts of members of other high-risk groups (chiefly IV drug abusers) constitute 4% of the patient population.

The epidemiology of HIV infection and AIDS is quite different in children younger than 13 years. Of the approximately 3000 cases of pediatric AIDS reported in the United States by mid-1991 more than 80% have resulted from transmission of the virus from mother to child (discussed later). The remaining 20% are hemophiliacs and others who received blood or blood products prior to 1985.

Based on epidemiologic studies and laboratory investigations, it is now established that transmission of HIV may occur through three routes: *sexual contact, parenteral inoculation,* and *passage of the virus from infected mothers to their newborns.*

Venereal transmission is clearly the predominant mode of infection worldwide. Because the vast majority of patients in the United States are homosexual or bisexual males, most sexual transmission has occurred among homosexual men. It is believed that the virus is carried in the lymphocytes present in the semen and enters the recipient's body through abrasions in rectal mucosa. Heterosexual transmission, although initially of less quantitative importance in the United States, is probably the most common mode by which HIV is spread outside the United States. Since 1985, however, even in the United States, *the rate of increase of heterosexual transmission is beginning to outpace transmission by other means.* Such spread is occurring most rapidly in female sex partners of male IV drug abusers. Not surprisingly therefore, the incidence of AIDS acquired by this route is highest in those areas with a high prevalence of IV drug abuse (e.g., metropolitan New York and Florida). In contrast to the United States experience, heterosexual transmission seems to be the dominant mode of HIV infection in Africa.

Although male-to-female transmission is firmly established, the frequency and risk of female-to-male spread is not as clear. This form of heterosexual spread is probably not common in the United States but may well occur frequently in Africa. The observation that the male-to-female case ratio in Africa is close to 1:1 as compared to 12:1 in the United States is consistent with the idea that female-to-male spread is important in Africa. The concomitant presence of other sexually transmitted diseases (and genital ulcerations) prevalent in many African locales may facilitate female-to-male transmission.

Parenteral transmission of HIV has occurred in three groups of individuals: intravenous drug abusers, hemophiliacs who received factor VIII concentrates, and random recipients of blood transfusion. Of these three, IV drug abusers constitute by far the largest group. Transmission occurs by sharing of needles, syringes, and other paraphernalia contaminated with HIV-containing blood. This group occupies a pivotal position in the AIDS epidemic because it represents the principal link in the transmission of HIV to other adult populations through heterosexual activity.

Transmission of HIV by transfusion of blood or blood products such as lyophilized factor VIII concentrates has been virtually eliminated in recent years. This happy outcome resulted from three public health measures: screening of donated blood and plasma for antibody to HIV, heat treatment of clotting factor concentrates, and screening of donors on the basis of history. However, this optimism has to be tempered by two facts. First, because antibodies may take 3 to 17 weeks to develop following HIV infection (the window period), an extremely small but definite risk of acquiring AIDS through transfusion of seronegative blood persists. Second, because of the long latent period, new cases of AIDS will continue to be detected among those who were infected by blood prior to 1985.

As alluded to earlier, mother-to-infant transmission is the major cause of pediatric AIDS. Infected mothers (most of whom are intravenous drug users), transmit HIV by the transplacental route. Other possible modes of transmission include exposure to maternal blood and other infected fluids during birth, and through breast milk.

Because of the uniformly fatal outcome of AIDS, there has been much concern in lay public and among health care workers regarding spread of HIV infection outside the high-risk groups. Extensive studies indicate that *HIV infection cannot be transmitted by casual personal contact in the household, workplace, or school.* No convincing evidence for spread by insect bites has been obtained. Regarding transmission of HIV infection to health care workers, there seems to be an extremely small but definite risk. Seroconversion has been documented following accidental needlestick injury or exposure of nonintact skin to infected blood in laboratory accidents. Following such accidents the risk of seroconversion is believed to be about 0.5%.

ETIOLOGY. There is little doubt that AIDS is caused by HIV, a human retrovirus belonging to the lentivirus family. Included in this group are feline immunodeficiency virus, simian immunodeficiency virus, visna virus of sheep, and the equine infectious anemia virus. These nontransforming retroviruses have several features in common:

- a long incubation period, followed by a slowly progressive fatal outcome
- tropism for hematopoietic and nervous system
- an ability to cause immunosuppression
- cytopathic effects in vitro.

Two genetically different but closely related forms of HIV, called HIV-1 and HIV-2, have been isolated from patients with AIDS. HIV-1 is the most common type associated with AIDS in the United States, Europe, and Central Africa, whereas HIV-2 causes a similar disease principally in West Africa. Although distinct, HIV-1 and HIV-2 share several antigens; because of the serologic cross-reactivity most (but not all) cases of HIV-2 infection can be detected by the enzyme-linked immunosorbent assay (ELISA) test for HIV-1 used by blood banks. The ensuing discussion relates primarily to HIV-1 and diseases caused by it; however, it is generally applicable to HIV-2 as well.

Like most C-type retroviruses, the HIV-1 virion is spherical and contains an electron-dense core surrounded by a lipid envelope derived from the host cell membrane. The virus core contains several core proteins, two strands of genomic RNA, and the enzyme reverse transcriptase (Fig. 6–31). Studding the viral envelope are two viral glycoproteins, gp 120 and gp 41, that are critical for HIV infection of cells. HIV-1 proviral genome contains the *gag, pol,* and *env*

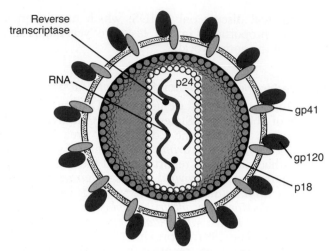

Figure 6–31. HIV virion. The virus particle is covered by a membrane that is derived from the host cell. Studding the membrane are viral glycoproteins, gp41 and gp120. Inside there is a core made up of proteins designated p18 and p24. The viral RNA and the enzyme reverse transcriptase are carried in the core.

genes that code for the core proteins, reverse transcriptase, and envelope proteins, respectively (Fig. 6–32). *In addition to these three standard retroviral genes, HIV and other lentiviruses contain several other genes* that exert regulatory functions. By using genetically manipulated viruses it has been found that some of these genes, such as *tat* (transactivator), *rev* (regulator of expression of virus), and *vif* (viral infectivity factor), enhance virus replication; others, such as *nef* (negative factor), suppress replication and may be responsible for latent infection (described later). It is conceivable that products of these regulatory genes may be suitable targets for potential anti-HIV drugs.

PATHOGENESIS. There are two major targets of HIV: the immune system and the central nervous system. The effects of HIV infection on each of these two will be discussed separately.

Immunopathogenesis of HIV disease. Profound immunosuppression, primarily affecting cell-mediated immunity, is the hallmark of AIDS. This results chiefly from a severe loss of CD4+ T cells as well as an impairment in the function of surviving helper T cells. Because depletion of CD4+ T cells is critical to the pathogenesis of AIDS, we will focus our attention first on the events that lead to the infection and destruction of T cells, after which HIV infection of monocytes and its consequences will be discussed.

There is abundant evidence that *the CD4 molecule is in fact a high-affinity receptor* for HIV. This explains the selective tropism of the virus for CD4+ T cells and its ability to infect other CD4+ cells, particularly macrophages (Fig. 6–33). The initial step in infection is the binding of gp 120 envelope glycoprotein to CD4 molecules. This is followed by fusion of the virus to the cell membrane and internalization. It is believed that fusion requires a postbinding step in which viral gp 41 makes contact with a yet to be identified component of the cell membrane. The binding of gp

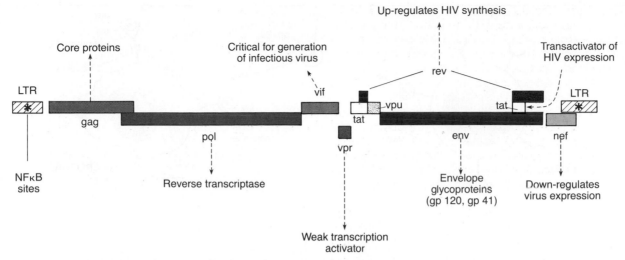

Figure 6–32. HIV proviral genome. Several viral genes and their recognized functions are illustrated. The genes outlined in red are unique to HIV; others are shared by all retroviruses. Like *vif*, *vpu* favors generation of infectious virus.

120 with the CD4 molecule has been scrutinized in great detail because this step provides a potential target for therapy designed to limit or even prevent HIV from infecting cells. For example, genetically engineered soluble CD4 molecules, or their fragments containing the gp120-binding domains, can bind free virus and thereby prevent infection of CD4+ T cells in vitro.

Whether CD4⁻ cells can be infected by HIV remains uncertain. According to some investigators, cells such as astrocytes, skin fibroblasts, and bowel epithelial cells (all lacking CD4) are infected through an entirely different receptor. In the central nervous system galactosyl ceramide, a myelin-associated glycolipid, has been implicated as a receptor.

Once internalized, the viral genome undergoes reverse transcription, leading to formation of proviral DNA that is then integrated into host genome. Following this the provirus may remain locked into the chromosome for months or years and hence the infection may become latent. Alternatively, proviral DNA may be transcribed with the formation of complete viral particles that bud from the cell membrane. Such productive infection when associated with extensive viral budding leads to cell death (Fig. 6–33). It is important to note that in T cells the initiation of proviral DNA transcription (and hence productive infection) occurs only when the infected cell is activated by an exposure to antigens or cytokines. It is obvious therefore that physiologic stimuli that promote activation and growth of normal T cells lead to the death of HIV-infected T cells.

It might be surmised from the preceding discussion that productive infection of T cells is the mechanism by which HIV causes lysis of CD4+ T cells. It is interesting to note, however, that in the peripheral blood of patients with AIDS only one in 10,000 to one in 1000 of the CD4+ cells shows evidence of active virus production, whereas 1 to 10% harbor latent HIV provirus. Because of the disparity between the number of

productively infected T cells and the severity of T-cell loss, it is suspected that mechanisms other than direct cytolysis are involved in the causation of profound T-cell deficiency that characterizes late stages of HIV infection. Three such mechanisms may be posited:

- Loss of immature precursors of CD4+ T cells, either by direct infection of thymic progenitor cells or by infection of accessory cells that secrete cytokines essential for CD4+ T-cell differentiation.
- Fusion of infected and uninfected cells, with formation of syncytia (giant cells) (Fig 6-34). In tissue culture the gp120 expressed on productively infected cells binds to CD4 molecules on uninfected T cells, followed by cell fusion. Fused cells develop "ballooning" and usually die within a few hours.
- Autoimmune destruction of both infected and uninfected CD4+ T cells. Soluble gp120 released from infected cells can bind to CD4 molecules on uninfected cells. Since many patients have circulating anti-gp120 antibodies, these gp120-coated cells could be destroyed by ADCC.

Loss of CD4+ cells by direct and indirect mechanisms leads to an inversion of the CD4-CD8 ratio in the peripheral blood. It may be recalled that the normal CD4-CD8 ratio is close to 2 whereas in patients with AIDS a ratio close to 0.5 is not uncommon. Such an inversion, although a consistent finding in AIDS, should not be considered diagnostic, because it may also occur with certain other viral infections.

Although marked reduction in CD4+ T cells, a hallmark of AIDS, can account for most of the immunodeficiency late in the course of HIV infection, there is compelling evidence for *qualitative defects in T cells that can be detected even in asymptomatic HIV-infected persons.* Such defects include a reduction in antigen-induced T-cell proliferation, impaired production of cytokines such as IL-2 and IFNγ, defects in intracellular signaling, and many more. There is also a selective loss of the memory subset of CD4+ helper T

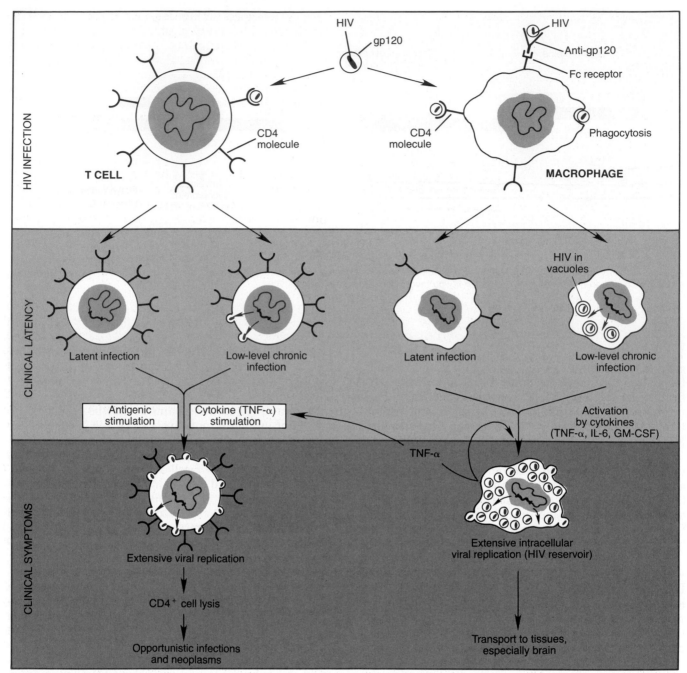

Figure 6–33. Immunopathogenesis of HIV infection. CD4+ T cells and macrophages are the major targets of HIV. Infection of these two cell types leads to somewhat distinctive events that eventually lead to a marked loss of CD4+ T cells and dissemination of HIV into various tissues, especially the central nervous system.

cells early in the course of disease. This observation explains the inability of peripheral blood T cells to be activated when challenged with common recall antigens.

In addition to infection and loss of CD4+ T cells, it is now apparent that *infection of monocytes and macrophages is also extremely important in the pathogenesis of HIV infection.* Several important differences between HIV infection of T cells and macrophages need to be emphasized:

• Unlike T cells, the majority of the *macrophages that*

are infected by HIV are found in the tissues and not in peripheral blood. A relatively high frequency (10 to 50%) of productively infected macrophages are detected in certain tissues such as brain, lymph nodes, and lungs.

• Since many macrophages express low levels of CD4, HIV may infect these cells by the gp120-CD4 pathway; in addition, HIV may enter macrophages by phagocytosis or by Fc receptor–mediated endocytosis of antibody-coated HIV particles (Fig. 6–33).

• Infected macrophages bud relatively small amounts

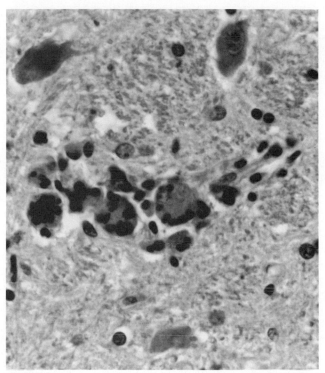

Figure 6-34. HIV infection. Formation of giant cells in the brain. (Courtesy of Dr. Dennis Burns, Department of Pathology, Southwestern Medical School, Dallas, TX.)

of virus from the cell surface, but these cells contain large numbers of virus particles located exclusively in intracellular vacuoles. Despite the fact that macrophages allow viral replication, unlike CD4+ T cells, they are quite resistant to the cytopathic effects of HIV.

HIV infection of macrophages has two important implications. First, monocytes and macrophages represent a veritable virus factory and reservoir, whose output remains largely protected from host defenses. Second, macrophages provide a safe vehicle for HIV to be transported to various parts of the body, particularly the nervous system.

Unlike tissue macrophages the number of monocytes in circulation infected by HIV is low; yet there are unexplained functional defects that have important bearing in host defense. These defects include impaired chemotaxis, decreased secretion of IL-1, and, most important, poor capacity to present antigens to T cells.

Low-level chronic or latent infection of T cells and macrophages is an important feature of HIV infection. Early in the course of HIV infection only rare CD4+ T cells in the blood express infectious virus, whereas 1 to 10% can be demonstrated to harbor HIV genome by polymerase chain reaction (PCR). It is widely believed that integrated provirus, without virus expression (latent infection), could remain in the cells from months to years. Completion of the viral life cycle in latently infected cells occurs only following cell activation, which in the case of CD4+ T cells results in cell lysis. To understand the molecular basis of release from

latency we must briefly consider the events that are associated with activation of CD4+ helper T cells. It is well known that antigen- or mitogen-induced activation of T cells is associated with transcription of genes encoding the cytokine IL-2 and its receptor (IL-2R). At the molecular level, this is accomplished in part by the induction of a nuclear binding factor called NF kB (nuclear factor kB), which binds to enhancer sequences (kB sites) within the promoter regions of IL-2 and IL-2R genes. Quite remarkably the LTR sequences that flank the HIV genome also contain similar kB sites that can be triggered by the same nuclear regulatory factors. Imagine now a latently infected CD4+ cell that encounters an environmental antigen. Induction of NF kB in such a cell (a physiologic response) activates the transcription of HIV proviral DNA (a pathologic outcome) and leads ultimately to the production of virions and to cell lysis. Furthermore, TNF-α, a cytokine produced by activated macrophages, also leads to transcriptional activation of HIV-mRNA by production of nuclear factors that bind to kB-enhancer elements of HIV. In effect, HIV thrives when the host macrophages and T cells are physiologically activated, an act that can be best described as "subversion from within." Such activation in vivo may result from antigenic stimulation, especially by other infecting microorganisms such as cytomegalovirus, EBV, hepatitis B virus, or herpes simplex virus. The life style of most HIV-infected patients in the United States places them at increased risk of recurrent exposure to other sexually transmitted diseases, and in Africa, socioeconomic conditions probably impose a higher burden of chronic microbial infections. It is easy to visualize how in patients with AIDS a vicious cycle of cell destruction may be set up. Multiple infections to which these patients are prone because of diminished helper T cell function lead to increased TNF-α production, which in turn stimulates more HIV production, followed by infection and loss of additional CD4+ T cells.

Although much attention has been focused on T cells and macrophages because they can be infected by HIV, patients with AIDS also display profound abnormalities of B cell function. Paradoxically, these patients have hypergammaglobulinemia and circulating immune complexes owing to polyclonal B-cell activation. This may result from multiple interacting factors such as infection with cytomegalovirus and EBV, both of which are polyclonal B-cell activators; gp120 itself can promote B-cell growth and differentiation, and HIV-infected macrophages produce increased amounts of IL-6, which favors activation of B cells. *Despite the presence of spontaneously activated B cells, patients with AIDS are unable to mount an antibody response to a new antigen.* This could in part be due to lack of T-cell help, but antibody responses against T-independent antigens are also suppressed, and hence there may be other defects in B cells as well. Impaired humoral immunity renders these patients prey to disseminated infections caused by encapsulated bacteria such as *Streptococcus pneumoniae* and *H. influenzae,* both of which require antibodies for effective opsonization.

In closing this discussion of immunopathogenesis it

must be recalled the CD4+ T cells play a pivotal role in regulating the immune response: they produce a plethora of cytokines such as IL-2, IL-4, IL-5, IFN-γ, macrophage chemotactic factors, and hematopoietic growth factors such as GM-CSF. Therefore loss of this "master cell" has ripple effects on virtually every other cell of the immune system, as illustrated in Figure 6–35 and summarized in Table 6–9.

Pathogenesis of Central Nervous System Involvement. The pathogenesis of neurologic manifestations deserves special mention because, in addition to the lymphoid system, the nervous system is a major target of HIV infection. Macrophages and cells belonging to the monocyte and macrophage lineage (microglia) are the predominant cell types in the brain that are infected with HIV. Hence it is widely believed that HIV is carried into the brain by infected monocytes. According to this view neuronal damage may be secondary to release of cytokines or other toxic products from infected macrophages. There is some evidence that HIV isolates from the brain constitute a special subgroup of the AIDS virus. These strains seem to grow equally well in macrophages and T cells, whereas those recovered from CD4+ lymphocytes seem to grow preferentially in T cells. Therefore it may well be that the risk of central nervous system damage is related to the strain of HIV. According to this view, those HIV strains that grow preferentially in T cells may be less

TABLE 6–9. MAJOR ABNORMALITIES OF IMMUNE FUNCTION IN AIDS

Lymphopenia
   Predominantly due to selective loss of the CD4+ helper-inducer T-cell subset; inversion of CD4-CD8 ratio
Decreased T-Cell Function in Vivo
   Susceptibility to opportunistic infections
   Susceptibility to neoplasms
   Decreased delayed-type hypersensitivity
Altered T-Cell Function in Vitro
   Decreased proliferative response to mitogens, alloantigens, and soluble antigens
   Decreased specific cytotoxicity
   Decreased helper function for pokeweed mitogen–induced B-cell immunoglobulin production
   Decreased IL-2 and IFN-γ production
Polyclonal B-Cell Activation
   Hypergammaglobulinemia and circulating immune complexes
   Inability to mount de novo antibody response to a new antigen
   Refractoriness to the normal signals for B-cell activation in vitro
Altered Monocyte or Macrophage Functions
   Decreased chemotaxis
   Decreased HLA class II antigen expression

prone to cause central nervous system disease. Some workers have reported that HIV is present in the brain in cell types other than macrophages, including astrocytes, oligodendrocytes, and endothelial cells. These

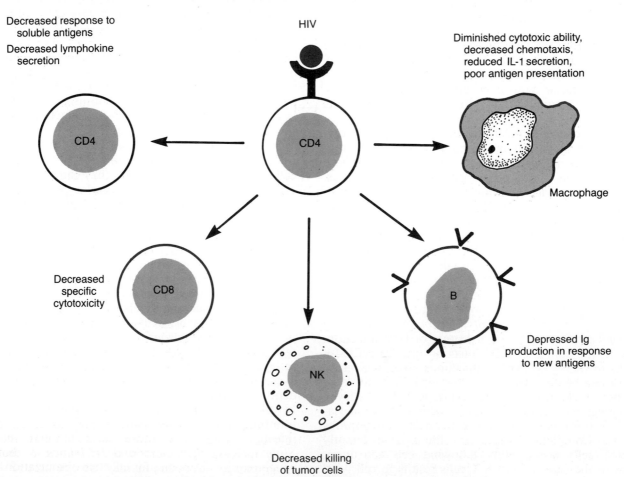

Figure 6–35. The multiple effects of loss of CD4+ T cells by HIV infection.

reports suggest a much wider tissue tropism for HIV as well as additional, possibly more direct, mechanisms for brain parenchymal injury. At present, however, pathways of HIV-induced brain damage that do not depend on macrophage transport must be considered "suggestoid" rather than proven.

NATURAL HISTORY OF HIV INFECTION. The course of HIV infection can be best understood in terms of an interplay between HIV and the immune system. *Three phases reflecting the dynamics of virus-host interaction can be recognized: an early, acute phase; a middle, chronic phase; and a final, crisis phase.* The four clinical subgroups of HIV infection, proposed by the Centers for Disease Control (CDC), can be reasonably assigned to the three phases of infection, as noted in Table 6–10. We first present the cardinal features of the three phases of HIV infection and their associated clinical syndromes and then recount the sequential virologic and immunologic findings during the course of HIV infection.

The early, acute phase represents the initial response of an immunocompetent adult to HIV infection. It is characterized initially by a high level of virus production, readily controlled by the development of an antiviral immune response. Clinically, this phase is associated with self-limited acute illness (CDC group I: Acute infection) that develops in 50 to 90% of adults infected with HIV. Nonspecific symptoms such as sore throat, myalgias, fever, rash, and sometimes aseptic meningitis develop three to six weeks after infection and resolve spontaneously two to three weeks later.

The middle, chronic phase represents a stage of immune containment of the virus. The immune system is largely intact and *there is smoldering, low-level HIV replication which may last for several years.* Patients are either asymptomatic (CDC group II) or develop persistent generalized lymphadenopathy (CDC group III). Constitutional symptoms are usually absent or mild. Persistent lymphadenopathy with significant constitutional symptoms (fever, rash, fatigue) reflects the onset of immune system decompensation, escalation of viral replication, and the onset of the "crisis" phase.

The final or crisis phase is characterized by a breakdown of host defense, resultant recrudescence of viral replication, and clinical disease referred to as AIDS-re-

lated complex followed by full-blown AIDS. Typically, patients with AIDS-related complex (CDC group IV, subgroup A) present with long-lasting fever (longer than a month), fatigue, loss of weight, and diarrhea; the CD4+ cell count is generally reduced. The borderline between advanced AIDS-related complex and AIDS is somewhat arbitrary. When serious opportunistic infections, secondary neoplasms, or clinical neurologic disease supervene, the patient is said to have developed AIDS (CDC group IV, B to E). In addition, according to recent CDC guidelines, any infected person with <200 CD4+ T cells/μl is considered to have AIDS. In the absence of treatment, most if not all patients with HIV infection will progress to AIDS after a chronic phase lasting from 7 to 10 years. This period, often referred to as the *clinical latent phase,* is shorter in those who receive a large parenteral inoculum of HIV, as occurs with blood transfusions, or may be especially long in those who receive prophylactic antiretroviral therapy.

With this overview of the three phases of HIV infection, we can consider some details of host-parasite relationships during the course of HIV infection. As mentioned earlier, when a normal immunocompetent adult is first exposed to HIV, there is a transient period of active viral replication associated with an abrupt, sometimes severe, reduction in CD4+ T cells. Soon, however, a virus-specific immune response develops, evidenced by seroconversion (usually within three to 17 weeks of presumed exposure), and more importantly, by development of virus-specific CD8+ cytotoxic T cells. *HIV-specific cytotoxic T cells are detected in blood at about the time viral titers begin to fall and are most likely responsible for the containment of HIV infection.* As viral replication abates, CD4+ T cells return to nearly normal numbers, signaling the end of the early acute phase. During the middle or chronic phase there is a continuing battle between HIV and the host immune system. The CD8+ cytotoxic T-cell response remains activated, *viral replication is restrained but not absent,* and the patients have few or mild symptoms. After an extended and variable period host defense begins to wane, the number of CD4+ cells begins to decline and the proportion of the surviving CD4+ cells infected with HIV increases, as does the viral burden per CD4+ cell. Not unexpectedly, HIV spillover into the plasma increases. From a practical standpoint, CD4+ T-cell counts in the blood are reasonably accurate prognosticators of disease progression. They decrease insidiously during the chronic phase, and more rapidly as decompensation begins. An absolute CD4+ T cell count below 150 cells per microliter or a rapidly falling cell count correlates with disease progression, while CD4+ cell counts above 400 cells per microliter have a much lower probability of rapid progression.

We are largely ignorant of the factors responsible for progression of HIV disease. As mentioned earlier, recurrent infections by other infecting microorganisms may increase HIV burden by activating T cells and macrophages. Progression may also be related to the "evolution" of HIV variants. It is well known that

TABLE 6–10. PHASES OF HIV INFECTION AND CORRESPONDING CDC CLASSIFICATION CATEGORIES

Phase	CDC Classification	
Early, acute	Group I:	Acute infection
Middle, chronic	Group II:	Asymptomatic infection
	Group III:	Persistent generalized lymphadenopathy
Final, "crisis"	Group IV	
	Subgroup A:	Constitutional disease
	Subgroup B:	Neurologic disease
	Subgroup C:	Secondary infection
	Subgroup D:	Secondary neoplasm
	Subgroup E:	Other conditions

numerous (possibly thousands) genetically related but distinct strains of HIV exist. They differ with respect to replication efficiency, cytopathic effects, sensitivity to neutralizing antibodies, and many other features that affect virulence. More recently it has been learned that a given virus strain can mutate within its host and gradually acquire the characteristics that favor increased virulence. For example, the viral isolates obtained from seropositive but asymptomatic patients are far less cytopathic in vitro, whereas mutants isolated from the same patients during later stages of the disease show increased virulence. In some careful studies detection of highly virulent strains preceded the development of AIDS by six months to two years. It may well be that highly virulent strains associated with low immunogenicity "evolve" owing to selective pressure exerted by an efficient immune system that eliminates less virulent variants during the protracted clinical latent phase.

It should be evident from our discussion that in each of the three phases of HIV infection variable degrees of viral replication continue to occur. Even in the middle chronic phase when the majority of infected cells have the provirus locked into the genome, productive infection of a small number of T cells is maintained. In other words *HIV infection lacks a phase of true microbiologic latency,* i.e., a phase during which *all* the HIV is in the form of proviral DNA and no cell is productively infected. Furthermore, because smoldering viral replication favors emergence of highly virulent variants, a strong case has been made for commencing antiretroviral therapy during the chronic asymptomatic period. Whether such therapeutic intervention will only postpone the inevitable or will truly alter the natural history of HIV infection remains to be tested.

CLINICAL FEATURES. The clinical manifestations of HIV infection can be readily surmised from the foregoing discussion. They range from a mild acute illness to severe disease. Because the salient clinical features of the acute early and chronic middle phases of HIV infection were described earlier, here we will summarize the clinical manifestations of the terminal phase, commonly known as AIDS.

In the United States the typical adult patient with AIDS is a young homosexual male or an IV drug abuser who presents with fever, weight loss, diarrhea, generalized lymphadenopathy, multiple opportunistic infections, neurologic disease, and, in many cases, secondary neoplasms. Pneumonia caused by the opportunistic fungus *P. carinii* (representing reactivation of a prior latent infection) is the presenting feature in about 50% of cases. The risk of developing this infection is extremely high in individuals with fewer than 200 CD4+ cells per microliter. Approximately 12% of patients present with an opportunistic infection other than *P. carinii* pneumonia (Table 6–11). Among the most common are recurrent mucosal candidiasis, disseminated cytomegalovirus infection (particularly enteritis and retinitis), severe ulcerating perianal herpes simplex, disseminated infection with atypical mycobacteria *(Mycobacterium avium-intracellulare),* cryptococcal meningitis, and central nervous system toxo-

TABLE 6–11. SELECTED OPPORTUNISTIC INFECTIONS FOUND IN PATIENTS WITH HIV INFECTION

Protozoal and Helminthic Infections
  Cryptosporidiosis or isosporidiosis (enteritis)
  Pneumocystosis (pneumonia or disseminated infection)
  Toxoplasmosis (pneumonia or central nervous system [CNS] infection)
  Strongyloidosis (pneumonia, CNS infection, or disseminated infection)
Fungal Infections
  Candidiasis (mouth, lung, skin or nails, disseminated)
  Cryptococcosis (CNS infection)
  Coccidioidomycosis (disseminated)
  Histoplasmosis (disseminated)
  Other opportunistic mycoses
Bacterial Infections
  Mycobacteriosis ("atypical," e.g., *M. avium-intracellulare* and *M. tuberculosis* infection, disseminated)
  Nocardiosis (pneumonia, meningitis, disseminated)
  Salmonella infections
  Shigella infections
Viral infections
  Cytomegalovirus (pulmonary, intestinal, or CNS infections)
  Herpes simplex virus (localized or disseminated)
  Varicella-zoster virus (localized or disseminated)
  Progressive multifocal leukoencephalopathy

plasmosis. Persistent diarrhea, so common in patients with AIDS, is often caused by *Cryptosporidium* or *Isospora belli* infections, but bacterial pathogens such as *Salmonella* and *Shigella* may also be involved. Because of depressed humoral immunity, AIDS patients are susceptible to infections with *S. pneumoniae* and *H. influenzae.*

About 20% of patients present with Kaposi's sarcoma, a vascular tumor that is otherwise extremely rare in the United States (p. 302). There are several peculiar features of this tumor in patients with AIDS. It is far more common among homosexual males than IV drug abusers or patients belonging to other risk groups. The lesions can arise early, before the immune system is compromised, or in advanced stages of HIV infection. Because its occurrence cannot clearly be related to host immune status, this tumor is not considered to be opportunistic. Instead, it seems that the product of the HIV-*tat* gene acts as a growth factor for the cells that make up the tumor. Unlike the lesions in sporadic cases of Kaposi's sarcoma, those that occur in patients with AIDS are multicentric and tend to be more aggressive.

Non-Hodgkin's lymphomas constitute the second most common type of AIDS-associated tumors. These tumors appear most frequently in severely immunosuppressed patients, involve many extranodal sites, and may occur as primary neoplasms of the brain in about 7% of cases. A large variety of other neoplasms, including Hodgkin's disease and squamous cell carcinomas, have also been reported.

Involvement of the central nervous system is a common and important manifestation of AIDS. *Seventy to ninety per cent of patients demonstrate some form of neurologic involvement at autopsy, and 30 to*

50% have clinically manifest neurologic dysfunction. Quite importantly, in some patients neurologic manifestations may be the sole or earliest presenting feature of HIV infection. In addition to opportunistic infections and neoplasms, several virally determined neuropathologic changes occur. These include a self-limited meningoencephalitis occuring at the time of seroconversion, aseptic meningitis, vacuolar myelopathy, peripheral neuropathies, and, most commonly, a progressive encephalopathy designated clinically as the AIDS-dementia complex (p. 711).

MORPHOLOGY. The anatomic changes in the tissues (with the exception of lesions in the brain) are neither specific nor diagnostic. In general the pathologic features of AIDS are those characteristic of widespread opportunistic infections, Kaposi's sarcoma, and lymphoid tumors. Most of these lesions have been discussed elsewhere, because they also occur in patients who do not have HIV infection. To appreciate the distinctive nature of lesions in the central nervous system, they are discussed in the context of other disorders affecting the brain (p. 711). Here we concentrate on changes in the lymphoid organs.

Biopsy specimens from enlarged lymph nodes in the early stages of HIV infection reveal nonspecific follicular hyperplasia with mild or minimal paracortical hyperplasia (p. 354). The medulla shows intense plasmacytosis. These changes, affecting primarily the B-cell areas of the node, are the morphologic counterparts of the polyclonal B-cell activation and hypergammaglobulinemia that is seen in patients with AIDS (p. 161). In addition to changes in the follicles, the sinuses show increased cellularity due primarily to an increase in histiocytes, but contributed to also by immunoblasts (B cells) and plasma cells.

With the onset of full-blown AIDS, the frenzy of B-cell proliferation subsides and gives way to a pattern of severe follicular involution and generalized lymphocyte depletion. These "burnt-out" lymph nodes are usually seen at autopsy and may harbor numerous opportunistic pathogens. Because of profound immunosuppression, the inflammatory response to infections both in the lymph nodes and at extranodal sites may be sparse or atypical. For example, mycobacteria do not evoke granuloma formation because CD4+ cells are deficient. In the empty-looking lymph nodes and in other organs the presence of infectious agents may not be readily apparent without the application of special stains. As might be expected, lymphoid depletion is not confined to the nodes; in later stages of AIDS, spleen and thymus also appear to be "wastelands."

Non-Hodgkin's lymphomas, involving the nodes as well as extranodal sites such as liver, gastrointestinal tract, and bone marrow, are primarily high-degree diffuse B-cell neoplasms (p. 358). It may well be that the origin of these tumors is related to long-term polyclonal B-cell proliferation in the face of deteriorating T-cell immunity, as has been postulated for the evolution of Burkitt's lymphoma (p. 202).

Since the discovery of AIDS in 1981, the concerted efforts of epidemiologists, immunologists, and molecular biologists have resulted in spectacular advances in our understanding of this disorder. Despite all this progress, however, the prognosis of patients with AIDS remains dismal. Of the 200,000 patients reported, over 100,000 were dead by late 1991. With time, true mortality figures are likely to be much higher, perhaps approaching 100%. Although a causative virus has been identified, many hurdles remain to be crossed before a vaccine can be developed. Molecular analyses have revealed an alarming degree of polymorphism in viral isolates from different patients; this renders the task of producing a vaccine remarkably difficult. Even if protective immune responses could be generated, only cells that express viral antigens would be eliminated. HIV that exists in a latent form in vivo would be immunologically silent and hence escape destruction. Despite these seemingly unsurmountable problems, intense research in vaccine development continues, and, in fact, some early vaccine trials in primates offer hope for the future.

AMYLOIDOSIS

Amyloid is an abnormal proteinaceous substance that is deposited between cells in many tissues and organs of the body in a variety of clinical disorders. Since its first recognition, it has been delineated by its morphologic appearance on light microscopy. With usual tissue stains, amyloid appears as an intercellular pink translucent material. At one time it was thought to be starch-like, hence the designation "amyloid"; however, it is now known to be composed largely of protein.

Despite the striking morphologic uniformity of amyloid in all cases, *it is quite clear that amyloid is not a single chemical entity.* There are two major and several minor biochemical forms. These are deposited by several different pathogenetic mechanisms, and therefore amyloidosis should not be considered a single disease; rather, it is a group of diseases that share in common the deposition of similar-appearing proteins. At the heart of the morphologic uniformity is the remarkably uniform physical organization of amyloid protein, which we will consider first. This will be followed by a discussion of the chemical nature of amyloid.

PHYSICAL NATURE OF AMYLOID. By electron microscopy, amyloid appears to be made up largely of nonbranching fibrils of indefinite length with a width of approximately 7.5 to 10 nm. X-ray crystallography and infrared spectroscopy demonstrate a characteristic pattern described as a "β-pleated sheet conformation," which is unique among fibrillar mammalian proteins. This conformation (Fig. 6–36), seen regardless of the clinical setting or the chemical composition, is responsible for the distinctive staining and optical properties of amyloid (to be discussed later). In other words, any fibrillar protein deposited in tissues that yields a β-pleated sheet will be recognized as amyloid. In addition to the fibrils, a nonfibrillar pentagonal substance

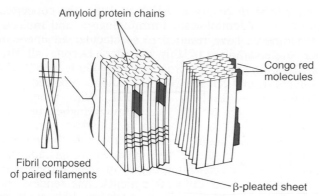

Figure 6–36. Structure of an amyloid fibril, depicting the β-pleated sheet structure and binding sites for the Congo red dye, which is used for diagnosis of amyloidosis. (After Glenner, G. G.: Amyloid deposit and amyloidosis. The β-fibrilloses. N. Engl. J. Med. *52*:148, 1980, by permission of The New England Journal of Medicine.)

(P component) is a minor component of all amyloid deposits.

CHEMICAL NATURE OF AMYLOID. *Two major chemical classes of amyloid have been identified: one composed of immunoglobulin light chains called AL (amyloid light chain), the other made up of a nonimmunoglobulin protein designated AA (amyloid-associated). These proteins are antigenically distinct and, as we shall discuss later, are deposited in different clinical settings.* Immunoglobulin amyloid fibril protein (AL) is made up of complete immunoglobulin light chains, the N-terminal fragment of light chains, or both. Most frequently it is the λ light chain that gives rise to AL. The AL amyloid protein is associated with B-cell dyscrasias and is produced by immunoglobulin-secreting cells. The other major form of amyloid fibril protein, AA, can be described as a unique nonimmunoglobulin protein with molecular weight of 8500 daltons. AA fibrils are derived from a larger precursor protein in the serum called SAA (serum amyloid–associated protein), which serves as the protein component (apoprotein) of a high-density lipoprotein. SAA behaves as an acute-phase reactant, its serum concentration increasing a thousandfold within 24 hours of an inflammatory stimulus. As will be pointed out, AA protein is the major component of the amyloid deposited secondary to chronic inflammatory diseases.

Several other biochemically distinct proteins have been found in amyloid deposits in a variety of clinical settings:

- *Transthyretin* is a normal serum protein that binds and *trans*ports *thy*roxine and *retin*ol, hence the name. *A mutant form of transthyretin (and its fragments) is deposited in a group of genetically determined disorders referred to as familial amyloid polyneuropathies.* Another variant form of transthyretin is deposited in *amyloidosis associated with aging.*
- *β_2-microglobulin,* a component of the MHC class I molecules (p. 166) and a normal serum protein, has been identified as the amyloid fibril subunit in the amyloidosis that complicates the course of patients receiving *long-term hemodialysis.*

- *β_2-amyloid protein,* a 4000-dalton peptide (also called A_4) constitutes the core of cerebral plaques found in Alzheimer's disease as well as the amyloid deposited in walls of cerebral blood vessels of patients with Alzheimer's disease. The A_4 protein is believed to be derived from a much larger (79,000-dalton) precursor that has the characteristics of a transmembrane glycoprotein.
- In addition to the foregoing types, amyloid deposits derived from diverse precursors such as hormones (procalcitonin, proinsulin) and keratin have also been reported.

The nonfibrillar P component described earlier is a normal serum α_1-glycoprotein that bears a striking structural homology to C-reactive protein, a well-known acute-phase reactant. Serum P component has an affinity for purified amyloid fibrils, and its presence in amyloid deposits is responsible for the staining with PAS that led early observers to believe that amyloid was a saccharide.

CLASSIFICATION OF AMYLOIDOSES. Classification of amyloidoses is based on the associated clinical setting, anatomic distribution, and chemical composition of amyloid (Table 6–12).

Immunocyte Dyscrasias with Amyloidosis. Amyloidosis in this category (sometimes called "primary") is systemic in distribution and results from deposition of immunoglobulin light chains (AL) or their fragments, produced by aberrant clones of B cells. *In the United States this is the most common form of amyloidosis.* The best example in this category is amyloidosis associated with multiple myeloma, a malignant neoplasm of plasma cells (p. 374). This disorder is characterized by proliferation of neoplastic cells in the bone marrow, often producing multiple osteolytic lesions in the skeleton. The malignant plasma cells are monoclonal and therefore secrete a single species of immunoglobulin (monoclonal gammopathy) producing an M (myeloma) protein spike on serum electrophoresis. In addition to complete immunoglobulin molecules, the plasma cells may also synthesize and secrete only the λ or κ light chains, also known as Bence Jones proteins. These are present in the blood of up to 70% of patients with multiple myeloma, but amyloidosis develops in only 6 to 15% of myeloma cases. Most of those who develop amyloidosis do have Bence Jones proteins. However, it is clear that free light chain production, although necessary, is not by itself sufficient to produce amyloidosis. It is believed that the quality of the light chain produced (amyloidogenic potential) and the subsequent handling (degradation?) are important factors that determine whether the Bence Jones proteins are deposited as amyloid.

Monoclonal gammopathy is another form of plasma cell dyscrasia. *The great majority of patients in this category do not have classic multiple myeloma but do* have Bence Jones proteins with or without monoclonal immunoglobulins found in the serum, and there is a modest increase in the number of plasma cells in the bone marrow. Unlike myeloma, however, there are no skeletal lesions. Clearly, these patients have an underlying dyscrasia of plasma cells, which has been dubbed

**TABLE 6-12. CLASSIFICATION
OF AMYLOIDOSIS**

Clinicopathologic Category	Associated Diseases	Major Fibril Protein	Chemically Related Precursor Protein
Systemic (Generalized) Amyloidosis			
Immunocyte dyscrasias with amyloidosis (primary amyloidosis)	Multiple myeloma and other monoclonal B-cell proliferations	AL	Immunoglobulin light chains, chiefly λ type
Reactive systemic amyloidosis (secondary amyloidosis)	Chronic inflammatory conditions	AA	SAA
Hemodialysis-associated amyloidosis	Chronic renal failure	β_2-microglobulin	β_2-microglobulin
Hereditary amyloidosis			
(1) Familial Mediterranean fever	—	AA	SAA
(2) Familial amyloidotic neuropathies (several types)	—	Transthyretin*	Transthyretin
Localized Amyloidosis			
Senile cardiac		Transthyretin	Transthyretin
Senile cerebral	Alzheimer's disease	A4 (β_2-protein)	?
Endocrine (e.g., medullary carcinoma of thyroid)	—	Procalcitonin	Calcitonin

* Transthyretin is also known as prealbumin. The transthyretins deposited as amyloid are mutant forms of normal transthyretin. Key: AL, amyloid light chain; AA, amyloid-associated (protein); SAA, serum amyloid-associated (protein).

"covert" myeloma by some experts. However, the exact relationship to multiple myeloma is not clear.

Reactive Systemic Amyloidosis. The amyloid deposits in this group are systemic in distribution and are composed of AA protein. This category is commonly referred to as *"secondary amyloidosis,"* because it is believed to be secondary to chronic inflammatory conditions. *The unifying feature of various conditions that predispose to reactive systemic amyloidosis is protracted breakdown of cells, resulting in most cases from a chronic inflammatory disorder.* Before the advent of antimicrobial chemotherapy, diseases such as tuberculosis, chronic osteomyelitis, and bronchiectasis were the common culprits, and in many parts of the world infectious disease is still the number one cause of amyloidosis. In the United States, however, it more commonly complicates RA, other connective tissue disorders, ulcerative colitis, neoplasms (e.g., Hodgkin's disease), and chronic skin infections associated with IV drug abuse. As mentioned, AA protein, which is deposited as amyloid, is derived from SAA, a precursor protein in the serum.

Heredofamilial Amyloidosis. This group includes several mendelian disorders characterized by widespread deposits of amyloid in the tissues. *Best-characterized is familial Mediterranean fever, which is inherited as an autosomal recessive trait.* Affected persons are of Armenian, Sephardic Jewish, or Arabic origins. The amyloid fibrils are composed of AA protein. This may be related to the recurrent bouts of inflammation of the joints and serosal surfaces that characterize this condition. Several other heredofamilial forms characterized by deposition of amyloid in the nerves have been recognized. These are extremely rare. As mentioned earlier, in these neuropathic forms mutant transthyretins are deposited as amyloid fibrils (see Table 6-12).

Localized Amyloidosis. Localized amyloidosis is a heterogeneous group, in terms of both chemical composition of amyloid and clinical presentation. One of the following sites may be involved in the form of nodular deposits: lungs, larynx, skin, urinary bladder, or tongue. Often infiltrates of plasma cells are found around the nodules, and in at least some cases the amyloid consists of AL protein. Local deposits of amyloid are also sometimes found within tumors of the endocrine system. Medullary carcinoma of the thyroid is one such example in which the amyloid is chemically related to calcitonin, a hormone secreted by the tumor cells.

Amyloid of Aging. Two well-documented forms of amyloidosis occur in aging persons. *Senile cardiac amyloidosis* affects elderly patients, most often in the eighth and ninth decades of life. In many cases the amyloid fibrils are formed of transthyretin. Senile cardiac amyloidosis may be asymptomatic or may produce serious cardiac dysfunction. *Senile cerebral amyloidosis* refers to the deposition of β_2-amyloid protein in the cerebral blood vessels and plaques of patients with Alzheimer's disease (p. 726).

PATHOGENESIS. Although the precursors of the two major amyloid proteins have been identified, several aspects of their origins still are not clear. In reactive systemic amyloidosis, it appears that longstanding tissue destruction and inflammation lead to elevated SAA levels (Fig. 6-37). SAA is synthesized by the liver cells under the influence of cytokines such as IL-6 and IL-1; however, increased production of SAA by itself is not sufficient for the deposition of amyloid. Elevation of serum SAA levels is common to inflammatory states but in most instances does not lead to amyloidosis. It is believed that SAA is normally degraded to soluble end products by the action of monocyte-derived enzymes. Conceivably, individuals who develop

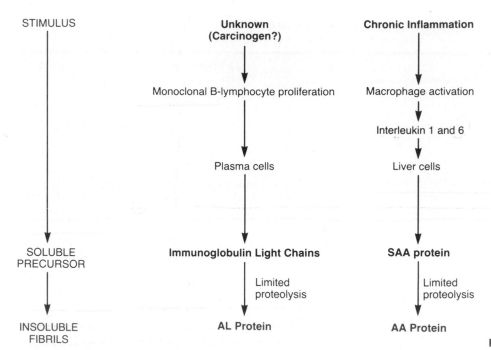

Figure 6-37. Proposed scheme of the pathogenesis of two major forms of amyloid fibrils.

amyloidosis have an enzyme defect that results in incomplete breakdown of SAA, thus generating insoluble AA molecules. In the case of immunocyte dyscrasias, the source of the precursor proteins is well defined, and amyloid material can be derived in vitro by proteolysis of immunoglobulin light chains. But we still do not know why only a fraction of persons who have circulating Bence Jones proteins develop amyloidosis. Again, defective proteolytic degradation has been invoked, but firm evidence is lacking.

MORPHOLOGY. There are no consistent or distinctive patterns of organ or tissue distribution of amyloid deposits in any of the categories cited. Nonetheless, a few generalizations can be made. Amyloidosis secondary to chronic inflammatory disorders tends to produce the most severe systemic involvements. Typically kidneys, liver, spleen, lymph nodes, adrenals, and thyroid, as well as many other tissues, are affected. Although immunocyte-associated amyloidosis cannot reliably be distinguished from the secondary form by its organ distribution, more often it involves the heart, gastrointestinal tract, respiratory tract, peripheral nerves, skin, and tongue. In addition, bizarre distributions, such as amyloidosis of the eye and musculoskeletal system, are encountered more often in patients with immunocyte-associated amyloidosis. However, the same organs affected by reactive systemic amyloidosis (secondary amyloidosis), including kidneys, liver, and spleen, may also contain deposits in the immunocyte-associated form of the disease.

The localization of amyloid deposits in the **heredofamilial syndromes** is quite varied. In familial Mediterra-

nean fever the amyloidosis may be widespread, involving the kidneys, blood vessels, spleen, respiratory tract, and rarely, liver. The localization of amyloid in the remaining hereditary syndromes can be inferred from the designation of these entities. **Localized organ amyloidosis** has already been characterized.

Whatever the clinical disorder, the amyloidosis may or may not be apparent on macroscopic examination. Often small amounts are not recognized until the surface of the cut organ is painted with iodine and sulfuric acid. This yields mahogany brown staining of the amyloid deposits. When amyloid accumulates in larger amounts, frequently the organ is enlarged, and the tissue appears gray with a waxy, firm consistency. **Histologically, the deposition always begins between cells,** often closely adjacent to basement membranes. As the amyloid accumulates, it encroaches on the cells. In time the depositions surround and destroy the trapped native cells. In the immunocyte-associated form, perivascular and vascular localizations are common.

The histologic diagnosis of amyloid is based almost entirely on its staining characteristics. The most commonly used staining technique utilizes the dye Congo red, which under ordinary light imparts a pink or red color to amyloid deposits. Under polarized light the Congo red-stained amyloid shows green birefringence. This reaction is shared by all forms of amyloid and is due to the crossed β-pleated configuration of amyloid fibrils. AA and AL amyloid can be distinguished in histologic sections. AA protein loses affinity for Congo red after incubation of tissue sections with potassium permanganate, whereas AL proteins and most other chemical forms of amyloid do not. Immunoperoxidase staining with monoclonal antibodies directed toward various chemical forms of amyloid is also useful in diagnosis.

Since the pattern of organ involvement in different clinical forms of amyloidosis is variable, each of the major organ involvements is described separately.

Amyloidosis of the kidney is the most common and the most serious involvement in the disease. Grossly, the kidney may appear unchanged; it may be abnormally large, pale, gray, and firm; or it may be reduced in size. Microscopically, the amyloid deposits are found principally in the glomeruli, but they are also present in the interstitial peritubular tissue as well as in the walls of the blood vessels. The glomerulus first develops focal deposits within the mesangial matrix and diffuse or nodular thickenings of the basement membranes of the capillary loops. With progression, the deposition encroaches on the capillary lumens and eventually leads to total obliteration of the vascular tuft (Fig. 6-38). The interstitial peritubular deposits frequently are associated with the appearance of amorphous pink casts within the tubular lumens, presumably of proteinaceous nature. Amyloid deposits may develop in the walls of blood vessels of all sizes, often causing marked vascular narrowing. It is this vascular narrowing that presumably leads to the contracture of the kidneys, mentioned previously.

Amyloidosis of the spleen often causes moderate or even marked enlargement (200 to 800 gm). For obscure reasons, one of two patterns may develop. The deposits may be virtually limited to the splenic follicles, producing tapioca-like granules on gross examination ("sago spleen"), or the involvement may affect principally the splenic sinuses and eventually extend to the splenic pulp, forming large, sheet-like deposits ("lardaceous spleen"). In both patterns, the spleen appears firm in consistency and often reveals on the cut surface, the pale, gray, waxy deposits in the distribution described.

Amyloidosis of the liver may cause massive enlargement, up to such extraordinary weights as 9000 gm. In such advanced cases, the liver is extremely pale, grayish, and waxy on both the external surface and the cut section. Histologically, the deposits appear first in the space of Disse and then progressively enlarge to encroach on the adjacent hepatic parenchyma and sinusoids. The trapped liver cells are literally squeezed to death and are eventually replaced by sheets of amyloid.

Amyloidosis of the heart may occur either as an isolated organ involvement or as part of a systemic distribution. When accompanied by systemic involvement, it is usually associated with immunocyte dyscrasias. The isolated form **(senile amyloidosis)** is usually confined to individuals of advanced age. The deposits may not be evident on gross examination, or they may cause minimal to moderate cardiac enlargement. The most characteristic gross findings are gray-pink, dew-drop-like subendocardial elevations, particularly in the atrial chambers. However, on histologic examination, in addition to these focal subendocardial accumulations, deposits are frequently found throughout the myocardium, beginning between myocardial fibers and eventually causing their pressure atrophy.

Amyloidosis of the endocrine organs, particularly of the adrenals, thyroid, and pituitary, is common in advanced systemic distributions. In this case also, the amyloid deposition begins in relation to stromal and endothelial cells and progressively encroaches on the parenchymal cells. Surprisingly, large amounts of amyloid may be present in any of these endocrine glands without apparent disturbance of function.

Other organs may be involved. Indeed, no organ or tissue of the body is exempt. Deposits may be encountered in the upper and lower respiratory passages, sometimes in nodular masses. The gastrointestinal tract is a relatively favored site, in which amyloid may be found at all levels, sometimes producing tumorous masses that must be distinguished from neoplasms. Depositions in the tongue may produce macroglossia. On the basis of the frequent involvement of the gastrointestinal tract in systemic cases, gingival, intestinal, and rectal biopsies are commonly employed in the diagnosis of suspected cases. Congo red staining and polarization microscopy should be employed in all cases to detect trace amounts, which may be limited to the vascular walls within the tissue examined. The skin, eye, and nervous system are also affected. Deposition of β_2-microglobulin amyloid in patients receiving long-term dialysis occurs most commonly in the carpal ligaments of the wrist, resulting in compression of the median nerve (carpal tunnel syndrome).

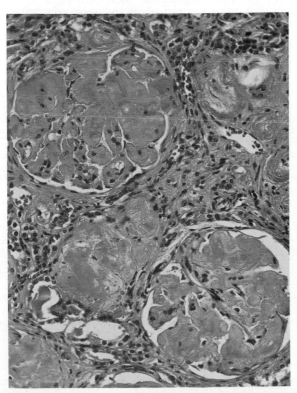

Figure 6-38. Amyloidosis of the kidney. The glomeruli are obliterated by the amorphous amyloid deposit. The vessels *(upper right)* are also virtually occluded by the deposition within their walls.

CLINICAL CORRELATION. Amyloidosis may be an unsuspected finding at autopsy in a patient who has no apparent related clinical manifestations, or it may be responsible for serious clinical dysfunction and even death. All depends on the particular sites or organs affected and the severity of the involvement. Nonspecific complaints such as weakness, fatigue, and weight loss are the most common initial symptoms. Later in the course, amyloidosis tends to manifest itself in one of several ways—by renal disease, hepatomegaly, splenomegaly, or cardiac abnormalities. Renal involvement is often the major cause of symptoms in reactive systemic amyloidosis (secondary amyloidosis). It is usually manifested by proteinuria that may be severe enough to induce the nephrotic syndrome (p. 444). Advancement of the renal disease may lead to renal failure, which is an important cause of death in these patients. The hepatosplenomegaly rarely causes significant clinical dysfunction, but it may be the presenting finding. Cardiac amyloidosis may manifest itself as conduction disturbances or an apparent cardiomyopathy. Cardiac arrhythmias are an important cause of death in cardiac amyloidosis. In one large series, 40% of the patients with AL amyloid died of cardiac disease.

The diagnosis of amyloidosis may be suspected from the clinical signs and symptoms and from some of the findings mentioned; however, more specific tests must often be employed for definitive diagnosis. Biopsy followed by Congo red staining is the most important tool in the diagnosis of amyloidosis. In general, biopsy is taken from the organ suspected to be involved. For example, renal biopsy is useful in the presence of urinary abnormalities. Rectal and gingival biopsy specimens contain amyloid in up to 75% of cases with generalized amyloidosis. Examination of abdominal fat aspirates stained with Congo red is a simple, low-risk method that is finding widespread use. In suspected cases of immunocyte-associated amyloidosis, serum and urinary protein electrophoresis and immunoelectrophoresis should be performed. Bone marrow in such cases usually shows plasmacytosis, even if skeletal lesions of multiple myeloma are not present.

The outlook for patients with generalized amyloidosis is poor, and the mean survival time after diagnosis ranges from one to three years. When the disease is associated with immunocytic dyscrasias, cytotoxic drugs have been used to treat underlying disorder.

Bibliography

Abbas, A. K., Lichtman, A. H., Pober, J. S.: Cellular and Molecular Immunology. Philadelphia, W. B. Saunders, 1991. (An excellent, up-to-date text covering the cellular and molecular aspects of the immune response and mechanisms of hypersensitivity diseases.)

Baltimore, D., Feinberg, M. B.: HIV revealed: Toward a natural history of the infection. N. Engl. J. Med. 321:1673, 1989. (This short editorial provides an excellent overview of the natural history of HIV infection.)

Buckley, R. M., Braffman, M. N., Stern, J. J.: Opportunistic infections in the acquired immunodeficiency syndrome. Semin. Oncol. 17:335, 1990. (This article focuses on the six most common infectious complications of AIDS.)

Fauci, A. S. (Moderator): NIH Conference: Immunopathogenic mechanisms in human immunodeficiency virus infection. Ann. Int. Med. 114:678, 1991. (A review that details the effects of HIV on the immune system.)

Geppert, T.: Southwestern Internal Medicine Conference: Clinical features, pathogenic mechanisms, and new developments in the treatment of systemic sclerosis. Am. J. Med. Sci. 299:193, 1990. (A short review of all major aspects of systemic sclerosis.)

Harris, E. D.: Rheumatoid arthritis: Pathology and implications for therapy. N. Engl. J. Med. 322:1277, 1990. (A succinct review of the current understanding of the nature of genetic and immunologic factors in the pathogenesis of rheumatoid arthritis.)

Haseltine, W. A.: Molecular biology of human immunodeficiency virus type I. FASEB J. 5:2349, 1991. (An excellent summary of the structure of HIV and the function of various viral genes.)

Joshi, V. V. (ed.): Pathology of AIDS and Other Manifestations of HIV Infection. New York, Igaku-Shoin, 1990. (This multiauthored monograph provides details of the organ pathology associated with HIV infections; also includes discussion of AIDS-related tumors.)

Krensky, A. M., Weiss, A., Crabtree, G., et al.: T-lymphocyte–antigen interactions in transplant rejection. N. Engl. J. Med. 322:510, 1990. (A brief and up-to-date discussion of HLA molecules and T-cell receptors and their interactions as they relate to rejection of solid tissue transplants.)

Lipsky, P. E., Davis, L. S., Cush, J. J., et al.: The role of cytokines in the pathogenesis of rheumatoid arthritis. Springer Semin. Immunopathol. 11:123, 1989. (A detailed review of the biology of cytokines, with special emphasis on their role in rheumatoid arthritis.)

McCune, J. M.: HIV-1. The infective process in vivo. Cell 64:351, 1991. (A broad overview of the host-parasite interactions following HIV infection.)

Meltzer, M. S., Skillman, D. R., Hoover, D. L., et al.: Macrophages and the human immunodeficiency virus. Immunol. Today 11:217, 1990. (This article is a part of the HIV series published in this journal in 1990. It details the mechanisms and consequences of HIV infection of macrophages; other articles in this series published between June and December 1990 are also excellent.)

Plotz, P. H. (moderator): NIH Conference: Current concepts in the idiopathic inflammatory myopathies: polymyositis, dermatomyositis, and related disorders. Ann. Intern. Med. 111:143, 1989. (A very good overview of the clinical features, histopathology, and immunology of inflammatory myopathies.)

Rosenberg, Z. F., Fauci, A. S.: Immunogenesis of HIV infection. FASEB J. 5:2382, 1991. (A short review of the interactions between HIV and cells of the immune system.)

Scleroderma. Rheum. Dis. Clin. North Am. 16(1):1990. (This entire monograph contains authoritative and current reviews of etiology, pathogenesis, pathology, and clinical features of systemic sclerosis.)

Stone, M. J.: Amyloidosis: A final common pathway for protein deposition in tissues. Blood 75:531, 1990. (An up-to-date review of the biochemistry, pathogenesis, and clinical features of amyloidosis.)

Systemic lupus erythematosus. Rhem. Dis. Clin. North Am. 14(1):1988. (This entire monograph contains several authoritative articles on epidemiology, etiology, pathogenesis, clinical features, and treatment of SLE.)

Valentine, F. T.: Pathogenesis of the immunologic deficiencies caused by infection with the human immunodeficiency virus. Semin. Oncol. 17:321, 1990. (A good, but not detailed, overview of how the immune system is affected by HIV.)

SEVEN

Neoplasia

DEFINITIONS
NOMENCLATURE
CHARACTERISTICS OF BENIGN AND
MALIGNANT NEOPLASMS
  Differentiation and Anaplasia
  Rate of Growth
  Local Invasion
  Metastasis
EPIDEMIOLOGY
  Cancer Incidence
  Geographic Factors
  Environmental Influences
  Age
  Heredity
  Acquired Preneoplastic Disorders
CARCINOGENESIS—THE MOLECULAR BASIS
OF CANCER
  Oncogenes and Cancer
    Protein Products of Oncogenes
    Activation of Oncogenes
  Cancer Suppressor Genes
    Biochemical Functions of Tumor
      Suppressor Genes
  Molecular Basis of Multistep Carcinogenesis
  Karyotypic Changes in Tumors
BIOLOGY OF TUMOR GROWTH
    Kinetics of Tumor Cell Growth
    Tumor Angiogenesis
    Tumor Progression and Heterogeneity
  Mechanisms of Local and Distant Spread
    Invasion of Extracellular Matrix
    Vascular Dissemination and Homing of
      Tumor Cells
    Molecular Genetics of Metastases
ETIOLOGY OF CANCER—CARCINOGENIC
AGENTS
  Chemical Carcinogens
    Direct-Acting Agents
    Indirect-Acting Agents
    Mechanisms of Action of Chemical
      Carcinogens
  Radiation Carcinogenesis

Viral Oncogenesis
    RNA Oncogenic Viruses
    DNA Oncogenic Viruses
HOST DEFENSE AGAINST TUMORS:
TUMOR IMMUNITY
  Tumor Antigens
  Antitumor Effector Mechanisms
  Immunosurveillance
  Immunotherapy of Human Tumors
CLINICAL FEATURES OF NEOPLASIA
  Effects of Tumor on Host
    Cancer Cachexia
    Paraneoplastic Syndromes
  Grading and Staging of Cancer
  Laboratory Diagnosis of Cancer
    Histologic and Cytologic Methods
    Biochemical Assays
SKIN TUMORS
  Squamous Cell (Epidermoid) Carcinoma
  Basal Cell Carcinoma
  Pigmented Nevi
  Melanoma (Malignant Melanoma,
    Melanocarcinoma)

Even laypersons are familiar with the gravity of a diagnosis of cancer, and most physicians, regardless of their specialty, come in contact with patients who have neoplasms. Hence the importance of the study of neoplasia needs no extensive documentation. Suffice it to note that malignant neoplasms (cancers) are the second leading cause of death in the United States; only cardiovascular disease exacts a higher toll. Even more anguishing than the mortality rate is the emotional and physical suffering inflicted by these neoplasms. The only hope for controlling this dreadful scourge lies in learning more about its molecular origins, and indeed in the past decade great strides have been made in understanding the origins of cancer. This chapter deals with the basic biology of neoplasia, namely, the nature of benign and malignant neoplasms as well as the agents that are known to cause cancers and their cellular interactions. We will also discuss the host response to tumors and the clinical features of neoplasia, including a brief description of some common cancers of the skin.

DEFINITIONS

Neoplasia literally means new growth. A neoplasm, as defined by Willis, is "an abnormal mass of tissue the growth of which exceeds and is uncoordinated with that of the normal tissues and persists in the same excessive manner after the cessation of the stimuli which evoked the change." *Fundamental to the origin of all neoplasms is loss of responsiveness to normal growth controls.* Neoplastic cells are said to be transformed; they continue to replicate, apparently oblivious to the regulatory influences that control normal cell growth. In addition, neoplasms have two other characteristics. They seem to behave as parasites and compete with normal cells and tissues for their metabolic needs. Thus, neoplasms may flourish in patients who are otherwise wasting. Neoplasms also enjoy a certain degree of autonomy, and more or less steadily increase in size regardless of their local environment and the nutritional status of the host. To an extent, then, they are uncontrolled growths. Their autonomy, however, is by no means complete. Some neoplasms require endocrine support, and, indeed, such dependencies can sometimes be exploited to the disadvantage of the neoplasm. Moreover, all are critically dependent on the host for their nutrition and blood supply.

In common medical usage a neoplasm is often referred to as a "tumor" and the study of tumors is called "oncology" (from *oncos,* tumor, and *logos,* study of). Strictly speaking, a tumor is merely a swelling which could be produced by, among other things, edema or hemorrhage into a tissue. Today, the term tumor is applied almost solely to neoplastic masses that may cause swellings on the body surface; use of the term for nonneoplastic lesions has almost disappeared. In oncology the division of neoplasms into benign and malignant categories is most important. This categorization is based on a judgment of a neoplasm's potential clinical behavior.

A tumor is said to be "benign" when its cytologic and gross characteristics are considered relatively innocent, implying that it will remain localized, cannot spread to other sites, and is, therefore, generally amenable to local surgical removal and survival of the patient. It should be noted, however, that benign tumors can produce more than localized lumps, and sometimes they are responsible for serious disease, as will be pointed out (p. 206).

Malignant tumors are collectively referred to as *cancers,* derived from the Latin word for crab—they adhere to any part that they seize upon in an obstinate manner, like the crab. "Malignant," as applied to a neoplasm, implies that it can invade and destroy adjacent structures and spread to distant sites (metastasize) to cause death. Obviously, not all cancers pursue so malignant a course. Some are discovered early and are successfully treated. But the designation "malignant" constitutes a red flag.

NOMENCLATURE

All tumors, benign and malignant, have two basic components: (1) the parenchyma, made up of transformed or neoplastic cells, and (2) the supporting stroma, made up of connective tissue, blood vessels, and possibly lymphatics. As will be seen, *it is the parenchyma of the neoplasm that largely determines its biologic behavior and is the component from which the tumor derives its name.* The stroma, however, carries the blood supply and provides support for the growth of parenchymal cells and is therefore crucial to the growth of the neoplasm.

BENIGN TUMORS. In general, these are designated by attaching the suffix "-oma" to the cell type from which the tumor arises. A benign tumor arising in fibrous tissue is a *fibroma;* a benign cartilaginous tumor is a *chondroma.* The nomenclature of benign epithelial tumors is more complex. They are classified sometimes on the basis of their microscopic and sometimes on the basis of their macroscopic patterns. Others are classified by their cells of origin. Some examples follow:

- *Adenoma.* This term is *applied to benign epithelial neoplasms producing gland patterns and to those derived from glands but not necessarily exhibiting gland patterns.* A benign epithelial neoplasm arising from renal tubule cells and growing in gland-like patterns would be termed an adenoma, as would a mass of benign epithelial cells that produces no glandular patterns but has its origin in the adrenal cortex.

- *Papilloma.* Papillomas are benign epithelial neoplasms, growing on any surface, that produce microscopic or macroscopic finger-like fronds (Fig. 7–1).

- *Polyp.* "Polyp" describes a neoplasm that projects above a mucosal surface, as in the gut, to form a macroscopically visible mass. Although this term is commonly used for benign tumors, some malignant tumors may also appear as polyps, but they are better characterized as polypoid cancers.

- *Cystadenomas.* Cystadenomas are hollow cystic masses; typically, they are seen in the ovary.

MALIGNANT TUMORS. The nomenclature of malignant tumors essentially follows that of benign tumors, with certain additions. *Malignant neoplasms arising in mesenchymal tissue or its derivatives are called sarcomas.* A cancer of fibrous tissue origin is a fibrosarcoma, and a malignant neoplasm composed of chondrocytes is a chondrosarcoma. Thus sarcomas are designated by their histogenesis—i.e., the cell type of which they are composed. *Malignant neoplasms of epithelial cell origin are called carcinomas.* It must be remembered that the epithelia of the body are derived from all three germ layers; thus, a malignant neoplasm arising in the renal tubular epithelium (mesoderm) is a carcinoma, as are the cancers arising in the skin (ectoderm) and lining epithelium of the gut (endoderm). It is evident, then, that mesoderm may give rise

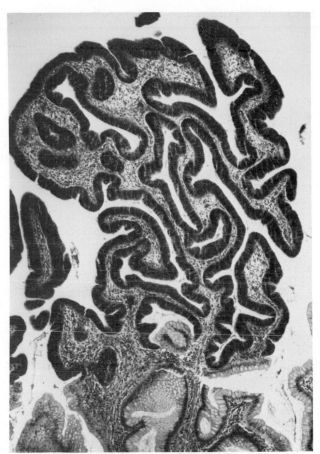

Figure 7-1. A papilloma of the colon with finger-like projections into the lumen. (Courtesy of Dr. Dennis Burns, Department of Pathology, Southwestern Medical School, Dallas, TX.)

to epithelial carcinomas and mesenchymal sarcomas. Carcinomas may be further qualified. *Squamous cell carcinoma* would denote a cancer in which the tumor cells resemble stratified squamous epithelium, and *adenocarcinoma,* a lesion in which the neoplastic epithelial cells grow in gland patterns. Sometimes the tissue or organ of origin can be identified, as for instance in the designation of renal cell adenocarcinoma, or in cholangiocarcinoma, which implies an origin from bile ducts. Sometimes the tumor grows in a very undifferentiated pattern and must be called poorly differentiated carcinoma.

The parenchymal cells in a neoplasm, benign or malignant, more or less resemble each other, as though all had been derived from a single progenitor. Indeed it appears that most neoplasms are of monoclonal origin, as will be documented later. However, in some instances, the stem cell may undergo *divergent differentiation, creating so-called mixed tumors.* The best example is the mixed tumor of salivary gland origin. These tumors have obvious epithelial components dispersed throughout an apparent fibromyxoid stroma sometimes harboring islands of cartilage or bone (Fig. 7-2). All of these diverse elements are thought to derive from epithelial or myoepithelial cells, or both, in the salivary glands, and hence the preferred designa-

tion of these neoplasms is *pleomorphic adenoma.* The schizophrenic mixed tumor should not be confused with a *teratoma, which contains recognizable mature or immature cells or tissues representative of more than one germ layer and sometimes all three.* Teratomas take origin from totipotential cells such as are normally present in the ovary and testis and sometimes abnormally present in sequestered midline embryonic rests. Such cells obviously have the capacity to differentiate into any of the cell types to be found in the adult body and so, not surprisingly, may give rise to neoplasms that mimic—in a helter-skelter fashion—bits of bone, epithelium, muscle, fat, nerve, and other tissues. When all the component parts are well differentiated, it is a *benign (mature) teratoma;* when less well differentiated, an *immature potentially or overtly malignant teratoma.*

The specific names of the more common forms of neoplasms are presented in Table 7-1. Some glaring inconsistencies may be noted. Witness the use of the terms lymphoma, mesothelioma, melanoma, and seminoma for malignant neoplasms. These inappropriate usages are firmly entrenched in medical terminology; perhaps it is irrational to expect humans to be rational.

melanoma, lymphoma, hepatoma

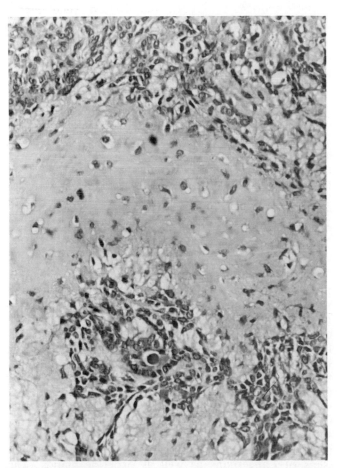

Figure 7-2. Mixed tumor of the parotid gland contains epithelial cells and a cartilage-like stroma, both derived from ductal epithelium. (Courtesy of Dr. Dennis Burns, Department of Pathology, Southwestern Medical School, Dallas, TX.)

TABLE 7–1. NOMENCLATURE OF TUMORS

Tissue of Origin	Benign	Malignant
I. Composed of One Parenchymal Cell Type		
A. Tumors of mesenchymal origin		SARCOMAS
1. Connective tissue and derivatives	Fibroma	Fibrosarcoma
	Lipoma	Liposarcoma
	Chondroma	Chondrosarcoma
	Osteoma	Osteogenic sarcoma
2. Endothelial and related tissues		
Blood vessels	Hemangioma	Angiosarcoma
Lymph vessels	Lymphangioma	Lymphangiosarcoma
Synovium		Synovioma (synoviosarcoma)
Mesothelium		Mesothelioma
Brain coverings	Meningioma	Invasive meningioma
3. Blood cells and related cells		
Hematopoietic cells		Leukemias
Lymphoid tissue		Malignant lymphomas
4. Muscle		
Smooth	Leiomyoma	Leiomyosarcoma
Striated	Rhabdomyoma	Rhabdomyosarcoma
B. Tumors of epithelial origin		CARCINOMAS
1. Stratified squamous	Squamous cell papilloma	Squamous cell or epidermoid carcinoma
2. Basal cells of skin or adnexa		Basal cell carcinoma
3. Epithelial lining		
Glands or ducts	Adenoma	Adenocarcinoma
	Papilloma	Papillary carcinoma
	Cystadenoma	Cystadenocarcinoma
4. Respiratory passages		Bronchogenic carcinoma
		Bronchial "adenoma"
5. Neuroectoderm	Nevus	Melanoma (melanocarcinoma)
6. Renal epithelium	Renal tubular adenoma	Renal cell carcinoma
7. Liver cells	Liver cell adenoma	Hepatocellular carcinoma
8. Urinary tract epithelium (transitional)	Transitional cell papilloma	Transitional cell carcinoma
9. Placental epithelium	Hydatidiform mole	Choriocarcinoma
10. Testicular epithelium (germ cells)		Seminoma
		Embryonal carcinoma
II. More Than One Neoplastic Cell Type— Mixed Tumors—Usually Derived From One Germ Layer		
1. Salivary glands	Pleomorphic adenoma (mixed tumor of salivary origin)	Malignant mixed tumor of salivary gland origin
2. Renal anlage		Wilms' tumor
III. More Than One Neoplastic Cell Type Derived From More Than One Germ Layer — Teratogenous		
1. Totipotential cells in gonads or in embryonic rests	Mature teratoma, dermoid cyst	Immature teratoma, teratocarcinoma

There are other instances of confusing terminology. The _hamartoma_ is a malformation that presents as a mass of disorganized tissue indigenous to the particular site. Thus, one may see a mass of mature but disorganized hepatic cells, blood vessels, and possibly bile ducts within the liver, or there may be a hamartomatous nodule in the lung containing islands of cartilage, bronchi, and blood vessels. Another misnomer is the term _choristoma_. This congenital anomaly is better described as a _heterotopic rest_ of cells. For example, a small nodule of very well-developed and normally organized pancreatic substance may be found in the submucosa of the stomach, duodenum, or even small intestine. This heterotopic rest may be replete with islets of Langerhans as well as exocrine glands. The term choristoma, connoting a neoplasm, imparts to the heterotopic rest a gravity far beyond its usual trivial significance. Regrettably, neither life nor the terminol-

ogy of neoplasms is simple, but the terminology has importance because it is the language by which the nature and significance of tumors are categorized.

CHARACTERISTICS OF BENIGN AND MALIGNANT NEOPLASMS

Nothing is more important to the patient with a tumor than being told "It is benign." In most instances such a prediction can be made with remarkable accuracy based on long-established clinical and anatomic criteria, but some neoplasms defy easy characterization. Certain features may point to innocence and others to malignancy. Moreover, in a few instances there is not perfect concordance between the appearance of a neoplasm and its biologic behavior. However, these problems are not the rule and there are generally reliable criteria by which benign and malignant tumors can be differentiated. These differences are discussed under the following headings: differentiation and anaplasia, rate of growth, local invasion, and metastasis.

DIFFERENTIATION AND ANAPLASIA _____

Differentiation and anaplasia refer only to the parenchymal cells that constitute the proliferating pool and bulk of most neoplasms. The stroma carrying the blood supply is critical to the growth of tumors but does not aid in the separation of benign from malignant ones. The amount of stromal connective tissue does, however, determine the consistency of a neoplasm. Certain cancers induce a dense, abundant fibrous stroma *(desmoplasia)* making them hard, so-called scirrhous tumors. It is the parenchyma that is the "cutting edge" of a neoplasm. *The differentiation of parenchymal cells refers to the extent to which they resemble their normal forebears, both morphologically and functionally.*

Benign neoplasms are composed of well-differentiated cells that resemble very closely their normal counterparts. Thus, the lipoma is made up of mature fat cells

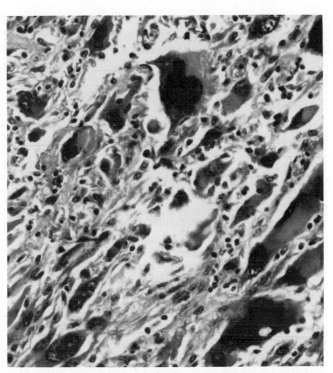

Figure 7–4. An anaplastic rhabdomyosarcoma. Note the marked cellular and nuclear pleomorphism, hyperchromatic nuclei, and tumor giant cells. (Courtesy of Dr. Dennis Burns, Department of Pathology, Southwestern Medical School, Dallas, TX.)

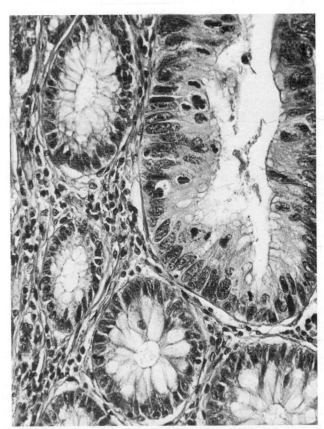

Figure 7–3. Histologic detail of well-differentiated adenocarcinoma of the colon. The normal colonic glands are at left and below, and the cancerous gland is at upper right. Compare the normal cells' basal small nuclei and apical vacuoles with the cancerous cells' pleomorphic nuclei and virtual lack of secretory vacuoles.

laden with cytoplasmic lipid vacuoles and the chondroma of mature cartilage cells that synthesize their usual cartilaginous matrix, evidence of both morphologic and functional differentiation. In well-differentiated benign tumors, mitoses are extremely scant in number and are of normal configuration.

Malignant neoplasms are characterized by a wide range of parenchymal cell differentiation, from surprisingly well-differentiated to completely undifferentiated (Fig. 7–3). Malignant neoplasms that are composed of undifferentiated cells are said to be "anaplastic." Indeed, lack of differentiation, or anaplasia, is considered a hallmark of malignancy. The term anaplasia literally means "to form backward." It implies dedifferentiation, or loss of the structural and functional differentiation of normal cells. However, we now appreciate that most, if not all, cancers arise from stem cells in tissues, so failure of differentiation, rather than dedifferentiation of specialized cells, accounts for undifferentiated tumors.

Anaplastic cells display marked pleomorphism, i.e., marked variation in size and shape (Fig. 7–4). Characteristically the nuclei are extremely *hyperchromatic and large.* The nuclear-cytoplasmic ratio may approach 1:1 instead of the normal 1:4 or 1:6. *Giant cells* may be formed that are considerably larger than their neighbors and possess either one enormous nucleus or several nuclei. *Anaplastic nuclei are variable and bizarre in size and shape.* The chromatin is coarse and clumped, and nucleoli may be of astounding size. More important, *mitoses are often numerous and distinctly atypical;* anarchic multiple spindles may be seen that sometimes can be resolved as tripolar or quadripolar forms, often with one spindle enormously large and the others puny and abortive (Fig. 7–5). Also, anaplastic cells usually fail to develop recognizable patterns of orientation to each other. They may grow in sheets, with total loss of communal structures, such as gland formations or stratified squamous architecture. Thus anaplasia is the most extreme disturbance in cell growth encountered in the spectrum of cellular proliferations. As mentioned at the outset, malignant tumors differ widely with respect to differentiation. At one extreme are extremely undifferentiated, anaplastic tumors, and at the other are cancers that bear striking resemblance to their tissue of origin. Well-differentiated tumors of the prostate, for example, may contain normal-looking glands. Such tumors may sometimes be difficult to distinguish from benign proliferations. Between the two extremes lie tumors loosely referred to as "moderately well differentiated."

Before we leave the subject of differentiation and anaplasia, we should discuss _dysplasia,_ a term used to describe disorderly but non-neoplastic proliferation. Dysplasia is encountered principally in the epithelia. _It is a loss in the uniformity of the individual cells, as well as a loss in their architectural orientation._ Dysplastic cells exhibit considerable pleomorphism (variation in size and shape) and often possess deeply stained (hyperchromatic) nuclei, which are abnormally large for the size of the cell. Mitotic figures are more abundant than usual, although almost invariably they conform to normal patterns. Frequently the mitoses

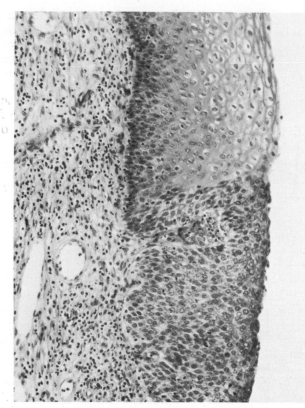

Figure 7–6. Dysplasia of the cervical mucosa. The normal squamous epithelium above changes relatively suddenly into the dysplastic epithelium below. The dysplastic cells have dark nuclei, are more crowded, and do not exhibit the orderly maturation of the surface layers.

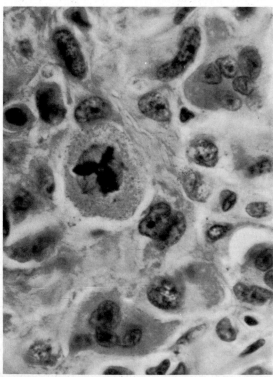

Figure 7–5. High-power detail of anaplastic tumor cells to show cellular and nuclear variation in size and shape. The prominent cell in the center field has an abnormal tripolar spindle.

appear in abnormal locations within the epithelium. Thus, in dysplastic stratified squamous epithelium, mitoses are not confined to the basal layers and may appear at all levels and even in surface cells. There is considerable architectural anarchy. For example, the usual progressive maturation of tall cells in the basal layer to flattened squames on the surface may be lost and replaced by a disordered scrambling of dark basal-appearing cells (Fig. 7–6). When dysplastic changes are marked and involve the entire thickness of the epithelium, the lesion is referred to as _carcinoma in situ,_ a preinvasive stage of cancer (p. 613). Although dysplastic changes are often found adjacent to foci of cancerous transformation and, in long-term studies of cigarette smokers, epithelial dysplasia almost invariably antedates the appearance of cancer, _dysplasia does not necessarily progress to cancer._ Mild to moderate changes that do not involve the entire thickness of epithelium may be reversible and, with removal of the putative inciting causes, the epithelium may revert to normal.

Turning to the functional differentiation of neoplastic cells, as you might presume, the better the differentiation of the cell, the more completely it retains the functional capabilities found in its normal counterparts. Thus, benign neoplasms and even well-differentiated cancers of endocrine glands frequently elaborate the hormones characteristic of their origin. Well-differentiated squamous cell carcinomas elaborate keratin

(Fig. 7–7) just as well-differentiated hepatocellular carcinomas elaborate bile. Indeed, there are few differences in the enzyme profiles of well-differentiated tumors vis-à-vis their normal counterparts. As one descends the scale of differentiation, enzymes and specialized pathways of metabolism are lost and the cells undergo functional simplification. Highly anaplastic undifferentiated cells, then, whatever their tissue of origin, come to resemble each other more than they do the normal cells from which they have arisen. However, in some instances unanticipated functions emerge. Some cancers may elaborate fetal proteins (antigens) not produced by the comparable cells in the adult (p. 210). On the other hand, cancers of nonendocrine origin may assume hormone synthesis to produce so-called ectopic hormones. For example, bronchogenic carcinomas may produce adrenocorticotropic hormone, parathyroid-like hormone, insulin, and glucagon, as well as others. More will be said about these phenomena later (p. 207). *Despite exceptions, the more rapidly growing and the more anaplastic a tumor, the less likely it is to have specialized functional activity.*

In summary, the *cells in benign tumors are almost always well differentiated and resemble their normal cells of origin; the cells in cancers are more or less differentiated but some loss of differentiation is always present.*

RATE OF GROWTH

It is common knowledge that most benign tumors grow slowly and that most cancers grow much faster to eventually spread locally and to distant sites (metasta-

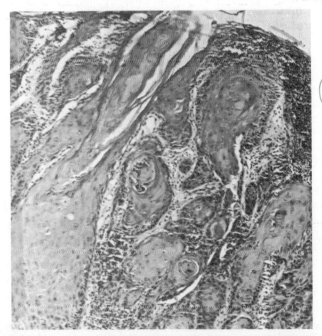

Figure 7–7. A well-differentiated squamous cell carcinoma of the oral cavity. The tumor cells clustered in squamoid nests form keratin pearls.

size) and cause death. There are many exceptions to this generalization, however, and some benign tumors grow more rapidly than some cancers. For example, the rate of growth of leiomyomas (benign smooth muscle tumors) of the uterus is influenced by the circulating levels of estrogens. Thus, they may rapidly increase in size during pregnancy and conversely cease growing or even atrophy and become largely fibrocalcific following menopause. Other influences such as adequacy of blood supply, and possibly pressure constraints, also may affect the growth rate of benign tumors. Adenomas of the pituitary gland locked into the sella turcica have been observed to suddenly shrink in size. Presumably they undergo a wave of necrosis as their progressive enlargement compresses their blood supply. Noting these variables, it is nonetheless true that most benign tumors under clinical observation for long periods of time increase in size slowly over the span of months to years, but there is some variation in rate of growth from one neoplasm to another.

The rate of growth of malignant tumors correlates in general with their level of differentiation. Thus there is wide variation. Some grow slowly for years and then enter a phase of rapid growth, signifying the emergence of an aggressive subclone of transformed cells. Others grow relatively slowly, and indeed there are exceptional instances when growth comes almost to a standstill. Even more exceptionally, cancers (particularly choriocarcinomas) have spontaneously disappeared as they have become totally necrotic, leaving only secondary metastatic implants. With the exception of these rarities, most cancers progressively enlarge over time, some slowly, others rapidly, but the notion that they "emerge out of the blue" is not true. Many lines of experimental and clinical evidence document that most, perhaps all, cancers take years, and sometimes decades, to evolve into clinically overt lesions. Rapidly growing malignant tumors often contain central areas of ischemic necrosis because the tumor blood supply, derived from the host, fails to keep pace with the oxygen needs of the expanding mass of cells.

LOCAL INVASION

A benign neoplasm remains localized at its site of origin. It does not have the capacity to infiltrate, invade, or metastasize to distant sites, as do cancers. As fibromas and adenomas, for example, slowly expand, *most develop an enclosing fibrous capsule that separates them from the host tissue.* This capsule is probably derived from the stroma of the native tissue as the parenchymal cells atrophy under the pressure of the expanding tumor. The stroma of the tumor itself may also contribute to the capsule (Figs. 7–8 and 7–9). However, it should be emphasized that *not all benign neoplasms are encapsulated.* The leiomyoma of the uterus, for example, is quite discretely demarcated from the surrounding smooth muscle by a zone of compressed and attenuated normal myometrium, but there is no well-developed capsule. Nonetheless, a well-defined cleavage plane exists around these lesions.

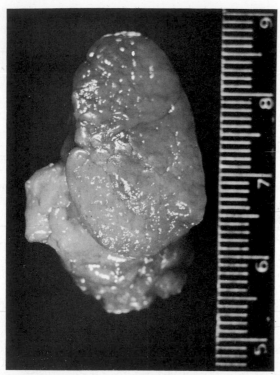

Figure 7–8. A gross view of a fibroadenoma of the breast. The discrete tumor bulges above the level of the surrounding breast substance as it extrudes from its tight encapsulation.

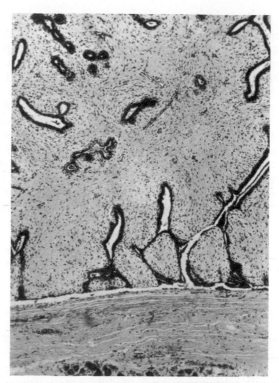

Figure 7–9. A microscopic view of the fibroadenoma of the breast seen in Figure 7–8. The fibrous capsule (*below*) separates the sharply delimited tumor mass from the surrounding breast substance.

A few benign tumors are neither encapsulated nor discretely defined. This is particularly true of some of the vascular benign neoplasms of the dermis. These exceptions are pointed out only to emphasize that

although encapsulation is the rule in benign tumors, the lack of a capsule does not imply that a tumor is malignant.

Cancers grow by progressive infiltration, invasion,

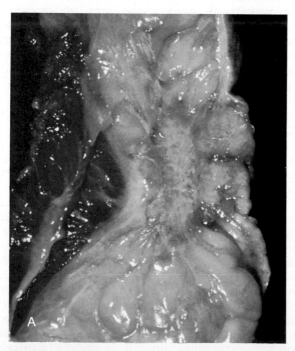

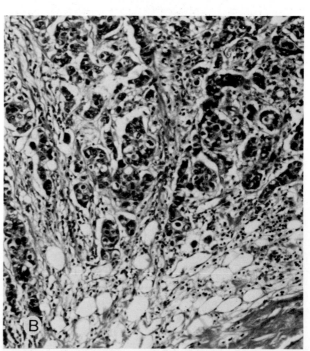

Figure 7–10. *A*, A close-up view of the cut surface of a cancer of the female breast. The infiltrative tumor has eroded through the skin (*right*) and its crab-like extensions pull on the adjacent fat and dark pectoral muscles (*left*). *B*, Microscopic view illustrates invasion of fat and breast stroma by nests of darkly stained tumor cells. (Courtesy of Dr. Dennis Burns, Department of Pathology, Southwestern Medical School, Dallas, TX.)

destruction, and penetration of the surrounding tissue (Fig. 7–10). They do not develop capsules. There are, however, occasional instances in which a slowly growing malignant tumor deceptively appears to be encased by the stroma of the surrounding native tissue, but usually microscopic examination reveals tiny, crab-like feet penetrating the margin and infiltrating adjacent structures. This invasion tends to occur along anatomic planes of cleavage. The infiltrative mode of growth makes it necessary to remove a wide margin of surrounding normal tissue when surgical excision of a malignant tumor is attempted. The surgeon must have knowledge of the invasive potential of the various forms of cancer, because there are striking differences among them.

Next to the development of metastases, local invasiveness is the most reliable feature that distinguishes malignant from benign tumors. We should note here that some (possibly all) epithelial cancers seem to evolve from a preinvasive stage referred to as carcinoma in situ. This is best illustrated by carcinoma of the uterine cervix (p. 613). In situ cancers display the cytologic features of malignancy (p. 175) without invasion of the basement membrane (Fig. 7–11). In time, however, almost all in situ cancers penetrate the basement membrane and invade the subepithelial stroma.

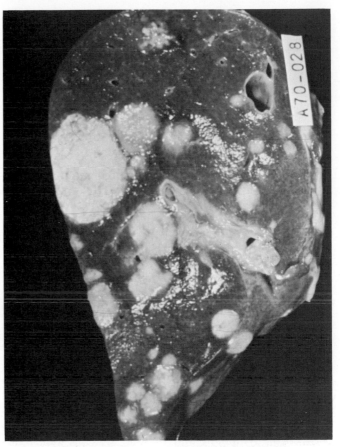

Figure 7–12. A liver studded with metastatic cancer.

METASTASIS

The term *metastasis* connotes the development of secondary implants *(metastases)* discontinuous with the primary tumor, possibly in remote tissues (Fig. 7–12). *The properties of invasiveness and, even more so, metastasis more unequivocally identify a neoplasm as malignant than any of the other neoplastic attributes. However, not all cancers have the ability to metastasize.* The notable exceptions are basal cell carcinoma of the skin and most primary tumors of the central nervous system. Although these neoplasms are highly invasive in their primary sites of origin, they rarely metastasize. It is evident, then, that the properties of invasion and metastasis are separable.

Approximately 30% of newly diagnosed patients with solid tumors (excluding skin cancers other than melanomas) present with metastases. An additional 20% have occult metastases at the time of diagnosis!

In general, the more anaplastic and the larger the primary neoplasm, the more likely metastatic spread. However, exceptions abound. For example, extremely small cancers have been known to metastasize, and conversely, some large, ugly lesions may not have spread. Dissemination strongly prejudices, if it does not preclude, the possibility of cure of the disease, so it is obvious that, short of prevention of cancer, no achievement would confer greater benefit on patients than methods to prevent metastasis.

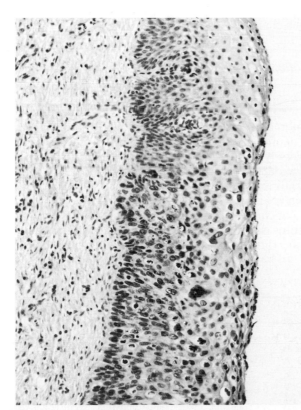

Figure 7–11. Carcinoma in situ of the uterine cervix. In the lower part of the section, the entire thickness of the epithelium is replaced by atypical, dysplastic cells, with loss of orderly differentiation. The basement membrane is intact, and there is no evidence of tumor cells in the subepithelial stroma.

Malignant neoplasms disseminate by one of three pathways: (1) *seeding within body cavities,* (2) *lymphatic spread, and* (3) *hematogenous spread.* Although direct transplantation of tumor cells, as, for example, on surgical instruments or on the surgeon's gloves, may theoretically occur, happily, in clinical practice it is exceedingly rare and, in any event, it is an artificial mode of dissemination.

Seeding of cancers occurs when neoplasms invade a natural body cavity. Carcinoma of the colon may penetrate the wall of the gut and reimplant at distant sites in the peritoneal cavity. A similar sequence may occur with lung cancers in the pleural cavities. This mode of dissemination is particularly characteristic of cancers of the ovary, which often cover the peritoneal surfaces widely. Strangely, the implants may literally glaze all peritoneal surfaces and yet not invade the underlying parenchyma of the abdominal organs. Here again is an instance of the ability to reimplant elsewhere that appears to be separable from the capacity to invade. Neoplasms of the central nervous system such as the medulloblastoma and ependymoma may penetrate the cerebral ventricles and be carried by the cerebrospinal fluid to reimplant on the meningeal surfaces, either within the brain or in the spinal cord.

Lymphatic spread is more typical of carcinomas, whereas the hematogenous route is favored by sarcomas. However, there are numerous interconnections between the lymphatic and vascular systems, and so all forms of cancer may disseminate through either or both systems. The pattern of lymph node involvement depends principally on the site of the primary neoplasm and the natural lymphatic pathways of drainage of the site. Thus lung carcinomas arising in the respiratory passages metastasize first to the regional bronchial lymph nodes and then to the tracheobronchial and hilar nodes. Carcinoma of the breast usually arises in the upper outer quadrant and first spreads to the axillary nodes. Medial lesions may drain through the chest wall to the nodes along the internal mammary artery. Thereafter, in both instances the supra- and infraclavicular nodes may be seeded. In some cases, the cancer cells appear to traverse the lymphatic channels within the immediately proximate nodes to be trapped in subsequent lymph nodes, producing so-called *skip metastases.* Indeed, the cells may traverse all of the lymph nodes to ultimately reach the vascular compartment via the thoracic duct.

It should be noted that enlargement of nodes in proximity to a primary neoplasm may not imply cancerous involvement. The necrotic products of the neoplasm and possibly tumor antigens (p. 203) often evoke reactive changes in the nodes, such as enlargement and hyperplasia of the follicles (lymphadenitis) and proliferation of reticulum cells and sinus reticuloendothelial cells (sinus histiocytosis).

Hematogenous spread is the most feared consequence of a cancer. It is the favored pathway for sarcomas, but carcinomas are by no means shy about using it. As might be expected, arteries are less readily penetrated than are veins. With venous invasion, the blood-borne cells follow the venous flow draining the site of the neoplasm. Understandably, the liver and lungs are the most frequently involved secondary sites in such hematogenous dissemination. All portal area drainage flows to the liver, and all caval blood flows to the lungs. Cancers arising in close proximity to the vertebral column often embolize through the paravertebral plexus, and this pathway is probably involved in the frequent vertebral metastases of carcinomas of the thyroid and prostate.

Certain carcinomas have a propensity for invasion of veins. The renal cell carcinoma often invades the renal vein to grow in a snake-like fashion up the inferior vena cava, sometimes reaching the right side of the heart. Hepatocarcinomas often penetrate portal and hepatic radicles to grow within them into the main venous channels. Remarkably, such intravenous growth may not be accompanied by widespread dissemination.

Many observations suggest that *mere anatomic localization of the neoplasm and natural pathways of venous drainage do not wholly explain the systemic distributions of metastases.* For example, prostatic carcinoma preferentially spreads to bone, bronchogenic carcinomas tend to involve the adrenals and the brain, and neuroblastomas spread to the liver and bones. Conversely, skeletal muscles are rarely the site of secondary deposits. The probable basis of such tissue-specific homing of tumor cells is discussed in a later section (p. 198).

In conclusion, the various features discussed in the preceding sections, as summarized in Table 7–2, permit the differentiation of benign and malignant neo-

TABLE 7–2. COMPARISON OF BENIGN AND MALIGNANT TUMORS

Characteristics	Benign	Malignant
Differentiation/anaplasia	Well-differentiated; structure may be typical of tissue of origin	Some lack of differentiation with anaplasia; structure is often atypical
Rate of growth	Usually progressive and slow; may come to a standstill or regress; mitotic figures are rare and normal	Erratic and may be slow to rapid; mitotic figures may be numerous and abnormal
Local invasion	Usually cohesive and expansile, well-demarcated masses that do not invade or infiltrate the surrounding normal tissues	Locally invasive, infiltrating the surrounding normal tissues; sometimes may seem cohesive and expansile
Metastasis	Absent	Frequently present; the larger and less differentiated the primary, the more likely are metastases

plasms. Against this background of the structure and behavior of neoplasms, we can turn to some considerations of their nature and origins.

EPIDEMIOLOGY

Because cancer is a disorder of cell growth and behavior its ultimate cause has to be defined at the cellular and molecular levels. However, cancer epidemiology can contribute substantially to knowledge about the origin of cancer. For example, the now well-established concept that cigarette smoking is causally associated with lung cancer arose primarily from epidemiologic studies. A comparison of the incidence of colon cancer and dietary patterns in the Western world and Africa led to the recognition that dietary fat and fiber content are important factors in the causation of this cancer. Thus major insights into the causes of cancer can be obtained by epidemiologic studies that relate particular environmental, racial (hereditary?), and cultural influences to the occurrence of specific neoplasms. In addition, certain diseases associated with increased risk of developing cancer (preneoplastic disorders) also provide clues to the pathogenesis of cancer. In the following discussion we first summarize the overall incidence of cancer to gain an insight into the magnitude of the cancer problem and then review some factors relating to the patient and environment that influence the predisposition to cancer.

CANCER INCIDENCE

Some perspective on the likelihood of developing a specific form of cancer can be gained from national incidence and mortality data. Overall, it is estimated that about 514,000 deaths were caused by cancer in the United States in 1991, accounting for approximately 23% of the total mortality. It is sobering to note that about one in four males and one in five females born in 1985 will eventually die of cancer. The incidence of the most common forms of cancer and the major killers is presented in Figure 7–13. It should be noted that some, such as cancer of the larynx in males, are eminently curable and hence they appear in Figure 7–13A but not in Figure 7–13B, whereas others, such as esophageal carcinomas, are less common but more frequently lethal.

The death rates of many forms of malignant neoplasia have changed in the past few decades (Fig. 7–14). To be particularly noted is the significant increase in the overall cancer death rate among males that is attributable largely to lung cancer. In contrast, the overall death rate among females has fallen slightly, owing mostly to the decline in death rates from cancers of the uterus, stomach, and liver. These welcome trends have more than counterbalanced the striking climb in the rate of lung cancer among females, not so long ago a relatively uncommon form of neoplasia in this sex. The declining death rate from uterine cancer can reasonably be attributed to the gratifying control of cervical carcinoma, made possible by the widespread use of cytologic smear studies for its early detection while still curable. The causes of decline in death rates for cancers of the liver and stomach are, however, obscure, but there have been speculations about decreasing exposure to dietary carcinogens.

GEOGRAPHIC FACTORS

Data on the death rates of specific forms of cancer among the nations of the world are also interesting;

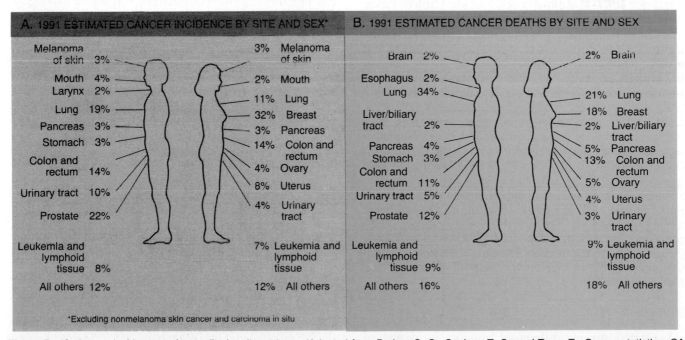

Figure 7–13. Cancer incidence and mortality by site and sex. (Adapted from Boring, C. C., Squires, T. S., and Tong, T.: Cancer statistics. CA 41:19, 1991.)

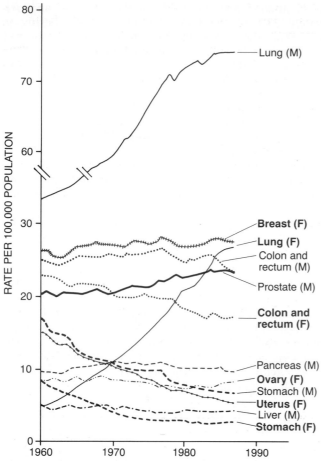

Figure 7–14. Age-adjusted cancer death rates for selected sites in the United States. M, male; F, female. (Adapted from Boring, C. C., Squires, T. S., and Tong, T.: Cancer statistics. CA *41*:26, 1991.)

sometimes there are striking differences. For example, the age-adjusted death rate in 1986 for cancer of the breast per 100,000 women was 27 in the United States, 36 in England and Wales, 32 in the Netherlands, but, in striking contrast, only 7 in Japan. Conversely, the death rate for stomach carcinoma in both males and females is about seven times higher in Japan than in the United States. Liver cell carcinoma is relatively infrequent in the United States but is the number one lethal cancer among many African native populations. Nearly all of the evidence indicates that these geographic differences are environmental rather than genetic in origin. For example, Nisei (second-generation Japanese living in the United States) have mortality rates for certain forms of cancer that are intermediate between those of natives of Japan and of Americans of native lineage, and the two rates come closer with each passing generation. Yet enigmas remain—the death rate from breast carcinoma in females is significantly higher in Denmark than in Sweden, yet environmental differences between these two countries are not immediately apparent.

ENVIRONMENTAL INFLUENCES _____

As stated above, differences in the incidence of cancer around the world usually can be traced to environmental influences. There is no paucity of environmental carcinogens. They lurk in the ambient environment, in the workplace, in food, and in personal practices. They can be as universal as sunlight (p. 201), be found particularly in urban settings (as, for example, asbestos), or be limited to a certain occupation (Table 7–3). Certain features of the diet have also been implicated as possible predisposing influences (p. 259). Among the possible environmental influences, the most distressing are those incurred in personal practices, notably cigarette smoking (described on p. 219 and p. 428) and chronic alcohol consumption. The risk of cervical cancer is also linked to age at first intercourse and the number of sex partners (pointing to a possible causal role for venereal transmission of an oncogenic virus). Suffice it that there is no escape; it seems that everything one does to earn a livelihood, to subsist, or for pleasure, turns out to be fattening, immoral, illegal, or—more disturbing—possibly carcinogenic.

AGE _____

In general, the frequency of cancer increases with age. Most of the mortality occurs between ages 55 and 75 years and then declines, along with the population base, after age 75. The rising incidence with age may be explained by the accumulation of somatic mutations associated with the emergence of malignant neoplasms (p. 192). The decline in immune competence that accompanies aging may also be a factor. However, cancer is no stranger among young people: it causes slightly more than 10% of all deaths among children younger than 15 years. The major lethal cancers in children, in approximate decreasing order of importance, are lymphoblastic leukemia, tumors of the central nervous system, lymphomas, soft tissue sarcomas, and bone sarcomas. Study of several childhood tumors, particularly retinoblastoma and Wilms' tumor,

TABLE 7–3. OCCUPATIONAL CANCERS

Agent (Persons at Risk)	Type of Cancer
Asbestos	Bronchogenic carcinoma, mesothelioma, others
β-naphthylamine (rubber, dye workers)	Bladder carcinoma
Benzene (rubber-cement workers, distillers, dye users)	Leukemia
Vinyl chloride (plastic industry workers)	Liver angiosarcoma
Arsenic (miners, insecticide makers and sprayers, chemical workers)	Skin, lung, liver carcinomas
Chromium (producers and processors exposed to volatilized gases)	Nasal cavity, sinuses, lung, and larynx cancers
Nickel (miners and processors exposed to volatilized gases)	Nasal, sinuses, lung cancers
Radioactive ores (miners exposed to dusts)	Lung and bone cancers, leukemia

has provided novel insights into the pathogenesis of malignant transformation (p. 189).

HEREDITY

Because cancer is destined to occur in one out of four or five individuals, nearly all families have at least one afflicted first- or second-degree relative. Understandably, a question often asked is, "Is cancer an inherited disease?" Regrettably, there is no simple answer. A predisposition to a few uncommon forms of cancer can be hereditary, transmitted in mendelian fashion (Table 7–4), and the suspicion grows that inherited susceptibility may also play a role in the genesis of several common cancers.

Childhood retinoblastoma is the most striking example of the role of heredity. Approximately 40% of the retinoblastomas are familial. The predisposition to this tumor shows an autosomal dominant pattern of inheritance. Carriers of this gene have a 10,000-fold greater risk of developing retinoblastoma, usually bilateral. They also have a greatly increased risk of developing a second cancer, particularly osteogenic sarcoma. As will be discussed later, a "cancer suppressor" gene has been implicated in the pathogenesis of retinoblastoma. Multiple polyposis coli is another hereditary disorder marked by an extraordinarily high risk of cancer. Individuals who inherit the autosomal dominant mutation have at birth, or soon thereafter, innumerable polypoid adenomas of the colon, and in virtually 100% of cases are fated to develop a carcinoma of the colon by age 50 years. Besides the dominantly inherited cancerous or precancerous disorders, there is a small group of autosomal recessive conditions collectively characterized by some defect in DNA repair. Homozygotes with xeroderma pigmentosum, for example, have a strong predisposition to sunlight-induced melanocarcinomas and basal cell and squamous cell carcinomas of the skin in addition to other nonneoplastic cutaneous and ocular abnormalities. All the well-defined conditions already discussed account for only a small fraction of the total burden of malignant neoplasia. What can be said about the influence of heredity on the large preponderance of malignant neoplasms? To begin with, as we point out in subsequent sections, the evidence is strong that carcinogenesis involves mutations in the genome. One or more such mutations may be inherited in this germ line. Such individuals are likely more predisposed to cancer than others. It is not surprising, therefore, that familial predisposition has also been noted with common neoplasms such as carcinoma of the breast, colon, ovary, prostate, and uterus, and with melanocarcinomas. Indeed, with each of these types of neoplasia, specific families have been identified in which there appear to be mendelian patterns of inheritance. Rare families have an increased predisposition to diverse forms of cancer, ranging from sarcomas of soft tissues and bone to breast carcinoma. However, *with most forms of malignancy, well-defined genetic influences can be identified in only a few instances.* The vast majority seem to develop spontaneously and are therefore presumed to be entirely or largely of environmental origin.

But are they really? It is highly likely that genetic predisposition contributes to at least a proportion of the so-called environmental or spontaneous cancers. The converse is equally true: environmental factors

TABLE 7–4. HEREDITARY NEOPLASMS AND PRENEOPLASTIC CONDITIONS

Disorder	Inheritance	Features
Hereditary Neoplasms		
Retinoblastoma	AD	Often bilateral; susceptibility to second tumors, especially osteosarcoma
Familial adenomatous polyposis coli	AD	Multiple adenomatous polyps and adenocarcinomas of the colon
Multiple endocrine neoplasia I	AD	Adenomas of the pituitary, parathyroid, and pancreatic islet cells
Multiple endocrine neoplasia II	AD	Medullary carcinoma of the thyroid, pheochromocytoma, and parathyroid tumors
Neurofibromatosis type I (von Recklinghausen's disease)	AD	Gliomas of the brain and optic nerve, acoustic neuroma, meningioma, pheochromocytoma
Wilms' tumor	AD	Wilms' tumor of kidney; other congenital malformations
Hereditary Preneoplastic Conditions		
Defective DNA repair–chromosomal instability		
Xeroderma pigmentosum	AR	Basal and squamous cell carcinoma of skin; malignant melanomas in patients exposed to UV light
Bloom's syndrome	AR	Acute leukemias, various carcinomas
Fanconi's anemia	AR	Acute leukemias, squamous cell carcinomas, and hepatomas
Ataxia-telangiectasia	AR	Acute leukemia, lymphoma, breast cancer in females
Immune deficiency syndromes		
X-linked agammaglobulinemia	XR	Lymphomas and leukemia
Wiskott-Aldrich syndrome	XR	Acute leukemias and lymphoma
X-linked lymphoproliferative syndrome	XR	Abnormal response to EBV; EBV-induced B-cell immunoblastic lymphomas
Cancer family syndrome	AD	Cancers of multiple organs: colon, endometrium, breast, lung

Key: AD, autosomal dominant; AR, autosomal recessive; XR, X-linked recessive.

contribute to the development of many hereditary neoplasms. For example, individuals with xeroderma pigmentosum develop primarily cancers of the skin, a tissue exposed to radiant energy.

Heredity and environment can be viewed then as the two ends of a spectrum of predisposing influences. At the extremes are neoplasms that develop because of a strong hereditary component and those related to heavy exposure to environmental carcinogens, but in between are the great majority that result from varying contributions of heredity and environment.

ACQUIRED PRENEOPLASTIC DISORDERS _____

Besides the genetic influences described above, certain clinical conditions are well-recognized predispositions to the development of malignant neoplasia. Sometimes they are referred to as *"preneoplastic disorders."* This designation is unfortunate because it implies a certain inevitability, but in fact although they may increase the likelihood, in most instances cancer does not develop. Brief citation of the chief conditions follows:

• *Persistent regenerative cell replication*—e.g., squamous cell carcinoma in the margins of a chronic skin fistula, or a long-unhealed skin wound; hepatocellular carcinoma in cirrhosis of the liver (particularly certain forms).

• *Hyperplastic and dysplastic proliferations*—e.g., endometrial carcinoma in atypical endometrial hyperplasia; bronchogenic carcinoma in the dysplastic bronchial mucosa of habitual cigarette smokers.

• *Chronic atrophic gastritis*—e.g., gastric carcinoma in pernicious anemia.

• *Chronic ulcerative colitis*—e.g., an increased incidence of colorectal carcinoma in long-standing disease.

• *Leukoplakia of the oral cavity, vulva, or penis*—e.g., increased risk of squamous cell carcinoma.

• *Villous adenomas of the colon*—e.g., high risk of transformation to colorectal carcinoma.

In this context it may be asked, what is the risk of malignant change in a benign neoplasm or, stated differently, are benign tumors precancerous? In general the answer is no, but inevitably there are exceptions and perhaps it is better to say that each type of benign tumor is associated with a particular level of risk, ranging from high to virtually nonexistent. For example, adenomas of the colon as they enlarge undergo malignant transformation in up to 50% of cases; in contrast malignant change is extremely rare in leiomyomas of the uterus.

CARCINOGENESIS—THE MOLECULAR BASIS OF CANCER _____

It could be justifiably argued that the proliferation of literature on the molecular basis of cancer has outpaced the growth of even the most malignant of tumors! Understandably, therefore, it is easy to get lost in the growing forest of information. It might then be profitable to list some fundamental principles before we delve into the details of the genetic basis of cancer.

• *Nonlethal genetic damage lies at the heart of carcinogenesis.* Such genetic damage (or mutation) may be acquired by the action of environmental agents such as chemicals, radiation, or viruses, or it may be inherited in the germ line. The genetic hypothesis of cancer implies that a tumor mass results from the clonal expansion of a single progenitor cell that has incurred the genetic damage, i.e., tumors are monoclonal. This expectation has been realized in the vast majority of tumors that have been analyzed. Clonality of tumors is assessed quite readily in women who are heterozygous for polymorphic X-linked markers such as the enzyme glucose-6-phosphate dehydrogenase (G6PD) or X-linked restriction fragment length polymorphisms (RFLPs). The principle underlying such an analysis is illustrated in Figure 7–15.

• *Two classes of normal regulatory genes—the growth-promoting protooncogenes and the growth-inhibiting cancer suppressor genes (antioncogenes)—are the principal targets of genetic damage.* Mutant

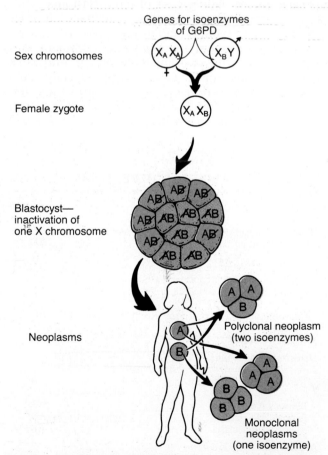

Figure 7–15. Diagram depicts the use of X-linked isoenzyme cell markers as evidence of the monoclonality of neoplasms. Because of random X inactivation, all females are mosaics with two cell populations (with G6PD isoenzyme A or B in this case). When neoplasms that arise in women who are heterozygous for X-linked markers are analyzed, they are made up of cells that contain the active maternal (X_A) or the paternal (X_B) X chromosome but not both.

alleles of protooncogenes are considered dominant because they transform cells despite the presence of their normal counterpart. In contrast, both normal alleles of the tumor suppressor genes must be damaged for transformation to occur, so this family of genes is sometimes referred to as recessive oncogenes.

- *Carcinogenesis is a multistep process at both the phenotypic and genetic level.* A malignant neoplasm has several phenotypic attributes, such as excessive growth, local invasiveness, and the ability to form distant metastases. These characteristics are acquired in a stepwise fashion—a phenomenon called *tumor progression (p. 195).* At the molecular level, progression results from accumulation of genetic lesions.

With this overview (Fig. 7–16) we can now address in some detail the molecular pathogenesis of cancer, and then discuss the carcinogenic agents that inflict genetic damage.

ONCOGENES AND CANCER

The discovery of *protooncogenes* and their potential to transform into cancer-causing *oncogenes* is one of the triumphs of modern molecular biology. In 1989, J. Michael Bishop and Harold Varmus received the Nobel Prize for their pioneering contributions to this field. As often happens in science, the discovery of protooncogenes was not straightforward. These cellular genes were first discovered as "passengers" within the genome of acute transforming retroviruses, which cause rapid induction of tumors in animals and can

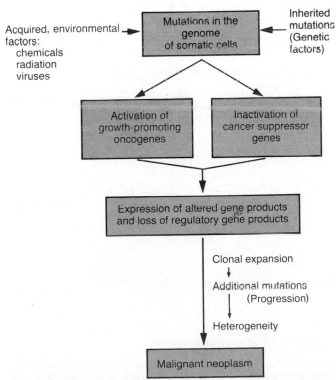

Figure 7–16. Flow chart depicts a simplified scheme of cancer pathogenesis.

also transform animal cells in vitro. Molecular dissection of their genomes revealed the presence of unique transforming sequences (viral oncogenes or v-*onc*s) not found in the genomes of nontransforming retroviruses. Most surprisingly, molecular hybridization revealed that the v-*onc* sequences were almost identical to sequences found in the normal cellular DNA. From this evolved the concept that during evolution retroviral oncogenes were *transduced* (captured) by the virus through a chance recombination with the DNA of a (normal) host cell that had been infected by the virus. Because they were discovered initially as "viral genes," protooncogenes are named after their viral homologs. Each v-*onc* is designated by a three-letter word that relates the oncogene to the virus from which it was isolated. Thus the v-*onc* contained in *fe*line *s*arcoma virus is referred to as v-*fes*, whereas the oncogene in *si*mian *s*arcoma virus is called v-*sis*. The corresponding protooncogenes are referred to as *fes* and *cis* by dropping the prefix.

Although the study of transforming animal retroviruses provided the first glimpse of protooncogenes, these investigations did not explain the origin of human tumors, which (with rare exceptions) are not caused by infection with retroviruses. Hence the question was raised: do nonviral tumors contain oncogenic DNA sequences? The answer was provided by experiments involving DNA-mediated gene transfer (DNA transfection). When DNA extracted from several different human tumors was transfected into mouse fibroblasts in vitro, the recipient cells underwent malignant transformation. The conclusion from such experiments was inescapable: DNA of spontaneously arising cancers contains oncogenic sequences, or oncogenes. Many of these transforming sequences have turned out to be homologous to the *ras* protooncogenes that are the forebears of v-*onc*s contained in Harvey (H) and Kirsten (K) sarcoma viruses. Others, such as the *neu* oncogene, represent novel transforming sequences that have never been detected in retroviruses. *To summarize, protooncogenes may become oncogenic by retroviral transduction (v-oncs) or by influences that alter their behavior in situ, thereby converting them into cellular oncogenes (c-oncs).* Two questions follow: (1) What are the functions of oncogene products? (2) How do the normally "civilized" protooncogenes turn into "enemies within"? These issues are discussed next.

Protein Products of Oncogenes

Oncogenes encode proteins called *oncoproteins,* which resemble the normal products of protooncogenes with the exception that oncoproteins are devoid of important regulatory elements and their production in the transformed cells is not dependent on growth factors or other external signals. To aid in the understanding of the nature and functions of oncoproteins it is necessary to briefly review the sequence of events that characterize normal cell proliferation. (These are discussed in more detail on p. 48.) Under physiologic conditions, cell proliferation can be readily resolved into the following steps:

- The binding of a growth factor to its specific receptor on the cell membrane
- Transient and limited activation of the growth factor receptor, which in turn activates several signal-transducing proteins on the inner leaflet of the plasma membrane
- Transmission of the transduced signal across the cytosol to the nucleus via second messengers
- Induction and activation of nuclear regulatory factors that initiate DNA transcription and ultimately cell division

With this background, we can readily identify oncogenes and oncoproteins as altered versions of their normal counterparts and group them on the basis of their role in the signal transduction cascade (Table 7–5).

GROWTH FACTORS. Beginning outside the cell, mutations of genes that encode growth factors can render them oncogenic. Such is the case with the protooncogene for platelet-derived growth factor (PDGF), which was initially discovered in the guise of the viral oncogene contained in the simian sarcoma virus (v-sis). Subsequently, several human tumor cell lines have been found to transcribe c-sis. Furthermore, it appears that several of the same tumors also possess receptors for PDGF and are hence subject to autocrine stimulation. Such an autocrine loop is not an uncommon characteristic of transformed cells. In many instances the growth factor gene itself is not altered or mutated, but the products of other oncogenes such as ras cause overexpression of growth factor genes, thus forcing the cell to secrete large amounts of growth factors such as transforming growth factor-α (TGF-α). This growth factor, you may recall, is related to the epidermal growth factor (EGF) and induces cell proliferation by binding to the EGF receptor.

In addition to c-sis, a group of related oncogenes that encode homologs of fibroblast growth factors (e.g., k-fgf, hst, FGF-3, and int-2) has also been detected in several gastrointestinal and breast tumors.

GROWTH FACTOR RECEPTORS. The next group in the sequence of signal transduction involves growth factor receptors, and several oncogenes that encode mutated forms of these receptors have been found. Many of them encode altered forms of known growth factor receptors, e.g., c-erbB-1 (EGF receptor) and c-fms (receptor for colony stimulating factor-1), whereas others, such as c-neu, encode receptor-like proteins with unknown ligands. To understand how mutations affect the function of these receptors it should be recalled that several growth factor receptors are transmembrane proteins with an external ligand-binding and a cytoplasmic tyrosine kinase domain. In the normal forms of these receptors the kinase activity is transiently activated by binding of their specific growth factors, followed rapidly by tyrosine phosphorylation of several substrates that are a part of the mitotic cascade. The oncogenic versions of these receptors are associated with persistent activation of the tyrosine kinase activity of the cytoplasmic domain without binding to the growth factor. Hence the mutant receptor proteins deliver continuous mitogenic signals to the cell.

In addition to mutations that derail the regulated function of these protooncogenes, overexpression of normal forms of their protein products occurs in many tumors including glioblastomas and cancers of breast, ovary, and stomach. These tumors, then, are exquisitely sensitive to growth-promoting effects of very small amounts of growth factors.

TABLE 7–5. SELECTED ONCOGENES, THEIR MODE OF ACTIVATION, AND ASSOCIATED HUMAN TUMORS

Category	Protooncogene	Mechanism of Activation	Associated Human Tumor
Growth Factors			
PDGF-β chain	sis	Overexpression	Astrocytoma
			Osteosarcoma
Fibroblast growth	hst-1	Overexpression	Stomach cancer
factors	int-2		Bladder cancer
			Breast cancer
Growth Factor Receptors			
EGF receptor	erb-B1	Amplification	Gliomas
EGF-like receptor	neu (erb-B2)	Amplification	Breast, ovarian, and stomach cancers
Proteins Involved in Signal Transduction			
GTP-binding	ras	Point mutations	A variety of human cancers including lung, colon, pancreas; many leukemias
Tyrosine kinase	abl	Translocation	Chronic myeloid leukemia
			Acute lymphoblastic leukemia
Nuclear Regulatory Proteins			
Transcriptional	myc	Translocation	Burkitt's lymphoma
activators	N-myc	Amplification	Neuroblastoma
			Small cell carcinoma of lung
	L-myc	Amplification	Small cell carcinoma of lung
Mitochondrial Protein	bcl-2	Translocation	Follicular B-cell lymphoma

SIGNAL-TRANSDUCING PROTEINS. Several examples of oncoproteins that mimic the functions of normal cytoplasmic signal-transducing proteins have been found. The subcellular location and the biochemical nature of such proteins are varied. Many are associated with the inner leaflet of the plasma membrane, e.g., products of c-*src*, *abl*, and *ras* genes, but some reside in the cytoplasm, e.g., *raf* proteins. Biochemically, *src* and *abl* are non–receptor-associated tyrosine kinases, whereas *ras* is a guanosine nucleotide-binding protein; *raf* product, on the other hand, is a serine-threonine kinase. Of the oncogenes that encode signal-transducing proteins, c-*ras* is commonly involved in human cancer and so will be discussed briefly.

Approximately 25% of all human tumors contain mutated versions of the *ras* gene. In some tumors, such as colon cancers, the incidence of *ras* mutations is even higher. The *ras* family of proteins binds guanosine nucleotides (GTP and GDP), as do the well-known G proteins. Normal *ras* proteins flip back and forth between an excited signal-transmitting state and a quiescent state. In the inactive state *ras* proteins (p21) bind GDP; when cells are stimulated by certain receptor-ligand interactions, p21 becomes activated by exchanging GDP for GTP (Fig. 7–17). The activated *ras* in turn activates downstream regulators of proliferation such as adenylate cyclase; however, the *excited signal-emitting stage of the normal* ras *protein is short lived because its intrinsic GTPase activity hydrolyzes GTP to GDP, thereby returning the protein to its quiescent ground state.* In contrast, *ras* oncoproteins (derived from the mutated *ras* gene) have greatly reduced GTPase activity, so the protein is "trapped" in its excited state, causing in turn pathologic activation of the mitogenic signaling pathway. In addition to *ras* proteins, mutant G proteins can also transform cells, and oncogenic versions of G proteins have been identified in several human endocrine tumors (involving the pituitary, ovary, and adrenals).

NUCLEAR REGULATORY FACTORS. Ultimately, all signal transduction pathways enter the nucleus and impact on a large bank of responder genes that orchestrate the cells' orderly advance through the mitotic cycle. Not surprisingly, therefore, mutations that affect genes that regulate transcription of DNA are associated with malignant transformation. A whole host of oncoproteins, including products of the *myc*, *myb*, *jun*, *fos*, and *rel* oncogenes, have been localized to the nucleus. The precise mechanisms by which these nuclear proteins deregulate cell proliferation are not entirely clear but two general principles seem to be emerging: (1) the products of *myc*, *jun*, and *fos* protooncogenes are believed to be regulators of nuclear transcription. A complex of *fos-jun* proteins binds specifically to DNA and functions as a transcriptional activator. During the normal cell cycle the expression of *fos* and *jun* is highly regulated. Oncogenic versions of these genes are associated with persistent expression and possibly sustained DNA transcription. (2) In contrast, mutant forms of *rel* and *Erb-A* protooncogenes *prevent* the expression of certain genes required for cell differentiation. Because differentiation is usually coupled with cessation of replication, an imbalance between proliferation and differentiation may occur. Of the various nuclear oncogenes, members of the *myc* family are most widely implicated in human tumors. In Burkitt's lymphoma c-*myc* is activated, whereas the related N-*myc* and L-*myc* are amplified in neuroblastomas and certain small-cell cancers of lung, respectively.

MITOCHONDRIAL ONCOGENE. A recent addition to the roster of oncogenes, *bcl-2*, has several unique features. First, its location is quite unusual—the inner mitochondrial membrane. (Recall that mitochondria are not believed to be in the signal transduction pathway.) Second, it operates in a completely different fashion: it does not cause cell proliferation but rather *prevents apoptosis or programmed cell death*. Overexpression of the *bcl-2* gene, brought about by translocation, is a characteristic feature of follicular B-cell lymphomas. Presumably by extending cell survival, *bcl-2* allows other mutations that affect protooncogenes and cancer suppressor genes to supervene. The functions of the *bcl-2* protein at the biochemical level remain to be elucidated. Some mechanisms by which oncogenes promote cell growth are summarized in Figure 7–18.

Activation of Oncogenes

In the preceding section we discussed how mutant forms of protooncogenes may provide gratuitous growth-stimulating signals. Next we focus on mechanisms by which protooncogenes are transformed into oncogenes. This is brought about by two broad categories of changes:

- Changes in the *structure* of the gene, resulting in the

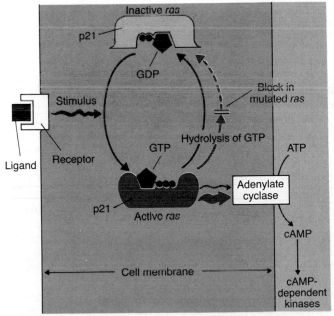

Figure 7–17. A model for action of *ras* genes. When a normal cell is stimulated through a receptor, inactive *ras* gene is activated, which in turn modulates the cellular activities by affecting cAMP levels. The mutant *ras* protein is permanently activated because of its inability to hydrolyze GTP, leading to continual stimulation of the cell without any external trigger.

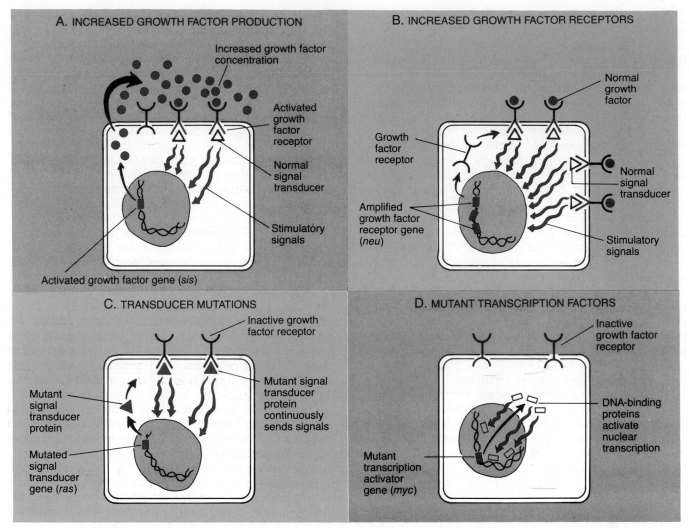

Figure 7–18. Mechanisms by which an oncogene may promote cell growth. *A*, It may code for a growth factor that stimulates the tumor cell by autocrine mechanisms. *B*, It may encode a growth factor receptor and be amplified, thus increasing the number of receptors on tumor cells. *C*, It may encode for defective signal transducers that transmit growth promoting signals without an external trigger. *D*, It may encode a transcription factor that binds to DNA and stimulates cell growth.

synthesis of an abnormal gene product (oncoprotein) having an aberrant function
● Changes in *regulation* of gene expression, resulting in enhanced or inappropriate production of the structurally normal growth-promoting protein.

We can now discuss the specific lesions that lead to structural and regulatory changes that affect protoon-cogenes.

POINT MUTATIONS. The *ras* oncogene represents the best example of activation by point mutations. Several distinct mutations have been identified, all of which affect a domain that is critical to the binding and hydrolysis of GTP; hence mutant *ras* proteins have reduced ability to hydrolyze GTP.

A very large number of human tumors carry *ras* mutations. The frequency of such mutations varies with different tumors, but in some types it is very high. For example, 90% of pancreatic adenocarcinomas contain a *ras* point mutation, as do about 50% of colon and thyroid cancers, and 30% of lung adenocarcinomas and myeloid leukemias. Interestingly, *ras* mu-

tations are very infrequent or even nonexistent in certain other cancers, particularly those arising in the ovary or breast, lending truth to the old belief that there is more than one way to skin a cat.

CHROMOSOMAL TRANSLOCATIONS. Rearrangement of genetic material brought about by *chromosomal translocation usually results in overexpression of protooncogenes, but in some cases the gene may incur structural changes as well*. Translocation-induced overexpression of a protooncogene is best exemplified by Burkitt's lymphoma. All such tumors carry one of three translocations, each involving chromosome 8q24, where the c-*myc* gene has been mapped. At its normal locus the expression of the *myc* gene is tightly controlled and is expressed only during certain stages of the cell cycle (p. 50). In Burkitt's lymphoma the most common form of translocation results in the movement of the c-*myc*-containing segment of chromosome 8 to chromosome 14q band 32 (Fig. 7–19). This places c-*myc* close to the immunoglobulin heavy chain (Cμ) gene, a region with hectic transcriptional activity.

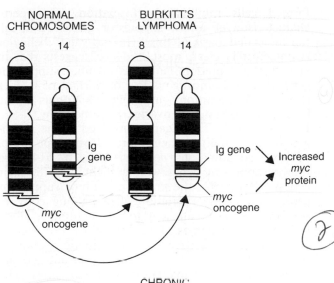

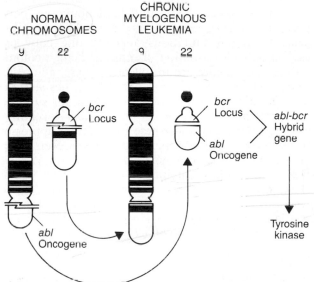

Figure 7–19. The chromosomal translocations and associated onco-genes in Burkitt's lymphoma and chronic myelogenous leukemia.

Detached from its normal regulatory elements, the c-*myc* gene responds to relentless stimulation by its excitable and evidently seductive neighbor and hence its product is expressed at a high level. Overexpression of the *bcl-2* gene occurs in an analogous fashion. In virtually all follicular B-cell lymphomas, the *bcl*-2 gene, mapped on 18q21, is shifted to chromosome 14 near the immunoglobulin heavy chain gene.

The Philadelphia chromosome, characteristic of chronic myeloid leukemia, provides an example of genetic damage wrought by translocation. In this case a reciprocal translocation between chromosomes 9 and 22 relocates a truncated portion of the protooncogene c-*abl* (from chromosome 9) to the breakpoint cluster (*bcr*) locus on chromosome 22. The hybrid c-*abl-bcr* gene encodes a chimeric protein that (like several other oncoproteins) has tyrosine kinase activity.

GENE AMPLIFICATION. Activation of protooncogenes resulting from overexpression of their products may result from reduplication and manifold amplification

of their DNA sequences. Such amplification may produce several hundred copies of the protooncogene in the tumor cell. Amplified genes can be detected by molecular studies or identified cytogenetically in the form of double minutes and homogeneous staining regions (Fig. 7–20). The most interesting cases of amplification involve N-*myc* (a member of the *myc* family of genes) in neuroblastoma and c-*neu* in breast cancers. These genes are amplified in 30 to 40% of these two tumors, and in both settings this amplification is associated with poor prognosis. Similarly amplification of L-*myc* and N-*myc* correlates strongly with disease progression in small-cell cancer of the lung.

CANCER SUPPRESSOR GENES

You may recall that the eminent physicist Newton predicted that every action has an equal and opposite reaction. Although Newton was not a cancer biologist his formulation holds true for cell growth. Whereas protooncogenes encode proteins that promote cell growth, the products of tumor suppressor genes apply brakes to cell proliferation. In this section we describe cancer suppressor genes, their products, and possible mechanisms by which loss of their function contributes to neoplastic transformation.

We begin our discussion with the retinoblastoma (*Rb*) gene, the first and prototypic cancer suppressor gene to be discovered. Like many advances in medicine, the discovery of cancer suppressor genes was accomplished by the study of a rare disease, in this case retinoblastoma, an uncommon childhood tumor. Approximately 60% of retinoblastomas are sporadic,

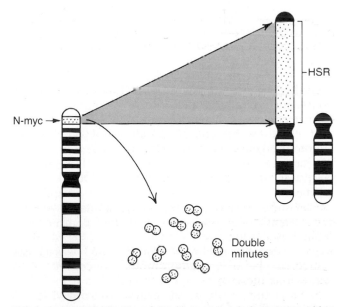

Figure 7–20. Amplification of the N-*myc* gene in human neuroblastomas. N-*myc* gene, present normally on chromosome 2p, becomes amplified and is seen either as extra chromosomal double minutes or as a chromosomally integrated homogeneous-staining region (HSR). The integration involves other autosomes such as 4, 9, or 13. (Modified from Brodeur, G.M., et al.: Clinical implication of oncogene activation in human neuroblastomas. Cancer 58:541, 1986.)

and the remaining ones are familial, the predisposition to tumor being transmitted as an autosomal dominant trait. To account for the sporadic and familial occurrence of an identical tumor, Knudson, in 1974, proposed his now famous two-hit hypothesis, which in molecular terms can be stated as follows:

- Two mutations ("hits") are required to produce retinoblastoma. These involve the *Rb* gene located on chromosome 13q14. Both normal alleles of the *Rb* locus must be inactivated (two hits) for the development of retinoblastoma (Fig. 7–21).
- In familial cases, children inherit one defective copy of the *Rb* gene in the germ line; the other copy is normal. Retinoblastoma develops when the normal *Rb* gene is lost in the retinoblasts as a result of somatic mutation. Because in retinoblastoma families only a single somatic mutation is required for expression of the disease, the familial transmission follows an autosomal dominant inheritance pattern.
- In sporadic cases, both normal *Rb* alleles are lost by somatic mutation in one of the retinoblasts. The end result is the same—a retinal cell that has lost both normal copies of the *Rb* gene becomes cancerous.

Although the loss of normal *Rb* genes was discovered initially in retinoblastomas, it is now evident that homozygous loss of this gene is a fairly common event in several tumors, including osteosarcomas, breast cancer, small cell cancer of the lung, and some brain tumors.

At this point we should clarify some terminology. It follows from our discussion that a cell heterozygous at the *Rb* locus is normal. *Cancer develops when the cell becomes homozygous for the mutant allele or in other words loses heterozygosity of the normal* Rb *gene.* Because neoplastic transformation is associated with loss of both normal copies of the *Rb* gene, this and other cancer suppressor genes are also often called recessive cancer genes.

The genetic damage that results in loss of the normal *Rb* gene may be a point mutation detected only by molecular analysis or a deletion of 13q14 (readily identified by cytogenetic studies). Indeed detection of consistent nonrandom deletions of chromosomes, with associated loss of heterozygosity, has provided important clues to the possible locations of other cancer suppressor genes. For example, such a search led to a cancer suppressor gene mapped to 18q21, referred to simply as "*d*eleted in *c*olon *c*arcinoma" (DCC).

The *Rb* gene stands as a paradigm for several other cancer suppressor genes that behave similarly. A list of the currently identified genes and brief comments relating to them follows:

- *p53*: Located on chromosome 17, p53 was considered to be a growth-promoting oncogene in its previous incarnation. Only recently has it joined the rank of tumor suppressor genes. Amazingly, it now appears that p53 can function both as an oncogene and a cancer suppressor gene—a hermaphrodite, so to speak. On the one hand, some *mutant* forms of p53 activate transcription and transform cells in vitro, as several oncogenes do. On the other hand transfection of a cloned *normal* p53 gene into trans-

formed cells inhibits transformation, a property characteristic of tumor suppressor genes. Although the molecular basis of this "yin-and-yang" behavior is not entirely clear, most evidence suggests that in vivo p53 acts predominantly as a tumor suppressor gene. Indeed, homozygous loss of normal p53 genes is extremely common—affecting carcinomas of the lung, colon, breast, and ovaries, to name a few.
- *NF-1* and *APC*: These genes, involved in the pathogenesis of hereditary neurofibromatosis type 1 (p. 88) and *a*denomatous *p*olyposis *c*oli (p. 514), are tumor suppressor genes with a slight twist to their action. Unlike *Rb,* the prototypic tumor suppressor gene, an *inherited* mutation affecting one copy of the NF-1 gene is sufficient to create tumors, albeit benign neurofibromas. Inactivation of the second allele (loss of heterozygosity) by somatic mutations reduces additional growth restraints, so affected patients develop (malignant) neurofibrosarcomas. The APC, previously called *f*amilial *a*denomatous *p*olyposis (FAP), gene behaves very much like the NF-1 gene. Germinal mutations affecting one copy are associated with formation of multiple benign colonic polyps; both copies are mutated in several colorectal cancers. The study of NF-1 and APC genes suggests that the original formulation that all tumor suppressor genes are "recessive" at the cellular level may have to be revised since these two tumor suppressor genes appear to exert phenotypic effects even when present in the heterozygous state.
- Deleted in colon carcinoma (DCC): This rather bland designation refers to a gene mapped on the long arm of chromosome 18, which is affected in the vast majority of colon carcinomas. As will be discussed later, the biochemical nature of its gene product sets it apart from other tumor suppressor genes.
- WT-1: This cancer suppressor gene is associated with the pathogenesis of another childhood neoplasm, Wilm's tumor, which, like retinoblastoma, occurs in both inherited and sporadic forms.

Biochemical Functions of Tumor Suppressor Genes

The signals and signal-transducing pathways for growth inhibition are much less well understood than those for growth promotion. Nevertheless, it is reasonable to assume that, like mitogenic signals, growth inhibitory signals may originate outside the cell and utilize receptors, signal transducers, and nuclear transcription regulators to accomplish their effects. The tumor suppressor genes seem to encode various components of this growth inhibitory pathway.

CELL SURFACE MOLECULES. The DCC gene encodes a protein that has structural similarity with cell-adhesion molecules, proteins involved in cell-to-cell communication. It is likely, therefore, that the DCC gene product is involved in transmission of negative signals responsible for phenomena such as contact inhibition, a property that is lost upon malignant transformation. The ligands of DCC and other similar genes may be

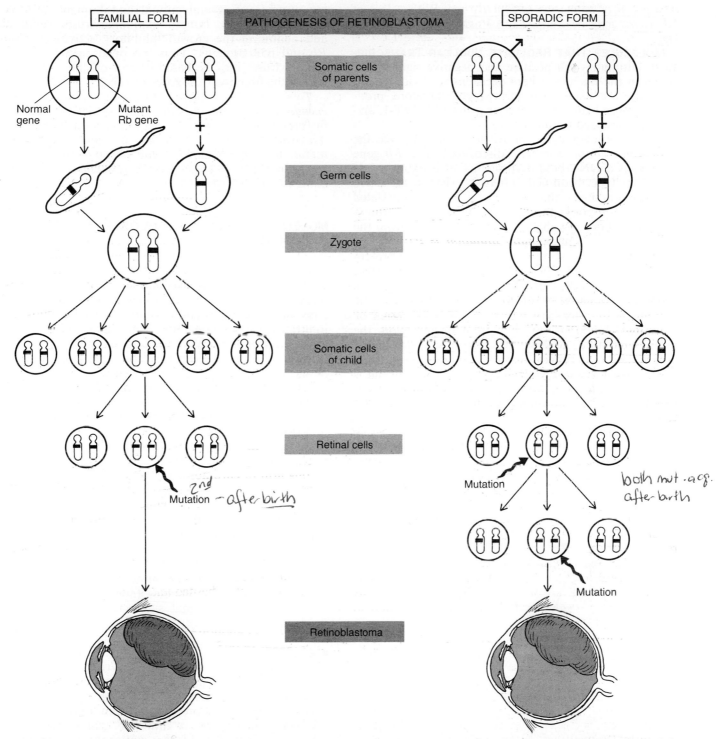

FAMILIAL FORM

PATHOGENESIS OF RETINOBLASTOMA

SPORADIC FORM

Somatic cells of parents

Normal gene   Mutant Rb gene

Germ cells

Zygote

Somatic cells of child

Retinal cells

2nd Mutation — after birth

Mutation

both mut. acg. after-birth

Mutation

Retinoblastoma

Figure 7–21. Pathogenesis of retinoblastoma. Two mutations of the *Rb* locus on chromosome 13q14 lead to neoplastic proliferation of the retinal cells. In the familial form, all somatic cells inherit one mutant *Rb* gene from a carrier parent. The second mutation affects the *Rb* locus in one of the retinal cells after birth. In the sporadic form, on the other hand, both mutations at the *Rb* locus are acquired by the retinal cells after birth.

expressed on the surface of neighboring cells or in extracellular matrix. Homozygous loss of the DCC gene is common in advanced colorectal cancers.

MOLECULES THAT REGULATE SIGNAL TRANSDUC- TION. Down-regulation of growth factor–derived sig- nals is another potential site at which products of

tumor suppressor genes may be operative. The product of the NF-1 gene falls in this category. Recall that the *ras* protein, involved in transmission of growth-pro- moting signals, flips back and forth between active and inactive states. *The normal NF-1 gene encodes a GTPase-activating protein (GAP) that facilitates the conversion of active* ras *to inactive* ras. With a loss of NF-1, *ras* may be trapped in its active, signal-emitting state.

MOLECULES THAT REGULATE NUCLEAR TRANSCRIPTION. Ultimately, all positive and negative signals converge on the nucleus, where decisions to divide or not to divide are made. Not surprisingly, therefore, products of several tumor suppressor genes (*Rb,* WT-1, and p53) are localized to the nucleus.

Much is known about the *Rb* gene since this was the first tumor suppressor gene discovered. The *Rb* gene product is a DNA-binding protein that is expressed in every cell type examined, where it exists in an active unphosphorylated and an inactive phosphorylated state. It is proposed that in its active state *Rb* protein serves as a brake on the advancement of cells from the G0/G1 to the S phase of the cell cycle (Fig. 7–22). When the cells are stimulated to divide, the *Rb* protein is inactivated by phosphorylation, the brake is released, and the cell undergoes mitosis. During mitosis the dephosphorylated form of *Rb* is regenerated, and the daughter cells enter G1. If the *Rb* protein is absent or its normal functions are suppressed by mutation, the cell may continue to cycle and may progress to malignancy. The p53 protein, like the *Rb* protein, is widely distributed in tissues, is localized to the nucleus, and is active in the unphosphorylated state. Through somewhat distinct mechanisms, the normal p53 also prevents cell cycling.

Rather striking evidence pointing to the critical role of *Rb* and p53 genes in neoplastic transformation has emerged quite unexpectedly from the study of DNA tumor viruses. It has been revealed that the transform-ing proteins of several animal and human DNA viruses (e.g., SV40, human papillomaviruses) bind to and neutralize the growth inhibitory activities of the *Rb* and p53 proteins. Thus the oncogenicity of such tumor viruses may be based in part on their ability to inhibit the function of suppressor genes.

To summarize, p53 and Rb tumor suppressor genes encode nuclear proteins that suppress cell proliferation by preventing the entry of cells into cycle. Loss or inactivation of these proteins—by gene deletion or mutation or by binding to the oncoproteins of DNA tumor viruses—releases growth restraints and favors malignant transformation.

MOLECULAR BASIS OF MULTISTEP CARCINOGENESIS

The notion that malignant tumors arise from a protracted sequence of events is supported by epidemiologic, experimental, and molecular studies. Many eons ago, before oncogenes and antioncogenes had infiltrated the scientific literature, cancer epidemiologists had suggested that the age-associated increase in cancers could best be explained by postulating that five or six independent steps were required for tumorigenesis. This idea received initial support from experimental models of chemical carcinogenesis (p. 199) in which the process of tumor formation could be divided into distinct steps such as initiation and promotion. In recent years the study of oncogenes and tumor suppressor genes has provided a firm molecular footing for the concept of multistep carcinogenesis:

- DNA transfection experiments reveal that no single oncogene (e.g., *myc, ras*) can fully transform cells in vitro but that together *ras* and *myc* can transform fibroblasts. Such cooperation is required because each oncogene is specialized to induce part of the phenotype necessary for full transformation. In this example, *ras* oncogene induces cells to secrete growth factors and enables them to grow without anchorage to a normal substrate (anchorage independence), whereas *myc* oncogene renders cells more sensitive to growth factors and immortalizes cells.

- *Every human cancer that has been analyzed reveals multiple genetic alterations involving activation of several oncogenes and loss of two or more cancer suppressor genes.* Each of these alterations represents crucial steps in the progression from a normal cell to a malignant tumor. A dramatic example of incremental acquisition of the malignant phenotype is documented by the study of colon carcinoma. These lesions are believed to evolve through a series of morphologically identifiable stages: colon epithelial hyperplasia followed by formation of adenomas that progressively enlarge and ultimately undergo malignant transformation (p. 515). The proposed molecular correlates of this adenoma-carcinoma sequence are illustrated in Figure 7–23. According to this scheme, inactivation of the APC tumor suppressor gene occurs first, followed by activation of *ras* and ultimately loss of DCC and p53 genes. Although

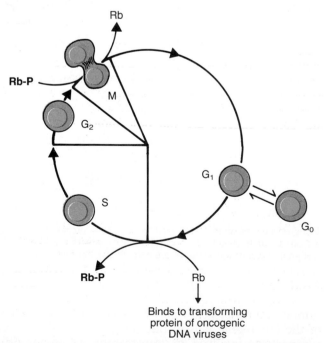

Figure 7–22. Proposed mechanism of action of the *Rb* protein in regulation of cell cycle. Oncoproteins of some DNA viruses (e.g., SV40, human papillomavirus) bind to unphosphorylated *Rb* and neutralize its action.

Figure 7–23 suggests a temporal sequence of mutations in specific genes, it should be noted that the order of mutations is considered less important than their total accumulation. Thus in some cases loss of APC genes precedes *ras* mutation; in others the sequence is reversed.

KARYOTYPIC CHANGES IN TUMORS

The genetic damage that activates oncogenes or inactivates tumor suppressor genes may be subtle (e.g., point mutations) or be large enough to be detected in a karyotype. In certain neoplasms karyotypic abnormalities are nonrandom and common. Specific abnormalities have been identified in most leukemias and lymphomas and in an increasing number of nonhematopoietic tumors. The common types of nonrandom structural abnormalities in tumor cells are (1) balanced translocations, (2) deletions, and (3) cytogenetic manifestations of gene amplification. In addition whole chromosomes may be gained or lost.

The study of chromosomal changes in tumor cells is important on two accounts. First, molecular cloning of genes in the vicinity of chromosomal breakpoints has been extremely useful in identification of oncogenes (e.g., *bcl*-2, *c-abl*) and tumor suppressor genes (e.g., DCC, *Rb*). Second, certain karyotypic abnormalities are specific enough to be of diagnostic value and in some cases they are predictive of clinical course. Several examples of karyotypic changes were provided in the discussion of carcinogenesis. Many others will be described with later considerations of specific forms of neoplasia. Only a few additional examples are presented here.

BALANCED TRANSLOCATIONS. Balanced translocations are extremely common, especially in hematopoietic neoplasms. Most notable is the Philadelphia (Ph¹) chromosome in chronic myelogenous leukemia (CML), comprising a reciprocal and balanced translocation between chromosomes 22 and, usually, 9. As a consequence, chromosome 22 appears somewhat abbreviated. *This change, seen in more than 90% of cases of CML, is a reliable marker of the disease. The few "Ph¹-negative" cases of CML are more resistant to therapy and tend to have a worse prognosis.* As another example, in more than 90% of cases of Burkitt's lymphoma, the cells have a translocation, usually between chromosomes 8 and 14. In follicular B-cell lymphomas, a reciprocal translocation between chromosomes 14 and 18 is extremely common.

DELETIONS. Chromosome deletions are the second most prevalent structural abnormality in tumor cells. As compared to translocations, deletions are more common in nonhematopoietic solid tumors. As discussed, deletions of chromosome 13q band 14 is associated with retinoblastoma. Deletions of 17p, 5q, and 18q, all noted in colorectal cancers, harbor three tumor suppressor genes. Deletion of 3p is extremely common in small-cell lung carcinomas, raising the suspicion that a cancer-suppressor gene will be found at this locale.

GENE AMPLIFICATIONS. There are two karyotypic manifestations of gene amplification: homogeneously staining regions (HSRs) on single chromosomes and double minutes (see Fig. 7–20), which are seen as very small paired fragments of chromatin. Neuroblastomas and breast cancers are the best-studied examples of gene amplification, involving the N-*myc* and c-*neu* genes, respectively (p. 189).

BIOLOGY OF TUMOR GROWTH

The natural history of a typical malignant tumor can be resolved into several steps: neoplastic transformation of a cell, clonal expansion of the transformed cell, local invasion, and ultimately distant spread. In this sequence, the molecular basis of transformation has already been considered. Next we discuss the factors that affect growth of transformed cells, and last the biochemical and molecular basis of invasion and metastasis.

The formation of a tumor mass by the clonal descendants of a transformed cell is a complex process that is influenced by many factors. Some, such as doubling time of tumor cells, are intrinsic to the

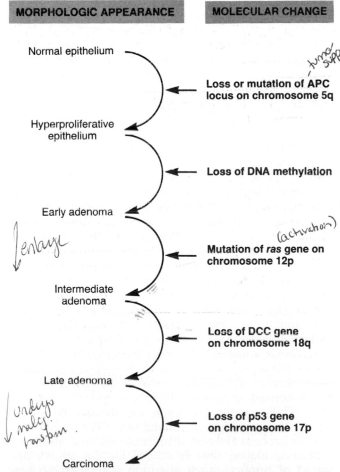

MORPHOLOGIC APPEARANCE	MOLECULAR CHANGE
Normal epithelium	Loss or mutation of APC locus on chromosome 5q
Hyperproliferative epithelium	Loss of DNA methylation
Early adenoma	
Intermediate adenoma	Mutation of *ras* gene on chromosome 12p
Late adenoma	Loss of DCC gene on chromosome 18q
Carcinoma	Loss of p53 gene on chromosome 17p

Figure 7–23. A molecular model for the evolution of colorectal cancers through the adenoma-carcinoma sequence. (Based on studies of Fearon, E. R., Vogelstein, B.: A genetic model of colorectal carcinogenesis. Cell 61:759, 1990.)

transformed cells, whereas others, such as angiogenesis, represent host responses elicited by tumor cells or their products. The multiple factors that influence tumor growth are considered under three headings: (1) kinetics of tumor cell growth, (2) tumor angiogenesis, and (3) tumor progression and heterogeneity.

Kinetics of Tumor Cell Growth

One can begin the consideration of tumor cell kinetics by asking the question, "How long does it take for the single transformed cell to produce a clinically overt mass?" This depends on three variables:

1. *The doubling time of tumor cells.* The cell cycle of the transformed cells has the same five phases observed in normal cells (G0, G1, S, G2, and M). While intuitively one may think that tumor cells divide more rapidly than normal cells, in reality the total cell cycle time for many tumors is equal to or longer than that of corresponding normal cells.
2. *Growth fraction.* The growth fraction is the proportion of cells within the tumor cell population that are in the replicative pool. Clinical and experimental studies suggest that during the early, submicroscopic phase of tumor growth the vast majority of transformed cells are in the proliferative pool (Fig. 7-24). As tumors continue to grow, cells leave the replicative pool in ever-increasing numbers due to shedding or lack of nutrients, by differentiating, and by reversion to G0. Indeed, most cells within cancers remain in the G0 phase. Thus by the time a tumor is clinically detectable most cells are not in the replicative pool. Even in some rapidly growing tumors the growth fraction is approximately 20%.
3. *Cell production and loss.* Ultimately, the progressive growth of tumors and the rate at which they grow is determined by the excess of cell production over cell loss. In some tumors, especially those with a relatively high growth fraction, the imbalance is large, resulting in more rapid growth than in those in which cell production exceeds cell loss by only a small margin.

An understanding of tumor cell kinetics has important clinical implications:

- *Cancer chemotherapy.* Almost all antineoplastic agents in current use are most effective on cycling cells. Hence tumors with high growth fractions (e.g., high-grade lymphomas) are very susceptible to anticancer agents. In contrast, common solid tumors such as colon cancer that have low growth fractions are relatively resistant. In such cases the treatment strategy is to first shift tumor cells from G0 into the cell cycle. This can be accomplished by debulking the tumor by surgery or radiation. The surviving tumor cells tend to reenter the cell cycle and thus become susceptible to drug therapy. Such considerations form the basis of combined-modality treatment.
- *Latent period of tumors.* If all descendants of an originally transformed cell remained in the replicative pool, most tumors would become clinically detectable within a few months after the first cell division, but because most tumor cells leave the replicative pool the accumulation of cells is a relatively slow process. This in turn results in a latent period of several months to years before a tumor becomes clinically detectable. Nevertheless, several cell doublings occur during the latent period, a fact that must be borne in mind in understanding tumor progression.

Tumor Angiogenesis

Factors other than cell kinetics modify the growth of tumors. Most important among these is blood supply. There is abundant experimental and clinical evidence that tumors cannot enlarge beyond 1 or 2 mm in diameter or thickness unless they are vascularized. Indeed it could be argued that the ability to induce angiogenesis is a necessary biologic correlate of malignancy, because without access to the vasculature the tumor would fail to metastasize. How do growing tumors develop a blood supply? Several studies indicate that tumors themselves secrete factors that are capable of effecting the entire series of events involved in the formation of new capillaries (p. 52). Tumor-associated angiogenic factors can be classified into two general groups: (1) those that are produced by tumor cells and (2) those that are derived from inflammatory cells (e.g., macrophages) that infiltrate tumors. The best-characterized members of the first group are heparin-binding fibroblast growth factors (FGF). These molecules *possess a triad of functions: they are chemotactic and mitogenic for endothelial cells and they induce the production of proteolytic enzymes that allow penetration of the stroma by endothelial sprouts.* Other tumor-derived angiogenic factors include TGF-α and EGF. TNF-α is the prototypic member of the second group. This macrophage-derived factor is mitogenic for endothelial cells and also stimulates their migration.

Because angiogenesis is critical for the growth and spread of tumors, much attention is focused on how angiogenesis is switched on and what can be done to retard it. In answer to the first question it should be recalled that several angiogenic molecules (growth fac-

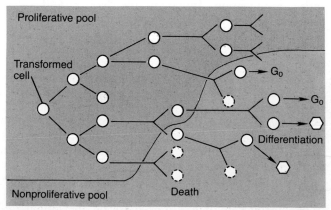

Figure 7-24. A schematic representation of tumor growth. As the cell population expands, a progressively higher percentage of tumor cells leaves the replicative pool by reversion to G0, differentiation, and death.

tors) are products of protooncogenes and are activated by mutations. Tumor angiogenesis may also involve loss of an angiogenesis-inhibiting factor encoded by a putative cancer suppressor gene. Thus angiogenesis and growth autonomy seem to be mediated by similar genetic events.

Can the basic knowledge about angiogenic factors be exploited for tumor therapy? In principle, inhibition of production of angiogenic molecules or prevention of endothelial cell response to them may be beneficial. Efforts directed toward these approaches are under way and may soon bear fruit.

Tumor Progression and Heterogeneity

It is well established that over a period of time many tumors become more aggressive and acquire greater malignant potential. This phenomenon is referred to as tumor *progression.* Careful clinical and experimental studies reveal that increasing malignancy (e.g., accelerated growth, invasiveness, and ability to form distant metastases) is often acquired in an incremental fashion. *This biologic phenomenon is related to the sequential appearance of subpopulations of cells that differ with respect to several phenotypic attributes such as invasiveness, rate of growth, metastatic ability, karyotype, hormonal responsiveness, and susceptibility to antineoplastic drugs. Thus, despite the fact that most malignant tumors are monoclonal in origin, by the time they become clinically evident their constituent cells are extremely heterogeneous.* At the molecular level tumor progression and associated heterogeneity most likely result from multiple mutations that accumulate independently in different cells, thus generating subclones with different characteristics.

What predisposes the original transformed cell to additional genetic damage is not entirely clear. Most investigators believe that transformed cells are genetically unstable. This renders them susceptible to a high rate of random, spontaneous mutations during clonal expansion (Fig. 7–25). Some of these mutations may be lethal; others may spur cell growth by affecting protooncogenes or cancer suppressor genes. The subclones so generated are subjected to immune and nonimmune selection pressures. For example, cells that are highly antigenic are destroyed by host defenses, whereas those with reduced growth factor requirements are positively selected. *A growing tumor, therefore,*

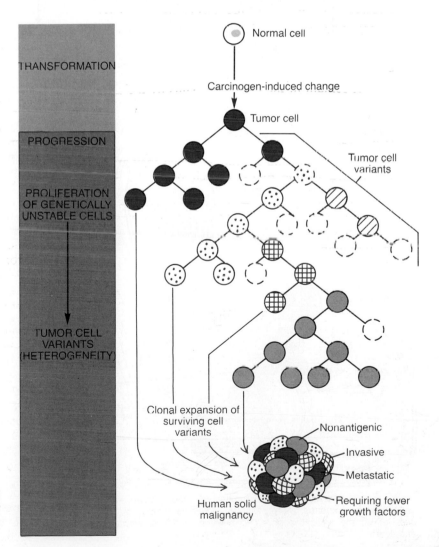

Figure 7–25. Tumor progression and generation of heterogeneity. New subclones arise from the descendants of the original transformed cell, and with progression the tumor mass becomes enriched for those variants that are more adept at evading host defenses and are likely to be more aggressive.

Normal cell

Carcinogen-induced change

Tumor cell

Tumor cell variants

Clonal expansion of surviving cell variants

Human solid malignancy

Nonantigenic

Invasive

Metastatic

Requiring fewer growth factors

TRANSFORMATION

PROGRESSION

PROLIFERATION OF GENETICALLY UNSTABLE CELLS

TUMOR CELL VARIANTS (HETEROGENEITY)

tends to be enriched for those subclones that "beat the odds" and are adept at survival, growth, invasion, and metastases. Although progression is most obvious after a tumor is diagnosed, it is important to remember that during the latent period many cell doublings occur and hence _generation of heterogeneity begins well before the tumor is clinically evident._

The rate at which mutant subclones are generated is quite variable. In some tumors such as osteosarcomas metastatic subclones are already present when the patient walks into the doctor's office. In others, typified by certain salivary gland tumors, aggressive subclones develop late and infrequently. Knowledge of such biologic differences is of obvious importance to the clinical potential of cancers and to the management of cancer patients.

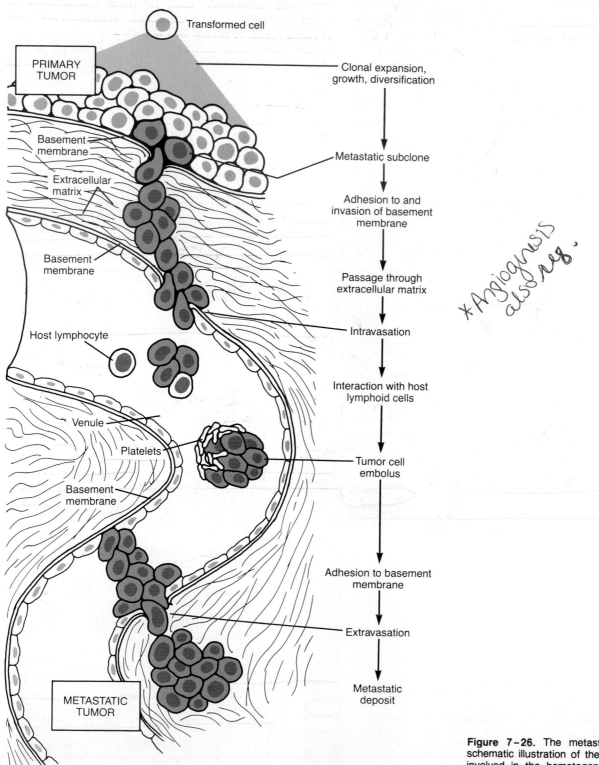

Transformed cell

PRIMARY TUMOR — Clonal expansion, growth, diversification

Basement membrane

Extracellular matrix — Metastatic subclone

Basement membrane — Adhesion to and invasion of basement membrane

*Angiogensis also reg.

Passage through extracellular matrix

Host lymphocyte — Intravasation

Venule — Interaction with host lymphoid cells

Platelets

Basement membrane — Tumor cell embolus

Adhesion to basement membrane

Extravasation

METASTATIC TUMOR — Metastatic deposit

Figure 7–26. The metastatic cascade. A schematic illustration of the sequential steps involved in the hematogenous spread of a tumor.

MECHANISMS OF LOCAL AND DISTANT SPREAD

In an earlier part of this chapter (p. 177) it was emphasized that invasion and metastasis are biologic hallmarks of malignancy. Here we will concentrate on the mechanisms by which tumors infiltrate locally and are transported to distant sites.

The spread of tumors is a complex process involving a series of sequential steps, diagrammed in Figure 7–26. (Angiogenesis, not shown in the figure, is also essential for the growth of both primary and metastatic tumors). Quite predictably, this sequence of steps may be interrupted at any stage by either host or tumor-related factors. As mentioned earlier, cells within a tumor are heterogeneous with respect to metastatic potential. Only certain subclones possess the right combination of gene products to complete all the steps outlined in Figure 7–26. For the purpose of discussion, the metastatic cascade can be subdivided into two

phases: invasion of extracellular matrix, and vascular dissemination and homing of tumor cells.

Invasion of Extracellular Matrix

As is well known, our tissues are organized into a series of compartments separated from each other by two types of extracellular matrix (ECM): basement membranes and interstitial connective tissue. Although organized differently, each of these components of ECM is made up of collagens, glycoproteins, and proteoglycans. A review of Figure 7–26 will reveal that tumor cells must interact with the ECM at several stages in the metastatic cascade. A carcinoma must first breach the underlying basement membrane, then traverse the interstitial connective tissue, and ultimately gain access to the circulation by penetrating the vascular basement membrane. This cycle is repeated when tumor cell emboli extravasate at a distant site. Invasion of the ECM is an active process that can be resolved into three steps (Fig. 7–27):

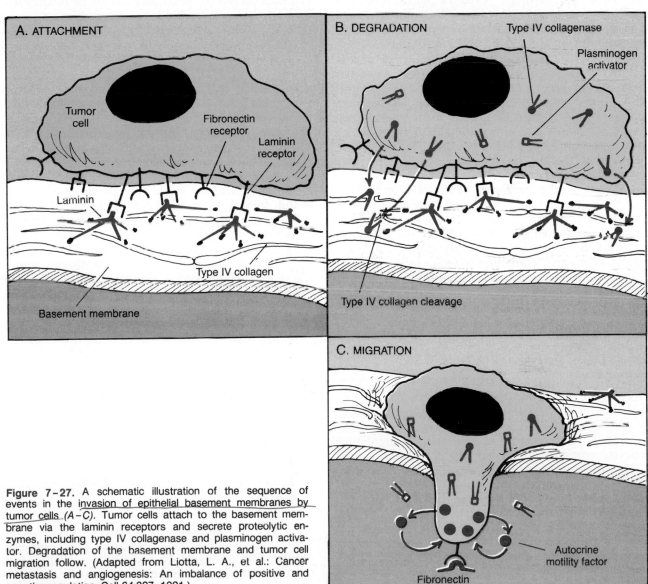

Figure 7–27. A schematic illustration of the sequence of events in the invasion of epithelial basement membranes by tumor cells (A–C). Tumor cells attach to the basement membrane via the laminin receptors and secrete proteolytic enzymes, including type IV collagenase and plasminogen activator. Degradation of the basement membrane and tumor cell migration follow. (Adapted from Liotta, L. A., et al.: Cancer metastasis and angiogenesis: An imbalance of positive and negative regulation. Cell *64*:327, 1991.)

- Attachment of tumor cells to matrix components
- Degradation of ECM
- Migration of tumor cells

There is substantial evidence that _attachment_ of tumor cells to laminin and fibronectin is important for invasion and metastasis. Normal epithelial cells have receptors for basement membrane laminin that are polarized at their basal surface. In contrast, carcinoma cells have many more receptors, and they are distributed all around the cell membrane. Further, there is a correlation between the density of laminin receptors on breast carcinoma cells and lymph node metastases. A similar correlation exists between the ability to bind fibronectin, the major glycoprotein of interstitial tissues, and invasiveness.

The second step in invasion is local _degradation of the basement membrane and interstitial connective tissue._ Tumor cells secrete proteolytic enzymes themselves, or induce the host cells (e.g., fibroblasts) to elaborate proteases. Several enzymes, including type IV collagenase, urokinase-type plasminogen activator, and cathepsin B, are involved. Type IV collagenase is a metalloproteinase that cleaves type IV collagen of the epithelial and vascular basement membranes. Benign tumors of the breast, colon, and stomach show very little type IV collagenase activity, whereas their malignant counterparts overexpress this enzyme. A similar correlation has been noted with cathepsin D and urokinase. Furthermore, in experimental animals chemical inhibitors of collagenase IV greatly reduce metastases. These observations not only highlight the importance of proteases in tumor invasion but also offer a glimmer of hope that therapeutic blockage of such enzymes may be beneficial.

Locomotion is the third step of invasion, propelling tumor cells through the degraded basement membranes and zones of matrix proteolysis. Migration seems to be mediated by tumor cell–derived cytokines such as _autocrine motility factors._ In addition, cleavage products of matrix components (e.g., collagen, laminin) and some growth factors (e.g., insulin-like growth factors I and II) have chemotactic activity for tumor cells. The latter could play a role in organ-selective homing of tumor cells.

Vascular Dissemination and Homing of Tumor Cells

Once in the circulation tumor cells are vulnerable to destruction by the host immune cells, a topic discussed later (p. 203). In the blood stream some tumor cells form emboli by aggregating and adhering to circulating leukocytes, particularly platelets; aggregated tumor cells are afforded some protection from the antitumor host effector cells. However, the majority of tumor cells circulate as single cells. Extravasation of free tumor cells or tumor emboli involves adhesion to the vascular endothelium, followed by egress through the basement membrane by mechanisms similar to those involved in invasion.

The site of extravasation, and hence the organ distribution of metastases, can generally be predicted by the location of the primary tumor and its vascular or lymphatic drainage. However, in many cases the natural pathways of drainage do not readily explain the distribution of metastases. As pointed out earlier, some tumors (e.g., lung cancers) tend to involve the adrenals with some regularity but almost never spread to skeletal muscle. Such organ tropism may be related to the following three mechanisms:

- Because the first step in extravasation is adhesion to the endothelium, tumor cells may express adhesion molecules whose ligands are expressed preferentially on the endothelial cells of the target organ.
- Some target organs may liberate chemoattractants that tend to recruit tumor cells to the site. Examples include insulin-like growth factors I and II.
- In some cases, the target tissue may be an unpermissive environment, unfavorable soil, so to speak, for the growth of tumor seedlings. For example, inhibitors of proteases could prevent the establishment of a tumor colony.

However, despite the foregoing considerations, the precise localization of metastases cannot be predicted with any form of cancer. Evidently many tumors have not read textbooks of pathology!

Molecular Genetics of Metastases

It can be asked: Are there oncogenes or tumor suppressor genes that elicit metastases as their principal or sole contribution to tumorigenesis? This question is of more than academic interest, because if altered forms of certain genes promote or suppress the metastatic phenotype, their detection in a primary tumor may have prognostic as well as therapeutic implications. At present no single "metastasis gene" has been found. Indeed, some have argued that since metastatic cells must acquire multiple properties (e.g., expression of adhesion receptors, production of collagenases, motility factors), no single genetic alteration is likely to render a cell metastasis prone. Nevertheless some intriguing correlations have emerged between the level of expression of a candidate tumor suppressor gene (nm23) and metastatic ability. In murine models, the expression of nm23 is high in lines with low metastatic potential and is reduced 10-fold in lines with high metastatic ability. In a series of human breast cancers, the nm23 levels were highest in the tumors that had three or fewer involved nodes and were uniformly low in tumors that had extensive nodal metastases. The generality of these findings and the causal association between the nm23 gene product and invasiveness are under active investigation.

ETIOLOGY OF CANCER—CARCINOGENIC AGENTS

Genetic damage lies at the heart of carcinogenesis. What agents inflict such damage? Three classes of carcinogenic agents can be identified: (1) chemicals, (2) radiant energy, and (3) oncogenic viruses. Chemicals and radiant energy are documented causes of cancer in humans, and oncogenic viruses are involved in the pathogenesis of at least some human tumors. In the following discussion each class of agents is considered separately, but it is important to note that several may act in concert or sequentially to produce the multiple genetic abnormalities characteristic of neoplastic cells.

CHEMICAL CARCINOGENS

It is now about 200 years since the London surgeon Sir Percival Pott correctly attributed scrotal skin cancer in chimney sweeps to chronic exposure to soot. A few years later, based on this observation, the Danish Chimney Sweeps Guild ruled that its members must bathe daily. No public health measure since that time has achieved so much in the control of a form of cancer! Nonetheless, these dramatic results lay unnoted for over a century, until Yamagiwa and Ichikawa in 1915 reawakened interest in Pott's observation by inducing cancer in a rabbit's ear with the repeated application of coal tar. Subsequently, Kennaway and Cook, in a monumental feat, extracted 50 grams of a chemically pure carcinogen, 3,4-benzpyrene, from *two tons* of crude coal tars. These pioneering observations documented the carcinogenicity of polycyclic aromatic hydrocarbons. Since then, hundreds of chemicals have been shown to be carcinogenic in animals.

The following pertinent observations have emerged from the study of chemical carcinogens:

1. They are of extremely diverse structure and include both natural and synthetic products.

2. Some are *direct-reacting* and require no chemical transformation to induce carcinogenicity, but others are *indirect-reacting* and become active only after metabolic conversion. Such agents are referred to as *procarcinogens* and their active end products are called *ultimate carcinogens*.

3. All chemical carcinogens, both the direct-reacting and the ultimate carcinogens, are highly reactive electrophiles (have electron-deficient atoms) that react with the electron-rich atoms in RNA, cellular proteins, and, mainly, DNA.

4. The carcinogenicity of some chemicals is augmented by agents that by themselves have little if any cancerous activity. Such augmenting agents have traditionally been called *promoters;* however, many carcinogens have no requirement for promoting agents.

5. Several chemical carcinogens may act in concert or with other types of carcinogenic influences (e.g., viruses or radiation) to induce neoplasia.

Some of the major agents are presented in Table 7–6. Only a few comments are offered on some.

Direct-Acting Agents

These substances as noted require no metabolic conversion to become carcinogenic. They are in general weak carcinogens and, depending on time-dose considerations, may not produce tumors. They are important because some of them are cancer chemotherapeutic drugs (e.g., alkylating agents) that have successfully

TABLE 7–6. MAJOR CHEMICAL CARCINOGENS

Direct-acting carcinogens
  Alkylating agents
    Anticancer drugs (cyclophosphamide, chlorambucil, nitrosoureas, and others)
  Acylating agents
    1-Acetyl-imidazole
    Dimethylcarbamyl chloride

Procarcinogens that require metabolic activation
  Polycyclic and heterocyclic aromatic hydrocarbons
    Benz(a)anthracene
    Benzo(a)pyrene
    Dibenz(a,h)anthracene
    3-Methylcholanthrene
    7,12-Dimethylbenz(a)anthracene

Aromatic amines, amides, azo dyes
    2-Naphthylamine (β-naphthylamine)
    2-Acetylaminofluorene
    Dimethylaminoazobenzene (butter yellow)

Natural plant and microbial products
    Aflatoxin B_1
    Griseofulvin
    Betel nuts

Others
    Nitrosamine and amides
    Vinyl chloride, nickel, chromium
    Insecticides, fungicides
    Polychlorinated biphenyls (PCBs)
    Arsenic
    Asbestos

cured, controlled, or delayed recurrence of certain types of cancer (e.g., leukemia, lymphoma, Hodgkin's disease, ovarian carcinoma) only to later evoke a second form of cancer, usually leukemia. This is even more tragic when their initial use has been for nonneoplastic disorders such as rheumatoid arthritis and Wegener's granulomatosis. The risk of induced cancer is low but the fact that it exists dictates judicious use of such agents.

Indirect-Acting Agents

This designation indicates that the chemicals require metabolic conversion before they become active. Some of the most potent indirect chemical carcinogens—the *polycyclic hydrocarbons*—are present in fossil fuels. Benz(a)anthracene produces cancer wherever it is applied—painted on the skin it induces skin cancers, injected subcutaneously it induces fibrosarcomas. Polycyclic agents are also produced in the combustion of organic substances. For example, benzo(a)pyrene and other carcinogens are formed in the high-temperature combustion of tobacco in cigarette smoking. These products are implicated in the causation of lung cancer in cigarette smokers. Polycyclic hydrocarbons may also be produced from animal fats in the process of broiling meats and are present in smoked meats and fish. The principal active products in many hydrocarbons are epoxides, which form covalent adducts (addition products) with molecules in the cell, principally DNA, but also with RNA and proteins.

Another class of indirect agents are the *aromatic amines and azo dyes*. Beta-naphthylamine was responsible, before its carcinogenicity was recognized, for a 50-fold increased incidence of bladder cancers in workers heavily exposed in the aniline dye and rubber industries. Many other occupational carcinogens are listed on page 182. Some of the azo dyes were developed to color food (e.g., butter yellow to make margarine more enticing, and scarlet red for maraschino cherries). What price esthetics? Most of the aromatic amines and azo dyes are converted into ultimate carcinogens in the liver by the cytochrome P-450 oxygenase system and therefore in experimental animals induce hepatocellular carcinomas.

A few *other agents* merit brief mention. *Nitrosamines* and *amides* have aroused great concern because of the evidence that they can be formed endogenously in the acidic conditions of the stomach. Various amines derived from food may undergo nitrosation with nitrites that have been added to food as preservatives or derived from nitrates by bacterial action. Repeatedly the question has been raised whether nitroso compounds could account for the increased incidence of gastric carcinoma in some populations. Nitroso compounds are also present in tobacco smoke and following absorption could lead to cancers in a variety of organs. *Aflatoxin B_1* is of interest because it is a naturally occurring agent produced by some strains of *Aspergillus,* a mold that grows on improperly stored grains and nuts. There is a strong correlation between the dietary level of this food contaminant and the incidence of hepatocellular carcinoma in some parts of Africa and the Far East. However, there is an even stronger correlation between the prevalence of infection with hepatitis B virus and hepatocellular carcinoma. Thus aflatoxin and hepatitis B virus may act in concert to produce hepatic cancers (see p. 559). This notion is strongly supported by recent studies that reveal mutational inactivation of the tumor suppressor gene p53 in liver cancers that occur in areas of the world where HBV and exposure to aflatoxins are endemic. *Saccharin* and *cyclamates* have been incriminated as carcinogens in experimental animals, but because induction of cancer with these artificial sweeteners requires extremely large doses, their role in human carcinogenesis remains in doubt. Finally, attention should be called to vinyl chloride, arsenic, nickel, chromium, insecticides, fungicides, and PCBs as potential carcinogens in the workplace and about the house.

Mechanisms of Action of Chemical Carcinogens

Because malignant transformation results from mutations that affect oncogenes and cancer suppressor genes, it will come as no surprise that the vast majority of chemical carcinogens are mutagenic. Although any gene may be the target of chemical carcinogens, *ras* gene mutations are particularly common in several chemically induced cancers in rodents. For example, in mammary cancers induced by nitrosomethylurea (NMU) in rats, 87% carried a *ras* mutation.

It was mentioned earlier that carcinogenicity of some chemicals is augmented by subsequent administration of "promoters" (such as phorbol esters, hormones, phenols, and drugs) that by themselves are nontumorigenic. To be effective, repeated or sustained exposure to the promoter must *follow* the application of the mutagenic chemical, or "initiator." The initiation-promotion sequence of chemical carcinogenesis raises an important question: *since promoters are not mutagenic, how do they contribute to tumorigenesis?* Although the effects of tumor promoters are pleiotropic, induction of cell proliferation is a sine qua non of tumor promotion. TPA, a phorbol ester and the best-studied tumor promoter, is a powerful activator of protein kinase C, an enzyme that is a critical component of several signal transduction pathways including those activated by growth factors. TPA also causes growth factor secretion by some cells. It seems most likely, therefore, that while the application of an initiator may cause the mutational activation of an oncogene such as *ras,* subsequent application of promoters leads to clonal expansion of initiated (mutated) cells. Such cells (especially after *ras* activation) have reduced growth factor requirements and may also be less responsive to growth inhibitory signals in their extracellular milieu. Forced to proliferate, the initiated clone of cells suffers additional mutations, developing eventually into a malignant tumor. The concept that sustained cell proliferation increases the risk of mutagenesis and hence neoplastic transformation is also applicable to human carcinogenesis. For example, pathologic hyperplasia of the endometrium (p. 617) and increased regenerative activity that accompanies chronic liver cell injury are associated with the development of cancer in these organs.

Before we leave the topic of chemical carcinogenesis, it must be emphasized that carcinogen-induced damage to DNA does not necessarily lead to initiation of cancer. Several forms of DNA damage (incurred spontaneously or through the action of carcinogens) can be repaired by cellular enzymes. Were this not the case, the incidence of environmentally induced cancer would in all likelihood be much higher. This is best exemplified by the rare hereditary disorder xeroderma pigmentosum, which is associated with defective DNA repair and a greatly increased risk of cancers induced by ultraviolet light and certain chemicals (p. 201).

RADIATION CARCINOGENESIS _____

Radiation, whatever its source—ultraviolet rays of sunlight, x-rays, nuclear fission, radionuclides—is an established carcinogen. The evidence is so voluminous that only a few examples will suffice. Many of the pioneers in the development of roentgen rays developed skin cancers. Among persons with fair skin, there is a linear correlation between intensity of exposure to sunlight and skin cancer—squamous cell carcinoma, basal cell carcinoma, and malignant melanoma. Miners of radioactive elements have suffered a 10-fold increased incidence of lung cancers. The follow-up of survivors of the atomic bombs dropped on Hiroshima and Nagasaki has disclosed a markedly increased incidence of leukemia—principally acute and chronic myelocytic leukemia—after an average latent period of about seven years. Decades later, the leukemia risk for those heavily exposed is still above the level for control populations, as is the mortality rate from thyroid, breast, colon, and pulmonary carcinoma and others. Even therapeutic irradiation has been documented to be carcinogenic. Thyroid cancers have developed in approximately 9% of those exposed during infancy and childhood to head and neck irradiation. Thus, it is abundantly clear that radiation is strongly oncogenic. The mutagenic effect of ionizing radiation is well established. Radiant energy causes chromosome breakage, translocations, and point mutations. Like chemical carcinogens, ionizing radiation is known to activate *ras* oncogenes and inactivate the *Rb* tumor suppressor gene. Thus the mutagenesis-carcinogenesis theme prevails. Because the latent period of irradiation-associated cancers is extremely long, it appears that cancer emerges only after the progeny of initially damaged cells accumulate additional mutations, induced possibly by other environmental factors.

The oncogenic effect of ultraviolet (UV) rays merits special mention because it highlights the importance of DNA repair in carcinogenesis. Natural UV radiation derived from the sun can cause skin cancers (melanomas, squamous cell carcinomas, and basal cell carcinomas). At greatest risk are fair-skinned people who live in locales that receive a great deal of sunlight. Thus, cancers of the exposed skin are particularly common in Australia and New Zealand. UV light has several biologic effects on cells. Of particular relevance to carcinogenesis is the ability to damage DNA by forming pyrimidine dimers. In normal persons, the altered DNA can usually be repaired by a series of repair enzymes, but in a small group of autosomal recessive disorders, one or more of the DNA repair enzymes is defective or deficient. Patients with such diseases, exemplified by xeroderma pigmentosum, have greatly increased predisposition to skin cancers, predominantly in the sun-exposed areas of skin. Three other "chromosomal instability syndromes"—ataxia telangiectasia, Fanconi's anemia, and Bloom's syndrome—are also characterized by an increased risk of cancer, possibly related to some inability to repair environmentally induced DNA damage.

VIRAL ONCOGENESIS

A large number of DNA and RNA viruses have proved to be oncogenic in animals as disparate as frogs and primates. However, despite intense scrutiny, only a few viruses have been linked with human cancer. Our discussion is limited mostly to human oncogenic viruses.

RNA Oncogenic Viruses

The study of oncogenic retroviruses in animals has provided spectacular insights into the genetic basis of cancer. Animal retroviruses transform cells by two mechanisms. (1) Some, called *acute transforming viruses,* contain a transforming viral oncogene such as *src, abl,* or *myb.* You may recall that v-*onc*s are transduced human protooncogenes. (2) Others, called *slow transforming viruses* (e.g., mouse mammary tumor virus) do not contain a v-*onc* but the proviral DNA is always found to be inserted near a protooncogene. Under the influence of the strong retroviral promoter, the adjacent normal or mutated protooncogene is overexpressed. With this brief summary of retroviral oncogenesis in animals, we can turn to the only known human retrovirus that is associated with cancer.

HUMAN T-CELL LEUKEMIA VIRUS TYPE 1. *Human T-cell leukemia virus-1 (HTLV-1)* is associated with a form of T-cell leukemia/lymphoma that is endemic in certain parts of Japan and the Caribbean basin but is found sporadically elsewhere, including the United States. Like the AIDS virus, HTLV-1 has tropism for CD4+ T cells, and hence this subset of T cells is the major target for neoplastic transformation. Human infection requires transmission of infected T cells via sexual intercourse, blood products, or breast feeding. Leukemia develops in only about 1% of the infected individuals after a long latent period of 20 to 30 years.

There is little doubt that HTLV-1 infection of T lymphocytes is necessary for leukemogenesis, but the molecular mechanisms of transformation are not entirely clear. Unlike acute transforming retroviruses, HTLV-1 does not contain a v-*onc*, and unlike slow transforming retroviruses, no consistent integration next to a protooncogene has been discovered. The genomic structure of HTLV-1 reveals the *gag, pol, env,* and long terminal repeat (LTR) regions typical of other retroviruses, but, unlike other leukemia viruses, it contains another region, referred to as *tax.* It seems that the secrets of its transforming activity are locked in the *tax* gene. The product of this gene is essential for viral replication because it stimulates transcription of viral m-RNA by acting on the 5' LTR. Recent findings indicate that the *tax* protein can also activate the transcription of several host cell genes including c-*fos*, c-*sis*, genes encoding the cytokine IL-2 and its receptor, and the gene for myeloid growth factor GM-CSF. From these and other observations the following scenario is emerging (Fig. 7–28): HTLV-1 infection stimulates proliferation of T cells. This is brought about by the *tax* gene, which turns on genes that encode a T-cell growth factor, IL-2, and its receptor, setting up an autocrine system for proliferation. At the same time, a paracrine pathway is activated by the increased production of GM-CSF. This myeloid growth factor, by acting on neighboring macrophages, induces increased secretion of other T-cell mitogens such as IL-1. Initially the T-cell proliferation is polyclonal, because the virus infects many cells. The proliferating T cells are at increased risk of secondary transforming events (mutations), which lead ultimately to the outgrowth of a monoclonal neoplastic T-cell population.

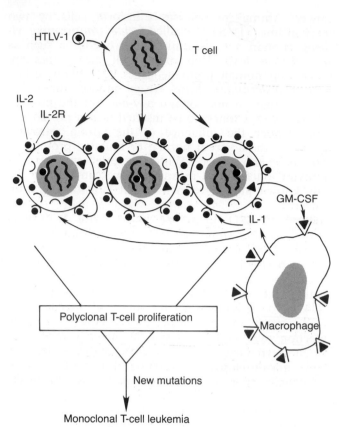

Figure 7–28. Pathogenesis of HTLV-1–induced T-cell leukemia/lymphoma. HTLV-1 infects many T cells and initially causes polyclonal proliferation by autocrine and paracrine pathways. Ultimately, a monoclonal T-cell leukemia/lymphoma results when one proliferating T cell suffers additional mutations.

DNA Oncogenic Viruses

As with RNA viruses, several oncogenic DNA viruses that cause tumors in animals have been identified. Three DNA viruses—papillomavirus, Epstein-Barr virus (EBV), and hepatitis B virus (HBV)—are of special interest because they have been accused of causing human cancer. Before we discuss the role of these viruses in carcinogenesis, a few general comments relating to transformation by DNA viruses are offered:

- Transforming DNA viruses form stable associations with the host cell genome. The integrated virus is unable to complete its replicative cycle because the viral genes essential for completion of replication are interrupted during integration of viral DNA.
- Those viral genes that are transcribed early (early genes) in the viral life cycle are important for transformation. They are expressed in transformed cells.

HUMAN PAPILLOMAVIRUS. Approximately 50 genetically distinct types of human papillomavirus (HPV) have been identified. Some types (e.g., 1, 2, 4, and 7) definitely cause benign squamous papillomas (warts) in humans. HPVs have also been implicated in the genesis of several cancers, particularly squamous cell carcinoma of the cervix and anogenital region. Epidemiologic studies suggest that carcinoma of the cervix is

caused by a sexually transmitted agent, and HPV is a prime suspect. DNA sequences of HPV types 16 and 18 are found in 75 to 100% of invasive squamous cell cancers and their presumed precursors (severe dysplasias and carcinoma in situ). In contrast with cervical cancers, genital warts with low malignant potential are associated with distinct HPV types, predominantly HPV-6 and -11. The oncogenic potential of HPV can be related to products of two early viral genes, E6 and E7. The proteins encoded by these genes bind to and neutralize the products of the *Rb* and p53 tumor suppressor genes. Quite remarkably the affinity of such interactions differs depending on the oncogenic potential of HPV. E6 and E7 proteins derived from high-risk HPVs (types 16, 18, and 31) bind to *Rb* and p53 with high affinity, whereas the E6 and E7 gene products of low-risk HPVs (types 6 and 11) bind with low affinity. When human keratinocytes are transfected with DNA from HPV 16, 18, or 31 in vitro they are immortalized, but they do not form tumors in experimental animals. Co-transfection with a mutated *ras* gene, however, results in full malignant transformation. These data strongly suggest that while HPV is very likely to play a role in human carcinogenesis, the virus does not act alone. In all likelihood other environmental factors must collaborate with the virus.

EPSTEIN-BARR VIRUS. EBV has been implicated in the pathogenesis of two human tumors, Burkitt's lymphoma and nasopharyngeal cancer.

Burkitt's lymphoma is a tumor of B lymphocytes that is endemic in certain parts of Africa and sporadic elsewhere. In endemic areas, tumor cells in virtually all patients carry the EBV genome. EBV exhibits strong tropism for B cells and infects many B cells, causing them to proliferate. In immunologically normal individuals EBV-driven polyclonal B-cell proliferation is readily controlled and the individual either remains asymptomatic or develops a self-limited episode of infectious mononucleosis (p. 359). In regions of the world where Burkitt's lymphoma is endemic, concomitant (endemic) malaria (or other infections) impairs immune competence, allowing sustained B-cell proliferation. Such B cells are at increased risk of acquiring mutations such as the t(8,14) translocation, which activates the *myc* oncogene and is a consistent feature of this tumor. The activation of c-*myc* causes further loss of growth control and the stage is set for additional gene damage that ultimately leads to the emergence of a monoclonal neoplasm. It should be noted that in nonendemic areas 80% of tumors do not harbor the EBV genome, but all tumors possess the specific translocation. This suggests that B cells triggered by other mechanisms may also suffer similar mutations and give rise to non-African Burkitt's lymphoma.

Nasopharyngeal carcinoma is endemic in Southern China and some other locales, and the EBV genome is found in all tumors. As in Burkitt's lymphoma, EBV acts in concert with other factors.

HEPATITIS B VIRUS. Although the epidemiologic evidence linking chronic HBV infection with hepatocellular carcinoma is strong (p. 559), the role of the virus in tumor production is unclear. The HBV genome does not encode any transforming proteins and there is no consistent pattern of integration in liver cells. The oncogenic effect of HBV appears to be multifactorial. First, by causing chronic liver cell injury and accompanying regeneration, HBV predisposes the cells to mutations, caused possibly by environmental agents (such as dietary toxins). Mutational inactivation of p53 has been noted in liver cancers that occur in areas of the world where HBV and exposure to aflatoxins is endemic. Second, an HBV-encoded regulatory element called x-protein disrupts normal growth control of infected liver cells by transcriptional activation of several host cell protooncogenes (recall *tax* proteins of HTLV-1, p. 201). This sequence is supported by the development of hepatocellular carcinomas in mice that are transgenic for the region of HBV DNA that encodes the x-protein. Third, in some patients viral integration seems to cause secondary rearrangements of chromosomes and possibly homozygous inactivation of the p53 gene (p. 190). Thus, it seems that virus-induced gene damage in regenerating liver cells may set the stage for multistep carcinogenesis.

HOST DEFENSE AGAINST TUMORS: TUMOR IMMUNITY

Malignant transformation, as we have discussed, is associated with complex genetic alterations, some of which may result in the expression of proteins that are seen as nonself by the immune system. The idea that tumors are not entirely self was conceived by Ehrlich, who proposed that immune-mediated recognition of autologous tumor cells may be a "positive mechanism" capable of eliminating transformed cells. Subsequently, Lewis Thomas and McFarlane Burnet formalized this concept by coining the term "immune surveillance" to refer to recognition and destruction of nonself tumor cells on their appearance. The very fact that cancers occur suggests that immune surveillance is imperfect; however, because some tumors escape such policing does not preclude the possibility that others may have been aborted. It is necessary therefore to explore certain questions about tumor immunity: What is the nature of tumor antigens? What host effector systems may recognize tumor cells? Is antitumor immunity effective against spontaneous neoplasms? Can immune reactions against tumors be exploited for immunotherapy?

TUMOR ANTIGENS

Antigens that elicit an immune response have been demonstrated in many experimentally induced tumors and in some human cancers. They can be broadly classified into two categories: *tumor-specific antigens* (TSA), which are present only on tumor cells and not on any normal cells, and *tumor-associated antigens* (TAA), which are present on tumor cells and also on some normal cells.

TUMOR-SPECIFIC ANTIGENS. TSAs are most clearly demonstrated in chemically induced tumors of rodents. In experimental model systems tumor antigenicity is usually assessed by (1) the ability of an animal to resist a live tumor implant following previous immunization with live or killed tumor cells, (2) the ability of tumor-free host animals to resist challenge when infused with immunocompetent cells from a tumor-immunized syngeneic donor, and (3) the demonstration in vitro of tumor cell destruction by cytotoxic T cells derived from a tumor-immunized animal. By these methods it has been found that many chemically induced tumors express "private" or "unique" antigens not shared by other (histologically identical) tumors induced by the same chemical, even in the same animal. Because the antigens expressed in such tumors induce resistance to a tumor transplant, they are referred to as tumor-specific transplantation antigens (TSTAs).

The molecular identity of TSTA expressed on chemically induced tumors has been revealed only recently by the genetic analysis of mouse tumor cell lines (Fig. 7–29). (Repeated reference to this figure will be helpful in understanding TSTA.) According to this scenario, in normal cells, peptide fragments derived from a diverse array of cellular proteins are presented on the

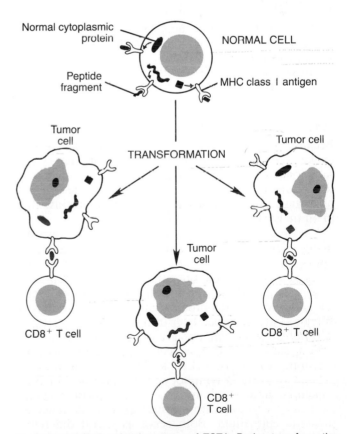

Figure 7-29. The molecular nature of TSTA. During transformation several normal cellular proteins may be altered due to mutations. A different protein is altered in each of the three transformed cells shown. Each mutant protein forms a distinct tumor antigen in association with MHC class I protein. The unique TSTAs so formed are recognized by different CD8+ cytotoxic T lymphocytes.

surface of cells in association with class I MHC molecules (p. 121). They do not induce an immune response, because T cells that recognize normal self peptide–class I complexes were clonally deleted during development (p. 136). During transformation, several mutations occur; some affect genes that encode normal cellular proteins and hence altered forms of these proteins are generated. The peptide–class I complex assembled from such mutant proteins is seen as non-self, just as a complex derived from a noncellular (e.g., viral) protein would be viewed as foreign (p. 121). This accounts for the antigenicity of tumor cells. The uniqueness of TSTA results from the fact that in each tumor a different array of normal cellular genes is randomly affected by mutations. Thus, in different neoplasms altered forms of distinct normal proteins are generated, each giving rise to a distinctive complex when bound by normal MHC antigens. Although there is no convincing evidence that such TSTAs exist on human tumors, this may reflect our inability to detect them rather than their absence. Indirect supporting evidence for the idea that some human tumors express specific antigens comes from the observation that certain tumors (e.g., testicular seminomas, melanomas, and medullary carcinomas of breast) evoke a significant lymphocytic infiltrate and that in general the prognosis for these tumors is better than for tumors of similar histologic type that lack a lymphocyte response. Furthermore, analyses of tumor-infiltrating lymphocytes in some human neoplasms suggest that they contain cytotoxic T lymphocytes that are specific for autologous tumor cells.

TUMOR-ASSOCIATED ANTIGENS. Most human tumor antigens are not unique to the individual tumors; rather, they are shared by similar tumors in other hosts. Such TAAs fall into two general categories: _differentiation-specific antigens_ and _oncofetal antigens._ Because TAAs are normal self proteins they do not evoke an immune response in humans and are of little functional significance in tumor rejection. Detection of these antigens is nevertheless of value in the diagnosis of certain tumors, and antibodies raised against them in animals can be useful for immunotherapy.

Oncofetal antigens, or embryonic antigens, are normally expressed in developing (embryonic) tissues but not in normal adult tissues. Their expression in some types of cancer cells is presumably due to derepression of genetic programs. The two best examples of oncofetal antigens—α-fetoprotein and carcinoembryonic antigen—are described later in this chapter (p. 210).

Differentiation antigens are peculiar to the differentiation state at which cancer cells are arrested. For example, CD10 (CALLA antigen), an antigen expressed in early B lymphocytes, is expressed in B-cell leukemias and lymphomas. Similarly, prostate-specific antigen is expressed on normal as well as cancerous prostatic epithelium. Both serve as useful differentiation markers in the diagnosis of lymphoid and prostatic cancers.

Of all human tumors, cutaneous melanomas have been investigated most extensively for tumor antigens and several melanoma antigens have been identified.

Although there is some evidence for the existence of TSAs in these tumors, the vast majority have turned out to be differentiation antigens or other molecules of diverse function. For example, a series of ganglioside (GD) antigens implicated in cell adhesion are expressed at high levels in advanced melanomas and have been targeted for antibody therapy. Another antigen, called S-100, is a calcium-binding cytoplasmic protein expressed not only in melanomas but also in several neural crest–derived tumors. It is used as a differentiation marker for these tumors.

ANTITUMOR EFFECTOR MECHANISMS _____

Both cell-mediated and humoral immunity can have antitumor activity. The cellular effectors that mediate immunity were described in Chapter 6, so it is necessary here only to characterize them briefly (Fig. 7–30):

- _Cytotoxic T lymphocytes._ The role of specifically sensitized cytotoxic T cells in experimentally induced tumors is well established. In humans they seem to play a protective role, chiefly against virus-associated neoplasms (e.g., EBV-induced Burkitt's lymphoma and HPV-induced tumors).
- _Natural killer cells._ Natural killer (NK) cells are lymphocytes that are capable of destroying tumor cells without prior sensitization. After activation with IL-2, NK cells can lyse a wide range of human tumors, including many that appear to be non-immunogenic for T cells. So NK cells may provide the first line of defense against many tumors. The target

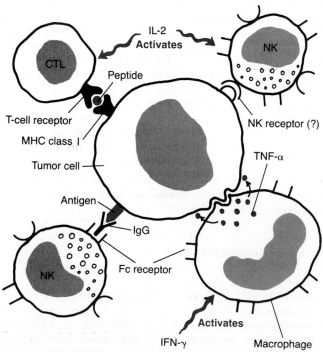

Figure 7–30. Cellular effectors of antitumor immunity and some cytokines that modulate antitumor activities. The nature of antigen recognized by T cells is depicted in Figure 7–29.

antigens recognized by NK cells or the relevant NK-cell receptors have not been identified. Because a wide variety of unrelated tumors can be lysed by NK cells without apparent specificity, it appears that the target antigens might be highly conserved tissue antigens whose expression is enhanced or altered on transformed cells. In addition to direct lysis of tumor cells, NK cells can also participate in antibody-dependent cellular cytotoxicity (ADCC), as described on page 127.

- *Macrophages.* Activated macrophages exhibit somewhat selective cytotoxicity against tumor cells in vitro. T cells and macrophages may collaborate in antitumor reactivity, since IFN-γ, a T cell–derived cytokine, is a potent activator of macrophages. These cells may kill tumors by mechanisms similar to those used to kill microbes (e.g., production of reactive oxygen metabolites; p. 40) or by secretion of TNF-α. In addition to its many other effects, this cytokine is lytic for several tumor cells.
- *Humoral* mechanisms may also participate in tumor cell destruction by two mechanisms: activation of complement and induction of ADCC by NK cells.

IMMUNOSURVEILLANCE

Given the host of possible and potential antitumor mechanisms, is there any evidence that they operate in vivo to prevent emergence of neoplasms? The strongest argument for the existence of immunosurveillance is the increased frequency of cancers in immunodeficient hosts. About 5% of persons with congenital immunodeficiencies develop cancers, about 200 times the expected prevalence. Analogously, immunosuppressed transplant recipients and patients with AIDS have more malignancies. It should be noted that most (but not all) of these neoplasms are lymphomas, often immunoblastic lymphomas. Particularly illustrative is the X-linked recessive immunodeficiency disorder termed XLP. When affected boys develop an EBV infection it does not take the usual self-limited form of infectious mononucleosis but instead evolves into a chronic or sometimes fatal form of infectious mononucleosis or, even worse, malignant lymphoma.

Most cancers occur in persons who do not suffer from any overt immunodeficiency. If immunosurveillance exists, how do cancers evade the immune system in immunocompetent hosts? To explain this, several escape mechanisms have been proposed.

- *Selective outgrowth of antigen-negative variants.* During tumor progression strongly immunogenic subclones may be eliminated.
- *Loss or reduced expression of histocompatibility antigens.* Tumor cells may fail to express normal levels of HLA class I antigens, thereby escaping attack by cytotoxic T cells.
- *Shedding or modulation of tumor antigens.* Sufficient shedding of tumor antigens may inhibit tumor cell recognition.
- *Sneaking through.* Emerging cancers may present too small an antigenic challenge to evoke an effec-

tive immune response. Later the mass becomes too large for destruction by the immune system.

- *Immunosuppression.* Many oncogenic agents (e.g., chemicals, ionizing radiation) suppress host immune responses. Tumors or tumor products may also be immunosuppressive. For example, TGF-β, secreted in large quantities by many tumors, is a potent immunosuppressant. In some cases the immune response induced by the tumor (e.g., activation of suppressor T cells) may itself inhibit tumor immunity.

While the increased occurrence of tumors in immunodeficient hosts supports the existence of immunosurveillance, the strongest argument against the concept of immunosurveillance also derives from the study of immunosuppressed patients. The commonest forms of cancers in immunosuppressed and immunodeficient patients are lymphomas, notably immunoblastic lymphomas, which could be the consequence of abnormal immunoproliferative responses to microbial infections or to the various therapeutic agents so often administered to these patients. Significantly, an increased incidence of the most common forms of cancer—lung, breast, gastrointestinal tract—and multiple neoplasms might be anticipated in immunologic cripples but does not occur.

IMMUNOTHERAPY OF HUMAN TUMORS

Even if immune surveillance exists, for the patient who develops cancer this protective mechanism has clearly failed. Can something be done to shore up defenses? The premise of immunotherapy is to either replace the suppressed components of the immune system or to stimulate endogenous responses. Three general approaches are being tested in humans.

ADOPTIVE CELLULAR THERAPY. Because incubation of peripheral blood lymphocytes with IL-2 generates lymphokine-activated killer (LAK) cells with potent antitumor activity in vitro, such cells are being utilized for adoptive immunotherapy. The patients' blood lymphocytes are cultured with IL-2 in vitro and the LAK cells (generated principally from expansion of blood NK cells) are reinfused along with additional IL-2. Human LAK trials are currently limited to advanced metastatic tumors.

Based on the assumption that tumor-specific cytotoxic T cells are likely to be enriched among tumor-infiltrating lymphocytes (TILs), investigators led by Steven Rosenberg are utilizing expanded and activated populations of TILs for immunotherapy. Lymphocytes harvested from surgically resected tumor masses are cultured in IL-2 and then reinfused into the patient. The efficacy of both these modalities of cell-based therapy is still being evaluated.

CYTOKINE THERAPY. Because cytokines can activate specific and nonspecific (inflammatory) host defenses, several cytokines, alone or in combination with other forms of treatment, are being evaluated for antitumor therapy. The use of IL-2 was mentioned above. In addition, IFN-α and -γ, TNF-α, and hematopoietic growth factors GM-CSF and G-CSF are also being tested in cancer patients. IFN-α has already shown considerable promise. It activates NK cells, increases expression of MHC molecules on tumor cells, and is also directly cytostatic. The most impressive results with IFN-α have been obtained in the treatment of hairy cell leukemia (p. 370).

ANTIBODY-BASED THERAPY. Although antibodies against TAA by themselves have not proven to be efficacious, current interest lies in using antibodies as targeting agents for delivery of cell toxins. In one approach, monoclonal antibodies against certain B-cell lymphomas are conjugated with ricin (a potent toxin) and the resulting "immunotoxin" is infused into patients. The efficacy of such "magic bullets" in the treatment of leukemias and lymphomas is under investigation.

CLINICAL FEATURES OF NEOPLASIA ____

Ultimately the importance of neoplasms lies in their effects on people. All tumors, even benign ones, may cause morbidity and mortality. Moreover, every new growth requires careful appraisal lest it be cancerous. This differential comes into sharpest focus with "lumps" in the female breast. Both cancers and many benign disorders of the female breast present as palpable masses. In fact, benign lesions are more common than cancers. Although clinical evaluation may suggest one or the other, "the only unequivocally benign breast mass is the excised and anatomically diagnosed one." This is equally true of all neoplasms. There are, however, instances when adherence to this dictum must be tempered by clinical judgment. Subcutaneous lipomas, for example, are quite common and readily recognized by their soft, yielding consistency. Unless they are uncomfortable, subject to trauma, or aesthetically disturbing, small lesions are often merely observed for significant increase in size. A few other examples might be cited, but it suffices that *with a few exceptions all masses require anatomic evaluation.* But besides the concern malignant neoplasms arouse, even benign ones may have many adverse effects. The sections that follow consider (1) the effects of a tumor on the host, (2) the grading and clinical staging of cancer, (3) the laboratory diagnosis of neoplasms, and (4) brief descriptions of common skin tumors not presented elsewhere in this text.

EFFECTS OF TUMOR ON HOST ____

Obviously, cancers are far more threatening to the host than are benign tumors. Nonetheless, both types of neoplasia may cause problems because of location and impingement on adjacent structures, functional activity such as hormone synthesis, and the production of bleeding and secondary infections when they ulcerate through adjacent natural surfaces. Any metastasis has the same potential. Cancers may also be responsible for cachexia (wasting) or paraneoplastic syndromes.

Location is of critical importance with both benign and malignant tumors. A small (1 cm) pituitary adenoma can compress and destroy the surrounding normal gland and give rise to hypopituitarism; a 0.5 cm leiomyoma in the wall of the renal artery may lead to renal ischemia and serious hypertension. A comparably small carcinoma within the common bile duct may induce fatal biliary tract obstruction.

The production of hormones is seen with both benign and malignant neoplasms arising in endocrine glands. The adenoma or carcinoma arising in the β cells of the islets of the pancreas often produces hyperinsulinism, sometimes fatal (Fig. 7–31). Analogously, some adenomas or carcinomas of the adrenal cortex elaborate corticosteroids (for example, aldosterone, which induces sodium retention, hypertension, and hypokalemia). Surprisingly, the functioning adenoma, wherever it arises, may induce a life-threatening endocrinopathy even though it may be less than 1 cm in diameter, and indeed such hormonal activity is more likely with a well-differentiated benign tumor than with a corresponding carcinoma.

Ulceration through a surface with consequent *bleeding or secondary infection* needs no further comment, but a few less obvious ramifications might be mentioned. The neoplasm, benign or malignant, that protrudes into the gut lumen may get caught in the peristaltic pull to telescope the neoplasm and its site of origin into the downstream segment of gut— intussusception (p. 519)—leading to ulceration of the mucosa or, even worse, intestinal obstruction or infarction.

It is evident that tumors create many problems, not only due to their need for removal or eradication but also in many other ways.

Cancer Cachexia ____

Many cancer patients suffer progressive loss of body fat and lean body mass, accompanied by profound

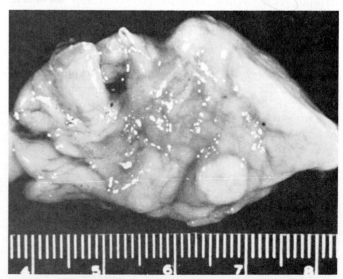

Figure 7–31. A graphic example of the potential significance of a benign tumor. An islet cell adenoma less than 1 cm in diameter was responsible for fatal hypoglycemia in a young adult.

weakness, anorexia, and anemia. This wasting syndrome is referred to as cachexia. Usually, an intercurrent infection brings a blessed end to the slow deterioration. There is in general some correlation between the size and extent of spread of the cancer and the severity of the cachexia. Small, localized cancers therefore are generally silent and produce no cachexia, but there are exceptions.

The origins of cancer cachexia are multifactorial. Anorexia is a common problem in patients who have cancer, even those who do not have tumors of the gastrointestinal tract. Reduced food intake has been related to abnormalities in taste and in the central control of appetite, but reduced calorie intake is not sufficient to explain the cachexia of malignancy. In patients with cancer, calorie expenditure remains high and basal metabolic rate is increased despite reduced food intake. This is in contrast to the lower metabolic rate that occurs as an adaptational response in starvation. The basis of these metabolic abnormalities is not fully understood. Perhaps circulating factors such as TNF-α and IL-1, released from activated macrophages, are involved. TNF-α suppresses appetite and inhibits the action of lipoprotein lipase, thereby inhibiting the release of free fatty acids from lipoproteins. Long-term administration of TNF-α to animals produces a state of cachexia. There is no satisfactory treatment for cancer cachexia other than removal of the underlying cause, the tumor.

Paraneoplastic Syndromes

Symptom complexes other than cachexia that appear in patients with cancer and that cannot be readily explained either by the local or distant spread of the tumor or by the elaboration of hormones indigenous to the tissue of origin of the tumor are referred to as paraneoplastic syndromes. They appear in 10 to 15% of patients with cancer and are important to recognize for several reasons:

- They may represent the earliest manifestation of an occult neoplasm.
- In affected patients they may represent significant clinical problems and may even be lethal.
- They may mimic metastatic disease and so confound treatment.

The paraneoplastic syndromes are diverse and are associated with many different tumors (Table 7-7). The most common syndromes are hypercalcemia, Cushing's syndrome, and nonbacterial thrombotic endocarditis; the neoplasms most often associated with these and other syndromes are bronchogenic and breast cancers and hematologic malignancies. Cushing's syndrome as a paraneoplastic phenomenon is usually related to ectopic production by the cancer of ACTH or ACTH-like polypeptides. The mediation of hypercalcemia, another common paraneoplastic syndrome, is less well understood. Some squamous cell carcinomas of the lung produce a parathyroid

TABLE 7-7. SOME PARANEOPLASTIC SYNDROMES

Clinical Syndromes	Major Forms of Underlying Cancer	Causal Mechanisms
Endocrinopathies		
Cushing's syndrome	Small cell cancer of the lung Pancreatic carcinoma Neural tumors	ACTH or ACTH-like substance
Hyponatremia	Small cell carcinoma of lung Intracranial neoplasms	Antidiuretic hormone or atrial natriuretic factor
Hypercalcemia	Squamous cell carcinoma of lung Breast carcinoma Renal carcinoma	PTH-like substance, TGF-α Vitamin D
Carcinoid syndrome	Bronchial carcinoid Pancreatic carcinoma Gastric carcinoma	Serotonin, bradykinin, ?histamine
Polycythemia	Renal carcinoma Cerebellar hemangioma Hepatocellular carcinoma	Erythropoietin
Nerve and muscle syndromes		
Disorders of the central and peripheral nervous systems	Small cell carcinoma of lung Breast carcinoma	?Immunologic, ?toxic
Myasthenia gravis	Thymoma	?Immunologic
Osseous, articular, and soft tissue changes		
Hypertrophic osteoarthropathy and clubbing of the fingers	Adenocarcinoma of lung	Unknown
Vascular and hematologic changes		
Venous thrombosis (Trousseau's phenomenon)	Pancreatic carcinoma Lung carcinoma Other cancers	Hypercoagulability
Nonbacterial thrombotic endocarditis	Advanced cancers	Hypercoagulability

hormone–like peptide. Also implicated are other tumor-derived factors such as TGF-α, a polypeptide factor that activates osteoclasts, and the active form of vitamin D. Another possible mechanism for hypercalcemia is widespread osteolytic metastatic disease of bone, but it should be noted that hypercalcemia as a paraneoplastic syndrome occurs in the absence of skeletal metastases. Sometimes one tumor induces several syndromes concurrently. Radioimmunoassays document, for example, that bronchogenic carcinomas may elaborate products identical to or having the effects of adrenocorticotropic hormone (ACTH), antidiuretic hormone (ADH), parathyroid hormone, serotonin, and human chorionic gonadotropin as well as other bioactive substances.

Paraneoplastic syndromes may take many other forms, such as hypercoagulability leading to venous thrombosis and nonbacterial thrombotic endocarditis (see p. 324) or the development of clubbing of the fingers and hypertrophic osteoarthropathy in patients with lung carcinomas (p. 432). Still others will be encountered in the consideration of the cancers of the various organs of the body.

GRADING AND STAGING OF CANCER _____

Methods to quantify the probable clinical aggressiveness of a given neoplasm and, further, to express its apparent extent and spread in the individual patient are necessary for comparisons of end results of various forms of treatment. The results of treating extremely small, highly differentiated thyroid adenocarcinomas that are localized to the thyroid gland are likely to be different from those obtained from treating highly anaplastic thyroid cancers that have invaded the neck organs.

The grading of a cancer attempts to establish some estimate of its aggressiveness or level of malignancy based on the cytologic differentiation of tumor cells and the number of mitoses within the tumor. The cancer may be classified as grade I, II, III, or IV, in order of increasing anaplasia. Criteria for the individual grades vary with each form of neoplasia and so are not detailed here. Moreover, difficulties in establishing clear-cut criteria have led increasingly to descriptive characterizations (e.g., well-differentiated adenocarcinoma with no evidence of vascular or lymphatic invasion, or highly anaplastic sarcoma with extensive vascular invasion, and so forth).

Staging of cancers is based on the size of the primary lesion, its extent of spread to regional lymph nodes, and the presence or absence of metastases. This assessment is usually based on clinical and radiographic examination, and in some cases surgical exploration. Two methods of staging are currently in use, the TNM system (T for primary tumor, N for regional lymph node involvement, and M for metastases) and the AJC (American Joint Committee) system. In the TNM system T1, T2, T3, and T4, respectively, describe the increasing size of the primary lesion; N0, N1, N2, or N3 indicates progressively advancing node involve-

ment; and M0 and M1 reflect the absence or presence of distant metastases. In the AJC method the cancers are divided into stages 0 to IV, incorporating the size of primary lesions as well as the presence of nodal spread and of distant metastases. Examples of the application of these two staging systems are cited in subsequent chapters. It is worth noting here, however, that the staging of neoplastic disease in the patient has assumed great importance in the selection of the best form of therapy for the patient and in multicenter treatment comparisons. Indeed, as compared with grading, staging has proved to be of greater clinical value.

LABORATORY DIAGNOSIS OF CANCER _____

Histologic and Cytologic Methods _____

In most instances, the laboratory diagnosis of cancer is not difficult. The two ends of the benign-malignant spectrum pose no problems; however, in the middle lies a "no-man's land" where the wise tread cautiously. This issue was aptly emphasized earlier in this chapter (p. 174); here the focus is on the roles of the clinician (often a surgeon) and the pathologist in arriving at the correct diagnosis.

Clinicians tend to underestimate the contributions they make to the diagnosis of a neoplasm. Clinical data are invaluable for optimal pathologic diagnosis. Radiation-induced changes in the skin or mucosa can be similar to those of cancer. Sections taken from a healing fracture can mimic remarkably an osteosarcoma. Moreover, the laboratory evaluation of a lesion can be only as good as the specimen submitted for examination. It must be adequate, representative, and properly preserved. Several sampling approaches are available: excision or biopsy, needle aspiration, and cytologic smears. When excision of a lesion is not possible, selection of an appropriate site for biopsy of a large mass requires awareness that the margins may not be representative and the center largely necrotic. Analogously with disseminated lymphoma (involving many nodes), those in the inguinal region draining large areas of the body often undergo reactive changes that may mask neoplastic involvement. The need for appropriate preservation of the specimen is obvious, yet it involves such issues as prompt immersion in a usual fixative (for example, formalin solution) or instead preservation of a portion in a special fixative (e.g., glutaraldehyde) for electron microscopy or prompt refrigeration to permit optimal hormone or receptor analysis. Requesting "quick-frozen section" diagnosis is sometimes desirable, for example in determining the nature of a breast lesion or in evaluating the margins of an excised cancer to ascertain that the entire neoplasm has been removed. This method, in which a sample is quick-frozen and sectioned, permits histologic evaluation within minutes. It is then possible with, for example, a breast biopsy to determine whether the lesion is malignant and may require wider excision or sampling of axillary nodes for possible spread. The patient is thereby spared the expense and trauma of a subsequent operation. In experienced, competent hands, frozen-section diagnosis is very accurate, but there are particular instances when the better histologic detail provided by the more time-consuming routine methods is needed—for example, when extremely radical surgery, such as the amputation of an extremity, may be indicated. Better to wait a few days despite the drawbacks than to perform inadequate or unnecessary surgery.

Fine-needle aspiration of tumors is another approach that is growing in popularity. This procedure is most commonly employed with readily palpable lesions affecting breast, thyroid, lymph nodes, and salivary glands. Modern imaging techniques enable the method to be extended to deeper structures such as liver, pancreas, and pelvic lymph nodes. It obviates surgery and its attendant risks. Although it entails some difficulties, such as small sample size and sampling errors, in experienced hands it can be extremely reliable, rapid, and useful.

Cytologic (Papanicolaou) smears provide yet another method for the detection of cancer. This approach is widely used for the discovery of carcinoma of the cervix, often at an in situ stage, but it is also used with many other forms of suspected malignancy, such as endometrial carcinoma, bronchogenic carcinoma, bladder and prostate tumors, and gastric carcinomas; for the identification of tumor cells in abdominal, pleural, joint, and cerebrospinal fluids; and, less commonly, with other forms of neoplasia. Neoplastic cells are less cohesive than others and so are shed into fluids or secretions (Fig. 7–32). The shed cells are evaluated for features of anaplasia indicative of their origin in cancer.

Cytologic interpretation requires a great deal of expertise but can yield, with cervical smears, nearly 100% true positive diagnosis; i.e., false positive results are rare. However, there is a significant fraction of false negative results, owing largely to sampling errors. It should be emphasized that *all positive findings are best confirmed by biopsy and histologic examination before therapy is instituted.* A negative report does not exclude the presence of a malignancy. The gratifying control of cervical cancer is the best testament to the value of the cytologic method.

It is well beyond our scope to delve into the technical details of the *anatomic diagnosis of cancer.* Only a brief "statement-of-the-art" will be made. Until relatively recently, it was in some part science and in large part art, depending much on subjective judgments of histologic appearance. Involved was, and to some extent still is, the solomonic judgment of when the level of cytologic atypia is sufficient to demand the diagnosis of cancer. Helpful diagnostic aids are the recent innovations in immunocytochemistry, flow cytometry, and DNA probe analyses that have added considerable objectivity to the laboratory diagnosis of cancer. These techniques can be applied to exfoliated cancer cells, tissue aspirates, or biopsy specimens. A few examples are illustrative. Monoclonal antibodies directed against intermediate filaments have proved to be valuable in the classification of otherwise poorly differentiated tumors. For example, detection of cytokeratin by immunoperoxidase staining allows distinction between poorly differentiated carcinoma and a large cell lymphoma. T- and B-cell neoplasms can be identified on the basis of clonal rearrangement of their antigen receptor genes by employing Southern blot analysis. Leukemias and lymphomas can be classified by flow

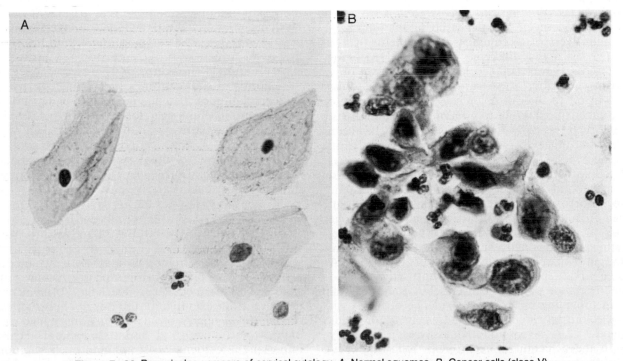

Figure 7–32. Papanicolaou smears of cervical cytology. *A,* Normal squames. *B,* Cancer cells (class V).

cytometric detection of differentiation-specific antigens (p. 355). Flow cytometry is also useful in assessing the DNA content of tumor cells. A relationship between DNA content (ploidy) and prognosis is becoming apparent for a variety of malignancies. Amplification of the N-*myc* and the c-*neu* oncogenes, detected by cytogenetic or molecular methods, has proven to be of prognostic value in neuroblastomas and breast carcinomas, respectively. Thus molecular biology has moved from the laboratory to the bedside, and the diagnosis of malignant neoplasia has progressed from the level of "eyeballing" to the precision offered by molecular genetics.

Biochemical Assays

Biochemical assays for tumor-associated enzymes, hormones, and other tumor markers in the blood cannot be construed as modalities for the diagnosis of cancer; however, they contribute to finding cases and in some instances are useful in determining the effectiveness of therapy. The application of these assays will be considered with many of the specific forms of neoplasia discussed in other chapters, so only a few examples suffice here. Prostatic carcinoma can be suspected when elevated levels of acid phosphatase are found in the blood. Regrettably, the levels become significantly raised only when the tumor is advanced, so the false negative rate is high. Radioimmunoassays for circulating hormones may point to the presence of tumors in the endocrine system and in some instances to the ectopic production of hormones by nonendocrine tumors (p. 207).

A host of circulating tumor markers have been described, and new ones are identified every year. Only a few have stood the test of time and proved to be clinically useful. *The two best-established are carcinoembryonic antigen (CEA) and α-fetoprotein.* CEA, normally produced in embryonic tissue of the gut, pancreas, and liver, is a complex glycoprotein that is elaborated by many different neoplasms. Depending on the serum level adopted as representative of a significant elevation, it is variously reported to be positive in 60 to 90% of colorectal carcinomas, 50 to 80% of pancreatic, and 25 to 50% of gastric and breast tumors. Much less consistently, elevated CEA has been described in other forms of cancer. Regrettably, in almost all types of neoplasia the level of elevation is correlated with the body burden of tumor, so highest levels are found in those with advanced metastatic disease. Moreover, CEA elevations have also been reported in many benign disorders, such as alcoholic cirrhosis, hepatitis, ulcerative colitis, Crohn's disease, and others. Occasionally levels of this antigen are elevated in apparently healthy smokers. Thus, CEA assays lack both specificity and the sensitivity required for the detection of early cancers, but they are still useful in providing presumptive evidence of the possibility of colorectal carcinoma because this tumor yields the highest CEA levels and the assay is particularly useful in the detection of recurrences following excision. With successful resection of the tumor, CEA disappears from the serum; its reappearance almost always spells the beginning of the end (p. 517).

The other well-established tumor marker is α-fetoprotein. Elevated circulating levels are encountered in adults with cancers arising principally in the liver and from yolk sac remnants. Less regularly it is elevated in teratocarcinomas and embryonal cell carcinomas of the testis, ovary, and extragonadal sites, and occasionally in cancers of the stomach and pancreas. As with CEA, benign conditions including cirrhosis, hepatitis, and pregnancy (especially with fetal distress or death) may cause modest elevations of α-fetoprotein. There is then a problem with both specificity and sensitivity, but the marker may still provide presumptive evidence of a hepatocellular carcinoma, for example, and is of value in the follow-up of therapeutic interventions. More details are found on page 561. This cursory overview suffices to indicate the many laboratory approaches in use for the detection and diagnosis of tumors.

SKIN TUMORS

Four types of lesions are considered here: squamous cell carcinoma, basal cell carcinoma, pigmented nevi, and melanomas.

Skin cancer in general is the most common form of malignant neoplasia. It has been estimated that almost half of all people who reach 65 years of age have had or will have at least one skin cancer. Fortunately, 90% of these lesions are curable by adequate local excision. Among the skin cancers, 20% are squamous cell carcinomas, about 70% are basal cell carcinomas, and approximately 2% are melanocarcinomas. The residual 8% include various uncommon forms of cancer too rare to merit description here. Over 90% of the common skin tumors (squamous and basal cell carcinomas) occur on the head and neck, regions most exposed to the sun, whereas melanomas tend to occur on the back, which also receives bouts of heavy sun exposure during vacation periods. The frequency of all these forms of skin cancer is higher in those living in southern latitudes than in inhabitants of the northern hemisphere. There is therefore epidemiologic evidence implicating the ultraviolet radiation of sunlight in their causation. Recall that certain hereditary conditions such as xeroderma pigmentosum, which are characterized by defective DNA-repair systems, predispose to sunlight-induced skin cancers.

SQUAMOUS CELL (EPIDERMOID) CARCINOMA ___

Squamous cell carcinomas may arise in any stratified squamous epithelium or mucosa that has undergone squamous metaplasia. Thus this form of cancer may occur, for example, in the tongue, lips, esophagus, cervix, vulva, vagina, bronchus, or urinary bladder. On oral or vulval mucosal surfaces, leukoplakia is an important antecedent. Most squamous cell carcinomas, however, arise in the skin (90 to 95%). Fair-skinned blonds who have outdoor occupations are particularly prone to develop this form of cancer. Often the tumors are preceded by so-called actinic (solar) keratoses, a form of dysplasia of the epidermal cells. Arsenic and coal tars have also been implicated in their causation. Protracted chronic inflammation constitutes yet another predisposing influence, so squamous cell carcinoma is sometimes encountered in the margins of long-standing draining sinuses and in old x-ray or burn scars. Sometimes the neoplasm does not appear until decades after the x-ray or thermal injury.

The earliest recognizable lesion, the carcinoma in situ, appears as a well-defined small (1- to 2-cm) red-brown plaque with slightly elevated firm margins. Often the surface is scaly owing to hyperkeratinization. On moist mucosal surfaces where keratinization is unusual, the patch may be red and oozing. The in situ stage is followed by progressive invasion and expansion of the tumor, creating a firm, elevated plaque. This is often followed by central ulceration yielding a necrotic crater, rimmed by firm margins. Histologically, the in situ stage reveals complete replacement of the normal epidermal thickness by atypical cells, showing the classic features of variation in cell and nuclear size and in morphology accompanied by hyperchromatic nuclei, which sometimes bear numerous and possibly abnormal mitotic figures well above the basal zone. Progressive penetration of the basement membrane and invasion of the dermis or underlying connective tissue follows in the form of tongue-like penetrations (Fig. 7–33).

Approximately 80% of these cancers are extremely well differentiated and are composed of readily recognized keratinocytes forming keratin pearls (concentric laminated keratinous layers). The burrowing, invasive strands and nests of cells in the well-differentiated lesions tend to replicate the organization of the normal epidermis; basal cells occupy the perimeter of these nests, and there is progressive maturation of the cells in the centers of the islands. Thus the central regions of these tumor nests are often keratinized and sometimes form "horn cysts." The residual 20% of squamous cell carcinomas show varying levels of loss of differentiation; some are totally undifferentiated with marked anaplasia, giant cell formation, numerous mitoses, and no keratinization.

The prognosis depends more on the location, size, and depth of penetration of the tumor than on the degree of anaplasia. Skin lesions tend to be discovered when relatively small, and fewer than 2 to 5% of patients have metastases to regional nodes. Resection then can be curative.

BASAL CELL CARCINOMA

Basal cell carcinomas almost never metastasize. These cancers arise in the basal cells of the pilosebaceous adnexa and occur only on the skin. Mucosal

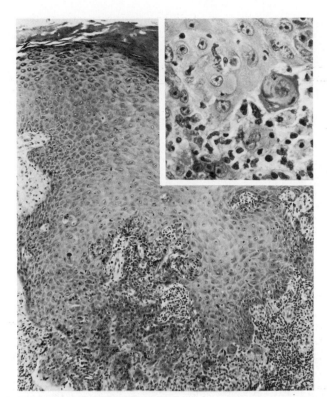

Figure 7–33. Squamous cell carcinoma of the skin. The penetrating tongues of tumor are seen below. Inset shows a keratinous pearl. (Courtesy of Dr. George F. Murphy, Brigham and Women's Hospital and Harvard Medical School, Boston, MA.)

surfaces lacking these adnexa, such as the lips, tongue, and cervix, are never primary sites. As with the squamous cell carcinoma, these cancers tend to occur after age 40 in those with fair skin. Blacks and Orientals are seldom affected. Although sunlight is considered to be a predisposing influence, for unexplained reasons these tumors are more frequent on the eyelids and bridge of the nose (rich in adnexal glands) than on the sun-exposed backs of hands and forearms. Use of arsenicals also increases the risk of basal cell carcinoma.

Grossly the tumors present as pearly papules, often displaying prominent dilated subepidermal blood vessels. Even small lesions (less than 1 cm) soon develop central ulcerations, which are characteristically rimmed by a pearly raised border (rodent ulcers). Some show varying degrees of pigmentation, which makes them superficially resemble nevi. Neglected lesions may be locally penetrating, ulcerative, and destructive, but in general their progression is slow and indolent, spanning many months to years.

Histologically, basal cell carcinomas usually appear as invasive clusters or strands of compact, darkly chromatic, spindled cells that in the plane of section may have no connection with the overlying epidermis or adnexa. On cross section the strands create numerous nests or islands having a peripheral array of palisaded basal cells that strongly resemble their normal forebears

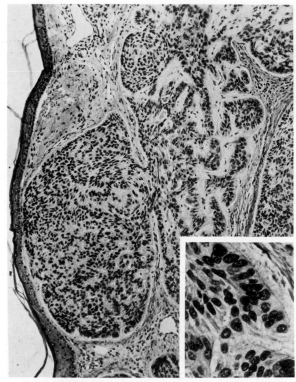

Figure 7–34. Basal cell carcinoma of the skin. Normal epidermis is at left. The nests and strands of invasive tumor cells are penetrating into the subcutaneous tissue. Inset reveals the peripheral palisade. (Courtesy of Dr. George F. Murphy, Brigham and Women's Hospital and Harvard Medical School, Boston, MA.)

and that enclose a uniform collection of spindled forms (Fig. 7–34). Giant cells, striking anaplasia, and mitotic figures are conspicuously absent. The tumor nests are embedded in a mucinous matrix that shrinks away from the tumor cells to create clefts or separation artifacts that are quite characteristic. Although most basal cell carcinomas are unicentric, on occasion multiple foci of tumor are separated by small zones of normal intervening epidermis. Usually, however, such multicentricity is confined to a localized area (1 to 3 cm) of the skin.

Surgical excision, irradiation, or adequate cauterization cures most basal cell carcinomas. Even when the neoplasm extends to the margins of surgical excision, only one third recur. These continue to extend and produce more difficult clinical problems. Ultimately, however, all are amenable to total cure. The presence of keratinization in a basal cell carcinoma does not alter its biologic behavior, and so basosquamous patterns do not assume the significance of the more ominous squamous cell carcinomas, which may metastasize.

PIGMENTED NEVI

Some clinicians refer to any colored lesion of the skin as a nevus, including those of vascular origin.

Here the term "nevus" is restricted to lesions composed of modified melanocytes (nevus cells) of neural crest origin. All types of nevi at some point in their course have excess melanin pigmentation, which makes them tan-brown distinctive skin lesions. *They can be divided into three categories: (1) common acquired nevi; (2) less frequent subtypes, including congenital giant nevus, blue nevus, and compound nevus of Spitz (spindle and epithelioid cell nevus, halo nevus); and (3) dysplastic nevi.* Although all may give rise to melanocarcinomas (more commonly referred to as melanomas), the risk is significantly greater with congenital giant nevi and dysplastic nevi. Only the common acquired and dysplastic nevi are described here.

Common acquired nevi are often referred to as "moles." They are extremely common lesions found in greater or lesser numbers (average 10 to 40) on most Caucasians. The evolution of acquired nevi strongly suggests that they are focal developmental aberrations of melanocytes rather than true neoplasms. Absent at birth, they first appear in early childhood and become more frequent in middle adult life (most on the trunk); then progressively disappear. Those on the extremities, particularly on the palms and soles, are apt to persist. The basis for this regional variation is unclear.

All common nevi begin as small (1 to 2 mm) uniformly tan to brown, almost black, macules. They gradually enlarge but rarely exceed 6 mm in diameter, and some become slightly elevated. **Characteristically they have distinct rounded borders.** Those on the trunk generally over the course of time become depigmented and transformed into pink or flesh-colored papules, whereas those on the extremities, as mentioned, often persist. Thus, to quote Greene and coworkers, "Most people enter life free of nevi and leave with relatively few."

An orderly histologic progression accompanies the macroscopic evolution, particularly with trunk nevi. At the outset the tiny lesions are composed of nests of nevus cells, which are basically rounded melanocytes having ovoid nuclei without prominent nucleoli, located within the epidermis at the dermoepidermal junction (**junctional nevus**). They usually contain cytoplasmic granules of melanin. As moles enlarge and become slightly raised, nests of neval cells appear in the dermis along with the intraepidermal nests (**compound nevus**) (Fig. 7–35). Over time, particularly in trunk nevi, the intraepidermal nests disappear (**intradermal nevus**). Concomitantly, the nevus cells in the dermis become more spindled and possibly dendritic; they differentiate along neural lines and simultaneously lose the ability to synthesize melanin. In this manner, the nevus becomes depigmented and transformed into a flesh-colored papule. Nevi on the extremities tend not to undergo this orderly "maturation" and persist as junctional or compound lesions.

Dysplastic nevi may arise de novo or in common acquired nevi when they fail to undergo orderly maturation. They have important differences from common

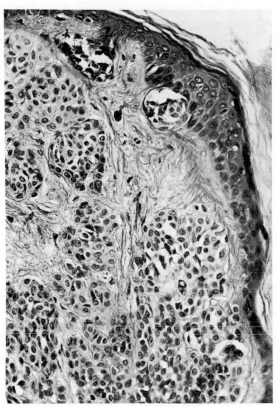

Figure 7–35. Compound nevus. Nests of nevus cells are present both at dermoepidermal junction and within dermis.

acquired nevi: (1) Although most do not progress to melanoma, the risk is significantly greater than with common nevi. (2) Other members of the family may have similar lesions, indicating that some individuals with these lesions have the *familial dysplastic nevus syndrome.* (3) They differ both macroscopically and microscopically from common nevi and may be difficult to differentiate from melanomas.

Dysplastic nevi occur on sun-exposed as well as unexposed skin surfaces. They tend to be larger macules (greater than 6 mm in diameter) and, unlike ordinary moles, have distinct irregular borders and a variegated tan to dark brown to pink color. This macroscopic appearance, as will become evident, is similar to that of some melanomas. Histologically, they appear to represent arrest of the evolution of the ordinary mole at the junctional or compound stage. But the melanocytes also have varying degrees of atypia and dysplasia, which in some instances borders on a superficial spreading melanoma (discussed later).

RELATIONSHIP OF NEVI TO MELANOMAS. Ask three dermatologists about the risk of transformation of a particular type of nevus into a melanoma and you will get four answers. Without going into the confusing controversy, the weight of evidence supports the following generalizations:

- Most melanomas arise de novo, but fully a third arise in preexisting nevi.
- Individuals who have many common acquired nevi have a significantly greater risk of melanoma

(roughly proportional to the number of nevi) than those who have no nevi. Nonetheless, only a small fraction of 1% of common moles become cancerous.
- Congenital giant nevi are more likely to undergo transformation than ordinary moles.
- Dysplastic nevi are the most ominous and most likely to undergo transformation to melanoma. The risk of melanoma is also increased in *clinically unaffected* skin and is proportional to the number of dysplastic nevi (hence the great risk with the familial nevus syndrome).

MELANOMA (MALIGNANT MELANOMA, MELANOCARCINOMA)

Uncommon forms of cancer, melanomas arise most often in the skin but infrequently are seen in the oral cavity, esophagus, anus, vagina, meninges, conjunctiva, or retina. Although persons of any age may be affected, the peak incidence is 40 to 60 years. An alarming increase in their incidence has been noted, particularly in the lower limbs of females, above the waist in males, and in the upper limbs of both sexes. This increase in frequency is attributed to the growing worship of a suntan with intense exposures to sunlight during the warm weather months.

The "melanomaniacs" who have intensively studied these lesions have evolved a complex classification and even more complex terminology for various subtypes. Only the two most frequent subtypes are described here. It is proposed that the development of melanomas involves two patterns of growth—radial and vertical. Radial growth implies lateral spread, largely confined to the epidermis and perhaps with minimal dermal penetration. Vertical growth implies tumor progression and the emergence of a new, more aggressive clone resulting in downward spread into the dermis and subjacent layers. These two patterns of growth have significantly different clinical consequences. In the radial phase the melanomas have little if any capacity for metastases, but unfortunately vertical growth brings with it the ugly potential of all anaplastic cancers. From the clinical standpoint, it is usually possible to distinguish these two growth phases macroscopically.

In the majority of melanocarcinomas radial growth predominates for months to years before becoming invasive, so these lesions have been called **superficial spreading melanomas.** They appear as flat to raised, brown to black lesions having several distinctive characteristics: (1) focal areas of red, white, or blue coloration and (2) irregular, ill-defined serpiginous margins, sometimes with tongue-like extensions or satellite lesions. This gross appearance should make them distinct from the sharply circumscribed, uniformly tan-brown common nevi with their regular rounded contours, but the shape and color closely approximate those of some dysplastic nevi. Histologically this pattern is marked by anaplastic, usually pigment-laden melanocytes confined to the epidermis. Distinctive are the occasional isolated cells enclosed by a clear halo (Paget's cells) resembling those seen in Paget's disease of the breast (p. 639). In time, individual and nested tumor cells penetrate all layers of the epidermis up to the surface, sometimes with ulceration of the surface. At the same time the cells invade the dermis and ultimately move more deeply, and with this vertical growth they acquire the potential to metastasize. A variable dermal infiltrate of lymphocytes may be present along with pigment-laden macrophages.

Some melanomas have a minimal radial phase and vertical growth is dominant (nodular melanomas). They appear as small (1 to 3 cm), firm, raised variegated lesions marked by total involvement of the full thickness of the epidermis, sometimes with ulceration through the surface accompanied by penetration into the dermis and deeper (Fig. 7–36). Rarely the anaplastic melanocytes do not form pigment (amelanotic melanomas). Pigmented or not, these are **nodular melanomas** having the capacity to metastasize widely to almost any organ or tissue in the body. The metastases are usually brown to black, but sometimes are nonpigmented with amelanotic primaries, on occasion even when the primary itself is deeply pigmented (attributed to the emergence of new clones that lack the ability to synthesize melanin).

Of major clinical importance are (1) early recognition of malignant melanomas before they have pene-

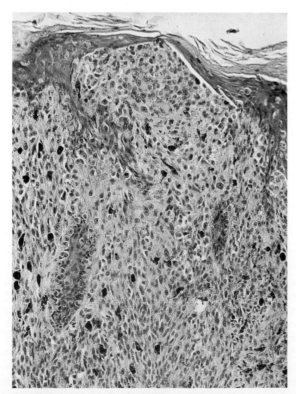

Figure 7–36. Nodular melanocarcinoma. The anaplastic cells have invaded the epidermis and have almost eroded through the surface. The dark cells are filled with melanin pigment.

trated deeply and acquired the potential to metastasize and (2) the maximum depth of penetration of the lesions. Early recognition requires their differentiation from common nevi, based on the distinctive margins and pigmentary changes already described. *Warning signs are changes in size, conformation, and pigmentation and ulceration with bleeding.* Much more difficult is their segregation from dysplastic nevi: usually biopsy is required. The prognosis following excision is largely determined by the vertical thickness (from granular layer to area of deepest penetration). For example, localized lesions that are less than 0.76 mm thick have a better than 95% 5-year survival rate, whereas lesions at least 4 mm thick are associated with a 50% survival rate. Although the thickness of a lesion is the most important prognostic index, other variables such as anatomic site of the lesion, mitotic rate, and lymphocytic response condition the outlook. Early recognition is critically important because when these lesions are invasive they are among the "ugliest" of cancers and may literally spray the body with implants.

Bibliography

Arends, M. J., Wyllie, A. H., and Bird, C. C.: Papilloma virus and human cancer. Human Pathol. *21*:686, 1990. (A short review of the oncogenicity of human papillomaviruses.)

Bishop, J. M.: Molecular themes in oncogenesis. Cell *64*:235, 1991. (An excellent overview of the molecular basis of cancer.)

Drinkwater, N. R.: Experimental models and biological mechanisms for tumor promotion. Cancer Cells *2*:8, 1990. (A brief and easy-to-read discussion of initiation and promotion sequence in chemical carcinogenesis.)

Fearon, E. R., and Vogelstein, B.: A genetic model of colorectal tumorigenesis. Cell *61*:759, 1990. (A detailed account of the molecular basis of multistep carcinogenesis.)

Fidler, I. J.: Critical factors in the biology of human cancer metastasis. Cancer Res. *50*:6130, 1990. (A broad overview of tumor cell heterogeneity and metastasis.)

Hunter, T.: Cooperation between oncogenes. Cell *64*:249, 1991. (A scholarly and detailed review of oncogene functions, classification, and interactions.)

Immunity to tumors. *In* Abbas, A. K., Lichtman, A. H., and Pober, J. S. Cellular and Molecular Immunology. Philadelphia, W. B. Saunders, 1991, p. 335. (A detailed discussion of tumor immunology, clinical as well as experimental.)

Joseph-Silverstein, J., and Silverstein, R. L.: Tumor angiogenesis. *In* Moosa, A. R., et al. Comprehensive Textbook of Oncology. 2nd ed. Baltimore, Williams & Wilkins, 1991, p. 138. (A short chapter that describes tumor angiogenesis, angiogenic factors, and their clinical implications.)

Liotta, L. A., Steeg, P. S., and Stetler-Stevenson, W. G.: Cancer metastasis and angiogenesis: an imbalance of positive and negative regulation. Cell *64*:327, 1991. (A review of the biochemical and molecular basis of tumor cell invasion and metastasis.)

Magrath, J.: The pathogenesis of Burkitt's lymphoma. Adv. Cancer Res. *55*:133, 1990. (A detailed review of the role of EBV and other factors in the causation of Burkitt's lymphoma.)

Marshall, C. J.: Tumor suppressor genes. Cell *64*:313, 1991. (An up-to-date review of tumor suppressor genes with emphasis on their biochemical functions.)

Sawyers, C. L., Denny, C. T., and Witte, O. N.: Leukemia and the disruption of normal hematopoiesis. Cell *64*:337, 1991. (A detailed account of the molecular basis of leukemogenesis including chronic myeloid leukemia and human T-cell leukemia.)

Tannock, I. F.: Tumor growth and cell kinetics. *In* Tannock, I. F., and Hill, R. P. (eds.). The Basic Science of Oncology. New York, Pergamon Press, 1987, p. 140. (An excellent chapter that details the kinetics of tumor cell growth and its clinical implications.)

Virji, M. A., et al.: Tumor markers in cancer diagnosis and prognosis.

CA *38*:104, 1988. (A classification and review of tumor markers, with emphasis on clinical use.)

Wands, J. R., and Blum, H. E.: Primary hepatocellular carcinoma. New Engl. J. Med. *325*:729, 1991. (This short editorial summarizes the current thinking on the relationship between HBV and liver cell cancer.)

Weinberg, R. A.: A short guide to oncogenes and tumor suppressor genes. J. NIH Res. *3*:45, 1991. (A succinct, easy-to-read summary of oncogenes and tumor suppressor genes and their interactions.)

Wigley, C., and Balmain, A.: Chemical carcinogenesis and precancer. *In* Franks, L. M., and Teich, N. M. (eds.): Introduction to Cellular and Molecular Biology of Cancer, 2nd ed., 1991. New York, Oxford University Press, p. 148. (An excellent discussion of chemical carcinogenesis in modern molecular terms.)

EIGHT

Environmental Diseases

MARY F. LIPSCOMB, M.D.

ENVIRONMENTAL POLLUTION
  Air Pollution
  Smoking
  Pneumoconioses
      Coal Workers' Pneumoconiosis
      Silicosis
      Asbestosis and Asbestos-Related
        Diseases
      Berylliosis
INJURY BY CHEMICAL AGENTS
  Injury by Therapeutic Agents
      Exogenous Estrogens and Oral
        Contraceptives
      Acetaminophen
      Aspirin (Acetylsalicyclic Acid)
  Injury by Nontherapeutic Toxic Agents
      Lead
      Carbon Monoxide (CO)
      Alcohol and Other Drugs of Abuse
INJURY BY PHYSICAL AGENTS
  Mechanical Trauma
  Thermal Injury
      Thermal Burns
      Hyperthermia
      Hypothermia
  Electrical Injury
  Injury by Ionizing Radiation
NUTRITIONAL DISEASES
  Protein-Energy Malnutrition
  Anorexia Nervosa and Bulimia
  Vitamin Deficiencies
      Vitamin A
      Vitamin D
      Vitamin E
      Vitamin K
      Thiamine
      Riboflavin
      Niacin
      Pyridoxine (Vitamin B_6)
      Vitamin C (Ascorbic Acid)
  Trace Elements

Obesity
Diet and Systemic Diseases
Diet and Cancer

Environmental pathology could encompass the study of all diseases that are not entirely genetic. Even the expression of inherited disorders can be influenced by environmental factors. Recognizing that very few diseases are purely environmental or genetic, we will limit our discussion to some general concepts and illustrative diseases that develop from (1) pollution of the environment, particularly of air, (2) use and abuse of drugs and physical agents, including radiation, and (3) over- or undernutrition. The discussion begins with an overview of environmental pollution and then turns to air pollution and its impact on the lungs.

ENVIRONMENTAL POLLUTION

Environmental medicine is rapidly becoming a major interest of physicians and biomedical scientists as well as a growing number of legal and governmental groups around the world. Microorganisms contaminating food and water have long been a major cause of morbidity and mortality in third world countries, and concerns about contamination of food and water by pesticides and industrial waste are increasing worldwide. Air is polluted in many communities by industrial waste or the products of automobile exhausts. Growing concern about the safety of food, water, and air has placed pressure on the scientific community to document the ill effects of pollutants and on governments to enact and enforce protective legislation.

Unfortunately, it is extremely difficult to acquire the data needed to accurately assess the risk associated with various levels of pollutants. Nevertheless, some data are available, and potentially beneficial legislative action has been taken to protect humanity from some of the perils of living in this populous, industrialized world. However, it is clear that more than scientific facts and legislative action are required to decrease the impact of some common environmental pathogens (i.e., tobacco smoke) on the incidence of disease.

TABLE 8–1. PATHOLOGIC EFFECTS OF ENVIRONMENTAL POLLUTANTS

Proximal (immediate) effects
direct Inflammation
Necrosis
indirect Hypersensitivity reactions
Distal (long-term) effects
Fibrosis
Degenerative changes
Teratogenesis
Cancer

A pollutant is defined as an agent in the environment the presence of which can cause disease in those who are exposed. Thus, agents that are "naturally" present but in abnormal quantities, such as ozone, may be considered pollutants as well as those that are not naturally present, such as polychlorinated biphenyls (PCBs). Pollutants produce disease by several mechanisms. Acute toxicity results directly when the agent induces inflammation or necrosis, or indirectly, when an immune response produces a hypersensitivity reaction. These acute reactions are referred to as "proximal" effects of the pollutant (Table 8–1). More difficult to study, and therefore to evaluate, are the distal effects of pollutants. These may take such forms as subclinical chronic inflammation and fibrosis, resulting from ongoing toxic effects and/or hypersensitivity reactions or degenerative changes that lead to organ malfunction, as might occur in the central nervous system of children with chronic lead toxicity. Pollutants can also cause congenital defects if the fetus is exposed during early embryogenesis or if germ cells are exposed during gametogenesis. Cancers may arise from pollutants that produce mutations or act as promoters (p. 199).

Most pollutants exist in quantities too small to produce proximal effects. When concentrations are sufficient to produce acute toxicity there is usually early awareness of the problem. Because small amounts are unlikely to produce changes for years, the connection between the pollutant and the disease often goes unappreciated. Several methods are used to study the effect of pollutants and to determine acceptable environmental concentrations. They include epidemiologic studies, experiments with normal human volunteers, and animal studies. The details of these methods are beyond the scope of our discussion. Suffice it to say that no method is perfect and so it is difficult to establish precise risks and causal relationships.

Infectious diseases resulting from contamination of food and water are discussed with gastrointestinal infections (p. 503) and hepatitis (p. 531). The effects of a number of chemicals that may contaminate food and water are discussed with nontherapeutic agents later in this chapter. A discussion of the health consequences of air pollution follows.

AIR POLLUTION

Air pollution has been a continuing problem in industrialized areas. Although levels of air pollution are monitored in many cities, only a limited number of specific pollutants are assessed, and data are incomplete as to whether some unmonitored pollutants may be harmful. Smog, the visible accumulation of air pollutants, is particularly heavy in cities where coal combustion is a source of energy and in certain communities where automobile exhaust fumes accumulate. Coal combustion results in release into the air of sulfur oxides and particulates (a so-called reducing smog). This form of smog is common in the northeastern United States and in some European cities. In the past, high levels of sulfur oxides and particulates have been clearly linked to increased morbidity and mortality, especially among persons with preexisting lung disease. "Photochemical oxidant" smog results when incompletely burned hydrocarbons release carbon monoxide (CO), carbon dioxide (CO_2), and nitrogen oxides. The action of sunlight on these primary pollutants leads to the release of secondary pollutants, including ozone and free radicals with oxidizing properties. This type of pollution occurs in cities like Los Angeles, California. The effects on morbidity and mortality of oxidant smog have been less clear-cut, but there is evidence that small decrements in pulmonary function occur in persons who inhabit areas where this form of pollution is heavy. Whether only a few or several specific pollutants are responsible for lung injury has been difficult to assess.

Although air pollutants can affect many organ systems (e.g., lead absorbed through the respiratory tract can produce extrapulmonary disease, p. 229), the lung itself usually bears the brunt and is particularly vulnerable when there is underlying lung disease, especially chronic obstructive lung disease (p. 391).

The pulmonary changes seen with various air pollutants range from minor irritation to the initiation of debilitating fibrotic disease to the induction of cancer (Table 8–2). Except for the pneumoconioses, which will be discussed in this chapter, and some general

TABLE 8–2. PATTERNS OF LUNG INJURY RELATED TO AIR POLLUTION

Lung Response	Pathogenic Mechanisms
Acute or chronic inflammation (e.g., chronic bronchitis)	Direct cell injury
Emphysema	Enhanced proteolysis
Asthma	Allergic or irritant effect
Hypersensitivity pneumonitis	Immunologic injury
Pneumoconiosis	Fibrotic reactions caused by cytokines released from macrophages and other recruited leukocytes
Neoplasia	Mutagenic and promoting effects

comments on smoking, all pollutant-caused lung diseases are discussed in Chapter 13.

Several factors determine whether an air pollutant causes lung injury and what form the injury takes.

- *Solubility in water.* A water-soluble molecule such as sulfur dioxide (SO_2) is dissolved readily in secretions in the upper air passages. This effect is referred to as the "scrubbing" action of the upper air passages and results in protection of the lower air passages.
- *Particle size and airway anatomy.* Particles greater than 5 or 10 μm are unlikely to reach distal airways, whereas particulates smaller than 0.5 μm tend to act like gases and move in and out of the alveoli, often without substantial deposition or injury. Particles that are 1 to 5 μm are the most dangerous because they impact at bifurcations of the distal airways.
- *Concentration and chemical reactivity.* Low concentrations of SO_2 (less than 0.1 ppm) produce only eye irritation. Concentrations in the range of 2 to 5 ppm (achieved in smog under some conditions) overcome the scrubbing action of the nose and cause increased airway resistance. Very high levels (more than 20 ppm), achieved under experimental conditions, result in decreased mucociliary clearance and even pulmonary edema.
- *Rate, depth, and type (nasal or oral) of respirations.* In addition to the absolute concentration of the pollutant in the inspired air, the mechanism of breathing can change the effective concentration. For example, deep, rapid pulmonary respiration, as would occur during heavy exertion (e.g., with coal miners at work), increases the exposure of the lower airways to an air pollutant.
- *Duration of exposure.* The longer the period of exposure to a pollutant continuously present in air, the greater the accumulation in the lungs. This is an important factor in occupational exposures that result in pneumoconiosis. Because even those who work outside the home spend more than 50% of their time in their homes, the pollution of the air inside the home can be an important problem. A list of the principal indoor air pollutants, their sources, and their major effects is provided in Table 8–3.
- *Host clearance mechanisms.* The decreased capacity to clear inhaled particles that occurs in lung diseases such as emphysema, chronic bronchitis, and cystic fibrosis leads to higher accumulations of potentially toxic substances in the lungs.

SMOKING

Of all air pollutants, tobacco smoke is the one associated with the highest prevalence of disease. For more than 25 years the United States Surgeon General has identified tobacco smoking as the single most common cause of preventable mortality. It is currently responsible for one in every six deaths! Happily, during this time the percentage of adults who smoke has decreased somewhat (from 43 to 32%). Nevertheless, the number of smokers remains large, and evidence exists that the smoke inhaled by nonsmoking bystand-

TABLE 8–3. THE PRINCIPAL INDOOR AIR POLLUTANTS AND THEIR SOURCES*

Pollutant	Typical Sources	Principal Effects
SO_2, respirable particles	Tobacco smoke, wood and coal stoves, fireplaces, outside air	Irritant to respiratory epithelium
NO, NO_2	Gas ranges and pilot lights	Irritant to respiratory epithelium
CO	Gas ranges and pilot lights, outside air	Forms carboxyhemoglobin
Infectious or allergenic biologic materials	Dust mites and cockroaches, pollens, animal dander, bacteria, fungi, viruses	Allergic reactions, infections
Formaldehyde	Urea formaldehyde foam insulation, glues, fiberboard, plywood, particle board	Allergic reactions
Radon and radon daughters	Ground beneath buildings	Lung cancer
Volatile organic compounds: benzene, styrene	Outgassing from water, solvents, paints, cleaning compounds; combustion	Respiratory toxin, cancer
Semivolatile organics: chlorinated hydrocarbons and polycyclic compounds such as benzopyrene, PCBs	Pesticides, herbicides, combustion of wood, tobacco, and charcoal	See Table 8–7 (p. 230)
Asbestos	Building insulation	Pneumoconiosis, cancer

* Exclusive of unique industrial pollutants that result in pneumoconioses.

ers also has adverse health effects. The following discussion summarizes the detrimental effects of cigarette smoking, the reversal of these effects upon cessation of smoking, and the evidence that passive smoking is also injurious to health.

The number of potentially noxious chemicals in tobacco smoke is extraordinary. Table 8–4 provides only a partial list and includes the likely mechanism by which each of these agents produces injury. This injury translates into a number of important diseases (Fig. 8–1), all of which are discussed in detail in later chapters. However, we should point out here the mechanisms for the most important diseases caused by cigarette smoke.

Emphysema, chronic bronchitis, and lung cancer are common lung diseases and cigarette smoking is by far the most common cause of these disorders. Agents in smoke have a direct irritant effect on the tracheobronchial mucosa, producing inflammation and increased mucus production (bronchitis). Cigarette smoke also results in the recruitment of leukocytes to the lung and increased local elastase production, with subsequent

TABLE 8-4. EFFECTS OF SELECTED TOBACCO SMOKE CONSTITUENTS

Substance	Effect
"Tar"	Carcinogenesis
Polycyclic aromatic hydrocarbons	Carcinogenesis
Nicotine	Ganglionic stimulation and depression, tumor promotion
Phenol	Tumor promotion and irritation
Benzopyrene	Carcinogenesis
CO	Impaired oxygen transport and utilization
Formaldehyde	Toxicity to cilia and irritation
Oxides of nitrogen	Toxicity to cilia and irritation
Nitrosamine	Carcinogenesis

injury to lung tissue and *emphysema*. Components of cigarette smoke, particularly the tars, are potent mutagens and promoters, such that 85% of cancers in the lung arising from the bronchial epithelium *(bronchogenic carcinoma)* are related to cigarette smoking. The risk for development of these three diseases is related

to the dose of exposure (i.e., the more cigarettes smoked the greater the risk). This is frequently expressed in terms of "pack years" (e.g., one pack daily for 20 years equals 20 pack years).

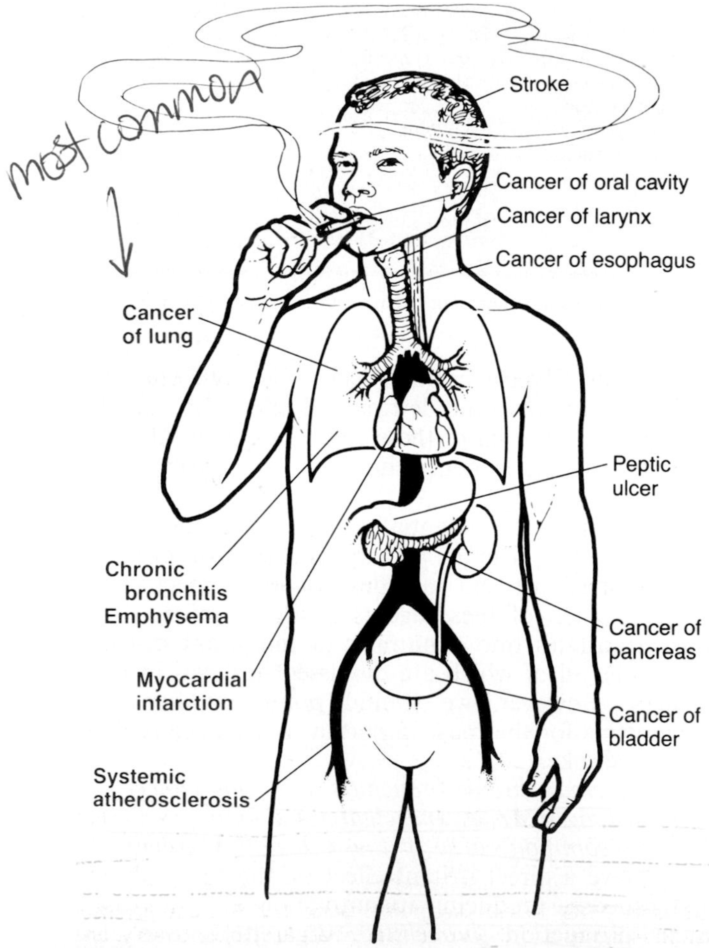

In addition to lung disease, *atherogenesis and myocardial infarction* have also been linked to cigarettes; causal mechanisms likely relate to several factors including increased platelet aggregation, a decreased myocardial oxygen supply (because of significant lung disease) accompanied by an increased oxygen demand, and a decreased threshold for ventricular fibrillation.

As might be expected, cessation of smoking leads to substantial benefits. The 1990 Surgeon General's report summarized the data on this issue. The overall risk of dying for individuals of all ages is increased if they smoke but is reduced somewhat within a year after quitting. The risk continues to decrease for at least 15 years, which is the extent of time for which data are currently available. Not shown in Figure 8-1 is the effect of smoking on the unborn fetus. Maternal smoking results in intrauterine growth retardation; birth weights of babies born to mothers who stopped smoking before pregnancy are normal.

In recent years evidence has accumulated that adults breathing sidestream smoke *(passive smoking)* also have an increased incidence of lung cancer. This is not surprising because it is estimated that in rooms where there is heavy cigarette smoking, passive smokers may inhale the equivalent of three cigarettes a day and the lung cancer risk for individuals who smoke one to nine cigarettes per day is greater than for nonsmoker controls. The precise increase in risk for cancer associated with passive smoking is difficult to quantitate. Most observers believe that passive smokers incur a risk that is significant but less than twice that of nonsmokers. Other effects of sidestream smoke on adults that have been less consistently demonstrated include irritant effects and decreased pulmonary function. In contrast, studies of children living in households with an adult who smokes show an increased incidence of respiratory illnesses and small but significant decreases in lung function. As might be expected, these effects are more closely linked to the mother's than the father's cigarette use.

Figure 8-1. Adverse effects of smoking. The more common are on the left and somewhat less common on the right.

PNEUMOCONIOSES _____

Pneumoconiosis is a term originally coined to describe the nonneoplastic lung reaction to inhalation of mineral dusts. The term has been broadened to include diseases induced by organic as well as inorganic particulates, and some experts also regard chemical fume- and vapor-induced nonneoplastic lung diseases as pneumoconioses.

The mineral dust pneumoconioses—the four most common result from exposure to coal dust, silica, asbestos, and beryllium—nearly always result from exposure in the workplace. However, the increased risk of cancer due to asbestos exposure extends to family members of asbestos workers and to other individuals exposed to asbestos outside the workplace. Table 8-5

TABLE 8–5. MINERAL DUST–INDUCED LUNG DISEASE

Agent	Disease	Exposure
Coal dust	Simple coal workers' pneumoconiosis: macules and nodules	Coal mining
	Complicated coal workers' pneumoconiosis: PMF, Caplan's syndrome	
Silica	Acute silicosis, chronic silicosis, PMF, Caplan's syndrome	Sandblasting, quarrying, mining, stone cutting, foundry work, ceramics
Asbestos	Asbestosis, Caplan's syndrome, pleural effusions, pleural plaques, or diffuse fibrosis, mesothelioma, carcinoma of the lung, larynx, stomach, colon	Mining, milling, and fabrication of ores and materials; installation and removal of insulation
Beryllium	Acute berylliosis, beryllium granulomatosis	Nuclear energy and aircraft industries

indicates the pathologic conditions associated with each mineral dust and the major industries in which the dust exposure is sufficient to produce disease. For all pneumoconioses, regulations limiting worker exposure have resulted in a decreased incidence of dust-associated diseases.

PATHOGENESIS. The reaction of the lung to mineral dusts depends on factors previously discussed, including size, shape, solubility, and reactivity of the particles. Coal dust is relatively inert and large amounts must be deposited in the lungs before lung disease is detectable clinically. Silica, asbestos, and beryllium are more reactive than coal dust, resulting in fibrotic reactions at lower concentrations. A unifying concept for the development of lesions in all pneumoconioses is depicted in Figure 8–2. The majority of inhaled dust is removed by entrapment in the mucous blanket and rapid removal from the lung by ciliary movement. However, some of the particles impact at alveolar duct bifurcations, where macrophages accumulate and endocytose the impacted particulates. The more reactive particulates trigger the macrophage to release a number of products that mediate an inflammatory response and initiate fibroblast proliferation and collagen deposition. Important macrophage mediators for tissue damage, cell recruitment, and fibroblast growth stimulation (p. 52) include: (1) oxygen radicals and proteases; (2) the leukotriene LTB4 and the cytokine interleukin 8 (IL-8), which are chemotactic for leukocytes; and (3) the cytokines IL-1, tumor necrosis factor alpha (TNF-$\propto$), fibronectin, platelet-derived growth factor (PDGF), and insulin-like growth factor-1 (IGF-1), which may play roles in fibrogenesis. Some of the particles may be taken up by epithelial cells or cross the epithelial cell lining and interact directly with fibroblasts and interstitial macrophages. Some may reach the lymphatics either by direct drainage or within migrating macrophages and thereby initiate an immune response to components of the particulates and/or to self proteins, modified by the particles. This then leads to an amplification and extension of the local reaction.

The concentration of the particulate and the length of exposure determine the course of the disease. A large bolus of particulate may cause an acute exudative reaction, whereas a smaller barrage over time, the more usual scenario, may lead to progressive fibrosis.

Tobacco smoking worsens the effects of all inhaled mineral dusts, asbestos in particular.

Coal Workers' Pneumoconiosis

A number of English novels, including D.H. Lawrence's *Sons and Lovers,* poignantly describe the

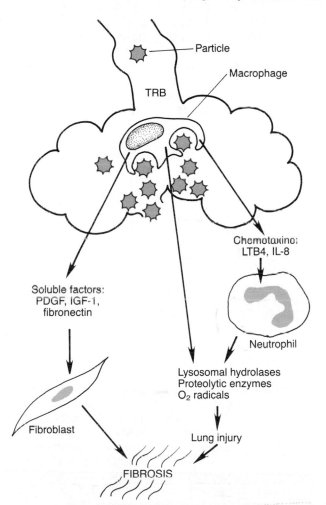

Figure 8–2. Pathogenesis of pneumoconiosis. Inhaled particulates usually impact at the bifurcations of terminal respiratory bronchioles (TRB) where they are engulfed by alveolar macrophages, which are then stimulated to secrete (1) various soluble growth factors for fibroblasts (PDGF; insulin-like growth factor 1, IGF-1; and fibronectin), (2) enzymes and O_2 radicals that initiate lung injury directly, and (3) chemotaxins that recruit additional inflammatory cells such as neutrophils.

tragedy of the coal miners at the turn of the century who toiled lifelong underground only to die of "black lung" complicated by tuberculosis. Dust reduction measures in the coal mines around the globe have drastically reduced the incidence of coal dust–induced disease. The spectrum of lung findings in coal workers is wide, from (1) asymptomatic anthracosis, in which pigment accumulates without a perceptible cellular reaction, to (2) simple coal workers' pneumoconiosis (CWP), in which cellular accumulations of macrophages occur with little to no pulmonary dysfunction, to (3) complicated CWP or progressive massive fibrosis (PMF), in which fibrosis is extensive and lung function is compromised (see Table 8–5). Although statistics vary, it appears that fewer than 10% of cases of simple CWP progress to PMF. It should be noted that *PMF is a generic term that applies to a confluent fibrosing reaction in the lung, which can be a complication of any one of the four pneumoconioses discussed here.*

The pathogenesis of both simple and complicated CWP is incompletely understood. In particular it is not clear what causes the lesions of simple CWP to progress to PMF. Contaminating silica in the coal dust and coexisting tuberculosis have been suggested to favor progressive disease. However, most of the evidence suggests that carbon dust itself is the major culprit. In studies in which the quantity of dust was measured in miners' lungs, complicated lesions contained considerably more dust than did simple lesions.

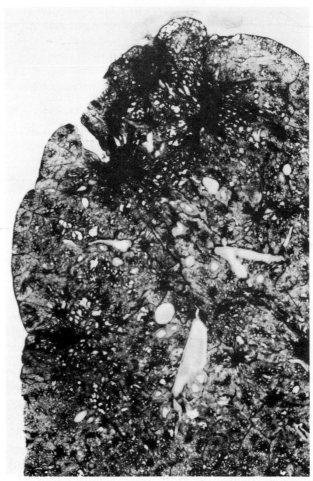

Figure 8–3. Progressive massive fibrosis superimposed on coal workers' pneumoconiosis. The large blackened scars are principally located in the upper lobe. Note extensions of scars into surrounding parenchyma and retraction of adjacent pleura. (Courtesy of Dr. Werner Laquer, Dr. Jerome Kleinerman, and the National Institute of Occupational Safety and Health.)

MORPHOLOGY. Pulmonary anthracosis is the most innocuous coal-induced pulmonary lesion in coal miners and is also commonly seen in all urban dwellers and tobacco smokers. Inhaled carbon pigment is engulfed by alveolar or interstitial macrophages, which then accumulate in the connective tissue along the lymphatics, including the pleural lymphatics, or in organized lymphoid tissue along the bronchi or in the lung hilus. At autopsy linear streaks and aggregates of anthracotic pigment readily identify pulmonary lymphatics and mark the pulmonary lymph nodes.

Simple CWP is characterized by **coal macules** and the somewhat larger **coal nodule.** The coal macule consists of dust-laden macrophages; the nodule also contains small amounts of a delicate network of collagen fibers. Although these lesions are scattered throughout the lung, the upper lobes and upper zones of the lower lobes are more heavily involved. They are primarily located adjacent to respiratory bronchioles, the site of initial coal dust accumulation. In due course dilatation of adjacent alveoli occurs, a condition sometimes referred to as centrilobular emphysema. However, by definition emphysema is associated with destruction of alveolar septa, and whether this occurs in primary CWP has not been clearly demonstrated.

Complicated CWP (PMF) occurs on a background of simple CWP and generally requires many years to develop. It is characterized by intensely blackened scars larger than 2 cm, sometimes up to 10 cm in greatest diameter. They are usually multiple (Fig. 8–3). Micro-scopically the lesions consist of dense collagen and pigment. The center of the lesion is often necrotic, resulting most likely from ischemia.

Caplan's syndrome is defined as the coexistence of rheumatoid arthritis with a pneumoconiosis, leading to the development of distinctive nodular pulmonary lesions that develop fairly rapidly. Like rheumatoid nodules (p. 146), the nodular lesions in Caplan's syndrome exhibit central necrosis surrounded by fibroblasts, macrophages, and collagen. This syndrome also occurs in asbestosis and silicosis.

CLINICAL COURSE. CWP is usually a benign disease with little decrement in lung function. Even mild forms of complicated CWP fail to demonstrate abnormalities of lung function. However, in a minority of cases PMF develops, leading to increasing pulmonary dysfunction, pulmonary hypertension, and cor pulmonale. Once PMF develops it may become progressive even if further exposure to dust is prevented. The incidence of clinical tuberculosis is increased in persons with CWP, but whether this reflects a greater vulnerability to infection or, instead, socioeconomic factors inherent in the life of miners is unclear. There is also some evidence that exposure to coal dust increases the incidence of chronic bronchitis and emphysema, independent of smoking, thus complicating the management of the patient with CWP. However, to date, there is no compelling evidence that CWP in the absence of smoking predisposes to cancer.

Silicosis

Silicosis is a lung disease caused by inhalation of crystalline silicon dioxide (silica). Currently the most prevalent chronic occupational disease in the world, it usually presents, after decades of exposure, as a slowly progressing, nodular, fibrosing pneumoconiosis. As shown in Table 8–5, workers in a large number of occupations are at risk, especially sandblasters and many mine workers. Less commonly, very heavy exposure over months to a few years can result in acute silicosis, a lesion characterized by the generalized accumulation of a lipoproteinaceous material within alveoli. In addition to silicosis, heavy exposure to silica-containing dusts causes chronic inflammation in the upper airways resulting in chronic cough and sputum production (chronic bronchitis).

Silica occurs in both crystalline and amorphous forms, but crystalline forms (including quartz, crystobalite, and tridymite) are biologically the most active. Of these, quartz is most commonly implicated in silicosis. In the earth, much of the silicon combines with oxygen and other elements to form silicates. Although amorphous silicates are biologically less active than crystalline silica, heavy lung burdens of these minerals may also produce lesions. Talc, vermiculite, and mica are examples of non-crystalline silicates that are less common causes of pneumoconioses.

Following inhalation, particles of quartz smaller than 5 μm may reach the terminal airways, and those around 1 μm are particularly apt to be retained and cause fibrosis. Animals exposed to silica demonstrate a steady increase in macrophages and lymphocytes in the alveolus and interstitium. There is substantial evidence that the recruited macrophages play a pivotal role by secreting factors that lead to fibroblast proliferation and collagen production. As with CWP, the initial lesions tend to localize in the upper lung zones although the reasons for this distribution are obscure. In contrast with CWP, however, early lesions of silicosis are more fibrotic and less cellular. It seems likely that factors secreted by macrophages ingesting coal dust have less potent fibroblast-stimulating capability than those secreted by macrophages that ingest silica. An interesting, perhaps related, phenomenon is that quartz, when mixed with other minerals, has a reduced fibrogenic effect. This is of practical importance because quartz in the workplace is rarely pure. Thus miners of the iron-containing ore hematite may have more quartz in their lungs than some quartz-exposed

workers and yet have relatively mild lung disease because the hematite provides a protective effect.

MORPHOLOGY. Silicosis is characterized grossly in its early stages by tiny, barely palpable, discrete pale to blackened (if coal dust is also present) nodules in the upper zones of the lungs. As the disease progresses these nodules may coalesce into hard collagenous scars (Fig. 8–4). Some nodules may undergo central softening and cavitation. This may be due to superimposed tuberculosis or to ischemia. The intervening lung parenchyma may be compressed or overexpanded and a honeycomb pattern may develop. Fibrotic lesions may also occur in the hilar lymph nodes and pleura. Sometimes thin sheets of calcification occur in the lymph nodes and are appreciated radiographically as "eggshell" calcification (e.g., calcium surrounding a zone lacking calcification). If the disease continues to progress, expansion and coalescence of lesions produces PMF. Histologically the nodular lesions consist of concentric layers of hyalinized collagen surrounded by a dense capsule of more condensed collagen (Fig. 8–5). Examination of the nodules by polarized microscopy reveals birefringent silica particles.

CLINICAL COURSE. The disease is usually detected when routine chest radiography is performed on an asymptomatic worker. The radiographs typically show a fine nodularity in the upper zones of the lung, but pulmonary functions are either normal or only moderately affected. Most patients do not develop shortness of breath until late in the course, after PMF is present. At this time, the disease may be progressive, even if the patient is no longer exposed. The disease is slow to kill, but impaired pulmonary function may severely limit activity.

There are several similarities between silicosis and CWP. First, an important complication in silicosis, as in CWP, is increased susceptibility to tuberculosis. Second, patients with either condition may develop PMF and Caplan's syndrome. Third, despite some suggestions, there is no clear evidence that either silicosis or CWP predisposes to the development of bronchogenic carcinoma.

Asbestosis and Asbestos-Related Diseases

Asbestos is a family of crystalline hydrated silicates with a fibrous geometry. Based on epidemiologic studies, occupational exposure to asbestos is linked to: (1) parenchymal interstitial fibrosis (asbestosis), (2) bronchogenic carcinoma, (3) pleural effusions, (4) localized fibrous plaques, or, rarely, diffuse pleural fibrosis, (5) mesotheliomas, and (6) laryngeal and perhaps other extrapulmonary neoplasms including colon carcinomas. An increased incidence of asbestos-related cancer in family members of asbestos workers has alerted the general public to the potential hazards of asbestos in the environment. For instance, asbestos is widely

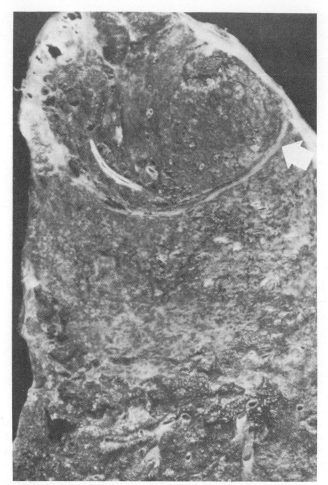

Figure 8-4. Advanced silicosis seen on transection of lung. Scarring is almost confluent, occupying most of upper lobe and contiguous region of lower lobe. Arrow indicates interlobar fissure. Several tuberculous cavities are present in apex. Note dense pleural thickening. (Courtesy of Dr. John Godleski, Brigham and Women's Hospital.)

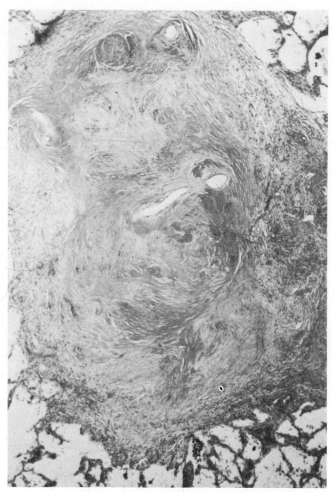

Figure 8-5. Several coalescent collagenous silicotic nodules. (Courtesy of Dr. John Godleski, Brigham and Women's Hospital.)

present in insulation and is detectable in water and air. The actual risk for the various asbestos-related diseases in the general population is unknown, and estimates to date have come from mathematical models. Nevertheless, the US government has mandated its Environmental Protection Agency (EPA) to inspect schools and to monitor and manage potential asbestos hazards.

PATHOGENESIS. Concentration, size, shape, and solubility of the different forms of asbestos dictate whether disease will occur. There are two distinct forms of asbestos: *serpentine* (the fiber is curly and flexible) and *amphibole* (the fiber is straight, stiff, and brittle). The serpentine chrysotile accounts for most of the asbestos used in industry. Amphiboles include crocidolite, amosite, tremolite, anthophyllite, and actinolyte. This confusing array of terms is important because amphiboles, even though less prevalent, are more pathogenic than chrysotiles, particularly with respect to induction of malignant pleural tumors (mesotheliomas). Indeed, some studies of mesotheliomas have shown the link is almost invariably to amphibole exposure. The relatively few cases of mesotheliomas arising in chrysotile workers are in all

likelihood due to contamination of chrysotile with the amphibole, tremolite. The greater pathogenicity of straight and stiff amphiboles is apparently related to their aerodynamic properties and solubility. Chrysotiles, with their more flexible, curled structure, are likely to become impacted in the upper respiratory passages and be removed by the mucociliary elevator. Furthermore, once trapped in the lungs chrysotiles are gradually leached from the tissues because they are more soluble than amphiboles. In contrast, the straight, stiff amphiboles may align themselves in the airstream and be delivered deeper into the lungs, where they can penetrate epithelial cells and reach the interstitium. The length of amphibole fibers also plays a role in pathogenicity, those longer than 8 mm and thinner than 0.5 mm being more injurious than shorter, thicker ones. Nevertheless, both asbestos forms are fibrogenic, and increasing doses are associated with a higher incidence of all asbestos-related diseases except mesothelioma. In contrast to other inorganic dusts that induce cellular and fibrotic lung reactions, experimental studies have indicated that asbestos can also act as both a tumor initiator and a promoter. However, potentially toxic chemicals adsorbed onto the asbestos fibers undoubtedly contribute to the pathogenicity of the fibers. *For example, the adsorption of carcinogens in tobacco smoke onto asbestos fibers may well be important* to the remarkable synergy between tobacco smoking and the development of bronchogenic carcinoma in asbestos workers.

Asbestosis, like the other pneumoconioses, depends on the interaction of inhaled fibers with lung macrophages and, perhaps more than for the other dusts, with other parenchymal cells. Release of mediators eventually leads to generalized interstitial pulmonary inflammation and interstitial fibrosis. It is not completely understood why silicosis is a nodular fibrosing disease and asbestosis a diffuse interstitial process. The more diffuse distribution may be related to the ability of asbestos to reach alveoli more consistently or its ability to penetrate epithelial cells, or to both.

> **MORPHOLOGY. Asbestosis** is marked by diffuse pulmonary interstitial fibrosis. These changes are indistinguishable from those resulting from other causes of diffuse interstitial fibrosis (p. 401), except for the presence of asbestos bodies, which are seen as **golden brown, fusiform or beaded rods with a translucent center. They consist of asbestos fibers coated with an iron-containing proteinaceous material** (Fig. 8–6). Asbestos bodies apparently arise when macrophages attempt to phagocytose asbestos fibers; the iron is presumably derived from phagocyte ferritin. Other inorganic particulates may become coated with similar iron-

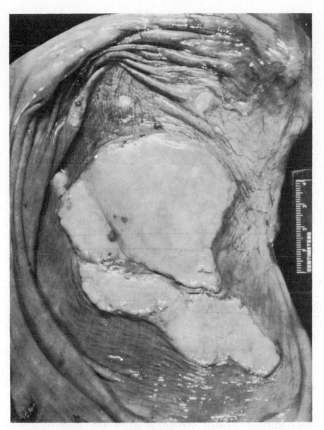

Figure 8–7. Asbestosis. Severe, discrete, characteristic fibrocalcific plaques on pleural surface of diaphragm. (Courtesy of Dr. John Godleski, Brigham and Women's Hospital.)

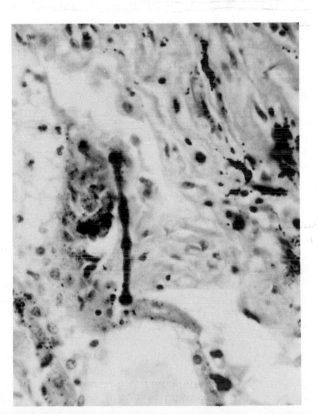

Figure 8–6. A high-power detail of an asbestos body, revealing the typical beading and knobbed ends.

protein complexes, and the term "ferruginous bodies" is better used where there is no evidence for an asbestos core. It should be noted that asbestos bodies can sometimes be found in lungs of normal persons, but usually in much lower concentrations and without an accompanying interstitial fibrosis.

Asbestosis begins as fibrosis around respiratory bronchioles and alveolar ducts and extends to involve adjacent alveolar sacs and alveoli. Contraction of the fibrous tissue distorts the native architecture, creating enlarged air spaces enclosed within thick fibrous walls. In this way the affected regions become honeycombed. In contrast to CWP and silicosis, asbestosis begins in the lower lobes and subpleurally, but the middle and upper lobes of the lungs become affected as fibrosis progresses. Simultaneously, the visceral pleura undergoes fibrous thickening and sometimes binds the lungs to the chest wall. Large parenchymal nodules typical of Caplan's syndrome may appear in a few patients who have concurrent rheumatoid arthritis. The scarring may trap and narrow pulmonary arteries and arterioles, causing pulmonary hypertension and cor pulmonale (p. 315).

Pleural plaques are the most common manifestation of asbestos exposure and are well-circumscribed plaques of dense collagen (Fig. 8–7), often containing calcium. They develop most frequently on the anterior and posterolateral aspects of the **parietal** pleura and over the domes of the diaphragm. They do not contain asbestos bodies and only rarely do they occur in persons who have no history or evidence of asbestos exposure. Uncommonly, asbestos exposure induces pleural effusions, which are usually serous but may be bloody. Rarely, diffuse visceral pleural fibrosis may occur and, in advanced cases, bind the lung to the thoracic cavity wall.

Both bronchogenic carcinomas and mesotheliomas develop in workers exposed to asbestos. The risk for bronchogenic carcinoma is increased about fivefold for asbestos workers; the relative risk for mesotheliomas, normally a very rare tumor (2 to 17 cases per 1,000,000 persons), is more than a thousandfold greater. Concomitant cigarette smoking greatly increases the risk of bronchogenic carcinoma, but not that of mesothelioma. These asbestos-related tumors are morphologically indistinguishable from cancers of other causes and are described on pages 428 and 432.

CLINICAL COURSE. The clinical findings in asbestosis are indistinguishable from those of any other diffuse interstitial lung disease (p. 402). Dyspnea is usually the first manifestation: at first it is provoked by exertion, later it is present even at rest. These manifestations rarely appear before 10 years after the first exposure, and more commonly after 20 years or more. The dyspnea is usually accompanied by a cough associated with production of sputum. The disease may remain static or progress to congestive heart failure, cor pulmonale (p. 315), and death. The development of Caplan's syndrome may accelerate the clinical course. Chest films reveal irregular linear densities, particularly in both lower lobes. With advancement of the pneumoconiosis, a honeycomb pattern develops. Pleural plaques are usually asymptomatic and are detected on radiographs as circumscribed densities. Asbestosis complicated by lung or pleural cancer is associated with a particularly grim prognosis.

Berylliosis

Heavy exposure to airborne dusts or to fumes of metallic beryllium or its oxides, alloys, or salts may induce acute pneumonitis; more protracted low-dose exposure may cause pulmonary and systemic granulomatous lesions that closely mimic sarcoidosis (p. 403). Recognition of the hazards of beryllium exposure in the workplace and enactment in the late 1940s of standards for limiting worker exposure resulted in the disappearance of acute berylliosis and marked reduction in reports of new cases of the chronic disease. Currently, workers in the nuclear and aerospace industries working with beryllium alloys are at highest risk for exposure, but new cases of chronic berylliosis are reported only occasionally.

Chronic berylliosis is caused by induction of cell-mediated immunity. Because only 2% of exposed workers develop disease, it appears that genetic suscep-

tibility is necessary for the initiation of an immune response. The development of delayed hypersensitivity leads to the formation of noncaseating granulomas in the lungs and hilar nodes—or less commonly in spleen, liver, kidneys, adrenals, and distant lymph nodes. The pulmonary granulomas become progressively fibrotic, giving rise to irregular, fine nodular densities detected on chest radiographs. Hilar adenopathy is present in about half the cases.

Chronic berylliosis may not result in clinical manifestations until many years after exposure, when the patient presents with dyspnea, cough, weight loss, and arthralgias. Some cases stabilize, others remit and relapse, still others progress to pulmonary failure. Epidemiologic evidence links heavy beryllium exposure to an increased incidence of cancer.

INJURY BY CHEMICAL AGENTS

There is a nearly endless list of chemical and biologic agents that can be injurious when inhaled, ingested, injected, or absorbed through the skin. Some may produce injury in the course of therapy for another disease _(therapeutic agents);_ others _(nontherapeutic agents)_ are introduced accidentally or intentionally into the body. Some of the latter agents (e.g., _alcohol and other drugs of abuse_) are used principally because of their psychotropic or mind-altering effects.

A perspective on the magnitude of the problem of chemical injury is gained by examining poison control center data, which have been collected and compiled annually since 1983. In 1989, about 2.1 million poison exposures resulted in calls to poison control centers. Of these exposures, 91% were in the home, 73% involved oral intake, and 61% of victims were children younger than six years. As might be expected, the most frequent offending agents were substances commonly available in the home; nearly 50% of reported episodes involved cleaning agents, analgesics, cosmetics, plants, or cold preparations. In 88% of cases the episode resulted in either minor or no toxic effects. Nevertheless, the problem is still enormous considering that 25% of the total number of callers were seen in health care facilities; 12% of the individuals suffered significant toxicity, and at least 590 died.

The spectrum of agents and victims involved in _serious_ poisonings differs from those of poison exposure in general. Again referring to 1989 data, the majority of poisoning deaths involved intentional rather than accidental exposure: 55% were suicides and 11% resulted from drug abuse. Analgesics were the culprits in 20% of deaths, but mood-altering drugs, all of which can be categorized as drugs of abuse (including illegal drugs), were by far the most important lethal agents (50% of cases).

There are a number of important principles in understanding the mechanisms of chemical injury.
● _Dose._ In general, the higher the dose, the greater the toxicity, although small doses may cause serious sequelae, particularly over a protracted period. An example is impairment of mental development in

children chronically exposed to low levels of lead. Widely debated is the risk of exposure to low levels of pesticides or food additives as causes of cancer.

- *Requirement for metabolic conversion.* An alkali (certain cleaning materials) may be *directly* toxic to cells and when swallowed injure the mucosa of the oral cavity, esophagus, and stomach. In contrast, many drugs, including alcohol, are converted in the liver to compounds that are more toxic than the parent compound. *Thus there may be little or no injury at the site of entry and the liver may bear the brunt of injury.*

- *Mode of action.* Many chemicals act directly on receptors or on physiologic receptor ligands and thus ordinarily affect only those cells that express the relevant receptor. For example, phenothiazines (used in treatment of major psychotic illnesses) act primarily on the extrapyramidal system; hence overdose leads to acute dystonic states, such as a Parkinson-like syndrome. This type of drug reaction is referred to as an expected (or predictable) drug reaction, in contrast with an unexpected or idiosyncratic reaction.

- *Sites of absorption, accumulation, or excretion.* For chemicals that are direct cell toxins, obviously the site of entry is important in determining the type of injury. The site of accumulation is also important. The aminoglycoside antibiotics, for instance, are particularly prone to accumulate in the endolymph and perilymph of the ear and in the renal cortex, thus explaining the propensity of these drugs (e.g., tetracycline) to cause ototoxicity and nephrotoxicity.

- *Individual variation.* The rates of absorption, metabolism, and excretion all determine the level of a chemical in plasma—and therefore in tissues. The liver is the major site at which many therapeutic agents are metabolized, and the kidney is the major organ of excretion; thus liver or kidney disease can affect plasma levels of toxicants. Another important determinant of the rate of drug metabolism is genetic polymorphisms in the enzymes that metabolize the drugs. For example, some drugs, including hydralazine (used in the treatment of hypertension), are acetylated in the liver in preparation for excretion. The rate of acetylation (rapid or slow) is genetically determined. Individuals who are slow acetylators are more likely to develop drug-induced lupus (an immune-mediated syndrome) than are rapid acetylators, possibly because prolonged elevation of the plasma level of native drug enhances its capacity to initiate an immune response. This type of drug reaction is an unexpected or idiosyncratic one.

- *Environmental agents or other drugs.* Environmental agents and other drugs may affect reactions to therapeutic agents. One of the most important metabolic pathways for drugs is the cytochrome P-450 enzyme (mono-oxidase) system in the liver. In children suffering protein-calorie malnutrition this system may be less active, and drugs inactivated by this system may accumulate and become more toxic. Commonly prescribed drugs, including cimetidine, used in the treatment of peptic ulcers, and the antibiotic erythromycin, block the P-450 enzyme system and can contribute to the toxicity of theophylline, a drug widely used in the treatment of asthma, that is detoxified by this enzyme system.

- *The capacity of the chemical to induce an immune response.* Many chemicals inflict injury by inducing an immune response. For example, penicillin may induce an immunoglobulin E (IgE)–mediated anaphylactic response or an IgG-mediated hemolytic anemia. The factors that determine whether a substance initiates an immune response relate to both the chemical and the host. Those related to the chemical include whether the molecule is a protein large enough to act as an immunogen or, if very small, whether it can bind to a self protein and act as a hapten. Host factors (i.e., immune response genes) are equally important.

INJURY BY THERAPEUTIC AGENTS _____

Adverse drug reactions refer to untoward effects of drugs that are given in conventional therapeutic settings. These reactions are extremely common in the practice of medicine. Several examples were given in the discussion of general principles above; Table 8–6 lists common pathologic findings in adverse drug reactions and the drugs most frequently involved. Because they are widely used, estrogens and oral contraceptives (OC) will be discussed in more detail. In addition, because acetaminophen and aspirin, so commonly used as over-the-counter drugs, are important causes of accidental or intentional overdose, they also merit additional comment. Sedatives and hypnotic and anxiolytic agents are also important causes of drug injury, but injury associated with their use is usually in the context of abuse.

Exogenous Estrogens and Oral Contraceptives _____

Estrogens and OCs are discussed separately because (1) estrogens for postmenopausal syndrome may be given alone and are usually natural estrogens, and (2) OCs contain synthetic estrogens, always with progesterone.

EXOGENOUS ESTROGENS. *Estrogen therapy,* once used primarily for the distressing symptoms of menopause, is now also used widely in postmenopausal women, with or without added progesterones, to prevent or slow the progression of osteoporosis (p. 682). Given the fact that endogenous hyperestrinism increases the risk of developing endometrial carcinoma and, likely, breast carcinoma, there is understandable concern about the use of exogenous estrogens as therapeutic agents. Current data support the following adverse effects of estrogen therapy:

- *Endometrial carcinoma.* Unopposed estrogen therapy (without accompanying progestin) increases the risk of endometrial carcinoma two to three times. The risk is reduced when progestins are added to the therapeutic regime; indeed, some studies indicate that combination therapy is protective.

TABLE 8–6. SOME COMMON ADVERSE DRUG REACTIONS AND THEIR AGENTS

Reaction	Major Offenders
Blood Dyscrasias (feature of almost half of all drug-related deaths)	
Granulocytopenia, aplastic anemia, pancytopenia	Antineoplastic agents, immunosuppressives, and chloramphenicol
Hemolytic anemia, thrombocytopenia	Penicillin, methyldopa, quinidine
Cutaneous	
Urticaria, macules, papules, vesicles, petechiae, exfoliative dermatitis, fixed drug eruptions	Antineoplastic agents, sulfonamides, hydantoins, many others
Cardiac	
Arrhythmias	Theophylline, hydantoins
Cardiomyopathy	Doxorubicin, daunorubicin
Renal	
Glomerulonephritis	Penicillamine
Acute tubular necrosis	Aminoglycoside antibiotics, cyclosporin, Amphotericin B
Tubulointerstitial disease with papillary necrosis	Phenacetin, salicylates
Pulmonary	
Asthma	Salicylates
Acute pneumonitis	Nitrofurantoin
Interstitial fibrosis	Busulfan, nitrofurantoin, bleomycin
Hepatic (p. 542)	
Fatty change	Tetracycline
Diffuse hepatocellular damage	Halothane, isoniazid, acetominophen
Cholestasis	Chlorpromazine, estrogens, contraceptive agents
Systemic	
Anaphylaxis	Penicillin
Lupus erythematosus syndrome (drug-induced lupus)	Hydralazine, procainamide
Central Nervous System	
Tinnitus and dizziness	Salicylates
Acute dystonic reactions and parkinsonian syndrome	Phenothiazine antipsychotics
Respiratory depression	Sedatives

● *Breast carcinoma.* Although it seems likely that postmenopausal estrogen therapy increases the risk of breast carcinoma, epidemiologic studies have yielded conflicting data, perhaps because physicians tend not to use estrogen supplementation in women with a strong family history of breast carcinoma and so have biased the data. A 1989 study of more than 23,000 Swedish women demonstrated a twofold increase in breast cancer in those who took the synthetic estrogen estradiol. (Whether the data would be the same with natural estrogen, the predominant form used in the United States, is uncertain.) Other recent studies have also demonstrated a significant, albeit smaller, risk. The effect of adding progestin to estrogen on the risk of breast cancer is also controversial; some studies suggest estrogen-progestin regimens protect against breast cancer, others indicate they increase the risk.

● *Thromboembolism.* Although estrogen replacement might be expected to increase the risk of this complication because synthetic estrogens stimulate the production of coagulation factors by the liver, statistics have not borne this out, perhaps because natural estrogens are used more frequently than synthetic estrogens and the former appear to be less thrombogenic.

● *Cardiovascular disease.* Myocardial infarction and stroke are among the leading causes of death in postmenopausal women, and hence there is considerable interest in the effects of estrogens on the incidence of cardiovascular disease. Estrogens absorbed through the gastrointestinal tract pass through the liver, where they tend to elevate the level of high-density lipoprotein (HDL) and reduce that of low-density lipoprotein (LDL). This lipid profile is protective against the development of atherosclerosis. Progestins on the other hand tend to lower HDL and elevate LDL, which counters the estrogen effect. Recent epidemiologic studies of the role of estrogens have shown a 40 to 50% decrease in the risk of ischemic heart disease in women who receive postmenopausal estrogen therapy as compared with those who did not receive estrogens. The general consensus seems to be that unopposed estrogens are likely to be beneficial; the effect of added progestins is still an open question. The risk of strokes seems unaltered by estrogen therapy.

ORAL CONTRACEPTIVES. Although OCs have been in use for about 30 years and despite innumerable analyses of their effects, experts continue to disagree about their safety and adverse effects. These drugs nearly always contain a *synthetic estradiol* and variable amounts of a progestin, but a few formulations contain only progestin. Currently prescribed oral contraceptives contain smaller amounts of estrogens (less than 50 μg per day) and are clearly associated with fewer side effects than were earlier formulations. This shift began after 1975, and results of epidemiologic studies have to be interpreted in the context of the dosage. Nevertheless, there is reasonable evidence to support the following conclusions about the effects of these drugs.

● *Breast carcinoma.* The issue of breast cancer risk is unresolved. Some studies indicate about a twofold increased risk, particularly with more than ten years of OC use and particularly when it is begun early in life and before the first pregnancy. Other studies, including one emanating from the Centers for Disease Control, reveal no increased risk. Possibly contributing to this conflict are variations in the estrogen content of the pill (both absolute and relative to the progestin content), duration of OC use, age at first use, and interval between first use and time of the study.

● *Endometrial cancer.* No increased risk and very likely a protective effect.

● *Cervical cancer.* Some increased risk, correlated with duration of use. More recent studies suggest the increased risk may be more strongly correlated with life style than with the drug (p. 613).

● *Ovarian cancer.* OCs protect against ovarian cancer;

the longer they are used, the greater the protection, which persists for some time after OC use stops.

- *Thromboembolism.* There is clearly an increased risk for venous thromboembolism with OC use. This effect relates to the role of synthetic estrogens (discussed above) in stimulating the liver to produce coagulation factors.
- *Hypertension.* Even the newer formulations of OC cause blood pressure elevations.
- *Cardiovascular disease.* As discussed, estrogens and progestins have opposing effects on HDL and LDL levels. The overall effect on the levels of these lipoproteins seems to depend on the preparations used, particularly the dose of progestin in the formulation. In the past there was considerable uncertainty regarding the risk of atherosclerosis and myocardial infarction in users of OCs. It is now apparent that several variables, such as the estrogen content of the formulation, age of the women, and the presence or absence of other risk factors for atherosclerosis, especially smoking, can influence the outcome of epidemiologic studies. Recent evidence seems to absolve OCs: it appears that nonsmoking, healthy women under the age of 45 years who use the newer formulations (low in estrogens) do not incur an increased risk of ischemic heart disease.
- *Gallbladder disease.* There was a slight increase with older formulations, none with the newer ones.

Obviously, the pros and cons of OC use must be viewed in the context of their wide applicability and acceptance as a form of contraception that protects against unwanted pregnancies with all their attendant hazards.

Acetaminophen

When taken in very large doses, this widely used (over-the-counter) analgesic and antipyretic causes hepatic necrosis. The window between the usual therapeutic dose (0.5 gm) and the toxic dose (15 to 25 gm) is large, however, and the drug is ordinarily very safe. Ingestion of massive toxic doses is accidental in children but generally is suicidal in adults or teenagers. Toxicity begins with nausea, vomiting, diarrhea, and sometimes shock, followed in a few days by evidence of jaundice; with serious overdosage, liver failure ensues, with centrilobular necrosis that may extend to the entire lobule. In some cases there is evidence of concurrent renal and myocardial damage.

Acetaminophen toxicity is attributable to the formation of a toxic metabolite by the hepatic mono-oxidase system. The metabolite is normally detoxified by binding to glutathione, but with massive overdoses glutathione is depleted and the reactive metabolite binds to critical hepatocyte macromolecules and results in the organ injury.

Aspirin (Acetylsalicylic Acid)

In the past aspirin overdose was frequently associated with accidental ingestion by young children. Education of parents and safer packaging has fortu-

nately reduced the incidence of such episodes. The major untoward consequences of massive aspirin overdose are metabolic; morphologic changes are sparse. Fluid and electrolyte imbalances are produced. At first respiratory alkalosis develops, followed by metabolic acidosis that often proves fatal before anatomic changes can appear. Ingestion of as little as 2 to 4 gm by children or 10 to 30 gm by adults may be fatal, but survival has been reported following doses five times larger. Overdose is often suicidal.

Chronic aspirin toxicity (salicylism) may develop in persons who take 3 gm or more daily, a dose required to treat chronic inflammatory conditions. Chronic salicylism is manifested by headache, dizziness, ringing in the ears (tinnitus), difficulty in hearing, mental confusion, drowsiness, nausea, vomiting, and diarrhea. The central nervous system changes may progress to convulsions and coma. The morphologic consequences of chronic salicylism are varied. Most often there is an acute erosive gastritis (p. 484), which may produce overt or covert gastrointestinal bleeding and may lead to gastric ulceration. Concurrently, in chronic toxicity a bleeding tendency may appear, because aspirin acetylates platelet cyclooxygenase and blocks the ability to make thromboxane A_2, an activator of platelet aggregation. Petechial hemorrhages may appear in the skin and internal viscera, and bleeding from gastric ulcerations may be exaggerated.

Proprietary analgesic mixtures of aspirin and phenacetin or its active metabolite acetaminophen, when taken over a span of years, have caused renal papillary necrosis, referred to as analgesic nephropathy (p. 456).

INJURY BY NONTHERAPEUTIC TOXIC AGENTS

Table 8–7 lists some of the more common agents involved in acute poisoning with a listing of their major pathologic effects. The purpose of this listing is to emphasize both the diversity of agents that may cause injury and the variety of responses that toxins can produce. A more detailed discussion of two common environmental pollutants, lead and CO, follows. Lung inhalation is the route of entry for CO and an important route for lead, but both manifest injury in extrapulmonary organs.

Lead

Acute lead poisoning may occur under unusual circumstances, e.g., battery burning. More commonly, lead compounds are accumulated slowly until they reach toxic levels. Adults usually present with colicky abdominal pain, fatigue, and perhaps headache, but in infants and children lead poisoning may remain unsuspected until it erupts in a catastrophic encephalopathic crisis. Poisoning by lead has proved to be one of the most difficult environmental health problems to control, and part of this difficulty is due to the lack of distinctive early manifestations.

There are innumerable sources of lead in our envi-

TABLE 8–7. SOME COMMON NONTHERAPEUTIC TOXIC AGENTS AND THE MAJOR ASSOCIATED PATHOLOGIC EFFECTS

Agent	Pathologic Effects
Carbon monoxide	Binds with hemoglobin with high affinity, causing systemic hypoxia
Cleaning compounds	
Bleach (sodium hypochlorite)	Local irritant, unlikely to scar
Caustic (acid or basic) agents	Local erosions with scarring
Chloroform, carbon tetrachloride	CNS depression, liver necrosis
Cyanide	Blocking of cytochrome oxidase activity, resulting in rapid death owing to pulmonary arrest
Ethylene glycol (antifreeze)	CNS depression, metabolic acidosis, acute tubular necrosis
Insecticides	
Chlorinated hydrocarbon (e.g., DDT)	CNS stimulant, accumulates in fat stores for long periods, ? carcinogenic
Organophosphates	Acetylcholinesterase inhibition: muscle weakness, cardiac arrhythmias, respiratory depression
Isopropanol (rubbing alcohol)	Similar to those of ethanol: gastritis, CNS depression
Mercurials	
High-dose mercury vapors	Pneumonitis
Low-dose exposure	Intention tremors, memory loss, gingivitis, skin rashes, nephrotic syndrome
Methanol (Sterno, antifreeze)	CNS depression, acidosis, blindness
Mushrooms	
Amanita muscaria	Parasympathomimetic symptoms, including bradycardia, hypotension
Amanita phalloides	Gastrointestinal symptoms with shock, convulsions, coma
Petroleum distillates (kerosene, benzene, gasoline)	Respiratory depression, gastrointestinal inflammation, severe pneumonitis
PCBs	Insidious development of chloracne, visual loss, impotence

ronment (Fig. 8–8). Indeed it is hard to avoid exposure to lead. Environmental lead is absorbed either through the gastrointestinal tract or through the lungs. In the United States, the acceptable upper limit of lead in blood has been established by the Centers for Disease Control as 25 μg/dl although there is accumulating evidence that this level may be too high. The average range found in contemporary urban dwellers is 10 to 15 μg/dl. Mass screening in the United States in the late 1970s disclosed that 1.9% of the population aged 6 months to 74 years had blood lead levels that exceeded the acceptable limit. What are the principal environmental sources of lead is a controversial question, but most agree that urban air, dirt, and food are the major conduits. Some years ago, automotive en-

gines and industries polluted the air with about 450,000 tons of lead per year. Control measures, particularly the use of unleaded gasoline, have significantly reduced the lead content of urban air and the level of lead in the blood. Volatilized lead is particularly hazardous, because most is absorbed in the lungs. By contrast, only a fraction of ingested lead is absorbed. Urban adults have a daily intake of 100 to 150 μg of lead in water and food, only about 10% of which is absorbed. Although children have, on average, a lower intake, they unfortunately absorb about 50%. Flaking lead paint in older houses and soil contamination pose major hazards to youngsters and ingestion of up to 200 μg per day is possible.

Most of the absorbed lead (80 to 85%) is taken up by bone; the blood accumulates about 5 to 10%; and the remainder is distributed throughout the soft tissues. In children, excess lead interferes with the normal remodeling of calcified cartilage and primary bone trabeculae in the epiphyses, leading to increased bone density that is detected as radiodense "lead lines" on radiographs (Fig. 8–9). Lead lines of a different sort may also occur in the gums, where excess lead stimu-

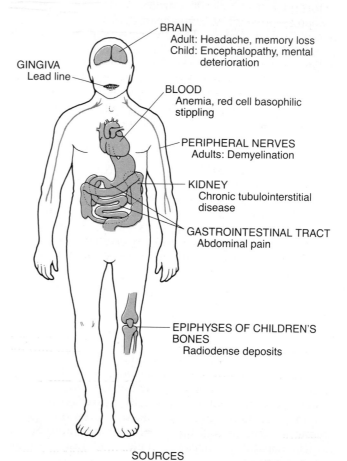

BRAIN
Adult: Headache, memory loss
Child: Encephalopathy, mental deterioration

GINGIVA
Lead line

BLOOD
Anemia, red cell basophilic stippling

PERIPHERAL NERVES
Adults: Demyelination

KIDNEY
Chronic tubulointerstitial disease

GASTROINTESTINAL TRACT
Abdominal pain

EPIPHYSES OF CHILDREN'S BONES
Radiodense deposits

SOURCES

OCCUPATIONAL
Spray painting
Foundry work
Mining and extracting lead
Battery burning

NONOCCUPATIONAL
Water supply
Paint dust and flakes
House dust
Urban soil
Newsprint
Automotive exhaust

Figure 8–8. Clinical and pathologic features of lead poisoning.

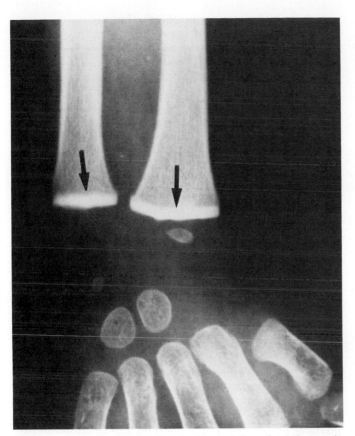

Figure 8–9. Lead poisoning. Impaired remodeling of calcified cartilage in the epiphyses (*arrows*) of the wrist has caused a marked increase in their radiodensity, so that they are as radiopaque as the cortical bone. (Courtesy Dietz, G. W., M.D., Department of Radiology, Southwestern Medical School, Dallas, TX.)

lates hyperpigmentation of the gum tissue adjacent to the teeth. Excretion of lead occurs via the kidneys, thereby exposing these organs to potential damage.

Lead causes injury by binding to disulfide groups in proteins, including enzymes, altering their tertiary structure. The major anatomic targets of lead are the blood, nervous system, gastrointestinal tract, and kidneys (see Fig. 8–8).

Blood changes resulting from lead accumulation occur fairly early and are characteristic. Lead interferes with normal heme biosynthesis by inhibiting the enzymes aminolevulinic acid dehydratase (ALA-D) and ferroketolase (involved in incorporation of iron into the protoporphyrin molecule to form heme). As a consequence of this latter enzyme defect, zinc-protoporphyrin is formed instead of heme. Thus the elevated blood level of zinc-protoporphyrin or its product, free erythrocyte protoporphyrin, is an important indicator of lead poisoning. Typically, a microcytic, hypochromic, mild hemolytic anemia appears and, even more distinctive, punctate basophilic stippling of the erythrocytes.

Brain damage is prone to occur in children. It may be very subtle, producing mild dysfunction, or massive and lethal. In young children, sensory, motor, intellectual, and psychologic impairments have been described, including reduced IQ, learning disabilities, re-

tarded psychomotor development, blindness, and in more severe cases, psychoses, seizures, and coma. The anatomic changes underlying the more subtle functional deficits are ill defined, but there is concern that some of the defects may be permanent. At the more severe end of the spectrum are (1) marked brain edema, (2) demyelination of the cerebral and cerebellar white matter, and (3) necrosis of cortical neurons accompanied by diffuse astrocytic proliferation. In *adults* the central nervous system is less often affected, but frequently a peripheral *demyelinating neuropathy* appears, typically involving the motor innervation of the most commonly used muscles. Thus the extensor muscles of the wrist and fingers are often the first to be affected, followed by paralysis of the peroneal muscles.

The *gastrointestinal tract* is also a major source of clinical manifestations. Lead "colic," characterized by extremely severe, poorly localized abdominal pain, is often associated with sufficient spasm and rigidity of the abdominal wall to create the impression of an acute "surgical abdomen." Other findings are shown in Figure 8–8.

The diagnosis of lead poisoning requires constant awareness of its prevalence. In children the only significant findings may be vague intellectual, behavioral, or motor abnormalities. In adults the symptoms are also relatively nonspecific. Sometimes the first clue is anemia and basophilic stippling of the red cells. In some children, the intense radiopacity of the deposits in and about the epiphyses of growing bones raises the suspicion of lead poisoning; however, the diagnosis requires the confirmatory findings of elevated blood lead and free erythrocyte protoporphyrin values (above 50 μg/dl) or, alternatively, zinc protoporphyrin levels. In view of the potential consequences of advanced intoxication, it is hardly necessary to point out the importance of early diagnosis.

Carbon Monoxide (CO)

This nonirritating, colorless, tasteless, odorless gas produced by the imperfect oxidation of carbonaceous materials continues to be a cause of accidental and suicidal death. Its sources include automotive engines, industrial processes using fossil fuels, home heating with fossil fuels (not natural gas), and cigarette smoke. The exhaust of automotive engines is about 5% CO; in a small, closed garage the average car exhaust will induce lethal coma within 5 minutes. CO kills by inducing CNS depression, which appears so insidiously that victims may not be aware of their plight and indeed may be unable to help themselves.

CO acts as a systemic asphyxiant. Hemoglobin has a 200-fold greater affinity for CO than for oxygen. The resultant carboxyhemoglobin is incapable of carrying oxygen and furthermore interferes with the release of oxygen from oxyhemoglobin. Systemic hypoxia appears when the hemoglobin is 20 to 30% saturated with CO, and unconsciousness and death are likely with 60 to 70% saturation. Depending on the rate of conversion to carboxyhemoglobin and the ultimate severity, one of two clinical patterns can be recognized.

Acute poisoning is marked by a characteristic generalized cherry-red color of the skin and mucous membranes resulting from the carboxyhemoglobin. If death occurs, depending on the rapidity of onset, morphologic changes may not be present; with longer survival the brain may be slightly edematous, with punctate hemorrhages and hypoxic neuronal changes. The morphologic changes are not specific for CO; they simply imply systemic hypoxia. When exposure has not been prolonged and only moderate hypoxia has occurred, complete recovery is possible; however, sometimes impairments of memory, vision, hearing, and speech remain.

Chronic poisoning may appear because the carboxyhemoglobin, once formed, is remarkably stable and, with low-level persistent exposure, may accumulate to a life-threatening concentration in the blood. The slowly developing hypoxia can insidiously evoke widespread changes in the central nervous system, particularly marked in the basal ganglia and lenticular nuclei. With cessation of exposure to CO the victim usually recovers, but often there are permanent neurologic sequelae. The diagnosis of CO poisoning is critically dependent on the identification of significant levels of carboxyhemoglobin in the blood.

The effects of carboxyhemoglobin levels of less than 10% are not clear. These levels may be attained in smokers and in some occupational or urban settings. There is evidence that incremental increases in blood carboxyhemoglobin can contribute to the onset of exercise-induced angina and may play a role in increased mortality associated with heavy urban pollution.

Alcohol and Other Drugs of Abuse

There is little need to elaborate extensively on the impact of drug abuse in our society. Countless lives have been lost as an indirect result of impaired motor coordination and judgment resulting from the use of mind-altering drugs. Our purpose here is to describe the pathology directly associated with the abuse of alcohol, therapeutic agents, and illicit drugs.

Drug abuse may be defined as the use of a mind-altering substance in a way that differs from generally approved *medical* or *social* practices. Ethanol is imbibed, at least partly, for its mood-altering properties but if used in moderation is socially acceptable. In excess, alcohol can cause marked physical and psychological damage. Table 8–8 provides a classification of drugs that are abused, with examples of each. Drugs of abuse are frequently implicated in suicide attempts and accidental drug overdoses, which are often fatal. Furthermore, these drugs have a propensity for inducing acute anxiety reactions and temporary psychosis in the abuser.

All drugs of abuse produce *psychological dependence* (a compulsion to use the agent), and the drug abuser comes to require the drug for feelings of well-being. The term *drug addiction,* in contradistinction to drug dependence, is used to convey a *pronounced* degree of psychological dependence. Many, but not all, drugs of abuse also produce variable degrees of *physical* depen-

TABLE 8–8. CLASSIFICATION OF DRUGS OF ABUSE*

Class	Examples
Sedatives and hypnotics	Alcohol, barbiturates, benzodiazepines
CNS sympathomimetics or stimulants	Cocaine, amphetamines, methylphenidate (ritalin), weight-loss products
Opioids	Heroin, morphine, methadone, and almost all prescription analgesics
Cannabinols	Marijuana, hashish
Hallucinogens or psychedelics	Lysergic acid diethylamide (LSD), mescaline, psilocybin, phencyclidine (PCP)
Inhalants	Aerosol sprays, glues, toluene, gasoline, paint thinner, amyl nitrite, nitrous oxide
Over-the-counter drugs	Ingredients: Atropine, scopolamine, weak stimulants, antihistamines, weak analgesics

* Modified from Schuckit, M.A. (ed.): *Drug and Alcohol Abuse,* A Clinical Guide to Diagnosis and Treatment. 3rd ed., New York, Plenum Press, 1989.

dence, which implies that (1) a state of physiologic *tolerance* exists that requires the user to take increasingly larger doses of the drug to derive the same benefit and/or (2) abstinence from the drug results in a physical *withdrawal reaction.* With the development of tolerance, habitual users may ingest quantities of drugs that might be lethal for a nonuser.

To understand the spectrum of physical effects of drugs of abuse it is necessary to understand that drug abusers may live in environments predisposed to additional abuse, including increased exposure to situations that result in trauma. In addition, abusers frequently mix drugs, many of which are adulterated with other toxins. Intravenous drug abusers (most frequently of heroin) may unknowingly inject a host of foreign substances that can cause direct toxicity, foreign body reactions, or infections.

ETHANOL. Eighty to ninety per cent of adults in many populations consume ethanol. Unfortunately, consumption is excessive in 5 to 10% of adult males and about 5% of adult females in most privileged societies. It is estimated that in the United States there are more than 10 million chronic alcoholics and an additional 7 million who drink enough to suffer adverse effects.

The major effects of acute alcohol intake are exerted on the CNS, but with chronic use other organs are also affected. Following ingestion, ethanol is absorbed unaltered in the stomach and small intestine. It is then distributed to all the tissues and fluids of the body in direct proportion to the blood level. Less than 10% of absorbed alcohol is excreted unchanged in the urine, sweat, and breath. The amount exhaled is proportional to the blood level and forms the basis of the breath test employed by law enforcement agencies.

Most of the alcohol in the blood is biotransformed to acetaldehyde in the liver through two pathways (Fig. 8–10). Acetaldehyde formed by either pathway is fur-

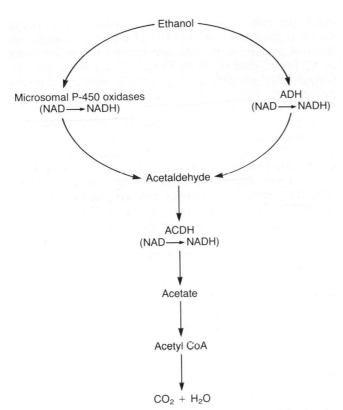

Figure 8-10. Metabolism of alcohol. With occasional intake the major pathway is via ADH. In chronic alcoholism the P-450 system is induced and plays a more important role. ADH = Hepatic alcohol dehydrogenase, ACDH = hepatic acetaldehyde dehydrogenase, NAD = nicotinamide adenine dinucleotide, NADH = reduced NAD.

ther metabolized by acetaldehyde dehydrogenase. With relatively low levels of alcohol intake this conversion is mediated primarily by alcohol dehydrogenase. At higher levels the microsomal P-450 system becomes more important. Indeed, high blood levels of alcohol enhance the activity of this system, so that other drugs metabolized by the same pathway are more rapidly oxidized (some, unfortunately, to more toxic products). This partially explains the enhanced toxicity of certain drugs in alcoholics. A man of average size and weight metabolizes about 9.0 gm of alcohol (about 3/4 ounce of whiskey) per hour irrespective of the blood level. However, genetic polymorphisms of liver alcohol and acetaldehyde dehydrogenases have been identified, some associated with more rapid metabolism of substrate than others. Moreover, chronic alcoholics develop a measure of tolerance due to enzyme induction (particularly of the microsomal P-450 system), leading to an increased rate of metabolism. In addition, they acquire a poorly defined adaptive capacity to perform motor and cognitive tasks at blood alcohol levels that would significantly affect the nonhabituated. Thus there is some individual variability in the ability to handle alcohol, but the variations are confined to a narrow range.

Acute alcoholism exerts its effects mainly on the central nervous system, but it may induce hepatic and gastric changes that are reversible in the absence of continued alcohol consumption. The hepatic changes

are described on page 545. The gastric changes constitute acute gastritis and ulceration (p. 484). *In the central nervous system, alcohol itself is a depressant,* first affecting subcortical structures (probably the high brain stem reticular formation) that modulate cerebral cortical activity. Consequently, there is stimulation and disordered cortical, motor, and intellectual behavior. At progressively higher blood levels, cortical neurons and then lower medullary centers are depressed, including those that regulate respiration. Respiratory arrest may follow.

Blood alcohol levels and the degree of impairment of central nervous system function in nonhabituated drinkers are closely correlated. In individuals of average size, consumption of 180 ml (6 ounces) of distilled spirits in a relatively brief time results in a blood alcohol level of approximately 100 mg/dl. This level will induce obvious ataxia and is usually considered the legal upper limit of sobriety. Drowsiness occurs at about 200 mg/dl, stupor at 300 mg/dl, and 400 to 500 mg/dl produces profound anesthesia, if not death. Fortunately, fatal levels are rarely encountered because stupor or vomiting of gastric contents intervenes.

Chronic alcoholism is responsible for morphologic alterations in virtually all organs and tissues in the body, particularly the liver and stomach. Only the gastric lesions that appear immediately after exposure can be related to the direct effects of ethanol on the mucosal vasculature. The origin of the other chronic changes is less clear. Acetaldehyde, a major oxidative metabolite of ethanol, is a very reactive compound and has been proposed as the mediator of the widespread tissue and organ damage. Although the catabolism of acetaldehyde is more rapid than that of alcohol, chronic ethanol consumption reduces the oxidative capacity of the liver, raising the blood level of acetaldehyde, which is augmented by the increased rate of ethanol metabolism in the habituated drinker. Other suggested mechanisms of injury include increased free radical activity and, possibly, immune reactions against hepatic neoantigens generated by acetaldehyde or free radical-induced alteration of proteins.

Whatever the basis, chronic alcoholics suffer significant morbidity and a shortened life span related principally to damage to the liver, stomach, brain, heart, and pancreas.

- *Liver.* Alcohol, the most common cause of hepatic injury, may lead to cirrhosis (p. 545). Cirrhosis of the liver is the ninth leading cause of death in the United States.
- *Gastrointestinal tract.* Massive bleeding from gastritis, gastric ulcer, or esophageal varices (associated with cirrhosis) may prove fatal.
- *Central nervous system.* A deficiency of thiamine is common in chronic alcoholics; the principal lesions of this deficiency are peripheral neuropathies and the Wernicke-Korsakoff syndrome (p. 253). Cerebral atrophy, cerebellar degeneration, and optic neuropathy may also occur, possibly directly related to alcohol or its products.
- *Cardiovascular system.* Direct injury to the myocardium may produce a dilated congestive cardiomyop-

athy (p. 327). Although *moderate* amounts of alcohol have been shown to increase the levels of HDL and decrease the incidence of coronary heart disease, heavy consumption with attendant liver injury results in a decrease in levels of HDL accompanied by an increase in the likelihood of coronary heart disease. Chronic alcoholism is associated with an increased incidence of hypertension.

- *Pancreas.* Excess alcohol intake increases the risk for acute and chronic pancreatitis (p. 581).
- *Other.* The heavy use of ethanol during pregnancy can cause fetal alcohol syndrome (growth retardation and some reduction in mental function in the child).

COCAINE. In the last decade cocaine has, along with its derivative "crack," become a major substance of abuse; it is estimated there are one to three million cocaine abusers in the United States. Cocaine, an alkaloid extracted from the leaves of the coca plant, is usually prepared in the form of a water-soluble powder, cocaine hydrochloride, but when sold on the street, it is liberally diluted with talcum powder, lactose, or other look-alikes. Crystallization of the pure alkaloid from cocaine hydrochloride yields nuggets of

crack (so called because of the cracking or popping sound it makes when heated). The pharmacologic actions of cocaine and crack are identical, but the latter is far more potent. Both forms of the drug are absorbed from all sites and so can be snorted, smoked mixed with tobacco, ingested, or injected subcutaneously or intravenously.

Cocaine produces an intense euphoria with so-called reinforcing qualities, making it one of the most addicting of all drugs. Experimental animals will press a lever more than 1000 times and forego food and drink in order to obtain the drug. In the cocaine abuser, although *physical dependence* appears not to occur, the psychologic withdrawal can be extremely difficult to treat. Recurrent intense cravings to reexperience drug-associated "highs" are particularly severe in the first several months following abstinence, but they can recur for years.

The most serious *physical* side effects of cocaine use relate to its acute toxic effects on the cardiovascular system and can be most readily understood by considering the sympathomimetic action of the drug (Fig. 8–11.) *Cocaine acts to facilitate neurotransmission both in the central nervous system, where it blocks the*

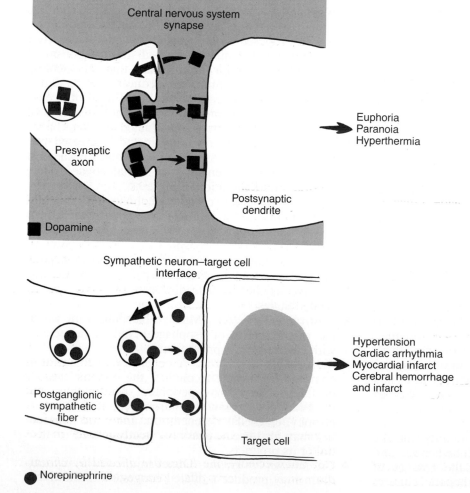

Figure 8–11. The effect of cocaine on neurotransmission. The drug inhibits reuptake of the neurotransmitters dopamine and norepinephrine by presynaptic neurons, leading to excess stimulation of postsynaptic fibers or effector cells.

reuptake of dopamine, and at adrenergic nerve endings, where it blocks the reuptake of norepinephrine. The net effect is the accumulation of these two neurotransmitters at adrenergic nerve endings, resulting in excess stimulation. In addition cocaine has a *direct toxic effect on the myocardium* and perhaps on skeletal muscle. These toxic effects are not necessarily dose-related and a lethal event may occur in a first-time abuser with what is a typical mood-altering dose. The following manifestations of *acute* cocaine toxicity are possible.

- Sympathetic nervous system stimulation resulting in dilated pupils, vasoconstriction, a rise in arterial blood pressure, and tachycardia.
- Lethal arrhythmias and myocardial infarction.
- Cerebral infarction and intracranial hemorrhage; the latter in persons who have preexisting vascular malformations and probably related to the sudden acute elevations in blood pressure. The most common CNS findings are hyperpyrexia (felt to be caused by aberrations of the dopaminergic pathways that control body temperature) and seizures.
- Rhabdomyolysis, sometimes accompanied by renal failure; the mechanism is not understood but may relate to intense vasoconstriction together with a direct effect of the drug on muscle.

In contrast to acute toxicity, *chronic* cocaine use may result in (1) perforation of the nasal septum in cocaine snorters, (2) decreased lung diffusing capacity in those who inhale the smoke from cocaine, and, rarely, (3) the development of dilated cardiomyopathy.

HEROIN. Heroin, although not as widely used as cocaine, is even more hazardous. It is an addicting opioid (closely related to morphine), derived from the poppy plant. It is sold on the street cut (diluted) with some agent, often talc or quinine, and the size of the dose is not only variable but is usually unknown to the buyer. The heroin, along with the contaminating substances, is usually self-administered intravenously or subcutaneously. It is short acting, so it must be taken every few hours to avoid withdrawal symptoms. Effects are varied and include euphoria, hallucinations, somnolence, and sedation. Heroin has a wide range of adverse physical effects: the pharmacologic action of the agent; reactions to the cutting agents or contaminants; hypersensitivity reactions to the drug or its adulterants (quinine itself has neurologic, renal, and auditory toxicity); and diseases contracted incident to the use of the needle.

- *Sudden death,* usually related to overdose, is an ever-present risk because drug purity is generally unknown and may range from 2 to 90%. Sudden death can also occur if tolerance for the drug built up over time is lost (as during a period of incarceration). The mechanisms of death include: profound respiratory depression, arrhythmia and cardiac arrest, and severe pulmonary edema.
- *Pulmonary complications* include moderate to severe edema, septic embolism, lung abscess, opportunistic infections, and foreign body granulomas from talc and other adulterants. Although *granulomas* occur principally in the lung, they are sometimes found in

the mononuclear-phagocyte system, particularly in the spleen, liver, and lymph nodes that drain the upper extremities. Examination under polarized light often highlights trapped talc crystals, sometimes enclosed within foreign body giant cells.

- *Infectious complications* are common. The four sites most commonly affected are the skin and subcutaneous tissue, heart valves, liver, and lungs. In a series of addicts admitted to the hospital, more than 10% had *endocarditis,* which often takes a distinctive form involving right-sided heart valves, particularly the tricuspid. Most cases are caused by *Staphylococcus aureus,* but fungi and a multitude of other organisms have been implicated. *Viral hepatitis* is the most common infection among addicts and is acquired by the casual sharing of dirty needles. In the U.S. this practice has also led to a very high incidence of acquired immunodeficiency syndrome (AIDS) in drug addicts, second only to that of homosexual men.
- *Cutaneous lesions* are probably the most frequent telltale sign of heroin addiction. Acute changes include abscesses, cellulitis, and ulcerations due to subcutaneous injections. Scarring at injection sites, hyperpigmentation over commonly used veins, and thrombosed veins are the usual sequelae of repeated intravenous inoculations.
- *Kidney disease* is a relatively common hazard. The two forms most frequently encountered are amyloidosis and focal glomerulosclerosis, and both induce heavy proteinuria and the nephrotic syndrome. Amyloidosis is secondary to chronic skin infections (p. 165).

MARIJUANA. Marijuana, or pot, is the most widely used illegal drug. It is made from the leaves of the *Cannabis sativa* plant, which contain the psychoactive substance delta-9-tetrahydrocannabinol (THC). When it is smoked, about 50% of the THC is absorbed; when ingested, only about 5 to 10%. According to several surveys, approximately 70% of 18- to 25-year-olds experiment with or regularly use this drug. Despite numerous studies, conflicting results still leave open the central question of whether the drug has persistent adverse physical and functional effects. Some of the untoward anecdotal effects may be allergic or idiosyncratic reactions, or may possibly be related to contaminants in the preparations rather than being directly related to marijuana's pharmacologic effects. On the other hand, two beneficial effects of THC are its capacity to decrease intraocular pressure in glaucoma and to combat intractable nausea secondary to cancer chemotherapy.

- *The functional and organic central nervous system consequences of cannabis* have received greatest scrutiny. Clearly, the use of pot distorts sensory perception and impairs motor coordination, but these acute effects generally clear in 4 to 5 hours. A recent study in Sweden indicated there was a sixfold increase in the incidence of schizophrenia in pot users.
- Not unexpectedly, *the lungs are affected by chronic pot smoking;* laryngitis, pharyngitis, bronchitis,

cough and hoarseness, and asthma-like symptoms have all been described, along with mild but significant airway obstruction. Smoking a marijuana cigarette, as compared with a cigarette, is associated with a threefold increase in the amount of tar inhaled and retained in the lungs. Presumably, the larger puff-volume, deeper inhalation, and longer breath holding are responsible. To date cannabis has not been shown to increase the incidence of bronchogenic carcinoma; recall, however, that it took more than 50 years to establish the carcinogenicity of tobacco.

- _Marijuana increases the heart rate and sometimes the blood pressure,_ and in a person with fixed coronary artery narrowing may cause angina.
- _Cannabis may induce chromosome damage in somatic and germ cells,_ but the evidence is not incontrovertible. A large study involving many thousands of women who were marijuana users revealed lower birth weights, shorter gestation periods, and an increased number of malformations among the offspring. Because the peak use of marijuana is among teenagers and young adults, these provocative findings require further study.

INHALANTS. These agents of abuse have achieved great popularity among very young persons; surveys indicate that about 15% of the general urban population younger than 25 years (some younger than 10 years) either experiment with or use them frequently. Favorites among the inhalants are glue, paint thinner, nail polish remover, and many substances in aerosol cans such as hairspray and room deodorizers. As a group the solvents and aerosolizers act as powerful central nervous system depressants; because they repress inhibitory pathways they produce a transient "high" much like that of acute alcoholism. For the most part the neurologic and psychologic effects (impairment in judgment, disorientation, and manic euphoria) are transitory, but deaths from heart failure have been reported, possibly because the solvents and fluorocarbons in aerosol cans intensify the effects of epinephrine on the heart.

INJURY BY PHYSICAL AGENTS _____

Injury induced by physical agents is divided into the following categories: mechanical, thermal, electrical, and ionizing radiation injury. Understanding the pathology of these forms of injury is clearly important to the physician who will undertake therapy, and also, when death is the outcome, to the forensic pathologist who may be required to determine the proximate cause of death and the medicolegal ramifications.

MECHANICAL TRAUMA _____

Mechanical forces may inflict damage in several ways. The impact of the body with a moving or stationary object can result in compression, stretching, torsion, or penetration of tissues. The type of injury depends on the type of object, the amount of energy discharged at impact, and the tissues or organs that bear the impact. With regard to particular tissues injured, bone and head injuries result in unique damage and are discussed elsewhere. All soft tissues react similarly to mechanical forces, and the patterns of injury can be summarized in the following terms:

- _Abrasion._ An abrasion is a wound produced by scraping or rubbing, resulting in removal of the superficial layer. Skin abrasions may remove only the epidermal layer.
- _Contusions._ A contusion, or bruise, is a wound usually produced by a blunt object and characterized by the damage to vessels and extravasation of blood into tissues.
- _Laceration._ A laceration is a tear or disruptive stretching of tissue due to the application of force by a blunt object. In contrast to an incision, most lacerations have jagged, irregular edges.
- _Incised wound._ An incised wound is one inflicted by a sharp instrument.
- _Puncture wound._ A puncture wound is caused by a long narrow instrument and is termed "penetrating" when the instrument pierces the tissue or "perforating" when it traverses a tissue to also create an exit wound. Gunshot wounds are special forms of puncture wounds which demonstrate distinctive features important to the forensic pathologist. For example the wound from a bullet fired at close range leaves powder burns, whereas one fired from more than 4 or 5 feet away does not.

One of the most common causes of mechanical injury is vehicular accidents; injuries sustained typically result from the driver or passenger (1) impacting a part of the interior of the vehicle or being hit by an object that enters the passenger compartment during the crash, such as the motor, (2) being thrown from the vehicle, or (3) being trapped in a burning vehicle. The pattern of injury relates to whether one or all of these three mechanisms are operative. For example, in a head-on collision a common pattern of injury sustained by a driver who is not wearing a seat belt includes trauma to the head (windshield impact), chest (steering column impact), and knees (dashboard impact). Under these conditions, common chest injuries include sternal and rib fractures, heart contusions, aortic lacerations (Fig. 8–12), and, less commonly, lacerations of the spleen and liver. Thus _in caring for an automobile injury victim it is essential to remember that the superficial abrasions, contusions, and lacerations are often accompanied by similar internal wounds. Indeed, in many cases external evidence of serious internal damage is completely absent._

A special category of mechanical injury is one that results in anoxia. An example is airway obstruction due to (1) external obstruction of the airways (smothering), (2) internal obstruction (as by an aspirated foreign body), or (3) crush injury (when an external object compresses the chest). In each of these, external evidence of the cause of hypoxia is accompanied by major pathologic changes in the brain (anoxia), described in Chapter 22.

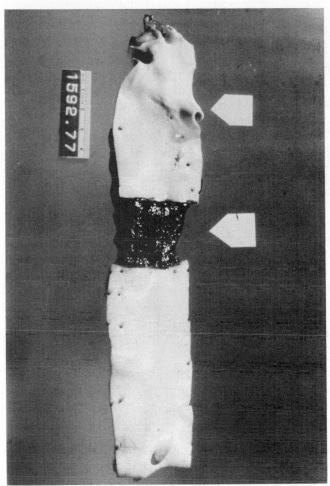

Figure 8-12. Transverse rupture of the descending thoracic aorta incurred in an automobile accident. (Courtesy of Dr. Charles Petty, Department of Pathology and Forensic Medicine, Southwestern Medical School, Dallas, TX).

THERMAL INJURY

Both excess heat and excess cold are important causes of injury. Burns are all too common, and are discussed first; a brief discussion of hyperthermia and hypothermia follows.

Thermal Burns

In the United States, burns cause 5000 deaths per year and result in the hospitalization of over ten times that many persons. Many victims are children, who are often *scalded* by hot liquids. Fortunately, marked decreases have been seen in both mortality rates and length of hospitalizations in the past 25 years. This improved prognosis results from a better understanding of the systemic effects of massive burns and discoveries of better ways to prevent wound infection and facilitate healing of skin surfaces.

The percentage of body surface involved and the depth of a burn dictates the approach to treatment. The depth of a burn is initially evaluated by the gross appearance. A *full-thickness* burn involves the total destruction of the epidermis and dermis with loss of the dermal appendages that would have provided cells for epithelial regeneration. Both *third- and fourth-degree* burns are in this category. In *partial-thickness* burns, at least the deeper portions of the dermal appendages are spared. Partial-thickness burns include *first-degree* burns (epithelial involvement only) and *second-degree* burns (both epidermis and superficial dermis).

Grossly, full-thickness burns are white or charred, dry, and anesthetic (because of nerve ending destruction), whereas, depending on the depth, partial-thickness burns are pink or mottled with blisters and are painful. Histologically, devitalized tissue demonstrates coagulative necrosis; adjacent vital tissue quickly develops inflammatory changes with an accumulation of inflammatory cells and marked exudation.

An immediate systemic consequence of burns of more than 20% of the body surface is a shift in body fluids into the interstitial compartments, both at the burn site and systemically, which can result in *hypovolemic shock* (p. 78). The mechanisms include an increase in local interstitial osmotic pressure (from release of osmotically active constituents of dying cells) and both neurogenic and mediator-induced increases in vascular permeability. Because protein from the blood is lost into interstitial tissue, generalized edema, including pulmonary edema, may become severe if fluids used for volume replacement are not osmotically active. Appreciation of these effects in the 1960s, followed by discovery of the advantage of early aggressive replacement of blood volume, has played an important role in salvaging patients with extensive burns.

A second important consideration in the early post-burn period is the degree of *injury to the airways and lungs*. Inhalation injury is frequent in persons trapped in burning buildings. This injury may result from direct effects of heat on the mouth, nose, and upper airways or from the inhalation of toxic components in smoke. Water-soluble gases such as chlorine, sulfur oxides, and ammonia may react with water to form acids or alkalis, particularly in the upper airways, and produce inflammation and swelling, which may lead to partial or complete airway obstruction. Lipid-soluble gases such as nitrous oxide and products of burning plastics are more likely to reach deeper airways, producing *pneumonitis*. Unlike shock, which develops within hours, pulmonary manifestations may not develop for 24 to 48 hours. Thus the initial absence of respiratory symptoms does not necessarily imply that there has been no respiratory injury.

Secondary *burn infection is an important complication* in all burn patients who have lost epidermis. Organ system failure resulting from burn *sepsis* continues to be the leading cause of death in burned patients. The burn site is ideal for growth of microorganisms; the serum and debris provide nutrients, and the burn injury compromises blood flow, blocking optimal inflammatory responses. The most common offender is the opportunist *Pseudomonas aeruginosa*, but antibiotic-resistant strains of other common hospital-acquired bacteria, such as *Staphylococcus aureus*, and fungi, particularly *Candida* species, may also be involved. Furthermore, cellular and humoral defenses against infections are compromised, and both lymphocyte and phagocyte functions are impaired. Direct bacteremic spread and release of toxic substances such as endotoxin from the local site exert dire consequences. *Pneumonia or septic shock with renal failure and/or the acute respiratory distress syndrome (ARDS, p. 399) are the most common serious sequelae.* Aggressive, early débridement of burn wounds is designed not only to provide a clean, vascular surface on which wound repair can proceed but also to provide phagocytes ready access to infecting microorganisms. Topical antibiotics may help, but burn infection continues to be an important problem.

Another very important pathophysiologic effect of burns is the development of a *hypermetabolic state with excess heat loss and an increased need for nutritional support.* It is estimated that when more than 40% of the body surface is burned the resting metabolic rate may approach twice normal. The consequence is breakdown of tissue, which may result in loss of essential protein stores reaching lethal proportions comparable to starvation within several weeks. Thus it is essential to keep room temperature elevated to reduce body heat loss and to implement appropriate nutritional supplementation.

Hyperthermia

Prolonged exposure to elevated ambient temperatures can result in heat cramps, heat exhaustion, and heat stroke.

- *Heat cramps* result from loss of electrolytes via sweating. Cramping of voluntary muscles, usually in association with vigorous exercise, is the hallmark. Heat-dissipating mechanisms are able to maintain normal core body temperature.
- *Heat exhaustion* is probably the most common heat syndrome. The onset is sudden, with prostration and collapse; it results from a failure of the cardiovascular system to compensate for hypovolemia, secondary to water depletion. After a period of collapse, which is usually brief, equilibrium is spontaneously reestablished.
- *Heat stroke* is associated with high ambient temperatures and high humidity. Thermoregulatory mechanisms fail, sweating ceases, and core body temperature rises. Temperatures of 112° to 113° F have been recorded in some terminal cases. Clinically, a rectal temperature of 106° F or higher is considered a grave prognostic sign, and the mortality rate exceeds 50%. The underlying mechanism is marked generalized peripheral vasodilatation with peripheral pooling of blood and a decreased effective circulating blood volume. Necrosis of muscles and myocardium may occur. Arrhythmias, disseminated intravascular coagulation, and other systemic effects are common. Elderly persons, those undergoing intense physical stress (including young athletes and military recruits), and those with cardiovascular disease are prime candidates for heat stroke.

Hypothermia

Prolonged exposure to low ambient temperature leads to hypothermia, a condition seen all too frequently in homeless persons. The lowering of body heat is hastened by high humidity in cold, wet clothing and dilatation of superficial blood vessels as a result of the ingestion of alcohol. At about 90° F loss of consciousness occurs, followed by bradycardia and atrial fibrillation at lower core temperatures.

ELECTRICAL INJURY

Electrical injuries, which may result in death, can arise from *low-voltage currents* (in the home and workplace), *high-voltage currents* from high-power lines, or *lightning*. Injuries are of two types: (1) burns and (2) ventricular fibrillation or cardiac and respiratory center standstill resulting from disruption of normal electrical impulses. The type of injury and the severity and extent of burning depend on the amperage and path of the electric current within the body.

It is important to remember that current flow (amperes) equals voltage (volts) divided by resistance (ohms). Obviously, current flow, and therefore injury, is less if voltage is low or resistance is high. Unfortunately, voltage in the household and workplace (120 or 220 volts) is high enough so that with low resistance at the site of contact (as when the skin is wet, much less so when dry), sufficient current can pass through the body to ground to cause serious injury, including ventricular fibrillation. If current flow continues long enough, it generates sufficient heat to produce burns at the site of entry and exit as well as in internal organs. An important characteristic of alternating current, the type available in most homes, is that it induces tetanic muscle spasm so that if an energized object is grasped, irreversible clutching is likely to occur, prolonging the period of current flow. This results in a greater likelihood of developing extensive electrical burns and in some cases, spasm of the chest wall muscles with death from asphyxia. Currents generated from high-voltage sources cause similar damage; however, because of the large current flows generated these are more likely to produce paralysis of medullary centers and extensive burns. Lightning also produces high-voltage electrical injury.

Before leaving the subject of electrical injury, a word about the health risk of exposure to electromagnetic fields (EMFs) is in order. Some, but not all, epidemiologic studies have linked exposure to EMFs among electrical workers (especially those who work on high-power lines) and children living near high-power lines to an increased risk for cancer, particularly leukemias, lymphomas, and cancers in the nervous system. Despite alarm in the lay press, much study is needed before a true assessment of risk can be made.

INJURY BY IONIZING RADIATION ___

Ionizing radiation is a double-edged sword: it provides an invaluable means of clinical diagnosis and sometimes a curative mode of therapy, but at the same time it is a potent mutagen and destroyer of cells. Cosmic radiation and emissions from naturally occurring terrestrial radionuclides (radon gas) are omnipresent; diagnostic x-ray procedures are common occurrences, as is radiotherapy for cancers. Public concern about the location of nuclear waste disposal sites and safety of nuclear reactors reflects a widespread awareness of the potential dangers of ionizing radiation.

Ionizing radiation occurs in two forms: (1) *electromagnetic waves* (x-rays and gamma rays) and (2) *high-energy neutrons and charged particles* (alpha, beta, and protons). All forms of ionizing radiation exert their effects on cells by displacing electrons from molecules and atoms with which they collide, causing ionization and inducing a cascade of events that may alter the cell transiently or permanently. The most important target molecule in living cells is DNA. *Ionizing radiation may directly damage DNA (direct target theory), but more often it indirectly damages it by inducing the formation of free radicals, particularly those that form from the radiolysis of water (indirect target theory).* Other cell molecules that may also be direct or indirect targets of radiant injury include lipids in cell membranes and proteins that function as critical enzymes. The transfer of energy to a target atom or molecule from the incident source of radiant energy occurs within microfractions of a second, yet its biologic effect may not become apparent for minutes or, if the effect is on DNA, even decades.

Several terms are used to express radiation dose.

- *Roentgen* (R) is a unit of x- or gamma irradiation defined by the quantity of induced ionization in air. Thus it is a measure of exposure.
- *Radiation absorbed dose* (rad) and *grays* (Gy) are units that express the energy *absorbed* by target tissue from gamma and x-rays. A rad or its equivalent centigray (cGy) is the dose that results in absorption of 100 ergs of energy per gram of tissue.
- *Curie* (Ci) defines the disintegrations per second of a spontaneously disintegrating radionuclide (radioisotope). One Ci is equal to 3.7×10^{10} disintegrations per second.

These three measurements do not directly quantify energy transferred per unit of tissue and therefore do not predict the biologic effects of radiation. The following terms provide a better approximation of such information:

- *Linear energy transfer* (LET) expresses energy loss per unit of distance traveled as electron volts per micrometer. This value depends on the type of ionizing radiation. LET is very high for alpha particles, less so for beta particles, and even less for gamma rays and x-rays. Thus, alpha and beta particles penetrate short distances and interact with many molecules within that short distance. Gamma rays and x-rays penetrate deeply but interact with relatively few molecules per unit distance. It should be evident that if equivalent amounts of energy entered the body in the form of alpha and gamma radiation, the alpha particles would induce heavy damage in a restricted area whereas gamma rays would dissipate energy over a longer course and produce considerably less damage per unit of tissue.
- *Relative biologic effectiveness* (RBE) is simply a ratio that represents the relationship of the LETs of various forms of irradiation to cobalt gamma rays and megavolt x-rays, both of which have an RBE of unity (1).

EFFECTS OF IONIZING RADIATION ON CELLS AND TISSUES. The primary target of ionizing radiation is DNA. Except at extremely high doses that impair DNA transcription, DNA damage is compatible with survival if the cell remains in the intermitotic phase; however, during mitosis, cells that have incurred irreparable DNA damage die because chromosome abnormalities prevent normal division. Understandably, therefore, tissues with a high rate of cell turnover, such as bone marrow and mucosa of the gastrointestinal tract, are extremely vulnerable to radiation and the injury is manifest early after exposure. Tissues with slower turnover rates such as liver and endothelium are not affected immediately after irradiation but are depopulated slowly because dividing cells cannot be replaced. Tissues with nondividing cells such as brain and myocardium do not demonstrate radiation effects except at doses that are so high that DNA transcription or some other molecule vital to the normal functioning of the cell is affected. In summary, within days of exposure to radiant energy, tissues containing many rapidly dividing cells show evidence of radiation injury, while tissues that contain few dividing cells show little injury.

Because tissues are made up of many cell types the effects of radiation are complex. For example, vascular injury can result in changes that interfere with repair, and therefore parenchymal cells may reveal manifestations of radiation injury months to years later. Endothelial cells, which are moderately sensitive to irradiation, may be damaged and the resultant narrowing or occlusion of the blood vessels may lead to impaired healing of parenchymal cells or chronic ischemic atrophy. Vascular changes in the central nervous system following irradiation can lead to late manifestations of radiation damage, although nerve cells were not directly affected by the ionizing radiation.

In addition to the number of replicating cells in a tissue, several other important parameters determine whether injury will occur in irradiated tissue. These include (1) rate of the dose delivered, (2) capacity of the cells to repair themselves, and (3) the effect of oxygen. An important practical application of this knowledge is in designing strategies for radiation treatment of cancer.

The rate of delivery significantly modifies the biologic effect. Although *the effect of radiant energy is cumulative,* delivery in divided doses may allow cells to repair some of the damage in the intervals. Thus fractional doses of radiant energy have a cumulative effect only to the extent that repair during the intervals is incomplete. Radiotherapy of tumors exploits the fact that, in general, normal cells are capable of more rapid repair and recovery and so do not sustain as much cumulative radiation injury as do tumor cells. Oxygenation amplifies radiation damage to cells and tissues. *Radiant energy may interact with molecular oxygen to induce free radicals, such as superoxide, which can then interact with atoms and molecules to compound the cellular injury.* The oxygen effect is significant in the radiotherapy of neoplasms. The center of rapidly growing tumors may be poorly vascularized and therefore somewhat hypoxic, making radiotherapy less effective. A summary of the biologic effects of ionizing radiation is provided in Figure 8–13.

MORPHOLOGY. At the **molecular level,** the DNA sustains a variety of alterations. These include the formation of pyrimidine dimers, cross-links, single-strand or double-strand breaks, and various rearrangements. Most single-strand breaks are rapidly repaired, often within minutes; double-strand breaks are more often irreparable. These alterations lead to a wide range of structural changes in chromosomes, including deletions, breaks, translocations, and fragmentation. The mitotic spindle often becomes disorderly, and polyploidy and aneuploidy may be encountered. At the **cellular level** there may be nuclear swelling and condensation and clumping of chromatin; sometimes the nuclear membrane breaks. All forms of abnormal nuclear morphology may be produced. Giant cells with pleomorphic nuclei or more than one nucleus may appear and persist for years after exposure. At extremely high dose levels of radiant energy, nuclear pyknosis or lysis appears quickly as a marker of cell death.

In addition to affecting DNA and nuclei, radiant energy may induce a variety of **cytoplasmic changes,** including cytoplasmic swelling, mitochondrial distortion, and degeneration of the endoplasmic reticulum. Plasma membrane breaks and focal defects may appear. The histologic constellation of cellular pleomorphism, giant cell formation, conformational changes in nuclei, and mitotic figures creates a more than passing similarity between radiation-injured cells and cancer cells, a problem that plagues the pathologist evaluating postirradiation tissues for the possible persistence of tumor cells.

At the light microscopic level, vascular changes are prominent in irradiated tissues. During the immediate postirradiation period, vessels may show only dilatation. Later, or with higher doses, a variety of degenerative changes appear, including endothelial cell swelling and vacuolation, or even dissolution with total necrosis of the walls of small vessels such as capillaries and venules. Affected vessels may rupture or may thrombose. Still later, endothelial cell proliferation and collagenous hyalinization with thickening of the media are seen in irradiated vessels, resulting in marked narrowing or even obliteration of the vascular lumina.

EFFECTS ON ORGAN SYSTEMS. Figure 8–14 depicts the organs that are particularly radiosensitive, together with common early and late manifestations.

The *hematopoietic and lymphoid* systems are extremely susceptible to radiant injury and deserve special mention here. With high dose levels and large exposure fields, severe lymphopenia may appear within hours of radiation, along with shrinkage of the lymph nodes and spleen. Radiation directly destroys lymphocytes, both in the circulating blood and in tissues (nodes, spleen, thymus, gut). With sublethal doses of irradiation, regeneration from viable precursors is prompt, leading to restoration of a normal lymphocyte count in the blood within weeks to months. The circulating granulocyte count may first rise but begins to fall toward the end of the first week. Levels near zero may be reached during the second week. If the patient survives, recovery of the normal granulocyte counts may require two to three months. Platelets are similarly affected, with the nadir of the count occurring somewhat later than that of the granulocytes, while recovery is similarly delayed. Hematopoietic cells in the bone marrow, including red cell precursors, are also quite sensitive to radiant energy. Erythrocytes are radioresistant, but anemia may nonetheless appear after two to three weeks and persist for months because of marrow damage.

Another effect of irradiation on organ systems that deserves special mention relates to *malignant transformation* (see Fig. 8–13, and p. 200). Any cell capable of division that has sustained a mutation has the potential to become cancerous. Thus an increased incidence

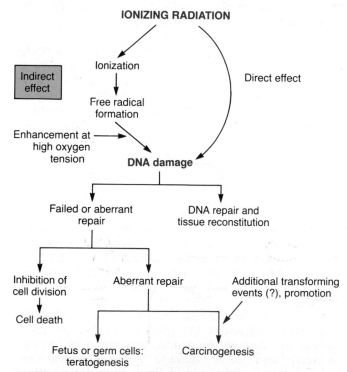

IONIZING RADIATION

Indirect effect

Ionization

Free radical formation

Direct effect

Enhancement at high oxygen tension

DNA damage

Failed or aberrant repair

DNA repair and tissue reconstitution

Inhibition of cell division

Aberrant repair

Additional transforming events (?), promotion

Cell death

Fetus or germ cells: teratogenesis

Carcinogenesis

Figure 8–13. Effects of ionizing radiation on DNA. The major effect is indirect, via free radical formation.

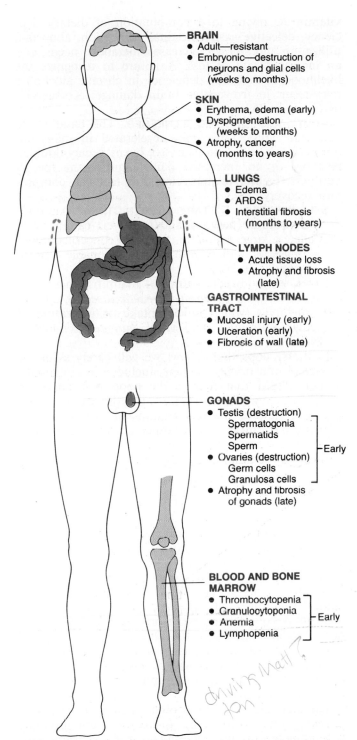

BRAIN
- Adult—resistant
- Embryonic—destruction of neurons and glial cells (weeks to months)

SKIN
- Erythema, edema (early)
- Dyspigmentation (weeks to months)
- Atrophy, cancer (months to years)

LUNGS
- Edema
- ARDS
- Interstitial fibrosis (months to years)

LYMPH NODES
- Acute tissue loss
- Atrophy and fibrosis (late)

GASTROINTESTINAL TRACT
- Mucosal injury (early)
- Ulceration (early)
- Fibrosis of wall (late)

GONADS
- Testis (destruction)
  Spermatogonia
  Spermatids
  Sperm ⎤ Early
- Ovaries (destruction)
  Germ cells
  Granulosa cells
- Atrophy and fibrosis of gonads (late)

BLOOD AND BONE MARROW
- Thrombocytopenia
- Granulocytopenia
- Anemia ⎤ Early
- Lymphopenia

Figure 8–14. An overview of the major morphologic consequences of radiation injury. Early changes occur in hours to weeks. Late changes occur in months to years.

of neoplasms may occur in any organ following radiation. The level of radiation required to increase the risk of cancer development is difficult if not impossible to determine. Radiation in very large doses kills cells and therefore is not associated with occurrence of tumors. Sublethal but relatively high doses are clearly associated with an increased risk. This is documented by the increased incidence of neoplasms in survivors of Hiroshima and Nagasaki, in radiologists of bygone years, and in miners of uranium ores (p. 200). Exposure to low-dose irradiation has its risks as well, as will be evident from the following discussion of the relationship of radon to bronchogenic carcinoma.

Radon is a ubiquitous alpha particle–emitting product of the spontaneous decay of uranium. Because radon is a gas, it moves freely in and out of the lungs and generally does not accumulate in tissues; nor does it cause damage, because, as discussed, alpha emitters penetrate tissues very poorly. In contrast, two of radon's decay by-products (or radon daughters) are alpha-emitting particulates. These particulates are more readily deposited in lung tissue and can accumulate, producing short-range DNA damage. Over a period of time, cells that suffer sufficient unrepaired DNA damage may become neoplastic and give rise to lung carcinomas. It is not currently known what levels of radon might be safe, but the question is of considerable importance because radon is ubiquitous and may accumulate in buildings, particularly where ventilation is poor. Fortunately, the levels of radon currently felt to be safe are only uncommonly exceeded except in those regions of the United States where uranium is closer to the surface and home construction practices facilitate leakage and entrapment of gases from the soil in basements.

TOTAL BODY RADIATION. Exposure of large areas of the body to even very small doses of radiation may have devastating effects. Although 10 to 50 rads of gamma or x-ray exposure may exert no discernible effects, 50 to 100 rads may cause as many as 10% of exposed individuals to manifest nausea and vomiting, fatigue, and transient decreases in lymphocytes and granulocytes. As little as 100 to 300 rads of radiant energy in total body exposure delivered in one dose may induce an "acute radiation syndrome." To place this radiation level in context, it must be appreciated that 4000 rads or more is often used in carefully shielded patients for radiotherapy of tumors. The lethal range in man for total body radiation begins at about 200 rads, and at 700 rads death is certain without medical intervention. Three often fatal acute radiation syndromes have been identified: (1) *hematopoietic,* (2) *gastrointestinal,* and (3) *cerebral* (Table 8–9).

NUTRITIONAL DISEASES

Adequate nutrition continues to be one of the most important concerns of humankind. In third world countries undernutrition or protein-energy malnutrition continues to be common, and in industrialized societies the most frequent diseases (atherosclerosis, cancer, diabetes, and hypertension) have all been linked to some form of dietary impropriety.

An adequate diet should provide: (1) energy, in the form of carbohydrates, fats, and proteins, (2) essential (as well as nonessential) amino acids and fatty acids to be utilized as building blocks for synthesis of structural and functional proteins and lipids, and (3) vitamins and minerals, which function as coenzymes or hor-

TABLE 8–9. SYNDROMES ASSOCIATED WITH VARIOUS LEVELS OF WHOLE BODY IRRADIATION

Syndrome	Dose (rads)	Clinical Manifestations
Hematopoietic	200–500	Nausea and vomiting; lymphopenia, thrombocytopenia, neutropenia, later anemia
Gastrointestinal	500–1000	Severe gastrointestinal symptoms including diarrhea, hemorrhage, emaciation; at higher doses death within days; at lower doses hematopoietic system manifestations
Cerebral	>5000	Listlessness and drowsiness, followed by convulsions, coma, and death within hours

mones in vital metabolic pathways or, as in the case of calcium and phosphate, as important structural components. In *primary* malnutrition one or all of these components is missing from the diet. However, malnutrition may result from nutrient malabsorption, impaired utilization or storage, excess losses, or increased need; in these circumstances, malnutrition is *secondary, or conditioned.*

In developing nations the incidence of overt hunger is high and of more subtle forms of undernutrition even higher. Even where there is sufficient food so that people can eat to satisfy hunger, vitamin and mineral deficiencies may exist. Vitamin A deficiencies are rampant in certain parts of Africa; iodine deficiencies occur in regions where iodized salt is not available; and iron deficiency is often seen in babies fed exclusively with milk diets. Thus, ignorance about the nutritional value of foods also plays an important role in malnutrition. In the United States, the National Research Council recommends daily allowances for protein, vitamins, and minerals for healthy adults, specifying ranges for both men and women. These standards represent the scientifically based general consensus of safe (not minimal) amounts of each nutrient necessary to maintain good health. Debates continue as to optimal levels of fat and fiber to prevent cardiovascular disease and cancer and this subject will be briefly discussed later.

It must be emphasized that affluent societies are not immune to a significant incidence of undernutrition. A listing of common causes in the United States highlights this point.

IGNORANCE AND POVERTY. The homeless, the aged, and children of the poor demonstrate effects of protein-energy malnutrition (PEM) as well as trace nutrient deficiencies. Even the affluent may fail to recognize the increased nutritional needs of growing infants and adolescents and of pregnant women.

CHRONIC ALCOHOLISM. Alcoholics may sometimes suffer PEM but are more frequently deficient in several vitamins, especially thiamine, pyridoxine, folate, and vitamin A, owing to a combination of dietary deficiency, defective gastrointestinal absorption, abnormal utilization and storage, increased metabolic needs, and an increased rate of loss. A failure to recognize the likelihood of thiamine deficiency in chronic alcoholics may result in irreversible brain damage (Korsakoff's psychosis, p. 253).

ACUTE AND CHRONIC ILLNESSES. The basal metabolic rate (BMR) becomes accelerated in many illnesses (in patients with extensive burns it may double), resulting in an increased daily requirement for all nutrients. Failure to appreciate this fact can compromise recovery.

SELF-IMPOSED DIETARY RESTRICTION. Anorexia nervosa, bulimia nervosa, and less overt eating disorders affect a large population who are concerned about body image or suffer from an unreasonable fear of cardiovascular disease.

Other, less common, causes of malnutrition include the *malabsorption syndromes, genetic diseases, specific drug therapies* (which block uptake or utilization of particular nutrients), and *total parenteral nutrition* (TPN).

In the sections that follow, we will barely skim the surface of nutritional disorders. Included in our discussion are PEM that ravages the poor, deficiencies of most of the vitamins and trace minerals, obesity, and a brief overview of the relationships of diet to atherosclerosis and cancer. Several other nutrients and nutritional issues are discussed in the context of specific disorders throughout the text.

PROTEIN-ENERGY MALNUTRITION

Severe PEM is a disastrous disease. It is far too common in third world countries, where up to 25% of children may be affected; in these countries it is a major factor in the high death rates among children under five years of age. PEM refers to a range of clinical syndromes characterized by an inadequate dietary intake of protein and calories to meet the body's needs. Before discussing the clinical presentations of severe malnutrition, e.g., marasmus and kwashiorkor, some general comments will be made on the clinical assessment of undernutrition and some of its general metabolic characteristics.

The diagnosis of PEM is obvious in its most severe forms; in mild to moderate forms the usual approach is to compare the body weight for a given height with standard tables; other parameters are also helpful, including evaluation of fat stores, muscle mass, and serum proteins. An important feature of PEM is loss of the major storage form of energy, fat, and, therefore, the thickness of skin folds (which includes skin and subcutaneous tissue) is reduced. In the face of malnutrition tissue protein is also catabolized, resulting in diminished muscle mass, which is reflected in reduced circumference of the midarm. Last, measurement of serum proteins (albumin, transferrin, and others), which are decreased because of the catabolic state, helps to assess the severity of PEM.

In general, when body weight falls to 20% below normal PEM is likely to be present. When calorie intake is restricted several adaptive hormonal mechanisms come into play. A decreased level of triiodothyronine (T_3) occurs, resulting in a lowered BMR. In addition levels of gonadotropin-releasing hormone (GnRH), follicle-stimulating hormone (FSH), and luteinizing hormone (LH) fall, resulting in loss of reproductive function. In the initial stages of starvation, when glucose and glycogen stores have been depleted, there is rapid catabolism of protein to utilize amino acids as a quick source of energy. In an effort to conserve protein, the body quickly adapts by metabolizing fatty acids and ketoacids and using proteins and amino acids more efficiently. Eventually, however, muscle mass and protein synthesis suffer.

The most common victims of PEM worldwide are children. A child whose weight falls to less than 80% of normal is considered malnourished. When the level falls to 60% of normal weight for sex and age, the child is considered to have marasmus. A marasmic child (Fig. 8-15) suffers growth retardation and loss of muscle and fat. The skin usually hangs loosely from emaciated extremities, the head appears too large for the body, and the abdomen may be bloated from a burden of parasites. Anemia and manifestations of multivitamin deficiencies are present, and there is evidence of immune deficiency, particularly of T cell–mediated immunity.

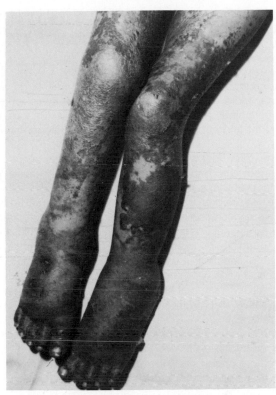

Figure 8-16. Kwashiorkor. Lower extremities of a child show the distinctive "flaky paint" skin lesions and dependent edema. (Courtesy of Dr. N. Scrimshaw, Massachusetts Institute of Technology; the Institute of Nutrition of Central America and Panama; and Science 133:2039, 1961. Copyright 1961 by the American Association for the Advancement of Science.)

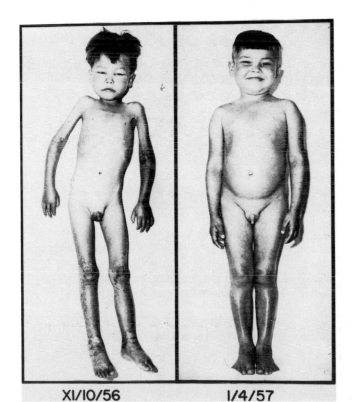

XI/10/56   1/4/57

Figure 8-15. Within every marasmic child (left) is a sturdy, smiling youngster; seen (right) after two months of adequate nutrition. (Courtesy of Dr. N. Scrimshaw, Massachusetts Institute of Technology; and the Institute of Nutrition of Central America and Panama.)

Kwashiorkor occurs when protein deprivation is relatively greater than the reduction in total calories. This is the most common form of malnutrition seen in African children who have been weaned (often too early owing to the arrival of another child) and are subsequently fed an exclusively carbohydrate diet. Less severe forms may occur worldwide in chronic diarrheal states when protein is not absorbed or in conditions where chronic protein loss occurs, such as in protein-losing enteropathies, the nephrotic syndrome, or following extensive burns. Children with severe kwashiorkor are typically 60 to 80% of normal weight. However, unlike marasmus, marked protein deprivation (accompanied by hypoalbuminemia) gives rise to generalized or dependent edema (Fig. 8-16). Indeed, the edema may mask loss of body fat and muscle mass. These children also have characteristic "flaky paint" skin lesions, with alternating zones of hyperpigmentation, areas of desquamation, and hypopigmentation. Hair changes include overall loss of color or alternating bands of pale and darker hair, straightening, fine texture, or loss of firm attachment to the scalp. Other features that differentiate kwashiorkor from marasmus include an enlarged fatty liver and a tendency to develop very early apathy, listlessness, and loss of appetite. As in marasmus, other vitamin deficiencies are likely to be present, as are defects in immunity, with increased susceptibility to infections. It should be emphasized that marasmus and kwashiorkor are two ends of a spectrum and that considerable overlap exists.

The central anatomic changes in PEM are (1) growth failure, more marked in marasmus than in kwashiorkor; (2) peripheral edema in kwashiorkor; and (3) loss of body fat and atrophy of muscle, more marked in marasmus.

The **liver** in kwashiorkor, but not in marasmus, is enlarged and fatty, owing to decreased synthesis of carrier proteins; superimposed cirrhosis is rare.

In kwashiorkor (rarely in marasmus) the **small bowel** shows a decrease in the mitotic index in the crypts of the glands, associated with mucosal atrophy and loss of villi and microvilli. In such cases, there is concurrent loss of small intestinal enzymes, most often manifested as disaccharidase deficiency. Hence, infants with kwashiorkor initially may not respond well to a full-strength, milk-based diet. With treatment, the mucosal changes are reversible.

The **bone marrow** in both kwashiorkor and marasmus may be hypoplastic, owing mainly to decreased numbers of red cell precursors. How much of this derangement is due to a deficiency of protein and folates, or to reduced synthesis of transferrin and ceruloplasmin is uncertain. Thus anemia is usually present, most often hypochromic-microcytic anemia, but a concurrent deficiency of folates may lead to a mixed microcytic-macrocytic anemia.

The **brain** in infants who are born to malnourished mothers and who suffer PEM during the first one or two years of life is reported by some observers to show cerebral atrophy, a reduced number of neurons, and impaired myelinization of the white matter, but there is no universal agreement on the validity of these findings.

Many **other changes** may be present, including (1) thymic and lymphoid atrophy (more marked in kwashiorkor than in marasmus), (2) anatomic alterations induced by intercurrent infections, particularly with all manner of endemic worms and other parasites, and (3) deficiencies of other required nutrients such as iodine and vitamins.

ANOREXIA NERVOSA AND BULIMIA _____

Anorexia nervosa is self-induced starvation, resulting in marked weight loss; bulimia is a condition in which the patient binges on food and then induces vomiting. These eating disorders occur primarily in previously healthy young women who have developed an obsession with attaining thinness. Although some consider the two disorders to be related, the more prevalent view is that bulimia (or bulimia nervosa) should be considered a separate entity for reasons that will become apparent.

Patients with *anorexia nervosa* have an intense fear of weight gain and see themselves as fat even in an advanced state of emaciation; as a result their diets are severely restricted. Some of them are also bulimic, i.e.,

they induce vomiting following meals and thus may have two causes for undernutrition. The clinical findings in anorexia nervosa are generally similar to those of severe PEM. In addition, because most of those affected are young women, the usual effects of PEM on the endocrine system are prominent. Amenorrhea resulting from decreased GnRH secretion (and subsequent decreased LH and FSH secretion) is so common that its presence is a diagnostic feature for the disorder. Other common findings, related to decreased thyroid hormone release, include cold intolerance, hypothermia, bradycardia, constipation, and changes in the skin and hair. The skin becomes dry and scaly and may be yellow owing to excess carotene in the blood. Body hair may be increased, but is usually fine and pale (lanugo). Bone density is decreased, most likely owing to low estrogen levels which mimic the postmenopausal acceleration of osteoporosis. As expected with severe PEM, anemia, lymphopenia, and hypoalbuminemia may be present. A major complication of anorexia nervosa is an increased susceptibility to cardiac arrhythmia with sudden death, resulting in all likelihood from hypokalemia.

In *bulimia,* binge eating is the norm. Huge amounts of food, principally carbohydrates, are ingested, only to be followed by vomiting. In contrast to patients with anorexia nervosa, patients with bulimia maintain a nearly normal weight-to-height ratio. Although menstrual irregularities are common, amenorrhea occurs in fewer than 50%, probably due to the maintenance of nearly normal weight and gonadotropin levels. The major medical complications relate to continual induced vomiting and include: (1) electrolyte imbalances (hypokalemia) which predispose the patient to cardiac arrhythmias, (2) pulmonary aspiration of gastric contents, and (3) esophageal and cardiac rupture.

VITAMIN DEFICIENCIES _____

Thirteen vitamins are necessary for health; four—A, D, E, and K—are fat soluble and the remainder water soluble. The distinction between the fat- and water-soluble vitamins is important because although the fat-soluble vitamins are more readily stored in the body, they are likely to be poorly absorbed in gastrointestinal disorders of fat malabsorption (p. 507). Small amounts of some vitamins can be synthesized endogenously—vitamin D from precursor steroids, vitamin K and biotin by the intestinal microflora, and niacin from tryptophan, an essential amino acid—but the rest must be supplied in the diet. A deficiency of vitamins may be primary (i.e., dietary in origin) or secondary, because of disturbances in intestinal absorption, transport in the blood, tissue storage, or metabolic conversion. In the following sections, the major vitamins together with their well-defined deficiency states are discussed individually (with the exception of B_{12} and folate) beginning with the fat-soluble vitamins. However, it should be emphasized that deficiencies of a single vitamin are uncommon and the expression of deficiency of a combination of vitamins may be submerged in concurrent PEM. A summary of all the essential vitamins, their functions, and deficiency syndromes are presented in Table 8–10.

Vitamin A

Vitamin A is actually a group of related natural and synthetic chemicals that exert a hormone-like activity or function. The relationship of some important members of this group is presented in Figure 8–17. *Retinol,* perhaps the most important form of vitamin A, is the transport form and, as the retinol ester, also the storage form. It is oxidized in vivo to the aldehyde *retinal* (the form used in visual pigment) and to the acid *retinoic acid.* Important dietary sources of vitamin A are animal derived (eggs, milk, butter). Yellow and leafy green vegetables such as carrots, squash, and spinach supply large amounts of carotenoids, many of which are provitamins that can be metabolized to active vitamin A in vivo; the most important of these is beta-carotene. A widely used term, *retinoids,* refers to both natural and synthetic chemicals that are structurally related to vitamin A but do not necessarily have vitamin A activity.

As with all fats, the digestion and absorption of carotenes and retinoids requires bile, pancreatic enzymes, and some level of antioxidant activity in the food. *Retinol,* whether derived from ingested esters or from beta-carotene (through an intermediate oxidation step involving retinal), is transported in chylomicrons to the liver for esterification and storage. More than

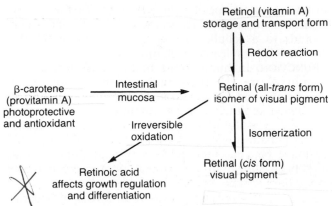

Figure 8–17. Interrelation of retinoids and their major functions.

90% of the body's vitamin A reserves are stored in the liver, predominantly in the perisinusoidal stellate (Ito) cells. In normal persons who consume an adequate diet, these reserves are sufficient for at least six months' deprivation. *Retinoic acid,* on the other hand, can be absorbed unchanged; it represents a small fraction of vitamin A in the blood and is active in epithelial differentiation and growth, but not in the maintenance of vision.

When the dietary intake of vitamin A is inadequate, the retinol esters in the liver are mobilized and released retinol is then bound to a specific retinol-binding protein (RBP), synthesized in liver. The uptake of retinol by the various cells of the body is dependent on

TABLE 8–10. VITAMINS: MAJOR FUNCTIONS AND DEFICIENCY SYNDROMES

Nutrient	Function	Deficiency Syndromes
Fat-Soluble Vitamins		
Vitamin A	Visual protein; hormonal regulation of cell growth	Night blindness, xerophthalmia, keratomalacia, metaplasia of columnar epithelium, immune deficiency
Vitamin D	Facilitates Ca and PO₄ absorption from intestine; helps maintain plasma Ca and PO₄ levels	Rickets in children, osteomalacia in adults, hypocalcemic tetany
Vitamin E	Antioxidant; maintenance of nervous system	Spinocerebellar syndrome
Vitamin K	Cofactor for hepatic carboxylation of prothrombin; factors VII, IX, and X; protein C and S	Bleeding diathesis
Water-Soluble Vitamins		
Thiamine (B₁)	As thiamine pyrophosphate functions as a coenzyme essential for maintaining nervous system	Wet and dry beriberi; Wernicke-Korsakoff syndrome
Riboflavin (B₂)	Cofactor in several enzymes, including FMN and FAD	Ariboflavinosis: cheilosis, glossitis, dermatitis, keratitis
Niacin	Component of coenzymes NAD and NADP	Pellagra: dementia, diarrhea, dermatitis
Pyridoxine (B₆)	Forms pyridoxal-5-phosphate, a coenzyme in many reactions	Cheilosis, glossitis, dermatitis, peripheral neuropathy
Pantothenic acid	Component of coenzyme A and acyl carrier protein	Recognized only under experimental conditions: constitutional and gastrointestinal symptoms, paresthesias, cramps, impaired coordination
Biotin	Cofactor in several carboxylation reactions	Deficiencies extremely rare: lassitude, anorexia, dermatitis, atrophic glossitis, myalgia, ECG changes, hypothermia, mild anemia
Folate (p. 347)	Coenzyme in transfer and utilization of 1-carbon units; essential step in nucleic acid synthesis	Megaloblastic anemia
Cyanocobalamin (B₁₂) (p. 347)	Role in utilization of folate in nucleic acid synthesis, also essential for maintenance of nervous system	Megaloblastic anemia, subacute combined degeneration
Vitamin C	Cofactor in hydroxylation and amidation reactions	Scurvy

surface receptors specific for RBP, not for the retinol. Retinol is transported across the cell membrane, where it binds to a cellular retinol-binding protein (CRBP) and the RBP is released back into the blood.

FUNCTION. In humans the best-defined functions of vitamin A are (1) maintaining normal vision in reduced light and (2) potentiating the differentiation of specialized epithelial cells, mainly mucus-secreting cells. A less well-understood effect of vitamin A relates to its enhancement of immunity. In addition, the retinoids, beta-carotene, and some related carotenoids have been shown to function as photoprotective and antioxidant agents.

The *visual process* involves four forms of vitamin A–containing pigments: rhodopsin in the rods, the most light-sensitive pigment and therefore important in reduced light; and three iodopsins in cone cells, each responsive to specific colors in bright light. The synthesis of rhodopsin from retinol involves (1) oxidation to all-*trans*-retinal, (2) isomerization to 11-*cis*-retinal, and (3) interaction with the rod protein, opsin, to form rhodopsin. When a photon of light impinges on the dark-adapted retina, rhodopsin undergoes a sequence of configurational changes to ultimately yield all-*trans*-retinal and opsin. In the process, a nerve impulse is generated (by changes in membrane potential) that is transmitted via neurons from the retina to the brain. During dark adaptation some of the all-*trans*-retinal is reconverted to 11-*cis*-retinal, but most is reduced to retinol and lost to the retina, dictating the need for continuous input of retinol.

Vitamin A plays an important role in the orderly *differentiation of mucus-secreting epithelium;* when a deficiency state exists, the epithelium undergoes squamous metaplasia and differentiation to a keratinizing epithelium. The mechanism is not precisely understood, but in cell culture systems retinoic acid (retinol is much less potent) regulates the gene expression of a number of cell receptors and secreted proteins, including receptors for growth factors.

There is accumulating evidence in both humans and experimental animals that vitamin A and the carotenoids may play roles in preventing cancer. The following mechanisms are proposed: (1) The regulatory effect of retinoic acid on growth and differentiation has an anticarcinogenic effect. (2) The immunity-enhancing function of vitamin A has a protective effect. (3) The antioxidant function of the carotenoids prevents oxidant-induced mutagenic effects. In a recent study pharmacologic (almost toxic) doses of retinoic acid prevented the development of second tumors in a group of high-risk patients following treatment of a first tumor. In contrast, a trial of carotenoids in patients at high risk for skin cancers failed to show any benefits. Thus the role of vitamin A compounds in the prevention or treatment of cancer is still uncertain, but carefully designed clinical trials are in progress and the results are eagerly awaited. There is no dispute, however, that certain nonneoplastic skin diseases, including severe acne and psoriasis, are controlled and often cured by some of the new synthetic retinoids.

DEFICIENCY STATE. Vitamin A deficiency occurs worldwide. It is most prevalent, on the basis of general undernutrition, in Southeast Asia, Indonesia, and the Philippines, but it is also common in many regions of Africa and Central and South America. In Asia as many as five million children a year develop eye disease, which results in blindness in 5% of them. The most serious eye manifestation relates to ulceration and destruction of the cornea, but night blindness and less severe forms of conjunctival changes may also occur (see below). Another very serious consequence of avitaminosis A is immune deficiency, the mechanisms of which are not well understood. This impairment of immunity leads to higher mortality rates from common infections such as measles, pneumonia, and infectious diarrhea. This observation is highlighted by recent studies from India and South Africa, which showed significantly decreased mortality rates from common childhood illnesses among children provided vitamin A supplements. Hypovitaminosis A is also seen sporadically in affluent societies among economically deprived persons who suffer from primary malnutrition, and as a conditioned deficiency among individuals having some cause for malabsorption of fats. In addition, extensive liver disease may lead to low circulating levels of vitamin A because of inadequate synthesis of RBP, just as the nephrotic syndrome may depress the levels of RBP because of excessive proteinuria. Not surprisingly, then, hypovitaminosis A is a global problem.

One of the earliest manifestations of vitamin A deficiency is impaired vision, particularly in reduced light (night blindness). If the deficiency persists, this condition is followed by a sequence of physical changes collectively referred to as *xerophthalmia* (dry eye). First there is dryness of the conjunctivae *(xerosis)* as the normal lachrymal and mucus-secreting epithelium is replaced by keratinized epithelium. This is followed by the build-up of keratin debris in small opaque plaques *(Bitot's spots),* and, eventually, erosion of the roughened corneal surface with softening and destruction of the cornea *(keratomalacia)* and total blindness (Fig. 8–18).

Because vitamin A and retinoids are involved in the differentiation of a variety of cells with a protracted deficiency, specialized epithelial cells, particularly in the eyes (as noted earlier), upper respiratory passages, and urinary tract, are replaced by keratinizing squamous cells. Loss of the mucociliary epithelium of the airways predisposes to secondary pulmonary infections. Desquamation of keratin debris in the urinary tract predisposes to renal and urinary bladder stones. Hyperplasia and hyperkeratinization of epidermis with plugging of the ducts of the adnexal glands may produce follicular or papular dermatosis. The pathologic effects of vitamin A deficiency are summarized in Figure 8–19.

VITAMIN A TOXICITY. Both short- and long-term excess of vitamin A may produce toxic manifestations, a point of some concern because clinical trials attempting to assess a therapeutic role for this vitamin in

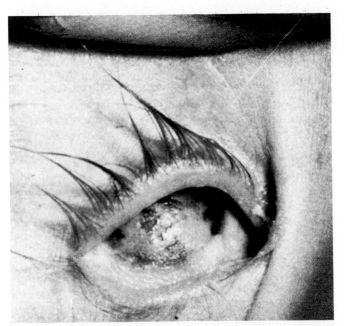

Figure 8–18. Advanced vitamin A deficiency with destruction of the eye, advanced keratomalacia. (Reproduced with the kind permission of Dr. Donald S. McLaren, Department of Medicine, Royal Infirmary, Edinburgh. From McLaren, D.: A Colour Atlas of Nutritional Disorders. London, Wolfe Medical Publications, Ltd., 1981, p. 26.)

cancer propose doses that are 50 to 100 times greater than the recommended daily allowance. The clinical consequences of acute hypervitaminosis A include headache, vomiting, stupor, and papilledema, all suggestive of brain tumor. Chronic toxicity is associated with weight loss, nausea, and vomiting; dryness of the mucosa of the lips; bone and joint pain; hyperostosis; and hepatomegaly with parenchymal damage and fi-

brosis. Although *synthetic* retinoids used for the treatment of acne are not associated with the complications listed above, their use in pregnancy should be avoided owing to a well-established increase in the incidence of congenital malformations. The consumption of large amounts of carrots or an inborn error of metabolism may result in hypercarotenemia and a benign yellowing of the skin, which can be confused with jaundice except that the sclerae are not icteric.

Vitamin D

The major function of vitamin D is the maintenance of normal plasma levels of calcium and phosphorus. In this capacity, it is *required for the prevention of bone diseases (rickets in growing children whose epiphyses have not already closed and osteomalacia in adults) and of hypocalcemic tetany.* With respect to tetany, vitamin D maintains the normal concentration of ionized calcium in the extracellular fluid compartment required for normal neural excitation and relaxation of muscle. Insufficient ionized calcium in the extracellular fluid results in continuous excitation of muscle leading to the convulsive state, hypocalcemic tetany. In passing, it should be mentioned that immunoregulatory functions have been ascribed to vitamin D, because receptors for a vitamin D metabolite have been demonstrated in activated and malignant lymphocytes, in macrophages, and in some leukemic cell lines.

Our attention here will be focused on the function of vitamin D in the regulation of serum calcium levels.

METABOLISM OF VITAMIN D. Humans have two possible sources of vitamin D—endogenous synthesis in the skin and the diet. There are large amounts of the precursor 7-dehydrocholesterol in the skin; ultraviolet light in sunlight converts it to vitamin D_3. Depending

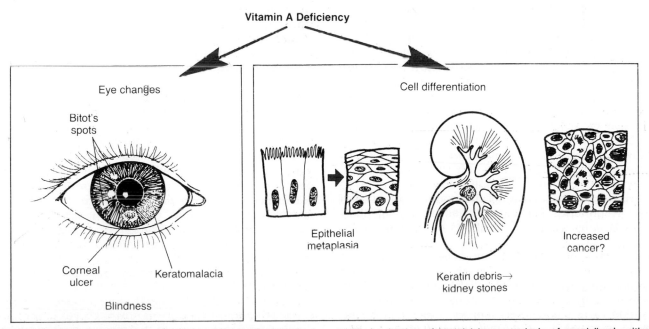

Figure 8–19. Vitamin A deficiency: its major consequences in the eye, in the production of keratinizing metaplasia of specialized epithelial surfaces, and its possible role in potentiating neoplasia.

on the skin's level of melanin pigmentation, which absorbs UV light, and the amount of exposure to sunlight, about 80% of the body's need can be endogenously derived. The remainder must be obtained from dietary sources such as deep-sea fish, plants, and grains. In the plant sources, vitamin D is present in its precursor form (ergosterol), which is converted to vitamin D_2 in the body. In many countries, various foods are fortified with vitamin D_2. Since D_3 and D_2 undergo identical metabolic transformations and have identical functions, both will hereafter be referred to as vitamin D.

The metabolism of vitamin D can be outlined as follows:

1. Absorption of vitamin D in the gut or synthesis from precursors in the skin.
2. Binding to a plasma α_1-globulin (D-binding protein or DBP) and transport to liver.
3. Conversion to 25-hydroxyvitamin D (25-OH-D) by a 25-hydroxylase in the liver.
4. Conversion of 25-OH-D to 1,25-$(OH)_2$-D by α_1-hydroxylase in the kidney. *Biologically this is the most active form of vitamin D.*

The production of 1,25-$(OH)_2$-D by the kidney is regulated by three mechanisms: (1) In a feedback loop, increased levels of 1,25-$(OH)_2$-D down-regulate synthesis of this metabolite by inhibiting the action of α_1-hydroxylase, and decreased levels have the opposite effect. (2) Hypocalcemia stimulates secretion of parathyroid hormone that, in turn, augments the conversion of 25-OH-D to 1,25-$(OH)_2$-D by activating the α_1-hydroxylase. (3) Hypophosphatemia directly increases formation of 1,25-$(OH)_2$-D.

FUNCTIONS OF VITAMIN D. 1,25-$(OH)_2$-D, the biologically active form of vitamin D, is best regarded as a steroid hormone. Like other steroid hormones it acts by binding to a high-affinity receptor that is widely distributed. However, the *essential functions of vitamin D — the maintenance of normal plasma levels of calcium and phosphorus — involve actions on the intestines, bones, and kidneys.* The active form of vitamin D (1) stimulates intestinal absorption of calcium and phosphorus; (2) collaborates with parathyroid hormone in the mobilization of calcium from bone; and (3) stimulates the parathyroid hormone (PTH)–dependent reabsorption of calcium in the distal renal tubules.

How 1,25-$(OH)_2$-D stimulates *intestinal absorption of calcium and phosphorus* is still somewhat unclear. The weight of evidence favors the view that it binds to epithelial receptors, activating the synthesis of calcium transport proteins. The increased absorption of phosphorus is independent of the effects on calcium transport.

The effects of vitamin D on *bone* depend on the plasma levels of calcium. On the one hand, with hypocalcemia, 1,25-$(OH)_2$-D collaborates with PTH in the resorption of calcium and phosphorus from bone to support the blood levels. On the other hand, vitamin D is required for *normal mineralization* of epiphyseal cartilage and osteoid matrix. It is still not clear how the resorptive function is mediated, but direct

activation of osteoclasts is ruled out. It is more likely that vitamin D favors differentiation of osteoclasts from their precursors (monocytes). Osteoblasts may also play a role, possibly by releasing an osteoclast-activating factor under the influence of vitamin D. The precise details of mineralization of bone when vitamin D levels are adequate are also uncertain. It is widely believed that the *main function of vitamin D is to maintain calcium and phosphorus at supersaturated levels in the plasma.* However, vitamin D–mediated increases in the synthesis of the calcium-binding proteins, osteocalcin and osteonectin, in the osteoid matrix may also play a role.

Equally unclear is the role of vitamin D in *renal reabsorption* of calcium. PTH is clearly necessary, but it is believed that vitamin D is, too. There is no substantial evidence that vitamin D participates in renal reabsorption of phosphorus. An overview of the normal metabolism of vitamin D and the consequences of a deficiency are depicted in Figure 8–20.

DEFICIENCY STATES. Rickets in growing children and osteomalacia in adults are worldwide skeletal diseases, but in developed countries they are rare on the basis of dietary deficiencies. Both forms of skeletal disease may result from deranged vitamin D absorption or metabolism or, less commonly, from disorders that affect the function of vitamin D or disturb calcium or phosphorus homeostasis. A summary of the causes of rickets and osteomalacia is given in Table 8–11. Whatever the basis, a deficiency of vitamin D tends to cause hypocalcemia. When hypocalcemia occurs, PTH production is increased, which (1) activates renal α_1-hydroxylase, thus increasing the amount of active vitamin D and calcium absorption, (2) mobilizes calcium from bone, (3) decreases renal calcium excretion, and (4) increases renal excretion of phosphate. Thus the serum level of calcium is restored to near normal, but hypophosphatemia persists, so mineralization of bone is impaired.

An understanding of the morphologic changes in rickets and osteomalacia is facilitated by a brief summary of normal bone development and maintenance. The development of flat bones in the skeleton involves intramembranous ossification, while the formation of the long tubular bones reflects endochondral ossification. With intramembranous bone formation, mesenchymal cells differentiate directly into osteoblasts, which synthesize the collagenous osteoid matrix upon which calcium is deposited. In contrast, with endochondral ossification, growing cartilage at the epiphyseal plates is provisionally mineralized and then progressively resorbed and replaced by osteoid matrix, which undergoes mineralization to create bone (Fig. 8–21).

MORPHOLOGY. The basic derangement in both rickets and osteomalacia is an excess of unmineralized matrix. The changes that occur in the growing bones of children with rickets, however, are complicated by inadequate provisional calcification of epiphyseal cartilage deranging

NORMAL VITAMIN D METABOLISM

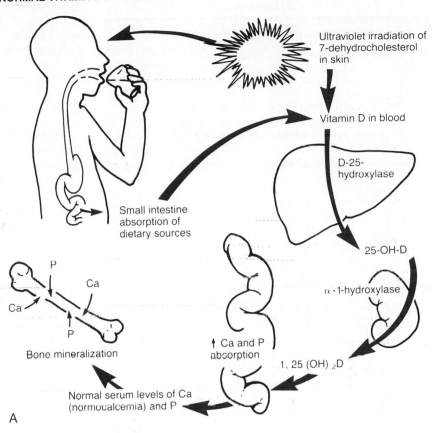

VITAMIN D DEFICIENCY

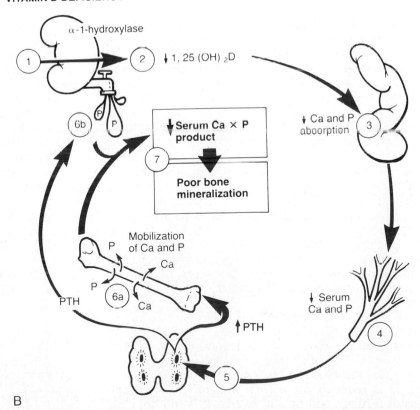

Figure 8–20. *A,* Schema of normal vitamin D metabolism. *B,* Vitamin D deficiency. There is inadequate substrate for the renal hydroxylase (1), yielding a deficiency of 1,25(OH)$_2$D (2), and deficient absorption of calcium and phosphorus from the gut (3), with consequent depressed serum levels of both (4). The hypocalcemia activates the parathyroid glands (5), causing mobilization of calcium and phosphorus from bone (6a). Simultaneously, the PTH induces wasting of phosphate in the urine (6b), and calcium retention. Consequently, the serum levels of calcium are normal or nearly normal but the phosphate is low; hence, mineralization is impaired (7).

TABLE 8-11. CAUSES OF RICKETS OR OSTEOMALACIA

Decreased Endogenous Synthesis of Vitamin D
Inadequate exposure to sunlight
Heavy melanin pigmentation of skin (blacks)

Decreased Absorption of Fat-Soluble Vitamin D in the Intestine
Dietary lack
Biliary tract, pancreatic, or intestinal dysfunction

Enhanced Degradation of Vitamin D and 25(OH)-D
Phenytoin, phenobarbital, rifampin induction of cytochrome P-450 enzymes

Impaired Synthesis of 25(OH)-D
Diffuse liver diseases

Decreased Synthesis of 1,25(OH)₂-D
Advanced renal disease with failure
Vitamin D–dependent rickets type I (inherited deficiency of renal alpha₁-hydroxylase)

Target Organ Resistance to 1,25(OH)₂-D
Vitamin D-dependent rickets type II (congenital lack of or defective receptors for active metabolite)

Phosphate Depletion
Poor absorption—long-term use of antacids, which bind phosphates and render them insoluble
Renal tubular disorders, acquired or genetic, causing increased excretion

endochondral bone growth. The following sequence ensues in rickets:

- Overgrowth of epiphyseal cartilage due to inadequate provisional calcification and failure of the cartilage cells to mature and disintegrate.

- Persistence of distorted, irregular masses of cartilage, many of which project into the marrow cavity (Fig. 8–21A).
- Deposition of osteoid matrix on inadequately mineralized cartilaginous remnants (see Fig. 8–21A).
- Disruption of the orderly replacement of cartilage by osteoid matrix, with enlargement and lateral expansion of the osteochondral junction (see Fig. 8–21A).
- Abnormal overgrowth of capillaries and fibroblasts in the disorganized zone because of microfractures and stresses on the inadequately mineralized, weak, poorly formed bone.
- Deformation of the skeleton due to the loss of structural rigidity of the developing bones.

The conformation of the gross skeletal changes depends on the severity of the rachitic process, its duration, and in particular the stresses to which individual bones are subjected. During the nonambulatory stage of infancy the head and chest sustain the greatest stresses. The softened occipital bones may become flattened and the parietal bones can be buckled inward by pressure, but with the release of the pressure, elastic recoil snaps the bones back into their original positions —**craniotabes.** An excess of osteoid produces **frontal bossing** and a **squared appearance to the head.** Deformation of the chest results from overgrowth of cartilage or osteoid tissue at the costochondral junction, producing the **"rachitic rosary."** The weakened metaphyseal areas of the ribs are subject to the pull of the respiratory muscles and thus bend inward, creating anterior protrusion of the sternum—**pigeon breast defor-**

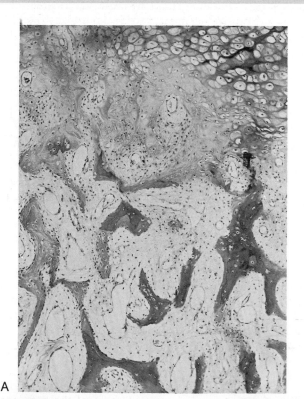
A

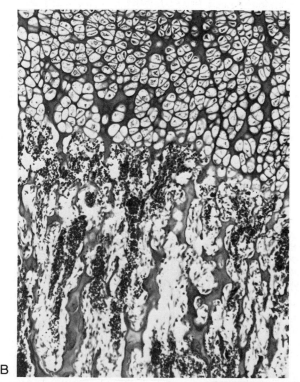
B

Figure 8–21. *A,* A detail of a rachitic costochondral junction. The palisade of cartilage is lost. Some of the trabeculae are old, well-formed bone, but the paler ones consist of uncalcified osteoid. *B,* For comparison, normal costochondral junction from a young child demonstrates the orderly transition from cartilage to new bone formation.

mity. The inward pull at the margin of the diaphragm creates **Harrison's groove,** girdling the thoracic cavity at the lower margin of the rib cage. The pelvis may become deformed. When an ambulating child develops rickets, deformities are likely to affect the spine, pelvis, and long bones (e.g., tibia), causing, most notably, **lumbar lordosis** and **bowing of the legs.**

In adults the lack of vitamin D deranges normal bone remodeling that occurs throughout life. As you know, trabecular bone is constantly being resorbed, but new bone formation exactly balances the trabecular resorption, to maintain the skeleton. The newly formed osteoid matrix laid down by osteoblasts is inadequately mineralized, thus producing the excess of persistent osteoid characteristic of **osteomalacia.** Although the contours of the bone are not affected, the bone is weak and vulnerable to gross fractures or microfractures, which are most likely to affect the vertebral bodies and femoral necks.

Histologically, the unmineralized osteoid can be visualized as a thickened layer of matrix (that stains pink in hematoxylin and eosin preparations) arranged about the more basophilic, normally mineralized trabeculae.

Persistent failure of mineralization in adults leads eventually to loss of skeletal mass, referred to as *osteopenia.* It is then difficult to differentiate osteomalacia from other osteopenias such as osteoporosis (p. 682). The distinction is important because therapy differs with the diagnosis. Ultimately, bone biopsy may be necessary to document excess unmineralized osteoid, but in the final analysis, in most instances the best way to make the diagnosis of osteomalacia is a therapeutic trial of vitamin D and calcium.

Vitamin E

A group of eight closely related fat-soluble compounds—four tocopherols and four tocotrienols—all exhibit vitamin E biologic activity, but α-tocopherol is the most active and most widely available. Vitamin E is so abundant in many foods—vegetables, grains, nuts and their oils, dairy products, fish, and meat—that a diet sufficient to sustain life is unlikely to be insufficient in vitamin E. The absorption of tocopherols, as of all fat-soluble vitamins, requires normal biliary tract and pancreatic function. After absorption, vitamin E is transported in the blood in the form of chylomicrons, which rapidly equilibrate with the plasma lipoproteins, mainly LDLs. Unlike vitamin A, which is stored predominantly in the liver, vitamin E accumulates throughout the body, mostly in fat depots but also in liver and muscle.

This essential nutrient is one of a group of *antioxidants that serve to scavenge free radicals formed in redox reactions throughout the body.* It plays a role in termination of free radical–generated lipid peroxidation chain reactions, particularly in cellular and subcellular membranes that are rich in polyunsaturated lipids. This action complements that of selenium, which as a constituent of glutathione peroxidase also metabolizes peroxides before they cause membrane damage. The nervous system is a particular target of vitamin E deficiency. Although reasons for this affinity are not entirely clear, it is speculated that neurons with long axons are particularly vulnerable because of their large membrane surface area. Mature red cells may also be vulnerable to vitamin E deficiency because they are at risk for oxidative injury imposed by the generation of superoxide radicals during oxygenation of hemoglobin. Accordingly, vitamin E, along with glutathione peroxidase and other free radical scavengers, protects against peroxide-induced hemolysis.

Hypovitaminosis E due to a deficient diet is uncommon in the Western world, and occurs almost exclusively in association with (1) *fat malabsorption,* including cholestasis, cystic fibrosis, and primary small intestinal disease, (2) *infant low birth weight* with immature liver and gastrointestinal tract, and (3) *abetalipoproteinemia,* a rare autosomal recessive disorder in which transport of vitamin E is abnormal because the apoprotein B component of chylomicrons, LDLs, and very–low density lipoproteins is not synthesized.

MORPHOLOGY. The anatomic changes found in the nervous system depend on the duration and severity of the deficiency state. Most consistent is **degeneration of the axons in the posterior columns of the spinal cord with focal accumulation of lipopigment and loss of nerve cells in the dorsal root ganglia, attributed to a dying-back type of axonopathy.** Myelin degeneration in sensory axons of peripheral nerves may also be present and, in more marked cases, degenerative changes in the spinocerebellar tracts may occur as well. Neuron pigmentation and loss have been observed in the sensory nuclei of the trigeminal, auditory, and vagus nerves. In occasional cases, features of both primary and denervation muscle disease have been observed in skeletal muscle.

Retinal pigmentary degeneration similar to that seen in severe vitamin A deficiency has also been observed in patients with abetalipoproteinemia. Whether this is due to an associated vitamin A deficiency is not certain. Vitamin E–deficient erythrocytes are more susceptible to oxidative stress and have a shorter half-life in the circulating blood.

The clinical manifestations of vitamin E deficiency depend on the distribution and severity of the neurologic lesions and vary somewhat among individuals. The most consistent ones are depressed (or, more often, absent) tendon reflexes, ataxia, dysarthria, loss of position and vibration sense, and loss of pain sensation. Muscle weakness is also common. In addition, there may be impaired vision and disorders of eye movement, sometimes progressing to total ophthalmoplegia. Anemia is not a feature of the deficiency state in adults but is often found in premature infants and is probably multifactorial in origin.

Vitamin K

Vitamin K is a required cofactor for a liver microsomal carboxylase that is necessary to convert glutamyl residues in certain protein precursors to γ-carboxyglutamates. The clotting factors II (prothrombin), VII, IX, and X all require carboxylation of glutamate residues for functional activity. Carboxylation provides calcium-binding sites and thus allows the calcium-dependent interaction of these clotting factors with a phospholipid surface involved in the generation of thrombin (p. 67). In addition, activation of anticoagulant proteins C and S also requires glutamate carboxylation.

In the course of the reaction of vitamin K with its substrate proteins its active (reduced) form is oxidized to an epoxide but then is promptly reduced back by a liver epoxide reductase (Fig. 8–22). Thus in a healthy liver vitamin K is efficiently recycled and the daily dietary requirement is low. Furthermore, endogenous intestinal bacterial flora readily synthesize the vitamin. Nevertheless, there is a small but definite need for exogenous vitamin, which fortunately is widely available in the usual Western diet. Deficiency usually occurs (1) in fat malabsorption syndromes, particularly with biliary tract disease, as with the other fat-soluble vitamins, (2) following destruction of the endogenous vitamin K–synthesizing flora, particularly with ingestion of broad-spectrum antibiotics, (3) in the neonatal period, when liver reserves are likely to be small and the bacterial flora is not yet developed, and (4) in diffuse liver disease even in the face of normal vitamin K stores, because hepatocyte dysfunction interferes with the synthesis of the vitamin K–dependent coagulation factors. In patients with thromboembolic disease therapeutically desirable vitamin K deficiency is induced by coumarin anticoagulants (e.g., warfarin). These agents block the activity of liver epoxide reductase and thereby prevent regeneration of reduced vitamin K (see Fig. 8–22).

The major consequence of vitamin K deficiency (or of inefficient utilization of vitamin K by the liver) is the development of a bleeding diathesis. In neonates the most serious manifestation is intracranial hemorrhage, but bleeding may occur at any site, including skin, umbilicus, and viscera. The estimated 3% prevalence of vitamin K–dependent bleeding diathesis among neonates warrants routine prophylactic vitamin K therapy for all newborns. However, in normal full-term infants, by one week of age endogenous flora provides sufficient vitamin K to correct any lingering deficit. In adults suffering from vitamin K deficiency or decreased synthesis of the vitamin K–dependent factors, a "bleeding diathesis" may occur, characterized by hematomas, hematuria, melena, ecchymoses, and bleeding from the gums.

Thiamine

Thiamine is widely available in the diet, although refined foods such as polished rice, white flour, and white sugar contain very little. During absorption from the gut, thiamine undergoes phosphorylation to produce thiamine pyrophosphate (TTP), the functionally active coenzyme form of the vitamin. TTP has three major functions: (1) it regulates oxidative decarboxylation of alpha-ketoacids leading to the synthesis of adenosine triphosphate (ATP), (2) it acts as a cofactor for transketolase in the pentose phosphate pathway, and, in a little-understood manner (3) it maintains neural membranes and normal nerve conduction (chiefly of peripheral nerves).

In underdeveloped countries when a large part of the scant diet consists of polished rice, as occurs in many areas of Southeast Asia, thiamine deficiency sometimes develops. In developed countries, although clinically evident thiamine deficiency is uncommon on a strictly dietary basis, it affects as many as a quarter of chronic alcoholics admitted to general hospitals. A thiamine deficiency state may also result from pernicious vomiting of pregnancy, long-term unsupplemented parenteral nutrition, or debilitating illnesses that impair the appetite, predispose to vomiting, or cause protracted diarrhea. Because a subclinical deficiency state may be converted into overt disease by extended intravenous glucose therapy or refeeding of chronically malnourished persons (particularly alcoholics), care must be taken that adequate amounts of thiamine are administered concurrently.

The major targets of thiamine deficiency are the peripheral nerves, the heart, and the brain, so persistent thiamine deficiency gives rise to three distinctive syndromes:

● a polyneuropathy (dry beriberi),
● a cardiovascular syndrome (wet beriberi),
● the Wernicke-Korsakoff syndrome.

Typically, these three syndromes appear in this sequence, but on occasion the deficiency manifests as only one of them. The polyneuropathy is *usually symmetric and takes the form of a nonspecific peripheral neuropathy with myelin degeneration and disruption of axons, involving motor, sensory, and reflex arcs.* It usually first appears in the legs, but it may extend to the arms, so classically these patients present

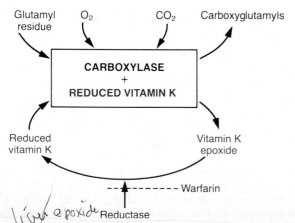

Figure 8–22. The biochemical events in the carboxylation of vitamin K–dependent proteins.

with toe, foot, and wrist drop. The progressive sensory loss is accompanied by muscle weakness and hypo- or areflexia.

Beriberi heart disease (wet beriberi) is associated with peripheral vasodilatation leading to more rapid arteriovenous shunting of blood, high-output cardiac failure, and eventually peripheral edema. The heart may be normal, have subtle changes, or be markedly enlarged and globular (owing to four-chamber dilatation) with pale, flabby myocardium. The dilatation thins the ventricular walls. Mural thrombi are often present, particularly in the dilated atria.

In protracted, severe deficiency states, most often encountered in chronic alcoholics in the Western world, *Wernicke-Korsakoff syndrome may appear.* It usually develops against a background of peripheral neuropathy and cardiac insufficiency, but in some instances it is the only manifestation of thiamine deficiency. Wernicke's encephalopathy is marked by opthalmoplegia, nystagmus, ataxia of gait and stance, and derangement of mental function characterized by global confusion, apathy, listlessness, and disorientation. About 10 to 20% of hospitalized patients with this encephalopathy die, usually of intercurrent infection, delirium tremens, liver failure, or sudden cardiovascular collapse. In the remainder, however, the initial manifestations clear in response to thiamine administration, only to reveal an underlying Korsakoff psychosis taking the form of serious impairment of remote recall (retrograde amnesia), inability to acquire new information, and confabulation. Despite thiamine therapy, only about 20% of patients who develop Korsakoff's psychosis recover completely, suggesting that the psychologic abnormality results from an irreversible anatomic lesion. Wernicke's encephalopathy and Korsakoff's psychosis are not distinct syndromes but rather successive stages of a single central nervous system disease that have the same pathophysiologic substrate.

The *central nervous system* lesions take the form of focal, symmetric areas of grayish discoloration, sometimes softening with congestion, and possibly punctate hemorrhages. These changes are particularly frequent in the paraventricular regions of the thalamus and hypothalamus; in the mammillary bodies (a favored location); about the aqueduct in the midbrain; in the floor of the fourth ventricle; and in the anterior region of the cerebellum. Histologically, there is variable hypertrophy and hyperplasia of small blood vessels, sometimes enclosed by fresh hemorrhage; degenerative changes in neurons extending to necrosis; and destruction of nerve fibers, accompanied by a surrounding glial reaction. The three major syndromes of thiamine deficiency are summarized in Figure 8–23.

Riboflavin B2

Riboflavin is a critical component of the coenzymes flavin mononucleotide (FMN) and flavin adenine dinucleotide (FAD), which participate in a wide range of oxidation-reduction reactions. In addition, flavin in covalent linkage is incorporated into succinic dehydro-

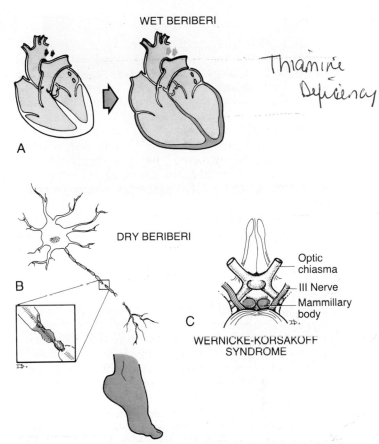

WET BERIBERI

A

Thiamine Deficiency

DRY BERIBERI

B

Optic chiasma
III Nerve
Mammillary body

C

WERNICKE-KORSAKOFF SYNDROME

Figure 8–23. *A,* The flabby, four-chambered, dilated heart of wet beriberi. *B,* The peripheral neuropathy with myelin degeneration leading to foot drop, wrist drop, and sensory changes in dry beriberi. *C,* Hemorrhages into the mammillary bodies in the Wernicke-Korsakoff syndrome.

genase and monoamine oxidase as well as into other mitochondrial enzymes. It is widely distributed in meat, dairy products, and vegetables as free riboflavin or riboflavin phosphate and is absorbed in the upper gastrointestinal tract. The conversion of riboflavin into its coenzymes (FMN and FAD) is influenced by many factors, notably hormones and drugs. For example, thyroid hormone and adrenal steroids augment synthesis of the coenzymes, whereas phenothiazines such as chlorpromazine and tricyclic antidepressants (imipramine and amitriptyline) are inhibitory.

Ariboflavinosis still occurs as a primary deficiency state among persons in economically deprived and developing countries. Under such circumstances, it is frequently accompanied by deficiencies of other vitamins and proteins. In industrialized nations, a deficiency is most likely to be encountered in alcoholics and in persons who have chronic infections, advanced cancer, or other debilitating diseases.

MORPHOLOGY. Ariboflavinosis is associated with changes at the angles of the mouth (known as cheilosis or cheilitis), glossitis, and ocular and skin changes.

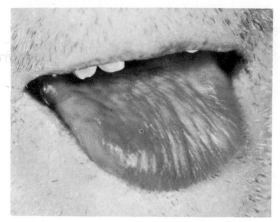

Figure 8-24. The glazed, shiny, atrophic tongue of riboflavin deficiency.

Cheilosis is usually the first and most characteristic sign of this deficiency state. It begins as areas of pallor at the angles of the mouth. Initially there is hyperkeratosis of the epidermis and a dermal inflammatory infiltrate. Later cracks or fissures may appear, radiating from the corners of the mouth, which tend to become secondarily infected.

With **glossitis** the **tongue** becomes atrophic, taking on a magenta hue strongly resembling the red-blue coloration of cyanosis (Fig. 8-24).

The **eye change** is a superficial interstitial keratitis. In the earlier stages the superficial layers of the cornea are invaded by capillaries. Interstitial inflammatory infiltration and exudation follow, producing opacities and sometimes ulcerations of the corneal surface.

A greasy, scaling **dermatitis** over the nasolabial folds may extend into a butterfly distribution to involve the cheeks and skin about the ears. Scrotal and vulvar lesions are common. In well-defined cases, atrophy of the skin may also develop. Erythroid hypoplasia in the **bone marrow** is typically present but is usually not marked.

Niacin

Niacin is the generic designation for nicotinic acid and its functionally active derivatives (e.g., nicotinamide). In the form of nicotinamide it is an essential component of two coenzymes, nicotinamide adenine dinucleotide (NAD) and nicotinamide adenine dinucleotide phosphate (NADP), both of which have central roles in cellular intermediary metabolism. NAD functions as a coenzyme for a variety of dehydrogenases involved in the metabolism of fat, carbohydrate, and amino acids. NADP participates in a variety of dehydrogenation reactions, particularly in the hexose-monophosphate shunt of glucose metabolism.

Niacin can be derived from the diet or may be synthesized endogenously. It is widely available in grains, legumes, and seed oils, and in much smaller quantities in meats. In some grains it is present in bound form and therefore not absorbable; the niacin in maize, in particular, is bound, so the niacin deficiency syndrome, pellagra, has appeared with unexpected frequency among native populations that subsist largely on maize. Niacin can also be synthesized endogenously from tryptophan. Thus pellagra may result from either a niacin or a tryptophan deficiency. In industrialized countries pellagra is encountered *sporadically (usually in combination with other vitamin deficiencies), principally among alcoholics and persons suffering from chronic debilitating illnesses.* It may also occur with protracted diarrheal states, with diets that are grossly deficient in protein, and with long-term administration of drugs such as isoniazid and 6-mercaptopurine.

MORPHOLOGY. The term pellagra, strictly speaking, refers to rough skin. The clinical syndrome, however, is classically identified by most clinicians as the three Ds—dermatitis, diarrhea, and dementia.

Dermatitis is usually bilaterally symmetric and is found mainly on exposed areas of the body. It may also occur in protected areas such as the elbows and knees and in the body folds. The changes comprise at first redness, thickening, and roughening of the skin, which may be followed by extensive scaling and desquamation, producing fissures and chronic inflammation (Fig. 8-25). Depigmentation or increased pigmentation may develop, resulting in a mottled rash. Similar lesions may occur in the mucous membranes of the mouth and vagina. The tongue often becomes red, swollen, and beefy, resembling the black tongue found in pellagrous animals.

Diarrhea is caused by atrophy of the columnar epithelium of the gastrointestinal tract mucosa, followed by submucosal inflammation. Atrophy may be followed by ulceration.

Dementia results from degeneration of the neurons in the brain accompanied by degeneration of the corresponding tracts in the spinal cord. The spinal cord lesions bear a close resemblance to the posterior column alterations observed in pernicious anemia, thus raising the question of whether a deficiency of another factor in the B complex, such as B_{12}, may also be implicated.

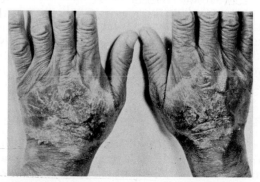

Figure 8-25. The sharply demarcated, characteristic scaling dermatitis of pellagra.

Pyridoxine (Vitamin B$_6$)

A primary, clinically overt deficiency of vitamin B$_6$ is rare in humans, but subclinical conditioned deficiency states, paradoxically, are thought to be quite common. Three naturally occurring substances, (1) pyridoxine, (2) pyridoxal, and (3) pyridoxamine, together with the phosphate forms of each, possess vitamin B$_6$ activity and are generically referred to as pyridoxine. All are equally active metabolically, and all are converted in the tissues to the coenzyme form, pyridoxal 5-phosphate. This coenzyme participates as a cofactor for a large number of enzymes involved in transaminations, carboxylations, and deaminations in the metabolism of lipids and amino acids and in the immune response.

Vitamin B$_6$ is present in virtually all foods; however, food processing may destroy the pyridoxine, and in the past it was responsible for severe deficiency in infants fed badly controlled dried milk preparations. Secondary hypovitaminosis B$_6$ is produced most often by long-term use of any of a variety of drugs that act as pyridoxine antagonists. These include isoniazid (used to treat tuberculosis), estrogens, and penicillamine. Alcoholics are also prone to develop vitamin B$_6$ deficiency because acetaldehyde, an alcohol metabolite, enhances pyridoxine degradation. Pregnancy is associated with increased demand. Thus, pyridoxine supplementation is required in these conditions.

Clinical findings in B$_6$-deficient patients resemble those of riboflavin and niacin deficiency. Patients may have seborrheic dermatitis, cheilosis, glossitis, peripheral neuropathy, and sometimes convulsions.

Vitamin C (Ascorbic Acid)

A deficiency of vitamin C leads to the development of scurvy, characterized principally by bone disease in growing children and hemorrhages and healing defects in both children and adults. Most mammals synthesize ascorbic acid from glucose via glucuronic acid because they possess a gluconolactone oxidase, but humans lack this oxidase. Ascorbic acid is present in milk and some animal products (liver, fish) and is abundant in a variety of fruits and vegetables. All but the most restricted diets provide adequate amounts of vitamin C.

With the abundance of ascorbic acid in so many foods, scurvy has ceased to be a global problem, although it is sometimes encountered even in affluent populations as a conditioned deficiency, particularly among elders, persons who live alone, and alcoholics —all groups that often have erratic and inadequate eating patterns. Occasionally scurvy appears in patients undergoing peritoneal dialysis and hemodialysis and among food faddists. Tragically, the condition sometimes appears in infants who are maintained on formulas of processed milk without supplementation.

Ascorbic acid functions in a variety of biosynthetic pathways by accelerating hydroxylation and amidation reactions. The most clearly established *function of vitamin C is the activation of prolyl and lysyl hydroxylases from inactive precursors, providing for hydroxylation of procollagen.* Inadequately hydroxylated precursors cannot acquire a stable helical configuration and cannot be adequately cross-linked, so they are poorly secreted from the fibroblast. Those that are secreted lack tensile strength, are more soluble and more vulnerable to enzymatic degradation. Collagen which normally has the highest content of hydroxyproline is most affected, such as in blood vessels, accounting for the predisposition to hemorrhages in scurvy. In addition it appears that a deficiency of vitamin C leads to *suppression of the rate of synthesis of collagen* peptides, independent of an effect on proline hydroxylation.

Scurvy in a growing child is far more dramatic than in an adult. **Hemorrhages** constitute one of the most striking features. Because the defect in collagen synthesis results in inadequate support of the walls of capillaries and venules, purpura and ecchymoses often appear in the skin, most prominently along the backs of the lower legs and in the gingival mucosa, particularly at the margins. Furthermore, the loose attachment of the periosteum to bone, together with the vascular wall defects, leads to extensive **subperiosteal hematomas** and **bleeding into joint spaces** following minimal trauma. Retrobulbar, subarachnoid, and intracerebral hemorrhages may prove fatal.

Skeletal changes may also develop in infants and children. The primary disturbance is in the formation of osteoid matrix, rather than in mineralization or calcification, such as occurs in rickets. Both membranous and endochondral bone formation may be severely disrupted. In scurvy, the palisade of cartilage cells is formed as usual and is provisionally calcified, but there is insufficient production of osteoid matrix by osteoblasts and what is laid down is unstable. Resorption of the cartilaginous matrix then fails or slows, and as a consequence there is cartilaginous overgrowth, with long spicules and plates projecting into the metaphyseal region of the marrow cavity, and sometimes widening of the epiphysis (Fig. 8–26). The epiphyseal region may be further disrupted by hemorrhage resulting from microfractures in the face of the poorly supported vessels. The scorbutic bone yields to the stresses of weight bearing and muscle tension, with bowing of the long bones of the lower legs and abnormal depression of the sternum with outward projection of the ends of the ribs (creating a so-called scorbutic rosary). The bone changes in adults are similar to those in children, with decreased formation of osteoid matrix, but deformation does not occur.

In severely scorbutic children and adults gingival swelling, hemorrhages, and secondary bacterial periodontal infection are common. A distinctive perifollicular, hyperkeratotic, papular rash that may be ringed by hemorrhage often appears. Wound healing and localization of focal infections are impaired because of the derangement in collagen synthesis. Anemia is a common finding. Most often it is normochromic and normocytic, related to bleeding into the various tissues and to de-

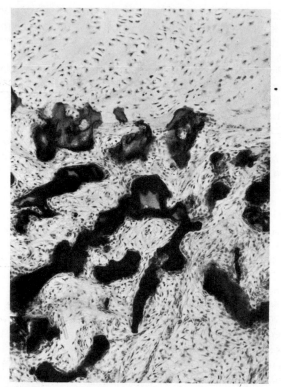

Figure 8-26. A detail of a scorbutic costochondral junction. The orderly transition from cartilage to new bone (Fig. 8-21*B*) is lost. There is dense mineralization of the spicules present but no evidence of newly formed osteoid.

creased iron absorption produced by a lack of ascorbic acid in the diet. The major features of scurvy are summarized in Figure 8-27.

Trace Elements

A number of minerals are essential for health. Calcium and phosphorus are required in large amounts and were considered in the discussion of vitamin D (p. 247). Trace elements are metals that occur at concentrations smaller than 1 μg per gram of wet tissue. Of the various trace elements found in the body only five—iron, zinc, copper, selenium, and iodine—have been associated with well-characterized deficiency states. In theory, a deficiency of a trace element might occur for many of the same reasons as does lack of a vitamin, but three influences are particularly relevant: (1) inadequate supplementation in preparations used for total parenteral nutrition, (2) interference with absorption by dietary constituents, and (3) inborn errors of metabolism leading to abnormalities of trace metal absorption. Dietary interference as a mechanism was first noted among inhabitants of Egypt and Iran who subsisted largely on unrefined cereals. Sufficient phytic acid and fiber were present in the diet to bind and block zinc absorption. *Genetic malabsorption syndromes* involving a trace element are very rare. In one, failure to synthesize metallothionein (a metal-binding protein) in intestinal mucosal cells blocks absorption of both copper and zinc.

Table 8-12 provides brief comments on the role of several trace elements in health and disease. Additional comments are offered only for zinc and selenium deficiency.

ZINC DEFICIENCY. A lack of zinc is very unusual because it is reasonably abundant in meats, fish, shellfish, whole-grain cereals, and legumes. Most cases of zinc deficiency have been related to either total parenteral nutrition unsupplemented by zinc or the aforementioned rare genetic syndrome that interferes with absorption.

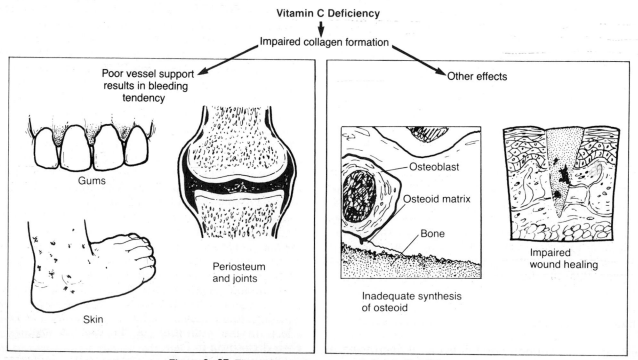

Figure 8-27. The major consequences of vitamin C deficiency.

TABLE 8–12. FUNCTIONS OF TRACE
METALS AND DEFICIENCY
SYNDROMES

Nutrient	Function	Deficiency Syndromes
Iron (p. 345)	Essential component of hemoglobin as well as a number of iron-containing metalloenzymes	Hypochromic, microcytic anemia
Zinc	Component of enzymes, principally oxidases	Acrodermatitis enteropathica, growth retardation, infertility
Iodine	Component of thyroid hormone	Goiter and hypothyroidism
Selenium	Component of glutathione peroxidase	Myopathy, rarely cardiomyopathy
Copper	Component of cytochrome C oxidase, dopamine β-hydroxylase, tyrosinase, lysyloxidase, and unknown enzyme involved in cross-linking keratin	Muscle weakness, neurologic defects, hypopigmentation, abnormal collagen cross-linking
Manganese	Component of metalloenzymes, including oxidoreductases, hydrolases, and lipases	No well-defined deficiency syndrome
Fluoride	Mechanism unknown	Dental caries

The essential features of zinc deficiency are (1) a distinctive rash, most often around the eyes, nose, mouth, anus, and distal parts, called *acrodermatitis enteropathica* (similar skin lesions may also occur in a variety of gastrointestinal diseases and chronic alcoholism); (2) anorexia, often accompanied by diarrhea; (3) growth retardation in children; (4) impaired wound healing; (5) hypogonadism with diminished reproductive capacity; (6) altered immune function; (7) impaired night vision related to altered vitamin A metabolism; (8) depressed mental function; and (9) an increased incidence of congenital malformations in infants of zinc-deficient mothers. Zinc deficiency should be suspected in any case of obscure growth retardation or infertility associated with a distinctive rash (acrodermatitis enteropathica). Oral zinc supplementation is promptly curative.

SELENIUM DEFICIENCY. Selenium deficiency is well known in China as Keshan disease, which presents as a congestive cardiomyopathy, mainly in children and young women. It results from a markedly low level of the metal in soil, water, and food. Rare instances of selenium deficiency have been described in the Western world, marked principally by skeletal myopathy rather than cardiomyopathy. Selenium is a component of glutathione peroxidase, which, like vitamin E, protects against peroxidative damage of membrane lipids. Whether this function relates to the myopathies is unclear.

OBESITY

Obesity is a common condition that is increasing in prevalence. Because it is highly correlated with an increased incidence of several diseases, it is important to define and recognize it, to understand its causes, and to be able to initiate appropriate measures to prevent it or to treat it.

Quite clearly, calories must be ingested daily to satisfy both basal metabolic needs and excess caloric needs (for metabolism of food and for energy expenditures). Calories consumed in excess of these required totals are stored, as glycogen to some extent but mainly as fat. (Fat is the most efficient form of stored energy: consider that 1 gm of fat provides nine calories while 1 gm of protein or carbohydrate provides only four). Obesity, then, is defined as an increased accumulation of body fat above a particular standard. Implicit in this definition, of course, is that the level of fat accumulation optimal for health be known.

How does one measure fat accumulation? There are several highly technical ways to approximate the measurement, but for practical considerations the following ones are commonly used:
- some expression of weight in relation to height, especially one referred to as the body mass index (BMI),
- skin fold measurements, and
- various body circumferences, particularly the ratio of the waist-to-hip circumference.

The BMI, expressed in kilograms per square meter, is closely correlated to body fat. A BMI of around 25 kg/m² is considered normal. As illustrated in Figure 8–27, persons with higher than normal BMI have an increased mortality rate. To be noted in this figure is that a BMI below 20 kg/m² is also associated with an increased mortality rate. This may be related to smoking and its attendant risks, because smoking is known to decrease appetite and subsequently the BMI.

A discussion of body fat assessment naturally leads to another question: What percentage of the body mass should be fat? Using the data in Figure 8–28 it seems reasonable to state that for maximal health the body weight should be no greater than 20% above the ideal BMI (i.e., no greater than 27 kg/m²), and that obesity is likely present when the BMI is greater than 30 kg/m². Even more important than total excess fat accumulation is the *site* of fat accumulation. *Central obesity* (when fat accumulates predominantly in the trunk and particularly in the abdomen) is associated with a much higher risk for a number of important diseases than is overall obesity (when fat also accumulates proportionally in the hips and limbs). Skin fold and waist-to-hip circumference measurements help determine these distinct types of obesity.

Causes of obesity and regulation of weight have been studied intensively and, as might be predicted, the mechanisms are complex. In studies of identical twins reared apart, genetic factors seem to be important determinants of the amount of excess fat. The genetic makeup may regulate mechanisms that determine satiety levels and thus the amount of food consumed. In addition there seems to be a genetically determined effect on the utilization of the calories ingested and their deposition in fat.

Obesity, particularly central obesity, increases the

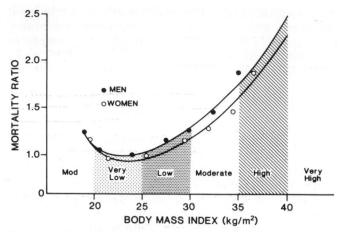

Figure 8-28. Mortality ratios are shown for men and women at different levels of body mass index. (Data from Lew EA, Garfinkel L: Variations in mortality by weight among 750,000 men and women. J. Chron. Dis. 32:563-576, 1979.)

risk for a number of conditions, including *diabetes, hypertension, hypertriglyceridemia, low HDL cholesterol* (p. 279), and, possibly, *coronary artery disease.* The mechanisms underlying these associations are complex and likely to be interrelated. Obesity, for instance, is associated with insulin resistance and hyperinsulinemia, important features of non–insulin-dependent or type II diabetes, and weight loss is associated with improvement. It has been speculated that excess insulin, in turn, may play a role in the retention of sodium, expansion of blood volume, production of excess norepinephrine, and smooth muscle proliferation that are hallmarks of hypertension. Whether or not these pathogenic mechanisms are actually operative, the risk of developing hypertension among previously normotensive persons increases proportionally with weight.

Obese persons are likely to have *hypertriglyceridemia and a low HDL cholesterol value,* and these factors may increase the risk of coronary artery disease in the *very* obese. It should be emphasized that the association between obesity and heart disease is not straightforward, and such linkage as there may be relates more to the associated diabetes and hypertension than to weight per se.

Cholelithiasis (gallstones) is six times more frequent in obese than in lean subjects. The mechanism is mainly an increase in total body cholesterol, increased cholesterol turnover, and augmented biliary excretion of cholesterol in the bile, which in turn predisposes to the formation of cholesterol-rich gallstones (p. 562).

Hypoventilation syndrome is a constellation of respiratory abnormalities in very obese persons. It has been called the *Pickwickian syndrome,* after the fat lad who was constantly falling asleep in Dickens' *Pickwick Papers.* Hypersomnolence, both at night and during the day, is characteristic and is often associated with apneic pauses during sleep, polycythemia, and eventual right-sided heart failure.

Marked adiposity predisposes to the development of

degenerative joint disease (osteoarthritis). This form of arthritis, which typically appears in older persons, is attributed in large part to the cumulative effects of wear and tear on joints. It is reasonable to assume that the greater the body burden of fat, the greater is the trauma to joints with passage of time.

The relationship between obesity and *stroke* is unclear, and opposing views can be found in the literature. According to some the true relationship to stroke is with hypertension, not with obesity per se (i.e., obese patients who are *not* hypertensive are not at higher risk for stroke).

Equally controversial is the relationship between obesity and *cancer,* particularly cancers arising in the endometrium and breast. Here the problem is complicated by the role of particular foods, such as animal fats, which may be independently associated with cancer and obesity. A summary of the relationship of obesity to these various diseases is shown in Figure 8-29.

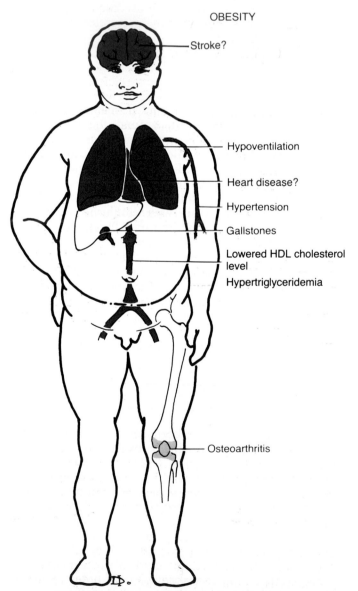

Figure 8-29. The major complications of obesity.

DIET AND SYSTEMIC DISEASES _____

The problems of under- and overnutrition, as well as specific nutrient deficiencies, have been discussed; however, the composition of the diet, even in the absence of any of these problems, may make a significant contribution to the causation and progression of a number of diseases. A few examples suffice here.

One of the most important and controversial issues today is the contribution of diet to atherogenesis. The central question is, Can dietary modification, specifically reduction in the consumption of cholesterol and saturated animal fats (e.g., eggs, butter, beef), reduce serum cholesterol levels and prevent or retard the development of atherosclerosis (most importantly coronary heart disease)? The average adult in the United States consumes an inordinate amount of fat and cholesterol daily, with a ratio of saturated fatty acids to polyunsaturated fatty acids of about 3:1. Lowering the saturates to the level of the polyunsaturates effects a 10 to 15% reduction in serum cholesterol level within a few weeks. Vegetable oils, such as corn and safflower oils, and fish oils contain polyunsaturated fatty acids and are good sources of such cholesterol-lowering lipids. Fish oil fatty acids belonging to the omega-3, or N-3, family have more double bonds than the omega-6, or N-6, fatty acids found in vegetable oils. Substitution of a portion of the saturated fat with a fish oil for a four-week period has been shown to effect a substantial reduction in serum lipid levels, particularly in triglycerides and very–low density lipoproteins, a reduction much greater than that produced with vegetable oils. Indeed, a study of Dutch men whose usual daily diet contained 30 gm of fish revealed a substantially lower frequency of death from coronary heart disease than that among comparable controls. The conclusion seems inescapable: diet modification can affect heart disease.

There are other examples of the effect of diet on disease: (1) Hypertension is beneficially affected by restricting sodium intake. (2) Dietary fiber, or roughage, resulting in increased fecal bulk, has a preventive effect against diverticulosis of the colon. (3) Even the lowly garlic has been touted to protect against heart disease (and also, alas, kisses), although research has yet to prove unequivocally this effect.

DIET AND CANCER _____

With respect to carcinogenesis, three aspects of the diet are of concern: (1) the possible content of exogenous carcinogens; (2) the potential that carcinogens might be endogenously synthesized from dietary components; and (3) a possible lack of protective factors. Relative to *exogenous carcinogens,* aflatoxins are clearly carcinogenic. There is increasing debate about the carcinogenicity of food additives, artificial sweeteners, and contaminating pesticides. The debate concerns the validity of the methods used in experimental animals to determine carcinogenicity. In order to hasten the accumulation of data or to induce sufficient numbers of cancers in experimental animals to attain significance, very high doses of the putative carcinogen are used. Whether these findings can be extrapolated to indicate an increased cancer risk for lower doses more akin to those usually used by humans is still not resolved.

The concern about *endogenous synthesis of carcinogens or promoters* from components of the diet relates principally to gastric carcinomas. With gastric carcinoma, nitrosamines and nitrosamides are believed by some to be carcinogens because they have been clearly shown to induce gastric cancer in animals. These compounds can be formed in the body from nitrites and amines or amides derived from digested proteins. Sources of nitrites include sodium nitrite, added to foods as a preservative, and nitrates, present in common vegetables, that are reduced in the gut by bacterial flora. There is, then, the potential for endogenous production of carcinogenic agents from dietary components, which might well have an effect on the stomach exposed to high concentrations.

High animal fat intake combined with low fiber intake has been implicated in the causation of colon cancer. The most convincing explanation of these associations is as follows: High fat intake increases the level of bile acids in the gut, which in turn modifies intestinal flora, favoring the growth of microaerophilic bacteria. The bile acids or bile acid metabolites produced by these bacteria might serve as carcinogens or promoters. The protective effect of a high-fiber diet might relate to (1) the increased stool bulk and decreased transit time, which decrease the exposure of mucosa to putative offenders, and (2) the capacity of certain fibers to bind carcinogens and thereby protect the mucosa. Attempts to document these theories in clinical and experimental studies have on the whole led to contradictory results.

Finally, *dietary components may also be anticarcinogenic.* For example, vitamins C and E, beta-carotenes, and selenium may be protective because of their antioxidant properties. Oxidants can cause mutations, the first step in carcinogenesis. It is theorized (but not proved) that antioxidants may play an important role in preventing cancers of all types, and their absence from the diet may potentiate the effect of carcinogens. Furthermore, the role of vitamin A in growth regulation may prove beneficial in preventing the emergence of neoplasms.

Despite much discussion in the lay press and proclamations by "diet gurus" we must conclude by saying that, to date, there is no definite proof that diet can cause or protect against cancer. Nonetheless concern persists that carcinogens lurk in things as pleasurable as a juicy steak and rich ice cream.

Bibliography _____

De Luca, L. M.: Retinoids and their receptors in differentiation, embryogenesis, and neoplasia. FASEB J. 5:2924, 1991. (An excellent review of the effects of retinoids on the regulation of normal and abnormal growth, with an extensive bibliography.)

Demling, R. H.: Burns. N. Engl. J. Med. *313:*1389, 1985. (A review of important recent advances in the care of patients with severe burns, including discussion of cardiopulmonary resuscitation, infections, metabolic and nutritional aspects, and local wound management.)

DiMaio, D. J., and DiMaio, V. J. M.: Forensic Pathology. New York, Elsevier, 1989, p. 253. (The chapter titled "Deaths due to motor vehicles" discusses with graphic illustrations the pathology of motor vehicle injury, with emphasis on fatal injury.)

Fielding, J. E., and Phenow, K. J.: Health effects of involuntary smoking. N. Engl. J. Med. 319:1452, 1988. (A summary of the data on the effects of passive smoking.)

Gawin, F. H.: Cocaine addiction: Psychology and neurophysiology. Science 251:1580, 1991. (A scholarly discussion of the neurochemical basis and clinical features of cocaine addiction.)

Gordon, I., Shapiro, H. A., and Berson, S. D.: Forensic Medicine: A Guide to Principles. New York, Churchill Livingstone, 1988, p. 221. (The chapter on wounds gives an overview of soft tissue wounds and their complications, with a brief discussion of the medicolegal ramifications of identifying the agent of injury.)

Hagen, U.: Biochemical aspects of radiation biology. Experientia 45:7, 1989. (A brief overview of the implications of DNA repair mechanisms in radiation injury.)

Harding, A. E.: Vitamin E and the nervous system. CRC Crit. Rev. Neurobiol. 3:89, 1987. (A brief review of the metabolism of vitamin E with emphasis on the clinical and pathological findings in the central nervous system in deficiency states.)

Hart, B. L., Mettler, F. A. Jr., and Harley, N. H.: Radon: Is it a problem? Radiology 172:593, 1989. (An examination of the relationship of level of radon exposure in a nonoccupational setting to an increased risk of lung cancer.)

Levine, M.: New concepts in the biology and biochemistry of ascorbic acid. N. Engl. J. Med. 314:892, 1986. (Overview of the biochemistry and physiologic effects of vitamin C.)

Mishell, D. R. Jr.: Contraception. N. Engl. J. Med. 320:777, 1989. (A review with bibliography weighs the evidence on the side effects of oral contraceptives.)

Obesity. Med. Clin. North Am. 73, 1989. (A collection of articles, each by an expert in a particular aspect, examining critical issues related to the causes, physiology, medical implications, prevention, and treatment of this common condition.)

Reichel, H., Koeffler, H. P., and Norman, A. W.: The role of the vitamin D endocrine system in health and disease. N. Engl. J. Med. 320:980, 1989. (An excellent discussion of the role of vitamin D in bone and mineral metabolism as well as possible effects on the hematopoietic system, immune system, growth regulation, and differentiation.)

Rom, W. N., Travis, W.D., and Brody, A. R.: Cellular and molecular basis of asbestos-related diseases. Am. Rev. Resp. Dis. 143:408, 1991. (A discussion of all the asbestos-related diseases, with an extensive bibliography.)

Stamper, M.J., Colditz, G.A., Willett, W.C., et al.: Postmenopausal estrogen therapy and cardiovascular disease. Ten-year follow up from nurses' health study. New Engl. J. Med. 325:756, 1991. (A comprehensive study that demonstrates the beneficial effects of estrogen therapy in reducing the incidence of and mortality from coronary artery disease.)

Upton, A. C.: Environmental medicine: Introduction and overview. Med. Clin. North Am. 74:235, 1990. (A collection of articles by experts in the field of environmental pathology and medicine. Many of the articles address the impact of environmental physical and chemical agents on specific organ systems. Of particular relevance to this chapter are the introduction and overview.)

U.S. Department of Health and Human Services: The Health Benefits of Smoking Cessation. Rockville, MD, 1990. (A compendium of the accumulated data supporting the benefits of discontinuing smoking, with a preface summarizing this data.)

U.S. Dept. of Health and Human Services. National Institute on Alcohol Abuse and Alcoholism. Seventh Special Report to the U.S. Congress on Alcohol and Health. 1990, Rockville, MD, p. 107. (A general review of the medical consequences of alcoholism.)

NINE

The Response to Infection

JOHN SAMUELSON, M.D., Ph.D.
ARLENE SHARPE, M.D., Ph.D.

CATEGORIES OF INFECTIOUS AGENTS
HOST BARRIERS TO INFECTION AND HOW
THEY BREAK DOWN
    Skin
    Respiratory Tract
    Intestinal Tract
    Spread of Microbes Throughout the Body
    Release of Microbes from the Body
HOW INFECTIOUS AGENTS CAUSE DISEASE
    Mechanisms of Virus-Induced Injury
    Mechanisms of Bacteria-Induced Injury:
        Bacterial Adhesins and Toxins
INFLAMMATORY RESPONSE TO INFECTIOUS
AGENTS

Modern industrial societies have made great progress in preventing and treating infectious diseases. Thanks to safe, uncontaminated water supplies, improved living conditions, widespread vaccination, and availability of effective antibiotics, death from infectious disease now occurs mainly in patients severely debilitated by other chronic diseases, infected with human immunodeficiency virus (HIV), or treated with immunosuppressive drugs. Instead, degenerative diseases such as atherosclerosis, cancer, and dementia are the most frequent causes of morbidity and mortality. By contrast, in the developing countries infectious diseases, aided and abetted by malnutrition and poor hygiene, continue to take their lethal toll. Most such deaths occur among children and are due to respiratory and diarrheal infections caused by common viruses and bacteria rather than by "exotic" tropical diseases.

Table 9–1 presents in chronologic sequence ten major breakthroughs in our understanding of infectious diseases and their causes, selected with the intent of providing a historical perspective for the concepts of microbial pathogenesis to be discussed here. For example, Jenner's discovery in 1798 that milkmaids working with cows were resistant to smallpox paved the way to our understanding of cross-reactive immunity; vaccinia virus induces cross-reactive immune reactions that neutralize subsequent infection with the much more virulent variola virus of smallpox. Because of a heroic vaccination campaign by the World Health Organization and others, *smallpox is the first and only disease of man that has been eradicated from the earth.* Similarly, Metchnikoff's discovery (1884) of the process of phagocytosis, whereby leukocytes ingest foreign particles, initiated the study of white cells and cell-mediated immunity in the protection against infection. Koch established the criteria for linking a specific microorganism to a specific disease: (1) the organism is regularly found in the lesions of the disease; (2) the organism can be isolated as single colonies on solid medium; (3) inoculation of this culture causes disease in an experimental animal; and (4) the organism can be recovered from the lesions in the animals. And more recently, the successful culture of polioviruses by Enders and Weller led to the development of a formalin-killed and attenuated live vaccines to prevent crippling infections by polio. Subsequently, viral cultures have been used to identify and dissect mechanisms of the pathogenesis of viral diseases.

The goal of this chapter is to discuss mechanisms by which infectious organisms cause disease. In discussing these mechanisms two separate but interrelated aspects must be considered: (1) the *specific properties of the organisms* causing the infection, and (2) *the host response to infectious agents.* Only a few of the many human infections will be used to illustrate concepts of microbial pathogenesis; greater coverage of particular organisms is found in the chapters that describe diseases by organ system (e.g., hepatitis B virus in Chapter 16 and *Mycobacterium tuberculosis* in Chapter 13). In addition, the role of the immune system and immunodeficiencies (including acquired immunodeficiency syndrome [AIDS]) in microbial infection are discussed in Chapter 6.

CATEGORIES OF INFECTIOUS AGENTS

Organisms that cause infectious diseases range in size from the 20-nm poliovirus to the 10-m tapeworm *Taenia saginata* (Table 9–2).

TABLE 9–1. TEN MAJOR DISCOVERIES IN MICROBIAL PATHOGENESIS

Year	Investigator	Discovery
1796	Jenner	Vaccination against smallpox
1865	Pasteur	Proof of germ theory and the beginning of modern biology
1882	Koch	Criteria for proof of causality in infectious disease
1884	Metchnikoff	Description of phagocytosis by macrophages
1902	Ross	Identification of mosquito vector for *Plasmodium falciparum* malaria
1906	Ehrlich	Description of chemotherapeutic agents
1908	Ellerman and Bang	Viral oncogenesis in chickens
1933	Lancefield	Serotyping of organisms and association of bacterial clones with disease
1945	Avery	Identification of DNA as genetic material and the start of the molecular biology revolution
1949	Enders	Culture of viruses and production of the polio vaccine

VIRUSES. Animal viruses are obligate intracellular agents that depend on the host metabolic machinery for their replication. Viruses are classified by the type of nucleic acid they contain—either DNA or RNA but not both—and by the shape of the surrounding protein coat or *capsid*. Viruses are the most common agents of human illness (more than 400 species), yet most human viral infections are asymptomatic and go unrecognized. Thus the distinction between viral infection (replication within the host) and viral disease (replication with tissue damage) is critical. Moreover, there are many infections in which viruses are not eliminated from the body but persist for years or for life, continuing to multiply and remaining demonstrable (chronic infection) or surviving in some *latent* noninfectious form with the potential to be reactivated

later; for example, the herpes zoster virus, the cause of chicken pox, may persist in a latent form in the dorsal root ganglia and be periodically activated to cause the painful skin condition called shingles. Different species of viruses can produce the same pathologic features (e.g., upper respiratory tract infections), and a single virus (e.g., cytomegalovirus—CMV) can produce different clinical manifestations depending on the host's resistance and age (p. 425).

Because viruses are only 20 to 300 nm large, individual viruses are best visualized with the electron microscope, where they may appear spherical or cylindrical, depending on whether the capsid proteins form an icosahedron or a helix. Some viral particles aggregate within the cells they infect and form characteristic inclusion bodies, which may be diagnostic with the light microscope. For example, CMV-infected cells are enlarged and show a large eosinophilic nuclear inclusion and smaller basophilic cytoplasmic inclusions; herpesviruses form a large nuclear inclusion surrounded by a clear halo (Fig. 9–1); smallpox and rabies viruses both form characteristic cytoplasmic inclusions. Viral inclusions are often difficult to find, and many viruses do not give rise to inclusions (e.g., HIV, Epstein-Barr virus).

BACTERIOPHAGES, PLASMIDS, AND TRANSPOSONS. Bacteriophages, plasmids, and transposons are mobile genetic elements that infect bacteria and indirectly cause human diseases by encoding bacterial virulence factors, including adhesins (see also p. 270), toxins, and enzymes that confer drug resistance. The addition of a bacteriophage or plasmid can instantly convert nonpathogenic bacteria into virulent ones, and plasmids encoding antibiotic resistance can quickly disseminate among many different microbial species.

BACTERIA. Bacteria are unicellular, prokaryotic cells that are distinguished from eukaryotic cells (e.g., mammalian cells) by the absence of a nucleus and an endoplasmic reticulum. However, bacteria contain

TABLE 9–2. CLASSES OF HUMAN ENDOPARASITES AND THEIR HABITATS

Taxonomic Class	Size	Site of Propagation	Sample Species and Its Disease	
Viruses	20–30 nm	Obligate intracellular	Poliovirus	Poliomyelitis
Chlamydiae	200–1000 nm	Obligate intracellular	*C. trachomatis*	Trachoma
Rickettsiae	300–1200 nm	Obligate intracellular	*R. prowazekii*	Typhus fever
Mycoplasmas	125–350 nm	Extracellular	*M. pneumoniae*	Atypical pneumonia
Bacteria, spirochetes, mycobacteria	0.8–15 μm	Cutaneous Mucosal Extracellular Facultative intracellular	*Staphylococcus epidermidis* *Vibrio cholerae* *Streptococcus pneumoniae* *M. tuberculosis*	Wound infection Cholera Pneumonia Tuberculosis
Fungi imperfecti	2–200 μm	Cutaneous Mucosal Extracellular Facultative intracellular	*Trichophyton* sp. *Candida albicans* *Sporothrix schenkii* *Histoplasma capsulatum*	Tinea pedis (athlete's foot) Thrush Sporotrichosis Histoplasmosis
Protozoa	1–50 mm	Mucosal Extracellular Facultative intracellular Obligate intracellular	*G. lamblia* *Trypanosoma gambiense* *Trypanosoma cruzi* *L. donovani*	Giardiasis Sleeping sickness Chagas' disease Kala-azar
Helminths	3 mm–10 m	Mucosal Extracellular Intracellular	*Enterobius vermicularis* *Wuchereria bancrofti* *Trichinella spiralis*	Oxyuriasis Filariasis Trichinosis

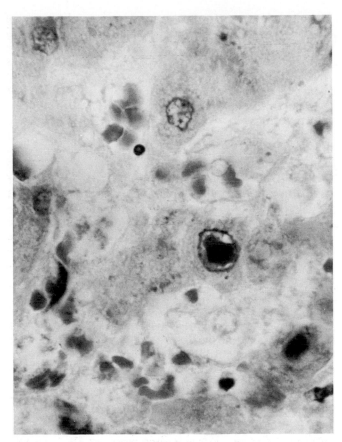

Figure 9–1. Herpes simplex inclusion body in a liver cell.

of the fallopian tubes, and (2) blindness, by trachoma, a chronic inflammation of the conjunctiva that eventually scars the cornea and makes it opaque.

Rickettsiae are transmitted by insect vectors, including lice (epidemic typhus), ticks (Rocky Mountain spotted fever, Q fever), and mites (scrub typhus). By injuring the endothelial cells, rickettsiae cause a hemorrhagic vasculitis that is often visible as a skin rash, but they may also cause a transient pneumonia or hepatitis (Q fever) or injure the central nervous system and cause death (Rocky Mountain spotted fever and epidemic typhus).

Mycoplasmas and the closely related ureaplasmas are the tiniest free-living organisms known (125 to 300 nm). Mycoplasmas spread from person to person in aerosols, bind to the surface of epithelial cells in the airways, and cause an atypical pneumonia characterized by peribronchiolar infiltrates of lymphocytes and plasma cells. Ureaplasmas are transmitted venereally and may cause nongonococcal urethritis (NGU).

FUNGI. Fungi are the most plant-like of human pathogens: they have thick cell walls, may have more than one single form in tissue or in culture, and frequently grow by extension and branching of filamentous structures. Fungi that infect man can be divided into those that remain superficial (i.e., dermatophytes restricted to the epidermal surface) and those that invade deep organs and tissues (deep fungi). Superficial fungi include *Tinea* species, which cause regional hair loss, depigmentation, "jock itch," and ath-

both DNA and RNA, synthesize proteins on ribosomes, and have cell walls composed of two phospholipid bilayer membranes separated by a peptidoglycan layer (gram-negative organisms) or an inner membrane surrounded by a peptidoglycan layer (gram-positive organisms). A normal healthy person is colonized by as many as 10^{12} bacteria on the skin, 10^{10} bacteria in the mouth, and 10^{14} bacteria in the alimentary tract. Bacteria colonizing the skin include *Staphylococcus epidermidis*, *Corynebacterium* species, and *Propionibacterium acnes* (the cause of acne among adolescents). Aerobic and anaerobic bacteria, particularly *Streptococcus mutans*, contribute to a dense microbial mass called dental plaque, a major cause of tooth decay. In the colon, more than 99.9% of bacteria are anaerobic, including *Bacteroides* species. When they invade the body, many bacteria remain extracellular, whereas *facultative intracellular bacteria* can survive and either replicate within host cells or outside of host cells (e.g., *Mycobacterium;* Fig. 9–2).

CHLAMYDIA, RICKETTSIA, AND MYCOPLASMA. These infectious agents are grouped together because they are similar to bacteria (they divide by binary fusion and are susceptible to antibiotics) but lack certain structures (for mycoplasmas a rigid cell wall) or metabolic capabilities (*Chlamydia* species cannot synthesize ATP). Chlamydiae and rickettsiae are obligate intracellular agents that replicate in phagosomes of epithelial cells and in the cytoplasm of endothelial cells, respectively. *Chlamydia trachomatis* is the leading infectious cause of (1) female sterility, by scarring and narrowing

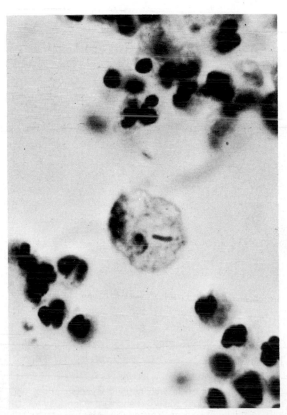

Figure 9–2. A mononuclear phagocyte with an engulfed tubercle bacillus.

lete's foot. Cutaneous fungi may also infect fingernails or subcutaneous tissues (*chromomycosis* or *mycetomas*). _Pathogenic deep fungi are geographic in their distribution_, because they depend on inhaled spores that are frequent in particular climates (e.g., *Histoplasma* in the Ohio River Valley, *Coccidioides* in the western United States, or *Blastomyces* in the tropics). These fungi often form localized granulomas in the lung but disseminate if a host becomes immunodeficient. _Opportunistic deep fungi_, in contrast, cause life-threatening infections only in immunosuppressed persons, producing widespread necrosis with minimal cellular infiltrates and frequent hemorrhages. AIDS patients with depressed cellular immunity and those receiving chemotherapy suffer recurrent oral infections with *Candida* (thrush) and systemic infections by these or other fungi such as *Aspergillus, Mucor,* and *Pneumocystis* (Fig. 9–3).

PROTOZOAN PARASITES. Parasitic protozoa are motile, single-celled eukaryotes that are among the foremost causes of disease and death in developing countries. In industrialized countries, protozoa are widely prevalent but are less often lethal. The simplest protozoan parasite is *trichomonas,* which has a single flagellated form, is sexually transmitted, and colonizes the vagina and the male urethra. Intestinal protozoa include the highly prevalent *Entamoeba histolytica* and *Giardia lamblia.* All have two forms: (1) motile trophozoites that attach to the intestinal epithelial wall and

may invade *(E. histolytica),* and (2) immobile cysts that are infectious when eaten because they have a chitin wall that is resistant to stomach acids. Protozoa that reside in the blood (*Trypanosoma brucei,* cause of African sleeping sickness) or in blood cells (*Plasmodia,* agents of malaria in erythrocytes, *Leishmania* and *Trypanosoma cruzi* in macrophages) are transmitted by insect vectors, in which they replicate extracellularly and are motile. *Toxoplasma* (an intracellular parasite) infection is acquired when humans ingest intramuscular cysts in undercooked meat.

HELMINTHS. Helminths are multicellular worms that have strict specificities for the *definitive host, in which* sexual reproduction takes place, or for the *intermediate host, or vector,* in which reproduction is asexual. Helminths do not themselves multiply within the host but instead make eggs, which must be cycled through the environment, insects, or snails before humans can be infected again. An exception to this scheme is *Strongyloides,* the larvae of which can become infectious while in the gut and cause overwhelming autoinfection. There are two important consequences of the lack of replication of adult worms: (1) disease is often caused by inflammatory responses to the eggs rather than to the adults (e.g., schistosomiasis) and (2) severity of disease is proportional to the number of organisms that have infected the host (e.g., 10 hookworms have little effect, whereas 1000 hookworms cause severe anemia by consuming 100 ml of blood per day). Fortunately, most persons in endemic areas harbor few worms and are free of disease and only a minority are heavily infected and ill.

There are three major classes of helminths: (1) the *roundworms (Nematodes)* including *Ascaris,* hookworms, and pinworms, which remain in the intestinal lumen, and *Trichinella* species, which invade tissues; (2) *flatworms (Cestodes)* including fish, beef, and pork tapeworms, and *Echinococcus* (hydatids); and (3) *flukes (trematodes)* including the important *schistosomes.* All human parasitic helminths are extracellular except for the larvae of *Trichinella spiralis,* which encyst for a very long time in skeletal muscles and so compensate for the short-lived existence of their adult parent (Fig. 9–4).

ECTOPARASITES. Ectoparasites are insects (lice, bedbugs, fleas) or arachnids (mites, ticks) that attach and live on or in the skin. These insects may cause itching and excoriations (e.g., pediculosis caused by lice attached to hair shafts or scabies caused by mites burrowing into the stratum corneum). Classically, at the site of the bite, mouth parts may be found in association with a mixed infiltrate of lymphocytes, macrophages, and eosinophils. In addition, attached arthropods can be vectors for other pathogens that produce characteristic skin lesions (e.g., the expanding erythematous plaque caused by the Lyme disease spirochete *Borrelia burgdorferi,* which is transmitted by deer ticks).

We will now turn to a discussion of the pathogenesis of infection and discuss first the normal host defenses against the entry and establishment of infectious agents and how these defenses can be overwhelmed.

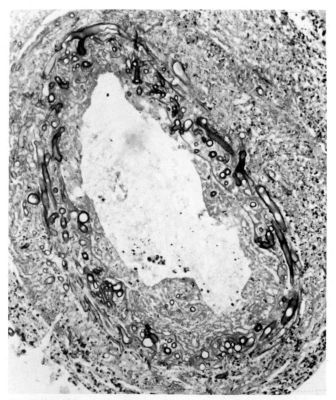

Figure 9–3. Mucormycosis with hyphae invading artery wall. Note irregular width and right-angled branching. (Courtesy of Dr. Jack Frenkel, University of Kansas, Kansas City, MO.)

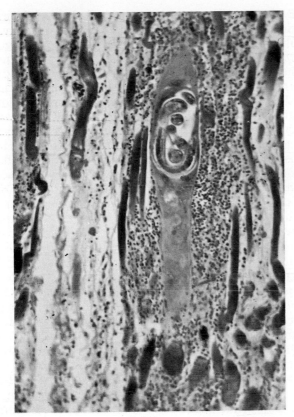

Figure 9–4. Trichinosis with a coiled, encysted parasite larva within skeletal muscle.

HOST BARRIERS TO INFECTION AND HOW THEY BREAK DOWN

Host barriers to infection prevent access of microbes to the body and their subsequent spread throughout the tissues. The first barriers are the intact skin and mucosal surfaces and the secretions that these surfaces produce; for example, lysozyme in tears degrades the peptidoglycan wall of bacteria. These are formidable defenses against most infections. Only four of every ten exposures to gonococci result in gonorrhea, and it takes 10^{11} vibrios to produce cholera in human volunteers with normal gastric juices. Still, some infectious agents are able to overcome these barriers, so that as few as 100 *Shigella* organisms, *Giardia* cysts or *M. tuberculosis* organisms, are sufficient to cause illness. In general, respiratory, gastrointestinal, and genitourinary tract infections occur in normal persons and are caused by relatively virulent organisms that are able to damage intact epithelial barriers. In contrast, most skin infections are caused by less virulent organisms entering through lesions caused by cuts or insect bites.

SKIN

Normal skin can be heavily colonized with a variety of bacteria, principally gram-positive cocci. Human skin, however, is covered by a relatively impermeable and dry outer layer of keratinocytes, many of which are shed each day along with attached colonies of bacteria. The low pH of the skin (about 5.5) and the presence of fatty acids also inhibit microbial growth, but wet skin is more permeable to microorganisms. Human papillomavirus, the cause of venereal warts, and *Treponema pallidum,* the agent of syphilis, both penetrate warm, moist skin during sexual intercourse. Superficial infections of the stratum corneum of the epidermis by *Staphylococcus aureus* (impetigo) or by cutaneous fungi are all aggravated by heat and humidity. Schistosome larvae released from fresh water snails penetrate the swimmer's skin by releasing collagenase, elastase, and other enzymes that dissolve the extracellular matrix. Most other microorganisms penetrate through lesions in skin, including superficial pricks (fungal infections), deep wounds (staphylococci), burns *(Pseudomonas aeruginosa),* and diabetic and pressure-related foot sores (multibacterial infections). Intravenous catheters in hospitalized patients frequently cause bacteremia with *Staphylococcus* species or gram-negative organisms. Needlesticks, intentional by drug abusers or unintentional by health care workers, expose the recipient to potentially infected blood and may transmit hepatitis B and HIV infection. However, the chance of the recipient becoming infected by a single needlestick varies greatly for these two viruses: up to 0.5% for HIV-1, and as much as 43% for "e" antigen–positive hepatitis B (p. 534).

Insect bites by fleas, ticks, mosquitoes, mites, and lice break the skin and transmit diverse infectious organisms, including arboviruses (causes of yellow fever and encephalitis), rickettsiae (typhus and Rocky Mountain spotted fever), bacteria (plague, Lyme disease), protozoa (malaria, leishmaniasis), and helminths (filariasis). The protozoans and helminths undergo important developmental changes in their insect vectors, and their infectivity may be much enhanced by the release from the insects of potent anticoagulants or vasodilators. For example, the infectivity of *Leishmania* in mice is increased 1000-fold by co-injection with saliva from the sandfly vector. Finally, animal bites may cause infections with anaerobic bacteria or with the deadly rabies virus.

RESPIRATORY TRACT

Some 10,000 microorganisms, including viruses, bacteria, and fungi, are inhaled daily by each city inhabitant. The distance these microorganisms travel into the respiratory system is inversely proportional to their size. Large microbes are trapped in the mucociliary blanket that lines the nose and the upper respiratory tract. Microorganisms are trapped in the mucus secreted by goblet cells and are then transported by ciliary action to the back of the throat, where they are swallowed and cleared. Organisms smaller than 5 μm travel directly to the alveoli, where they are phagocytosed by alveolar macrophages or by neutrophils recruited to the lung by cytokines. Damage to the mucociliary defense results from repeated insults in smokers and in patients with cystic fibrosis, while acute injury occurs in intubated patients and in those who aspirate gastric acid. Virulent respiratory pathogens escape the intact mucociliary defense by attaching via hemagglutinins to carbohydrates on epithelial cells in the lower respiratory system and pharynx (e.g., influenza virus). Further, it is thought that influenza, parainfluenza, and mumps viruses use viral neuraminidase to lower the viscosity of mucus and free themselves from entrapment. Certain organisms (e.g., *Haemophilus influenzae*) release factors that inhibit ciliary motion. Secondary respiratory infections with *Streptococcus pneumoniae* or *Staphylococcus* species, which lack specific adherence factors, occur after viral damage to epithelial cells. *M. tuberculosis* causes respiratory infection because it is able to escape phagocytotic killing by the macrophage. Finally, opportunistic fungi infect the lungs when cellular immunity is depressed and leukocytes are deficient in number (e.g., *Pneumocystis carinii* in AIDS and *Aspergillus* in patients receiving chemotherapy.)

INTESTINAL TRACT

Most gastrointestinal pathogens are transmitted by food or drink contaminated with human feces so that exposure can be reduced by washing hands, obtaining clean water, and using proper cooking methods. Defenses against microbial invasion through the gastrointestinal tract include: (1) the mucus covering of epithelial cells; (2) acid in gastric juice; (3) pancreatic enzymes; (4) the detergent bile salts; and (5) secreted antibodies (IgA). In addition, pathogenic organisms must compete for nutrients with nonpathogenic bacteria already growing within the intestinal lumen (mostly anaerobes), and all organisms are passed from the body each day with the stool.

Like many respiratory infections, most gastrointestinal infections occur in healthy persons who are exposed to relatively virulent organisms that can escape the normal host defenses. Several conditions interfere with these gastrointestinal defenses:

- *Decrease of gastric acid.* This can be caused by chronic disease or ingestion of antacids. For example, the infectious dose of cholera bacteria is reduced from 10^{11} organisms to 10^4 if gastric pH is increased.
- *Treatment with antibiotics.* Antibiotics alter the normal flora so that it is overrun by pathogenic bacteria (e.g., *Clostridium difficile,* an important cause of pseudomembranous enterocolitis, p. 506).
- *Interference with normal bowel motion or outright obstruction* (e.g., blind loop syndrome).

VIRUSES. Most enveloped viruses are killed by secretions and so cannot enter via the gut, but nonenveloped *enteropathic viruses,* such as hepatitis A virus, are resistant to stomach acids, intestinal proteases, and bile. Rotaviruses infect and damage intestinal epithelia; reoviruses pass through mucosal M cells into the blood without causing any detectable local injury.

BACTERIA. Some enteropathogenic bacteria release toxins that can damage the host without invading or multiplying in the gut wall (e.g., food poisoning by *Staphylococcus* species, and *Clostridium botulinum*). Other bacteria (e.g., *Vibrio cholerae* and toxigenic *E. coli*) use their flagellae to move along a chemotactic gradient through the mucus layer covering colonic epithelial cells, and attach via specific adhesins to sugars in the brush border of epithelial cells. There the bacteria multiply and release toxins (see p. 271) that cause epithelial cells to secrete large volumes of fluid into the lumen. The result is a watery diarrhea by which the physiology of the intestinal epithelium and of the host is dramatically affected, although histopathologic changes are relatively slight. In contrast, other bacteria (e.g., *Shigella, Salmonella* species, *Campylobacter*) invade and disrupt the intestinal epithelium and so cause ulcerations, inflammation, and hemorrhage, which present clinically as dysentery (p. 504). Finally, some bacteria (e.g., *Salmonella typhi* and *Yersinia*) pass through the epithelium and enter Peyer's patches, where they multiply and cause pathologic changes.

PARASITES. Intestinal parasites break the intestinal barrier by a number of different mechanisms. The cyst forms of protozoan parasites *E. histolytica* and *G. lamblia* are infectious because they are resistant to stomach acids, while the motile trophozoite forms cause injury by attaching via parasite lectins to sugars on the intestinal epithelium cells (Fig. 9–5). *Giardia*

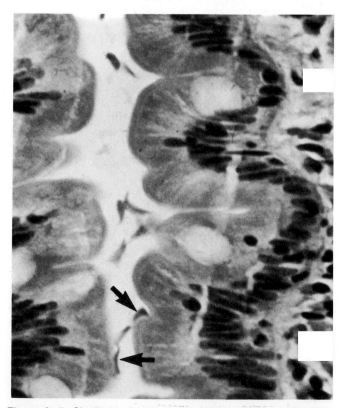

Figure 9–5. Giardiasis of jejunum. Parasites *(arrows)* show sickle-shaped profile; some are sitting on the epithelial brush border.

and *Cryptosporidium* species damage the epithelium without stromal invasion, while *Entamoeba* organisms cause contact-mediated cytolysis by releasing a channel-forming pore protein (similar to that of cytotoxic lymphocytes) that inserts into the target epithelial cell plasma membrane and depolarizes it. Some helminth parasites can damage the host by remaining in the intestinal lumen and consuming essential nutrients (e.g., the fish tapeworm, which depletes the host of vitamin B_{12}) or by mechanically obstructing the bile duct (*Ascaris*). Ancylostomas (hookworms) suck the blood from the intestinal vessels and so may cause severe iron-deficiency anemia. Finally, some helminth larvae pass innocuously through the intestines and then encyst in muscle (*Trichinella*) or the central nervous system (*Cysticerca*).

SPREAD OF MICROBES THROUGHOUT THE BODY

Microbes spread rapidly along the wet epithelial surfaces of the intestines, lungs, and genitourinary tract and, slowly, if at all, on the dry surface of the skin. Many microbes do not travel beyond the epithelium because they proliferate only in superficial layers of epithelia (e.g., HPV), but others are able to penetrate (e.g., streptococci and staphylococci, which secrete hyaluronidase that degrades the extracellular matrix between host cells). The routes of microbial spread initially follow tissue planes of least resistance and the regional lymphatic and vascular anatomy. For example, staphylococci cause a locally expanding skin abscess (furuncle), followed by regional lymphadenitis, that sometimes leads to bacteremia (blood-borne infection) and colonization of distant organs deep to the body's surfaces (heart, liver, brain, spleen, bones). Invasive parasites secrete proteolytic enzymes (e.g., collagenase and elastase) that also degrade the extracellular matrix. Once in the blood, organisms are transported by a variety of means. Hepatitis B and polioviruses, most bacteria and fungi, and all helminths are transported *free in the plasma.* Herpesviruses, HIV, CMV, and *Mycobacterium, Leishmania,* and *Toxoplasma* organisms are carried by leukocytes. Certain viruses (Colorado tick fever virus) and parasites (plasmodia, agents of malaria) are carried by red cells.

Dissemination of the pathogens in the blood can lead to systemic signs of infection, including fever, which is caused by host cytokines released in response to bacterial endotoxin (p. 45). Massive sustained bloodstream invasion by pyogenic bacteria and certain parasites (e.g., malaria) may be fatal. Infectious foci disseminated by blood are called secondary and usually have a widespread distribution, either in a single organ (e.g., the miliary or seedlike distribution of secondary *tuberculosis* within the lung) or through many tissues (e.g., microabscesses throughout the kidneys, intestines, and skin caused by septic emboli shed from a staphylococcal aortic valve infection). Invasive microbes quickly spread within fluid-lined cavities such as

pleura, peritoneum, and meninges. Frequently, organisms cause the major disease manifestations at sites distant from the point of entry. For example, the chicken pox virus enters through the lungs (Fig. 9–6) but causes rashes in the skin; polioviruses enter through the intestine but selectively cause damage to motor neurons; and *Schistosoma mansoni* penetrate the skin but eventually localize in blood vessels of the portal system and the mesentery, causing damage to the liver and intestines. Rabies viruses track to the brain in a retrograde fashion along nerves, while varicella-zoster virus, after its viremic phase, hides in dorsal root ganglia, whence it may travel along the nerves and cause shingles.

Severe damage to the developing fetus occurs when infectious organisms circulate in the mother's blood or reach the uterus from the vagina to infect the placenta and the baby. Placental or fetal infections with bacteria frequently cause premature birth or stillbirth, while viral infections can also cause maldevelopment of the fetus, depending on the time of infection. Rubella infection in the first trimester may cause congenital heart disease, mental retardation, cataracts, or deafness in the baby, whereas little damage is caused by rubella infection in the third trimester. In contrast, transmission of treponemes gives rise to syphilis only when they invade the fetus late in the second trimester, but then they cause a severe fetal osteochondritis and periostitis that leads to multiple bony lesions. Treponemes, CMV, herpesviruses, and toxoplasmas all infect and damage the fetal nervous system. Because these infections persist at birth, their diagnosis and subsequent treatment is important. During the birth process, infants can also become infected with the mother's viruses and bacteria, which may subsequently cause acquired immunodeficiency (HIV), chronic hepatitis or liver cancer (hepatitis B virus), blindness (chlamydia), and multisystem organ failure (herpesviruses).

RELEASE OF MICROBES FROM THE BODY _____

For transmission of disease, the exit of infectious agents from the host's body is as important as their entry into it. Many of the mechanisms by which infectious organisms are cleared from the infected individual are responsible for their spread from one person to another, including skin shedding, coughing, sneezing, urination, and defecation. Stool pathogens that are resistant to drying (e.g., bacterial spores, protozoan cysts, helminth eggs) survive in the environment for a long time, whereas certain viruses must be quickly passed from person to person, often by direct contact. Stool-contaminated food and water are important vehicles for spread of epidemic and endemic pathogens. Viruses that infect the salivary glands (e.g., herpesvirus, mumpsvirus) are released during talking, singing, spitting, and kissing. All classes of organisms are transmitted by intimate mucosal or venereal contact, including viruses (e.g., herpesvirus, human papillomavirus, hepatitis B virus, HIV), chlamydia, bacteria

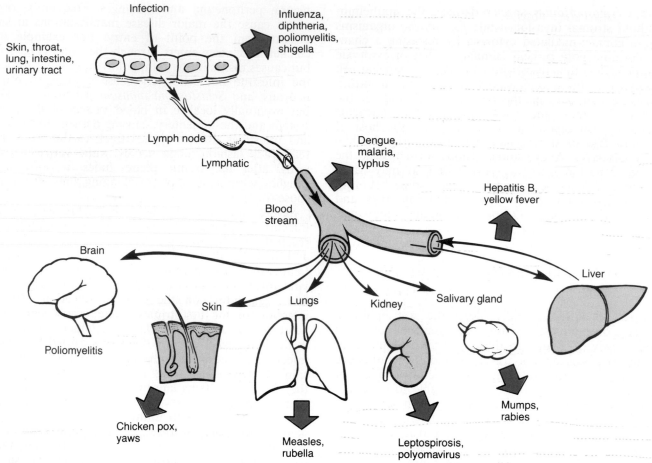

Figure 9-6. Routes of entry, dissemination, and release of microbes from the body. (Adapted from Mims, C. A.: The Pathogenesis of Infectious Disease. Orlando, FL, Academic Press, 1987.)

(*T. pallidum* and *Neisseria gonorrhoeae*), fungi *(Candida),* protozoa *(Trichomonas),* and insects *(Phthiris pubis* or crab lice). Microorganisms transmitted by blood-sucking arthropods must be in the blood to infect the next insect that feeds, even when the major lesions caused by them are in the brain (viral encephalitis), liver, spleen *(Leishmania donovani),* or heart *(Trypanosoma cruzi* in Chagas' disease).

HOW INFECTIOUS AGENTS CAUSE DISEASE

Having reviewed the manner by which infectious agents break host barriers, we will examine how they injure cells and cause tissue damage. There are three general mechanisms:

1. Infectious agents contact or enter host cells and directly cause cell death.
2. Pathogens can release endotoxins or exotoxins that kill cells at a distance; release enzymes that degrade tissue components; or damage blood vessels and cause ischemic necrosis.
3. Pathogens can induce host cell responses that may

cause additional tissue damage, usually by immune-mediated mechanisms.

Immune-mediated injury is discussed in Chapter 6. Here we describe some of the specific mechanisms whereby viruses and certain bacteria cause cell and tissue injury.

MECHANISMS OF VIRUS-INDUCED INJURY

Viruses damage host cells by entering the cell and replicating at the host's expense. They have specific surface viral proteins (ligands) that bind to particular host proteins (receptors), many of which have known functions. For example, HIV binds to the protein involved with T-cell activation (CD4) on helper lymphocytes, Epstein Barr virus binds to the complement receptor (CR2) on macrophages, and rhinoviruses bind to the adherence protein ICAM-1 on mucosal cells. For several viruses, x-ray crystallographic studies have identified the specific part of the viral attachment protein that binds to a particular segment of the host cell receptor, and this knowledge may lead eventually to the rational design of antiviral drugs and vaccines.

The presence or absence of host cell proteins that allow the virus to attach is one reason for *viral tropism*—the tendency of certain viruses to infect specific cells but not others. Similarly, some paramyxoviruses are not infectious until their envelope glycoproteins undergo proteolytic cleavage by tissue proteases to reveal the cryptic viral attachment sites that bind to host cells. A second major cause of viral tropism is the ability of the virus to *replicate* inside some cells but not in others. Viral enhancer or promoter sequences determine this specificity. For example, the JC papovavirus infection of leukoencaphalopathy is restricted to oligodendroglia in the central nervous system (p. 712). Studies of foreign DNA expression in cultured cells show that the JC virus promoter and enhancer DNA sequences upstream from the viral genes are active in cultured glial cells but not in other cell types. Similarly, when JC virus genes are injected into transgenic mice, oligodendroglial dysfunction is dependent on the presence of particular JC virus promoter and enhancer sequences that are recognized by glial cell–specific proteins involved in mRNA synthesis.

Once attached, the entire virion, or a portion containing the genome and essential polymerases, penetrates into the cell cytoplasm by (1) translocation of the entire virus across the plasma membrane, (2) fusion of the viral envelope with the cell membrane, or (3) receptor-mediated endocytosis and fusion with endosomal membranes. Within the cell the virus uncoats, separating its genome from its structural components and losing its infectivity. Viruses then replicate, using enzymes that are distinct for each virus family. For example, RNA polymerase is used by negative-sense RNA viruses to generate positive-sense mRNA, while reverse transcriptase is used by retroviruses to generate DNA from their RNA template. These virus-specific enzymes provide points at which drugs may be used to inhibit viral replication. Viruses also use host enzymes for viral synthesis, and such enzymes may be present in some but not all of the tissues. Newly synthesized viral genomes and capsid proteins are assembled into progeny virions in the nucleus or cytoplasm and are either released directly (unencapsulated viruses) or bud through the plasma membrane (encapsulated viruses).

Viruses kill host cells and cause tissue damage in a number of ways (Fig. 9–7).

- Viruses may inhibit host cell DNA, RNA, or protein synthesis. For example, the poliovirus inactivates "cap-binding protein," a protein essential for translation of host cell mRNAs, but leaves translation of poliovirus mRNAs unaffected.
- Viral proteins may insert into the host cell's plasma membrane and directly damage its integrity or promote cell fusion (HIV, measles, and herpesviruses).
- Viruses replicate efficiently and lyse host cells. For example, respiratory epithelial cells are killed by explosive rhinovirus or influenza virus multiplication; liver cells by yellow fever virus; and neurons by poliovirus or rabies viruses.
- Virus-dictated proteins on the surface of the host

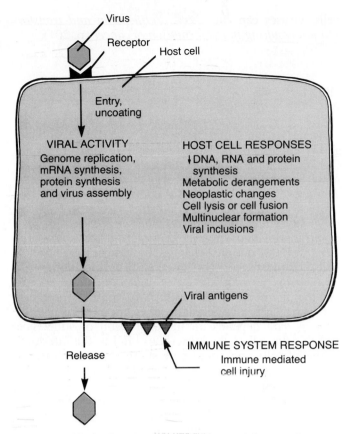

Figure 9–7. Mechanisms by which viruses cause injury to cells.

cells may be recognized by the immune system, and the host lymphocytes attack the virus-infected cells (e.g., liver cells infected with hepatitis B virus). Some persistent viruses escape immune recognition by reducing the expression of viral peptides or MHC class I antigens on the cell surface.

- Viruses may also damage cells involved in host antimicrobial defense, leading to secondary infections. For example, viral damage to respiratory epithelium predisposes to the subsequent development of pneumonia caused by the pneumococci or *Haemophilus* organisms, while HIV depletes CD4+ helper lymphocytes and opens the floodgates for many opportunistic infections.
- Viral killing of cells of one type may cause damage to other cells that are dependent on their integrity. Denervation by the attack of poliovirus on motor neurons causes atrophy, and sometimes death, of distal skeletal muscle cells.
- *Slow virus infections* (e.g., subacute sclerosing panencephalitis caused by measles virus) culminate in severe progressive disease after a long latency period. The precise mechanism of injury under these conditions is unknown but is now under intensive study.

In addition to all the potential mechanisms of killing

cells, viruses can cause *cell proliferation and transformation resulting in the formation of cancer* (p. 201).

MECHANISMS OF BACTERIA-INDUCED INJURY: BACTERIAL ADHESINS AND TOXINS _____

Bacterial damage to host tissues depends on their ability to adhere to host cells and to deliver toxins. Certain bacteria also enter the cell (see below), though most extracellular bacteria also cause tissue damage. *The coordination of bacterial adherence and toxin delivery is so important to bacterial virulence that the genes encoding adherence proteins and toxins are frequently regulated together by specific environmental signals.* For example, changes in temperature, osmolarity, or pH trigger the synthesis by *Bordetella pertussis* of some 20 different genes, including those encoding the filamentous hemagglutinin, fimbrial proteins, and pertussis toxin. Similarly, the virulence of enterotoxic *E. coli* depends on the expression of adherence proteins that allow the bacteria to bind to the intestinal epithelial cells and coordinate synthesis and release of heat-labile or heat-stable toxins that cause intestinal cells to secrete isotonic fluids.

BACTERIAL ADHESINS. Bacterial adhesins that bind bacteria to host cells are limited in type but have a broad range of host cell specificity. The surface of gram-positive cocci such as streptococci is covered with lipotechoic acids and M-protein–bearing fibrilla (Fig. 9–8). Lipoteichoic acids are hydrophobic and bind to the surface of all eukaryotic cells, although with a higher affinity to particular receptors on blood cells and oral epithelial cells. Fimbriae or pili on the surface of gram-negative rods and cocci are nonflagellar filamentous structures composed of repeating subunits. While sex pili are used to exchange genes carried on plasmids or transposons from one bacterium to another, most pili mediate adherence of bacteria to host cells. The base of the subunit that anchors the pilus to the bacterial cell wall is similar for widely divergent bacteria (e.g., *Mycobacterium, Pseudomonas, Neisseria*). At the tips of the pili are minor protein components that determine to which host cells the microbes will attach (bacterial tropism). In *E. coli* these minor proteins are antigenically distinct and are associated with particular infections (e.g., type I bind mannose and cause lower urinary tract infections, type P bind galactose and cause pyelonephritis, type S bind sialic acid and cause meningitis). A single bacterium can express more than one type of pilus as well as adhesins not located in pili (e.g., proteins I and II of gonococci).

Unlike viruses, which infect a broad range of host cells, facultative intracellular bacteria are more restricted and infect epithelial cells (*Shigella* and enteroinvasive *E. coli*), macrophages (*M. tuberculosis, Mycobacterium leprae*), or both (*Salmonella typhi*). Most of these bacteria attach to host cell integrins, plasma membrane proteins that bind complement, or extracellular matrix proteins, including fibronectin, laminin, and collagen (p. 55). For example, *Legionella* organisms, *M. tuberculosis,* and the protozoan *Leishmania* all bind to CR3, the cell receptor for complement C3bi. In contrast to rickettsiae, the facultative intracellular bacteria are unable to directly penetrate the host cells but are endocytosed by the epithelial cells or phagocytosed by the macrophages. *Shigella* and enteroinvasive *E. coli* use a plasmid-encoded hemolysin to escape from the endocytic vacuole into the cytoplasm. Once in the cytoplasm, *Shigella* and *E. coli* inhibit host protein synthesis, rapidly replicate, and within 6 hours lyse the host cells. In contrast, *Salmonella, Mycobacterium,* and *Yersinia* organisms replicate within the phagolysosome of the macrophage, while *Legionella* organisms inhibit the acidification that normally

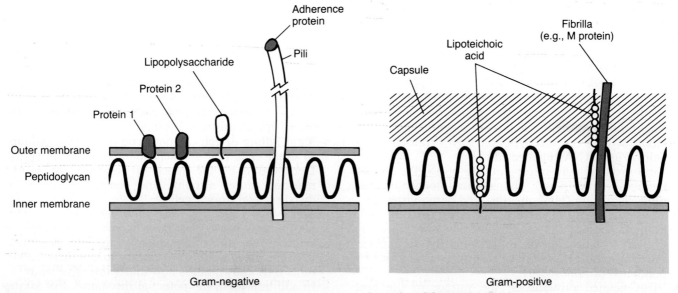

Figure 9–8. Some molecules on the surface of gram-negative and gram-positive bacteria involved in pathogenesis.

occurs after endosome fusion with the lysosome. In the absence of a host cellular immune response, many replicating organisms persist within the macrophages (e.g., lepromatous leprosy, *Mycobacterium avium* infection in AIDS patients), but activated macrophages can kill these organisms or limit their growth.

BACTERIAL ENDOTOXIN. Bacterial endotoxin is a lipopolysaccharide (LPS) that is a structural component of the outer cell wall of gram-negative bacteria. LPS is composed of a long-chain fatty acid anchor (lipid A) connected to a core sugar chain, both of which are the same in all gram-negative bacteria. Attached to the core sugar is a variable carbohydrate chain (0 antigen), which is used to serotype and distinguish different bacteria. The many biologic activities of endotoxins are discussed elsewhere in this book. They include induction of fever (p. 45), septic shock (p. 78), disseminated intravascular coagulation (p. 378), the acute respiratory distress syndrome (p. 399), and a variety of effects on cells of the immune system. All the biologic activities of endotoxin come from lipid A and the core sugars. They are mediated both by direct effects of endotoxin and by the induction of host cytokines such as interleukin 1 (IL-1), tumor necrosis factor (TNF), and others.

BACTERIAL EXOTOXINS. Many potentially harmful products are secreted by bacteria, yet relatively few have been proved to have defined deleterious effects in vivo. Leukocidins, hemolysins, hyaluronidases, coagulases, fibrinolysins, and other enzymes extracted from bacterial cultures act on their respective substrates in vitro, but their role in human disease is unproven. In contrast, *certain bacterial exotoxins directly cause cellular injury and determine disease manifestations,* and the molecular mechanisms underlying such injury have been well studied. The effects of diphtheria toxins, for example, are well-established. When diphtheria toxin binds via its carboxyl end to glycoproteins on the surface of target cells, it is composed of fragment B (the carboxyl end) and fragment A (the amino end), which are held together by a disulfide bridge (Fig. 9–9). Bound diphtheria toxin enters the acidic endosome, where it fuses with the endosomal membrane and enters the cell cytoplasm. Within the cytoplasm the disulfide bond of diphtheria toxin is reduced and broken, releasing the enzymatically active amino fragment A of the toxin that catalyzes the covalent transfer of ADP-ribose from NAD to EF-2, inactivating it. (EF-2 is an elongation factor in polypeptide synthesis). One toxin molecule can kill a cell by ADP-ribosylating more than 10^6 EF-2 molecules. The effect of the toxin is to create a layer of dead cells in the throat, on which *Corynebacterium diphtheriae* bacteria outgrow competing bacteria. Subsequently, wide dissemination of diphtheria toxin causes neural and myocardial dysfunction. The heat-labile enterotoxins of *V. cholerae* and of *E. coli* also have an A-B structure and are ADP-ribosyl transferases, but these enzymes catalyze transfer from NAD to the guanyl nucleotide–dependent regulatory component of adenylate cyclase. This generates excess cAMP, which causes intestinal epithelial cells to secrete isoosmotic fluid, resulting in volu-

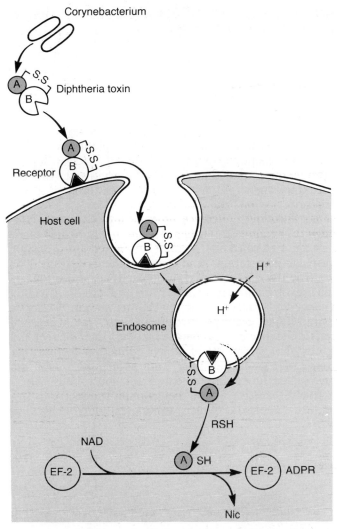

Figure 9–9. Inhibition of cellular protein synthesis by diphtheria toxin. (Adapted from Collier, R. J.: Corynebacteria. *In* Davis, B. D., Dulbecco, R., Eisen, H. N., Ginsberg, H. S. (eds.): Microbiology. New York, Harper & Row, 1990.)

minous diarrhea and loss of water and electrolytes. The gram-positive anaerobic *Clostridium perfringens,* the agent of gas gangrene, literally digests host tissues, including the relatively resistant collagens. Its α-toxin is a lecithinase that disrupts plasma membranes, including those of red and white blood cells.

More selective and subtle are the exotoxins of *Clostridium tetani,* a wound contaminant, and of *Clostridium botulinum,* which grows in poorly preserved food rather than in human tissue. Tetanospasmin finds its way to the presynaptic terminals of the spinal interneurons, where it inferferes with the release of inhibitory transmitter substance, thus inducing the violent muscle contractions that characterize tetanic spasm. *C. botulinum* toxins block the release of cholinergic neurotransmitters, particularly at the neuromuscular junctions, resulting in progressive paralysis of the limbs, breathing muscles, and cranial motor nerves.

INFLAMMATORY RESPONSE TO INFECTIOUS AGENTS

We conclude this chapter by summarizing the most common histologic patterns of host responses induced by infectious agents. In contrast to the vast molecular diversity of parasites, the patterns of inflammatory response to these agents are limited, as are the mediator mechanisms that direct these responses. At the microscopic level, therefore, many pathogens evoke identical reaction patterns, and few of the features are unique to or pathognomonic of each agent. Broadly speaking, there are five histologic patterns of tissue reaction:

SUPPURATIVE POLYMORPHONUCLEAR INFLAMMATION. This is the familiar reaction to acute tissue damage described in Chapter 2, marked by increased vascular permeability and neutrophilic exudation. The neutrophils are attracted to the site of infection by release of chemoattractants from the rapidly dividing "pyogenic" bacteria that evoke this response, mostly extracellular gram-positive cocci and gram-negative rods. The bacterial chemoattractants include secreted bacterial peptides, all of which contain N-formyl methionine residues at their amino terminals that are recognized by specific receptors on neutrophils. Alternatively, bacteria attract neutrophils indirectly by releasing endotoxin, which stimulates macrophages to

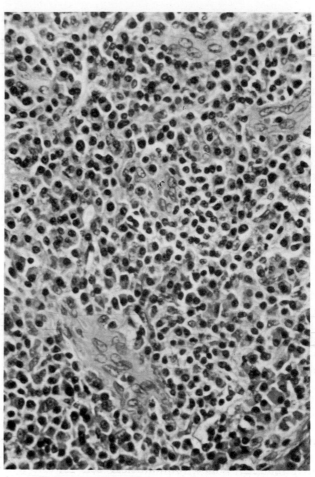

Figure 9-11. Syphilitic chancre: diffuse plasmacytic infiltration and endothelial proliferation.

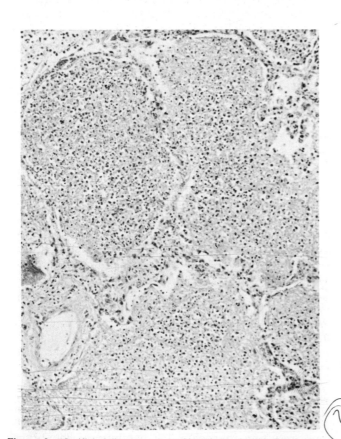

Figure 9-10. *Klebsiella* pneumonia. Note intra-alveolar exudate and destruction of alveolar septa.

secrete interleukin 1 or tumor necrosis factor, or by cleaving complement into the chemoattractant peptide C5b. Massing of neutrophils results in the formation of pus. The size of exudative lesions may vary tremendously, from tiny microabscesses formed in multiple organs during sepsis secondary to a colonized heart valve, to distended pus-filled fallopian tubes caused by *N. gonorrhoeae* (the gonococcus), to diffuse involvement of the meninges during *H. influenzae* infection, to pneumonia in which many entire lobes of the lung are involved. How destructive the lesions are depends on their location and the organism involved. For example, pneumococci usually spare pulmonary alveolar walls and cause lobar pneumonia permitting resolution (p. 411), while staphylococci and *Klebsiella* species destroy them and form abscesses, which can only be followed by scarring (p. 424; Fig. 9-10). Bacterial pharyngitis heals without sequelae, whereas untreated acute bacterial inflammation can destroy a joint in a matter of days.

MONONUCLEAR INFLAMMATION. Diffuse, predominantly mononuclear interstitial infiltrates are a common feature of all chronic inflammatory processes, but when they occur acutely, they are often in response to

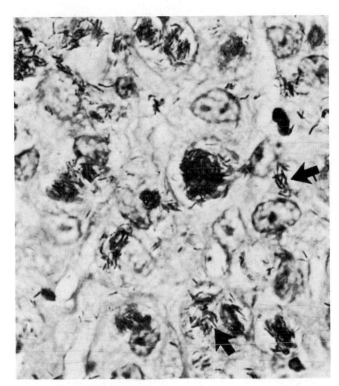

Figure 9–12. Leprosy. High-power view of acid-fast bacilli *(arrows)* proliferating in foamy macrophages.

viruses, intracellular bacteria, or intracellular parasites. In addition, spirochetes and helminths cause chronic inflammation. Which mononuclear cell predominates within the inflammatory lesion depends on the host immune response to the organism. For example, mostly plasma cells are seen in the chancres of primary syphilis (Fig. 9–11), but lymphocytes with active hepatitis B infection, or in viral infections of the brain. These lymphocytes represent cell-mediated immunity against the pathogen or the pathogen-infected cells. At the other extreme, macrophages filled with *M. avium* are present in many tissues of AIDS patients, who have no helper T cells left and can mount no immune response to the organisms. For *M. leprae* infection and for cutaneous leishmaniasis, some persons mount a strong immune response so that their lesions contain few organisms, few macrophages, and many lymphocytes; others with a weak immune response have lesions that contain many organisms, many macrophages, and few lymphocytes (Fig. 9–12). *Granulomatous inflammation* (described in detail on p. 42) is a distinctive form of mononuclear inflammation usually evoked by relatively slow-dividing infectious agents (e.g., *M. tuberculosis)* and by those of relatively large size (e.g., schistosome eggs); they almost always reflect a cell-mediated immune reaction (p. 130).

CYTOPATHIC-CYTOPROLIFERATIVE INFLAMMATION. These reactions, usually produced by viruses, are characterized by damage to individual host cells with little or no host inflammatory response. Some viruses replicate within cells and make viral aggregates that are visible as inclusion bodies (e.g., CMV, adenovirus) or induce cells to fuse and form polykaryons (e.g.,

measles, herpesviruses). Focal cell damage may cause epithelial cells to become "discohesive" and form blisters (e.g., chicken pox virus). Viruses can also cause epithelial cells to proliferate and take unusual forms (e.g., venereal warts by human papillomavirus or the umbilicated papules of molluscum contagiosum by pox viruses). Finally, viruses can cause dysplastic changes and cancers in epithelial cells and lymphocytes (Chapter 7).

NECROTIZING INFLAMMATION. *C. perfringens* and other organisms that secrete very strong toxins cause such rapid and severe tissue damage that cell death is the dominant feature. Because so few inflammatory cells are involved these lesions resemble infarct necrosis, with disruption or loss of basophilic nuclear staining and preservation of cellular outlines. Often clostridia are opportunistic pathogens introduced into muscle tissue by penetrating trauma or by infection of the bowel in a neutropenic host. Similarly, the parasite *E. histolytica* causes colonic ulcers and liver abscesses characterized by extensive tissue destruction with liquefactive necrosis in the absence of an inflammatory infiltrate. Occasionally viruses can cause necrotizing inflammation when host cell damage is particularly widespread and severe (for example, there may be total destruction of the temporal lobes of the brain by herpesvirus or of the liver by hepatitis B virus).

CHRONIC INFLAMMATION AND SCARRING. The final common pathway of many infections is chronic inflammation, which may lead to complete healing but extensive scarring (e.g., chronic gonococcal salpingitis). For some organisms that are relatively inert the exuberant host scarring response is the major cause of disease (e.g., the "pipestem" fibrosis of the liver caused by schistosome eggs [Fig. 9–13] or the scars at the apices of the lungs in tuberculosis). These patterns of

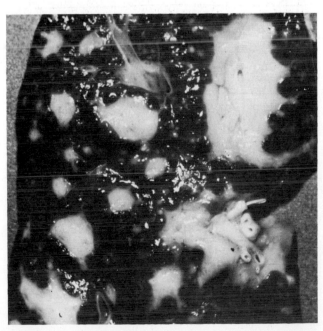

Figure 9–13. Liver pipe-stem fibrosis due to chronic *Schistosoma japonicum* infection.

tissue reaction are useful for analyzing the infective processes but they frequently overlap.

It is evident that many factors that relate to the invader and the host modify the development and nature of the microbe-induced disease and its outcome. In this chapter we have emphasized the structural and molecular mechanisms relevant to the interaction between microbe and host. But it should also be remembered that, considering the multiplicity of potential invaders, the majority of infectious diseases are caused by a relatively small number of agents that differ in geographic locales and are determined largely by environmental, socioeconomic, and public health factors.

Bibliography

Baddour, L. M., Christensen, G. D., Simpson, W. A., Beachey, E. H.: Microbial adherence. *In* Mandell, G. L., Douglas, R. G., Bennet, J. E. (eds.): Principles and Practice of Infectious Disease. New York, Churchill Livingstone, 1990.

Binford, C. H., O' Connor, D. H.: Pathology of Tropical and Extraordinary Diseases. Vols. I and II. Washington, DC, Armed Forces Institute of Pathology, 1976. (To date, some of the best descriptions and illustrations of the histopathology of infectious diseases).

Collier, R. J.: Corynebacteria. *In* Davis, B. D., Dulbecco, R., Eisen, H. N., Ginsberg, H. S. (eds.): Microbiology. New York, Harper & Row, 1990. (Review of the mechanisms of action of the best-understood toxin.)

Enders, J. F., Weller, T. H., Robbins, F. C.: Cultivation of the Lansing strain of poliomyelitis virus in culture of various human embryonic tissues. Science *109*:85, 1949. (Report of the Nobel prize–winning work that led to the polio vaccines).

Finlay, B. B., Falkow, S.: Common themes in microbial pathogenicity. Microbial Rev. *53*:210, 1989. (Overview of bacterial pathogenesis.)

Fischetti, V. A.: Streptococcal M Protein. Sci. Am. *264*:58, 1991.

Marsh, M., Helenius, A.: Virus entry into animal cells. Adv. Viral Res. *36*:107, 1989.

Miller, J. F., Mekalanos, J. J., Falkow, S.: Coordinate regulation and sensory transduction in the control of bacterial virulence. Science *243*:916, 1989. (Review of mechanisms of global regulation of pathogenicity of bacteria.)

Mims, C. A.: The Pathogenesis of Infectious Disease. Orlando, FL, Academic Press, 1987. (An extensive discussion of the mechanisms of microbial pathogenesis).

Sharpe, A. H., Fields, B. N.: Pathogenesis of viral infections: Basic concepts derived from the reovirus model. N. Engl. J. Med. *312*:486, 1985.

von Lichtenberg, F.: Pathology of Infectious Disease. New York, Raven Press, 1991. (An authoritative and concise presentation of the broad gamut of microbial diseases with excellent coverage of the resultant morphologic lesions.)

Walsh, J.: Estimating the burden of illness in the tropics. *In* Warren, K. S., Mahmoud, A. A. F. (eds.): Tropical and Geographical Medicine. New York, McGraw-Hill, 1990. (An overview of the epidemiology of infectious diseases in the developing world.)

2

DISEASES OF
ORGAN SYSTEMS

TEN

Diseases of Blood Vessels

ARTERIAL DISORDERS

ARTERIOSCLEROSIS
  Atherosclerosis
VASCULITIS
  Hypersensitivity (Leukocytoclastic) Vasculitis
  Polyarteritis Nodosa
  Wegener's Granulomatosis
  Churg-Strauss Syndrome
  Temporal (Giant Cell, Cranial) Arteritis
  Takayasu's Arteritis (Pulseless Disease)
  Kawasaki's Disease (Mucocutaneous Lymph
    Node Syndrome)
  Thromboangiitis Obliterans (Buerger's Disease)
RAYNAUD'S DISEASE
ANEURYSMS
  Atherosclerotic Aneurysm
  Syphilitic (Luetic) Aortitis and Aneurysm
  Dissecting Aneurysm (Dissecting Hematoma,
    Aortic Dissection)

VENOUS DISORDERS

VARICOSE VEINS
PHLEBOTHROMBOSIS AND
THROMBOPHLEBITIS
OBSTRUCTION OF SUPERIOR VENA CAVA
(SUPERIOR VENA CAVAL SYNDROME)
OBSTRUCTION OF INFERIOR VENA CAVA
(INFERIOR VENA CAVAL SYNDROME)

LYMPHATIC DISORDERS

LYMPHANGITIS
LYMPHEDEMA

TUMORS

HEMANGIOMAS
HEMANGIOENDOTHELIOMA AND
ANGIOSARCOMA
GLOMANGIOMA (GLOMUS TUMOR)
KAPOSI'S SARCOMA

Vascular disorders are responsible for more morbidity and mortality than any other category of human disease. Among them arterial diseases are the most important. They achieve this unenviable preeminence by (1) narrowing vessels, (2) damaging the endothelial lining to promote intravascular thrombosis (processes that contribute to critical ischemia of vital organs such as the heart and brain), and (3) weakening the walls of vessels, predisposing to dilatation, or possibly rupture. Although disorders of veins are by no means trivial, they are dwarfed in significance by the diseases of arteries, in particular atherosclerosis. In the following discussions, the various conditions are divided into those that affect the arteries, the veins, and the lymphatics; this is followed by a brief consideration of vascular tumors, because whatever their origin they are quite similar clinically and anatomically.

Arterial Disorders

ARTERIOSCLEROSIS

Arteriosclerosis is the generic term for three patterns of vascular disease, all of which cause thickening and inelasticity of arteries. The dominant pattern is atherosclerosis, characterized by the formation of intimal fibrofatty plaques that often have a central grumous core rich in lipid, hence the term "atherosclerosis" from the Greek stem *athera* meaning "gruel or

porridge." The second morphologic form of arteriosclerosis is the rather trivial *Mönckeberg's medial calcific sclerosis,* characterized by calcifications in the media of muscular arteries. It is encountered in medium-sized muscular arteries in persons usually over the age of 50 years. The calcifications take the form of irregular medial plates or discrete transverse rings, which create a nodularity on palpation and are readily visualized radiographically. Occasionally, the calcific deposits undergo ossification. Since these medial lesions do not encroach on the vessel lumen, medial calcific sclerosis is largely of anatomic interest alone; however, arteries so affected may also develop atherosclerosis. Disease of small arteries and arterioles— *arteriolosclerosis*—is the third pattern. Small vessel sclerosis is most often associated with hypertension and diabetes mellitus. There are two anatomic variants, hyaline and hyperplastic, depending on the cause and rate of progression of disease. Both cause thickening of vessel walls with luminal narrowing and may in the aggregate induce ischemic injury to tissues or organs. Since the lesions are often prominent in the kidneys, where they induce distinctive forms of nephropathy, they are described on pages 462 and 463. Thus, only atherosclerosis requires further consideration here. Indeed, atherosclerosis is so clearly the dominant form of arteriosclerosis that it is often loosely referred to as arteriosclerosis.

ATHEROSCLEROSIS _____

No disease in the United States (or other developed countries) is responsible for more deaths, has stimulated more research, and has engendered more controversy about how best to control it than atherosclerosis (AS). Basically it is characterized by intimal plaques called *atheromas* that protrude into the lumen, weaken the underlying media, and undergo a series of complications that predispose to overlying thrombosis. Alone AS accounts for more than half of all the deaths in the Western world. Although any artery may be affected, the major targets are the aorta and the coronary and cerebral arteries. Coronary atherosclerosis induces ischemic heart disease (IHD) and when the arterial lesions are complicated by thrombosis, the most serious form of IHD, myocardial infarction (MI), which alone is responsible for 20 to 25% of all deaths in the United States. Atherothrombotic disease of the cerebral vessels is the major cause of brain infarcts, so-called strokes, one of the commonest forms of neurologic disease. Were this not sufficient, atherosclerosis often produces critical ischemia of the intestines and lower extremities, and it is a major cause of abdominal aortic aneurysms (abnormal dilatations) that sometimes rupture to produce massive fatal hemorrhage. The disease begins in early childhood and progresses slowly over the decades. Thus, in some measure AS is a pediatric disease, and if its toll is to be reduced, measures must be instituted early before it rears its ugly head and provokes one of its unfortunate consequences.

EPIDEMIOLOGY. AS is virtually ubiquitous among the populations of North America, Europe, Australia, New Zealand, the Soviet Union, and other developed nations. In contrast, as judged by the number of deaths attributable to IHD (including MI), it is much less prevalent in Central and South America, Africa, Asia, and the Orient. For example, the mortality rate for IHD in the United States is six times higher than in Japan. Indeed, in most developed nations AS and its sequelae have assumed nearly epidemic proportions. But happily in the United States there is convincing evidence that the epidemic has been brought under control. Between 1968 (the peak year) and 1984 there was a nearly 40% decrease in the death rate from IHD and a 53% decrease in that from strokes. The basis for this happy trend is not entirely clear, but has reasonably been attributed to changes in living habits including reduced cigarette smoking, altered dietary habits with reduced consumption of cholesterol and other saturated animal fats, better control of hypertension, and improved methods of treatment of nonfatal myocardial infarcts. Without proof, there is a strong suspicion that such influences, rather than genetic predispositions, underlie the striking geographic contrasts mentioned earlier.

RISK FACTORS. The prevalence and severity of the disease, and therefore age when it is likely to cause tissue or organ injury, are related to a number of factors, some constitutional and therefore immutable, but others acquired and potentially controllable. The *constitutional factors* include age, sex, and familial background.

- *Age.* Age is a dominant influence. Although early lesions of AS appear in childhood, clinically significant disease, as judged by the death rates from IHD, rises with each decade, even into advanced age. For example, from age 40 to age 60 there is a greater than fivefold increase in the incidence of myocardial infarction. It is an exceptional adult in the United States who is older than 20 years and does not have at least mild AS.

- *Sex.* Other factors being equal, males are much more prone to AS than females. Females are more or less sheltered from advanced, disease-producing AS until menopause, so myocardial infarction is uncommon in premenopausal women unless they are predisposed by diabetes or some unusual (possibly familial) form of hyperlipidemia or have severe hypertension. After menopause the protection slowly dwindles until the frequency of MI becomes the same in both sexes by the seventh to eighth decade of life. Between ages 35 and 55 years, white women have one fifth the mortality from IHD of white males.

- *Familial Predisposition.* There is a well-defined familial predisposition to AS and to IHD. In some instances it relates to familial clustering of other risk factors, such as hypertension and diabetes. In other instances, it involves well-defined hereditary genetic derangements in lipoprotein metabolism that result in excessively high blood lipid levels. The prototype of these conditions is familial hypercholesterolemia, but in addition there is a growing number of familial dyslipoproteinemias, most of which result from mutations that yield defective apolipoproteins. You may recall, these are proteins bound to the various blood lipid fractions, which have many functions, among them activation or inhibition of particular enzymes, facilitating transmembrane transport of certain lipoproteins, and serving as ligands to high-affinity cellular receptors that guide the lipoproteins to specific sites of catabolism.

There are four major acquired risk factors that are at

least in some part amenable to control: (1) acquired hyperlipidemia, (2) hypertension, (3) cigarette smoking, and (4) diabetes (as well as a number of less important "soft" risks).

Hyperlipidemia is virtually universally acknowledged to be a major risk factor for AS. Most of the evidence specifically implicates hypercholesterolemia, but hypertriglyceridemia may also play a role, although it is not as significant as hypercholesterolemia. You recall from an earlier discussion (p. 86) that the various classes of blood lipids are transported as lipoproteins complexed to specific apoproteins (Table 10–1).

The major evidence implicating hypercholesterolemia in the genesis of AS includes the following:

- High-cholesterol diets can produce atherosclerotic plaques in rabbits, guinea pigs, dogs, and other nonhuman animals that are nearly identical to those observed in the human disease.
- The major lipids in atheromas (plaques) are cholesterol and cholesteryl esters derived from the plasma. Triglycerides and fatty acids are present in small amounts.
- Many large-scale analyses (notably the Framingham study) have demonstrated a nearly linear correlation between the total plasma cholesterol or low-density lipoprotein (LDL) level and the severity of AS as judged by the mortality rate from IHD. The higher the total cholesterol level the greater the risk of symptomatic and fatal atherosclerotic disease. No threshold clearly separates persons at risk from those free of risk, but in general, atherosclerotic events are very uncommon with total serum cholesterol levels below 150 mg/dl. Hypertriglyceridemia, as manifested by elevated very–low density lipoprotein (VLDL) levels, is also associated with some increased risk, but the association is much weaker than for LDL.

- Genetic or acquired disorders (e.g., diabetes mellitus, hypothyroidism) that cause hypercholesterolemia lead to premature and rampant atherosclerosis; witness familial hypercholesterolemia, which in the homozygous state is often associated with myocardial infarction before age 20 years.
- When levels of serum cholesterol are lowered, there is substantial evidence in animals and suggestive evidence in humans that some (?many) atherosclerotic plaques regress, or fail to progress, within months.

It is important at this point to emphasize the *inverse relationship* between symptomatic AS and the high-density lipoprotein (HDL) level. HDL participates in reverse transport of cholesterol and is believed to mobilize this lipid from cells and presumably from atherosclerotic plaques and transport it to the liver for excretion in the bile. *The higher the levels of HDL 3 and HDL 2 the lower the risk of IHD.* Hence the great interest in methods of lowering the serum LDL and raising the HDL level. A heavy dietary intake of saturated animal fat, including cholesterol-laden butter, other dairy products, and eggs, raises the serum cholesterol level. Conversely, diets in which saturated fats are replaced by monounsaturated (e.g., olive oil) or

TABLE 10–1. LIPOPROTEINS

Lipid Class	Description	Major Lipid Content	Major Complexed Apoproteins
Chylomicron	Transports dietary triglyceride from gut to liver, adipose tissue, and muscle	Dietary triglyceride and cholesterol	B48, C, E
Chylomicron remnant	Chylomicrons after most of triglyceride is removed within the capillary beds of muscle and adipose tissue by the action of lipoprotein lipase	Dietary cholesterol	B48, C, E
Very–low density lipoprotein (VLDL)	Transports mostly triglyceride, some cholesterol, from liver to periphery	Endogenous triglyceride	B100, C, E
Intermediate-density lipoprotein (IDL)	Transient; derived from VLDL in the capillaries of adipose tissue and muscle by the lipoprotein lipase extraction of most of the triglyceride	Endogenous cholesterol	B100, E
Low-density lipoprotein (LDL)	Derived from VLDL via the intermediate IDL. It is the fraction most strongly correlated with AS	Endogenous cholesterol	B100
High-density lipoprotein 3 (HDL 3)	Involved in "reverse transport" of cholesterol from cells and tissues to the liver	Cholesterol	A-1, A-2, E
High-density lipoprotein 2 (HDL 2)	Derived from HDL 3 and transports cholesterol to liver cells, which have receptors for specific attached apoprotein	Cholesterol	A-1, A-2, E

polyunsaturated fats (e.g., fish, corn oil) lower the LDL levels, but may concurrently modestly reduce the HDL level. In particular, the Ω-3 polyunsaturated fatty acids derived mostly from fish and fish oils have a well-defined hypolipidemic effect. Vegetarians and habitual fish eaters (e.g., Greenland Eskimos) with diets high in unsaturated fats relative to saturated fats have low levels of LDL and a low risk of IHD. Nondietary influences may also affect the level of the blood lipids. Exercise and moderate consumption of ethanol both raise the HDL level, whereas obesity and smoking lower it. Many more observations could be cited, but it suffices that blood cholesterol and LDL levels are major contributors to atherogenesis.

Hypertension is at all ages a major risk factor for atherosclerosis and may well be more important than hypercholesterolemia after age 45. In the Framingham study, men aged 45 to 62 whose blood pressure exceeded 160/95 mm Hg had a more than fivefold greater risk of IHD than those with blood pressures of 140/90 or lower. The diastolic level appears to be more important than the systolic.

Smoking is also a major risk factor and is thought to account for the recent increase in the incidence and severity of AS in women. When one or more packs of cigarettes are smoked per day for years, the death rate from IHD increases up to 200%. Cessation of smoking dramatically reduces this increased risk in time.

Diabetes mellitus induces hypercholesterolemia and a markedly increased predisposition to atherosclerosis. Other factors being equal, the incidence of myocardial infarction is twice as high in diabetics as in nondiabetics. There is also an increased risk of strokes and even more striking, perhaps, a hundredfold increased risk of atherosclerosis-induced gangrene of the lower extremities. Indeed, in the absence of diabetes, atherosclerotic gangrene of the lower extremities is uncommon.

Other risk factors are sometimes called "soft" risk factors because their impact on atherogenesis is less clearly defined and in some instances is controversial. There is substantial evidence that physical activity increases the serum level of HDL, having a protective effect against IHD, and conversely inactivity favors the development of AS. Moreover, physical activity appears to reduce the risk of sudden death, which is most often a consequence of IHD. Analogously, in the Framingham study, _being more than 30% overweight increased the mortality rate from IHD._ The risk appears to be mainly connected to weight gain in the abdominal region, in contrast to adiposity located mainly in the gluteal region or proximal extremities. Genetic metabolic factors may determine this variable distribution of adiposity because with abdominal obesity there is frequently concomitant hypertriglyceridemia, impaired glucose tolerance, and hypertension not seen with the other forms of obesity. Some of the other less significant ("softer") risk factors include type A personality behavior, hyperuricemia, and the use of former oral contraceptives. There have been claims of a direct association between coffee consumption and increased serum cholesterol levels, particularly the consumption of coffee brewed by boiling. To the great relief of "coffeeholics," the drinking of filtered coffee is reported to have no effect on the blood lipids, removing the stigma from one of life's simpler but cherished pleasures.

In closing this discussion of risk factors it is important to note that _multiple factors impose more than an additive effect._ The Framingham study documented that when three risk factors were present (hyperlipidemia, hypertension, and smoking), the heart attack rate was seven times greater than when none was present. Two risk factors increased the risk fourfold. However, the converse is equally important: AS may develop in the absence of any apparent risk factors, so even those who live "the prudent life" and have no genetic predispositions are not immune to this killer disease.

PATHOGENESIS. Understandably, the commanding importance of AS has stimulated enormous efforts to discover its cause. A mountain of evidence has accumulated, but unfortunately it is strewn with claims and counterclaims and has led to numerous pathogenic theories. Comments will be restricted to only three of these theories. Favored today and receiving the greatest attention is the response-to-injury hypothesis. It best accommodates the various risk factors discussed. Central to this thesis are the following features:

1. The development of focal areas of chronic endothelial injury, usually very subtle, with resulting increased endothelial permeability or other evidence of endothelial dysfunction.
2. Increased imbibition (insudation) of lipoprotein, mainly LDL or modified LDL with its high content of cholesterol, and also VLDL.
3. A series of cellular interactions in these foci of injury involving endothelial cells, monocytes/macrophages, T lymphocytes, and smooth muscle cells of intimal or medial origin.
4. Proliferation of smooth muscle cells in the intima with the formation of connective tissue by the smooth muscle cells (Fig. 10–1).

Each of these aspects of the atherogenic process will now be considered.

Chronic or repeated endothelial injury is the keystone of the response-to-injury hypothesis. Although endothelial denuding injuries will certainly initiate atherosclerotic changes in experimental animals, the naturally occurring disease of humans begins with some form of nondenuding, subtle injury. Circulating endotoxins, anoxia, carbon monoxide or other products derived from cigarette smoke, viruses, and specific endotheliotoxins such as homocysteine (accounting for the premature and severe atherosclerosis of homocystinurics) could be involved, but thought to be much more likely are hemodynamic disturbances (shear stress, turbulent flow) and adverse affects of hypercholesterolemia, perhaps acting in concert. Shear stress and turbulent flow have been shown experimentally to increase endothelial permeability and cell turnover and to enhance receptor-mediated LDL endocytosis. The complex geometry of the arterial system, with its twists and turns and branchings, could give rise to turbulent

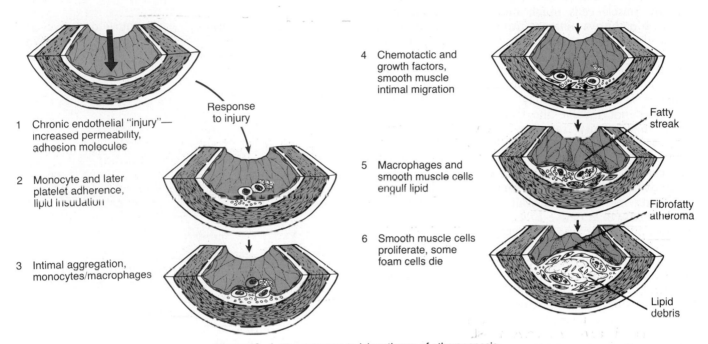

1 Chronic endothelial "injury"—increased permeability, adhesion molecules

2 Monocyte and later platelet adherence, lipid insudation

3 Intimal aggregation, monocytes/macrophages

Response to injury

4 Chemotactic and growth factors, smooth muscle intimal migration

5 Macrophages and smooth muscle cells engulf lipid

6 Smooth muscle cells proliferate, some foam cells die

Fatty streak

Fibrofatty atheroma

Lipid debris

Figure 10–1. The response-to-injury theory of atherogenesis.

flow patterns with variable levels of shear stress capable of causing focal areas of endothelial injury. In support of this notion is a well-defined tendency for plaques to occur at mouths of exiting vessels, branch points, and along the posterior wall of the descending and abdominal aorta, which is caught between the anvil of the vertebral column and the hammer of the arterial pulse. Whether hemodynamic stress can account for the widespread involvement often seen in the aorta with advanced disease remains to be established.

The possibility that chronic hyperlipidemia, and particularly hypercholesterolemia, may itself initiate endothelial injury has enticed many investigators. Much evidence suggests that hypercholesterolemia has a variety of adverse effects.

• It increases the cholesterol-phospholipid ratio of endothelial cell membranes, rendering them more rigid and less able to maintain their normal intercellular associations, potentially increasing permeability and in effect causing a subtle form of endothelial injury.

• It favors the adherence of monocytes and lymphocytes to the focus of injury, in part owing to the stimulation of endothelial cell synthesis of adhesion molecules.

• It induces changes in platelet membrane composition, leading to activation and increased adhesiveness of platelets.

• With chronic hyperlipidemia, lipoproteins accumulate within the intima at sites of endothelial injury or dysfunction. Although significant amounts may enter the arterial wall, there is some concurrent efflux, perhaps mediated by HDL.

• Most important, it provides the opportunity for oxidation of lipoproteins, yielding modified LDL.

Oxidative modification of LDL is currently thought to be an important aspect of the atherogenic process. It is proposed that LDL in the microenvironment of interadherent monocytes and endothelial cells is exposed to free radicals generated by these activated cells. Oxidized LDL is itself toxic to endothelial cells, compounding the endothelial injury. It is also chemotactic to monocytes and immobilizes macrophages, favoring their accumulation at sites of atheroma formation. Further, it is also taken up by macrophages and smooth muscle cells much more avidly than native LDL, by pathways different from those used by native LDL. The earlier discussion of lipoproteins (p. 86) indicated that hepatocytes and other cells had specific receptors for native LDL, accounting for the removal of about two thirds of plasma LDL. Oxidized LDL, however, is taken up through a "scavenger pathway" that does not involve the usual LDL receptors but rather high-affinity receptors specific for modified LDL. Other modifications of LDL may also facilitate its uptake. LDL within arterial walls may complex with certain proteoglycans to form insoluble complexes that are avidly taken up by macrophages. Still other complexes may be formed, all of which are taken up more rapidly than native LDL. Thus much of the lipid content of atheromas is thought to be oxidized LDL, and indeed it has been shown that it is possible to confer some protection against atherosclerosis in rabbits by treating them with antioxidants. Another variant of LDL (a complex of LDL linked to ApoA by disulfide oxides) called lipoprotein A (LPA) has also been identified. Elevated levels are genetically determined, and low-fat diets, lipid-lowering drugs, and other interventions have no effect on the blood levels. LPA's precise role in atherogenesis is now under study.

A complex series of cellular events are involved in the formation of atheromatous plaques. Following adhesion to endothelial cells, monocytes migrate between endothelial cells to localize subendothelially. There they become transformed into macrophages and avidly engulf lipoproteins, largely oxidized LDL, to become foam cells (Fig. 10-2). You recall that oxidized LDL is chemotactic to monocytes and immobilizes macrophages at sites where it accumulates. In addition, early in the evolution of the lesion, smooth muscle cells (SMCs), some of medial origin, gather in the intima, where they multiply and some take up lipids to also be transformed into foam cells. As long as the hypercholesterolemia persists, monocyte and lymphocyte adhesion, subendothelial migration of SMCs, and accumulation of lipids within the macrophages and SMCs continue to eventually yield aggregates of foam cells in the intima, which are apparent macroscopically as *fatty streaks.* These, many believe, are the forerunners of fully evolved atheromas. Should the hypercholesterolemia be ameliorated, these fatty streaks may regress, but if they persist they continue to evolve.

Proliferation of SMCs about the focus of foam cells converts the fatty streak into a mature fibrofatty atheroma. It has been clearly shown that arterial SMCs can synthesize collagen, elastin, and glycoproteins. A number of growth factors have been implicated in the

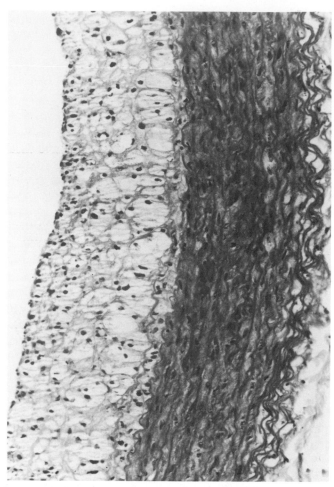

Figure 10-2. A fatty streak composed of intimal lipid-laden foam cells in experimental atherosclerosis in a rat. (Courtesy of Dr. Myron Cybulsky, Brigham and Women's Hospital, Boston, MA.)

proliferation of SMCs, most importantly "platelet-derived growth factor" (PDGF), released from platelets adherent to the focus of endothelial injury but also produced by macrophages, endothelial cells, and SMCs in response to the release of cytokines (e.g., tumor necrosis factor [TNF], interleukin-1 (IL-1), and interferon [IFN]-γ) generated by macrophage-lymphocyte interactions. Additional candidate mitogens are fibroblast growth factor, epidermal growth factor, and transforming growth factor-α (TGF-α). Indeed, the evolving atheroma has been likened to a chronic inflammatory reaction, with activated T cells, monocyte/macrophages, endothelial cells, and SMCs all expressing or contributing a variety of cytokines, which could play roles in cell adhesion, locomotion, and replication. Theoretically, SMC proliferation might also result from loss of growth inhibitors such as heparin-like molecules present in endothelial and smooth muscle cells or TGF-β derived from endothelial cells or macrophages.

At this stage in atherogenesis, the intimal plaque represents a central aggregation of foam cells of macrophage and SMC origin, some of which may have died and released extracellular lipid and cellular debris surrounded by SMCs, and possibly fibroblasts of arterial wall origin embedded within a scant connective matrix.

With progression, the cellular-fatty atheroma is modified by the further deposition of collagen, elastin, and proteoglycans. This connective tissue is particularly prominent on the intimal aspect, where it produces the so-called *fibrous cap.* Thus evolves the fully mature *fibrofatty atheroma.* Some atheromas undergo considerable cellular proliferation and connective tissue formation to yield *fibrous plaques.* Others retain a central core of lipid-laden cells and fatty debris. Whether the cellular atheromas represent the end stage of fibrofatty lesions is not clear. *End theory 1*

Two other theories of atherogenesis merit brief mention. These theories, including the response-to-injury proposal, are not mutually exclusive, and conceivably all proposed *(2) mechanisms* may collaborate in atherogenesis. The *monoclonal hypothesis* proposes that so-called fibrous plaques are monoclonal or at least oligoclonal (i.e., are composed of the progeny of a single SMC or a few cells) stimulated to proliferate by mutagens, possibly viruses, or fractions derived from cholesterol or tobacco smoke. Thus, in effect the cellular plaque is likened to a smooth muscle tumor. In theory such cellular lesions might then accumulate lipoproteins in hypercholesterolemic persons. Subsequent studies have disproven the monoclonality of cellular plaques and have contended that their oligoclonal makeup simply reflects the overgrowth of more vigorous cells in the area of arterial wall injury. Yet another hypothesis might be termed the *(3) thrombogenic or encrustation theory* (i.e., plaques arise from mural thrombi formed over foci of endothelial injury). Organization and reendothelialization of the thrombi, in effect, incorporate them into the intimal layer, and it is the breakdown of the blood constituents that yields the lipid content. While thrombi may well form over preexisting ulcerated atheromas and be incorporated into the evolving lesion and may also worsen the luminal narrowing, it is doubtful that they constitute the *origins* of atheromatous lesions.

Each of the several pathogenic sequences cited has theoretically attractive features that could participate in atherogenesis, so it may well be that "more than one road leads to Rome."

MORPHOLOGY. Atherosclerotic lesions evolve over time, so it is necessary to characterize them from their origins to their ultimate configurations.

Many experts believe that at least some atheromas arise as **fatty streaks** in the first years of life. These subendothelial lesions begin as 1-mm, soft, yellow, intimal discolorations that progressively enlarge by becoming thicker and slightly elevated while they elongate in the long axis of the vessel to produce typical fatty streaks 1 to 3 mm wide and up to 1.5 cm long (Fig. 10–3). Some may not be elevated and so are better seen after staining the aortic surface with oil red O, a stain for lipid. Early in their evolution fatty streaks tend

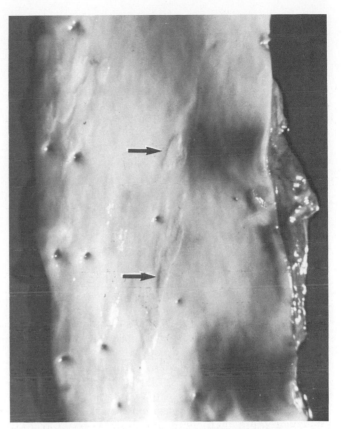

Figure 10–3. Atherosclerosis of the aorta. The barely elevated early lipid-laden fatty streaks *(arrows)* seen on reflected light.

to be located in the region of the aortic valve ring, in the posterior wall of the descending thoracic aorta, and adjacent to the orifices of the intercostal arteries in the thoracic aorta. With age they increase in number and at the same time progress down the aorta to involve the abdominal portion. At about ten years of age fatty streaks also appear in the coronary arteries, most abundantly in the proximal segment of the left coronary artery.

Histologically they constitute intimal aggregations of foam cells with finely vacuolated cytoplasm derived from both macrophages and SMC (see Fig. 10–2). A few marginal T lymphocytes may be present. In larger aggregates there may be some extracellular lipid debris derived from the death of foam cells, but there is little cellular proliferation in the margins, little enclosing connective tissue, and only a very delicate fibrous cap intervening between the lesion and the overlying intact endothelial surface. Although fatty streaks may be the forerunners of fully evolved atheromas, some undoubtedly regress because many fatty streaks are located at sites in the aorta that typically are little involved in the fully developed disease (e.g., the arch of the aorta). Moreover, fatty streaks are equally prevalent in all children, regardless of race, geography, and predisposition to the later development of atherosclerosis. Thus although many atheromatous plaques probably arise out of fatty streaks, all fatty streaks do not necessarily evolve into atheromatous plaques.

The atheromatous plaque is the hallmark of AS. It may have a rich content of lipid, more usually it is a fibrofatty lesion, and sometimes is almost solidly cellular and fibrotic. Plaques range up to several centimeters in largest dimension, and depending on the content of lipid, may be bright yellow to gray, intimal lesions raised several millimeters above the surface of the surrounding intima. Irregular in shape they may coalesce to form map-like configurations. On transection there is usually a central core of yellow grumous debris enclosed within a firmer, poorly defined wall and covered by a tough, gray-white, fibrous cap. As noted earlier, in some plaques there is scant lipid and only a tough, elevated, gray-white lesion.

Plaques tend to be found in certain locations, in descending order of extent and severity of involvement: lower abdominal aorta, coronary arteries, popliteal arteries, descending thoracic aorta, internal carotid arteries, and circle of Willis. Other medium-sized muscular arteries may also be affected, but the vessels of the upper extremities, mesenteric arteries, and renal arteries are largely spared save for their ostia. The aortic arch also tends to be spared, except when the patient has underlying syphilitic aortitis. As the disease evolves, there is a tendency for more plaques to be formed and in severe cases they may virtually coat the abdominal aorta. Similarly, they become more numerous in the coronary arteries but are usually most abundant in the first 6 cm. Although their protrusion into the lumen of the aorta does not significantly threaten the patency of this vessel, in smaller arteries, particularly the coronaries and those of the brain, atherosclerosis may significantly impair blood flow, particularly when the lesions become complicated, as will soon be detailed.

Microscopically, **plaques have essentially three components: (1) cells, including vascular SMC, blood-derived monocytes/macrophages, and a scattering of lymphocytes; (2) connective tissue fibers and matrix; and (3) lipids.** Some plaques contain relatively small amounts of lipid and are composed almost entirely of smooth muscle cells together with collagen and elastin fibers and proteoglycans to create the so-called **fibrous plaque** (Fig. 10–4). In others, the cellular and matrix elements create a luminal "fibrous cap" overlying a soft grumous center containing a variable mixture of proteoglycans, cellular debris, fibrin and other plasma proteins, and, most important, cholesterol (which may form needle-like crystals) and cholesteryl esters—the classic **fibrofatty atheroma** (Fig. 10–5). In the margins of this soft center are a few or many lipid-laden foam cells. As the plaques enlarge, they cause atrophy and fibrosis of the underlying media, impairing wall elasticity and strength, evoke a lymphocytic infiltrate in the contiguous adventitia, and develop vascularization about their margins, initially by the ingrowth of vessels from the vasa vasorum. Mural thrombi may form on plaques and become organized and incorporated into them; canalization of the organizing thrombi is an additional mechanism of vascularization of the plaques.

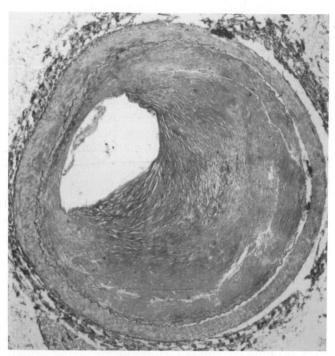

Figure 10–4. An eccentric fibrous atheroma markedly narrowing the lumen of the coronary artery.

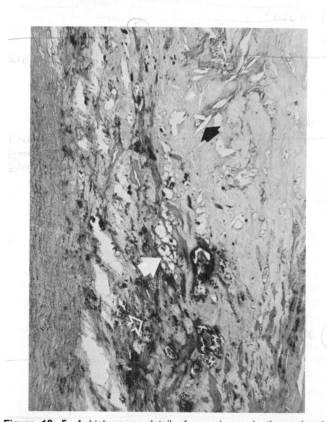

Figure 10–5. A high-power detail of an advanced atherosclerotic plaque. The media is to the left. The pale atheroma *(upper right)* contains cholesterol clefts *(black arrow)*, a few remaining foam cells *(white arrow)*, and granular black precipitates of calcium *(open arrow)*.

The typical atheroma may undergo one of four changes, giving rise to so-called **complicated plaques:**

- In advanced disease, **plaques frequently undergo patchy or massive calcification,** and arteries may be converted to virtual pipestems.
- **Fissuring or ulceration of the luminal surface** with rupture of the plaque may discharge debris into the bloodstream **(cholesterol emboli).**
- Fissured or ulcerated lesions may develop **superimposed thrombosis** (Fig. 10–6).
- **Hemorrhage** into a plaque may result from loss of endothelial integrity (early ulceration), leading to progressive influx of blood from the vessel lumen, or the hemorrhage may arise from the periplaque capillaries described. The hemorrhage may balloon the plaque and lead to its rupture.

Plaques may develop the four complications in any combination. It is evident that **ulceration, thrombosis, and intraplaque hemorrhage have serious consequences in smaller vessels such as those of the heart and brain, because they may cause total vascular occlusion.** In larger vessels (e.g., the aorta), such complications have little effect on the luminal diameter, but damage to the underlying media may yield an **atherosclerotic aneurysm** (p. 294) typically located in the distal aorta below the renal arteries.

CLINICAL SIGNIFICANCE. The clinical implications and potential consequences of AS have already been amply emphasized. Understandably, then, there are intensive efforts to devise means to reduce its toll. These involve *primary prevention* programs for persons who have never suffered an acute atherosclerotic event, aimed at preventing or delaying the formation of atheromatous plaques or possibly causing regression in persons who have never suffered an acute atherosclerotic event, and *secondary prevention* programs intended to prevent recurrence of acute atherosclerotic events such as MI. The media are filled with advice (some of it quite sound) on primary prevention: cessation of cigarette smoking, treatment of hypertension, weight reduction by control of total calorie intake coupled with increased exercise, moderating alcohol consumption, and most important, lowering blood cholesterol levels, particularly LDL and VLDL, while increasing HDL. Thus the great current interest in replacing saturated fats (red meat, eggs, butter, and other fat-laden dairy products) with mono- or polyunsaturated fats such as are in olive, corn, and safflower oils and the Ω-3 fatty acids derived from fish. If such methods are not successful in lowering high blood levels of cholesterol, there is growing interest in the use of lipid-lowering drugs and particularly in the genetic hyperlipidemias. A large number of agents have been developed, such as clofibrate, cholestyramine, and lovastatin to name only a few, that lower lipoprotein levels either by diminishing their production or by augmenting their removal from plasma.

Although the controversy persists, most of the evidence indicates that treatment of hypercholesterolemia, whether by diet or drugs, reduces the mortality rate from IHD. Moreover, it is also hoped that lipid-lowering regimens will favor the regression of already developed atherosclerotic plaques, as has been documented in animals. In addition, several angiographic studies in humans strongly suggest that lipid-lowering diets retard the progression of coronary arterial narrowing and even reduce the size of plaques. Analogously (as we will point out in the discussion of myocardial infarction), secondary prevention programs based on attempts to lower blood lipid levels and prevent thrombotic complications using antiplatelet drugs have successfully reduced the frequency of recurrent myocardial infarcts (p. 313). Despite all the encouraging results, a minority of investigators decry the preoccupation with blood lipids, pointing out that the pathogenesis of this disease is undoubtedly multifactorial. But if we wait until all the pieces of the puzzle have been put together, thousands of possibly preventable deaths may have occurred.

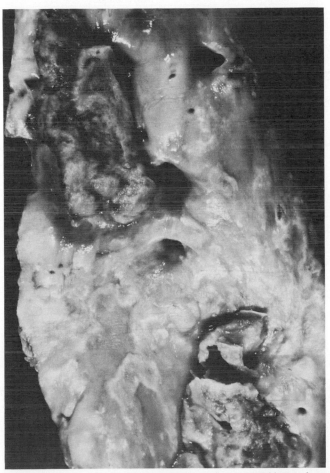

Figure 10–6. Advanced atherosclerosis of the aorta with two large mural thrombi overlying atheromatous plaques. (Courtesy of Dr. Frederick Schoen, Brigham and Women's Hospital and Harvard Medical School, Boston, MA.)

VASCULITIS

The term *vasculitis* is applied to any inflammatory involvement of an artery, vein, or venule; when the aorta is affected it is referred to as aortitis. One or a relatively few vessels may be affected, as for example in a localized area of infection, irradiation, mechanical trauma, or in the Arthus reaction, but in a few more or less distinctive conditions, the vasculitis is more widespread. Some of these systemic disorders have been described previously, such as the connective tissue diseases, e.g., systemic lupus erythematosus (p. 139) and serum sickness. There remains for consideration here the *systemic necrotizing vasculitides* cited in Table 10–2. Because the morphologic changes in some of these disorders are very similar, the clinical setting and distribution of lesions assume great importance in the differential diagnosis.

HYPERSENSITIVITY (LEUKOCYTOCLASTIC) VASCULITIS

This designation may be applied in a generic sense to any form of immune-mediated vasculitis, but most often it refers to immune complex–mediated postcapillary venulitis involving solely or predominantly the microvenules in the skin, and occasionally also those in various internal organs such as lungs, brain, kidneys, and gastrointestinal tract. This form of vasculitis occurs in Henoch-Schönlein purpura, serum sickness, systemic lupus erythematosus and other connective tissue diseases, mixed cryoglobulinemia, chronic active hepatitis B, and sometimes lymphoproliferative diseases, but in the majority of cases it is encountered in the absence of a background disease, as a hypersensitivity response to some exogenous antigen such as bacteria, viruses, drugs, or chemicals. The presumed pathogenesis of the venulitis is as follows:

TABLE 10–2. MAJOR VASCULITIS SYNDROMES

Syndrome	Vessels Involved	Distribution of Vascular Involvement	Principal Morphologic Features
Hypersensitivity (leukocytoclastic) vasculitis	Venules, capillaries, arterioles	Widespread, but particularly skin	Necrosis and neutrophilic infiltration of venules with leukocytoclasis "nuc dust"
Polyarteritis nodosa	Medium-sized and small arteries	GI tract, liver, kidney, pancreas, muscles, other sites	Panmural acute necrotizing arteritis with fibrinoid necrosis, neutrophil and eosinophil infiltration, and extension into adventitia
Wegener's granulomatosis	Small to medium-sized arteries	Upper and lower respiratory tracts; occasionally eye, skin, heart	Acute and chronic (sometimes granulomatous) angiitis with prominent eosinophils and occasional giant cells in association with extravascular granulomas
Churg-Strauss allergic angiitis and granulomatosis	Medium-sized and small arteries and veins	Systemic, with pulmonary involvement in many cases	Same as for Wegener's with more eosinophils
Temporal (cranial) arteritis	Elastic tissue–rich major arteries	Head, including ocular and intracranial vessels; uncommonly systemic	Chronic mononuclear inflammatory infiltration, mostly in inner half of the media, with giant cells and granuloma formation
Kawasaki's arteritis	Small and medium-sized arteries	Skin, ocular and oral mucosa, coronary arteries, but may be widespread	Acute and chronic infiltration, mainly with lymphocytes and macrophages, and with endothelial cell necrosis and immunoglobulin deposition
Thromboangiitis obliterans (Buerger's disease)	Medium-sized and small arteries and veins	Extremities	Acute and chronic inflammatory infiltration of arteries and veins, often with giant cells, granulomas, intravascular thrombi containing microabscesses, and later perivascular fibrosis trapping nerve trunks

1. Antibody response to an inciting antigen.
2. Formation of circulating immune complexes.
3. Deposition of these complexes in venules.
4. Activation in situ of complement with the formation of C3a and C5a.
5. Chemotactic accumulation of neutrophils within the vessel walls.
6. Release of lysosomal enzymes from neutrophils and macrophages, particularly elastase and collagenase, and possibly also toxic free radicals, with necrosis of the vessel wall (Fig. 10–7).

Rupture of dermal venules leads to the classic finding of *palpable purpura,* which may become confluent to produce large macules, vesicles, and even necrotic ulcerations.

The classic histologic features are the aggregation of neutrophils within and about venules followed by karyorrhexis of some nuclei to produce nuclear dust (leukocytoclasis; Fig. 10–8). In severe cases, there is deposition of fibrinoid in vessel walls and necrosis or thrombosis of venules. Immunofluorescence of early lesions often reveals mural granular deposits of immunoglobulin G (IgG), IgM, and C3. Infrequently, and possibly later, lymphocytic infiltration of the venule walls predominates.

In Henoch-Schönlein purpura, which usually occurs in children but occasionally in adults, the hypersensitivity vasculitis produces not only palpable purpura

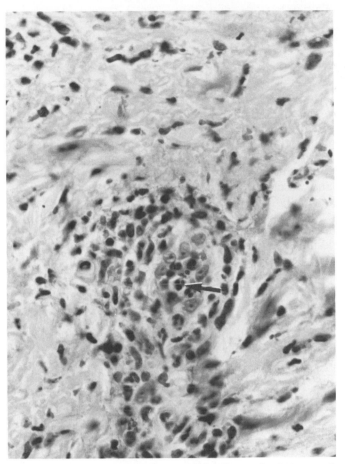

Figure 10–8. Leukocytoclastic vasculitis. The wall of the small venule is infiltrated with neutrophils and nuclear debris and is markedly thickened with near obliteration of the lumen *(arrow).*

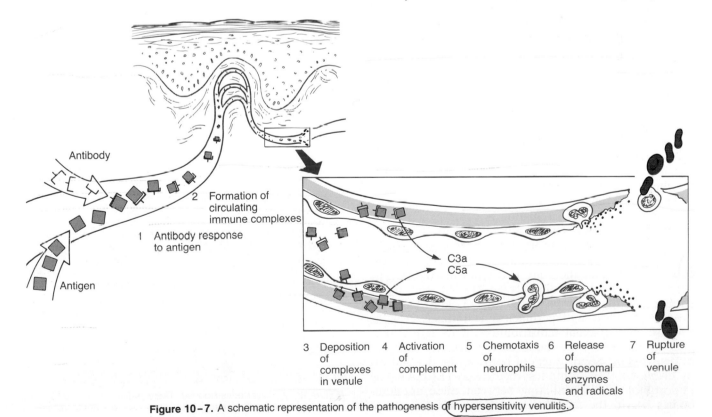

Antibody

2 Formation of circulating immune complexes

1 Antibody response to antigen

Antigen

C3a
C5a

3 Deposition of complexes in venule
4 Activation of complement
5 Chemotaxis of neutrophils
6 Release of lysosomal enzymes and radicals
7 Rupture of venule

Figure 10–7. A schematic representation of the pathogenesis of hypersensitivity venulitis.

but also abdominal pain, arthralgia, and hematuria and proteinuria as manifestations of glomerulopathy.

POLYARTERITIS NODOSA _____

Polyarteritis nodosa (PAN), formerly called "periarteritis nodosa," classically is a disease of medium- to small-sized arteries characterized by transmural acute necrotizing inflammation of these vessels. The involvement is peculiarly focal, random, and episodic, often producing irregular aneurysmal dilatation, nodularity, and vascular obstruction, and sometimes infarctions. Virtually any organ or tissue of the body may be affected, with the striking exception of the lungs and the aorta with its primary branches. In some cases the lesions are entirely microscopic, in which case the disease is called microscopic PAN. The unpredictability of the organ involvement leads to a variety of signs and symptoms that often challenge clinical diagnosis.

When there is systemic vasculitis with very similar vascular histologic changes but involvement of the lungs the condition is likely to represent the Churg-Strauss syndrome (p. 289). Analogously, Wegener's granulomatosis (p. 289) is associated with necrotizing arteritis virtually identical to that in PAN, but in both Churg-Strauss syndrome and Wegener's granulomatosis the acute arterial lesions are often accompanied by granulomatous inflammation in extravascular sites and sometimes within the vessel walls, as well as other distinctive features that distinguish these conditions from PAN.

PAN appears most often in middle-aged adults, although any age may be affected from infancy to the advanced years of life; the male-female ratio is 2:1 or 3:1. No familial distribution or particular human leukocyte antigen (HLA) phenotype has been observed.

The *cause and pathogenesis* of PAN remain uncertain, although there are strong hints that the vascular lesions are immune complex mediated. PAN is often associated with hepatitis B antigenemia, and the resultant immune complexes have been identified within the foci of vascular inflammation. Moreover, the lesions of PAN resemble those seen in the Arthus reaction. However, the basis for the peculiarly quixotic segmental involvement is unknown. Of recent date another possible mechanism has been proposed. Antineutrophil cytoplasmic autoantibodies (ANCA) have been identified in the circulation of some patients with polyarteritis nodosa. These antibodies were first identified in, and are far more importantly related to, Wegener's granulomatosis. Immunofluorescence microscopy revealed that there are two types of ANCA: one stains the cytoplasm diffusely (c-ANCA) and reacts with a recently described proteinase-3, and a second produces nuclear and perinuclear staining (p-ANCA) because of artifactual redistribution of its target antigen, myeloperoxidase, found in the primary granules of neutrophils. Serum titers of both can be determined by enzyme-linked immunosorbent assay (ELISA). The importance of differentiating between these autoantibodies lies in the fact that c-ANCA is almost always present in patients with Wegener's granulomatosis, but infrequently in the other vasculitides, including PAN. Either or both types of ANCA may appear in some patients with PAN. It has been speculated that these antibodies, which appear for uncertain reasons but possibly as an autoimmune reaction, interact with and activate neutrophils and monocytes causing the release of toxic oxygen radicals and lytic enzymes that damage endothelial cells and lead to the vascular necrosis. Intercurrent infections amplify the leukocyte activation by releasing cytokines. Plausible as this hypothesis may be, it needs documentation.

In the classic case, PAN involves arteries of medium to small size in any organ, with the possible exception of the lung. The distribution of lesions in descending order of frequency is: kidneys, heart, liver, gastrointestinal tract, followed by pancreas, testes, skeletal muscle, nervous system, and skin. Individual lesions are sharply segmental, and indeed on microscopic evaluation may not involve the entire circumference of the vessel. They tend to be located at branch points and bifurcations. Aneurysmal dilatation and nodularity may appear in the area of involvement; however, as noted earlier, sometimes the lesions are exclusively microscopic and produce no visible gross changes. Whatever the gross appearance, the vasculitis during the acute phase is characterized by transmural inflammation of the arterial wall with a heavy infiltrate of neutrophils, eosinophils, and mononuclear cells, frequently accompanied by fibrinoid necrosis of the inner half of the vessel wall (Fig. 10–9). Typically the inflammatory reaction permeates the adventitia. The lumen may become thrombosed. In some lesions only a portion of the circumference is affected, leaving segments of normal arterial wall juxtaposed to areas of vascular inflammation. At a later stage the acute inflammatory infiltrate begins to disap-

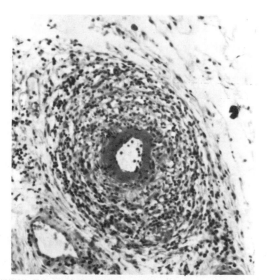

Figure 10–9. Polyarteritis nodosa. There is fibrinoid necrosis of the intima and severe inflammatory infiltration in and about the vessel.

pear and is replaced by fibrous thickening of the vessel wall accompanied by a mononuclear infiltrate. The fibroblastic proliferation may extend into the adventitia, contributing to the firm nodularity that sometimes marks the lesions. At a still later stage, all that remains is marked fibrotic thickening of the affected vessel devoid of significant inflammatory infiltration. **Particularly characteristic of PAN is that all stages of activity may co-exist in different vessels or even within the same vessel.** Thus, whatever the inflammatory insult, it is apparently recurrent and strangely haphazard.

The clinical signs and symptoms of this disease are as varied as the sites of vascular involvement. The onset may be acute or insidious, but in most cases it pursues a protracted course with recurrent flare-ups of activity. Malaise, fever, weakness, and weight loss may usher in the disease. Eventually organ damage appears. Renal involvement is one of the prominent manifestations of PAN and a major cause of death. Hypertension is common and may precede the apparent renal disease. Vascular lesions in the gastrointestinal tract produce a wide variety of symptoms, including abdominal pain, diarrhea, and melena. Peripheral neuropathy or spinal cord involvement is sometimes encountered. Indeed, except for the lungs, no organ is spared.

The presentations are so diverse that clinical diagnosis can be established only by biopsy of suspected areas of involvement, favored sites being kidney and skeletal muscle. The anatomic evaluation of the biopsy must take into consideration the close similarities among PAN, Churg-Strauss syndrome, and Wegener's granulomatosis. Death may occur during an acute fulminant attack, but more often the course is protracted, with recurrent relapses spaced by intervals of months to years. Some success has been achieved in producing remissions and possibly cures with the use of steroids or cyclophosphamide.

WEGENER'S GRANULOMATOSIS

Wegener's granulomatosis (WG) is classically characterized by the triad of (1) necrotizing granulomas of the upper respiratory tract (ear, nose, throat) or lower respiratory tract or both, (2) necrotizing or granulomatous vasculitis of small arteries and veins dominantly in the lungs but possibly elsewhere, and (3) necrotizing, often crescentic, glomerulonephritis. There are, however, instances of "limited WG" in which the kidneys are unaffected and the involvement is restricted to the respiratory tract, and conversely more widespread WG with vasculitis involving the eye, skin, and rarely other organs, notably the heart. These systemic distributions may produce clinical syndromes very similar to PAN save that the lungs are involved. Males are affected somewhat more often than females—at an average age of about 40 years.

Morphologically, the upper respiratory tract lesions range from inflammatory sinusitis due to the development of mucosal granulomas to ulcerative lesions of the nose, palate, or pharynx rimmed by necrotizing granulomas and accompanying vasculitis. In the lungs, dispersed focal necrotizing granulomas may coalesce to produce radiographically visible nodules that may undergo cavitation. Microscopically, the granulomas reveal a geographic pattern of necrosis rimmed by lymphocytes, plasma cells, macrophages, and variable numbers of giant cells. In association with such lesions there is a necrotizing or granulomatous vasculitis of small, and sometimes larger, arteries and veins (Fig. 10-10). The necrotizing pattern produces a vasculitis that is indistinguishable from that in polyarteritis. Scattered eosinophils may be present in the inflammatory foci. With severe disease, involvement of the vessels extends down to the level of alveolar capillaries, sometimes producing large areas of alveolar hemorrhage. Focal segmental necrotizing glomerulonephritis is present in most but not all cases (p. 451).

The pathogenesis of WG is unknown, although many hints point to autoimmunity. Immune complexes have been identified in the circulation and in the glomeruli and vessel walls in occasional patients. Frequently rheumatoid factor can be identified in the serum and hypergammaglobulinemia is present (elevated levels of serum IgG and IgA). Recently the previously described (p. 288) autoantibodies, termed ANCAs, particularly the c-ANCA directed against specific cytoplasmic targets in neutrophils and monocytes, have been identified in more than 95% of these patients. In the absence of p-ANCA, the cytoplasmic type c-ANCA, appears to be quite specific for WG. What role the ANCAs play in the pathogenesis of the granulomatous lesions remains unknown, but their possible contribution to the necrotizing vasculitis was pointed out on page 288.

The clinical features of WG can be deduced from the anatomic findings, so it remains only to point out that the course of untreated disease is progressive with a two-year mortality rate of over 90%. When the diagnosis is established—usually by biopsy of a respiratory lesion to confirm the presence of granulomas and arteritis—appropriate therapy (cyclophosphamide, possibly prednisone, and sometimes antibacterial drugs) produces a gratifying response in the great majority of patients with only occasional relapses.

CHURG-STRAUSS SYNDROME

Churg-Strauss syndrome (CSS), also known as *allergic granulomatosis and angiitis,* is an uncommon condition, the clinical features of which overlap those of PAN and WG. *In the classic case of CSS there is a systemic vasculitis in association with fever, severe asthma, and marked eosinophilia.* The vasculitis involves both arteries and veins, particularly in the lungs,

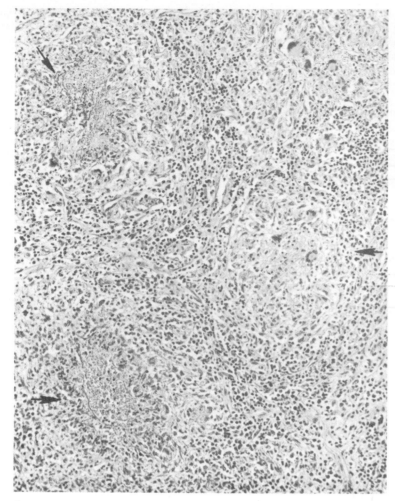

A

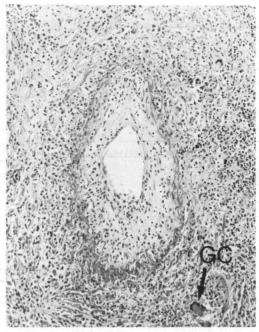

B

Figure 10–10. *A,* Multiple granulomas in lungs in Wegener's granulomatosis *(arrows).* Note central necrosis and multinucleate giant cells. *B,* Small artery in lung in Wegener's granulomatosis. The wall is markedly thickened, fibrotic, and infiltrated with white cells. There is perivascular inflammation and a giant cell (GC).

spleen, gastrointestinal tract, and heart, and only rarely in the kidney (in contrast to WG). The vasculitis may be granulomatous, resembling the changes in WG, or on the other hand may be nonspecific and necrotizing, resembling the lesions of PAN. Extravascular necrotizing granulomas replete with giant cells and eosinophils are also present. Distinctive in all vascular and extravascular lesions is the striking number of eosinophils, more than are seen in WG or PAN.

The pathogenesis of this condition is obscure, but some form of hypersensitivity reaction very likely to an exogenous antigen is suspected and consistent with the induction of the asthma and the morphologic changes. Moreover, the vasculitis of CSS usually responds dramatically to steroid therapy, which is also consonant with an immune cause, but unlike WG, such cytotoxic agents as cyclophosphamide often are not effective. Thus, to differentiate CSS from WG is rather important, and in this regard testing for antineutrophil antibodies may be very helpful. Whereas c-ANCA can be demonstrated in most patients with WG, they are not found in CSS.

It must be evident from the preceding discussions that there are many similarities among PAN, WG, and CSS, and while distinguishing features have been em-

phasized, some cases "fall into the cracks," defying clear-cut categorization.

TEMPORAL (GIANT CELL, CRANIAL) ARTERITIS

The most common of the arteritides, temporal arteritis is characterized by segmental acute and chronic (most often granulomatous) vasculitis involving predominantly the larger arteries in the head, particularly the branches of the carotid artery. Favored locations are the temporal arteries and the terminal branches of the ophthalmic artery, involvements that may lead to unilateral, rarely bilateral, blindness. Other vessels may be affected, including the aorta and arteries to the brain and the breast, but almost never are heart and lungs involved. Temporal arteritis usually occurs in elders (after age 50) with a 2:1 or 3:1 female-male ratio. The incidence increases with age. In about half of cases the arteritis develops on a background of polymyalgia rheumatica, a disorder common in elders, marked by pain and stiffness in the proximal muscles of the hip and shoulder girdles, neck, and buttocks, but in the remaining cases it arises de novo.

Characteristically, short segments of one or more affected arteries develop nodular thickenings with reduction of the lumen, possibly to a slit-like orifice, which may become thrombosed. Histologically, two patterns are seen. In the more common variant there is granulomatous inflammation of the inner half of the media centered on the internal elastic membrane marked by a mononuclear infiltrate, multinucleate giant cells of both foreign body and Langhans type, and fragmentation of the internal elastic lamina (Fig. 10–11). The lymphocytes in the infiltrate have been shown to bear T-cell markers, but there is disagreement as to whether helper or suppressor T cells predominate. In the other pattern, granulomas are rare or absent and there is only a nonspecific panarteritis with a mixed inflammatory infiltrate largely of lymphocytes and macrophages admixed with some neutrophils and eosinophils but no giant cells. Occasionally in this variant there is some fibrinoid necrosis. The later healed stage of both of these patterns reveals only collagenous thickening of the vessel wall; organization of the luminal thrombus sometimes transforms the artery into a fibrous cord.

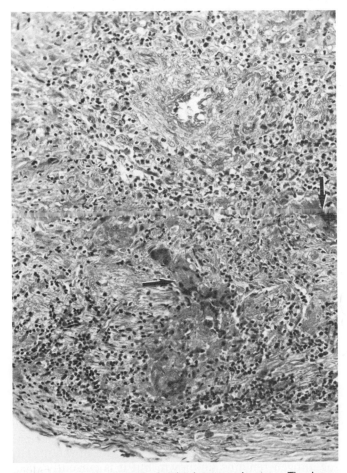

Figure 10–11. A markedly involved temporal artery. The lumen above is severely narrowed by the inflammation and there are numerous giant cells (arrows) at the inner boundary of the media, but the elastic membrane cannot be seen.

The pathogenesis of temporal arteritis is unknown, but on the basis of the granulomatous nature of the inflammation, immune mechanisms are suspected. T cells reactive to arterial wall have been described in a few cases, but the particular antigenic target remains unknown. Although in the past attention was focused on some modification of the elastica as the inciting trigger, more recently emphasis has been placed on some basis for increased expression of HLA-DR antigens on smooth muscle cells in the media. Familial aggregations and predominance of the disease among whites suggest a genetic predisposition.

Clinically this condition may begin with only vague constitutional symptoms—fever, fatigue, weight loss—without localizing signs or symptoms, but in the great majority of instances there is facial pain or headache, which is severe, sometimes unilateral, and often most intense along the course of the superficial temporal artery. The vessel itself may be nodular and painful to palpation. More serious are ocular symptoms, which sometimes appear quite abruptly in about half of all patients, ranging from diplopia to transient to complete vision loss. Hence the urgency in establishing the diagnosis promptly, as treatment with steroids is remarkably effective. The diagnosis rests on biopsy and histologic confirmation, but because of the segmental nature of the involvement, adequate biopsy requires at least a 2- to 3-cm length of artery. Obviously, a negative biopsy result does not rule out the condition. Hematologic malignancies appear in 2 to 4% of those who have concurrent polymyalgia rheumatica.

TAKAYASU'S ARTERITIS (PULSELESS DISEASE)

Takayasu's arteritis (pulseless disease) is a chronic vasculitis that affects principally the aorta and its main branches and sometimes the pulmonary arteries. The aortic involvement may be restricted to the arch alone, may spare the arch and affect the rest of the aorta, or in some cases involves the entire aorta. Uncommonly, the major branches of the aortic arch are more severely affected than the aorta. This condition occurs predominantly in persons younger than 40 years and shows a strong female preponderance. Although previously it was reported most often in Asians, Takayasu's arteritis is global in distribution. Genetic predisposition has been proposed, based on an increased frequency of HLA-DR4 genes among those affected.

Gross morphologic changes, when present, are thickening of the aortic wall with intimal wrinkling and narrowing of the orifices of the great vessels that arise from areas of involvement, accounting for the name **pulseless disease.** The origins of the coronary and renal arteries may be similarly affected. Sometimes the vasculitis extends some distance into the aortic branches, and in about half the cases it also involves the pulmonary arteries. The histologic changes evolve over time. In the earlier active stage there is a prominent granulomatous arteritis, principally restricted to the media and adventitia but sometimes extending throughout the thickness of the vessel wall with patchy destruction of the musculoelastic lamellae of the media. At this stage of Takayasu's disease the histologic changes are reminiscent of those in temporal arteritis, and indeed both conditions are sometimes included under the rubric **giant cell aortitis or arteritis.** Prominent in the inflammatory infiltrate are lymphocytes and plasma cells, confined mainly to the media and adventitia. There are in addition numerous giant cells of both Langhans and foreign body types. Later or after treatment with steroids the inflammatory reaction is predominantly marked by collagenous fibrosis involving all layers of the vessel wall, but particularly the intima, accompanied by lymphocytic infiltration (Fig. 10–12). Still later only the collagenous thickening persists. When the root of the aorta is affected, it may undergo dilatation, producing aortic valve insufficiency. Narrowing of the coronary ostia may lead to myocardial infarction.

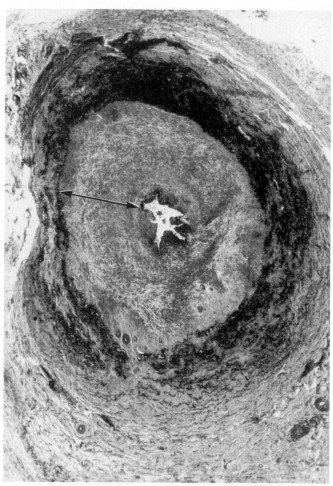

Figure 10–12. Takayasu's arteritis involving the common carotid artery — end-stage disease. There is striking intimal thickening *(arrow)*. The preceding mural inflammation has left areas of medial fibrosis and inflammation, and other areas of marked reduplication of the elastica (black in the elastic tissue stain).

The *cause and pathogenesis* of this disease remain obscure, although immune mechanisms have been suspected for many years. Reports of circulating antibodies directed against arterial wall antigens have not been confirmed, and attention is currently directed to some form of cell-mediated mechanism, the existence of which is supported by the demonstration of an increased prevalence of the HLA-DR4 haplotype and blast transformation of T cells on exposure to extracts of aortic wall. However, none of the immunologic findings to date are very convincing.

Most patients (usually young women) have symptoms of vascular insufficiency of the extremities, mainly in the upper extremities, with coldness or numbness of the fingers. In time a pulse discrepancy between the left and right arms of more than 30 mm Hg sometimes appears. Involvement of the more distal aorta may lead to claudication of the legs. Other features include a bruit, most frequently heard over the carotid artery and abdominal aorta but possibly elsewhere; postural dizziness; visual disturbances; and in some cases manifestations of coronary artery insufficiency or aortic valve regurgitation. Involvement of pulmonary arteries may lead to pulmonary hypertension and manifestations of cor pulmonale (p. 315). The diagnosis rests mainly on angiographic or sonographic documentation of the aortic thickening. The course of the disease is variable. In some persons there is rapid progression, but in others a quiescent stage is reached in 1 or 2 years, permitting long-term survival albeit sometimes with visual or neurologic deficits.

KAWASAKI'S DISEASE (MUCOCUTANEOUS LYMPH NODE SYNDROME)

An acute febrile illness of infancy and early childhood, Kawasaki's disease is self-limited in many instances but in most cases vasculitis of the coronary arteries appears, sometimes leading to aneurysm formation and possibly superimposed thrombosis. Thus 0.5 to 1% of patients die of myocardial infarction.

The cause of the condition is unknown, but there is increasing evidence that the vasculitis is based on an immunoregulatory defect characterized by T-cell and macrophage activation, the secretion of cytokines, polyclonal B-cell hyperactivity, and the formation of autoantibodies to endothelial cells leading to their destruction and subsequent acute vasculitis. The following scenario is proposed: Some unknown antigenic agent leads to activation of the immune system with the formation of high serum levels of IL-1, TNF, and IFN-γ. These cytokines induce the expression of endothelial cell activation antigens, which in turn stimulate the production of antibodies to the antigens that are cytotoxic to endothelial cells. The nature of the initiating antigen remains unknown, but it is currently speculated that in genetically susceptible persons a variety of common infectious agents (more likely viral) may trigger the sequence of changes described.

The acute phase of disease begins with vasculitis and perivasculitis of small vessels—arterioles, venules, and capillaries. Small vessel changes resemble those of "microscopic PAN" save that the inflammation is maximal in the intima. Later, larger arteries in the body, including the coronaries, may be affected with changes similar to those of polyarteritis. At this time, myocarditis, pericarditis, or valvulitis may appear. The acute phase eventually begins to subside spontaneously or in response to treatment, but it is during this subsiding phase that the acute vasculitis of the coronary arteries often leads to aneurysm formation, and sometimes associated thrombosis with myocardial infarction.

Thromboangiitis is characterized by sharply segmental acute and chronic vasculitis of medium-sized and small arteries with secondary spread to contiguous veins and nerves. Often the vascular supply to the extremities, upper as well as lower, is affected. By contrast, atherosclerosis affects predominantly the larger arteries, and mostly those in the lower extremities. Microscopically acute and chronic inflammation permeates the arterial walls accompanied by thrombosis of the lumen, which may undergo organization and recanalization. Characteristically, the thrombus contains small microabscesses marked by a central focus of neutrophils surrounded by granulomatous inflammation. The inflammatory process extends into and about the accompanying veins and nerves, and in time all three structures become encased in fibrous tissue.

The characteristic clinical features are fever, bilateral nonpurulent conjunctivitis, erythema of the palms of the hands and soles of the feet accompanied by edema and later desquamation, followed by the development of a rash composed of erythematous plaques or even pustules. Lymphadenopathy, frequently present at this time, is usually limited to a single node in the neck. All these manifestations are relatively inconsequential compared to the involvement of the heart leading to arrhythmias, cardiac dilatation with mitral insufficiency, congestive heart failure, and most ominously myocardial infarction.

Often clinically manifest Buerger's disease is preceded by Raynaud's phenomenon (below) or recurrent episodes of migratory thrombophlebitis of superficial veins. Eventually the classic manifestations of vascular insufficiency appear: claudication, and color and temperature changes. In contrast to the insufficiency caused by atherosclerosis, in Buerger's disease it tends to be accompanied by severe pain, even at rest, related undoubtedly to the neural involvement. Chronic ulcerations of the toes, feet, or fingers may appear, perhaps followed in time by frank gangrene. Abstinence from cigarette smoking in the early stages of the disease often brings dramatic relief from further attacks.

THROMBOANGIITIS OBLITERANS (BUERGER'S DISEASE)

Buerger's disease is a remitting, relapsing, inflammatory disorder that often leads to thrombosis of medium-sized vessels principally the tibial and radial arteries with secondary extension to the adjacent veins and nerves. Mainly it is a disease of male cigarette smokers aged 25 to 50 years but the recent increase among females is attributed to the changing smoking practices in the past two decades. This condition is very important because it often leads to vascular insufficiency in the extremities and sometimes gangrene, so it must be differentiated from other potential causes of peripheral vascular disease such as atherosclerosis and thromboembolism.

The cause and pathogenesis of Buerger's disease are unknown, but they are clearly related in some way to the use of tobacco products. Many patients show hypersensitivity to intradermally injected tobacco extracts. Conceivably some derivative of tobacco or tobacco smoke might have direct endothelial toxicity or incite an immunologic reaction in predisposed persons. In this connection there is an increased prevalence of HLA-A9 and -B5 in these patients, and the condition is far more common in Israel, Japan, and India than in the United States and Europe, all hinting at genetic influences.

RAYNAUD'S DISEASE

Unlike the vasculitis syndromes, which have well-defined organic lesions, Raynaud's disease (as opposed to Raynaud's phenomenon) refers to paroxysmal pallor or cyanosis of acral parts (usually the digits of the hands, sometimes those of the feet, and infrequently the tip of the nose or the ears) caused by intense spasm of local small arteries and arterioles. It is an idiopathic disease, principally of otherwise healthy young women. In contrast, Raynaud's phenomenon refers to arterial insufficiency of the acral parts secondary to some other disorder that is responsible for arterial narrowing, for example, systemic lupus erythematosus, systemic sclerosis, atherosclerosis, or Buerger's disease. Indeed, Raynaud's phenomenon may be the first manifestation of any of these conditions. Although the cause of Raynaud's disease is unknown, it appears to be based on an exaggeration of normal central and local vasomotor responses to cold or to emotion. Anatomically, the involved vessels are normal until late in the course, when prolonged vasospasm may cause secondary intimal thickening. The course of Raynaud's disease is variable. Often it remains static for years and is no more than a nuisance for the patient, who must avoid situations that are likely to precipitate an attack. In some cases the disorder subsides spontaneously. Occasionally patients develop progressive disease and have some degree of cyanosis at all times. Eventually trophic changes and ulcerations appear in the skin, and even areas of gangrene at the fingertips.

ANEURYSMS

Abnormal dilatations of arteries or veins are called aneurysms. They are described here because they are much more frequent and important in arteries, especially the aorta. They develop wherever there is marked weakening of the wall of a vessel. Any vessel may be affected by a wide variety of disorders, including congenital defects, local infections (mycotic aneurysms), trauma (traumatic aneurysms or arteriovenous aneurysms), or systemic diseases that weaken arterial walls. The principal causes of aortic aneurysms are atherosclerosis, syphilis, and medionecrosis leading to dissecting and nondissecting aneurysms. Congenital defects of the intracranial arteries, _berry aneurysms,_ are also fairly frequent; they represent an important cause of cerebrovascular accidents (CVA) (see p. 715). Much has been made in the past about the following terms in relation to the gross appearance of an aneurysm—saccular, fusiform, cylindroid, and berry-shaped. Actually, these are merely descriptors that require no further comment save that many aneurysms have not heard about them and refuse to conform to these classical patterns. Having made these comments, we can deal with the three major etiologic forms of aortic aneurysms.

ATHEROSCLEROTIC ANEURYSM

Atherosclerosis is by far the most common cause of aortic aneurysms. They are most frequent in males (5:1 ratio) after the fifth decade of life. The major risk factors for atherosclerosis (p. 278) are the risk factors for these aneurysms. Although any site in the aorta may be affected, including the thoracic aorta, the great preponderance occur in the abdominal aorta, usually below the renal arteries. _Until proved otherwise, an abdominal aneurysm is assumed to be atherosclerotic in origin._ Occasionally, several separate dilatations occur, and not infrequently abdominal aortic lesions are accompanied by additional aneurysms in the iliac arteries.

Atherosclerotic aneurysms take the form of saccular (balloon-like), cylindroid, or fusiform swellings, sometimes up to 15 cm in greatest diameter and of variable length (up to 25 cm). As would be expected, at these sites there is severe complicated atherosclerosis, which destroys the underlying tunica media and thus weakens the aortic wall. Mural thrombus frequently is found within the aneurysmal sac. In the saccular forms, the thrombus may completely fill the outpouching up to the

level of the surrounding aortic wall (Fig. 10–13). The elongated fusiform or cylindroid patterns more often have layers of mural thrombus that only partially fill the dilatation.

The clinical consequences of these aneurysms depend principally on their location and size. Occlusion of the iliac, renal, or mesenteric arteries may result either from pressure by the aneurysmal sac or from propagation of the thrombus. The thrombus may embolize. As enlarging pulsatile masses, these aneurysms not only simulate tumors but also progressively erode adjacent structures such as the vertebral bodies. They have been known to erode the wall of the gut or, when they occur in the thorax, the wall of the trachea or esophagus. Rupture is the most feared consequence and is related to the size of the dilatation. In general, when they are smaller than 6 cm in diameter these

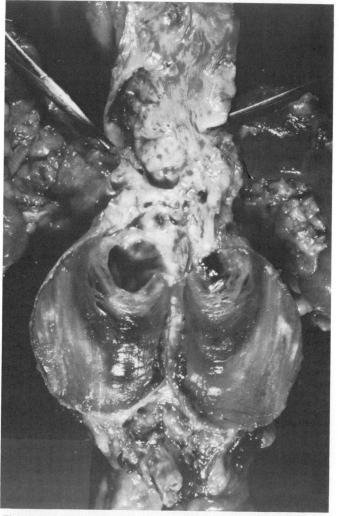

Figure 10–13. An atherosclerotic aneurysm of the abdominal aorta below the renal arteries (marked by clamps). The saccular dilatation with its laminated thrombus has been transected to reveal the layered clot.

aneurysms rarely rupture, whereas 50% of patients with larger lesions die of rupture within ten years of the diagnosis. Fortunately, since most such aneurysms occur below the level of the renal arteries, many can be replaced with prosthetic arterial channels with excellent results. The operative mortality before rupture is about 5%; after rupture it rises sharply, to 50%.

SYPHILITIC (LUETIC) AORTITIS AND ANEURYSM

As we pointed out in the general discussion of syphilis in Chapter 18, the tertiary stage of the disease shows a predilection for the cardiovascular and nervous systems. Fortunately, with better control and treatment of syphilis in its early stages, these involvements are becoming rare. Before discussing the cardiovascular lesion, which is termed *syphilitic (luetic) aortitis,* reference should be made to Chapter 18 for the basic tissue reactions incited by *Treponema pallidum* (i.e., *obliterative endarteritis, perivascular cuffing,* and *gumma formation*).

Although obliterative endarteritis in tertiary syphilis may involve small vessels in any part of the body, it is clinically most devastating when it affects the vasa vasorum of the aorta. Such involvement gives rise to thoracic aortitis, which in turn leads to the aneurysmal dilatation of the aorta and aortic valve ring characteristic of full-blown cardiovascular syphilis. Propensity for involvement of the proximal thoracic aorta may be related to the greater density of vasa vasorum in this region. Since this sequel to infection by *T. pallidum* does not manifest itself until 15 to 20 years later, it is seen most frequently in the age range of 40 to 55 years. Males are involved three times as often as females.

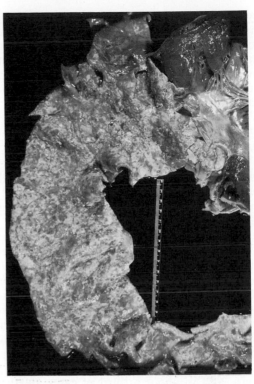

Figure 10–14. Syphilitic aortitis with superimposed florid atherosclerosis. The aortic root shows marked involvement beginning at the heart (barely visible at top right), with aneurysmal dilatation of the arch.

Syphilitic aortitis is almost always confined to the thoracic aorta, usually to the ascending and transverse portions, and rarely extends below the diaphragm. The earliest changes are obliterative endarteritis with perivascular cuffing of the vasa vasorum by plasma cells. The narrowing of these nutrient arteries leads to ischemic destruction of the elastic tissue and muscle of the media and to subsequent development of stellate fibrous scars in the media and fibrous thickening of the adventitia. With contraction of the irregular medial scars, longitudinal wrinkling or "tree barking" of the intimal surface ensues. More important, the scarring may envelop and narrow the ostia of vessels arising from the aorta, including those of the coronary arteries.

With destruction of the tunica media, the aorta loses its elastic support and tends to become dilated, producing a syphilitic aneurysm (Fig. 10–14). Secondary atherosclerotic involvement of these damaged areas is almost invariable and may contribute to the weakening of the aortic wall. The end result is diffuse involvement by calcified atherosclerotic plaques, which obliterate the intimal tree bark pattern. **Even when these aneurysms** are complicated by atherosclerosis, their location in the thorax tends to distinguish them from typical atherosclerotic aneurysms, which rarely affect the aortic arch and never involve the root of the aorta. Calcification of the ascending aorta on chest radiographs is diagnostic of luetic aortitis. Syphilitic aneurysms are sometimes enormous, achieving a diameter of 15 to 20 cm. They may contain mural thrombus. When the aneurysmal dilatation includes the aortic valve ring, the valvular commissures are widened and the valve leaflets are stretched, so that their free margins tend to roll and become thickened. Incompetence of the valve leads to marked, sometimes extraordinary, hypertrophy and dilatation of the left ventricle with resultant heart weights of up to 1000 gm (such a heart is known as **cor bovinum**).

Syphilitic aortitis with aneurysmal dilatation may give rise to (1) respiratory difficulties as a result of encroachment on the lungs and airways; (2) difficulty in swallowing, due to compression of the esophagus; (3) persistent brassy cough, from pressure on the recurrent laryngeal nerve; (4) pain, caused by erosion of bone (ribs and vertebral bodies); and (5) cardiac disease. As the aneurysm leads to dilatation of the aortic root, signs of aortic valvular insufficiency develop; these typically include a loud, diastolic murmur and widening of the pulse pressure to produce a bounding pulse (Corrigan's pulse). Most patients with syphilitic aneurysms die of heart failure due to aortic valvular incompetence. Myocardial ischemia (or infarction) from coronary ostial stenosis may contribute to cardiac dysfunction. Other causes of death include rupture of the aneurysm (with fatal hemorrhage) and erosion of vital contiguous structures such as the bronchi or esophagus by the expanding pulsatile mass.

DISSECTING ANEURYSM (DISSECTING HEMATOMA, AORTIC DISSECTION) _____

Dissecting aneurysms, as they have been called for decades, arise from intimal defects that permit blood to penetrate into the wall of the aorta with propagation of the hemorrhage along the laminar planes of the media for variable distances. Sometimes these hematomas dissect back and rupture into the pericardium, and at other times they dissect the length of the aorta to rupture into the peritoneal cavity or elsewhere. Even though the intramural hematoma produces moderate expansion of the aorta, there is rarely aneurysmal dilatation and hence a growing trend to the alternative terms "dissecting hematoma" or "aortic dissection." The development of an aortic dissection is a catastrophic event for the patient, producing sudden, severe pain, and in about a third of cases, death within the first day of the acute onset of symptoms. The male-female ratio is 3:1 at virtually any age. Half of all dissections in women under the age of 40 occur during pregnancy, usually in the third trimester. These catastrophies also appear in the first and second decades of life when there is an underlying genetic disorder of connective tissue such as Marfan's syndrome or Ehlers-Danlos syndrome. Indeed, aortic rupture is the commonest cause of death in both conditions. Other predispositions include bicuspid aortic valves and aortic coarctation. Hypertension is an almost invariable antecedent and as we will see may well play an important role in the pathogenesis of this condition.

Based on the origin and extent of the dissection, these aortic involvements have been variously subclassified. DeBakey recognized three types. Types I and II arise in the ascending aorta. In type I, the dissection extends beyond the ascending aorta (sometimes it involves the entire aorta). In type II, it is confined to the ascending aorta. The intimal tears in both types I and II are almost always in the ascending aorta. Type III dissections, on the other hand, originate in distal tears in the descending thoracic section of the vessel, some extending down to the iliac or further, but others confined to the descending thoracic aorta (Fig. 10–15). More recently the classification has been simplified into two subsets: type A includes all dissections involving the ascending aorta and type B all others. The importance of these subsets will become evident in the consideration of their natural history and management.

CLASSIFICATION. Dissections almost always originate with intimal tears, although in about 5% of cases none are found. Although these tears may occur anywhere in the aorta, 90% are located within 10 cm of the aortic valve. The next most common site of origin is

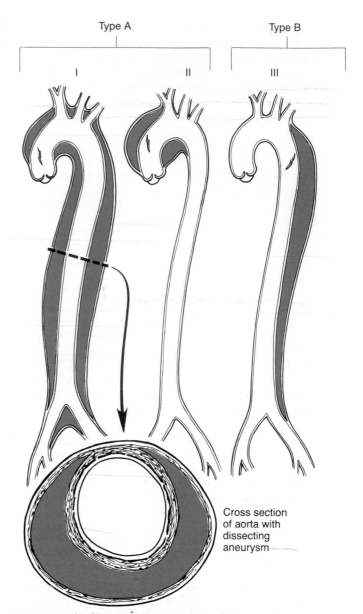

Figure 10–15. Classification of aortic dissections into types A and B and I, II, and III (see text).

Type A   Type B

I   II   III

Cross section of aorta with dissecting aneurysm

in the descending thoracic aorta just distal to the origin of the left subclavian artery.

MORPHOLOGY. The tear is usually longitudinal or oblique and 4 to 5 cm long with sharp, clean, possibly irregular edges. Blood entering this defect usually penetrates into the media and propagates generally in the medial laminar planes, typically between the outer and the middle third of the media. Concurrent atherosclerosis is usually present, consonant with the patient's age and risk factors, but only infrequently does an ulcerated plaque constitute the site of origin of the intimal tear—and usually only with dissections that arise distally. The hemorrhage may dissect proximally toward the heart, sometimes into the coronary arteries, or it may rupture into the pericardial sac or pleural cavity. In other instances, it dissects distally for some distance, sometimes into the iliac and femoral arteries. In long dissections, the hemorrhage may re-rupture back into the aortic lumen through a second distal intimal tear to produce a false lumen, or double-barrelled aorta, through which blood may flow, thus protecting against rupture into one of the body cavities or periaortic structures. The false lumen over the course of years may become endothelialized and indeed develop atherosclerosis. While the entire circumference of the aorta or other vessel may be involved, in some instances the hematoma is confined to one arc of the circumference, sparing a portion. With dissection into the smaller branches of the aorta, the inner layers may collapse upon themselves causing significant vascular obstruction.

Histologically, in the great majority of cases there are few abnormal findings in the aortic walls save for the dissection and its content of blood, which may be unchanged if the victim dies abruptly or may have undergone more or less organization depending on how long the patient survives. Overall, in fewer than 20% of cases are there focal areas of medial degeneration producing so-called cystic or laminar medionecrosis. These ill-defined lesions constitute focal clefts or irregular defects created by loss of elastica and smooth muscle cells that are filled with amorphous basophilic ground substance (Fig. 10–16). There is no accompa-

nying inflammatory reaction and the media separating these random lesions may be entirely normal. Such changes are present in the majority of patients with Marfan's syndrome, but in fewer than 20% of others.

The pathogenesis of aortic dissection remains a mystery. Its well-defined association with Marfan's syndrome points to a possible role for some connective tissue defect in all patients, but none has been identified in non-Marfan's cases. Yet in the experimental setting, copper deficiency (impairing the function of copper-dependent enzymes) and the administration of β-aminopropionitrile (producing lathyrism) block the formation of cross-linkages in collagen and elastic fibrils and lead to aortic dissections. However, the facts that the great majority of non-Marfan's patients have no cystic or laminar medionecrosis in the dissected aorta and that medionecrosis is sometimes encountered in elders as an incidental finding both indicate that such medial lesions are not critical to the development of dissection. Hypertension is present in the great majority of patients (70 to 90%) and conceivably could in some manner predispose to medial degeneration, but well-defined hypertensive changes in the vasa vasorum are infrequent. Nonetheless the elevated blood pressure may well favor propagation of the dissection. It is equally unclear whether the intimal tears initiate the dissection or occur as a secondary phenomenon, nor is the basis for the tear clear. The fact that no tear can be found in a few cases indicates that it is not a requisite initiating event.

CLINICAL COURSE. The clinical manifestations of aortic dissection derive from (1) the dissection itself and its extent, (2) the impact of the mural hematoma on aortic branches such as the coronary, renal, mesenteric, or other arteries, (3) the impact of the dissection on the aortic valve, possibly producing insufficiency, and ultimately (4) the site of the external rupture and amount of hemorrhage. Typically the onset of dissection is marked by excruciating chest pain in the great majority of patients. The differential diagnosis includes mainly acute myocardial infarction, but in aortic dissection the patients may categorize the pain as tearing or ripping with a tendency for the pain to shift or migrate as the dissection advances. The pain may be episodic and recurrent, with bouts of advancing dissection. A murmur of aortic valvular regurgitation may be present, owing to extension of the dissection into the aortic root. As the aortic branches become involved a multitude of findings may evolve: sensory and motor changes in the lower half of the body reflect compression of the vertebral branches; abdominal pain reflects compromise of the mesenteric circulation; and sudden changes or inequalities in blood pressures between the two arms reflect unequal compression of the major aortic trunks. Radiography may disclose some subtle, but not aneurysmal, widening. More effective is computed tomography (CT) or magnetic resonance imaging (MRI), which in most cases accurately reveals the abnormal thickening of the aortic wall in the area

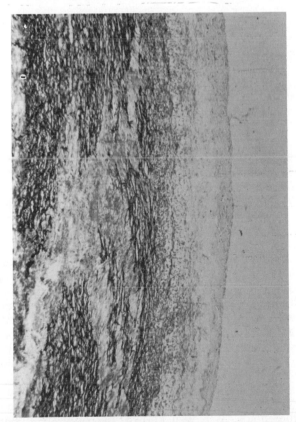

Figure 10–16. Cystic medionecrosis of the aorta. The intima is to the right. An elastic tissue stain accentuates the elastica of the media. The irregular cleft-like areas devoid of elastica represent the foci of medionecrosis. Note the absence of inflammatory reaction.

of dissection. The natural history and prognosis of this condition are extremely dependent on the promptness of diagnosis and institution of therapy. As noted earlier, without treatment about a third of patients die within the first day, and 90% within the first three months. However, this outlook has been dramatically improved by the prompt institution of effective antihypertensive treatment, optimally within minutes to hours of the onset of symptoms, followed by replacement of the ascending aorta with its intimal tear by a prosthetic graft for patients with type A dissections and long-term antihypertensive medical therapy for those with type B dissections who are at lower risk of rupture. With these regimens, the overall ten-year survival rate is now in the range of 40%, and for those who survive the acute event and leave the hospital, approximately 60%.

Venous Disorders

Although none of the disorders of veins has the impressive frequency of atherosclerosis, several, such as varicose veins and phlebothrombosis, are extremely common. Varicose veins induce a great deal of discomfort and morbidity but are rarely life threatening. On the other hand, phlebothrombosis, although somewhat less prevalent, may have lethal consequences. Discussions of these two venous disorders, as well as of the relatively rare involvements of the superior and inferior venae cavae, follow.

VARICOSE VEINS

Varicose veins are abnormally dilated, tortuous veins; this condition is caused by increased intraluminal pressure, and to a lesser extent by loss of support of the vessel wall. _Although any vein in the body may be affected, the superficial veins of the leg are by far the most frequently involved._ This predilection is due to the high venous pressure in the legs when they are dependent, coupled with the relatively poor tissue support for the superficial, as opposed to the deep, veins. Even in otherwise normal persons, these factors produce a tendency toward the development of varices with advancing age and its attendant loss of tissue tone, atrophy of muscles, and degenerative changes within the vessel walls followed by sufficient dilatation of veins to render their valves incompetent. Indeed, this disorder is seen in approximately 50% of persons after age 50 years. There is a familial tendency to develop varicose veins relatively early in life. Because of the venous stasis in the lower legs caused by pregnancy, females are more often afflicted than males. In addition, any impediment to venous flow, such as an encroaching neoplasm or encircling surgical dressing, promotes the development of varicosities, in the legs or elsewhere.

Attention should be called to two special sites of varix formation. _Hemorrhoids_ result from varicose dilatation of the hemorrhoidal plexus of veins at the anorectal junction. The causative mechanism is presumed to be prolonged pelvic congestion resulting, for example, from repeated pregnancies or chronic constipation and straining at stools. An important cause of hemorrhoids is portal hypertension, due usually to cirrhosis of the liver (p. 545).

The second and more important special site of varicosities is the esophagus, and this form is encountered virtually only in patients who have cirrhosis of the liver and its attendant portal hypertension. Rupture of an esophageal varix may be more serious than the primary liver disease itself (p. 480).

MORPHOLOGY. The affected veins are dilated, tortuous, and elongated. Characteristically, the dilatation is irregular, with nodular or fusiform distentions and even aneurysmal pouchings. Accompanying this asymmetric dilatation is marked variation in the thickness of the vessel wall. Thinning is seen at the points of maximal dilatation, whereas compensatory hypertrophy of the media and fibrosis of the wall may produce thickening in a neighboring segment. Valvular deformities (thickening, rolling, and shortening of the cusps) are common, as is intraluminal thrombosis. Microscopically, the changes are quite minimal and consist of variations in the thickness of the wall of the vein. Smooth muscle hypertrophy and subintimal fibrosis are apparent in the areas of compensatory hypertrophy. Frequently there is degeneration of the elastic tissue in the major veins and spotty calcifications within the media (**phlebosclerosis**).

CLINICAL COURSE. Sometimes distention of the veins in the legs is painful, although most often early varicose veins are asymptomatic. As the valves become incompetent, a vicious circle is established, and the resultant venous stasis further increases intraluminal pressure. Marked venous congestion with edema may occur. Such edema impairs circulation, rendering the affected tissues extremely vulnerable to injury. In these severe cases, trophic changes, stasis dermatitis, cellulitis, and varicose ulcerations are common. _Although varicose veins frequently thrombose, embolization to the lungs is uncommon from the superficial leg veins._ Hemorrhoids, as is well known, not only are uncomfortable but also may be a source of bleeding. Sometimes they thrombose and in this distended state are prone to painful ulceration.

PHLEBOTHROMBOSIS AND THROMBOPHLEBITIS

These two designations are synonyms for thrombus formation in veins. This condition was described in some detail on page 65. Here we need only recall that the thrombi most often arise in the deep veins of the lower extremities, particularly the muscular veins of the calf. Frequently they are silent clinically but have the distressing potential of giving rise to emboli that lodge in the lungs to produce pulmonary embolism and infarction, which are extremely important causes of morbidity and mortality. You may recall that phlebothrombosis is most often associated with cardiac failure, prolonged bed rest or immobilization of an extremity, postoperative and postpartal states, neoplasia, and any form of severe trauma, particularly extensive burns. In cases of cancer, particularly those primary in the abdominal cavity, the venous thromboses have a tendency to appear spontaneously in one site, only to dissappear and be followed by thromboses in other veins, giving rise to the entity referred to as *migratory thrombophlebitis (Trousseau's sign);* (p. 72). Because of the clinical settings in which phlebothrombosis appears, pulmonary embolization often constitutes the final mortal blow to those already gravely ill.

OBSTRUCTION OF SUPERIOR VENA CAVA (SUPERIOR VENA CAVAL SYNDROME)

This dramatic entity is usually caused by neoplasms that compress or invade the superior vena cava. Most commonly, a primary bronchogenic carcinoma or a mediastinal lymphoma is the underlying lesion. Occasionally, other lesions, such as an aortic aneurysm, may impinge on the superior vena cava. Regardless of the cause, the consequent obstruction produces a distinctive clinical complex referred to as the *superior vena caval syndrome.* It is manifested by dusky cyanosis and marked dilatation of the veins of the head, neck, and arms. Commonly the pulmonary vessels are also compressed, and consequently respiratory distress may develop.

OBSTRUCTION OF INFERIOR VENA CAVA (INFERIOR VENA CAVAL SYNDROME)

This is analogous to the superior vena caval syndrome and may be caused by many of the same processes. Neoplasms may either compress or penetrate the walls of the inferior vena cava. In addition, one of the most common causes of inferior vena caval obstruction is upward propagation of a thrombus from the femoral or iliac vein. Certain neoplasms, particularly hepatocellular carcinoma and renal cell carcinoma, show a striking tendency to grow within the lumens of the veins, extending ultimately into the inferior vena cava.

As would be anticipated, obstruction to the inferior vena cava induces marked edema of the legs, distention of the superficial collateral veins of the lower abdomen, and, when the renal veins are involved, massive proteinuria.

Lymphatic Disorders

Disorders of the lymphatic channels fall into two categories: primary diseases, which are extremely uncommon, and secondary processes, which develop in association with inflammation (lymphangitis) or cancer. In both patterns, there is frequently obstruction to the lymphatic channels followed by lymphedema, entirely analogous to the edema that develops distal to venous obstructions.

LYMPHANGITIS

Infections that spread into the lymphatics may either drain through these channels without causing any reaction or may produce acute inflammatory involvement—lymphangitis. The most common causative agents of lymphangitis are the group A β-hemolytic streptococci, although any virulent pathogen may be responsible. The inflammation is marked by redness and dilatation of the channels (red streaks) as well as local tenderness. An acute leukocytic exudate is found within the lumens. Almost inevitably the lymph nodes of drainage are involved with acute lymphadenitis. When these barriers to further spread are overwhelmed, infection may eventually drain into the venous system and initiate bacteremia or septicemia.

LYMPHEDEMA

Lymphedema is divided into primary and secondary forms. *Secondary lymphedema* may develop from (1) postinflammatory scarring of lymphatic channels, (2) spread of malignant neoplasms with obstruction of either the lymphatic channels or nodes of drainage, (3) radical surgical procedures with excision of regional lymph nodes (as, for example, the removal of axillary nodes in radical mastectomy), (4) postradiation fibrosis, or (5) filariasis.

In contrast, *primary lymphedema* may occur as an isolated congenital defect *(simple congenital lymphedema),* or it may be familial, in which case it is known as *Milroy's disease* or *heredofamilial congenital lymphedema.* Both entities are presumed to be caused by faulty development of lymphatic channels, possibly with poor structural strength, permitting abnormal dilatation and incompetence of the lymphatic valves. Classically, these disorders involve the lower extremities, although they may affect other areas, sometimes in a rather sharply limited, bizarre distribution. Both simple congenital lymphedema and Milroy's disease are present from birth. In contrast, a third form of primary lymphedema, known as *lymphedema praecox,* appears between the ages of 10 and 25 years, usually in females. The cause is unknown. This disorder begins in one or both feet, and the edema slowly accumulates throughout life, so that the involved extremity may swell to many times its normal size; the process may extend upward to affect the trunk. Although the size of the limb may produce some disability, more serious complications such as superimposed infection or chronic ulcerations may occur.

> With lymphedema from any cause, the morphologic changes in the lymphatics consist of dilatation distal to the point of obstruction accompanied by increases of interstitial fluid. Persistence of edema leads to interstitial fibrosis, which is most evident subcutaneously. The thickened skin assumes the texture of orange peel, a finding termed *peau d'orange;* often this is seen in the female breast when there is widespread lymphatic dissemination of a primary cancer. Enlargement of the affected part, brawny induration, infection (cellulitis), and chronic skin ulcers are common sequelae to persistent primary lymphedema.

Tumors

Tumors of vessels (blood or lymphatic) run the gamut from benign lesions that usually produce vascular channels to borderline, more cellular tumors referred to as hemangioendotheliomas, to overtly malignant neoplasms termed hemangiosarcomas or angiosarcomas. Although the well-differentiated benign tumor can be readily distinguished from the anaplastic cancer, the line in the middle of the spectrum dividing the benign from the malignant is poorly defined, but in general the following criteria apply:

- Benign tumors produce readily recognized vascular channels filled with blood cells, or in the case of lymphatics filled with transudate. The lining cells of the channels are identical to normal endothelial cells.
- Malignant tumors are much more solidly cellular and form few or no vascular channels.
- Solidly cellular neoplasms often have cytologic anaplasia, including mitotic figures.

The differentiation of solidly cellular angiosarcomas from other spindle cell neoplasms (e.g., fibrosarcoma or leiomyosarcoma) is at times difficult. Helpful in this regard is the finding, by electron microscopy, of endothelium-specific Weibel-Palade bodies (rod-like cytoplasmic inclusions made up of several interadherent tubules), or factor VIII–related antigens by immunocytochemistry.

There are in addition a few vascular lesions that lie in the gray area between non-neoplastic and neoplastic. The majority of benign angiomas—capillary and cavernous—are present from birth and expand along with the growth of the child. Many regress spontaneously at or before puberty. Are these true neoplasms or merely hamartomatous congenital anomalies? Which-ever, the common angiomatous birthmark so distressing to mothers of infants may well disappear spontaneously at puberty. Other interface lesions are the *granuloma pyogenicum* and the *pregnancy tumor.* The former usually is secondary to some chronic localized infection and is an exuberant overgrowth of granulation tissue rich in vascular channels. The latter is a granuloma pyogenicum occurring in the gingiva of pregnant women. Pregnancy tumors almost always regress spontaneously after delivery, but the granuloma pyogenicum may require excision or cauterization.

Another vascular lesion more clearly non-neoplastic is the *spider telangiectasia.* It is a more or less radial array of somewhat dilated subcutaneous arteries or arterioles about a central core. Because they have arteriolar or arterial connections they may pulsate. They tend to be located on the face, neck, or upper chest and are most frequent in pregnant women and in patients with diffuse liver disease, notably cirrhosis. The hyperestrinism found in these two settings is believed in some way to play a role in the development of these telangiectases. However, in the autosomal dominant Osler-Weber-Rendu disease, these telangiectases are clearly genetic malformations present from birth. In this condition they are distributed widely over the skin and mucous membranes of the oral cavity, lips, respiratory, gastrointestinal, and urinary tracts, as well as in the liver, brain, and spleen. Any one of these innumerable lesions may rupture to cause such problems as nosebleeds, hematuria, or bleeding into the gut, but only rarely are these bleeding episodes serious. Now we can turn to the undoubted vascular neoplasms.

HEMANGIOMAS

Benign

Hemangiomas may be composed of masses of cavernous or capillary-like channels filled with either blood or lymph.

MORPHOLOGY. Cavernous angiomas may arise in blood vessels or in lymphatics. The cavernous hemangiomas often occur on the skin and mucosal surfaces of the body but may also arise in viscera, particularly in the liver, spleen, pancreas, and, rarely, the brain. In the rare autosomal dominant von Hippel–Lindau disease, these vascular tumors may occur within the cerebellum, brain stem, retina, and sometimes in the pancreas and liver along with other visceral neoplasms. In infants, cavernous hemangiomas sometimes constitute large lesions of the skin of the face or scalp, the so-called port wine stains or birthmarks. Cavernous hemangiomas are generally red-blue, compressible, spongy lesions, 2 to 3 cm in diameter, sharply defined at their margins, and composed of large cavernous spaces filled with fluid blood; they sometimes have partially thrombosed channels (Fig. 10–17). In most instances, these cavernous lesions have little clinical significance, and in children they may regress. When picked up in internal organs by CT or MRI scans, they must be differentiated from more ominous lesions. Those in the brain are most threatening, since they may cause pressure symptoms or rupture.

A capillary hemangioma is an unencapsulated tangle of closely packed capillaries separated by a scant connective tissue stroma. The channels are usually filled with fluid blood; however, thrombosis and fibrous organization within some of the component capillaries are common. The endothelial cells of the lining appear normal. Although any organ or tissue may be involved— liver, spleen—capillary hemangiomas usually occur in the skin, subcutaneous tissues, or mucous membranes of the oral cavity and lips. On gross inspection, they appear as bright red to blue lesions, ranging from a few millimeters to several centimeters in diameter. They may be level with the surface of the surrounding tissue, slightly elevated, or—occasionally—even pedunculated. Uncommonly, capillary hemangiomas take the form of large, flat, map-like discolorations that cover large areas of the face or upper parts of the body, producing port wine stains analogous to those caused by cavernous hemangiomas.

Capillary hemangiomas, because they are usually located on the skin or mucous membranes, are significant only because they are vulnerable to traumatic ulceration and bleeding.

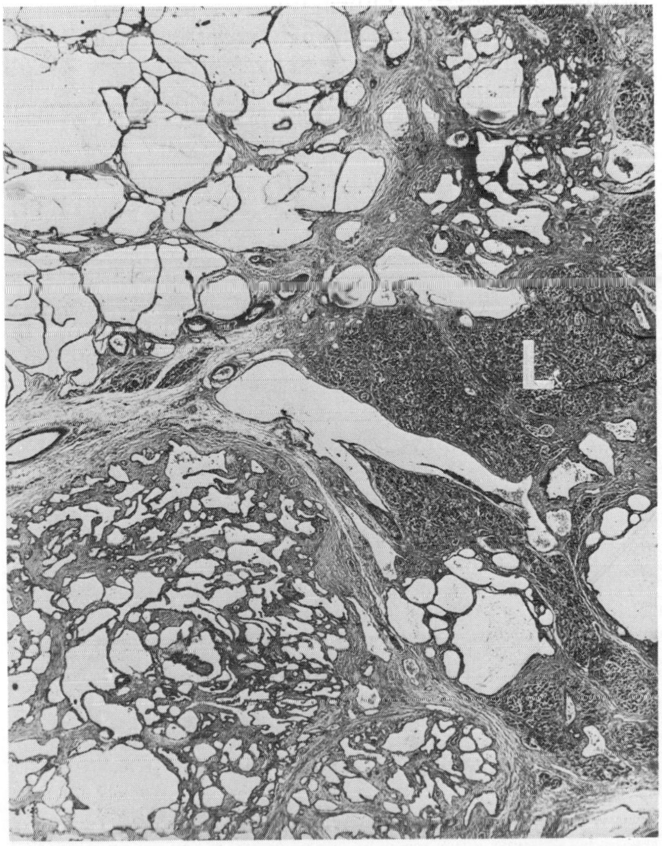

Figure 10–17. Cavernous hemangioma of liver (L). The dilated spaces are lined by endothelium.

HEMANGIOENDOTHELIOMA AND ANGIOSARCOMA

middle *malignant*

Both of these neoplasms represent the malignant counterparts of the benign angiomatous lesions. The hemangioendothelioma constitutes an intermediate grade between the benign hemangiomas and the unmistakably malignant anaplastic angiosarcoma.

In the hemangioendothelioma, vascular channels are usually readily discernible within the masses of proliferating, reasonably well-differentiated endothelial cells. In the angiosarcoma, vascular channels may be virtually inapparent. Thus, the angiosarcoma is composed of masses of anaplastic spindle cells with sparsely scattered, poorly formed vascular channels, themselves lined by tumorous endothelial cells. Both patterns of tumors are found in the same locations as their benign counterparts and tend to be larger, more solid, less obviously vascular, and more unmistakably invasive. In some cases the tumor cells contain Weibel-Palade bodies and/or factor VIII–related antigens, products of normal endothelium (p. 381).

The angiosarcomas are of interest because there is now good evidence that exposure to arsenic compounds, polyvinylchloride (used in plastics industries), or the radioactive Thorotrast (formerly used in radiography) predisposes to the development of these neoplasms in the liver.

GLOMANGIOMA (GLOMUS TUMOR) _____

This uncommon but curious benign lesion, which arises from the modified smooth muscle cells of a glomus body, is invariably small, red-blue, and exquisitely painful to the slightest pressure. They are most commonly encountered in the distal fingers and toes, especially under the nails. The tumors are small and on the order of 5 mm in diameter. When in the skin, they are slightly elevated, rounded, red-blue, firm nodules. Under the nail, they appear as minute foci of fresh hemorrhage. Histologically, they are composed of branching vascular channels enclosed within a stroma bearing nests or larger aggregates of glomus cells, which are small, round to cuboidal, and regular in size and shape with central dark nuclei. On electron microscopy they have features of modified smooth muscle cells.

They are usually readily excised and cured.

KAPOSI'S SARCOMA _____

At one time thought to be an uncommon neoplasm of elderly, mostly Jewish, men of European extraction, Kaposi's sarcoma (KS) has come into prominence because several variant forms have been identified. The form that affects elderly men is referred to as "classic KS." Another pattern, called "endemic KS," is endemic among black African young men and children. Another variant occurs in immunosuppressed transplant patients, and yet another highly virulent variant, called "epidemic KS," is particularly common in AIDS patients. A few details of these four subsets are provided in Table 10–3.

Classic KS is an indolent disease that typically begins with red-blue inflamed-looking lesions (one or more) on the distal lower extremities. Over the course of years, the lesions tend to become more numerous centripetally, more nodular, and are sometimes complicated by involvement of lymph nodes, gastrointestinal tract, lung, liver, and other viscera. Rarely the visceral lesions precede the cutaneous ones. Even with dissemination, the course of the disease is indolent, only occasionally fulminant, and 90% of the patients die of intercurrent disease. About a third have a history of or develop lymphoma.

Endemic KS, particularly prevalent among the Bantus of South Africa, has the same geographic distribution as Burkitt's lymphoma. Whites in this same locale have no increased prevalence of KS. Among young males the disease may be benign and resemble the classic pattern or be extremely aggressive. Occasionally the virulent form is largely restricted to lymph nodes, sparing the skin but occasionally involving the viscera. This "lymphadenopathic pattern" is particularly likely to occur in children with KS, often in the first years of life.

KS in immunosuppressed patients tends to be indolent but is sometimes aggressive and more or less resembles the classic pattern. The lesions sometimes regress when immunosuppressive therapy is discontinued.

Epidemic KS seen in AIDS may begin with a nodular skin or mucosal lesion but spreads rapidly to nodes and viscera. Despite the spread of the disease, most patients die of opportunistic infections (as do most patients with AIDS) or of an intercurrent lymphoma. For completely obscure reasons, 90 to 95% of all AIDS-asssociated KS occurs in homosexual men, far

TABLE 10–3. KAPOSI'S SARCOMA VARIANTS*

Type	Population	Clinical Characteristics	Course
Classic	Older men (aged 50–80 yr) of Jewish and Mediterranean heritage	Usually confined to lower extremities, often with venous stasis and lymphedema; M-F ratio 10–15:1	Indolent: Survival 10–15 yr; 37% associated with other lymphoid malignancies
African	Young adult (aged 25–40 yr) black men in Central Africa	Localized nodular lesions (57%); large aggressive exophytic tumors or invasive to underlying bone (38%); M-F ratio 13:1	Indolent if nodular; otherwise slowly progressive and fatal within 5–8 yr
	Children (aged 2–13 yr)	Generalized lymphadenopathy (5%); M-F ratio 3:1	Rapidly progressive; fatal within 2–3 yr
Renal transplant	Iatrogenically immunosuppressed patients	May be localized to skin or widespread with systemic involvement; M-F ratio 2–3:1	Can be indolent or rapidly progressive; may regress when immunosuppressive therapy is discontinued; fatal in 30%
Epidemic	AIDS patients; primarily homosexual men; few intravenous drug users and Africans	Disseminated mucocutaneous lesions often involving lymph nodes and visceral organs, especially gastrointestinal tract and lungs	Fulminant; less than 20% survival at 2 yr if associated with opportunistic infections

* Modified from Krigel, R. L., Friedman-Kien, A. E.: Kaposi's sarcoma. *In* DeVita, V., et al. (eds.): AIDS. Philadelphia, J.B. Lippincott, 1988, p. 245, as reproduced in Krigel, R. L., and Friedman-Kien, A. E.: Epidemic Kaposi's sarcoma. Semin. Oncol. *17*:350, 1990.

out of proportion to their representation in the AIDS population, but the incidence of KS among these homosexual men has declined dramatically—from about 40% to now about 20%.

ETIOLOGY AND PATHOGENESIS. The etiology, and indeed the very nature of KS, are unknown. The disorder begins with multifocal, red to violet patches that histologically resemble granulation tissue or some form of inflammatory dermatitis and then progresses at varying rates to unmistakable tumorous nodules or masses. The question arises, Is KS a neoplasm that arises in a non-neoplastic disease or, instead, are the multifocal lesions vasoproliferative responses to angiogenic growth factors such as IL-1 or TNF-α produced by T cells in stimulated lymph nodes? Equally uncertain is the histogenesis of these lesions. Despite a persistent minority view favoring origin from multipotential mesenchymal cells, the weight of evidence favors an endothelial cell origin for KS, but whether it is derived from blood or lymphatic channels is still uncertain. If neoplastic, what is the nature of the oncogenic influence? Investigations of genetic predisposition, oncogenes or suppressor genes, immunoregulatory derangements, and microbiologic infection, mainly viral, have all produced equivocal findings. The fact that the disease is endemic among black males in Africa and epidemic among homosexual males would seem to suggest an infectious agent, and, when all else fails, perhaps a virus. However, no viral genome or telltale fragments are consistently identified in KS cells. There are suggestive pieces of evidence that HIV may play a role in the epidemic disease. When the transactivating gene *(tat)* of HIV was introduced into transgenic mice, about 15% of the males developed KS-like lesions. It is thought that the *tat* gene codes for a growth factor for the cells that make up the tumor. Intriguing as this observation may be, it is hard to relate it to the non-AIDS disease, so to date the cause of KS is still unknown.

MORPHOLOGY. In the relatively indolent, classic disease of older men, and sometimes in the other variants, three stages can be identified that have been termed "patch, plaque, nodule." The patches comprise pink to red to purple solitary or multiple macules, in the classic disease usually confined to the distal lower extremities or feet. On section, these disclose only dilated, perhaps irregular and angulated blood vessels lined by normal-looking endothelial cells with an interspersed infiltrate of lymphocytes, plasma cells, and macrophages (sometimes containing hemosiderin). Such lesions are difficult to distinguish from granulation tissue. Over time, in the classic disease the lesions spread proximally and usually convert into larger, violaceous, raised plaques that reveal dermal, dilated, jagged vascular channels lined by somewhat plump spindle cells accompanied by perivascular aggregates of similar spindled cells. Scattered between the vascular channels are red cells, hemosiderin-laden macrophages, lymphocytes, and plasma cells. Pink hyaline globules of uncertain nature may be found in the spindled cells and macrophages. Occasional mitotic figures may be present.

At a still later stage the skin and mucous membrane lesions may become nodular, more distinctly neoplastic, and composed of sheets of plump, proliferating spindle cells, mostly in the dermis or subcutaneous tissues (Fig. 10–18). Particularly characteristic in this cellular background are scattered small vessels and slit-like spaces that often contain rows of red cells characteristically arranged in a "boxcar" pattern. More marked hemorrhage, hemosiderin pigment, lymphocytes, and occasional macrophages may be admixed with this cellular

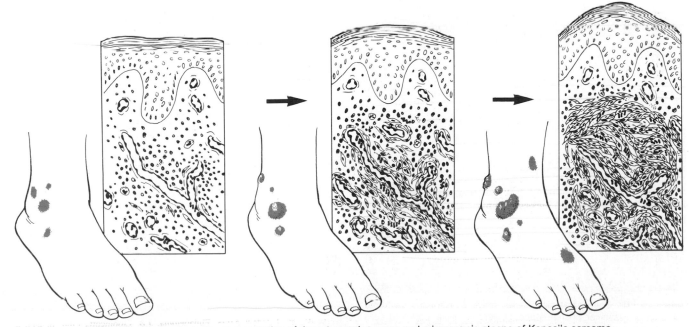

Figure 10–18. A schematic representation of the progressive gross and microscopic stages of Kaposi's sarcoma.

background. Mitotic figures are common, as are the round, pink, cytoplasmic globules. At this stage the lesion comes to resemble an angiosarcoma or fibrosarcoma (Fig. 10–19). The nodular stage is often accompanied by involvement of lymph nodes and of viscera, particularly in the African and AIDS-associated diseases.

CLINICAL COURSE. The presentation and natural course of KS vary widely and are significantly affected by the setting in which it occurs. Some of these details were presented earlier. Whereas the classic form is at the outset largely restricted to the surface of the body, in the endemic and epidemic subsets, the condition at presentation tends to be more widespread, particularly in persons who have AIDS. Visceral involvement is often present when the cutaneous manifestations appear. Whereas the classic disease is relatively indolent and compatible with long survival, both the endemic and epidemic patterns are much more aggressive and usually fatal within two to five years. Regrettably, no form of therapy has proven to be very effective.

Bibliography

Barron, K. S., Murphy, D. J.: Kawasaki syndrome: Still a fascinating enigma. Hosp. Pract. 24:49, 1989. (A simplified but accurate and complete coverage.)

DeSanctis, R. W., et al.: Aortic dissection. N. Engl. J. Med. 317:1060, 1987. (An overview of the condition with brief consideration of the pathogenesis, but good clinical details.)

Friedman-Kien, A. E., Saltzman, B. R.: Clinical manifestations of classical, endemic, African, and epidemic AIDS–associated Kaposi's sarcoma. J. Am. Acad. Dermatol. 22:1237, 1990. (An excellent review of the several forms of Kaposi's sarcoma with considerations of etiology and morphology.)

Ginsberg, H. N.: Lipoprotein physiology and its relationship to atherogenesis. Endocrinol. Metab. Clin. North Am. 19:211, 1990. (Detailed exposition of the pathophysiology of lipoproteins in the genesis of atherosclerosis.)

Hall, S., Buchbinder, R.: Takayasu's arteritis. Rheum. Dis. Clin. North Am. 16:411, 1990. (A comprehensive description that includes epidemiology, pathogenesis, pathology, and clinical features.)

Hunder, G. G.: Giant cell (temporal) arteritis. Rheum. Dis. Clin. North Am. 16:399, 1990. (A succinct, general presentation with epidemiologic, clinical, and morphologic coverage.)

Leung, D. Y. M.: Clinical and immunologic aspects of Kawasaki disease. Immunodeficiency Rev. 1:261, 1989. (An excellent overview of this disease with good morphologic details.)

Libby, P., Hansson, G. K.: Involvement of the immune system in human atherogenesis: Current knowledge and unanswered questions. Lab. Invest. 64:5, 1991. (An interesting and provocative view of atherogenesis.)

Lie, J. T.: Illustrated histopathologic classification criteria for selected vasculitis syndromes. Arthritis Rheum. 33:1074, 1990. (A summary of the essential morphologic features of the various forms of vasculitis prepared by a committee of experts.)

Ross, R.: Mechanisms of atherosclerosis—a review. Adv. Nephrol. 19:79, 1990. (An excellent delineation of atherogenesis with particular emphasis on the response-to-injury hypothesis by its originator.)

Schwartz, C. J., et al.: Pathophysiology of the atherogenic process. Am. J. Cardiol. 64:23G, 1989. (A multiauthor consideration of the complex events contributing to the development of atheromatous lesions.)

Sams, W. M.: Hypersensitivity angiitis. J. Invest. Dermatol. 93:78S, 1989. (A brief but very good characterization including morphologic and clinical features.)

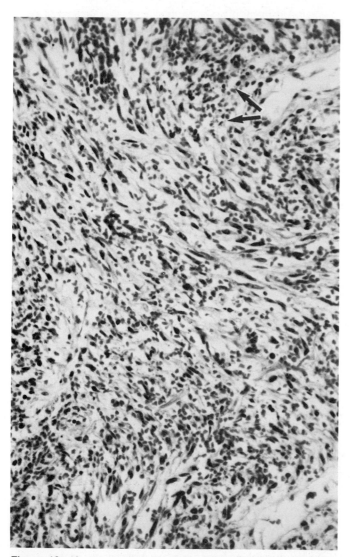

Figure 10–19. The anaplastic cellular stage of Kaposi's sarcoma. Compressed vascular channels and numerous small, dark red cells (*arrows*) are discernible.

ELEVEN

The Heart

CONGESTIVE HEART FAILURE
    Left-Sided Heart Failure
    Right-Sided Heart Failure
ISCHEMIC HEART DISEASE
    Angina Pectoris
    Myocardial Infarction
    Chronic Ischemic Heart Disease
    Sudden Cardiac Death
HYPERTENSIVE HEART DISEASE
COR PULMONALE (PULMONARY HEART DISEASE)
CONGENITAL HEART DISEASE
    Left-to-Right Shunts (Late Cyanosis)
        Ventricular Septal Defect
        Atrial Septal Defect
        Patent Ductus Arteriosus
    Right-to-Left Cyanotic Shunts
        Tetralogy of Fallot
    Obstructive Noncyanotic Congenital Anomalies
        Coarctation of the Aorta
        Valvular Anomalies
    Malpositions of the Heart
ENDOCARDIAL AND VALVULAR DISEASE
    Calcific Aortic Valve Stenosis
    Mitral Valve Prolapse
    Rheumatic Fever and Rheumatic Heart Disease
    Infective Endocarditis
    Nonbacterial Thrombotic Endocarditis, Marantic Endocarditis
    Endocarditis of Systemic Lupus Erythematosus (Libman-Sacks Disease)
    Calcification of Mitral Anulus
    Carcinoid (Argentaffinoma) Heart Disease
    Complications of Artificial Valves
MYOCARDIAL DISEASE
    Myocarditis
    Cardiomyopathy
        Dilated (Congestive) Cardiomyopathy
        Hypertrophic Cardiomyopathy
        Restrictive or Obliterative Cardiomyopathy
PERICARDIAL DISEASE
    Accumulations of Fluid in Pericardial Sac
    Pericarditis
        Chronic or Healed Pericarditis
MISCELLANEOUS DISORDERS
    Rheumatoid Heart Disease
    Metastatic Tumors
    Primary Tumors

Heart disease is the principal cause of disability and death in all industrialized nations. Currently in the United States it causes about 700,000 deaths annually, almost 40% of the total mortality. Four categories account for 85 to 90% of these deaths: ischemic heart disease, hypertensive and pulmonary hypertensive heart disease (cor pulmonale), congenital heart disease, and certain valvular diseases—aortic valve calcific sclerosis, mitral valve prolapse, infective endocarditis, and rheumatic heart disease. These major disorders are considered first, followed by the less common disorders grouped into endocardial-valvular, myocardial, and pericardial categories. A few random entities that refuse categorization are remanded to the rear, but first a brief characterization of congestive heart failure, the end point of all forms of significant heart disease.

CONGESTIVE HEART FAILURE

Congestive heart failure (CHF) occurs when the heart cannot maintain an output adequate for the metabolic needs of the tissues and organs of the body or can do so only at abnormally elevated filling pressures. The various significant cardiac diseases lead to failure either because they impair the contractility of the myocardium owing to some intrinsic damage to myocytes (systolic or forward failure, also called "pump failure"), or because they impair the ability of the heart to accommodate the volume of venous return (diastolic or backward failure). Sometimes both derangements coexist.

A variety of compensatory mechanisms come into play; for example, expansion of the blood volume and vasodilatation, but these further burden an already taxed heart. Decreased cardiac output and failure of ventricular emptying lead to dilatation and stretching of the myofibers, thereby enhancing contractility and ultimately inducing myocardial hypertrophy, but these changes impose new burdens and eventually failure ensues. Thus, at autopsy the heart is often dilated and usually hypertrophic, but these changes also may be present in a "compensated heart," so that it is impossible from examination of the heart to judge its competence. *The definitive morphologic changes of CHF are found away from the heart.*

Although the heart is a single organ, under various pathologic stresses one side may fail before the other, so that, from the clinical standpoint, left-sided and right-sided failure may occur separately, but ultimately in a closed system biventricular failure eventuates. It is helpful to consider failure of each side separately.

LEFT-SIDED HEART FAILURE _____

Left-sided failure is most often caused by (1) ischemic (coronary) heart disease, (2) hypertension, (3) aortic valvular disease and mitral regurgitation (rheumatic heart disease, mitral valve prolapse), or (4) primary myocardial disease. Except with narrowing of the mitral valve or other processes that restrict overload or reduce compliance of the left ventricle, this chamber is usually dilated. The lungs are most markedly affected, but to a lesser extent other organs as well, mainly the brain and kidneys.

LUNGS. As the left ventricle fails to keep pace with the venous return from the lungs, pressure in the pulmonary circuit builds. Pulmonary congestion and edema result.

At first the transudate is limited to perivascular "cuffing." In time it overflows into the alveoli **(pulmonary edema).** Not infrequently, transudate accumulates in the pleural space, producing a gross pleural effusion. Persistent elevation of pulmonary venous pressure with repeated episodes of pulmonary edema leads to changes of **chronic passive congestion** of the lungs.

The edema at first appears as an intra-alveolar granular precipitate, with widening of the alveolar septa. The congestion causes dilatation of the alveolar capillaries. In more advanced cases, the capillaries may become tortuous with small aneurysmal outpouchings, and rhexis may produce small hemorrhages into the alveolar spaces. As a result of alveolar hemorrhages, hemosiderin-laden macrophages, termed "heart failure cells," appear in the alveolar spaces. Long persistence of septal edema often induces fibrosis within the alveolar walls, which together with the accumulation of hemosiderin produces **brown induration of the lungs.** The weight of each lung increases to 700 or 800 gm (normal, 350 to 400 gm). The most severely affected areas, principally the lower lobes, are soggy and subcrepitant. Sectioning of such lungs permits the free escape of a frothy hemorrhagic fluid. All these changes predispose to secondary bacterial invasion with resultant bronchopneumonia.

These anatomic changes account for the major manifestations of left-sided failure: *dyspnea* (breathlessness), *orthopnea* (dyspnea on lying down that is relieved by sitting or standing), and *paroxysmal nocturnal dyspnea* (attacks of extreme dyspnea when the patient has been asleep for some time). *Cough* is common in left-sided failure, and may produce frothy, blood-tinged sputum.

OTHER ORGANS. The failing circulation may induce *cerebral hypoxia,* leading to irritability, restlessness, and even stupor and coma (hypoxic encephalopathy; p. 713). Reduced *renal perfusion* and compensatory mechanisms such as activation of the renin-angiotensin-aldosterone axis lead to retention of salt and water, and possibly peripheral edema and concurrently impaired excretion of nitrogenous products, so-called *prerenal azotemia.*

RIGHT-SIDED HEART FAILURE _____

Right-sided heart failure most often follows left-sided failure; however, it may occur in relatively pure form with (1) mitral stenosis; (2) congenital left-to-right shunts, which produce great increases in right heart pressure; or (3) intrinsic disease of the lungs or pulmonary vasculature that increases resistance in the pulmonary circulation (cor pulmonale). Less common causes of right-sided heart failure include the various forms of cardiomyopathy and diffuse myocarditis, which often affect the thinner right ventricle more than the left.

The major organs affected are the liver, spleen, kidneys, subcutaneous tissues, brain, and the portal drainage system. The lungs are little affected.

LIVER. The so-called *nutmeg liver* is created by congestive changes and accentuation of the centrilobular areas surrounded by paler hypoxic peripheral regions (Fig. 11–1). With more severe central hypoxia, *centrilobular necrosis* appears along with sinusoidal congestion. If the right-sided failure develops rapidly, rupture of sinusoids produces *central hemorrhagic necrosis.* With persistence, the central areas in time become fibrotic, creating *cardiac sclerosis.*

SPLEEN. Acute congestion produces tense, cyanotic, modest enlargement (200 to 250 gm; normal, 150 gm) secondary to marked sinusoidal dilatation and foci of hemorrhage. With chronic congestion—*congestive splenomegaly* (p. 383)—there is greater enlargement (500 to 600 gm) caused by fibrous thickening of chronically distended sinusoidal walls.

KIDNEYS. Congestion and hypoxia of the kidneys are more marked with right- than with left-sided heart failure, leading to greater fluid retention, peripheral edema, and more pronounced prerenal azotemia.

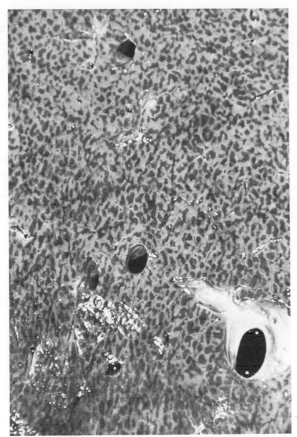

Figure 11–1. A close-up view of the transected surface of the liver with marked chronic passive congestion—the so-called nutmeg pattern.

OTHER INVOLVEMENTS. Some degree of *peripheral edema* of dependent portions of the body occurs regularly, and it may be severe enough to produce *anasarca* (p. 63). *Pleural effusions* may appear, particularly on the right side. Symptoms emanating essentially from venous congestion and hypoxia of the brain may appear analogous to those described in left-sided failure. Right-sided failure may eventually lead to moderate portal hypertension with splenic congestion, abnormal accumulation of transudate in the peritoneal cavity *(ascites),* and congestion of the gut.

The consideration of heart failure has been somewhat artificially divided. Most patients present with full-blown CHF, encompassing the clinical manifestations of both right- and left-sided heart failure.

ISCHEMIC HEART DISEASE _____

Ischemic heart disease (IHD), also called coronary heart disease, is the generic designation for a group of closely related syndromes that result from an imbalance between the cardiac need for oxygenated blood and its supply. Although ischemia also implies reduced nutrient substrates and inadequate removal of metabolites, the critical factor is the insufficiency of oxygen. The societal importance of IHD as a cause of death cannot be overemphasized; alone it causes about a third of all deaths in the United States.

The principal basis of the deficiency of oxygen is severe coronary atherosclerosis (AS) with stenosing plaques, which cause a more than 75% reduction in the cross-sectional area of the arterial lumen (hence the term "coronary heart disease"), but superimposed on these fixed stenoses in many cases is *intraluminal thrombosis overlying a ruptured or fissured plaque. Vasospasm and platelet aggregation* also contribute to the ischemia in some (perhaps many) instances. Rarely, increased myocardial demand, reduction in the oxygen transport capacity of the blood (e.g., anemia), an abrupt drop in blood pressure (e.g., with shock), or some form of nonatherosclerotic coronary disease such as coronary emboli or arteritis play a role in the perfusion deficit. Despite all these possibilities, until it is proven otherwise, IHD implies advanced stenosing coronary AS.

Depending on the rate of development of the ischemia and its ultimate severity, one of four syndromes may result: (1) angina pectoris (AP), of which there are three variants; (2) myocardial infarction (MI), the predominant form of IHD; (3) chronic ischemic heart disease (CIHD, ischemic cardiomyopathy); and (4) sudden cardiac death (SCD), which may be superimposed on any of the other three conditions (Fig. 11–2). Before any of these overt disorders becomes manifest, there is a decades-long prodrome of silent, slowly progressive coronary atherosclerosis.

Against this background we can turn to the various clinicopathologic patterns of IHD, beginning with AP, before turning to myocardial infarction, the "main event."

ANGINA PECTORIS _____

AP can be characterized briefly because it is basically a clinical condition associated with only modest anatomic changes. *It is the form of IHD characterized by paroxysmal attacks of substernal or precordial chest pain or discomfort caused by myocardial ischemia that falls precariously short of inducing infarction.* The only anatomic changes are possibly myocardial damage from previous infarctions, interstitial fibrosis, and myocyte atrophy and necroses from long-standing marginal ischemia and coronary changes (described below) responsible for the myocardial ischemia.

There are three overlapping patterns of AP:

- Stable or typical angina, usually provoked by exertion and tachycardia.
- Prinzmetal's, or variant, angina, which typically occurs at rest.
- Unstable, or crescendo, angina, the most serious form with the most intense and prolonged pain that augurs serious ischemia bordering on myocardial infarction, hence the synonym "preinfarction angina."

All three patterns are caused by varying combinations of fixed stenosing lesions, vasospasm, platelet aggregation, and increased myocardial demand.

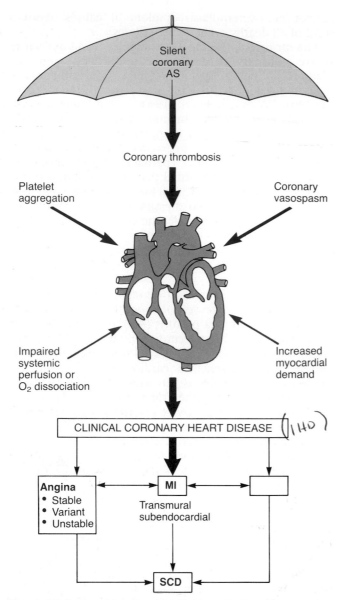

Figure 11-2. A schematic representation of the multiple mechanisms that lead to clinical coronary heart disease and the interrelationships of the various clinical patterns.

Typical angina generally implies fixed atherosclerotic narrowings that induce sufficient stenosis and luminal narrowing to render the supply inadequate whenever the myocardial demand is increased. Typically this form of angina is precipitated by exertion or emotional stress and is relieved by rest.

Prinzmetal's angina is generally attributed to vasospasm, usually but not invariably superimposed on fixed stenoses. This pattern of angina may appear even at rest and in most instances is relieved by vasodilators such as nitroglycerin.

The basis for the perfusion deficit in *unstable angina* is not always clear and is likely to be multifactorial (i.e., coronary AS with progressive luminal narrowing; thrombosis of coronary branches; vasospasm; and platelet activation). As will be seen, these are the same changes that underlie MI, except that "twigs" rather

than the major trunks are occluded. Whatever the mechanism, unstable angina forewarns of the imminent danger of a subsequent acute MI. In the spectrum of ischemic heart syndromes, then, it is intermediate between stable angina on the one hand and MI on the other.

MYOCARDIAL INFARCTION ___

Acute MI (AMI) alone is the leading cause of death in the United States and other industrialized nations. It is responsible for the majority of deaths attributable to IHD. Every year about 1.5 million persons in the United States suffer an AMI: more than 500,000 die, many more than succumb to all forms of cancer collectively. More than half these fatalities occur before the patient reaches the hospital, owing largely to the unfortunate onset of some form of fatal arrhythmia; however, there is also some good news. As we pointed out in the discussion of AS, the mortality from IHD has been declining remarkably and is now 40% below the peak level reached only about two decades ago. To what is this welcome trend owed? Probably to a combination of factors: improved medical management of MI and better control of the "big four" atherogenic factors—cigarette smoking, hypertension, diabetes mellitus, and hypercholesterolemia.

EPIDEMIOLOGY. *An AMI may occur any time from youth to advanced age; the incidence progressively increases throughout life.* At 45 to 54 years of age, there is a four- to fivefold male preponderance; this drops to about twofold in the eighth decade. Only at age 80 and thereafter does the difference disappear. *Except for those who have some predisposing atherogenic condition such as diabetes mellitus, women are remarkably protected against MI during reproductive life.* Although oral contraceptives (as they were formulated in the past) increased the risk of MI, especially in women past age 35 who were smokers, the newer formulations with less estrogen appear to be free of risk.

Other variables may influence the incidence of MI: personality, regular exercise, and alcohol consumption. There is a belief that so-called type A persons—hard-driving, impatient, competitive, compulsive—are coronary prone, but recent studies have challenged this conventional wisdom. There is, however, nearly universal agreement that regular exercise reduces the likelihood of developing an MI, other factors being equal, reduces the risk of dying from IHD, and lowers the susceptibility to fatal cardiac arrhythmias following an MI. So the joggers may well inherit the earth. Moderate alcohol consumption has likewise been accorded a protective role. Attractive as this idea may be to sedentary authors, the evidence is fragile, and there is no dispute that heavy use of alcohol increases the risk of coronary heart disease.

PATHOGENESIS. *There are in fact two types of myocardial infarction, which have somewhat different origins and clinical significance.* The more common and serious type is the *transmural infarct,* in which the ischemic necrosis involves the full thickness, or nearly that, of the ventricular wall. In contrast, the *subendocardial infarct* involves not more than the inner one third to half the thickness of the wall.

First the transmural infarct is considered. *The overwhelming majority of transmural infarcts are caused by a dynamic interaction among: (1) marked stenosing coronary AS; (2) plaque fissure, rupture, or intraplaque hemorrhage with superimposed thrombus; (3) platelet activation and aggregation; and (4) vasospasm.* Any one of these changes may predominate in the individual case, but whichever ones are involved the end result is marked coronary narrowing or occlusion and critical myocardial ischemia. The major villain in the causation of most MIs is coronary atherosclerosis.

- More than 90% of patients who sustain a myocardial infarction have advanced coronary atherosclerosis with one or more stenotic lesions, causing at least 75% luminal reduction in at least one of the major subepicardial arteries. A 75% reduction prevents the increase in coronary flow needed to meet even moderate increases in myocardial demand.
- Although only a single major coronary trunk may be affected, more often two or all three—left anterior descending (LAD), left circumflex (LC), right coronary (RC) or a first-order branch—are involved.
- Thrombosis overlying a stenosing plaque, usually ulcerated, fissured, or ballooned by an intraplaque hemorrhage, with complete luminal occlusion is found in 90 to 95% of AMIs. Platelet aggregation and vasospasm often play contributing roles and rarely are solely responsible even in the absence of severe atherosclerosis.

The following sequence of events is proposed: *Spontaneously, or perhaps triggered by vasospasm, intraplaque hemorrhage, or a sudden increase in heart rate, a large atheroma ruptures or fissures, initiating superimposed occlusive thrombosis.* Platelet adherence and activation contribute to the build-up of the thrombus, and release of vasoactive products such as thromboxane from the activated platelets may exacerbate the vasospasm. The significant contributions of platelets and vasospasm are documented by many observations. Diets rich in fish, with their polyunsaturated Ω-3 fatty acids, substantially lower the incidence of and mortality from ischemic heart disease; this effect is attributed at least in part to reduced platelet aggregation. Most infarcts occur in the morning, when platelet aggregability is greatest and released platelet products can be identified in the blood immediately after an infarct. Relevant to vasospasm, acute MIs have occurred in the absence of atherosclerotic narrowing, which has been related to angiographically documented vasospasm. More often the vasospasm worsens the luminal narrowing of fixed stenoses to precipitate the rupture of a plaque or further slows the flow, precipitating the thrombus.

Other conditions sometimes produce an imbalance —a hypotensive crisis (as with spinal anesthesia or shock); marked tachycardia with greatly increased demand in a heart with even moderate atherosclerosis; emboli to coronary arteries; arteritis triggering thrombosis of the coronary arteries (e.g., Kawasaki's syndrome); aortic stenosis or an arrhythmia that impairs coronary filling; narrowing of the ostia by a dissecting aneurysm; and thrombosis induced by traumatic injury to the coronary arteries.

The ultimate configuration of an MI evolves over a period of minutes to hours. Depending on variations in the level of ischemia introduced by collateral flow and possible reflow through collaterals or lysed thrombi (fibrinolytic therapy), certain zones of cells die before others. The window of minutes to perhaps a few hours between the onset of ischemia and irreversible injury is of obvious relevance to the current use of fibrinolytic agents for reperfusion of the ischemic area (Table 11–1). "Teetering" cells conceivably may be "rescued"; although, despite the reflow, myocytes may have sustained sufficient biochemical injury to be dysfunctional ("stunned") for one or two days even though they remain viable. Moreover, reflow itself may cause hemorrhage into the injured area, compressing microvessels, and the reperfusion of reversibly injured cells that have already sustained membrane injury may hasten their demise or even jeopardize reversibly injured cells. The precise basis for this reflow injury is uncertain, but it probably involves excess inflow of calcium, development of explosive cellular edema, and release of free radicals by the neutrophils attracted to the site of the infarct; according to recent studies, it may also be mediated by activated complement with its membrane attack complex (C5–9).

In animals, and possibly in humans, most transmural MIs begin as subendocardial lesions. The subendocardial myocardium is the least well-perfused zone of the left ventricular wall because it and its microcirculation are subject to the compressive forces of the outer layers of the ventricular wall during systole. Thus, this zone undergoes ischemic injury first. If the ischemia is sufficiently severe, the ischemic necrosis may extend in a "wave front" across the wall. *The ultimate size of the infarct depends then on (1) the extent, severity, and duration of ischemia, (2) the magnitude of the collateral flow, (3) the metabolic demands of the myocardium at risk, and (4) the complicating influence of "reperfusion injury."*

The *pathogenesis of the subendocardial infarct* differs somewhat from that of the transmural infarct. As pointed out, the subendocardium is most vulnerable to any reduction in coronary blood flow. With these lesions almost always there is advanced stenosing three-vessel coronary atherosclerosis, but *a major trunk is thrombosed in only about 20% of cases.* Some of these lesions represent developing transmural lesions,

TABLE 11–1. TIME SEQUENCE OF CHANGES IN MYOCARDIAL CELLS WITH ACUTE ISCHEMIA

Beginning depletion of ATP	Almost immediate
Loss of contractility	1–2 min
50% depletion of ATP	10 min
Irreversible cell injury	20–40 min

ATP = adenosine triphosphate.

the evolution of which is halted by death. For the remaining 80%, four possible mechanisms may trigger the acute ischemic event:

- Thrombosis of a large artery followed within a few hours by spontaneous fibrinolysis.
- Thrombosis of branches of the major trunks that induce ischemia severe enough to cause the death of only the most vulnerable inner zone of the left ventricular wall.
- A hypotensive episode (shock, an arrhythmia, surgery—especially cardiac).
- An increase in myocardial demand (tachycardia) in a person who has preexisting global cardiac ischemia.

MORPHOLOGY. Virtually all transmural infarcts involve the left ventricle (including the interventricular septum). Sometimes those in the posterior wall and septum extend into the adjacent right ventricular wall. Isolated infarction of the right ventricle is rare and occurs only in association with chronic right ventricular strain and hypertrophy. Atrial infarction occurs in 1 to 2% of acute myocardial infarcts (AMIs), in conjunction usually with a large posterior left ventricular infarct.

The **transmural left ventricular infarct** may be small (a few centimeters) in transverse dimension but may be

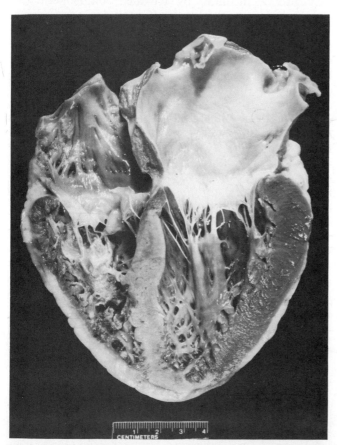

Figure 11–3. Acute myocardial infarct involving most of the interventricular septum and apex and extending into the contiguous right ventricle near the apex. The pale infarction is approximately 10 days old, and its definition has been highlighted by triphenyl-tetrazolium chloride, which colors the noninfarcted myocardium red-brown.

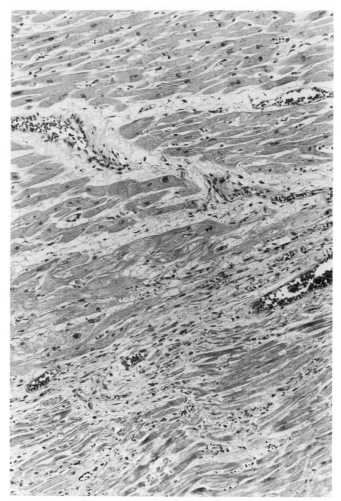

Figure 11–4. Acute myocardial infarct. The coagulated necrotic fibers below have retained their basic shape but have lost their nuclei. Compare with viable fibers above. The infarcted area reveals a heavy neutrophilic infiltrate.

circumferential. An occlusive coronary thrombus can usually (but not always) be identified in the trunk that supplies the ischemic lesion in the following distribution:

Left anterior descending coronary artery (40 to 50%)	Anterior wall of left ventricle near apex; anterior two thirds of interventricular septum
Right coronary artery (30 to 40%)	Posterior wall of left ventricle; posterior one third of interventricular septum
Left circumflex coronary artery (15 to 20%)	Lateral wall of left ventricle

Because of intercoronary anastomoses, occasionally a thrombus is present in the absence of an MI.

Although most transmural infarcts occur singly, several of varying age may be present. Occasionally, more and more myocardium is jeopardized by propagation of a thrombus **(stuttering infarct)** or as a consequence of repetitive ischemic episodes.

The appearance of the AMI changes with time. **When fewer than 8 to 12 hours old,** they may be slightly paler than normal or inapparent grossly; however, the area of ischemia can be visualized within the first 3 to 6 hours by immersing tissue slices in a solution of triphenyl-tetrazolium chloride (TTC), which imparts a red-brown color to **noninfarcted** myocardium (where the oxidative enzymes are preserved) revealing pale, unstained, infarcted areas depleted of enzymes. **By 18 to 24 hours** the infarct becomes apparent because of its pallor or cyanotic hue. Progressively, over the succeeding days, it becomes more sharply defined, yellow, and softened. By the **end of the first week** it is rimmed by a hyperemic, moist zone of highly vascularized reactive connective tissue (Fig. 11–3), and over the succeeding weeks, it is progressively replaced by fibrous, vascular scar tissue. In most instances the scarring is well advanced by the end of the sixth week, but the time required for total replacement depends on the size of the original lesion.

Many morphologic complications are associated with transmural MIs:

- The **anterior or posterior papillary muscle may undergo infarction** when the contiguous free wall is affected, possibly rendering the mitral valve incompetent.
- The **acutely infarcted papillary muscle may rupture transversely** to cause catastrophic incompetence of the mitral valve.

- **A fibrinous or fibrinohemorrhagic pericarditis** usually develops about the second or third day. This may be localized to the region overlying the necrotic area or it may be generalized. It does not impair the cardiac function and usually resolves.
- **Mural thrombosis** is frequent with involvement of the ventricular endocardium, producing a risk of **peripheral embolism.** Later it may give rise to dense fibrous endocardial thickening.
- **Rupture of the infarct** occurs in 4 to 15% of cases, usually between days 2 and 10. Rupture of the free wall (90% of cases) causes massive **cardiac tamponade.** The less common rupture of the interventricular septum produces a left-to-right shunt.
- **Ventricular aneurysms** may develop with large infarcts as the necrotic area balloons out, or much later by stretching of large fibrous scars. Mural thrombosis is common in such aneurysms.

The histopathologic changes also pursue a more or less predictable progression, as outlined in Table 11–2. Basically, the irreversibly injured cells first sustain biochemical and submicroscopic changes and then undergo typical ischemic coagulative necrosis with increasing eosinophilia and pyknosis (condensation of nuclei) followed eventually by resorption and replacement by scar (Fig. 11–4). Note, **with routine tissue stains, the coagulative necrosis may not be detectable for the first 4 to**

TABLE 11–2. SEQUENCE OF CHANGES IN MYOCARDIAL INFARCTION

| Time | Changes | | | |
	Electron Microscope	Histochemistry	Light Microscope	Gross
$0-\frac{1}{2}$ hr	Reversible injury: Mitochondrial swelling, distortion of cristae, matrix densities, relaxation of myofibrils	↓ Dehydrogenases, ↓ oxidases, ↓ phosphorylases, ↓ glycogen, ↓ K, ↑ Na$^+$, ↑ Ca^{++}	Waviness of fibers at border	
1–2 hr	Irreversible injury: Sarcolemmal disruption, mitochondrial amorphous densities		Fine cytoplasmic lipid droplets, cell swelling, contraction bands in areas of reflow	
4–12 hr	Margination of nuclear chromatin		Myocytolysis, beginning coagulation necrosis, edema, hemorrhage, beginning neutrophilic infiltrate	
18–24 hr			Continuing coagulation necrosis (pyknosis of nuclei, shrunken eosinophilic cytoplasm, marginal contraction band necrosis)	Pallor
24–72 hr			Total coagulative necrosis with loss of nuclei and striations; heavy interstitial infiltrate of neutrophils	Pallor, sometimes hyperemia
3–7 d			Beginning disintegration of dead myofibers and resorption of sarcoplasm by macrophages; onset of marginal fibrovascular response	Hyperemic border, central yellow-brown softening
10 d			Well-developed cellular disintegration; prominent fibrovascular reaction in margins	Maximally yellow and soft, red-brown and depressed margins
7th wk				Scarring complete

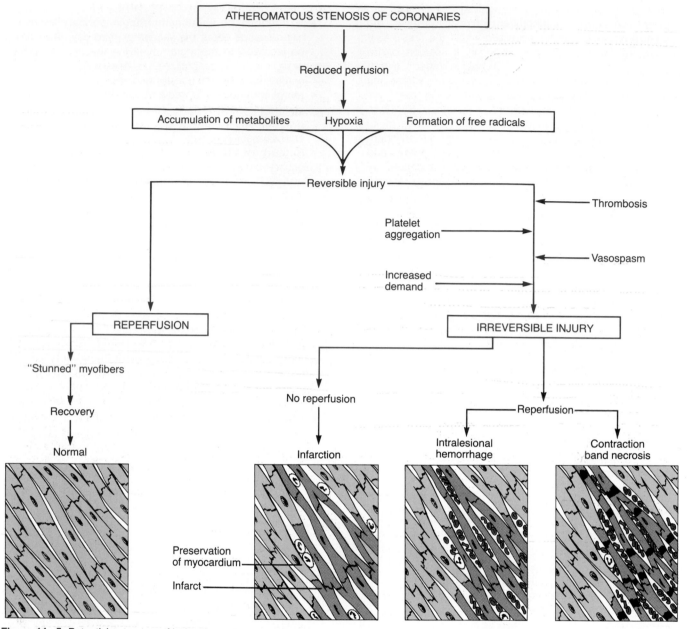

Figure 11-5. Potential outcomes of ischemia.

8 hours; however, within the hour after the onset of ischemia, the viable fibers immediately adjacent to the noncontractile dead fibers may become stretched and wavy because of the abnormal strains imposed on them. Also visible in the injured marginal cells or in the cells throughout the infarct when reperfusion has occurred are dense transverse **contraction bands** and sometimes **intercellular hemorrhage.** The various consequences of ischemic injury to the myocardium are depicted in Figure 11-5.

The morphology of the **subendocardial infarct** is analogous qualitatively to that of transmural lesions. By definition, however, the areas of necrosis are limited to the inner third of the left ventricular wall. The lesion may be multifocal, cover an arc of the circumference of the left ventricle, or sometimes totally encircle it. The temporal sequence of macroscopic and microscopic changes that follows has already been described, though in subendocardial infarction the changes in gross appearance may not be as sharply defined as in larger lesions. Although mural thrombi may supervene over the endocardial surface of these lesions, pericarditis, ventricular aneurysms, and rupture rarely follow.

CLINICAL COURSE. The clinical diagnosis of acute MI is based on three sets of data: (1) symptoms, (2) electrocardiographic (ECG) changes, and (3) elevations of specific serum enzymes. Typically, the onset is sudden, with severe precordial pain that may radiate to the left shoulder, arm, or jaw. The pain is often accompanied by sweating, nausea, vomiting, or breathlessness. Occasionally, the clinical manifestations are less typical. In about 20% of patients the onset is entirely asymptomatic and the disease is uncovered only by ECG changes, elevations of serum enzymes, or both. Most valuable are the serum levels of lactic dehydrogenase (LDH) and creatine kinase (CK). As soluble cytoplasmic enzymes, they leak out of fatally damaged myocardial cells. LDH-1 isoenzyme is mainly a cardiac enzyme; its level peaks in 18 to 36 hours and returns to baseline within three or four days. The CK serum level, particularly its MB fraction, is more specific. It rises above baseline within 4 to 8 hours and may peak very early or not for several days, falling to baseline in about four days.

After the onset of an acute ischemic event, one of several pathways may be followed. Regrettably, one is very brief—sudden coronary death (SCD) (25% of patients) caused by a ventricular arrhythmia. Indeed, SCD accounts for more than half of all deaths caused by IHD. If the patient reaches the hospital, the spectrum is as follows*:

1. Uncomplicated cases (10 to 20%).
2. Complicated cases (80 to 90%).
   A. Cardiac arrhythmias occur in 75 to 95% of complicated cases.
   B. Left ventricular congestive failure with mild to severe pulmonary edema (60%).
   C. Cardiogenic shock (10%).
   D. Rupture of free wall, septum, papillary muscle (4 to 8%).
   E. Thromboembolism (15 to 40%).

Among these post-MI complications, cardiac rupture and cardiogenic shock are the most life threatening. The former is almost invariably fatal, and severe cardiogenic shock has about a 70% mortality rate, accounting for two thirds of in-hospital deaths. Approximately 10% of patients die during hospitalization and an equal proportion during the remainder of the first year.

Before closing, brief mention should be made of two therapeutic advances that have become available to patients with advanced coronary artery disease: coronary artery bypass grafting (CABG) and transluminal coronary angioplasty (TCA). CABGs have undoubtedly prevented many first MIs and recurrences, but regrettably when veins are used as the bypass vessels, in 5 to 10 years they develop intimal thickening and stenosing plaques, changes that do not appear in internal mammary artery bypasses. TCA was developed as a simpler method of opening stenoses by balloon dilatation. This procedure, too, has its darker side, being impossible in 15 to 20% of cases, causing local dissections of the vessels as the stenoses are stretched, and in approximately 30% of cases restenosing within the next 2 to 3 years.

---

*Modified from Yu, P.N.: The acute phase of myocardial infarction. Cardiovasc. Clin. 7:45, 1975.

CHRONIC ISCHEMIC HEART DISEASE ___

CIHD, also termed "ischemic cardiomyopathy" and "coronary cardiomyopathy," is the diagnosis applied to the form of heart disease that appears insidiously in elders who develop ECG changes and congestive heart failure as a consequence of long-term, progressive ischemic myocardial damage. In most instances there is a history of angina—and sometimes previous episodes of myocardial infarction, often years before the onset of the congestive failure. Whatever its name, CIHD implies the slow attrition of myocardial reserve by protracted ischemia, sometimes hastened by intercurrent infarctions.

MORPHOLOGY. The heart may be normal in weight, but it is often smaller and dark brown (i.e., brown atrophy) with modest left ventricular dilatation. Invariably there is moderate to severe stenosing atherosclerosis of the coronary arteries and sometimes total occlusions. The myocardium generally has patchy foci of gray-white fibrosis or larger healed infarcts. The leaflets of the mitral valve may be slightly thicker than normal, and sometimes there is calcification of the mitral anulus (p. 325), but these changes are attributed to wear and tear and are not clearly related to ischemia.

The major microscopic findings are a diffuse myocardial atrophy, often with dense deposits of perinuclear lipofuscin within myocytes; a diffuse, mainly perivascular, interstitial fibrosis; patchy foci (smaller than 1 cm) of fibrous scar; myocytolysis of single cells or clusters of cells; and in some instances large healed scars of previous acute infarctions (Fig. 11–6).

CLINICAL COURSE. The clinical diagnosis of CIHD is made largely by exclusion of other causes for cardiac failure in an elderly patient who may have other stigmata of IHD such as a history of angina, conduction disturbances, or infarction. A major item in the differential diagnosis is dilated cardiomyopathy (p. 327). Generally in CIHD the congestive failure progresses slowly over the course of many years, and it may eventually be fatal. Most patients, however, die of unrelated problems, and some of a serious cardiac arrhythmia or an infarction.

SUDDEN CARDIAC DEATH ___

SCD is variously defined as unexpected death from cardiac causes within 1 to 24 hours of the onset of acute symptoms, but many investigators favor (as do we) the 1-hour time limit, to which the following data apply. It is the cause of about 300,000 deaths annually in the United States, and as noted earlier is responsible for more than half of all mortality related to IHD.

Many forms of heart disease may cause sudden death, including hypertrophic cardiomyopathy, mitral valve prolapse, aortic valve stenosis, and hereditary or acquired anomalies of the cardiac conduction systems,

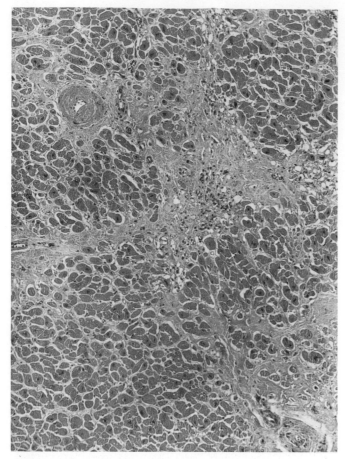

Figure 11-6. Patchy fibrous myocardial scarring with loss of many myocytes. Note the marked thickening of the wall and narrowing of the lumen of the intramyocardial vessel in the upper left.

but in 75 to 90% of cases it is the consequence of IHD. In these victims the great majority (approximately 80%) had marked stenosing atherosclerosis of at least one major coronary trunk. A recent thrombus was found in 10 to 35% of these victims. In those who were successfully resuscitated (providing an opportunity for characteristic changes to occur), 20 to 46% had an MI. Uncommonly, platelet aggregates have been identified in the small intramural vessels as the presumed basis for an acute ischemic event. In about 5 to 10% no cause can be established. Obesity and hypertension are well-recognized predisposing influences. The ultimate mechanism of death is almost always a lethal arrhythmia (e.g., systole, ventricular flutter, or fibrillation); however, the precise trigger remains uncertain, possibly an episode of worsening ischemia (increased myocardial demand, an acute coronary event, an evolving myocardial injury). For those who are rescued by prompt intervention, paradoxically, the risk of recurrence is lower for those who sustained an infarct than for those who did not suffer infarction.

HYPERTENSIVE HEART DISEASE _____

The minimal anatomic criteria for the diagnosis of hypertensive heart disease (HHD) are: (1) a history of hypertension and (2) left ventricular hypertrophy in the absence of other conditions that might reasonably induce it (e.g., aortic valve stenosis, aortic coarctation). Idiopathic asymmetric septal hypertrophy, which may mimic the morphologic changes of HHD, must also be ruled out on clinical grounds (e.g., no history of hypertension, younger age). In hypertension (p. 459) the stimulus to hypertrophy is pressure overload. The stress leads to production within myocytes of new myofilaments, myofibrils, mitochondria, and ribosomes and to a switch in the type of myosin synthesized. In this manner the load carried by individual cellular elements is reduced. Intriguingly, activation of the protooncogene c-myc may be involved in these cytologic changes.

With hypertrophy, the heart may maintain adequate output for decades, but as the heart wall thickens, the oxygen demand is increased, the left ventricular compliance is reduced, and myofiber enlargement increases the distance for diffusion of oxygen and nutrients from adjacent capillaries. Moreover, hypertension, as is well known, strongly predisposes to atherosclerosis, which undoubtedly adds an element of ischemia. Whatever the basis, eventually these enlarged hearts fail.

MORPHOLOGY. The essential feature of compensated HHD is concentric hypertrophy of the left ventricular wall in the absence of lesions that might account for it. The wall thickens, sometimes to more than 2.0 cm. The heart usually weighs more than 450 gm. In time, the increased stiffness of the left ventricular wall impairs diastolic filling and reduces the stroke volume output. With the onset of decompensation there may be dilatation of the ventricular chamber that neutralizes the thickening and expands the size of the heart.

The earliest microscopic changes (which may be subtle) are myocyte enlargement with enlarged nuclei that are often polyploid, because despite the enlargement these cells cannot divide. In the late stages, random cell atrophy and dropout lead to increased interstitial fibrosis.

CLINICAL COURSE. Compensated HHD can be asymptomatic and may be suspected only in the appropriate clinical setting when there is radiographic, electrocardiographic, or echocardiographic evidence of left ventricular enlargement. Note that the dilatation rather than the concentric hypertrophy is more readily detected radiographically. In many patients it comes to attention by the onset of atrial fibrillation or cardiac decompensation. Often there are other manifestations frequently associated with hypertension (e.g., headache, dizziness, nosebleed, and occasionally postural unsteadiness). Depending on the severity and duration of the hypertension, its effect on vital organs (brain, kidney, heart), and the effectiveness of therapeutic control of the hypertension, the patient may enjoy normal longevity and die of unrelated causes, may develop progressive IHD owing to the development of coronary atherosclerosis, may suffer progressive renal damage or cerebrovascular "stroke," or may enter a phase of progressive cardiac dilatation and heart failure. The risk of SCD is also increased. There is evidence that effective control of the hypertension by some therapeutic agents (e.g., methyldopa) in time leads to regression of the cardiac hypertrophy, but surprisingly other equally effective antihypertensives (e.g., vasodilators) have no effect on the heart.

COR PULMONALE (PULMONARY HEART DISEASE)

Cor pulmonale constitutes right ventricular enlargement secondary to the pulmonary hypertension resulting from disorders that affect either the structure or function of the lungs. According to this definition, right ventricular enlargement secondary to diseases of the left side of the heart and congenital heart diseases is excluded. *The cor pulmonale may be acute or chronic.*

Acute cor pulmonale refers to the right ventricular *dilatation* that follows right heart strain owing to massive pulmonary embolization. *Chronic cor pulmonale* implies right ventricular *hypertrophy* secondary to prolonged pressure overload, but with congestive failure, dilatation may mask the increased wall thickness. The major disorders that lead to pulmonary hypertension are cited in Table 11–3. Whatever the pulmonary disorder, the vasoconstrictive effects of hypoxemia and acidosis contribute significantly to the pulmonary hypertension. Moreover, in time the increase in pressure leads to so-called pulmonary vascular sclerosis (p. 408), worsening the situation and creating a vicious cycle. *The right ventricular wall thickens, sometimes to 1.0 cm or more, and sometimes is almost as thick as the left ventricular wall.* There is concurrent thickening of the trabeculae carneae and papillary muscles.

Because of its association with such widespread disorders as chronic bronchitis and emphysema (chronic

TABLE 11–3. DISORDERS THAT PREDISPOSE TO COR PULMONALE

Diseases of the lungs
  Chronic obstructive lung disease
  Diffuse pulmonary interstitial fibrosis
  Extensive persistent atelectasis
  Cystic fibrosis
Diseases of pulmonary vessels
  Pulmonary embolism
  Primary pulmonary vascular sclerosis
  Extensive pulmonary arteritis (e.g., Wegener's granulomatosis)
  Drug-, toxin-, or radiation-induced vascular sclerosis
Disorders affecting chest movement
  Kyphoscoliosis
  Marked obesity ("pickwickian syndrome")
  Neuromuscular diseases
Disorders inducing pulmonary arteriolar constriction
  Metabolic acidosis
  Hypoxemia
    Chronic altitude sickness
    Obstruction to major airways
    Idiopathic alveolar hypoventilation

TABLE 11–4. RELATIVE FREQUENCIES OF SOME CARDIAC MALFORMATIONS

Malformation	% of Congenital Heart Disease	M:F Ratio
VSD	30	1:1
PDA	10	1:2.5
ASD	10	1:3
Pulmonic stenosis	7	1:1
Coarctation of aorta	7	3–4:1
Aortic stenosis	6	3–5:1
Tetralogy of Fallot	6	1:1
Transposition of great arteries	4	3:1
Persistent truncus arteriosus	2	1:1
Tricuspid atresia	1.5	1:1

ASD = atrial septal defect; PDA = patent ductus arteriosus; VSD = ventricular septal defect.

obstructive pulmonary disease, COPD), cor pulmonale is said to be responsible for 10 to 30% of admissions to hospitals for cardiac decompensation. In most instances, it is overshadowed by the diseases that led to the pulmonary hypertension.

CONGENITAL HEART DISEASE

Cardiac anomalies are major forms of heart disease in the first decade of life. Some may be incompatible with intrauterine survival; others permit live birth but are soon fatal or produce manifestations early in life; still others become evident only in adult life. Here our attention is directed to anomalies that cause disease at birth or soon after. Those that do not cause problems until adult life, such as bicuspid aortic valves, are not included in our present consideration, nor are the cardiovascular abnormalities encountered in specific genetic syndromes, such as Marfan's, Ehlers-Danlos, and Hunter-Hurler disease (many are covered elsewhere).

EPIDEMIOLOGY. The ten most common anomalies and their relative frequencies are presented in Table 11–4, but only the more important ones are described. They fall into three functional categories:

1. *Shunts that produce left-to-right flow at the outset.* The most common of these are ventricular and atrial septal defects (ASD) and patent ductus arteriosus (PDA). At first they are acyanotic, but in time the pressure overload of the right heart and pulmonary system leads to reversal of flow; unoxygenated blood is then shunted into the left side of the heart *(cyanose tardive or late cyanosis).*
2. *Shunts that produce right-to-left flow and are associated with cyanosis from the outset.* Included here are tetralogy of Fallot, truncus arteriosus, and some instances of transposition of the great arteries. These right-to-left shunts also permit emboli arising in peripheral veins to bypass the normal filtration action of the lungs and thus enter the systemic

circulation. Septic emboli have produced brain abscesses.

3. *Obstructions to flow with no cyanosis.* These are coarctation of the aorta, aortic valvular stenosis, and pulmonary valvular stenosis.

About 60% of patients with untreated congenital heart disease die in infancy, 25% in the newborn period, and only 15% survive to adolescence or adulthood. But even the survivors suffer many untoward complications, further stressing the need for appropriate surgical intervention. Long-standing cyanosis, whatever its cause, eventually leads to clubbing of the tips of the fingers and toes, hypertrophic osteoarthropathy (p. 688), and polycythemia. Cerebral thrombosis sometimes occurs in children, presumably related to the polycythemia and increased blood viscosity, with perhaps some contribution from dehydration during a febrile illness. Moreover, congenital anomalies producing jet streams are vulnerable to the development of infective endocarditis (IE) at the site where the jet impinges. In addition to these specific problems, children with significant congenital defects may fail to thrive, suffer from retarded development, and are at greater risk of developing diseases of childhood.

ETIOLOGY. The cause of congenital heart disease is rarely known; however, multifactorial inheritance with both genetic and environmental influences is suspected. On the one hand, siblings of an affected patient or children of an affected parent have an increased incidence of similar anomalies, but despite identical genes, monozygotic twins have only a 10% concordance rate for ventricular septal defects. On the other hand, some cases are strongly associated with environmental influences. Best documented is maternal rubella in the first trimester of pregnancy, which sometimes results in PDA, pulmonic valvular and/or arterial stenosis, and VSD and ASD, either alone or in combination, often accompanied by cataracts, deafness, and microcephaly. In addition, there is substantial evidence that maternal diabetes mellitus, phenylketonuria, alcohol abuse, long-term use of lithium, and possibly excessive cigarette smoking may also contribute. It is important to note that the basic development of the heart occurs between the second and eighth weeks of embryogenesis; environmental insults, then, must occur during this vulnerable period to cause anomalies.

LEFT-TO-RIGHT SHUNTS (LATE CYANOSIS) _____

Ventricular Septal Defect _____

VSD is the most common congenital cardiac anomaly. For reasons unknown, there has been a significant increase in the frequency of this defect in the United States. Frequently it is associated with other anomalies, particularly tetralogy of Fallot but also PDA, ASD, coarctation of the aorta, and transposition of the great arteries. About 30% are isolated anomalies. Larger lesions may produce difficulties virtually from birth; smaller lesions may not be recognized until later.

VSDs vary enormously in size and location. They range from probe patencies to lesions sufficiently large to create virtually a single ventricle (cor triloculare biatriatum). About 90% lie just below the aortic valve, within or immediately adjacent to the membranous septum. The remainder are below the pulmonic valve or are located within the muscular septum. Though generally they are single those in the muscular septum may be multiple.

The clinical significance of a VSD depends on its size. Defects smaller than 0.5 cm in diameter (known as Rogers' disease) tend to close spontaneously or are well tolerated for years, although they induce a loud systolic murmur, sometimes accompanied by a systolic thrill. A particular risk for persons who have small or moderate-sized defects that produce jet lesions in the right ventricle is superimposed infective endocarditis. Larger defects remain patent and permit a significant left-to-right flow with all of its consequences (p. 315). Surgical closure of persisting defects is indicated before pulmonary vascular disease develops.

Atrial Septal Defect _____

An ASD usually goes unnoticed in infants and children until the left-to-right flow leads to pulmonary hypertension with reversal of flow, cyanosis, or right-sided heart failure. *The three types of ASD—ostium primum, ostium secundum, and sinus venosus—*are distinguished by their location in the septum. All represent developmental failures in the primary or secondary septa. During fetal development the common atrial canal is divided by an incomplete septum primum. Among its defects, the ostium secundum at the midregion is most important and permits right-to-left flow during development. Later this defect is partially closed by a septum secundum, which develops to the right of the septum primum. The second septum is itself incomplete at the foramen ovale but normally is apposed to an intact region of the septum primum. Right-to-left flow continues then through the foramen ovale as long as the pressure on the right is greater than that on the left. At birth, with reversal of the pressure relationship, left-to-right flow is blocked by the flap covering the foramen ovale (Fig. 11–7). Normally, fusion of this flap over the foramen ovale closes the septum, leaving only the fossa ovalis to mark the site.

Inadequate development of the membrane that normally closes the foramen ovale produces an ASD. It should be differentiated from a persistent patent foramen ovale that constitutes an oblique probe patency that does not permit interatrial flow after birth because, owing to the higher pressure in the left atrium, the fully developed membrane acts as a flap valve to close the communication.

ASDs are tolerated well if they are less than 1 cm in diameter. Even larger defects do not constitute serious problems during the first years of life, when the low-pressure flow is from left to right. Eventually, however, pulmonary hypertension appears, with reversal of flow, cyanosis, and possibly cardiac failure. Rarely, rheu-

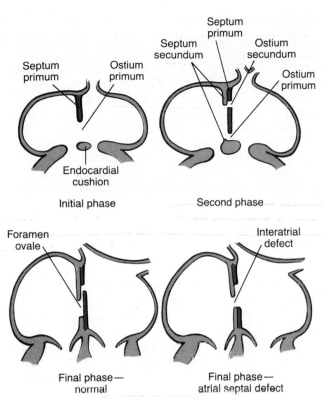

Figure 11–7. The embryogenesis of an atrial septal defect.

matic mitral stenosis combines with an ASD *(Lutem-bacher's syndrome)* to greatly raise the left-sided pressure and hasten the development of pulmonary hypertension. Infective endocarditis is rare with ASDs because the low-pressure, sluggish flow does not produce jet lesions, but paradoxical embolism or brain abscesses (from infected emboli) are risks. Operative closure of these defects is advised early in life to prevent the development of pulmonary hypertension.

Patent Ductus Arteriosus

The ductus arteriosus is a normal channel that courses between the pulmonary artery and the aorta just distal to the origin of the left subclavian artery. Although anatomic patency may persist for weeks, in full-term infants functional closure occurs within the first day or two of life. In premature infants, especially those with respiratory distress syndrome, ductal flow persists longer.

The basis for abnormally persistent patency is not well understood. During fetal life, low oxygen tension and circulating prostaglandin E_2 (PGE$_2$, most of it synthesized in the placenta) maintain its patency. After birth, with left-to-right flow, the increased levels of oxygen and lowered levels of PGE$_2$, owing to loss of the placental component, stimulate muscular contraction.

In about 85 to 90% of cases, PDA is an isolated defect. The remainder are most often associated with VSD, coarctation, or pulmonary or aortic stenosis. The length and diameter of the connection vary widely.

Sometimes the communication consists of only a defect between the approximated pulmonary artery and the aorta. In most instances, it is a channel several centimeters in length and up to 1 cm in diameter. Commonly, the left ventricle is hypertrophic and the pulmonary artery dilated.

Most often, PDA does not produce functional difficulties at birth, but it produces a continuous, harsh, machine-like murmur, and often a systolic thrill. Since the shunt is at first left to right, there is no cyanosis; however, reversal of flow, pulmonary hypertension, and pulmonary vascular disease eventually ensue, with their associated consequences. There is also a risk of infective endocarditis, so early closure is recommended if the child is not dependent on ductal flow for survival (e.g., concurrent pulmonary valve atresia).

RIGHT-TO-LEFT CYANOTIC SHUNTS _____

Tetralogy of Fallot   DROV

The four features of this disorder are (1) VSD, (2) a dextroposed aorta that overrides the ventricular defect, (3) obstruction to the right ventricular outflow, and (4) right ventricular hypertrophy (Fig. 11–8). The VSD is usually large. It sometimes approximates the diameter of the aortic orifice and often abuts on the aortic valve ring. The aortic origin is dextroposed so that it straddles the septal defect. The obstruction to right ventricular outflow is most often due to narrowing of the infundibulum of the right ventricle but sometimes to pulmonary stenosis. *The severity of the clinical manifestations is directly related to the degree of obstruction to right ventricular outflow, producing the right-sided hypertension, right ventricular hypertrophy, and right-to-left flow.* An atrial septal defect, PDA, tricuspid atresia, or other anomaly is present in about 40% of cases.

The clinical consequences of the tetralogy depend on its precise conformation. With a large septal defect and

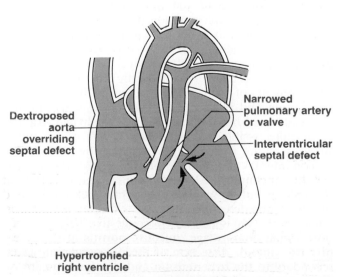

Figure 11–8. Tetralogy of Fallot.

mild pulmonic stenosis there is a left-to-right shunt without cyanosis, but with some obstruction to right ventricular outflow right-sided hypertension appears, causing right-to-left shunt, hypoxemia, dyspnea, and cyanotic or hypoxic spells. Ultimately pulmonary hypertension appears with the consequences cited earlier. Infective endocarditis is a risk; usually it develops at the site of pulmonic stenosis. Moreover, as the infant grows and the heart increases in size, the pulmonic orifice does not expand, making the obstruction and right-to-left shunt ever worse. Surgical repair, or at least partial correction, is now possible in almost all instances.

OBSTRUCTIVE NONCYANOTIC CONGENITAL ANOMALIES

Coarctation of the Aorta

Coarctation (narrowing or constriction) of the aorta is a common anomaly. Males are affected three to four times more often than females, but the condition is frequent in Turner's syndrome (p. 110). Although coarctation may occur as the sole defect, in 50% of instances it is associated with other anomalies—PDA, bicuspid aortic valve, congenital aortic stenosis, ASD, VSD, mitral regurgitation, and berry aneurysms of the circle of Willis. The narrowings have been subdivided into preductal (infantile) and postductal (adult) categories. Most are of the postductal type, located alongside or just distal to the usually obliterated ductus arteriosus (ligamentum arteriosum).

Preductal coarctation often involves large segments of the aortic root. Usually there is PDA, which produces manifestations and leads to death in early life. Indeed, many infants with this anomaly have concurrent hypoplasia of the left side of the heart and do not survive the neonatal period.

Postductal coarctations tend to be localized, ridge-like constrictions. The encroachment on the aortic lumen varies: sometimes it leaves only a very small channel; at other times it produces only minimal narrowing. Most often the children are asymptomatic and disease goes unrecognized until adult life.

Typically, there is hypertension in the upper extremities but weak pulses and lower pressure in the lower extremities associated often with claudication and coldness. Particularly characteristic in adults is the development of collateral circulation between precoarctation and postcoarctation arteries. Thus, the intercostals may become enlarged and palpable. Radiographically, visible erosions ("notching") of the inner surfaces of the ribs may be produced by abnormally dilated internal mammary arteries.

With uncomplicated coarctation, surgical resection or replacement by a prosthetic graft yields excellent results. Untreated, the mean life expectancy is about 40 years. Death is caused by congestive heart failure, intracranial hemorrhage, infective aortitis at the point of narrowing, or dissection of the precoarctation aorta secondary to the hypertension and the development of cystic medial necrosis (p. 297).

Valvular Anomalies

Any one of the valves may be imperfectly formed, creating a partial (stenosis) or complete occlusion of the lumen (atresia). The pulmonic and aortic valves are more often involved. In the more extreme narrowings, some concomitant anomaly must be present to permit blood flow to bypass the obstruction and prevent early death. Less severe are malformations of the leaflets (e.g., bicuspid aortic valve). Such malformations may have no functional importance, but as we will see (p. 323) they may predispose to infective endocarditis (IE) or, decades later, to degenerative changes.

MALPOSITIONS OF THE HEART

Positional anomalies are, fortunately, uncommon. Some are extraordinary and are encountered only in fetal monsters, such as the heart situated outside of the body (ectopia cordis). Other malpositions, such as dextrocardia when it occurs as an isolated anomaly, are important only as curiosities imposed on unsuspecting nurses or medical students, but they may be accompanied by inversion of all of the viscera in the genetically recessive situs inversus totalis.

ENDOCARDIAL AND VALVULAR DISEASE

A number of acquired disorders are characterized principally by valvular involvement: calcific aortic valve stenosis; mitral valve prolapse; rheumatic heart disease (RHD); calcification of the mitral anulus; carcinoid heart disease; and three forms of vegetative endocarditis (infective endocarditis [IE], nonbacterial thrombotic endocarditis [NBTE], and the endocarditis of systemic lupus erythematosus). The aortic valve involvement of tertiary syphilis was discussed on page 295. Increasingly often today, diseased valves are replaced by prostheses. These interventions have engendered their own pathology, which is considered later in this section. The most important causes of heart valve dysfunction are summarized in Table 11–5 and are discussed in the following sections.

CALCIFIC AORTIC VALVE STENOSIS

Aortic valve stenosis may be congenital or acquired. The congenital deformities take the form of stenosis resulting from incomplete formation and fusion of leaflets, leaving a minimally or markedly reduced lumen, unicuspid valves with fusion of the commissure, and bicuspid valves with fused commissures. In the absence of the congenital commissural adhesions, the bicuspid and even the unicuspid valves may be functionally satisfactory.

Acquired aortic stenosis is rarely as severe as some of the congenital lesions. When it is rheumatic in origin

TABLE 11-5. MAJOR CAUSES OF ACQUIRED VALVULAR HEART DISEASE*

Mitral Valve Disease	Aortic Valve Disease
Mitral stenosis 　Postinflammatory scarring 　　(RHD)	*Aortic stenosis* 　Postinflammatory scarring 　　(RHD) 　Senile calcific aortic steno- 　　sis 　Calcification of congenitally 　　deformed valve
Mitral regurgitation 　Abnormalities of leaflets 　　and commissures 　　　Postinflammatory scar- 　　　　ring 　　　IE 　　　Floppy mitral valve 　Abnormalities of tensor ap- 　　paratus 　　　Rupture of papillary 　　　　muscle 　　　Papillary muscle dys- 　　　　function (fibrosis) 　　　Rupture of chordae 　　　　tendineae 　Abnormalities of left ven- 　　tricular cavity and/or 　　anulus 　　　LV enlargement (myo- 　　　　carditis, congestive 　　　　CMP) 　　　Calcification of mitral 　　　　ring	*Aortic regurgitation* 　Intrinsic valvular disease 　　Postinflammatory scar- 　　　ring (rheumatic heart 　　　disease) 　　IE 　Aortic disease 　　Syphilitic aortitis 　　Ankylosing spondylitis 　　RA 　　Marfan's syndrome

* From Schoen, F. J. Jr.: Symposium on cardiovascular pathology, part II. Surgical pathology of removed natural and prosthetic valves. Hum. Pathol. *18*:558, 1987.

CMP = cardiomyopathy; IE = infective endocarditis; LV = left ventricle; RA = rheumatoid arthritis; RHD = rheumatic heart disease.

(p. 322) it is almost always accompanied by mitral stenosis; more often (90%) it is the consequence of age-related calcification of either a congenital bicuspid valve or a normal one. In bicuspid valves degenerative calcifications come to clinical attention in the sixth or seventh decade of life, but not until the eighth and ninth decades in previously normal valves.

MORPHOLOGY. The hallmarks of acquired nonrheumatic, calcific aortic stenosis are heaped-up, calcified masses at the cuspal bases, behind the aortic cusps, protruding into the sinuses of Valsalva and distorting the cuspal architecture (Fig. 11-9). The cusps are frequently fibrosed and thickened, but usually the commissures remain largely unaltered to permit differentiation of bicuspid from tricuspid valves and calcific aortic stenosis from calcific rheumatic aortic stenosis with its commissural fusion.

The obstruction to left ventricular outflow leads to a pressure gradient across the valve that gradually increases over the course of years. The left ventricular output is sustained by the development of concentric left ventricular hypertrophy (pressure overload). Eventually, as the stenosis worsens, angina or poorly under-

stood attacks of syncope may appear that carry the risk of sudden death. Eventually, cardiac decompensation ensues that can be benefited by valve replacement or balloon valvuloplasty.

MITRAL VALVE PROLAPSE ___

In this curious valvular abnormality, "floppy" enlarged mitral leaflets prolapse (balloon back) into the left atrium during systole. Other names include floppy valve or Barlow's syndrome and myxomatous degeneration of the mitral valve. Whatever the name, it is an extremely common condition, variously reported in up to 38% of populations, representing the commonest valve disorder in the United States. The female-to-male ratio is 6:4, and the condition is most often discovered between 20 and 40 years of age. In some cases, the condition is familial (autosomal dominant). Whether sporadic or hereditary, the lesions are usually incidental findings on physical examination, but they may have serious import. Sometimes the valvular abnormality is one feature of Marfan's or Ehlers-Danlos syndromes (p. 86).

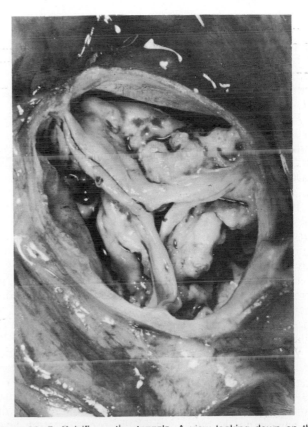

Figure 11-9. Calcific aortic stenosis. A view looking down on the markedly deformed unopened valve with thickened cusps and calcific masses within the sinuses of Valsalva.

MORPHOLOGY. The essential anatomic change is floppiness and enlargement of the mitral leaflets, most evident in the posterior leaflet with ballooning of the leaflet(s) into the left atrium during systole (Fig. 11–10). Sometimes the chordae tendineae are elongated or attenuated, and occasionally they rupture, creating a flail leaflet. The tricuspid valve is also involved in 20 to 40% of cases, and the pulmonary valve in about 10%. There is no commissural fusion.

Histologically, the normal zona fibrosa on which the structural integrity of the cusp depends is attenuated and more or less replaced by an enlarged and myxomatous spongiosa, accounting for the weakness despite the thickening of the leaflets. The chordae tendineae are similarly affected.

PATHOGENESIS. The basis for the myxomatous changes is not known, but a developmental anomaly is proposed involving connective tissue throughout the body, as in Marfan's syndrome. Yet the collagen genes are not abnormal.

CLINICAL COURSE. Patients with milder mitral valve prolapse have no symptoms or regurgitation, and the condition is discovered only on routine examination by the detection of a midsystolic click as the prolapsing leaflets snap taut or is visualized on echocardiography. Such patients usually suffer no untoward consequences throughout a long life. However, with the

more marked valvular involvements, there is mitral valve regurgitation and with it a number of potential unpleasant consequences: (1) the development of chest pain, (2) an arrhythmia, (3) eventual CHF, (4) superimposed IE, (5) thrombosis behind the cusps with embolism, and (6) sudden death precipitated by arrhythmia. Thus valve replacement is frequently performed for more severe involvement—so frequently that it accounts for 25% of all mitral valve surgery.

RHEUMATIC FEVER AND RHEUMATIC HEART DISEASE

Rheumatic fever (RF) is an acute, nonsuppurative, immune-mediated, inflammatory disease, principally of children, that follows after a few weeks an infection, usually pharyngeal, with group A β-hemolytic streptococci. A major virulence factor, an M protein, present on the surface of specific strains of rheumatogenic streptococci evokes antibodies that although cross-reactive with human cardiac epitopes (some found in myocardial myosin) may not be directly responsible for the tissue lesions. Possibly these antibodies, in concert with other immune mechanisms, evoke an acute disease that is systemic in distribution and characterized principally by polyarthritis, skin lesions, and carditis. Although the arthritis, skin lesions, and other systemic disturbances of the acute disease resolve, the cardiac involvement sometimes leads, decades later, to permanent valvular fibrocalcific deformity. So it is said, "Rheumatic fever licks the joints but bites the heart" (Fig. 11–11).

The incidence of acute RF and the mortality rate from rheumatic heart disease (RHD) have steadily declined in the United States and other developed countries, a finding that is attributed to several factors —better control of spread of streptococcal throat infections owing to improved socioeconomic conditions, prompter treatment or prevention of primary and particularly secondary streptococcal infections by penicillin or other agents, and, for mysterious reasons, some apparent reduction in the virulence of the pathogens. Nonetheless, the condition is endemic among economically deprived persons throughout the world and periodically flares up in the United States.

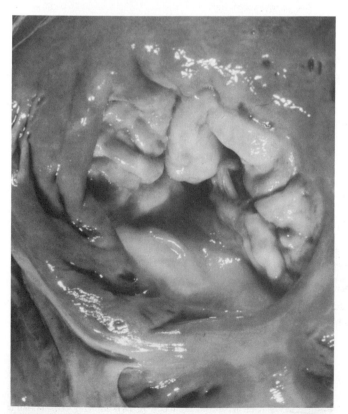

Figure 11–10. Floppy mitral valve as viewed from the left atrium. The redundant posterior leaflet mushrooms into the valvular orifice.

MORPHOLOGY. In acute RF, widely scattered focal inflammatory lesions are found in various sites. Within the heart they are pathognomonic of RF and are called Aschoff bodies (Fig. 11–12). They constitute foci of necrosis of collagen with fibrin deposition, surrounded by lymphocytes, macrophages, and occasional plump modified histiocytes (called variously Anitschkow cells or Aschoff cells), which sometimes form multinucleated giant cells. With time (years to decades), the Aschoff bodies are replaced by fibrous scar.

During acute RHD, Aschoff bodies may be found in any of the three layers of the heart—hence the term, pancarditis. In the pericardium they are accompanied

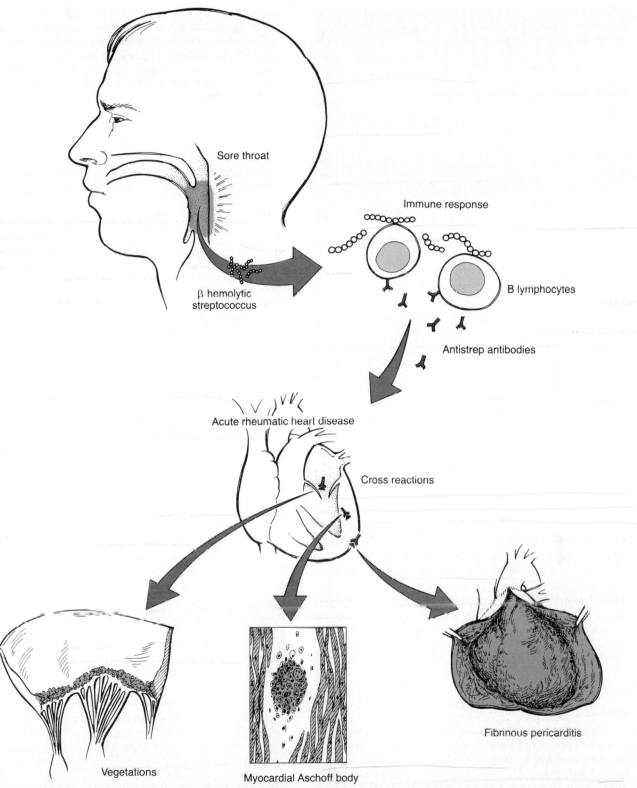

Sore throat

β hemolytic
streptococcus

Immune response

B lymphocytes

Antistrep antibodies

Acute rheumatic heart disease

Cross reactions

Vegetations

Myocardial Aschoff body

Fibrinous pericarditis

Figure 11–11. The presumed pathogenesis of acute rheumatic fever and rheumatic heart disease with the major cardiac consequences below.

by a serofibrinous "bread-and-butter" pericarditis (p. 330). The **myocardial involvement** takes the form of scattered Aschoff bodies within the interstitial connective tissue, often in relation to intramyocardial blood vessels, producing a myocarditis that may lead to dilatation of the heart and mitral valve ring. **There is usually concurrent inflammatory involvement of the endocardium, mainly the left-sided valves—mitral alone (70**

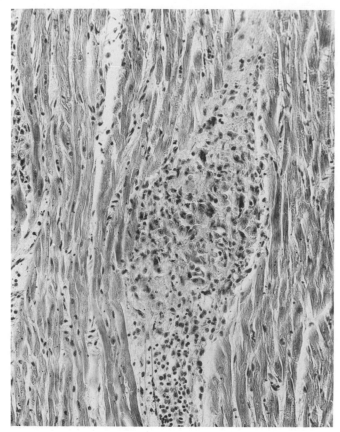

Figure 11–12. Acute rheumatic heart disease with prominent Aschoff body composed of modified histiocytes, scattered lymphocytes, and occasional giant cells.

with RF and less often in children. The large joints are most often affected, but the inflammation is transitory, leaving no residua. **Lesions of the skin** occur in less than half of patients and take the form of **subcutaneous nodules** or **erythema marginatum**. The **subcutaneous nodules,** most often located overlying the extensor tendons of the extremities at the wrists, elbows, ankles, and knees, are essentially giant Aschoff bodies with large central areas of fibrinoid necrosis enclosed by a palisade of fibroblasts and mononuclear inflammatory cells. **Erythema marginatum** begins as flat, slightly reddened maculopapules that progressively enlarge while the centers clear. **Rheumatic arteritis** has been described in the coronary, renal, mesenteric, and cerebral arteries as well as in the aorta and pulmonary vessels during the height of an attack. The morphologic alterations are characteristic of hypersensitivity angiitis, described on page 129. **Rheumatic interstitial pneumonitis** and **fibrinous pleuritis** are rare complications of the acute disease. In the late chronic stages of RHD with tight mitral stenosis, marked pulmonary congestive changes may develop, turning into dense interstitial fibrosis with siderotic pigmentation.

CLINICAL COURSE. Typically, acute RF appears about 2 to 3 weeks after streptococcal tonsillitis or pharyngitis in children between 5 and 15 years of age, but some first attacks occur in middle life or later. By

to 75%), mitral and aortic (25%)—**and sometimes also the tricuspid and pulmonic valves.** The inflammatory valvular involvement predisposes to the formation of small (1- to 2-mm) vegetations (verrucae) along the lines of closure. These acute changes may resolve leaving little or no fibrosis or be transformed into chronic RHD.

Chronic RHD usually does not appear for at least 10 years, sometimes not for several decades. It is characterized by fibrocalcific thickening with intercommissural adhesions of the valves involved in acute disease to produce marked stenoses (which may also be regurgitant). This unfortunate sequence is more likely (1) when the first acute attack occurs in early childhood, (2) when the initial attack of RF is severe, and (3) with recurrent attacks. The mitral valve is most commonly affected, resulting possibly in "fish mouth" or "buttonhole" stenoses. Simultaneously the chordae tendineae become thickened, fused, and shortened (Fig. 11–13). The same basic changes occur in the other chronically involved valves, often accompanied in the aortic valve by prominent nodular calcifications behind the leaflets, simulating to some degree degenerative calcific aortic stenosis (p. 318).

Other organs and tissues may be involved. **Acute nonspecific arthritis** appears in about 90% of adults

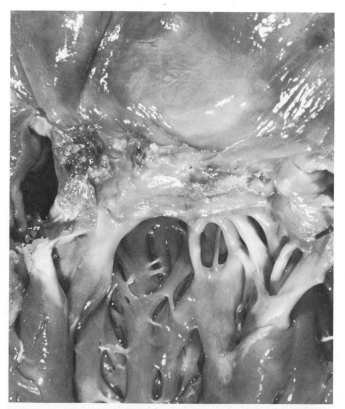

Figure 11–13. Chronic (healed) rheumatic mitral valvulitis with fibrocalcific thickening of the valvular leaflets and marked thickening, fusion, and shortening of the chordae tendineae.

the time manifestations appear it is usually impossible to find organisms on throat culture, but telltale antibodies (e.g., antistreptolysin O [ASO] and antistreptokinase [ASK]) are present in the serum. During the initial acute attack it is the myocarditis that is most threatening, causing arrhythmias, particularly atrial fibrillation (which predisposes to auricular thrombi), or cardiac dilatation with possibly insufficiency of the mitral valve. These changes usually resolve as the acute disease subsides. Rarely is the acute disease fatal.

Following an initial attack, there is increased vulnerability to reactivation of the disease with subsequent streptococcal infections and the likelihood of worsening carditis with each recurrence. Hence, long-term antistreptococcal therapy is administered to anyone who has had RF. Even with chronic mitral stenosis (and possibly regurgitation), the heart may remain compensated for many years but may in time decompensate and require valve replacement. Other hazards include respiratory failure from advanced congestive changes incident to a tight mitral stenosis, embolization from mural thrombi within the atrial appendages, and IE superimposed on chronically deformed valves.

from p. 74

INFECTIVE ENDOCARDITIS _____

IE is characterized by colonization or invasion of the heart valves (or the mural endocardium) by a microbiologic agent, leading to the local formation of thrombotic masses laden with organisms—so-called infective vegetations. A similar phenomenon may occur within the aorta (infective endaortitis), aneurysmal sacs, or other vessels. Virtually every microbe has at one time or another been implicated, but most cases are caused by certain bacteria. IE has particular clinical importance because prompt diagnosis and early effective antimicrobial treatment significantly alter the outlook for the patient.

It has been conventional to subdivide IE into acute and subacute forms based largely on the severity of the disease and its course. *Subacute endocarditis* usually is caused by less virulent organisms; the heart has some underlying predisposing lesion; the course tends to be protracted (months); and most patients survive with appropriate therapy. *Acute endocarditis,* on the other hand, occurs with highly virulent organisms capable of attacking even normal hearts to produce hectic, febrile, erosive infections that sometimes cause death within days to weeks. There is, however, no sharp delineation between acute and subacute IE, and the infective vegetations are more alike than dissimilar.

EPIDEMIOLOGY AND PATHOGENESIS. A variety of cardiac abnormalities predispose to IE: congenital heart disease (most often anomalies with high pressure, small shunts or tight stenoses creating jet streams, e.g., a small interventricular septal defect), chronic RHD (at one time preeminent), mitral valve prolapse, degenerative calcific valvular stenosis, bicuspid aortic valve, and notably at the present time intravenous (IV) drug abuse, artificial valves, and indwelling arterial cath-

eters. However, as noted some cases occur in normal hearts, usually caused by highly virulent organisms.

Virtually every bacterial species, as well as (rarely) chlamydia, fungi, and other agents, have caused IE. Overall, about 50 to 60% of cases are attributable to various alpha streptococci; usually these cause subacute disease. *Staphylococcus aureus* (10 to 20% of all cases) is the leading cause of acute endocarditis. The roster of other pathogens is very large and includes *Streptococcus pneumoniae, Enterobacter* species, *Neisseria gonorrhoeae,* as well as every conceivable commensal and saprophyte in immunocompromised and otherwise vulnerable hosts (transplant recipients, cancer chemotherapy, and cardiac surgery patients and persons who have acquired immunodefiency syndrome [AIDS]). IV drug abusers account for about 10 to 15% of all cases; the right-sided valves are often affected, and the major offenders are *S. aureus, Candida,* and *Aspergillus* species. In about 10 to 15% no organism can be isolated (so-called "culture-negative" endocarditis).

The portal of entry of the agent into the bloodstream may be overt, as when there is an infection elsewhere, IV drug abuse, or a previous dental, surgical, or other interventional procedure (catheterization); however, it may be covert, presumably emanating from transient bacteremia from the gut, oral cavity, or a trivial injury. Predisposing influences are (1) the sterile fibrin-platelet valvular deposits (i.e., nonbacterial thrombotic endocarditis); (2) agglutinating antibodies that produce bacterial clumps likely to attach to developing vegetations; and (3) adhesion factors on the endocardium and on bacteria. Fibronectin, a component of the extracellular matrix of endothelium, has been shown to have specific receptors for various bacteria, some among the commonest causes of IE, favoring their implantation on the endocardium.

MORPHOLOGY. The diagnostic findings in both subacute and acute forms of the disease are irregular, friable, bulky (0.2- to 2.0-cm), microbe-laden vegetations attached most often near the lines of closure of the leaflet(s). They may occur singly or multiply on one or more valves (most commonly the mitral, followed closely by the aortic valve, Fig. 11–14). As noted, in drug addicts the tricuspid is mainly affected. **The vegetations in acute endocarditis tend to be bulkier than those in subacute disease, occur more often on previously normal valves, more often cause perforation or erosion of the underlying valve leaflet, and sometimes erode into the underlying myocardium to produce paravalvular abscesses** (Fig. 11–15). With nonvalvular congenital defects the vegetations tend to be located on the low-pressure side of the defect (e.g., on the right ventricular margins of an interventricular septal defect. With mechanical prostheses the vegetations are usually located on the margin of the sewing ring, causing a ring abscess and sometimes paravalvular perforation.

The histologic changes are not distinctive. The vegetations constitute tangled masses of fibrin, blood cells, platelets, and usually masses or colony formations of

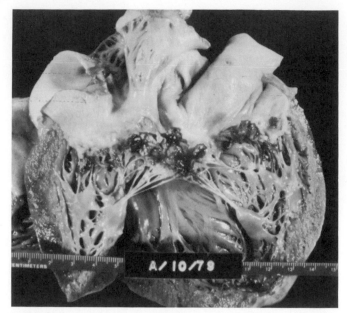

Figure 11–14. Infective endocarditis of the mitral valve with large attached vegetations.

organisms overlying inflamed and sometimes ulcerated or perforated valve leaflets. Essential is the culture of the vegetation to identify the offending agent.

CLINICAL COURSE. The presentation of subacute disease is quite different from that of acute disease. In the former, the fever may be low grade, and particularly in elders fever may be slight or absent. Often the only manifestations are nonspecific,—fatigue, loss of weight—with little to point to the heart. Murmurs are absent in about 10% of patients with subacute disease and moreover may merely relate to a preexisting cardiac abnormality. Only rarely do they "change" with time (reflecting build-up or fragmentation of vegetations). Petechiae, subungual hemorrhages, clubbing of the fingertips, and Roth's spots in the eyes have now become uncommon clinical findings owing to the aborted clinical course produced by effective therapy.

In contrast, *acute endocarditis* has a stormy onset with rapidly developing, often spiking fever, chills, weakness, and lassitude. A murmur is more likely to be present with acute endocarditis because of the large size of the vegetations, and often it changes as the vegetations build up and fragment. The spleen is more often enlarged in the acute form of the disease than in the subacute.

Sometimes complications involving the heart (valvular erosions or perforations with insufficiency, suppurative pericarditis), kidneys (focal or diffuse glomerulonephritis, multiple abscesses), or embolism (to spleen, kidneys, brain) call attention to the underlying disease. Confirmation of the diagnosis of IE depends on positive blood culture, but to wait too long (recall the culture-negative cases) runs the risks of allowing the

vegetations to get too large to be sterilized with therapy or of developing one of the complications. The prognosis depends mostly on the promptness of diagnosis, the virulence of the organism, and its susceptibility to therapy. Overall, more than 70% of patients survive the infection; the range is 30 to 90%, depending on the factors mentioned.

NONBACTERIAL THROMBOTIC ENDOCARDITIS, MARANTIC ENDOCARDITIS

NBTE is characterized by the deposition of small masses of fibrin and other blood elements on the leaflets of the valves of either side of the heart. In contrast to infective endocarditis, the vegetations are sterile, not associated with inflammatory changes in the involved leaflet(s), usually arise on previously normal valves (more often the mitral or aortic), and tend to be small (1 to 5 mm). Consequently, they are only loosely attached to the underlying valve. They resemble those of acute rheumatic endocarditis and Libman-Sacks disease quite closely. In NBTE the vegetations occur along the lines of closure of the leaflets, as single isolated lesions on any one of the valves or multiply on one valve or several valves simultaneously.

The vegetations are thought to reflect a hypercoagulable state, usually induced by a disease such as metastatic cancer, renal failure, or chronic sepsis. Thus they often occur along with venous thromboses or pulmonary embolization. Endocardial trauma, as from an indwelling pulmonary artery (Swan-Ganz) catheter, is also a predisposing condition; however, *this form of thrombotic endocarditis has occurred in otherwise healthy persons of all ages who are not marantic.*

The lesions are generally of little significance but they may provide a soil for the implantation of microorganisms to yield infective endocarditis (p. 323), and those on the left side of the heart may embolize.

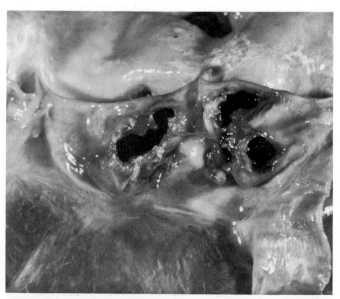

Figure 11–15. Infective endocarditis of the aortic valve with several perforations of the valve leaflets.

ENDOCARDITIS OF SYSTEMIC LUPUS ERYTHEMATOSUS (LIBMAN-SACKS DISEASE) ___

The cardiac lesions of lupus take many forms. Best known are sterile small vegetations (similar to those of NBTE, p. 324) on the leaflets of any one of the valves on *either the exposed or undersurface of the leaflets.* In addition, in chronic disease the leaflets may become thickened and fibrotic but rarely sufficient to cause serious dysfunction. Fibrinous pericarditis, and rarely myocarditis (p. 326), are other possible patterns of cardiac involvement. All are described in more detail later.

CALCIFICATION OF MITRAL ANULUS _____

In elders, calcific deposits may accumulate in the anulus of the mitral valve, often in association with but not related to IHD. The calcification, which takes the form of irregular beading (2 to 5 mm thick) within the anulus and behind the leaflets, rarely affects valve function. It is more readily palpable (as stony hard thickening of the valve ring) than visible, no inflammatory change is associated, and it is postulated to reflect the degenerative changes of aging. Occasionally the calcific masses penetrate the underlying myocardium, and sometimes they impinge on the conduction system to produce arrhythmias.

CARCINOID (ARGENTAFFINOMA) HEART DISEASE _____

Involvement principally of the mural endocardium and valves of the right heart is one of the major features of the *carcinoid syndrome (p. 518), which is characterized by* (1) *distinctive episodic flushing of the skin;* (2) *cramps, nausea, vomiting, and diarrhea in almost all patients;* (3) *bronchoconstrictive episodes resembling asthma in about a third of cases; and* (4) *cardiac lesions in about half.* The changes are attributed to the tumorous elaboration and absorption into the circulation of a variety of bioactive products, including serotonin (5-hydroxytryptamine), kallikrein, bradykinin, histamine, prostaglandins, and the newly described tachykinins neuropeptide K and substance P. Which of these products is implicated is still not clear, but favored are serotonin and the tachykinins (the latter known to stimulate fibroblast proliferation).

The carcinoid syndrome is mostly associated with midgut carcinoids (i.e., in the small intestine) but occasionally with foregut and hindgut tumors. Even with midgut carcinoids it appears in only 25 to 50% of cases that *have hepatic metastases.* In the absence of hepatic metastases, gastrointestinal carcinoids may not induce the syndrome because there is rapid breakdown of bioactive products in the portal circulation during traversal of the liver. In contrast, tumors primary in organs outside the portal system (e.g., ovary, lung) may induce the carcinoid syndrome without hepatic metastases.

In the majority of cases, plaque-like thickenings composed of a cellular fibrous tissue are superimposed on the endocardium of the cardiac chambers, *mainly on the outflow tract of the right ventricle, and on the cusps of the right-sided valves (principally tricuspid), producing thickening of the leaflets and sometimes stenosis.* Right ventricular and atrial enlargements frequently accompany the valvular changes. Uncommonly, there is also left-sided involvement, but it rarely induces valvular dysfunction, and even more rarely fibrous thickenings within the aortic or arterial intima, capsule of liver (overlying tumor implants), and elsewhere.

COMPLICATIONS OF ARTIFICIAL VALVES _____

Replacement of damaged cardiac valves with prostheses has now become a common and often life-saving mode of therapy; however, 6 to 9% per patient year of prostheses develop problems. Artificial valves fall into two categories: mechanical valves (e.g., caged balls, tilting disks, hinged flaps) and bioprostheses, pretreated animal (usually porcine or bovine) valves. Whether mechanical or biologic, all are subject to the following complications.

Paravalvular leaks are on the whole uncommon, are often insignificant, and usually result from a defect in the sewing of the ring of the valve into the cardiac bed or from postsurgical loss of one or more stitches secondary to infection.

Thromboembolic complications are major causes of prosthesis-related morbidity and mortality, more often with mechanical valves than with bioprostheses. The thrombi may block the function of valves and bioprostheses, embolize (most often to the brain), or become secondarily infected. In addition, hemorrhagic complications may arise because of the long-term anticoagulation required to prevent thrombosis.

IE develops in about 6% of patients within five years of valve replacement (see p. 323).

Deterioration. Mechanical valves are remarkably resistant to wear and tear, but rarely some structural component succumbs to the ravages of time (e.g., erosion of a ball valve occluder, breakage of a strut). However, within ten years 20 to 30% of glutaraldehyde-pretreated porcine aortic valves undergo sufficient sterile tissue degeneration followed by calcification to require replacement.

Other complications may develop: hemolysis induced by mechanical injury to red cells as they pass through the valves, and dysfunctional ingrowth of fibrous tissue. Although these complications are not common, they may be serious in the individual instance, so, overall, valve replacement, life-saving as it often is, has its risks.

MYOCARDIAL DISEASE _____

Many major forms of myocardial involvement have already been discussed (e.g., infarction, hypertrophy, rheumatic involvement); here our focus is on diffuse heart muscle disease, broadly separable into (1) myocarditis characterized by inflammatory changes and (2) noninflammatory myocardial disease called cardiomyopathy (CMP). In general myocarditis is of acute onset and often produces the fairly rapid onset of cardiac failure, but in most cases it resolves after a relatively short course, leaving little or no significant myocardial deficit. Most important, it is characterized by changes indicative of myocardial inflammation such as myofiber necrosis and well-defined inflammatory infiltrates. In contrast, the CMPs typically are of insidious onset, do not have evidence of active inflammation comparable to that in myocarditis, and often run a protracted, unrelenting downhill course. Regrettably, the two patterns do not always behave typically and occasional cases resist categorization. For example, some hearts with apparent CMP have minimal inflammatory myocardial changes that may readily be misinterpreted as incompletely resolved myocarditis. Nonetheless, the two categories are for the most part distinctive.

MYOCARDITIS

When the diagnosis is restricted to those instances of myocardial inflammation that are sufficient to cause clinical manifestations, myocarditis is an uncommon condition seen most often in young to middle-aged adults, but no age is immune. It is an important form of heart disease because although usually benign, it may induce rapidly progressive, sometimes fatal cardiac failure, potentially lethal arrhythmias, or sudden death.

There is a large number of potential causes of myocarditis (Table 11–6). Viruses, particularly the enteroviruses Coxsackie A and B, influenza, cytomegalovirus, and human immunodeficiency virus (HIV), are the major causes of myocarditis in the United States and Europe, but in rare cases other agents are involved. It is frequently difficult to document a viral

TABLE 11–6. CAUSES OF MYOCARDITIS

Infectious
  Viruses
  Bacteria
  Rickettsiae
  Mycoplasmas
  Fungi
  Protozoa
  Parasites
Noninfectious
  Drug hypersensitivity
  Collagen-vascular diseases
  Radiation
  Heavy metals
  Insect stings
  Transplant rejection
Idiopathic
  Sarcoidosis
  Fiedler's
  Giant cell

pathogen because by the time manifestations appear the agent is generally no longer isolable even from endomyocardial biopsy specimens. Recourse is often made to rising serum titers of antibodies, but more specific is immunohistochemical documentation of viral antigens or, using molecular probes, viral nucleic acid sequences in biopsies. With the latter approach enteroviral RNA has been identified in almost half of all cases of dilated cardiomyopathy, implying presumably a prior episode of viral myocarditis. Whether the viruses are directly injurious to the cells they infect or instead initiate an immune response that is cross-reactive with myocardial antigens remains uncertain.

In South America, the major cause of myocarditis is the *Trypanosoma cruzi* of Chagas' disease. Among the many other possible causes cited in Table 11–6, special mention should be made of trichinosis and cardiac transplant rejection. With the latter, endomyocardial biopsy to estimate the severity of the inflammatory rejection reaction assumes great importance in adjusting the level of immunosuppressive therapy.

There are several forms of idiopathic myocarditis. Myocardial lesions are found at autopsy in about 20% of patients with sarcoidosis, although most often it is of little clinical significance. Another idiopathic disorder is so-called giant cell myocarditis, closely related (if not identical) to Fiedler's myocarditis. Both merit attention because they are often fatal. The general features of these and other forms of myocarditis are now described.

MORPHOLOGY. The heart may appear normal or enlarged, with dilatation usually of all chambers. The ventricular myocardium is typically thinned out by the dilatation, flabby, and sometimes mottled by widespread or patchy pale foci or minute hemorrhagic lesions. Strangely, the involvement may be more severe in some areas than in others, creating the need for caution in the interpretation of endomyocardial biopsies. The endocardium and valves are unaffected except that mural thrombi may be present in dilated chambers.

The histologic changes vary with the specific pathogen. Only some generalizations can be offered. **With viral myocarditis typically there is only isolated myofiber necrosis, but there also may be prominent interstitial edema and mononuclear infiltration of lymphocytes, macrophages, and occasional plasma cells** (Fig. 11–16). With other forms of microbial invasion, the histologic pattern mirrors the changes produced by the same organism in extracardiac locations. Thus, **pyogens (e.g., staphylococci) induce a patchy, focal, suppurative reaction, and sometimes microabscesses, whereas streptococci cause more diffuse, spreading reactions. In trichinosis, although the parasite often invades the heart, it rarely encysts within its myofibers.** Usually only infiltrates of lymphocytes, macrophages, and eosinophils can be identified in foci of myocytolysis. **The myocarditis of Chagas' disease is rendered distinctive by parasitization of scattered myofibers by trypanosomes accompanied by an in-**

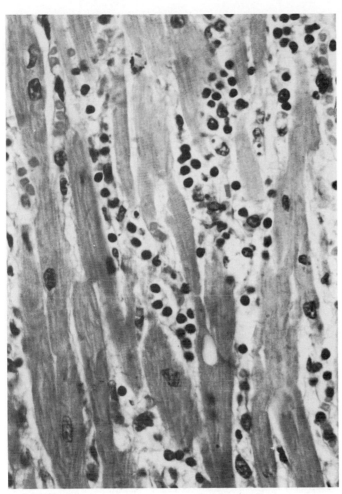

Figure 11–16. Viral myocarditis: edema and a mononuclear inflammatory infiltrate separate many of the myocardial fibers.

flammatory infiltrate of neutrophils, lymphocytes, macrophages, and occasional eosinophils.

Hypersensitivity and rejection reactions induce spotty myofiber necrosis and interstitial infiltrates that are principally perivascular, composed of lymphocytes, plasma cells, macrophages, and eosinophils. Occasionally with a severe rejection reaction, acute myofiber necrosis, neutrophils, and acute vasculitis can be seen.

There remain two morphologically distinctive forms of myocarditis: **Fiedler's** and **idiopathic giant cell myocarditis**, both characterized by focal areas of myocardial necrosis surrounded by a granulomatous reaction, often bearing giant cells. There is a strong likelihood that both entities are, in fact, a single disease of unknown, possibly viral or immunologic origin.

If the patient survives any form of myocarditis, the changes resolve leaving no residua or possibly an interstitial fibrosis.

CLINICAL FEATURES. All forms of myocarditis produce similar clinical manifestations. At one end of the clinical spectrum the disease is entirely asymptomatic and suspected only when an arrythmia or more subtle ECG change points to a myocardial lesion. At the other end, the myocarditis announces itself by the acute onset of CHF. In such cases systolic murmurs related to dilatation of the atrioventricular valve rings or arrhythmias often appear. Most patients recover completely without sequelae. Occasionally, years later, when the attack, particularly of viral myocarditis, is forgotten, the patient is diagnosed as having dilated (congestive) cardiomyopathy of unknown cause. The rare severe attack, particularly characteristic of the giant cell myocarditides, may take a rapid downhill course to death in cardiac failure.

CARDIOMYOPATHY

It is fruitless to delve into the ever-changing definition of CMP. It is sufficient to say that currently the term generally implies a noninflammatory myocardial disease that is not attributable to pressure or volume overload (i.e., HHD, cor pulmonale, valvular heart disease, congenital heart disease). Some would also exclude ischemia as a basis for the myocardial dysfunction, but increasingly the designation "ischemic CMP" is being used. Analogously, at one time the term CMP was restricted to conditions of unknown cause, the remainder being referred to as specific heart muscle disease. The present usage includes such specific conditions, indicating the cause when it is known (e.g., cobalt cardiomyopathy) to distinguish it from those that remain idiopathic.

The various CMPs have been divided into three clinicopathologic categories (Fig. 11–17): (1) dilated (congestive) CMP; (2) hypertrophic CMP; and (3) restrictive/obliterative CMP.

Dilated (Congestive) Cardiomyopathy

This diagnosis is applied to markedly dilated hearts with impaired contractile function that lack all stigmata of myocarditis. This condition probably reflects a large variety of insults, including past episodes of viral myocarditis, alcohol abuse, some pregnancy-related conditions, selenium deficiency, and toxic injury by such agents as cobalt, nickel, lithium, and anthracycline drugs. A genetic basis, or at least predisposition, may exist because familial clustering of cases has been reported. Only some limited comments will be made about a few of the potential causes.

Enteroviral traces have been identified by RNA hybridization in the myofibers of 30 to 50% of patients with dilated CMP. Coxsackie B, one of the enteroviruses, is likely to be the commonest viral cause of myocarditis. It thus appears that a significant fraction of cases of dilated CMP represent the end-stage of previous viral injury to the myocardium.

Alcohol, or one of its metabolites, has been strongly implicated as a possible cause of dilated CMP because a history of alcohol abuse is sometimes present in these patients and alcohol has been shown to impair myocardial contraction and induce regressive morpho-

328 ___ THE HEART

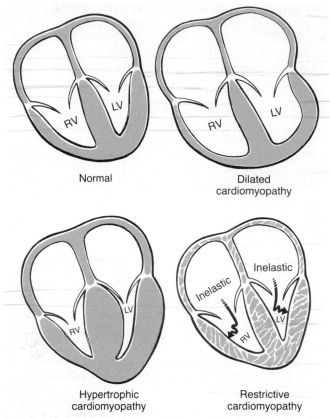

Normal

Dilated
cardiomyopathy

Hypertrophic
cardiomyopathy

Restrictive
cardiomyopathy

Figure 11–17. Representations of the three clinicopathologic categories of cardiomyopathy.

logic changes within the myocardium in animals. Conceivably in the chronic alcoholic, concomitant thiamine deficiency may contribute to the myocardial dysfunction, as is well known in so-called wet beriberi.

Pregnancy and *peripartum CMP* is a nebulous name applied to the onset of CHF in the third trimester of pregnancy or first six months of the puerperium. The basis for this association is unclear but has been vaguely ascribed to an underlying subclinical viral myocarditis predisposed to by some pregnancy-related immune dysfunction. Conceivably the physiologic, metabolic, or nutritional stresses of multiple pregnancies contribute in some ill-defined manner. Whatever the basis, this pattern of the disease is distinctive because, unlike most forms of dilated CMP, about half of the patients spontaneously recover in time but nonetheless are at increased risk with a subsequent pregnancy.

Much better established is the cardiotoxicity of such agents as cobalt, lithium, emetine, the anthracycline drugs (adriamycin and daunorubicin), and cyclophosphamide. With most the cardiac reaction is unpredictable, but with the anthracyclines the hazard is dose-dependent (total dose above 500 mg/m²) and attributed to peroxidation of lipids in myofiber membranes. Also to be included here is the potential cardiotoxicity of large amounts of catecholamines, such as may be released by a pheochromocytoma. Increasingly, cocaine has come to the forefront as a threat to the heart. Although this drug may act to produce coronary

spasm, arrhythmias, and MI, in a number of instances it has caused direct myocyte necrosis and changes consistent with dilated cardiomyopathy.

Despite all the potential causes mentioned, most cases remain idiopathic, but there is a strong suspicion that they may represent previous episodes of viral myocarditis that have initiated a continuing autoimmune response. Histologic traces of myocarditis have been observed in some cases of dilated CMP, and a large variety of immune system abnormalities have been demonstrated as well as a dramatic increase in the expression of both class I and class II histocompatibility antigens in the myocytes.

MORPHOLOGY. The gross changes are more distinctive than the microscopic ones. The heart is always increased in weight (up to 900 gm), but dilatation of the chambers may neutralize the thickening of the ventricular walls. The poor cardiac contraction and stasis of blood often lead to mural thrombi, particularly in dilated atria. The walls are usually flabby.

Histologic examination may disclose few specific alterations, but in many instances there is variation in myofiber size owing to stretching of some, atrophy of others, and focal myocytolysis. There may be an increase in interstitial fibrous tissue and a sparse focal infiltrate of mononuclears reminiscent of a past episode of viral myocarditis.

CLINICAL COURSE. This condition may occur at any age including during childhood. It presents with slowly developing CHF caused by a poorly contracting heart with markedly reduced cardiac output. About 35% of patients die within five years and 70% within ten. Frequently, the diagnosis is one of exclusion. Death is usually attributable to progressive failure, embolism from dislodgement of intracardiac thrombi, or a fatal arrhythmia. Cardiac transplantation may be the only hope.

Hypertrophic Cardiomyopathy

This form of CMP is also known as asymmetric septal hypertrophy (ASH), idiopathic hypertrophic subaortic stenosis (IHSS), and hypertrophic obstructive cardiomyopathy. It is characterized by a heavy, muscular *hyper*contracting heart in striking contrast to the flabby, *hypo*contracting heart of dilated CMP. In more than half the patients, the disease is familial and is transmitted by autosomal dominant inheritance. Recently, mutations in the myosin heavy chain genes on chromosome 14 bands q11–13 have been identified in two kindreds, so the time is fast approaching when molecular probes will make it possible to determine whether similar mutations (some perhaps sporadic) are present in all cases of hypertrophic CMP. The identified mutations affect the synthesis of certain myosin heavy chains and could conceivably derange the formation of myofibrils, producing myofiber enlargement and the overall cardiac hypertrophy.

MORPHOLOGY. The essential feature is cardiac enlargement with an increase in weight (up to a kilogram) disproportionate to the increase in size owing to marked myocardial hypertrophy, most evident in the left ventricle and interventricular septum. Uncommonly the increase in weight is modest. Although classically the septum is disproportionately thickened (2.5 to 3 cm) as compared with the free wall of the left ventricle, sometimes the entire left ventricle is uniformly affected or the basal or apical septum is disproportionately involved. On cross section, the ventricular cavity may be compressed into a banana-like configuration by bulging of the interventricular septum into the lumen (Fig. 11-18). In such hearts, the subaortic septal thickening comes into contact with the anterior leaflet of the mitral valve in systole, narrowing the aortic outflow to induce an obstructive element. With less basal thickening of the septum and less systolic anterior movement of the mitral leaflet, the outflow is not obstructed, so the designations that use the term "obstructive CMP" are misleading.

Microscopically, there are the changes of myocyte hypertrophy (p. 314), but the most distinctive feature is disorganization of the hypertrophic myofibers so that they are arrayed haphazardly rather than in parallel bundles. Disarray of the myofibrils within sarcomeres is also present. This disorganization typically is more evident in the septum than in the left ventricular free wall, but not in all cases. **Not all hearts with hypertrophic CMP have significant myofiber disorganization, however, and similar changes may appear with other forms of myocardial hypertrophy, though they are far more widespread and prominent in hypertrophic CMP. It is the quantitative aspect that is important.**

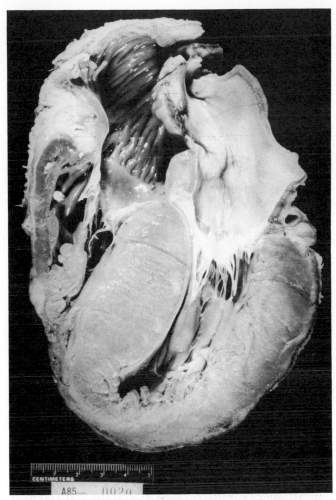

Figure 11-18. Hypertrophic cardiomyopathy with marked thickening of the left ventricular wall and particularly of the interventricular septum. The banana-shaped left ventricular cavity is markedly reduced in size and the bulging interventricular septum encroaches on the outflow tract.

CLINICAL COURSE. Hypertrophic CMP occurs most often in young adults but may first appear in elders as dyspnea on exertion, angina, or attacks of syncope. Sudden death may occur. The symptoms of cardiac insufficiency are related more to reduced ventricular compliance and reduced stroke volume output than to outflow obstruction. Paradoxically then, dilatation of the heart and impairment of systolic contraction account for the spontaneous improvement often seen with cardiac failure. With the recognition that outflow obstruction is not the major problem, most patients can be significantly helped by medical therapy alone.

Restrictive or Obliterative Cardiomyopathy

Restrictive or obliterative CMP is the least common form. A number of disparate entities induce this form of CMP, including cardiac amyloidosis, sarcoidosis, endocardial fibroelastosis, endomyocardial fibrosis, and Loeffler's endocarditis. Common to all is reduced ventricular compliance and diastolic ventricular filling. Most of these conditions are either very rare or have been described elsewhere (amyloidosis, sarcoidosis). Only endocardial fibroelastosis will be characterized here.

Endocardial fibroelastosis is an uncommon heart disease characterized by focal or diffuse cartilage-like fibroelastic thickening of the mural endocardium restricting diastolic compliance and often obliterating some of the apical ventricular cavity. Most often only the left side of the heart is affected, but occasionally both sides or (least commonly) only the right. The nature of this disorder is obscure but it has been related to past episodes of myocardial eosinophilia of obscure origin with secondary endocardial damage caused by factors released from activated eosinophils.

PERICARDIAL DISEASE

Pericardial lesions are almost always associated with disease in the heart or surrounding structures or with a systemic disorder. Rarely, pericardial involvement may occur as a primary isolated process. Despite the large number of causes (infectious and noninfectious) there are relatively few anatomic forms of pericardial involvement.

ACCUMULATIONS OF FLUID IN PERICARDIAL SAC

PERICARDIAL EFFUSION. The term "pericardial effusion" is restricted to accumulations of *noninflammatory* fluids in the pericardial sac, as distinguished from collections of blood or exudate (discussed later). Normally, there is about 30 to 50 ml of thin, clear, straw-colored fluid in the pericardial space. Under a variety of circumstances effusions, rarely larger than 500 ml, may appear. The various types of effusion and their common causes are as follows:

Serous: congestive heart failure; hypoproteinemia (renal, hepatic, nutritional).

Serosanguineous: blunt chest trauma; cardiopulmonary resuscitation.

Chylous: lymphatic obstruction (benign or malignant mediastinal neoplasms).

Cholesterol: myxedema; idiopathic (possibly previous hemorrhage).

Because most effusions accumulate slowly, they are usually without clinical significance except for producing enlargement of the heart shadow on x-ray. Rarely, a large volume may embarrass diastolic filling, requiring withdrawal.

HEMOPERICARDIUM. The term hemopericardium should be limited to the accumulation of pure blood in the pericardial sac, as distinct from hemorrhagic pericarditis. The former is almost always due to rupture of the heart secondary to MI or rupture of the intrapericardial aorta. Quite rarely, it may follow traumatic perforation of the heart or penetration of a myocardial abscess or tumor. The blood that escapes rapidly fills the sac under greatly increased pressure and produces cardiac tamponade. As little as 200 to 300 ml may be sufficient to cause death.

PERICARDITIS

Primary pericarditis is a rarity and almost always of viral origin. The most common causes of secondary pericarditis are myocardial infarction, uremia, and cardiac surgery. In a second category of importance are systemic lupus erythematosus, rheumatic fever, rheumatoid disease, microbial seeding, cancerous invasion, and radiation.

The many causes mentioned usually evoke an acute fibrinous pericarditis, but bacterial seeding may produce suppuration; both patterns usually resolve without residua if the patient survives. Tuberculosis and fungi, on the other hand, produce chronic reactions. On occasion the acute reaction is hemorrhagic, raising the suspicion of cancerous invasion, which can sometimes be confirmed by identification of the tumor cells in the exudate. The chronic reactions often lead to disabling fibrous encasement of the heart (see below).

Chronic or Healed Pericarditis

The term chronic pericarditis is a misnomer, since it refers in reality to a healed stage of some form of pericardial inflammation. One pattern comprises the formation of pearly, thickened, nonadherent epicardial plaques ("soldier's plaque"). Alternatively, thin, delicate adhesions may develop, which are termed diffuse or focal obliterative pericarditis, according to their distribution. These adherences rarely hamper cardiac contraction or impair function even when the entire pericardial sac is obliterated (obliterative pericarditis).

Two forms of healed pericarditis are of clinical importance: adhesive mediastinopericarditis and constrictive pericarditis.

Adhesive mediastinopericarditis may follow a suppurative or tuberculous caseous pericarditis but can also be the consequence of previous cardiac surgery or high-dose irradiation to the mediastinum (e.g., radiotherapy of a neoplasm). Only rarely is it a sequela to fibrinous or suppurative exudation. The pericardial sac is obliterated with adherence of the external aspect of the parietal layer to surrounding structures. With each systolic contraction, the heart pulls not only against the parietal pericardium, but also against the surrounding structures. *The increased workload causes cardiac hypertrophy and dilatation, which may be quite massive.*

CONSTRICTIVE PERICARDITIS. The heart may be encased in a dense fibrous or fibrocalcific scar (often 0.5 to 1.0 cm thick) that limits diastolic expansion and seriously restricts cardiac output, mimicking the restrictive CMPs discussed earlier (p. 329). In extreme cases, it appears as if the heart were enclosed within a plaster mold *(concretio cordis).* Sometimes there is a well-defined history of suppurative or caseous pericarditis, but more often the cause is buried in the remote past. Fibrinous or serofibrinous inflammatory reactions rarely lead to this form of damage.

Unlike the case with mediastinopericarditis, *cardiac hypertrophy and dilatation cannot occur,* and as a consequence the volume output and pulse pressure are reduced. Constriction of the venae cavae as they drain into the right atrium blocks the venous return, adding to the cardiac dysfunction.

MISCELLANEOUS DISORDERS

RHEUMATOID HEART DISEASE

The heart is affected in 20 to 40% of cases of prolonged rheumatoid arthritis (p. 145). Most common is a fibrinous pericarditis that may progress to fibrous thickening of the visceral and parietal pericardium with dense fibrous adhesions. In the early stages of this process rheumatoid inflammatory granulomatous nodules may be identifiable, resembling those that occur subcutaneously (p. 146). Much less frequently, rheumatoid nodules involve the myocardium, atrioventricular valve rings, endocardium, valve leaflets, and the root of the aorta. These inflammatory lesions are particularly damaging when they are located in the valves, because they lead to marked fibrous thickening and secondary calcifications, producing changes resembling those of chronic rheumatic valvular disease but lacking the intercommissural adhesions.

METASTATIC TUMORS

Although primary tumors of the heart are extremely rare, cardiac metastases occur in about 5% of patients who die of cancer. Implicated neoplasms, in descending order of frequency, are carcinoma of the lung, breast, malignant melanoma, lymphoma, and leukemia. The implants most often involve the pericardium and sometimes produce manifestations of pericarditis, but they may directly seed the myocardium, sometimes to invade the endocardium and evoke thrombosis.

PRIMARY TUMORS

The most common primary tumors, in descending order of frequency, are myxomas, lipomas, papillary fibroelastomas, rhabdomyomas, angiosarcomas, and rhabdomyosarcomas. Note that the four most common are all benign and account collectively for about 70% of all primary tumors of the heart. Only myxoma, fibroelastoma, and rhabdomyoma will be described.

Myxomas are by far the most common primary tumor of the heart. Although they may arise in any chamber (or, rarely, on the heart valves) about 90% are located in the atria, in a left-to-right ratio of approximately 4:1. The region of the fossa ovalis is a favored site of origin. They range from small (less than 1 cm), usually pedunculated masses to large (up to 10 cm) often sessile ones, and from soft, gray, myxoid to firm, gray-red tumors. All are covered by an intact endocardium, but fragmentation and embolization of papillary lesions are sometimes encountered. In some locations the pedunculated type may be sufficiently mobile to move into or sometimes through the atrioventricular valves during diastole, either blocking it or exerting a wrecking ball effect on the leaflets (Fig. 11–19). Histologically, myxomas are composed of stellate or globular myxoma cells, endothelial cells, macrophages, mature or immature smooth muscle cells, and a variety of intermediate forms embedded within an abundant acid mucopolysaccharide ground substance.

These neoplasms may be encountered at any age, even in infants, with a predominance in females. Because of valvular obstructions they sometimes cause unanticipated syncope attacks, cardiac insufficiency, and even sudden death. Visualization by echocardiography often permits life-saving surgical excision.

Papillary fibroelastomas are curious (usually incidental) paint brush–like clusters, about 2 to 5 mm in length, attached by a short pedicle to the underlying endocardial surface, generally on valves. These curiosities are thought to represent organized fibrinous deposits.

Rhabdomyomas are much less common than myxomas. They are, however, the most frequent primary tumor of the heart in infants and children and are

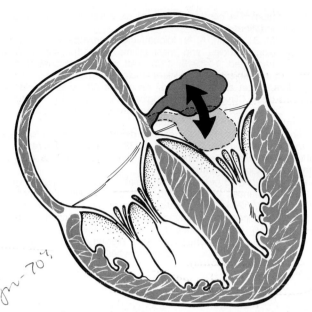

Figure 11–19. A representation of a pedunculated left atrial myxoma attached to the interatrial septum. Its mobility permits it to possibly occlude the mitral orifice.

frequently discovered in the first years of life because of obstruction of a valvular orifice or cardiac chamber. They are generally small, gray-white myocardial masses up to several centimeters in diameter located on either the left or right side of the heart and protruding into the cardiac chamber. Histologically, they are composed of a mixed population of cells, prominent among which are large, rounded or polygonal cells that have numerous glycogen-laden vacuoles separated by strands of cytoplasm running from the plasma membrane to the more or less centrally located nucleus— so-called "spider cells." These cells can be shown to have myofibrils and actin and desmin intermediate filaments marking them as muscle cells. In addition there may be spindle cells, histiocytic-appearing cells, and an abundant mucopolysaccharide matrix. The nature of these lesions is not clear, but the high frequency of tuberous sclerosis in patients with cardiac rhabdomyomas supports the notion that they are developmental anomalies rather than neoplasms.

Bibliography

Barst, R. J., Gersony, W. M.: The pharmacologic treatment of patent ductus arteriosus. A review of the evidence. Drugs 38:249, 1989. (A brief review of the anatomic and clinical features with emphasis on medical management approaches.)

Bisno, A. L.: Group A streptococcal infections and acute rheumatic fever. N. Engl. J. Med. 325:783, 1981. (A detailed account of the epidemiology of rheumatic fever and possible factors influencing the prevalence.)

Cheng, T. O.: Mitral valve prolapse. Ann. Rev. Med. 40:201, 1989. (A concise discussion mainly of the potential complications of this condition.)

Collins, P., Fox, K. M.: Pathophysiology of angina. Lancet 355:94, 1990. (Concise discussion of the complex dynamics of myocardial ischemia underlying the various patterns of angina pectoris.)

Davies, M. J.: The cardiomyopathies: A review of terminology, pathology, and pathogenesis. Histopathology 8:363, 1984. (A clear presentation of a complex group of disorders with fine morpho-logic descriptions.)

Gravanis, M. B., Ansari, A. A.: Idiopathic cardiomyopathies. A review of pathologic studies and mechanisms of pathogenesis. Arch. Pathol. Lab. Med. *111:*915, 1987. (An excellent discussion of a complicated subject. Good clinicopathologic correlations.)

Hollanders, G., et al.: A six years' review on 53 cases of infective endocarditis: Clinical, microbiological and therapeutic features. Acta Cardiol. *43:*121, 1988. (A comprehensive overview of the salient etiologic and clinical features.)

Kemers, M. S., et al.: Sudden cardiac death: Etiologies, pathogene-sis, and management. Dis. Month *35:*383, 1989. (A large review of the subject with more emphasis on the clinical aspects than on the pathogenesis or pathology.)

Lundin, L.: Carcinoid heart disease: Relationship of circulating vaso-active substances to ultrasound-detectable cardiac abnormalities. Circulation *77:*264, 1988. (An overview of the subject with good discussion of possible pathogeneses and diagnostic approaches.)

Markowitz, M: Reappearance of rheumatic fever. Adv. Pediatr. *36:*39, 1989. (A comprehensive review placing particular emphasis on changing epidemiology and pathogenesis with a detailed bibli-ography.)

Mitral valve prolapse. Lancet *1:*1173, 1989. (A brief presentation of the major features with emphasis on the relationship between the severity of the process and its clinical significance.)

Pepine, C. J.: New concepts in the pathophysiology of acute MI. Am. J. Cardiol. *64:*2B, 1989. (An excellent overview of the factors leading to myocardial infarction and its evolution.)

Reimer, K. A., Ideker, R. E.: Myocardial ischemia and infarction. Anatomic and biochemical substrates for ischemic cell death and ventricular arrhythmias. Hum. Pathol. *18:*462, 1987. (A detailed consideration of the biochemical, metabolic, and ultrastructural consequences of myocardial ischemia.)

Selzer, A. S.: Changing aspects of the natural history of valvular aortic stenosis. N. Engl. J. Med. *317:*91, 1987. (Succinct but thorough review of pathogenetic, anatomic, and clinical aspects.)

Waller, B. F.: The pathology of acute myocardial infarction: Defini-tion, location, pathogenesis, effects of reperfusion, complications, and sequelae. Cardiol. Clin. *6:*1, 1988. (An excellent detailed presentation of the morphology, complications, and consequences of myocardial infarction.)

TWELVE

The Hematopoietic and Lymphoid Systems

RED CELL DISORDERS

HEMORRHAGE—BLOOD LOSS ANEMIA

INCREASED RATE OF RED CELL
DESTRUCTION—THE HEMOLYTIC ANEMIAS

- Hereditary Spherocytosis
- Sickle Cell Anemia
- Thalassemia
- Glucose-6-Phosphate Dehydrogenase
  Deficiency
- Paroxysmal Nocturnal Hemoglobinuria
- Immunohemolytic Anemias
- Erythroblastosis Fetalis (Hemolytic Disease of
  the Newborn)
- Hemolytic Anemias Resulting from Mechanical
  Trauma to Red Cells
- Malaria

ANEMIAS OF DIMINISHED ERYTHROPOIESIS

- Iron Deficiency Anemia
- Anemia of Chronic Disease
- Megaloblastic Anemias
  - Folate (Folic Acid) Deficiency Anemia
  - Vitamin B_{12} (Cobalamin) Deficiency
    Anemia—Pernicious Anemia
- Aplastic Anemia
- Myelophthisic Anemia

POLYCYTHEMIA

WHITE CELL DISORDERS

NONNEOPLASTIC DISORDERS OF WHITE
CELLS

- Leukopenia
  - Neutropenia—Agranulocytosis
- Reactive Leukocytosis
  - Infectious Mononucleosis
- Reactive Lymphadenitis
  - Acute Nonspecific Lymphadenitis
  - Chronic Nonspecific Lymphadenitis
  - Cat Scratch Disease

NEOPLASTIC PROLIFERATIONS OF WHITE
CELLS

- Malignant Lymphomas

  - Non-Hodgkin's Lymphomas
  - Hodgkin's Disease
- Leukemias and Myeloproliferative Diseases
  - Acute Leukemias
  - Myelodysplastic Syndromes
  - Chronic Myeloid Leukemia
  - Chronic Lymphocytic Leukemia
  - Hairy Cell Leukemia
  - Myeloproliferative Disorders
- Plasma Cell Dyscrasias and Related Disorders
- Histiocytoses
  - Langerhans' Cell Histiocytosis

BLEEDING DISORDERS

DISSEMINATED INTRAVASCULAR
COAGULATION

THROMBOCYTOPENIA

- Idiopathic Thrombocytopenic Purpura
- Thrombotic Thrombocytopenic Purpura

COAGULATION DISORDERS

- Deficiencies of Factor VIII–von Willebrand's
  Factor Complex
  - von Willebrand's Disease
  - Factor VIII Deficiency (Hemophilia A,
    Classic Hemophilia)
- Factor IX Deficiency (Hemophilia B, Christmas
  Disease)

DISORDERS THAT AFFECT THE SPLEEN

Disorders of the hematopoietic and lymphoid systems encompass a wide range of diseases. They may affect primarily the red cells, the white cells, or the hemostatic mechanisms. *Red cell disorders* are usually reflected in *anemia*. *White cell disorders,* in contrast, most often involve overgrowth, usually malignant. Hemostatic derangements result in *hemorrhagic diatheses*. Finally, splenomegaly, a feature of several hematopoietic diseases, is discussed at the end of the chapter.

Red Cell Disorders

Disorders of the red cells usually result in some form of anemia, or sometimes in erythrocytosis (an increase in the number of red cells). Anemia is a reduction in the oxygen transporting capacity of blood, usually due to a reduction below normal limits of the total circulating red cell mass. This is reflected by subnormal hematocrit and hemoglobin concentrations. In most anemias, erythropoietin production and erythropoiesis are increased, causing erythroid marrow hyperplasia. Increased erythropoiesis can also occur in the spleen and liver of infants (extramedullary hematopoiesis).

TABLE 12–1 CLASSIFICATION OF ANEMIA ACCORDING TO MECHANISM OF PRODUCTION

I. Blood loss
  A. Acute: Trauma
  B. Chronic: Lesions of GI tract, gynecologic disturbances
II. Increased rate of destruction (hemolytic anemias)
  A. Intrinsic (intracorpuscular) abnormalities of red cells
    Hereditary
    1. Disorders of red cell membrane cytoskeleton, e.g., spherocytosis, elliptocytosis
    2. Red cell enzyme deficiencies
      a. Glycolytic enzymes: Pyruvate kinase, hexokinase
      b. Enzymes of hexose monophosphate shunt: G6PD, glutathione synthetase
    3. Disorders of hemoglobin synthesis
      a. Deficient globin synthesis: Thalassemia syndromes
      b. Structurally abnormal globin synthesis (hemoglobinopathies): Sickle cell anemia, unstable hemoglobins
    Acquired
    1. Membrane defect: Paroxysmal nocturnal hemoglobinuria
  B. Extrinsic (extracorpuscular) abnormalities
    1. Antibody mediated
      a. Isohemagglutinins: Transfusion reactions, erythroblastosis fetalis
      b. Autoantibodies: Idiopathic (primary), drug-associated, SLE
    2. Mechanical trauma to red cells
      a. Microangiopathic hemolytic anemias: Thrombotic thrombocytopenic purpura, DIC
      b. Cardiac traumatic hemolytic anemia
    3. Infections: Malaria
III. Impaired red cell production
  A. Disturbance of proliferation and differentiation of stem cells: Aplastic anemia, pure red cell aplasia, anemia of renal failure, anemia of endocrine disorders
  B. Disturbance of proliferation and maturation of erythroblasts
    1. Defective DNA synthesis: Deficiency or impaired utilization of vitamin B_{12} and folic acid (megaloblastic anemias)
    2. Defective hemoglobin synthesis
      a. Deficient heme synthesis: Iron deficiency
      b. Deficient globin synthesis: Thalassemias
    3. Unknown or multiple mechanisms: Sideroblastic anemia, anemia of chronic infections, myelophthisic anemias due to marrow infiltrations

Classification of anemias is based on the mechanism of production (Table 12–1).

HEMORRHAGE — BLOOD LOSS ANEMIA

With acute blood loss the immediate threat to the patient is hypovolemia (shock) rather than anemia (see p. 78). If the patient survives, hemodilution begins at once and achieves its full effect within two to three days, unmasking the extent of the red cell loss. If body iron stores are adequate, after several days there is increased erythropoiesis in the marrow with complete replacement of red cells. Marrow compensation is reflected by release of reticulocytes in the blood.

With chronic blood loss, iron stores are gradually depleted, resulting in anemia of iron deficiency. Because iron deficiency anemia can occur in other clinical settings as well, it is described later in this chapter along with other anemias of diminished erythropoiesis (p. 345).

INCREASED RATE OF RED CELL DESTRUCTION — THE HEMOLYTIC ANEMIAS

Shortened survival of red cells may be due either to inherent defects in the erythrocyte (intracorpuscular hemolytic anemia), which are usually inherited, or to external influences (extracorpuscular hemolytic anemia), which are usually acquired. Several examples are listed in Table 12–1.

Before proceeding to discuss the various disorders individually, we will describe certain general features of hemolytic anemias. All are characterized by (1) *increased rate of red blood cell destruction* and (2) *retention by the body of the products of red cell destruction, including iron.* Since the iron is conserved and recycled readily, red cell regeneration can keep pace with the hemolysis. Consequently, these *anemias are almost invariably associated with marked hypercellularity within the marrow due to an increase in erythropoiesis.* Sometimes there is also extramedullary hematopoiesis in the liver and spleen. *Red cell regeneration is reflected by an increase in the reticulocyte count in peripheral blood.* The destruction of red cells may occur within the vascular compartment *(intravascular hemolysis)* or within the cells of the mononuclear phagocyte, or reticuloendothelial (RE), system *(extravascular hemolysis).*

Intravascular hemolysis is seen in red cells subjected to mechanical trauma or damaged by fixation of complement, as occurs in hemolytic transfusion reactions and in paroxysmal nocturnal hemoglobinuria. Whatever the cause, intravascular hemolysis results in he-

THE HEMATOPOIETIC AND LYMPHOID SYSTEMS _____ **335**

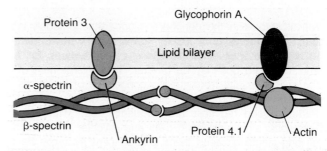

Figure 12–2. Schematic view of the proteins that form the cytoskeleton of the red cell membrane. Spectrin consists of α- and β-chains that lie on the inner surface of the cell membrane and are connected to it through ankyrin, actin, and protein 4.1.

moglobinemia, hemoglobinuria, and hemosiderinuria. Conversion of the heme pigment to bilirubin may give rise to unconjugated hyperbilirubinemia and jaundice. Massive intravascular hemolysis sometimes leads to acute tubular necrosis (p. 457). Levels of serum haptoglobin, a protein that binds free hemoglobin, are characteristically low.

Extravascular hemolysis, the more common mode of red cell destruction, takes place largely within the phagocytic cells of the spleen and liver. The mononuclear phagocyte system removes erythrocytes from the circulation whenever red cells are injured or immunologically altered. Since extreme alterations of shape are necessary for red cells to successfully navigate the splenic sinusoids, reduction in deformability makes this passage difficult and leads to splenic sequestration, followed by phagocytosis (Fig. 12–1). This is believed to be an important factor in the pathogenesis of red cell destruction in a variety of hemolytic anemias. Extravascular hemolysis is not associated with hemoglobinemia and hemoglobinuria, but jaundice may result and in long-standing cases lead to gallstone formation. In most forms of hemolytic anemia there is hyperactivity of the RE system, which results in splenomegaly.

Because the pathways for the excretion of excess iron are limited, there is a tendency in hemolytic anemias for abnormal amounts of iron to accumulate, giving rise to systemic hemosiderosis (p. 19) or in very severe cases secondary hemochromatosis (p. 554).

HEREDITARY SPHEROCYTOSIS _____

This disorder is characterized by an inherited (intrinsic) defect in the red cell membrane that renders the erythrocytes spheroidal, less deformable, and vulnerable to splenic sequestration and destruction. Hereditary spherocytosis (HS) is transmitted as an autosomal

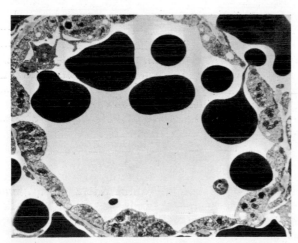

Figure 12–1. Splenic sinus (electron micrograph). An erythrocyte is in the process of squeezing from the cord into the sinus lumen. Note the degree of deformability required for the red cell to pass through the wall of the sinus. (From Enriquez, P., Neiman, R. S.: The Pathology of the Spleen. A Functional Approach. Chicago, American Society of Clinical Pathologists, © 1976, p. 7. Used by permission.)

dominant trait; however, in 20% of the cases there is no family history, indicating that the mutation can arise de novo.

PATHOGENESIS. Although the exact defect has not yet been clarified, *it is generally accepted that the primary abnormality resides in the proteins that form the skeleton of the red cell membrane.* Several such proteins (Fig. 12–2) form an interlocking but flexible structure on the intracellular face of the cell membrane. Together they are responsible for the normal shape, strength, and flexibility of the red cell. Although a quantitative or qualitative defect in any one of the membrane skeletal proteins could adversely affect the shape of red cells, most available evidence points to deficiency of spectrin molecules. Spectrin-deficient red cells have reduced membrane stability and consequently lose membrane fragments as the cells are exposed to shear stresses in the circulation. Reduction in the membrane substance (and surface area) forces the cells to assume the smallest possible diameter for a given volume, namely, a sphere.

Regardless of the precise molecular defect in HS, there is no doubt that *the spleen plays a major role in the destruction of spherocytes.* Red cells must undergo extreme degrees of deformation to leave the cords of Billroth and enter the splenic sinusoids. The discoid shape of normal red cells allows considerable latitude for changes in cell shape. In contrast, because of their spheroidal shape and reduced membrane plasticity, spherocytes have great difficulty leaving the splenic cords. The abnormal red cells are sequestered and eventually destroyed by macrophages, which are plentiful in the splenic cords. *The critical role of the spleen in this process is illustrated by the invariably beneficial effect of splenectomy. The red cell defect persists but the anemia is corrected.*

MORPHOLOGY. On smears the red cells lack the central zone of pallor because of their spheroidal shape. Spherocytosis, although distinctive, is not diagnostic since it is also seen in immune hemolytic anemias. To compensate for the excessive red cell destruction, erythropoiesis in the marrow is stimulated. As with other hemolytic anemias, red cell regeneration is reflected by reticulocytosis in the peripheral blood. Splenomegaly is greater and more common in HS than in any other form of hemolytic anemia. The weight is usually between 500 and 1000 gm but may be greater. The enlargement of the spleen results from striking congestion of the cords of Billroth, leaving the splenic sinuses virtually empty. Phagocytosed red cells are frequently seen within hypertrophic sinusoidal lining cells and reticular cord cells. In long-standing cases there is prominent systemic hemosiderosis.

The other general features of hemolytic anemias described earlier are present with this disorder. In particular, cholelithiasis occurs in 40 to 50% of these patients.

CLINICAL COURSE. The characteristic clinical features are anemia, splenomegaly, and jaundice. The severity of this disorder is highly variable. Asymptomatic cases occur, as well as those characterized by a profound anemia, but in general the anemia is moderate. Since the red cells are spheroidal in shape, there is little margin for expansion of volume when cells are exposed to hypotonic salt solution. As a result, *increased osmotic fragility is a characteristic finding that is helpful in diagnosis.* The more or less stable clinical course may be punctuated by two kinds of "crises." A *hemolytic crisis* may develop, consisting of a wave of increased hemolysis accompanied by a transient increase in jaundice, splenomegaly, and anemia. These episodes, often triggered by infection, are usually self-limited. Less commonly, a life-threatening "*aplastic crisis*" associated with complete cessation of marrow function with consequent leukopenia and thrombocytopenia may appear. Transfusions may be necessary to support the patient. HS is cured by splenectomy.

SICKLE CELL ANEMIA _____

The hemoglobinopathies are a group of hereditary disorders characterized by the presence of a structurally abnormal hemoglobin. More than 300 hemoglobins have been discovered, a third of which are associated with significant clinical manifestations. The prototype and most prevalent hemoglobinopathy results from a mutation in the gene coding for the β-globin chain that causes the formation of the sickle hemoglobin (HbS). The associated disease, sickle cell anemia, is discussed here; other hemoglobinopathies are far too infrequent for our consideration.

HbS, like 90% of other abnormal hemoglobins, results from a single amino acid substitution in the globin chain. Hemoglobin, as you may recall, is a tetramer of four globin chains comprising two pairs of similar chains. In the normal adult, hemoglobin is composed of 96% HbA ($\alpha_2\beta_2$), 3% HbA$_2$ ($\alpha_2\delta_2$), and 1% fetal hemoglobin (HbF, $\alpha_2\gamma_2$). *Substitution of valine for glutamic acid at the sixth position of the β chain produces HbS.* In homozygotes all HbA is replaced by HbS, whereas in heterozygotes only about half is replaced.

INCIDENCE. Approximately 8% of American blacks are heterozygous for HbS. In parts of Africa where malaria is endemic, the gene frequency approaches 30%, attributed to the slight protective effect of HbS against *Plasmodium falciparum* malaria. In the United States, sickle cell anemia affects approximately one of every 600 blacks; worldwide, sickle cell anemia is the most common form of familial hemolytic anemia.

ETIOLOGY AND PATHOGENESIS. Upon deoxygenation, HbS molecules undergo polymerization, a process sometimes called gelation or crystallization. The change in the physical state of HbS distorts the red cells, which assume an elongated crescent, or sickle, shape (Fig. 12–3). Sickling of red cells is initially reversible by oxygenation; however, membrane damage occurs with each episode of sickling and eventually the cells accumulate calcium, lose potassium and water, and become irreversibly sickled despite adequate oxygenation.

Many factors influence sickling of red cells. The two most important ones are as follows:

- *The amount of HbS and its interaction with other hemoglobin chains in the cell.* In heterozygotes approximately 40% of hemoglobin is HbS; the rest is HbA, which interacts only weakly with HbS during the processes of aggregation. Therefore heterozygotes have little tendency to sickle and are said to have the *sickle cell trait*. In contrast, *homozygotes have all HbS, and thus full-blown sickle cell anemia.*
- *The mean corpuscular hemoglobin concentration (MCHC) per cell.* The higher the HbS concentration within the cell, the greater are the chances of contact and interaction between HbS molecules. Thus, de-

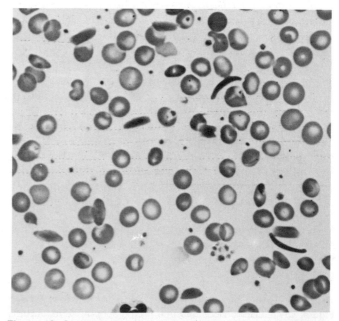

Figure 12–3. Peripheral blood smear from a patient with sickle cell anemia. Low magnification shows sickle cells, anisocytosis, and poikilocytosis. (Courtesy of Dr. Robert W. McKenna, Department of Pathology, University of Texas, Southwestern Medical School, Dallas, Texas).

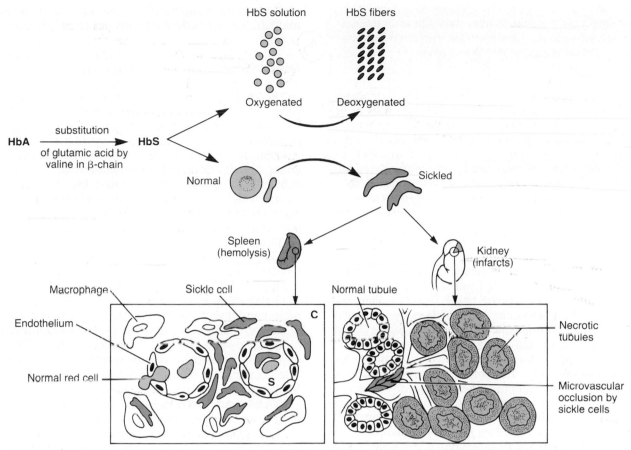

Figure 12-4. Pathophysiology and morphologic consequences of sickle cell anemia. Key: S, splenic sinusoids; C, splenic cords.

hydration, which increases the MCHC, greatly facilitates sickling and may trigger occlusion of small blood vessels. Conversely, the coexistence of α-thalassemia (described later), characterized by reduced synthesis of globin chains, reduces the MCHC and therefore the severity of sickling.

Two major consequences stem from the sickling of red cells (Fig. 12-4). *Sickled red cells become rigid and therefore susceptible to sequestration and hemolysis within the spleen, as already discussed* (p. 335). Their mean life span is reduced from 120 days to approximately 20 days. In addition to hemolytic anemia, *sickle cell disease is associated with widespread microvascular obstructions and resulting ischemic damage.* It is generally assumed that occlusion of small blood vessels results from rigidity and log-jamming of the sickled cells; however, recent observations suggest that the presence of HbS is associated with other abnormalities (such as increased stickiness of red cells to endothelium) that play a significant role in the pathogenesis of vascular occlusion.

MORPHOLOGY. The anatomic alterations stem from the following three aspects of the disease: (1) hemolysis with resultant anemia, (2) increased release of hemoglobin with bilirubin formation, and (3) capil-

lary stasis with thrombosis. When tissue sections are fixed in formalin so that anaerobiosis develops before complete fixation, sickled red cells are evident as bizarre, elongated, spindled, or boat-shaped structures. Both the severe anemia and the vascular stasis lead to hypoxic fatty changes in the heart, liver, and renal tubules. Fatty marrow is activated. The hypercellularity of the marrow occurs principally at the level of the normoblasts. Expansion of marrow may lead to resorption of bone with appositional new bone formation on the external aspect of the skull, leading to a "crew cut" appearance on radiographs. Extramedullary hematopoiesis may appear in the spleen and liver.

In children there is moderate splenomegaly (up to 500 gm) caused by congestion of the red pulp with masses of red cells sickled and jammed together. Eventually this splenic erythrostasis leads to enough hypoxic tissue damage, sometimes with frank infarction, to create a shrunken, fibrotic spleen. This process, termed **autosplenectomy,** is seen in all long-standing adult cases. Ultimately, only a small nubbin of fibrous tissue remains of the spleen.

Vascular congestion, thrombosis, and infarction may affect any organ, including bones, liver, kidney, and retina. Approximately 50% of adult patients develop leg ulcers because of hypoxia of the subcutaneous tissues.

Cor pulmonale may result from thromboses in the pulmonary vessels. As with the other hemolytic anemias, hemosiderosis and gallstones are common.

CLINICAL COURSE. Homozygous sickle cell disease usually becomes apparent after the sixth month of life, as fetal hemoglobin (HbF) is gradually replaced by HbS. The anemia is severe, with hematocrit values ranging between 18 and 30% (normal 35 to 45%). The chronic hemolysis is associated with marked reticulocytosis and hyperbilirubinemia. From the time of onset, the process runs an unremitting course, punctuated by sudden episodes of so-called crises. The most serious of these are the *vasoocclusive, or painful, crises.* The pain in these crises is usually localized to the abdomen (sometimes simulating "acute abdomen") or to some portion of the skeletal system. The painful crises are believed to result from microvascular occlusions and associated hypoxic tissue injury. Ischemia of the central nervous system is manifested by headaches, convulsions, or hemiplegia. In the course of the disease virtually any organ may be damaged by such ischemic injury. The other form, *aplastic crisis,* represents a sudden but usually temporary cessation of bone marrow activity. Reticulocytes disappear from the blood and anemia worsens. Both types of crises may appear without any warning or be triggered by infections, to which these patients are very susceptible. The increased susceptibility to infections is probably multifactorial: (1) impaired spleen function—the erythrophagocytosis interferes with bacterial killing; (2) in later stages total splenic fibrosis removes an important biologic filter of blood-borne microorganisms; and (3) defects in the alternate complement pathway impair opsonization of encapsulated bacteria such as pneumococci. For reasons not entirely clear, patients with sickle cell disease are particularly predisposed to *Salmonella* osteomyelitis.

With the full-blown *sickle cell disease,* at least some sickled erythrocytes can be seen on an ordinary peripheral blood smear. Ultimately, the diagnosis depends on the electrophoretic demonstration of HbS. Prenatal diagnosis of sickle cell anemia can be performed by analyzing the DNA in fetal cells obtained by amniocentesis or biopsy of chorionic villi. The sickle mutation abolishes the recognition site for a restriction endonuclease enzyme, Mst II. When DNA extracted from fetal cells is digested with Mst II, the presence of the sickle mutation leads to the generation of DNA fragments of abnormal sizes. These can be detected by Southern blot analysis, as described in detail on page 112.

The clinical course of patients with sickle cell anemia is highly variable. As a result of improvements in supportive care, an increasing number of patients are surviving into adulthood and producing offspring. A variety of antisickling agents have been proposed, but none has stood the test of time. At present the therapeutic approach is largely symptomatic. *Sickle cell*

trait, in contrast, generally remains entirely asymptomatic unless the patient becomes extremely hypoxic.

THALASSEMIA

The thalassemias are a heterogeneous group of genetic disorders of hemoglobin synthesis characterized by a lack of or decreased synthesis of globin chains. In α-thalassemia, α-globin chain synthesis is reduced, whereas in β-thalassemia, β-globin chain synthesis is either absent (designated β^0-thalassemia) or markedly deficient (β^+-thalassemia). Unlike the hemoglobinopathies, which represent qualitative abnormalities, thalassemias result from quantitative abnormalities of globin chain synthesis. The consequences of reduced synthesis of one globin chain derive not only from the low level of intracellular hemoglobin but also from the relative excess of the other globin chain, as will be discussed later.

Thalassemia is inherited as an autosomal codominant condition. The heterozygous form (*thalassemia minor* or *thalassemia trait*) may be asymptomatic or mildly symptomatic. The homozygous form, *thalassemia major,* is associated with severe hemolytic anemia. The mutant genes are particularly common among Mediterranean, African, and Asian populations.

MOLECULAR PATHOGENESIS. A complex pattern of molecular defects underlying the thalassemias has emerged in recent years. To understand these, we must first review the structure and expression of normal globin genes. Here we will summarize only the salient features; more details are available in specialized texts. The adult hemoglobin, or HbA, contains two α-chains and two β-chains (coded by two β-globin genes located on each of the two chromosomes 11). In contrast, one pair of functional α-globin genes is located on each of the two chromosomes 16. With recombinant DNA techniques it has been possible to clone all the human globin genes, and their nucleotide sequences have been determined. The basic structure of the α- and β-globin genes as well as the steps involved in the biosynthesis of globin chains are similar. Each β-globin gene has three coding sequences, or *exons,* that are interrupted by two intervening sequences, or *introns.* Flanking the 5′ extremity of the globin gene are a series of untranslated *promoter sequences* that are required for the initiation of β-globin mRNA synthesis.

β-Thalassemia. As mentioned earlier, β-thalassemia syndromes can be classified into two categories: (1) β^0-*thalassemia,* associated with total absence of β-globin chains in the homozygous state, and (2) β^+-*thalassemia,* characterized by reduced (but detectable) β-globin synthesis in the homozygous state. Sequencing of cloned β-globin genes obtained from thalassemic patients has revealed more than 90 different mutations responsible for β^0- or β^+-thalassemia. Most of these result from single base changes. In contrast to α-thalassemias, described later, *gene deletions rarely underlie β-thalassemias.*

Details of these mutations and their effects on β-glo-

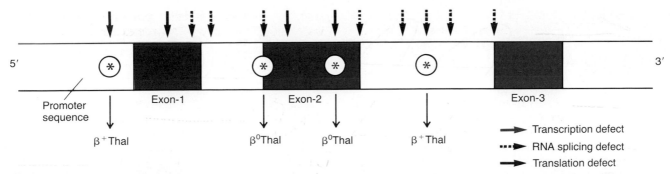

Figure 12–5. Diagrammatic representation of the β-globin gene and some sites where point mutations giving rise to β-thalassemia have been localized. (Modified from Wyngaarden, J. B., Smith, L. H. (eds.): Cecil Textbook of Medicine. 17th ed. Philadelphia, W. B. Saunders, 1985, p. 919).

bin synthesis are beyond our scope, but a few illustrative examples will be cited (Fig. 12–5).

- The promoter region controls the initiation and rate of transcription, and therefore mutations affecting promoter sequences usually lead to reduced globin gene transcription. Because some β-globin is synthesized, the patients develop β⁺-thalassemia.

- Mutations in the coding sequences are usually associated with more serious consequences. For example, in some cases a single nucleotide change in one of the exons leads to the formation of a termination or "stop" codon, which interrupts translation of β-globin mRNA. Premature termination generates nonfunctional fragments of the β-globin, leading to β⁰-thalassemia.

- *Mutations that lead to aberrant mRNA processing are the commonest cause of β-thalassemia.* Most of these affect introns but some have been located within exons. If the mutation alters the normal splice junctions, splicing does not occur and all of the mRNA formed is abnormal. Unspliced mRNA is degraded within the nucleus, and β⁰-thalassemia results. However, some mutations affect the introns at locations away from the normal intron-exon splice junction. These mutations create new sites that are sensitive to the action of splicing enzymes at abnormal locations—within an intron, for example. Because normal splice sites remain unaffected, both normal and abnormal splicing occur, giving rise to normal as well as abnormal β-globin mRNA. These patients develop β⁺-thalassemia.

Two factors contribute to the pathogenesis of anemia in β-thalassemia. Reduced synthesis of β-globin leads to inadequate HbA formation, so that the overall hemoglobin concentration per cell is lower and the cells appear hypochromic. Much more important is the hemolytic component of β-thalassemia. This is due not to lack of β-globin but to the relative excess of α-globin chains, whose synthesis remains normal. Free α-chains form insoluble aggregates that precipitate within the erythrocytes (Fig. 12–6). These inclusions damage the cell membranes, reduce their plasticity, and render the red cells susceptible to phagocytosis by the mononuclear phagocyte system. Not only are mature red cells susceptible to premature destruction but also a majority of the erythroblasts within the marrow are destroyed, owing to the presence of the inclusions. Such intramedullary destruction of red cells *("ineffective erythropoiesis")* has another untoward effect: it is associated with increased absorption of dietary iron, which contributes to the iron overload in these patients.

α-Thalassemia. The molecular basis of α-thalassemia is quite different from that of β-thalassemia. Most important, *most of the α-thalassemias are due to deletions of α-globin gene loci.* Since there are four functional α-globin genes, there are four possible degrees of α-thalassemia based on loss of one to four α-globin genes from the chromosomes. These cover a wide spectrum of clinical disorders, the severity of which is related to the number of deleted α-globin genes (Table 12–2). On one end, loss of a single α-globin gene is associated with a silent carrier state, whereas deletion of all four α-globin genes is associated with fetal death in utero, since the blood has virtually no oxygen-carrying capacity. The basis of the hemolysis is similar to that in β-thalassemia. With loss of three α-globin genes there is a relative excess of β-globin or other non-α-globin chains, which form insoluble tetramers within red cells and render the cells vulnerable to phagocytosis and destruction. It should be noted, however, that non-α-chains in general form more soluble and less toxic aggregates than do those derived from α-chains. Hence the hemolytic anemia and ineffective erythropoiesis tend be less severe in α-thalassemia.

MORPHOLOGY. Only the morphologic changes in β-thalassemia, which is more common in the United States, will be described. Typically, in thalassemia major the peripheral blood smear shows microcytic, hypochromic red cells. Some red cells have an abnormal distribution of hemoglobin, giving them a target-like appearance (target cells). In addition, there is severe poikilocytosis, anisocytosis, and reticulocytosis. Normoblasts are present in the peripheral blood.

In β-thalassemia major, the anatomic changes are those of all hemolytic anemias, but especially prominent

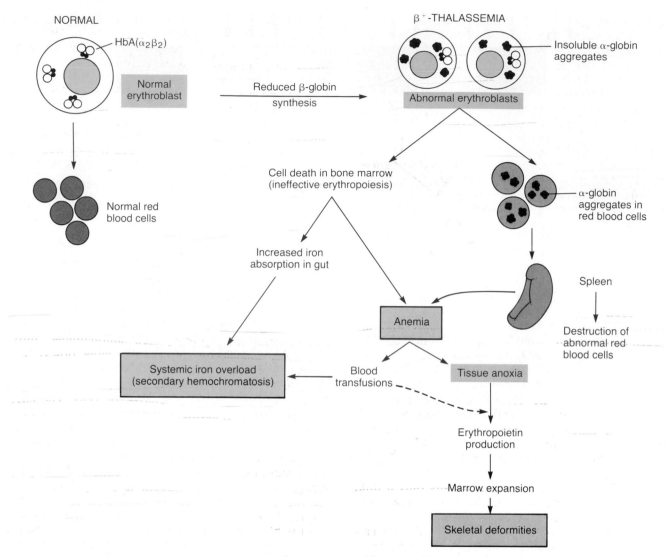

Figure 12–6. Pathogenesis of β-thalassemia major. Note that aggregates of excess α-globin are not visible on routine blood smears. Blood transfusions, on the one hand, correct the anemia and reduce stimulus for erythropoietin secretion and deformities induced by marrow expansion; on the other hand, they add to systemic iron overload.

TABLE 12–2. CLINICAL AND GENETIC CLASSIFICATION OF THALASSEMIAS

Clinical Nomenclature	Genotype	Disease	Molecular Genetics
β-Thalassemias			
Thalassemia major	Homozygous β⁰-thalassemia (β^0/β^0); Homozygous β⁺-thalassemia (β^+/β^+)	Severe, requires blood transfusions regularly	Rare gene deletions in β^0/β^0 Defects in transcription, processing, or translation of β-globin mRNA
Thalassemia minor	β^0/β β^+/β	Asymptomatic with mild anemia or none; red cell abnormalities seen	
α-Thalassemia			
Silent carrier	$-\alpha/\alpha\alpha$	Asymptomatic; no red cell abnormality	
α-Thalassemia trait	$--/\alpha\alpha$ (Asian); $-\alpha/-\alpha$ (black African)	Asymptomatic, like thalassemia minor	Gene deletions mainly
HbH disease	$--/-\alpha$	Severe anemia, tetramers of β-globin (HbH) formed in red cells	
Hydrops fetalis	$--/--$	Lethal in utero	

are hyperactivity of the bone marrow and splenomegaly. The marrow is expanded to the fetal level, so all the fatty marrow may be reactivated. In the red cell series there is a striking shift toward primitive forms. Massive erythropoiesis within the bone invades the bony cortex, impairs bone growth, and produces skeletal deformities. Splenomegaly and hepatomegaly result from marked extramedullary hematopoiesis as well as RE cell hyperplasia. Over the span of years, excessive breakdown of red cells and ineffective erythropoiesis result in severe hemosiderosis, and, rarely, a form of hemochromatosis (p. 554). The iron overload is due in part to excessive dietary iron absorption that is associated with ineffective erythropoiesis and to the repeated blood transfusions these patients need to survive (see Fig. 12–6).

CLINICAL COURSE. Thalassemia major manifests itself as soon as HbF is normally replaced by HbA. Affected children fail to develop normally and are retarded almost from birth. They are sustained only by repeated blood transfusions, which not only improve the anemia but also reduce the skeletal deformities associated with excessive erythropoiesis. With transfusions, survival into the second or third decade is possible, but gradually systemic iron overload develops. Cardiac failure resulting from secondary hemochromatosis is an important cause of death in those who reach adolescence. The average age at death is 17 years.

With thalassemia minor there is usually only a mild microcytic hypochromic anemia, and in general these patients have a normal life expectancy. Since iron deficiency anemia is associated with a similar appearance of red cells, it should be excluded by appropriate laboratory tests, described later in this chapter. The diagnosis of β-thalassemia minor is made by hemoglobin electrophoresis. In addition to reduced amounts of HbA ($\alpha_2\beta_2$), the level of HbA$_2$ ($\alpha_2\delta_2$) is increased. The diagnosis of β-thalassemia major can generally be made on clinical grounds. Hemoglobin electrophoresis shows profound reduction or absence of HbA and increased levels of HbF. The HbA$_2$ level may be normal or increased. Prenatal diagnosis of both forms of thalassemia can be made by DNA probe analysis.

GLUCOSE-6-PHOSPHATE DEHYDROGENASE DEFICIENCY

The erythrocyte and its membrane are vulnerable to injury by endogenous and exogenous oxidants. Normally, intracellular reduced glutathione (GSH) inactivates such oxidants. *Abnormalities of enzymes that participate in the hexose monophosphate shunt or glutathione metabolism reduce the ability of red cells to protect themselves from oxidative injury and lead to hemolytic anemias.* The prototype and most prevalent

of these anemias is caused by a deficiency of glucose-6-phosphate dehydrogenase (G6PD). The G6PD gene is located on the X chromosome, and there is considerable polymorphism at this locus. More than 250 G6PD genetic variants, most of which are not associated with disease, have been identified. In the United States, the G6PD A⁻ variant is associated with hemolytic anemia. It is encountered primarily in blacks. Approximately 10% of the black males in the United States are affected. To explain such a high frequency of a deleterious gene, it has been suggested that some G6PD variants, like HbS, confer protection against malaria. The molecular basis of the defect in the A⁻ type deficiency is not entirely clear. A normal amount of enzyme is synthesized in the red cell precursors, but it decays more rapidly than normal during the life span of the red cells, so older red cells become progressively more deficient in enzyme activity and are most vulnerable to oxidant stress.

This disorder produces no symptoms unless the red cells are subjected to oxidant injury by exposure to certain drugs or toxins. The drugs incriminated include antimalarials (e.g., primaquine), sulfonamides, nitrofurantoin, phenacetin, aspirin (in large doses), and vitamin K derivatives. *Even more important are infections that presumably trigger hemolysis owing to release of free radicals from phagocytic cells.* The effect of these offending agents is to cause oxidation of GSH to glutathione through the production of hydrogen peroxide. Because regeneration of GSH is impaired in G6PD-deficient cells, hydrogen peroxide accumulates and denatures globin chains by oxidation of sulfhydryl groups. Denatured hemoglobin is precipitated within the red cells in the form of inclusions called *Heinz bodies.* Not only are inclusion-bearing red cells less deformable, their cell membranes are further damaged when splenic phagocytes attempt to "pluck" out the inclusions. All these changes predispose the red cells to becoming trapped in the splenic sinuses and destroyed by the phagocytes.

The drug-induced hemolysis is acute and of variable clinical severity. Typically, the patients develop evidence of intravascular hemolysis after a lag period of two or three days. Since the G6PD gene is located on the X chromosome, all the erythrocytes of affected males are deficient in enzyme activity. However, owing to random inactivation of one X chromosome in women (p. 109), heterozygous females have two distinct populations of red cells, some normal, others deficient in G6PD activity. Indeed, females heterozygous for G6PD enzymes have two populations of all somatic cells. Thus affected males are more vulnerable to oxidant injury whereas most carrier females are asymptomatic. Only when heterozygous females have a very large proportion of deficient red cells ("unfavorable lyonization") are they susceptible to induced hemolysis. Because the enzyme deficiency is most marked in older red cells, they are more susceptible to lysis. As the marrow compensates by producing new (young) red cells, hemolysis tends to abate even if drug exposure continues.

PAROXYSMAL NOCTURNAL HEMOGLOBINURIA ___

This rare disorder of unknown etiology is mentioned here because it is the *only form of hemolytic anemia that results from an acquired membrane defect secondary to a mutational event of unknown cause that affects myeloid stem cells*. Proliferation of the abnormal clone of myeloid stem cells yields red cells, granulocytes, and platelets that are inordinately sensitive to the lytic activity of complement. The affected cells are deficient in a membrane glycoprotein called decay-accelerating factor (DAF), which limits the spontaneous activation in vivo of the alternate complement pathway. These patients have intravascular hemolysis and a striking predisposition to infections and intravascular thromboses. Because paroxysmal nocturnal hemoglobinuria (PNH) is an acquired disorder of stem cells, it sometimes transforms into other stem cell disorders such as acute leukemia and aplastic anemia.

IMMUNOHEMOLYTIC ANEMIAS ___

In these uncommon disorders the hemolytic anemia is caused by antibodies reactive against normal or altered red cell membranes. Anti–red cell antibodies may arise spontaneously in *autoimmune hemolytic anemias,* or their formation may be initiated by exogenous agents such as drugs or chemicals. *Immunohemolytic anemias* are classified on the basis of the nature of the antibody involved and possible associated predisposing conditions, which are presented in simplified form in Table 12–3.

Whatever the cause of antibody formation, the diagnosis of immunohemolytic anemias depends on the demonstration of anti–red cell antibodies. *The method most commonly used to detect such antibodies is the Coombs' antiglobulin test, which is based upon the capacity of antihuman antibodies (prepared in animals) to agglutinate red cells.* A positive result indicates that the patient's red cells are coated with human antibodies that can react with the antihuman globulin serum. This is called the *direct Coombs' test.* The *indirect Coombs' test* is used to detect antibodies in the patient's serum and involves incubating normal red cells with the patient's serum, followed by a direct Coombs' test on these incubated red cells.

TABLE 12–3. CLASSIFICATION OF IMMUNOHEMOLYTIC ANEMIAS

Warm Antibody Type
   Primary (idiopathic)
   Secondary: Lymphomas and leukemias (CLL and non-Hodgkin's lymphomas)
          SLE
          Drugs (e.g., α-methyldopa, penicillin, quinidine)
Cold Antibody Type
   Acute: Mycoplasma infection, infectious mononucleosis
   Chronic: Idiopathic
          Associated with lymphomas

WARM ANTIBODY IMMUNOHEMOLYTIC ANEMIAS. These are characterized by the presence of immunoglobulin G (IgG) (rarely IgA) antibodies, which are active at 37° C. A great majority of cases (more than 60%) are idiopathic (primary) and so belong to the category of autoimmune diseases. Approximately one fourth of the cases are so-called secondary because there is an underlying disease (such as systemic lupus erythematosus) affecting the immune system or the anemia is induced by drugs. The pathogenesis of hemolysis in most instances involves opsonization of the red cells by the IgG antibodies and subsequent phagocytosis by splenic macrophages. Spheroidal cells resembling those found in hereditary spherocytosis are often found in idiopathic immune hemolytic anemia. Presumably, bits of cell membrane are injured and removed during attempted phagocytosis of antibody-coated cells; this reduces surface area and induces spheroidal conformation. The spherocytes are then sequestered and destroyed in the spleen, as we described earlier (p. 335). The clinical severity of immunohemolytic anemia is quite variable. Most patients have chronic mild anemia with moderate splenomegaly and often require no treatment.

The mechanisms of hemolysis induced by drugs are varied and in some cases poorly understood:

- Drugs such as α-methyldopa induce an anemia indistinguishable from the primary idiopathic form of hemolytic anemia. Autoantibodies directed against intrinsic red cell antigens, in particular Rh blood group antigens, are formed. How α-methyldopa induces autoantibody formation is not clear.
- Drugs such as penicillin are believed to act as haptens. They bind to the red cell membrane, evoking the formation of antidrug antibodies. These antibodies attach to the cell-bound penicillin and predispose the cells to phagocytic destruction, as outlined previously.
- Drugs such as quinidine bind to plasma proteins and evoke an antibody response. Immune complexes composed of protein-bound drug and antibody molecules then become deposited on the red cell membranes and damage the erythrocytes as "innocent bystanders."

COLD ANTIBODY IMMUNOHEMOLYTIC ANEMIAS. These anemias are characterized by the presence of IgM antibodies, which have enhanced activity at temperatures below 30° C. The hemolytic process occurs because of fixation of complement on IgM-coated red cells. This interaction occurs best in the distal body parts, where the temperature may drop below 30° C. Once the red cells are coated with antibody and complement, they are removed from the circulation by the mononuclear phagocytic cells, particularly Kupffer cells. Cold agglutinins occur acutely during recovery from mycoplasma pneumonia and infectious mononucleosis. The resulting anemia is mild, transient, and of no clinical import. Chronic cold agglutinin formation and associated hemolytic anemia may also occur in association with lymphoproliferative disorders or as an idiopathic condition. In addition to anemia, Raynaud's phenomenon may occur in these patients owing to agglutination of red cells in the capillaries of exposed parts of the body.

ERYTHROBLASTOSIS FETALIS (HEMOLYTIC DISEASE OF THE NEWBORN) _____

Erythroblastosis fetalis may be defined as an antibody-induced hemolytic disease in the newborn that is caused by blood group incompatibility between mother and fetus. Obviously, such an incompatibility can occur only when the fetus inherits red cell antigenic determinants from the father that are foreign to the mother. Important in this respect are the ABO and Rh blood group antigens. Although the incidence of hemolytic disease due to Rh incompatibility has declined remarkably in recent years, it is necessary to discuss Rh hemolytic disease since successful prophylaxis of this disorder has resulted chiefly from an understanding of its pathogenesis.

ETIOLOGY AND PATHOGENESIS. The underlying basis of erythroblastosis fetalis is the immunization of the mother by blood group antigens on fetal red cells and the free passage of antibodies from mother through the placenta to the fetus. Fetal red cells may reach the maternal circulation during the last trimester of pregnancy, when the cytotrophoblast is no longer present as a barrier, or during childbirth itself. The mother thus becomes sensitized to the foreign antigen.

Of the numerous antigens included in the Rh system, only the D antigen is the major cause of Rh incompatibility. Several factors influence the immune response to Rh-positive fetal red cells that reach the maternal circulation.

- *Concurrent ABO incompatibility protects the mother against Rh immunization* because the fetal red cells are promptly coated by isohemagglutinins and removed from the maternal circulation.
- The antibody response depends on the *dose of immunizing antigen,* hence hemolytic disease develops only when the mother has experienced a significant transplacental bleed (more than 1 ml Rh-positive red cells).
- The *isotype of the antibody* is important because IgG (but not IgM) antibodies can cross the placenta. The initial exposure to Rh antigen evokes the formation of IgM antibodies, so Rh disease is very uncommon with the first pregnancy. Subsequent exposure during the second or third pregnancy generally leads to a brisk IgG antibody response.

Appreciation of the role of *prior sensitization* in the pathogenesis of Rh erythroblastosis has led to its remarkable control in recent years. Currently, Rh-negative mothers are administered anti-D globulin soon after the delivery of an Rh-positive baby. The anti-D antibodies mask the antigenic sites on the fetal red cells that may have leaked into the maternal circulation during childbirth, thus preventing long-lasting sensitization to Rh antigens.

Owing to the remarkable success achieved in prevention of Rh hemolytic disease, fetomaternal ABO incompatibility is currently the most common hemolytic disease of newborns. *Although ABO incompatibility occurs in approximately 20 to 25% of pregnancies, only a small fraction of infants subsequently born develop hemolytic disease, and in general the disease is much milder than Rh hemolytic disease.* It occurs almost exclusively in infants of group A or B who are born of group O mothers. The normal anti-A and anti-B isohemagglutinins in group O mothers are usually of the IgM type and so do not cross the placenta. However, for reasons not well understood, certain group O women possess IgG antibodies directed against group A or B antigens (or both) even without prior sensitization. Therefore, the first-born may be affected. Fortunately, even with transplacentally acquired antibodies, lysis of the infant's red cells is minimal. Two factors seem to be responsible for this happy circumstance: neonatal red cells express group A and B antigens poorly, and the widespread presence of these antigens on other tissue cells serves to "soak up" some of the transferred antibodies. There is no effective method of preventing hemolytic disease resulting from ABO incompatibility.

MORPHOLOGY. The anatomic findings in erythroblastosis fetalis vary with the severity of the hemolytic process. Infants may be stillborn, die within the first few days, or recover completely. In its mildest form, the anemia may be only slight and the child may survive without further complication. More severe hemolysis gives rise to jaundice and other features associated with hemolytic anemias (p. 334). Hypoxic injury to the heart and liver may lead to circulatory and hepatic failure with resultant generalized edema. This pattern is known as **hydrops fetalis.** In most cases the liver and spleen are enlarged, the degree depending on the severity of the hemolytic process and the compensatory extramedullary erythropoiesis. In all forms, the bone marrow is hyperactive and extramedullary hematopoiesis is present in the liver, spleen, and possibly other tissues such as the kidneys, lungs, and even the heart. The increased hematopoietic activity accounts for the presence in the peripheral circulation of large numbers of immature red cells, including reticulocytes, normoblasts, and erythroblasts (hence the name erythroblastosis fetalis).

When hyperbilirubinemia is marked (usually above 20 mg/dl in full-term infants, often less in premature babies), the central nervous system may be damaged **(kernicterus).** The circulating unconjugated bilirubin is taken up by the brain tissue, on which it apparently exerts a toxic effect. The brain becomes enlarged and edematous and, when sectioned, has a bright yellow pigmentation of the basal ganglia, thalamus, cerebellum, cerebral gray matter, and spinal cord. This pigmentation is evanescent and fades within 24 hours despite prompt fixation. It is interesting that adults are protected from this effect of hyperbilirubinemia by the blood-brain barrier.

CLINICAL COURSE. The clinical patterns of erythroblastosis fetalis vary from fetal hydrops fetalis to extremely mild degrees of anemia in otherwise healthy children. Kernicterus may manifest itself by apathy and poor feeding, and later by mental retardation, cerebral irritability, extrapyramidal signs, and cranial nerve palsies.

Because severe erythroblastosis fetalis can be treated, early recognition of the disorder is imperative. That which results from Rh incompatibility may be more or less accurately predicted, since it correlates well with rapidly rising Rh antibody titers in the mother during pregnancy. Amniotic fluid obtained by amniocentesis may show high levels of bilirubin. As might be expected, the result of a direct Coombs' test is positive on fetal cord blood if the red cells have been coated by maternal antibody. Exchange transfusion of the infants is an effective form of therapy. Postnatally, phototherapy is helpful since visible light converts bilirubin to readily excreted dipyrroles. As already discussed, administration of anti-D globulins to the mother can prevent the occurrence of Rh erythroblastosis.

Group ABO erythroblastosis fetalis is more difficult to predict, but it is readily monitored by awareness of the blood incompatibility between mother and father and by hemoglobin and bilirubin determinations on the vulnerable newborn infant.

HEMOLYTIC ANEMIAS RESULTING FROM MECHANICAL TRAUMA TO RED CELLS _____

Red blood cells may be disrupted by physical trauma in a variety of circumstances. *Clinically important are the hemolytic anemias associated with cardiac valve prostheses and with narrowing or obstruction of the vasculature.* Traumatic hemolytic anemia is more severe with artificial valves than with porcine valves. In the case of prosthetic valves, the red cells are damaged by the shear stresses resulting from the turbulent blood flow and abnormal pressure gradients caused by the mechanical valves. Because pressure gradients across aortic valves are greater, cardiac hemolysis is more frequently encountered after replacement of the aortic valve than replacement of the mitral valve. *Microangiopathic hemolytic anemia*, on the other hand, is characterized by mechanical damage to the red cells as they squeeze through abnormally narrowed vessels. Most often the narrowing is caused by widespread deposition of fibrin in the small vessels, in association with disseminated intravascular coagulation (p. 378). Other causes of microangiopathic hemolytic anemia include malignant hypertension, systemic lupus erythematosus, thrombotic thrombocytopenic purpura (TTP), hemolytic uremic syndrome, and disseminated cancer. Most of these disorders are discussed elsewhere in this book. It suffices to say that common to all these disorders is the presence of vascular lesions that predispose the circulating red cells to mechanical injury. The morphologic alterations in the injured red blood cells may be striking. Thus "burr cells," "helmet cells," and "triangle cells" may be seen in the peripheral blood film. It should be pointed out that, except for TTP and the related hemolytic uremic syndrome,

the extent of hemolysis is not a major clinical problem in most instances.

MALARIA _____

It has been estimated that 200 million persons suffer from this infectious disease; it is one of the most widespread afflictions of mankind. Malaria is endemic in Asia and Africa, but with widespread jet travel cases are now reported from all over the world. The fact that the eradication of malaria is theoretically feasible makes its prevalence even more unfortunate. Malaria is caused by one of four types of protozoa. *Plasmodium vivax* causes benign tertian malaria. *Plasmodium malariae* causes quartan malaria, another benign form; *Plasmodium ovale* causes ovale malaria, a relatively uncommon and benign form similar to vivax malaria; and *P. falciparum* causes malignant tertian malaria (falciparum malaria), which has a high fatality rate. All forms are transmitted only by the bite of female *Anopheles* mosquitoes, and humans are the only natural reservoir.

ETIOLOGY AND PATHOGENESIS. The life cycle of the plasmodia is a well understood but complex process, which may require review.

Briefly, it consists of two phases: (1) asexual reproduction, or schizogony, which occurs in humans, and (2) sexual reproduction, or sporogony, which occurs in the mosquito. When the sporozoites are introduced into human blood by the mosquito, they circulate only briefly then invade the liver cells (exoerythrocytic cycle). This represents the incubation period of malaria. For P. vivax and P. ovale, it is about 14 days; for P. malariae, 24 days; and for P. falciparum, 8 to 20 days. Within the liver, the parasites develop into schizonts, which rupture the liver cells and yield free merozoites that in turn enter red cells. During the erythrocytic cycle, further development of the parasites occurs, yielding trophozoites, which are somewhat distinctive for each of the four forms of malaria. Thus, the specific form of malaria can be recognized in appropriately stained thick smears of the peripheral blood. For details on such parasitology, reference should be made to specialized texts. When the trophozoites are fully grown within the red cells, they divide into merozoites, which rupture the erythrocytes and may then enter other red cells, where they develop into gametocytes that infect the next hungry mosquito.

The distinctive clinical and anatomic features of malaria are related to the following events: (1) Showers of new merozoites are released from the red cells at intervals of approximately 48 hours for *P. vivax, P. ovale* and *P. falciparum,* and 72 hours for *P. malariae.* The clinical spikes of fever and chills coincide with this release. (2) The parasites destroy large numbers of red cells and thus cause hemolytic anemia. (3) A characteristic brown malarial pigment, probably a derivative of hemoglobin that is identical to hematin, is released from the ruptured red cells along with the merozoites, discoloring principally the spleen but also the liver, lymph nodes, and bone marrow. (4) Activation of the phagocytic defense mechanisms of the host leads to marked hyperplasia of the mononuclear phagocyte system throughout the body, reflected in massive splenomegaly. Less frequently the liver may also be enlarged.

CLINICAL COURSE. Benign malaria is characterized by recurrent paroxysms of shaking chills, high fever, and drenching sweats, correlated with the release of merozoites from the ruptured red cells. Occasionally jaundice is evident. There is progressive hepatosplenomegaly, particularly in those long-standing, smoldering cases associated with partial immunity. In the usual course of events, spontaneous recovery ensues or the patient benefits dramatically from antimalarial drugs.

Fatal falciparum malaria is characterized by prominent involvement of the brain. Cerebral blood vessels are full of parasitized red cells and are often occluded by microthrombi. The disease may begin suddenly or slowly, but it is rapidly progressive, with the development of high fever, chills, convulsions, shock, and death, usually within days to weeks. In other cases, falciparum malaria may pursue a more chronic course but may be punctuated at any time by a dramatic complication known as *blackwater fever*. This uncommon syndrome is characterized by the sudden onset of severe chills, fever, jaundice, vomiting, and the passage of dark red to black urine. The trigger for this complication is obscure, but it is associated with massive hemolysis, leading to jaundice, hemoglobinemia, and hemoglobinuria. With appropriate chemotherapy, the prognosis with most forms of malaria is good; however, treatment of falciparum malaria is much more difficult owing to the emergence of drug-resistant strains. Because of the potentially serious consequences of this disease, early diagnosis and treatment are particularly important but are sometimes delayed in non-endemic settings.

ANEMIAS OF DIMINISHED ERYTHROPOIESIS

In this category are included anemias that are caused by an inadequate supply to the bone marrow of some substance necessary for hematopoiesis. The most common deficiencies are those of iron, folic acid, or vitamin B$_{12}$. Infrequently, there is a *pyridoxine-responsive anemia* or a *thiamine-dependent anemia*. Another important cause of impaired erythropoiesis is suppression of marrow stem cells, exemplified by aplastic anemia and myelophthisic anemia. In the following section some common examples of anemias resulting from nutritional deficiencies and marrow suppression are discussed individually.

IRON DEFICIENCY ANEMIA

It is estimated that 10% of the population in developed countries and as many as 25 to 50% in develop-ing countries are anemic. Iron deficiency accounts for most of this prevalence. *It is without question the commonest form of nutritional deficiency.* The factors responsible for iron deficiency differ somewhat in various populations and can be best considered in the context of normal iron metabolism.

Total body iron content is in the range of 2 gm for women and 6 gm for men. Approximately 80% of functional body iron is found in hemoglobin; the remainder of this pool represents myoglobin and iron-containing enzymes (e.g., catalase and cytochromes). The iron storage pool, represented by hemosiderin and ferritin-bound iron, contains approximately 15 to 20% of total body iron. Stored iron is found in all tissues but particularly in liver, spleen, bone marrow, and skeletal muscle. Because serum ferritin is largely derived from the storage pool of iron, its level is a good indicator of the adequacy of body iron stores. Staining bone marrow for iron-containing histiocytes is another useful and simple method for estimating body iron content. Iron is transported in the plasma by an iron-binding protein called transferrin. In normal persons transferrin is about 33% saturated with iron, yielding serum iron levels that average 120 μg/dl in men and 100 μg/dl in women. Thus the total iron-binding capacity of serum is in the range of 300 to 350 μg.

Body iron losses are extremely and rigidly limited, ranging from 1 to 2 mg per day lost by shedding of mucosal and skin epithelial cells. Iron balance therefore is maintained largely by regulating the absorption of dietary iron. The normal daily Western diet contains approximately 10 to 20 mg of iron, most of which is in the form of heme contained in animal products. The remainder is inorganic iron in vegetables. About 20% of heme iron (in contrast to 1 to 2% of nonheme iron) is absorbable, so the average Western diet contains sufficient iron to balance fixed daily losses. The duodenum is the primary site of absorption, where dietary heme iron enters the mucosal cells directly. In contrast, nonheme iron is transported into the cell by mucosal transferrin. A fraction of the absorbed iron is rapidly delivered to plasma transferrin. The remainder is bound to mucosal ferritin, some to be transferred more slowly to plasma transferrin and some to be lost with exfoliation of mucosal cells. When the body is replete with iron, most of the iron that enters the duodenal epithelium is bound to ferritin and lost with exfoliation; *in iron deficiency, or when there is increased effective or ineffective erythropoiesis, transfer to plasma transferrin is enhanced.*

Negative iron balance and consequent anemia may result from low dietary intake, malabsorption, excessive demand, and chronic blood loss.

- *Low dietary intake alone is rarely the cause of iron deficiency in the United States* because the average daily dietary intake of 10 to 20 mg is more than enough for males and about adequate for females. In other parts of the world, however, low intake and poor bioavailability from predominantly vegetarian diets is an important cause of iron deficiency.

- *Malabsorption* may occur with sprue and celiac disease or following gastrectomy (p. 507).

• *Increased demands* not met by normal dietary intake may occur around the world in pregnancy and infancy.
• *Chronic blood loss is the most important cause of iron deficiency anemia in the western world;* this loss may occur from the gastrointestinal tract (e.g., peptic ulcers, colonic cancer, hemorrhoids, hookworm disease) or the female genital tract (e.g., menorrhagia, metrorrhagia, cancers).

Regardless of the cause, the development of the deficient state occurs insidiously. At first there is depletion of the stored iron, which is marked by a decline in serum ferritin and depletion of stainable iron in the bone marrow. There follows a decrease in circulating iron, with a low level of serum iron and a rise in the serum transferrin iron-binding capacity. Ultimately, the inadequacy makes its impact on the hemoglobin, myoglobin, and other iron compounds. With more significant deficits, impaired work performance and brain function and reduced immunocompetence may develop.

MORPHOLOGY. Except in unusual circumstances, iron deficiency anemia is relatively mild. The red cells are microcytic and hypochromic, reflecting the reduced mean corpuscular volume (MCV) and mean corpuscular hemoglobin concentration (MCHC). Although there is normoblastic hyperplasia, it is limited by the availability of iron, and hence active marrow is usually only slightly increased in volume. Extramedullary hematopoiesis is uncommon.

The skin and mucous membranes of these patients are pale, and the nails may become spoon-shaped and have longitudinal ridges. In some cases, atrophic glossitis is present, giving the tongue a smooth, glazed appearance. When this is accompanied by dysphagia and esophageal webs, it constitutes the **Plummer-Vinson syndrome** (see p. 479).

CLINICAL COURSE. In most instances, iron deficiency anemia is asymptomatic. Nonspecific indications, such as weakness, listlessness, and pallor, may be present in severe cases. Rarely, in the United States and more often in Scandinavia and Great Britain, the *Plummer-Vinson syndrome* occurs. With long-standing severe anemia, thinning, flattening, and eventually "spooning" of the fingernails sometimes appears.

Diagnostic criteria include low hemoglobin concentration, low hematocrit, low mean corpuscular volume, hypochromic microcytic red cells, low serum ferritin, low serum iron levels, low transferrin saturation, increased total iron-binding capacity, and, ultimately, response to iron therapy. *Persons frequently die with this form of anemia, but rarely of it.* It is well to remember that in reasonably adequately nourished persons microcytic hypochromic anemia is not a disease but rather a symptom of some underlying disorder.

ANEMIA OF CHRONIC DISEASE

This common but poorly understood form of anemia is discussed here because it is associated with a defect in iron utilization and may therefore mimic anemia of iron deficiency. It occurs in a variety of chronic illnesses that include:
• Chronic microbial infections such as osteomyelitis, bacterial endocarditis, and lung abscess
• Chronic immune disorders such as rheumatoid arthritis and regional enteritis
• Neoplasms such as Hodgkin's disease and carcinomas of the lung and breast.
The common features that characterize anemia in these diverse clinical settings are *low serum iron and reduced total iron-binding capacity in association with abundant stored iron in the mononuclear phagocytic cells.* This combination suggests that there is a defect in the reutilization of iron due to some impediment in the transfer of iron from the storage pool to the erythroid precursors. In addition, defects in erythropoietin production and shortened red cell survival have also been documented. The red blood cells may be normocytic and normochromic or may be hypochromic and microcytic as in anemia of iron deficiency. *The presence of increased storage iron in the marrow macrophages, a high serum ferritin level, and reduced total iron-binding capacity readily rule out iron deficiency as the cause of anemia.* Treatment of the underlying condition corrects the anemia.

MEGALOBLASTIC ANEMIAS

There are two principal types of megaloblastic anemia, one caused by a folate deficiency and the other by a lack of vitamin B_{12}. The megaloblastic anemias may be caused by a nutritional deficiency of folic acid (folate) or, in many cases, the deficiency reflects impaired absorption, as is the case with vitamin B_{12} (p. 347). Both have in common enlargement of proliferating cells, in particular erythroid precursors that create megaloblasts and correspondingly abnormally large red cells (macrocytes). Other proliferating cells such as granulocyte precursors are enlarged (giant metamyelocytes), yielding enlarged *hypersegmented neutrophils.* Underlying the cellular gigantism, paradoxically, is impairment of DNA synthesis, so that proliferating cells laboriously synthesize DNA and enlarge their nuclei but the ultimate mitotic division is delayed. However, synthesis of RNA and cytoplasmic elements proceeds at a normal pace. The nuclei are thus immature, whereas the cytoplasm is fully mature, a situation referred to as *nuclear-cytoplasmic asynchrony.* Because of these maturational derangements there is an accumulation of megaloblasts in the bone marrow, yielding too few erythrocytes, hence the anemia. Two concomitant processes further aggravate the anemia: (1) ineffective erythropoiesis (a predisposition of megaloblasts to undergo autohemolysis), and (2) increased hemolytic destruction of the abnormally large red cells. This increased breakdown of red cells and precursors leads to iron accumulation, mostly in the mononuclear phagocytic cells of the bone marrow. Increased intramedullary destruction may also affect granulocyte and platelet precursors, giving rise to pancytopenia.

Folate (Folic Acid) Deficiency Anemia

Megaloblastic anemia secondary to a lack of folate is not common, but precarious folate levels in the body are surprisingly common among economically deprived persons of all countries who live on marginal diets; among pregnant women, whose dietary inadequacies combine with increased metabolic requirements; and among alcoholics and drug addicts, whose diet is typically grossly inadequate. Although reserves of this nutrient are relatively modest in the body, a negative balance does not become evident for months unless there is an increased demand, as occurs during rapid growth, pregnancy, or chronic disease. Ironically, folate is widely prevalent in nearly all raw foods, but it is readily destroyed by 10 to 15 minutes' cooking. Thus the best sources of folate in the diet are fresh or fresh-frozen vegetables and fruits eaten either uncooked or lightly cooked. Food folates are predominantly in the polyglutamate form, and most must be split into monoglutamates for absorption. Acidic foods and conjugase inhibitors found in beans and other legumes hamper absorption by inhibiting intestinal conjugases that catalyze the formation of monoglutamates from polyglutamates. Dilantin and a few other drugs also inhibit folate absorption. Others, such as methotrexate, inhibit folate metabolism (see below). The principal site of intestinal absorption is the upper third of the small intestine, so malabsorptive disorders such as celiac disease and tropical sprue, which affect this level of the gut, impair absorption.

The metabolism and physiologic functions of folic acid after absorption are complex. It suffices for our purposes that after absorption, folic acid is transported in the blood mainly as a monoglutamate. Within cells it undergoes conversion to several derivatives, but of principal importance is that it must be reduced to tetrahydrofolate (THF) by a reductase. (This reductase is sensitive to inhibition by folate analogs such as methotrexate, which deprives cells of folate and the capacity to rapidly divide—a property that is the basis for the use of folic acid antagonists as antineoplastic agents.) The primary function of THF is as an acceptor and donor of one-carbon units in a variety of steps involved in DNA synthesis. Several one-carbon transfers are critical to the synthesis of purines, thymidylate, and therefore thymine. Thus it should be apparent why a deficiency of folate causes the slow DNA synthesis that accounts for megaloblastic anemia.

MORPHOLOGY. The principal anatomic changes are seen in the bone marrow and blood; secondary alterations are referable to the anemia in severe cases. The bone marrow is markedly hypercellular owing to increased numbers of megaloblasts (i.e., abnormal erythroblasts). These cells are larger than normoblasts and have a delicate, finely reticulated nuclear chromatin (suggestive of nuclear immaturity) and an abundant, strikingly basophilic cytoplasm. As the megaloblasts differentiate and begin to acquire hemoglobin, the nucleus retains its finely distributed chromatin and fails to undergo the chromatin clumping typical of an orthochromatic normoblast. Similarly, the granulocytic precursors also demonstrate nuclear-cytoplasmic asynchrony, yielding giant metamyelocytes. Megakaryocytes, too, may be abnormally large, with bizarre multilobed nuclei.

In the peripheral blood, the earliest change is usually the appearance of hypersegmented granulocytes. These appear even before the onset of anemia. Although the normal number of lobes in a granulocyte nucleus is two or three, with megaloblastic anemias it may be markedly increased, to five or six. Erythrocytes are typically large and oval (macroovalocytes) with mean corpuscular volumes over 100 μ^3 (normal 82 to 92 μ^3). Large, misshapen platelets may also be seen. Although macrocytes appear hyperchromic because of their large size, in reality the MCHC is normal. Morphologic changes in other systems, especially the gastrointestinal tract, may also occur, giving rise to some of the clinical features discussed next.

CLINICAL COURSE. Typically, patients with folate deficiency anemia are rather sick and present a complex clinical picture, since the malnutrition that is responsible for folic acid deficiency produces other deficiencies as well. In most cases, a clearly inadequate diet is discovered by history, and the patient may appear obviously malnourished. The onset of the anemia is insidious and is associated with nonspecific symptoms such as weakness and easy fatigability. Since the gastrointestinal tract, like the hematopoietic system, is a site of rapid cell turnover, symptoms referable to the alimentary tract are common and often severe. These include sore tongue and cheilosis. *It should be stressed that in contrast to vitamin B$_{12}$ deficiency, neurologic abnormalities do not occur.*

The diagnosis of a megaloblastic anemia is readily made from examination of a smear of peripheral blood and the bone marrow. The important differentiation between the anemia of folate deficiency and that of vitamin B$_{12}$ deficiency is best accomplished by assays for serum folate and vitamin B$_{12}$ and red cell folate levels.

Vitamin B$_{12}$ (Cobalamin) Deficiency Anemia — Pernicious Anemia

Inadequate levels of vitamin B$_{12}$, or cobalamin, in the body result in a megaloblastic macrocytic anemia similar hematologically to that of folate deficiency. However, a deficiency of vitamin B$_{12}$ causes at the same time a demyelinating disorder involving the peripheral nerves and, ultimately and most important, the spinal cord. Thus, unlike the megaloblastic anemia of folate deficiency, that of B_{12} deficiency, when sufficiently prolonged and severe, is marked by neurologic dysfunction (hence the designation "combined systems disease"). The term "pernicious anemia" (PA) is a relic of the days when the pathogenesis and therapy of the condition were unknown. Today we appreciate that there are many potential causes for a B_{12} deficiency state, including inadequate diet, increased requirement, and impaired absorption. *Only the vitamin B_{12} deficiency resulting from inadequate gastric production or defective function of intrinsic factor (IF) necessary to absorb B_{12} constitutes pernicious anemia.* Intrinsic factor (IF) plays a critical role in the absorption of vitamin B_{12}, as will be evident from the following sequence of events involved in B_{12} absorption.

- Peptic digestion releases dietary vitamin B_{12}, which is then bound to salivary and gastric B_{12}-binding proteins called R binders.
- R-B_{12} complexes, transported to the duodenum, are split by pancreatic proteases, and the released B_{12} attaches to IF secreted by the parietal cells of the gastric fundic mucosa.
- The IF-B_{12} complex passes to the distal ileum, where it attaches to the epithelial IF receptors, followed by absorption of vitamin B_{12}.
- The absorbed B_{12} is bound to a transport protein, transcobalamin I, which then delivers it to the liver and other cells of the body.

PATHOGENESIS. Among the many potential causes of cobalamin deficiency, malabsorption is the most common and important. A dietary deficiency of cobalamin is virtually limited to strict vegetarians. This nutrient is abundant in all animal foods, including eggs and dairy products. Indeed, bacterial contamination of nonanimal foods and water may provide adequate amounts of B_{12}; it is stored in the liver and efficiently reabsorbed from the bile, so it would require 20 to 30 years to deplete the normal reserves. Moreover, it is resistant to cooking and boiling. A tiny daily supply, therefore, suffices. *Thus, a dietary lack of B_{12} is uncommon; until proven otherwise, a deficiency of this nutrient implies PA secondary to inadequate production or function of IF.* The deranged synthesis of IF appears to be caused by an autoimmune reaction against parietal cells and IF itself, producing gastric mucosal atrophy. Several findings favor the concept of gastric autoimmunity. (1) Autoantibodies are present in the serum and gastric juice of most patients with PA. Three types of antibodies have been found: *parietal canalicular antibodies* bind to the mucosal parietal cells; *blocking antibodies* block the binding of B_{12} to IF; and *binding antibodies* react with IF-B_{12} complex and prevent it from binding to the ileal receptor. (2) The association of PA with other autoimmune diseases such as Hashimoto's thyroiditis, Addison's disease, and type I diabetes mellitus is well documented. (3) There is an increased frequency of serum antibodies to IF in patients who have other autoimmune diseases. It should be noted that in a small minority of patients, mostly elders whose production of IF is inadequate, no

autoantibodies can be demonstrated. Perhaps in these patients age-related gastric mucosal atrophy is the root problem. Conversely, low titers of parietal canalicular antibodies have been identified in elders who do not have pernicious anemia. However, these patients do not possess antibodies to IF. *In addition to PA, malabsorption of vitamin B_{12} may result from gastrectomy,* which leads to loss of IF-producing cells; resection of ileum, the site of absorption of the IF-B_{12} complex; and disorders that involve the distal ileum such as regional enteritis, tropical sprue, and Whipple's disease.

The precise metabolic defects induced by a cobalamin deficiency that eventually lead to the megaloblastic anemia are still somewhat uncertain. However, it seems established that B_{12} deficiency leads to an "internal folate deficiency" by affecting some critical step in folate metabolism. Although folates are abundant, they are not available in a metabolically useful form, so DNA synthesis is impaired. The nature of the B_{12}-folate interaction that is deranged remains controversial. Even more uncertain is the biochemical basis of the neuropathy in B_{12} deficiency. Although both folate and B_{12} deficiency give rise to megaloblastic anemia, neurologic disease does not occur in patients with folate deficiency. It is likely therefore that the function of vitamin B_{12} in the nervous system is independent of its effects on folate metabolism.

MORPHOLOGY. Pernicious anemia is characterized by changes in the bone marrow, alimentary tract, and nervous system. The appearance of the bone marrow is similar to that described with folate deficiency anemia. It is soft, red, jelly-like, and extremely hypercellular, with extension into the formerly inactive areas. A maturation arrest at the megaloblastic level is seen, with nests of megaloblasts and relatively few normoblasts and maturing red cells (Fig. 12–7).

The peripheral blood picture is also very similar to that of folate deficiency anemia, with macroovalocytes and hypersegmented granulocytes as the hallmarks.

The atrophic gastric mucosa of pernicious anemia is described on page 485. In addition, atrophic glossitis may be present in these patients. The tongue is beefy red and slightly swollen and has a glazed appearance. Histologically, there is nonspecific submucosal chronic inflammation, with atrophy of the overlying epidermis and papillae. The neurologic lesions associated with PA comprise, in essence, demyelination of the posterior and lateral columns of the spinal cord, sometimes beginning in the peripheral nerves. In time axonal degeneration may supervene. Uncommonly, the neurologic disease occurs in the absence of megaloblastic anemia.

An element of hemolysis, discussed earlier, contributes to the hemosiderosis that is frequently seen within the liver, spleen, and bone marrow.

CLINICAL COURSE. In general, these patients are less sick than those with folate deficiency anemia. Nonspecific indications of severe anemia include weakness, dyspnea, and syncope. Since most of these patients are

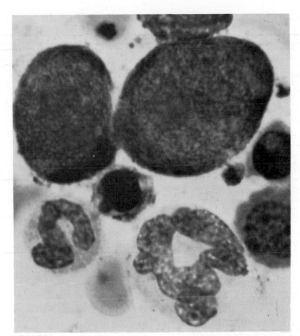

Figure 12-7. A marrow smear from a patient with pernicious anemia. Two megaloblasts are seen above and a "macropoly" (macropolymorphonuclear neutrophil) appears below.

elderly, the anemia and hypovolemia (which is present for obscure reasons) often lead to angina pectoris, palpitations, and high output cardiac failure. Gastrointestinal symptoms similar to those described under folate deficiency may also be present. Of particular concern is the appearance of neurologic changes such as symmetric numbness, tingling, and burning in feet or hands followed by unsteadiness of gait and loss of position sense, particularly in the toes. *Although the anemia responds dramatically to parenteral vitamin B_{12}, the neurologic manifestations may persist.*

The diagnostic features of PA include (1) low serum vitamin B_{12} levels, (2) normal or elevated serum folate levels, (3) histamine-fast gastric achlorhydria (due to loss of gastric parietal cells), (4) inability to absorb an oral dose of cobalamin (the Schilling test), (5) moderate to severe megaloblastic anemia, (6) leukopenia with hypersegmented granulocytes, and, most critically, (7) dramatic reticulocytic response (within 2 to 3 days) to parenteral administration of vitamin B_{12}.

It is frequently stated that patients with long-standing pernicious anemia have a three to five times greater risk of gastric carcinoma, but relatively recent studies place the increased risk at a significantly lower level.

APLASTIC ANEMIA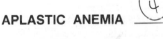

Suppression of bone marrow function occurs in a variety of clinical forms. Most often there is a failure or suppression of stem cells leading to a hypocellular marrow, anemia, thrombocytopenia, and agranulocytosis *(pancytopenia)*. Although all the formed elements are affected, this condition is usually called *aplastic anemia*. In some cases, however, marrow suppression

may be selective, affecting erythroid stem cells *(pure red cell aplasia)*, granulocytic stem cells *(agranulocytosis)*, or megakaryocytes *(thrombocytopenia)*. The following discussion is restricted largely to aplastic anemia, the most common expression of marrow failure. Agranulocytosis and thrombocytopenia are discussed later.

ETIOLOGY AND PATHOGENESIS. In more than half the cases, aplastic anemia appears without any apparent cause and so is termed *idiopathic*. In other cases, exposure to a known myelotoxic agent can be identified, such as *whole body irradiation* (as may occur in nuclear plant accidents) or use of *myelotoxic drugs*. Drugs and chemicals are the commonest causes of secondary aplastic anemia. With some agents, the marrow damage is predictable, dose related, and usually reversible. Included in this category are antineoplastic drugs (alkylating agents, antimetabolites), benzene, and chloramphenicol. In other instances marrow toxicity occurs as an apparent "idiosyncratic" or sensitivity reaction to small doses of known myelotoxic drugs (such as chloramphenicol) or following the use of such agents as phenylbutazone, sulfonamides, or methylphenylethylhydantoin, which are not myelotoxic in other persons.

Aplastic anemia has been reported in patients who have had viral infections. Although several viruses, including HIV, have been implicated, it most often follows viral hepatitis of non-A, non-B type. Marrow aplasia develops insidiously several months after recovery from non-A, non-B hepatitis and follows a relentless course.

The pathogenetic events leading to marrow failure are obscure, even when a cause can be identified. Several studies suggest that aplastic anemia is not a single entity but a heterogeneous group of pathogenetically distinct disorders. It can result from (1) defective or deficient hematopoietic stem cells, (2) a defect in the bone marrow stroma ("hematopoietic microenvironment") that causes it to be unable to support normal stem cell function, or (3) suppression of marrow stem cells by immune mechanisms. Each of these mechanisms is supported by some evidence. Restoration of normal hematopoiesis, in many cases by bone marrow transplantation, suggests that defective stem cells may be the cause of aplasia. In other cases, administration of antilymphocytic globulin has led to recovery of marrow function, implicating suppressor T cells as the cause of stem cell failure.

> **MORPHOLOGY.** The bone marrow typically is hypocellular, with an increase in the amount of fat. Small foci of lymphocytes and plasma cells may be seen in the fibrous stoma. Scattered islands of primitive hematopoietic cells are seen in less severe cases. A number of secondary changes may accompany marrow failure. Hepatic fatty change may result from anemia, and thrombocytopenia and granulocytopenia may give rise to hemorrhages and bacterial infections, respectively. Multiple transfusions may cause hemosiderosis.

CLINICAL COURSE. Aplastic anemia usually occurs insidiously; it affects persons of all ages and both sexes. Anemia may cause the progressive onset of weakness, pallor, and dyspnea. Petechiae and ecchymoses may herald thrombocytopenia. Granulocytopenia may manifest itself only by frequent and persistent minor infections or by the sudden onset of chills, fever, and prostration. *Splenomegaly is characteristically absent; if it is present the diagnosis of aplastic anemia should be seriously questioned.* Typically, the red cells are normocytic and normochromic, although occasionally slight macrocytosis is present; *reticulocytosis is absent.*

The diagnosis rests on examination of bone marrow biopsy and peripheral blood. It is important to distinguish aplastic anemia from other causes of pancytopenia, such as "aleukemic leukemia" and myelodysplastic syndromes (p. 368). Because pancytopenia is common to these conditions, their clinical manifestations are often indistinguishable; however, with aplastic anemia the marrow is hypocellular owing to stem cell failure, whereas in leukemias and myelodysplasia the marrow is populated by abnormal and immature myeloid cells. The prognosis of marrow aplasia is quite unpredictable. As mentioned earlier, withdrawal of toxic drugs may lead to recovery in some cases. The idiopathic form has a poor prognosis. Bone marrow transplantation is an extremely effective form of therapy, especially in patients younger than 40 years. Older patients benefit from immunosuppressive therapy (e.g., antithymocyte globulin).

MYELOPHTHISIC ANEMIA

This form of marrow failure is caused by extensive replacement of the marrow by tumors or other lesions. This is most commonly associated with metastatic cancer arising from a primary lesion in the breast, lung, prostate, or thyroid. Multiple myeloma, lymphomas, leukemias, advanced tuberculosis, lipid storage disorders, and osteosclerosis are less commonly implicated. Myelophthisic anemia is also seen with progressive fibrosis of the bone marrow (myelofibrosis), to be discussed later (p. 373). The manifestations of marrow infiltration include anemia and thrombocytopenia. The white cell series is less affected. Characteristically, mis-

TABLE 12–4. PATHOPHYSIOLOGIC CLASSIFICATION OF POLYCYTHEMIA

Relative
  Reduced plasma volume (hemoconcentration) dehydration
Absolute
  Primary: Abnormal proliferation of myeloid stem cells, normal or low erythropoietin levels (polycythemia vera)
  Secondary: Increased erythropoietin levels
    Appropriate: Lung disease, high-altitude living, cyanotic heart disease
    Inappropriate: Erythropoietin-secreting tumors (e.g., renal cell carcinoma, hepatoma, cerebellar hemangioblastoma)

shapen and immature red cells are seen in the peripheral blood, along with a slightly elevated white cell count ("leukoerythroblastosis"). The treatment obviously involves the management of the underlying condition.

POLYCYTHEMIA

Polycythemia, or *erythrocytosis,* as it is sometimes referred to, denotes an increased concentration of red cells, usually with a corresponding increase in hemoglobin level. Such an increase may be *relative,* when there is hemoconcentration due to decreased plasma volume, or *absolute,* when there is an increase in total red cell mass. Relative polycythemia results from any cause of dehydration, such as deprivation of water, prolonged vomiting, diarrhea, or excessive use of diuretics. *Absolute polycythemia* is said to be *primary* when the increase in red cell mass results from an autonomous proliferation of the myeloid stem cells and *secondary* when the red cell progenitors are normal but proliferate in response to increased levels of erythropoietin. Primary polycythemia (polycythemia vera) is one of several expressions of clonal, neoplastic proliferation of myeloid stem cells and is therefore best considered with other myeloproliferative disorders (p. 372). Secondary polycythemias may be caused by an increase in erythropoietin secretion that is physiologically appropriate or by an inappropriate (pathologic) secretion of erythropoietin (Table 12–4).

White Cell Disorders

Disorders of white cells may be associated with a deficiency of leukocytes (leukopenias) or proliferations that may be reactive or neoplastic. Reactive proliferation in response to an underlying primary, often microbial, disease is fairly common. Neoplastic disorders, although less common, are more ominous; they cause approximately 9% of all cancer deaths in adults and a staggering 40% in children younger than 15 years. In the following discussion we first describe some non-

neoplastic conditions and then consider in some detail malignant proliferations of white cells.

NONNEOPLASTIC DISORDERS OF WHITE CELLS

Under this heading are included leukopenias and nonspecific as well as specific reactive proliferations.

LEUKOPENIA ①

A decrease in the peripheral white cell count may occur because of decreased numbers of any of the specific types of leukocytes, but most often it involves the neutrophils (neutropenia). Lymphopenias are much less common; they are associated with congenital immunodeficiency diseases or are acquired in association with specific clinical states such as treatment with corticosteroids. Only the more common leukopenias that affect granulocytes are discussed here.

Neutropenia — Agranulocytosis

A reduction in the number of granulocytes in blood is known as neutropenia or sometimes, when severe, as agranulocytosis. Characteristically the total white cell count is reduced to 1000 cells per microliter of blood, and in some instances as low as 200 to 300 cells. Affected persons are extremely susceptible to infections, which may be severe enough to cause death.

ETIOLOGY AND PATHOGENESIS. The mechanisms that cause neutropenia can be broadly divided into two categories:

- *Inadequate or ineffective granulopoiesis.* Reduced granulopoiesis may be a manifestation of generalized marrow failure, such as occurs in aplastic anemia and a variety of leukemias. Alternatively only the committed granulocytic precursors may be affected, most commonly by certain drugs. Like aplastic anemia, granulocytopenia is predictably produced by cancer chemotherapeutic agents; it may also be an idiosyncratic and unpredictable reaction to drugs such as chloramphenicol, sulfonamides, or chlorpromazine.

- *Accelerated removal or destruction of neutrophils.* This may be encountered with immune-mediated injury to neutrophils, triggered in some cases by drugs such as aminopyrine, or it may be idiopathic. In some idiopathic cases there is proliferation of CD8+ large granular lymphocytes, which seem to suppress myelopoiesis. An enlarged spleen may also lead to accelerated removal of neutrophils by sequestration.

MORPHOLOGY. Anatomic alterations in bone marrow depend on the underlying basis of the neutropenia. Marrow hypercellularity due to increased numbers of immature granulocytic precursors is seen when the neutropenia is caused by excessive destruction of the mature neutrophils, or in ineffective granulopoiesis such as occurs in megaloblastic anemia. In contrast, marrow hypocellularity is noted when agranulocytosis is caused by agents that affect the committed granulocytic precursors. Erythropoiesis and megakaryopoiesis usually remain at normal levels, but with certain myelotoxic drugs all marrow elements may be affected.

CLINICAL COURSE. The initial symptoms are often malaise, chills, and fever, followed in sequence by marked weakness and fatigability. Infections constitute the major problem; they commonly present as ulcerating, necrotizing lesions of the gingiva, floor of the mouth, buccal mucosa, pharynx, or other sites within the oral cavity (agranulocytic angina). All these lesions often show massive growth of microorganisms with a relatively poor leukocyte response. The prognosis is most unpredictable. Before the advent of antibiotics, the mortality rate ranged between 70 and 90%. At present, antibiotics, steroids, and other supportive measures such as neutrophil transfusions allow better survival.

REACTIVE LEUKOCYTOSIS ②

An increase in the number of white blood cells is a common reaction in a variety of inflammatory states caused by microbial and nonmicrobial stimuli. Leukocytoses are relatively nonspecific and can be classified on the basis of the particular white cell series affected (Table 12–5). Infectious mononucleosis (IM), a form of lymphocytosis caused by Epstein-Barr virus (EBV) infection, merits separate consideration because it gives rise to a distinctive syndrome.

Infectious Mononucleosis

In the Western world IM is an acute, self-limited disease of adolescents and young adults (it delights in college students) that is caused by the B lymphocytotropic EBV, a member of the herpes virus family. The infection is characterized mainly by fever, sore throat, generalized lymphadenitis, peripheral lymphocytosis many with atypical morphology, and a humoral antibody response to EBV. In passing it should be noted that the cytomegalovirus may induce a similar syndrome that can be differentiated only by serologic methods.

EPIDEMIOLOGY AND IMMUNOLOGY. EBV is ubiquitous in all human populations. Where economic depri-

TABLE 12–5. CAUSES OF LEUKOCYTOSIS

Polymorphonuclear Leukocytosis	Acute bacterial infections, especially caused by pyogenic bacteria; sterile inflammations caused, for example, by tissue necrosis (myocardial infarction, burns)
Eosinophilic Leukocytosis (Eosinophilia)	Allergic disorders such as asthma, hay fever, allergic skin disease (e.g., pemphigus); parasitic infestations; drug reactions
Monocytosis	Chronic infections (e.g., tuberculosis), bacterial endocarditis, rickettsiosis and malaria; collagen vascular diseases (e.g., systemic lupus erythematosus)
Lymphocytosis	Accompanies monocytosis in many disorders associated with chronic immunologic stimulation; viral infections (e.g., hepatitis, CMV infection, infectious mononucleosis)

vation results in inadequate living standards, EBV infection early in life is nearly universal. At this age symptomatic disease is uncommon, and despite the fact that infected hosts develop an immune response (described below), more than half of the population continues to be virus shedders, explaining the dissemination of infection. In contrast, in developed countries that enjoy better standards of hygiene, infection is usually delayed until adolescence or young adulthood. Perhaps better standards of health and less underlying intercurrent chronic disease permit a more effective immune response to the EBV, so only about 20% of healthy seropositive persons shed the virus. Concomitantly, only about 50% of those exposed acquire the infection. Transmission to a seronegative "kissing cousin" usually involves direct intimate oral contact. The virus initially penetrates nasopharyngeal, oropharyngeal, and salivary epithelial cells, which are known to possess receptors for EBV, and persists as a subclinical productive infection in the oropharyngeal region. Thus the agent is shed in the saliva. Simultaneously, it spreads to underlying oropharyngeal lymphoid tissue and, more specifically, to B lymphocytes, all of which have receptors for EBV. Infection of B cells may take one of two forms: in a minority of B cells there is productive infection with lysis of infected cells and release of virions; in the vast majority of cells however, the virus associates with the host cell genome, giving rise to a latent infection. B cells that harbor the EBV genome undergo polyclonal activation and proliferation. They disseminate in the circulation and secrete antibodies with several specificities, including the well-known heterophil anti–sheep red blood cell antibodies used for the diagnosis of IM.

A normal immune response is extremely important in controlling the proliferation of EBV-infected B cells and cell-free virus. Early in the course of the infection IgM, and, later, IgG, antibodies are formed against viral capsid antigens. The latter persist for life. More important in the control of polyclonal B-cell proliferation are cytotoxic CD8+ T cells, and natural killer (NK) cells. Curiously, however, a large number of activated T cells with the phenotypic attributes of suppressor cells are also generated. They are not specific for EBV-infected B cells, so their role in recovery from EBV infection is not clear. Together with the virus-specific cytotoxic T cells, these suppressor T cells appear as atypical lymphocytes in the circulation, so characteristic of this disease. It is significant to note that in otherwise healthy persons the fully developed humoral and cellular responses to EBV act as brakes on viral shedding, limiting the number of infected B cells rather than eliminating them. Latent EBV remains in a few B cells as well as in oropharyngeal epithelial cells. As will be seen, impaired immunity in the host can have disastrous consequences.

MORPHOLOGY. The major alterations involve the blood, lymph nodes, spleen, liver, central nervous system, and, occasionally, other organs. The **peripheral blood** shows absolute lymphocytosis with a total white cell count between 12,000 and 18,000 per microliter, more than 60% of which are lymphocytes. Many of these are large, **atypical lymphocytes,** 12 to 16 μm in diameter, characterized by an abundant cytoplasm containing multiple clear vacuolations and an oval, indented, or folded nucleus. These atypical lymphocytes, most of which bear T-cell markers, are usually sufficiently distinctive to permit the diagnosis from examination of a peripheral blood smear.

The **lymph nodes** are typically discrete and enlarged throughout the body, principally in the posterior cervical, axillary, and groin regions. Histologically, the lymphoid tissue is flooded by atypical lymphocytes, which occupy the paracortical (T-cell) areas. There is in addition some B-cell reaction, with enlargement of follicles. Although the underlying architecture is usually preserved, it may be blurred by intense lymphoproliferation. Occasionally cells resembling Reed-Sternberg (RS) cells (p. 362) may also be found in the nodes. Together these features sometimes make it difficult to distinguish the nodal morphology from that seen in malignant lymphomas, particularly Hodgkin's disease. Differentiation then depends on recognition of the atypical lymphocytes. Similar changes commonly occur in the tonsils and lymphoid tissue of the oropharynx.

The **spleen** is enlarged in most cases, weighing between 300 and 500 gm. It is usually soft and fleshy, with a hyperemic cut surface. The histologic changes are analogous to those of the lymph nodes, showing a heavy infiltration of atypical lymphocytes, which may result either in prominence of the splenic follicles or in some blurring of the architecture. These spleens are especially vulnerable to rupture, possibly in part resulting from infiltration of the trabeculae and capsule by the lymphocytes.

Liver function is almost always transiently impaired to some degree, although hepatomegaly is at most moderate. Histologically, atypical lymphocytes are seen in the portal areas and sinusoids, and scattered, isolated cells or foci of parenchymal necrosis filled with lymphocytes may be present. This histologic picture may be difficult to distinguish from that of viral hepatitis.

The **central nervous system** may show congestion, edema, and perivascular mononuclear infiltrates in the leptomeninges. Myelin degeneration and destruction of axis cylinders have been described in the peripheral nerves.

CLINICAL COURSE. Although classically IM presents with fever, sore throat, lymphadenitis, and the other features mentioned earlier, quite often it is more aberrant in behavior. It may present with little or no fever and only malaise, fatigue, and lymphadenopathy, raising the spectre of leukemia-lymphoma; as a fever of unknown origin without significant lymphadenopathy or other localized findings; as hepatitis that is difficult to differentiate from one of the hepatotropic viral syndromes; or as a febrile rash resembling rubella. *Ultimately, the diagnosis depends on the following* *findings (in increasing order of specificity):* (1) *lympho-cytosis with the characteristic atypical lymphocytes in the peripheral blood,* (2) *a positive heterophil reaction (Monospot test), and* (3) *specific antibodies for EBV antigens (viral capsid antigens, early antigens, or Epstein-Barr nuclear antigen).* In the great majority of patients, IM resolves within four to six weeks, but sometimes the fatigue lasts longer. Occasionally, one or more complications supervene. They may involve virtually any organ or system in the body. Perhaps most common is marked hepatic dysfunction with jaundice, elevated hepatic enzyme levels, disturbed appetite, and, rarely, even liver failure. Other complications involve the nervous system, kidneys, bone marrow, lungs, eyes, heart, and spleen (splenic rupture has been fatal). A more serious complication in those suffering from some form of immunodeficiency such as acquired immunodeficiency syndrome (AIDS) or receiving immunosuppressive therapy (perhaps posttransplant) is that the polyclonal B-cell proliferation may run amok, leading to death. True monoclonal B-cell lymphomas have also appeared, sometimes preceded by polyclonal lymphoproliferation. These unfortunate consequences were described in a family suffering from an X-linked recessive T-cell defect, and so the condition has been designated Duncan disease or X-linked lymphoproliferation (XLP) syndrome.

REACTIVE LYMPHADENITIS

Infections and nonmicrobial inflammatory stimuli not only cause leukocytosis but also involve the lymph nodes, which act as defensive barriers. Here an immune response against foreign antigens develops, a process often associated with lymph node enlargement (lymphadenopathy). The infections that cause lymphadenitis are numerous and varied. In most instances the histologic picture in the nodes is entirely nonspecific, designated acute or chronic nonspecific adenitis. A somewhat distinctive form of lymphadenitis that occurs with cat scratch disease will be described separately.

Acute Nonspecific Lymphadenitis

This form of lymphadenitis may be confined to a local group of nodes draining a focal infection or it may be *generalized,* when there is systemic bacterial or viral infection.

Macroscopically, acutely inflamed nodes are swollen, gray-red, and engorged. Histologically, there are large germinal centers containing numerous mitotic figures. When the condition is caused by pyogenic organisms, a neutrophilic infiltrate is seen about the follicles and within the lymphoid sinuses. With severe infections the centers of follicles may undergo necrosis, resulting in the formation of an abscess.

Affected nodes are tender and, when abscess formation is extensive, become fluctuant. The overlying skin is frequently red, and penetration of the infection to the skin may produce draining sinuses. With control of the infection the lymph nodes may revert to their normal appearance, or scarring may follow the more destructive disease.

Chronic Nonspecific Lymphadenitis

This condition may assume one of three patterns, depending on the causative agent:

- **Follicular hyperplasia.** This pattern is often associated with chronic infections caused by organisms that represent B-cell antigens. Large germinal centers develop that contain lymphocytes in varying stages of "blast" transformation (Fig. 12-8). Plasma cells, immunoblasts, histiocytes, and occasionally neutrophils or eosinophils may be found in the parafollicular regions. Some causes of follicular hyperplasia are rheumatoid arthritis, toxoplasmosis, and early stages of human immunodeficiency virus (HIV) infection. This form of lymphadenitis may be confused morphologically with follicular (nodular) lymphomas (p. 357). Findings that favor a diagnosis of follicular hyperplasia are: (1) preservation of the lymph node architecture with

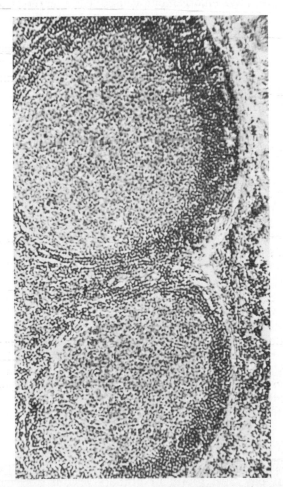

Figure 12-8. Chronic follicular hyperplasia, demonstrating marked enlargement and prominence of germinal follicles.

normal lymphoid tissue between germinal centers; (2) marked variation in the shape and size of the lymphoid nodules; (3) a mixed population of lymphocytes in different stages of differentiation; and (4) prominent phagocytic activity in germinal centers.

- **Paracortical lymphoid hyperplasia.** This pattern is characterized by reactive changes within the T-cell regions of the lymph node. Parafollicular T cells undergo proliferation and transformation to immunoblasts that may efface the germinal follicles. Paracortical lymphoid hyperplasia is encountered, particularly, in viral infections or following smallpox vaccination, and in immune reactions induced by certain drugs (especially phenytoin [Dilantin]).
- **Sinus histiocytosis.** This reactive pattern is characterized by distention and prominence of the lymphatic sinusoids due to marked hypertrophy of lining endothelial cells and infiltration with histiocytes. Sinus histiocytosis is often encountered in lymph nodes draining cancers and may represent an immune response to the tumor or its products.

Cat Scratch Disease

Cat scratch disease is a specific form of self-limited lymph node enlargement caused by a gram-negative bacterium. It is primarily a disease of childhood, with 90% of patients being younger than 18 years. It takes the form of regional lymphadenopathy, most frequently in the axilla and neck. The nodal enlargement appears approximately two weeks following a feline scratch or, uncommonly, following a splinter or thorn injury. A raised, inflammatory nodule, vesicle, or eschar may or may not be visible at the site of skin injury. In most patients the lymph node enlargement regresses over the next two to four months. Systemic manifestations such as fever and mild neutrophilia or eosinophilia are usually minimal. Rarely, patients develop encephalitis, osteomyelitis, or thrombocytopenia.

The major anatomic changes involve the nodes of drainage, which may become significantly enlarged and sometimes fluctuant. Early in the condition there is a nonspecific reactive lymphadenitis (p. 353). Thereafter, sarcoid-like granulomas (p. 403) may develop throughout the lymph node, around its capsule, and in the walls of draining veins. Coalescence of these granulomas produces the most distinctive phase of the disease, with the formation of so-called **stellate abscesses,** irregular, central accumulations of vital and disintegrating neutrophils surrounded by a prominent rim of palisaded epithelioid macrophages. Although such abscesses are distinctive, they are not pathognomonic and are similar to the lesions of lymphogranuloma venereum (p. 605).

An unclassified pleomorphic gram-negative bacterium has been found in primary lesions and lymph nodes. It is extracellular and can be visualized only with silver stains or electron microscopy. Diagnosis is based on history of exposure to cats, clinical findings, positive skin test to the bacterial antigen, and the distinctive morphologic changes in the lymph nodes.

NEOPLASTIC PROLIFERATIONS OF WHITE CELLS

These represent the most important of the white cell disorders. They can be divided into somewhat overlapping categories that can be briefly defined as follows:

1. *Malignant lymphomas* take the form of cohesive tumorous lesions, composed usually of neoplastic lymphocytes, and rarely of histiocytes, that typically arise in lymphoid tissue.
2. *Leukemias and myeloproliferative disorders* are neoplasms of the hematopoietic stem cells that arise in the bone marrow and secondarily flood the circulating blood or other organs.
3. *Plasma cell dyscrasias and related disorders,* usually arising in the bones, take the form of localized or disseminated proliferations of antibody-forming cells (plasma cells).
4. *The histiocytoses* are proliferative lesions of histiocytes and include the rare histiocytic neoplasms that present as malignant lymphomas, mentioned above. A special category of histiocytes referred to as Langerhans' cells gives rise to a spectrum of disorders, some of which behave as disseminated malignant tumors and others as localized benign proliferations. This special group is called Langerhans' cell histiocytoses.

MALIGNANT LYMPHOMAS

Lymphomas are malignant neoplasms of cells native to lymphoid tissue (i.e., lymphocytes and histiocytes and their precursors and derivatives). The term lymphoma is somewhat of a misnomer because all these disorders are malignant, and, unless controlled by therapy, ultimately lethal.

Two broad groups of lymphomas are recognized: Hodgkin's disease (Hodgkin's lymphoma) and non-Hodgkin's lymphomas (NHL). Although both arise in the lymphoid tissue, Hodgkin's disease is set apart by the presence in the lesions of the distinctive Reed-Sternberg giant cells (p. 362) and by the fact that in the involved nodes nonneoplastic inflammatory cells frequently outnumber the neoplastic element represented by the Reed-Sternberg cell.

Non-Hodgkin's Lymphomas

NHL arises in lymphoid tissue, usually in the lymph nodes (65% of cases), or less frequently in the lymphoid tissue of parenchymal organs (35%). *All variants have the potential for spread to other lymph nodes and into various tissues throughout the body, especially the liver, spleen, and bone marrow.* In some cases, bone marrow involvement is followed by a spillover of the proliferating cells into the peripheral blood, creating a leukemia-like picture. Although we speak of NHL as a group, we should recognize that it encompasses a wide spectrum of disorders, differing in patient age at onset, the cells of origin, and response to therapy. It is therefore necessary to classify NHL into various subgroups.

Few areas of pathology have evoked as much controversy and confusion as the classification of NHL. We will not attempt to discuss all previous classifications but will present the Working Formulation of Clinical Usage, which is now widely accepted. Before the details of this classification are presented, three important principles relevant to the subgrouping of NHL need to be emphasized.

(1) As tumors of the immune system, NHLs may originate in T cells, B cells, or histiocytes; distinction can be made on the basis of phenotypic and molecular characteristics of the tumor cells. The vast majority of NHL (65 to 70%) are of B-cell origin, the remainder are in large part T-cell tumors. Tumors of histiocytes or macrophages are quite uncommon. Tumors of T

and B cells may represent cells arrested at any stage along their differentiation pathways (Fig. 12–9). This figure also illustrates the genotypic and phenotypic characteristics of differentiating T and B cells that are useful in subdividing this group of tumors.

(2) Histologically, the lymphoma cells exhibit two different growth patterns: *they are either clustered into identifiable nodules (nodular lymphoma) or spread diffusely throughout the node (diffuse lymphoma;* Figs. 12–10, 12–11). With either pattern the normal lymph node architecture is completely destroyed. The distinction between nodular and diffuse lymphomas, proposed initially by Rappaport, has proven to be an important and reliable indicator of tumor behavior. In general, *nodular (or follicular) architecture is associated with a significantly superior prognosis to that of diffuse pattern.*

(3) It may be recalled that normal B cells form follicles within lymph nodes; malignant B cells tend to recapitulate this behavior with nodule formation. *Not surprisingly, therefore, nodular lymphomas are composed exclusively of B cells.* Lukes first pointed out that during antigen-induced differentiation within germinal centers of lymph nodes normal B cells undergo

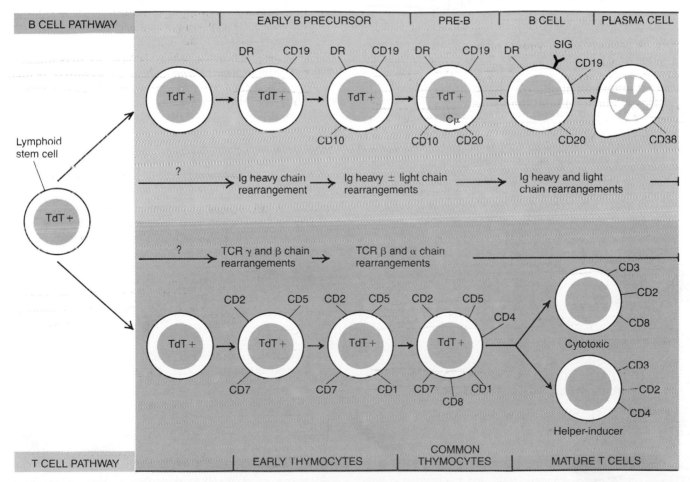

Figure 12–9. Schematic illustration of the phenotypic and genotypic changes associated with the differentiation of B cells and T cells. Not shown are some CD4 + CD8 + cells (common thymocytes) that also express CD3, and some B cells that express CD10. Key: CD, cluster designation; TdT, terminal deoxynucleotidyl transferase; Ig, immunoglobulin; TCR, T-cell receptor.

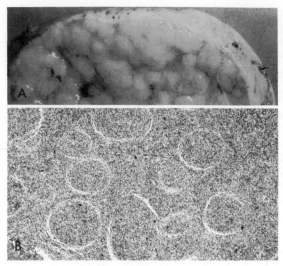

Figure 12–10. Non-Hodgkin's lymphoma, nodular pattern. *A,* A view of the cut surface of an involved lymph node. *B,* A low-power microscopic view showing the prominent nodules.

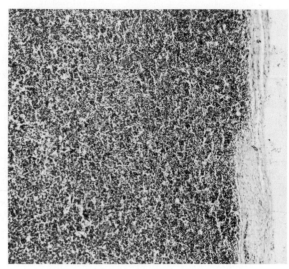

Figure 12–11. Non-Hodgkin's lymphoma, diffuse pattern of involvement. The capsule of the node is on the right. The architecture of the node is obliterated by the monotonous cells, which have obscured the sinusoids.

a series of morphologic changes, diagrammed in Figure 12–12. Such transformation of small B cells to activated immunoblasts is characterized by changes in cell and nuclear size and in nuclear configuration (clefts or folds). One suggested sequence of changes is as follows: small cleaved cell to large cleaved cell to small noncleaved cell to large noncleaved cell. Nodular lymphomas that arise from these follicular center cells are composed of any of these differentiation patterns, as though they had been arrested at a particular stage of transformation. It should be remembered, however,

that neoplastic follicular center cells can also spread diffusely in the lymph nodes and therefore give rise to diffuse lymphomas as well.

With this background we can discuss the Working Formulation for Clinical Usage. Under this scheme *NHLs are divided into three prognostic groups, designated as low-, intermediate-, and high-grade, based on survival statistics* (Table 12–6). The ten-year survival rates for tumors classified as low-grade, intermediate, and high-grade lymphomas, respectively, are approxi-

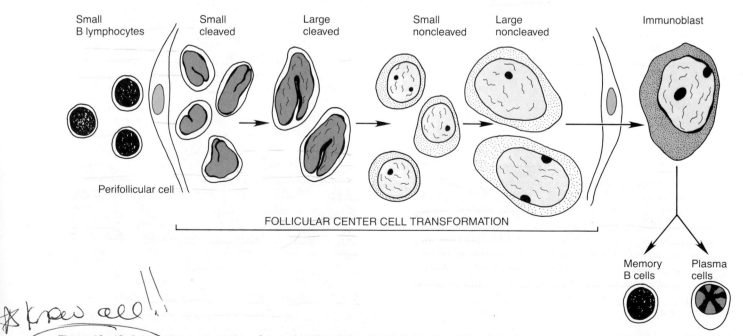

Figure 12–12. Schematic representation of normal antigen-induced transformation of B cells in the germinal centers of lymphoid follicles. (The sequence of morphologic changes is drawn after Lukes, R. J., et al. Semin. Hematol. *15*:322, 1978.) Some authors (Weisenburger, D. D. et al.: Pathol. Ann. *25*:99, 1990) consider noncleaved cells to be the precursors of cleaved cells.

TABLE 12–6. A WORKING FORMULATION OF NON-HODGKIN'S LYMPHOMAS FOR CLINICAL USAGE

Low-Grade
  Small lymphocytic
  Follicular, predominantly small cleaved cell
  Follicular, mixed small cleaved and large cell
Intermediate-Grade
  Follicular, predominantly large cell
  Diffuse, small cleaved cell
  Diffuse, mixed small and large cell
  Diffuse, large cell
High-Grade
  Large cell immunoblastic
  Lymphoblastic
  Small noncleaved cell — *Burkitt's*
Miscellaneous

mately 45, 26, and 23%. Within each prognostic group are several morphologic categories based on the architecture (follicular or diffuse) and the cytologic appearance of cells. No attempt is made to classify malignancies by their cell of origin, since in general immunophenotyping has not proven to have significant prognostic value. The Working Formulation also contains a miscellaneous group to encompass the rare histiocytic tumors and two unusual forms of T-cell neoplasia. It will be noted that in Table 12–6 there are ten histologic categories in this scheme of classification. However, on the basis of clinicopathologic features, NHLs most commonly seen in the United States can be grouped into five categories:

- Small lymphocytic lymphomas
- Follicular lymphomas (includes all three follicular subtypes of the Working Formulation)
- Diffuse large cell lymphomas (includes diffuse mixed large and small cell, diffuse large cell, and diffuse immunoblastic subtypes of Working Formulation)
- Lymphoblastic lymphomas
- Small noncleaved (Burkitt's) lymphoma.

SMALL LYMPHOCYTIC LYMPHOMA

Small lymphocytic lymphoma (SLL) makes up approximately 4% of all NHLs and is the only low-grade lymphoma that does not have a follicular architecture.

MORPHOLOGY. Cells are compact, small, apparently unstimulated lymphocytes with dark-staining round nuclei, scanty cytoplasm, and little variation in size. Mitotic figures are rare and there is little or no cytologic atypia. Bone marrow is involved in almost all cases, and in about 40% of patients the neoplastic cells spill over into blood, evoking a chronic lymphocytic leukemia-like picture. SLL overlaps with chronic lymphocytic leukemia (CLL) both clinically and morphologically, and in some cases with Waldenström's macroglobulinemia.

CLINICAL FEATURES. SLL (and the related CLL) occur primarily in older age groups. Patients have

generalized lymphadenopathy with mild to moderate enlargement of the liver and spleen; the associated symptoms are mild, and prolonged survival is usual.

IMMUNOPHENOTYPE. These are tumors of mature B cells, so they display surface IgM, IgD, and the pan-B cell antigen CD19. However, they also express CD5, an antigen found on all T cells and only on rare normal B cells. The significance of this unusual phenotype, shared by CLL, is discussed later (p. 369).

FOLLICULAR LYMPHOMAS

These tumors, characterized by a nodular or follicular architecture, are extremely common and constitute 40% of adult NHLs in the United States. They include three histologic subtypes of the Working Formulation, described below.

MORPHOLOGY. These are tumors of follicular center cells (FCC) and hence they are made up of cells that resemble normal FCC but in varying proportions. Follicular small cleaved cell lymphoma is the most common form of follicular NHL. The neoplastic B cells resemble small cleaved cells seen within normal germinal centers. However, they are slightly larger than normal lymphocytes, with an irregular "cleaved" nuclear contour characterized by prominent indentations and linear infoldings (Fig. 12–13). Nuclear chromatin is coarse and con-

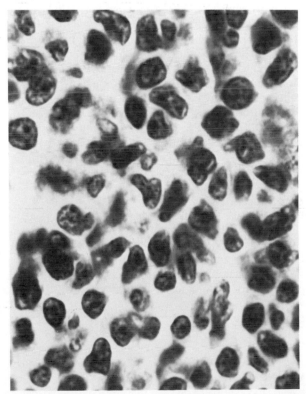

Figure 12–13. Non-Hodgkin's lymphoma, follicular small cleaved cell type. At this magnification the follicular architecture is not seen. Nuclei are irregular with indentations and marked angularity. (Courtesy of Dr. Jose Hernandez, Department of Pathology, Southwestern Medical School, Dallas, Texas).

densed, and nucleoli are indistinct. Mitoses are infrequent. When the small cleaved cells are admixed with approximately equal numbers of large cleaved or noncleaved cells, the tumors are referred to as **follicular, mixed small cleaved and large cell.** Least common is the third variant, **follicular, predominantly large cell lymphoma,** in which the large cleaved and noncleaved cells predominate.

CLINICAL FEATURES. The follicular lymphomas have the following distinctive clinical characteristics:

- They occur predominantly in older persons (rarely before age 20 years).
- They affect males and females equally.
- They present with painless lymphadenopathy, which is frequently generalized. Involvement of extranodal (e.g., visceral) sites is uncommon, but bone marrow is frequently involved (75% of cases) at the time of diagnosis.
- Peripheral blood involvement in the form of frank leukemia is less common than in SLL, but small clonal B-cell populations can be detected in most cases by flow cytometry or molecular techniques.
- In almost all patients, tumor cells reveal a characteristic translocation t(14;18). The break point on chromosome 18 involves 18q21, where the proto-oncogene *bcl*-2 has been mapped (p. 189).
- They have a long natural history (median survival seven to nine years) that appears to be largely unaffected by treatment.
- In some patients the follicular lymphomas progress to a diffuse high-grade histologic type, with or without treatment. Such a transition, reflecting the emergence of an aggressive subclone of neoplastic B cells, occurs most commonly in tumors composed predominantly of large cells.

IMMUNOPHENOTYPE. As neoplasms of follicular center cells, these tumors express the pan–B cell markers such as CD19 and CD20 and the more restricted B-cell marker CD10. Like SLL, they also express surface immunoglobulins, but unlike SLL they do not express CD5.

DIFFUSE LARGE CELL LYMPHOMAS

This clinicopathologic grouping includes three histologic subtypes of the working formulation: diffuse mixed small and large cell, diffuse large cell, and diffuse immunoblastic lymphomas. Although phenotypically and histologically heterogeneous, they share several clinical features and an aggressive natural history. They account for approximately 50% of all NHLs.

MORPHOLOGY. Two tumors in this group (diffuse mixed and diffuse large cell) may be considered diffuse counterparts of follicular mixed and follicular large cell lymphomas. Accordingly they contain either a mixture of small cleaved and large (cleaved or noncleaved) cells or

predominantly large cells. The small cleaved cell component of the mixed tumors is similar to that described in follicular small cleaved lymphomas. The nuclei of large cleaved cells are irregular in contour, indented, and larger compared with nuclei of normal histiocytes. The nuclear chromatin is dispersed and nucleoli are inconspicuous. Cytoplasm is scant and pale. Large noncleaved cells are up to four times the size of normal lymphocytes, with a round or oval nucleus and one or two prominent nucleoli. The nuclear chromatin is vesicular and mitoses are prominent. The amount of cytoplasm is greater than in large cleaved cells (Fig. 12–14).

The cells of the large cell immunoblastic variant are distinct from follicular center cells. They are four to five times larger than a small lymphocyte and have a round or multilobated large vesicular nucleus with one or two centrally placed prominent nucleoli. The cytoplasm is either deeply staining and pyroninophilic or clear.

CLINICAL FEATURES. These tumors share the following clinical features that differentiate them from follicular lymphomas:

- Although they occur mainly in older persons (median age about 60 years), unlike follicular lymphomas, the age range is much wider, and diffuse large cell NHLs constitute about 20% of childhood lymphomas.

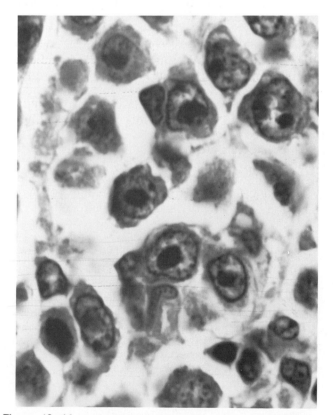

Figure 12–14. Non-Hodgkin's lymphoma, diffuse large cell type. Tumor cells in this example have large nuclei and prominent nucleoli. (Courtesy of Dr. Jose Hernandez, Department of Pathology, Southwestern Medical School, Dallas, Texas.)

- In contrast to patients with follicular lymphomas, patients with these tumors typically present with a rapidly enlarging, often symptomatic mass at a single nodal or extranodal site. Localized disease and extranodal manifestations are more common than in follicular lymphomas. Indeed, involvement of the gastrointestinal tract, skin, bone, or brain may be the presenting feature. The Waldeyer's ring of oropharyngeal lymphoid tissue is involved in about 50% of these cases.

- Involvement of liver and spleen is not common at the time of diagnosis, but when it occurs, the lymphoma cells form large destructive masses rather than the uniform miliary nodules that involve B-cell areas in low-grade follicular lymphomas.

- Bone marrow involvement is relatively uncommon in these patients, especially at the time of diagnosis. With progressive disease, however, the marrow may be involved, and, rarely, a leukemic picture may emerge.

- These three diffuse large cell lymphomas are aggressive tumors that are rapidly fatal if untreated. With intensive combination chemotherapy, however, complete remission can be achieved in 60 to 80% of the patients and approximately 50% remain free of disease for several years and may be considered cured. In contrast, it should be recalled that although follicular lymphomas follow an indolent course, they are very difficult to cure.

IMMUNOPHENOTYPE. Immunologically, these lymphomas are heterogeneous. Many (85%, including all tumors composed of follicular center cells, and some immunoblastic large cell lymphomas) are of B-cell origin. Approximately 15% have T-cell surface markers or contain rearranged T-cell–receptor genes indicative of T-cell origin. Rare tumors have markers of macrophages. Currently, subclassification based on immunophenotype is not considered useful for therapy or prognostication. Future refinements may change this impression.

LYMPHOBLASTIC LYMPHOMA
This high-grade tumor represents 4% of all NHLs in adults but 40% of childhood lymphomas. It is closely related to T-cell acute lymphoblastic leukemia (T-ALL).

MORPHOLOGY. Tumor cells are fairly uniform in size, with scanty cytoplasm and nuclei somewhat larger than those of small lymphocytes. The nuclear chromatin is delicate and finely stippled, and nucleoli are either absent or inconspicuous. The nuclear membrane shows deep subdivision imparting a convoluted (lobulated) appearance in some, but not all, cases. A high mitotic rate with a "starry sky" pattern produced by the interspersed benign macrophages is typically seen.

CLINICAL FEATURES. Lymphoblastic lymphoma predominantly affects males under the age of 20 years. The presence of a prominent mediastinal mass in 50 to 70% of patients is very characteristic and suggests a thymic origin for this tumor. The disease is rapidly progressive; early dissemination to the bone marrow and thence to blood and meninges leads to the evolution of a picture resembling T-ALL. The prognosis is generally poor, but recent attempts to treat this tumor aggressively by utilizing protocols effective in ALL have produced encouraging results.

IMMUNOPHENOTYPE. Tumor cells resemble intrathymic T cells. Terminal deoxynucleotidyl transferase (TdT), an enzyme associated with primitive lymphoid cells, is expressed in all cases.

SMALL NONCLEAVED (BURKITT'S) LYMPHOMA
Burkitt's lymphoma is endemic in some parts of Africa and sporadic in other areas, including the United States. Histologically, the African and nonendemic disease are identical, although there are clinical and virologic differences. The relationship of these disorders to EBV is discussed on p. 202.

MORPHOLOGY. Tumor cells are monotonous, intermediate in size between small lymphocytes and large noncleaved cells, and have round or oval nuclei containing two to five prominent nucleoli. The nuclear size approximates that of benign macrophages within the tumor. There is a moderate amount of faintly basophilic or amphophilic cytoplasm, which is intensely pyroninophilic and often contains small, lipid-filled vacuoles. A high mitotic rate is very characteristic of this tumor, as is cell death, accounting for the presence of numerous tissue macrophages with ingested nuclear debris. Because these benign macrophages are often surrounded by a clear space, they create a "starry sky" pattern (Fig. 12–15).

CLINICAL FEATURES. Both the endemic and non-African cases mainly affect children or young adults, accounting for approximately 30% of childhood NHLs in the United States. In both forms, the disease rarely arises in lymph nodes. In African patients, involvement of the maxilla or mandible (Fig. 12–16) is the common mode of presentation, whereas abdominal tumors (bowel, retroperitoneum, ovaries) are more common in North America. Leukemic transformation is uncommon, especially in African cases. Burkitt's lymphoma is a high-grade tumor that may be the fastest-growing human neoplasm; however, with aggressive modern chemotherapy 50% long-term survival can be expected.

IMMUNOPHENOTYPE. These are tumors of B cells that express surface IgM and pan–B cell markers such as CD19, as well as the CD10 (previously called the CALLA) antigen.

MISCELLANEOUS NON-HODGKIN'S LYMPHOMAS
This group includes several uncommon tumors, but only two, both of T-cell origin, are described here, because each is associated with a distinctive clinical presentation.

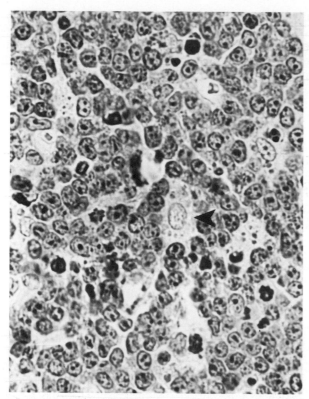

Figure 12–15. Burkitt's lymphoma. Tumor cells have multiple small nucleoli and a high mitotic index. Lack of significant variation in nuclear shape and size lends a monotonous appearance interrupted by pale-staining, benign tissue macrophages *(arrow)*, which impart a "starry sky" appearance better appreciated at a lower magnification. (Courtesy of Dr. Jose Hernandez, Department of Pathology, Southwestern Medical School, Dallas, Texas.)

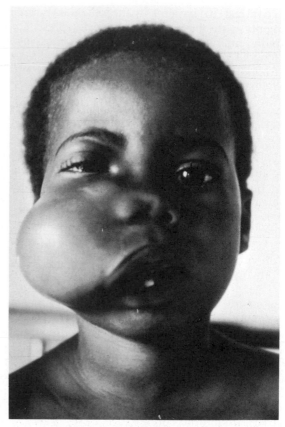

Figure 12–16. Burkitt's lymphoma in a nine-year-old child. The maxillary tumor mass is a characteristic presentation of the African form of this disease.

MYCOSIS FUNGOIDES AND SÉZARY'S SYNDROME. These tumors of peripheral CD4+ T cells are characterized by involvement of the skin and therefore belong to the group of *cutaneous T-cell lymphomas.*

Mycosis fungoides presents with an inflammatory premycotic phase and progresses through a plaque phase to a tumor phase. Histologically, there is infiltration of the epidermis and upper dermis by neoplastic T cells, which often have a cerebriform nucleus characterized by marked infolding of the nuclear membrane. With progressive disease, nodal and visceral dissemination appear. Sézary's syndrome is a related condition in which skin involvement is manifested clinically as a generalized exfoliative erythroderma along with an associated leukemia of "Sézary" cells, which also have a cerebriform nucleus. Circulating Sézary cells can also be identified in as many as 25% of cases of mycosis fungoides in the plaque or tumor, phase. These are indolent tumors with a median survival time of eight or nine years.

ADULT T-CELL LEUKEMIA/LYMPHOMA. This T-cell neoplasm caused by infection with a retrovirus, human T-cell leukemia virus type-I (HTLV-1), is endemic in southern Japan and the Caribbean basin, but similar cases have been found sporadically elsewhere, including the southeastern United States. The pathogenesis of this tumor was discussed on p. 201. It should be noted that in addition to causing lymphoid malignancies, HTLV-1 infection can also give rise to a progressive demyelinating disease that affects the central nervous system and the spinal cord.

Adult T-cell leukemia/lymphoma is characterized by skin lesions, generalized lymphadenopathy, hepatosplenomegaly, hypercalcemia, and an elevated leukocyte count with multilobed CD4+ lymphocytes. The leukemic cells constitutively express high levels of receptors for interleukin 2 (IL-2). Therefore targeting of the IL-2 receptor with antibody-toxin conjugates is being tested as a therapeutic approach to this malignancy. In the vast majority of cases this is an extremely aggressive disease, with a median survival time of about eight months. Approximately 15 to 20% of patients follow a chronic course; their disease is clinically indistinguishable from cutaneous T-cell lymphomas.

MORPHOLOGY OF ALL LYMPHOMAS. The cellular details of the various types of lymphomas have already been presented in the consideration of the classification. Further remarks are limited to some of the morphologic features common to all.

The fundamental anatomic changes occur first in the lymph nodes. As the disease advances, there is involvement of the liver, spleen, and other viscera. In a large series of cases, the cervical lymph nodes were the initial site of involvement in about 40% of cases and the axillary nodes in 20%. Following them in importance were the inguinal, femoral, iliac, and mediastinal nodes. Unusual patterns of presentation such as primary involvement of the mediastinum, visceral organs, and other extranodal sites have already been mentioned. Grossly, the affected nodes are variably enlarged in all forms, sometimes up to 10 cm in diameter. They vary in consistency from soft to moderately firm, depending on the amount of fibrous tissue present. In the less aggressive processes, the nodes remain discrete and freely moveable, but in other instances, invasion of the capsule and extension into the pericapsular tissues may lead to interadherence and fixation of the nodes, resulting in a matted, irregularly nodular mass of lymphoid tissue. The cut surface in diffuse lymphomas is usually fairly homogeneous, yellow-white to pearl gray. Nodular

forms usually reveal vague nodularity, sometimes striking enough to be visible on gross inspection. Microscopically, the nodular or diffuse infiltrate of the tumor cells completely effaces the normal architecture of the lymph nodes.

DIAGNOSIS. The diagnosis of NHL can be suspected from the clinical features, but histologic examination of a node is required for confirmation. Definite assignment of lymphomas to the T- or B-cell lineage is accomplished by immunophenotyping and by analysis of T- and B-cell antigen-receptor gene rearrangements (see Fig. 12–9). DNA hybridization studies also aid in the distinction between monoclonal (neoplastic) and polyclonal (reactive) lymphoid proliferations.

A summary of the salient clinicopathologic features of the five major categories of lymphomas is presented in Table 12–7.

TABLE 12–7. SUMMARY OF NON-HODGKIN'S LYMPHOMAS

Lymphoma Type or Group	% (In Adults)	Salient Morphology	Immunophenotype	Comments
Small Lymphocytic Lymphoma (SLL)	3–4	Small, unstimulated lymphocytes in a diffuse pattern	>95% B cells	Occurs in old age; generalized lymphadenopathy with marrow involvement and a blood picture resembling CLL; indolent course with prolonged survival
*Follicular Lymphomas**	40	Germinal center cells arranged in a follicular pattern	B cells	Follicular small cleaved cell type most common; occur in older patients; generalized lymphadenopathy; associated with t(14;18); leukemia less common than in SLL; indolent course but difficult to cure
Diffuse Large Cell Lymphomas†	40–50	Various cell types; predominantly large germinal center cells; some mixed with smaller cells; others with immunoblastic morphology	~80% B cells ~20% postthymic T cells	Occur in older patients as well as pediatric age group; greater frequency of extranodal, visceral disease; marrow involvement and leukemia very uncommon at diagnosis and poor prognostic sign; aggressive tumors but up to 60% are curable
Lymphoblastic Lymphoma	4	Cells somewhat larger than lymphocytes; in many cases nuclei markedly lobulated; high mitotic rate	>95% immature intrathymic T cells	Occurs predominantly in children (40% of all childhood lymphomas); prominent mediastinal mass; early involvement of bone marrow and progression to T-cell ALL; very aggressive
Small Noncleaved (Burkitt's) Lymphoma	<1	Cells intermediate in size between small lymphocytes and immunoblasts; prominent nucleoli; high mitotic rate	B cells	Endemic in Africa; sporadic elsewhere; predominantly affects children; extranodal visceral involvements presenting features; rapidly progressive but responsive to therapy; t(8;14)

* Includes all three follicular subtypes of Working Formulation.
† Includes diffuse large cell, diffuse mixed, and large cell immunoblastic lymphomas of the Working Formulation. Other NHLs with diffuse pattern, e.g., lymphoblastic lymphomas, that form distinct clinicopathologic categories not included.

HODGKIN'S DISEASE _____

Hodgkin's disease, like NHL, is a disorder involving primarily the lymphoid tissues. It arises almost invariably in a single node or chain of nodes and spreads characteristically to the anatomically contiguous nodes. Nevertheless, it is separated from NHL for several reasons. First, it is characterized morphologically by the presence of distinctive neoplastic giant cells called Reed-Sternberg (RS) cells admixed with a variable inflammatory infiltrate. Second, it is often associated with somewhat distinctive clinical features, including systemic manifestations such as fever. Finally, the target cell of neoplastic transformation has yet to be identified with certainty. Although overall it is an uncommon form of cancer, its importance stems from the fact that it is one of the most common forms of malignancy in young adults, with an average age at diagnosis of 32 years. Happily, tremendous progress has been made in the treatment of this disease in the last two decades, and it is now considered to be curable in most cases.

CLASSIFICATION. It should be some relief to the student to know that, unlike NHL, there is nearly universal acceptance of a single classification of Hodgkin's disease—the Rye classification. Basically, there are four subtypes: (1) *lymphocyte predominance,* (2) *mixed cellularity,* (3) *lymphocyte depletion,* and (4) *nodular sclerosis.* Before delineating them, however, we should describe the common denominator among all—the RS cell—and the method used to characterize the extent of the disease in a patient—namely, the staging system.

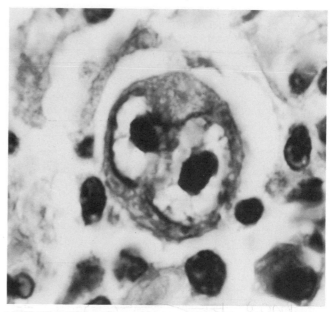

Figure 12-17. Reed-Sternberg cell. Note the prominent inclusion-like nucleoli with a clear halo around them. (Courtesy of Dr. Patrick Ward, Department of Pathology and Laboratory Medicine, University of Minnesota School of Medicine, Duluth, Minnesota.)

The sine qua non for the histologic diagnosis of Hodgkin's disease is the **RS cell** (Fig. 12-17). However, although necessary, it is not specific for Hodgkin's disease, since it is sometimes found in infectious mononucleosis, mycosis fungoides, and, occasionally, in NHLs, as well as in other settings. The RS cell has abundant, usually slightly eosinophilic, cytoplasm and ranges in diameter from 15 to 45 μm. It is distinguished principally either by having a multilobate nucleus or by being multinucleate with large, round, prominent nucleoli. **Particularly characteristic are two mirror-image nuclei, each containing a large ("inclusion-like") acidophilic nucleolus surrounded by a distinctive clear zone; together they impart an owl-eyed appearance. The nuclear membrane is distinct. Other abnormal cells, possibly variant RS cells, may also be present in Hodgkin's disease.**

The staging of Hodgkin's disease (Table 12-8) is of great clinical importance, since the course, choice of therapy, and prognosis are all intimately related to the distribution of the disease. Staging involves not only a careful physical examination but also several investigative procedures, including lymphangiography, chest radiography, biopsy of the liver and bone marrow, scan of liver and spleen, and computed tomography. In selected cases a laparotomy, which allows direct visualization of the intraabdominal nodes, liver biopsy, and removal of the spleen, is part of the staging protocol. It will become apparent that the more aggressive the variant of the disease the more likely it is to be in a more advanced stage at the time of diagnosis.

With this background we can turn to the morphologic classification of Hodgkin's disease into its subgroups

TABLE 12-8. CLINICAL STAGES OF HODGKIN'S AND NON-HODGKIN'S LYMPHOMAS (ANN ARBOR CLASSIFICATION)*†

Stage	Distribution of Disease
I	Involvement of a single lymph node region (I) or involvement of a single extralymphatic organ or site (I$_E$)
II	Involvement of two or more lymph node regions on the same side of the diaphragm alone (II) or with involvement of limited contiguous extralymphatic organ or tissue (II$_E$)
III	Involvement of lymph node regions on both sides of the diaphragm (III), which may include the spleen (III$_S$), limited contiguous extralymphatic organ or site (III$_E$), or both (III$_{ES}$)
IV	Multiple or disseminated foci of involvement of one or more extralymphatic organs or tissues with or without lymphatic involvement

* All stages are further divided on the basis of the absence (A) or presence (B) of the following systemic symptoms: significant fever, night sweats, unexplained loss of more than 10% of normal body weight.

† From Carbone, P. T., et al.: Symposium (Ann Arbor): Staging in Hodgkin's disease. Cancer Res. *31*:1707, 1971.

TABLE 12-9. PERCENTAGE OF PATIENTS IN EACH PATHOLOGIC STAGE ACCORDING TO HISTOLOGIC SUBTYPE*

Histologic Subtype	Number of Patients	Pathologic Stage (%)		
		I and II	III	IV
Lymphocyte predominance	55	76	22	2
Mixed cellularity	215	44	47	9
Lymphocyte depletion	21	19	62	19
Nodular sclerosis	628	60	35	5

* From Desforges, J. F., et al.: Hodgkin's disease. N. Engl. J. Med. *301*:1212, 1979. Reprinted by permission of the New England Journal of Medicine.

and point out some of the salient clinical features of each. Later the manifestations common to all will be presented. The essential morphologic feature that serves to differentiate three subgroups (lymphocyte predominance, mixed cellularity, and lymphocyte depletion) is the frequency of the neoplastic elements (RS cells) relative to the reactive elements, represented by small lymphocytes. The extent of spread and the natural history of untreated Hodgkin's disease appear to be directly related to the ratio of RS cells to lymphocytes. The fourth subgroup, nodular sclerosis, appears to represent a special expression of the disease that has distinctive clinicopathologic features. The relative frequency of the four histologic subtypes may be gleaned from Table 12-9.

Lymphocyte-Predominance Hodgkin's Disease. This uncommon subgroup is characterized by a large number of mature-looking lymphocytes admixed with a variable number of benign histiocytes (Fig. 12-18). The cells may diffusely flood the lymph nodes and obliterate the normal architecture or may occur within poorly defined nodular areas. Typical RS cells are extremely difficult to find. More common are variant cells that have a delicate multilobed, puffy nucleus that has been likened in appearance to popcorn ("popcorn cell"). Other cells, such as eosinophils, neutrophils, and plasma cells, are scanty or absent, and there is little evidence of necrosis or fibrosis. The nodular form of lymphocyte-predominance Hodgkin's disease has a more than superficial resemblance to nodular NHLs and may well be more closely related to follicular lymphomas than to other variants of Hodgkin's disease. Regardless of the precise nosology the prognosis of this variant is excellent.

Mixed-Cellularity Hodgkin's Disease. This is a common form of Hodgkin's disease, second only to the nodular sclerosis type in frequency. It occupies an intermediate clinical position between the lymphocyte-predominance and the lymphocyte-depletion patterns. Typical RS cells are plentiful, but there are fewer lymphocytes than in lymphocyte-predominance disease. This pattern of Hodgkin's disease is rendered distinctive by its heterogeneous cellular infiltrate, which includes eosinophils, plasma cells, and benign histiocytes. Small areas of

necrosis and fibrosis may be present, but usually they are not as prominent as in the lymphocyte-depletion type. The mixed-cellularity form of Hodgkin's disease is more common in males than in females.

Although the disease may be diagnosed in any of the clinical stages, as compared with the lymphocyte-predominance pattern more patients present with disseminated disease, and these patients more often have systemic manifestations (Table 12-9).

Lymphocyte-Depletion Hodgkin's Disease.. This is the least common form of Hodgkin's disease. It is characterized by a paucity of lymphocytes and a relative abundance of RS cells or their pleomorphic variants. It presents in two morphologic forms, the so-called **diffuse fibrosis** and the **reticular variants.** In the former, the node is hypocellular and is replaced largely by a proteinaceous fibrillar material that represents a disorderly nonbirefringent connective tissue. Pleomorphic histiocytes, a few typical and atypical RS cells, and some lymphocytes are scattered within the fibrillar material (Fig. 12-19). The reticular variant is much more cellular and is composed of highly anaplastic, large, pleomorphic cells that resemble RS cells. Only a few typical RS cells can be recognized. A majority of patients with the lymphocyte-depletion pattern are older, have disseminated involvement (Table 12-9), present with systemic manifestations, and have an aggressive form of the disease.

Nodular Sclerosis Hodgkin's Disease. This is by far the most common histologic form of Hodgkin's disease. It is distinct from the other three forms, both clinically and histologically. It is characterized morphologically by two features: (1) The presence of a particular variant of the RS cell, the **lacunar cell** (Fig. 12-20). This cell is large and has a single hyperlobate nucleus with multiple small nucleoli and an abundant, pale-staining cytoplasm with well-defined borders. In formalin-fixed tissue, the cytoplasm of these cells often retracts, giving rise to the appearance of cells lying in clear spaces, or lacunae. (2) The presence in most cases of collagen bands that divide the lymphoid tissue into circumscribed nodules (Fig. 12-21). The fibrosis may be scant or abundant, and the cellular infiltrate may show varying proportions of lymphocytes and lacunar cells. Classic RS cells are infrequent. In instances in which collagen bands are scanty, the diagnosis may depend on the identification of lacunar cells. Clinically, nodular sclerosis Hodgkin's disease has several distinctive features: it is the only form more common in women, and it has a striking propensity to involve the lower cervical, supraclavicular, and mediastinal lymph nodes. Most of the patients are adolescents or young adults, and they have an excellent prognosis, especially when their disease is in clinical stages I and II.

It is apparent that Hodgkin's disease spans a wide range of histologic patterns and that certain forms, with their characteristic fibrosis, eosinophils, neutrophils, and plasma cells, come deceptively close to simulating an inflammatory reactive process. **The diagnosis, then, of**

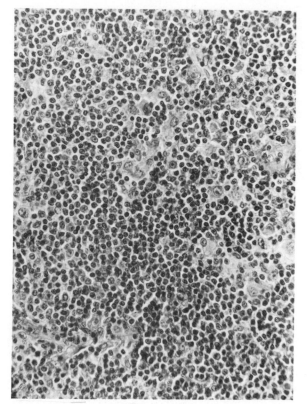

Figure 12–18. Lymphocyte-predominance Hodgkin's disease. (From Neiman, R. S.: Current problems in histopathologic diagnosis and classification of Hodgkin's disease. *In* Sommers, S. C. and Rosen, P. P. (eds.): Pathology Annual. Vol. 13, Part 2. East Norwalk, CT, Appleton-Century-Crofts, 1978, p. 289.)

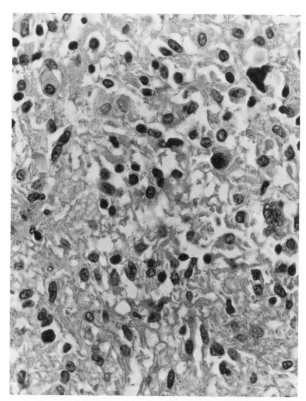

Figure 12–19. Lymph node in diffuse fibrosis Hodgkin's disease. All cellular elements are greatly diminished, and granular, proteinaceous interstitial material is prominent. A few highly atypical polyploid cells that lack the cytologic features of Reed-Sternberg cells are present. (From Neiman, R. S.: Current problems in histopathologic diagnosis and classification of Hodgkin's disease. *In* Sommers, S. C. and Rosen, P. P. (eds.): Pathology Annual. Vol. 13, Part 2. East Norwalk, CT, Appleton-Century-Crofts, 1978, p. 289.)

> **Hodgkin's disease rests solely on the unmistakable identification of the RS cells in most variants and of the lacunar cells in the nodular sclerosis pattern.**
>
> In all forms, involvement of the spleen, liver, bone marrow, and other organs and tissues may appear in due course and take the form of irregular, tumor-like nodules of tissue resembling that present in the nodes. At times the spleen is much enlarged and the liver is moderately enlarged by these nodular masses. At other times, the involvement is more subtle and becomes evident only on microscopic examination.

ETIOLOGY AND PATHOGENESIS. The origins of Hodgkin's disease are unknown. There are some who believe that Hodgkin's disease is an unusual inflammatory reaction (possibly to an infectious agent) that behaves like a neoplasm. However, it is now widely accepted that it is a neoplastic disorder and that the RS cells are the transformed cells. But the origin of RS cells remains an enigma. By both immunohistochemical and molecular analysis, RS cells appear to be of diverse origins. In some cases they seem to arise from B cells, in others from T cells. No specific markers can be detected in many instances; however, there is consensus that RS cells are *not* of monocyte-macrophage lineage. Indeed Hodgkin's disease may be a group of

histogenetically distinct disorders that share a common clinicopathologic expression. In all variants there is defective cell-mediated immunity. This is considered to be secondary to dysregulation of the immune system rather than to transformation of a particular cell type.

Given that RS cells represent the malignant component of Hodgkin's disease, what causes the neoplastic transformation? For years an infective cause of Hodgkin's disease has been suspected. Some reports have linked infection with EBV to Hodgkin's disease. However, EBV is found in the genome of RS cells in only a minority of patients. Interest in the possible infective nature of Hodgkin's disease has nevertheless been sustained by reports that suggested a "clustering" of Hodgkin's disease among certain high school students. Other studies, however, have failed to confirm the suggested horizontal spread of Hodgkin's disease. The question of an infectious origin therefore remains unresolved.

CLINICAL COURSE. Hodgkin's disease, like NHLs, usually presents with a painless enlargement of lymph nodes. Although a definitive distinction between Hodgkin's and NHLs can be made only by examination of a lymph node biopsy, several clinical features favor the diagnosis of Hodgkin's disease (Table 12–10). Younger patients, with the more favorable histo-

THE HEMATOPOIETIC AND LYMPHOID SYSTEMS ——— 365

logic types, tend to present in clinical stage I or II (see Table 12–9) and are usually free of systemic manifestations. Patients with disseminated disease (stages III and IV) are more likely to present with systemic complaints such as fever, unexplained weight loss, pruritus, and anemia. As mentioned earlier (p. 362), these patients generally have the histologically less favorable variants. The outlook following aggressive radiotherapy and chemotherapy for patients with this disease, including those with disseminated disease, has changed considerably. With current modalities of therapy the histologic picture has very little impact on the prognosis; instead, the clinical stage appears to be the important prognostic indicator. The five-year survival rate of patients with stage I-A or II-A disease is close to 100%. Even with advanced disease (stage IV-A or IV-B), 50% five-year disease-free survival can be achieved. However, the recent therapeutic advances have also brought new problems. Long-term survivors of combined chemotherapy-radiotherapy protocols are at much higher risk of developing acute leukemia, lung cancer, melanomas, and some forms of NHLs.

LEUKEMIAS AND MYELOPROLIFERATIVE DISEASES

The leukemias are malignant neoplasms of the hematopoietic stem cells characterized by diffuse replacement of the bone marrow by neoplastic cells. In most cases, the leukemic cells spill over into the blood,

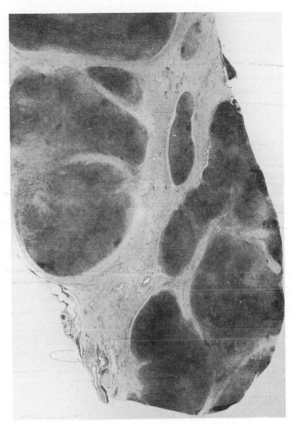

Figure 12–21. Hodgkin's disease, nodular sclerosing pattern. The low-power view shows the division of the node into well-defined nodules by wide, fibrous trabeculae.

where they may be seen in large numbers. These cells may also infiltrate the liver, spleen, lymph nodes, and other tissues throughout the body. Although the presence of excessive numbers of abnormal cells in the peripheral blood is the most dramatic manifestation of leukemia, it should be remembered that the leukemias are primary disorders of the bone marrow. Indeed, some patients with a diffusely infiltrated bone marrow may present with leukopenia rather than leukocytosis.

CLASSIFICATION. Traditionally, leukemias are classified on the basis of the cell type involved and the state of maturity of the leukemic cells. Thus *acute leuke-*

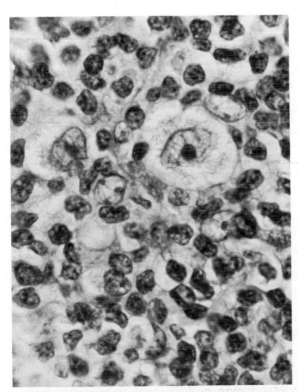

Figure 12–20. Hodgkin's disease, nodular sclerosing pattern. The distinctive "lacunar cell," so called because the cell appears to lie within a cleared space, is apparent.

TABLE 12–10. CLINICAL DIFFERENCES BETWEEN HODGKIN'S AND NON-HODGKIN'S LYMPHOMAS

Hodgkin's Disease	Non-Hodgkin's Lymphoma
More often localized to a single axial group of nodes (cervical, mediastinal, para-aortic)	More frequent involvement of multiple peripheral nodes
Orderly spread by contiguity	Noncontiguous spread
Mesenteric nodes and Waldeyer's ring rarely involved	Waldeyer's ring and mesenteric nodes commonly involved
Extranodal involvement uncommon	Extranodal involvement common

mias are characterized by the presence of very immature cells (called blasts) and by a rapidly fatal course in untreated patients. On the other hand, *chronic leukemias* are associated, at least initially, with well-differentiated (mature) leukocytes and with a relatively indolent course. Two major variants of acute and chronic leukemias are recognized: *lymphocytic* and *myelocytic* (myelogenous). Thus, a simple classification would have four patterns of leukemia: acute lymphocytic leukemia (ALL), chronic lymphocytic leukemia (CLL), acute myelocytic (myeloblastic) leukemia (AML), and chronic myelocytic leukemia (CML). This simple and time-honored classification raises several difficulties when dealing with "chronic leukemias." Acute leukemias, despite differences in their cell of origin, share important morphologic and clinical features. They are associated with replacement of normal marrow elements by a sea of proliferating blast cells that do not seem to undergo normal maturation. Consequently, there is a loss of mature myeloid elements such as red cells, granulocytes, and platelets, and hence clinical features of acute leukemias are dominated by anemia, infections, and hemorrhages. In contrast, the grouping together of chronic lymphocytic and myelogenous leukemias is problematic. A characteristic shared by these two disorders is that they are not rapidly fatal, but the clinical and morphologic features that seem to unite the acute leukemias are absent. Furthermore, this traditional grouping of chronic leukemias has become less tenable with recent advances in our knowledge of the origins of chronic myelogenous leukemia and related disorders. *It is now widely accepted that CML, polycythemia vera, essential thrombocythemia, and myeloid metaplasia represent clonal neoplastic proliferations of the multipotent myeloid stem cells.* If the erythrocyte precursors dominate, the resulting clinical disorder is classified as *polycythemia vera;* on the other hand, the dominance of granulocytic series is manifested as *CML.* It seems that the term *"chronic myeloproliferative disorders,"* coined by Dameshek over 40 years ago, best describes these neoplasms of the myeloid stem cell. Although the individual chronic myeloproliferative disorders have distinctive clinical features, interconversions and overlaps between some members of this group are well known and further attest to their relatedness. For example, a patient may present initially with polycythemia vera, but over the years the disorder may "convert" to myeloid metaplasia with myelofibrosis.

In analogy with chronic myeloproliferative disorders, it is possible to segregate chronic lymphoproliferative disorders. This group would include *chronic lymphocytic leukemia* and *hairy cell leukemia,* both neoplastic proliferations of lymphoid cells, most often of B-cell lineage. It will be apparent that as proliferative disorders of lymphoid cells they are related to the NHLs already discussed. Indeed there is very little clinical or anatomic difference between CLL and small lymphocytic lymphomas.

It should be obvious from the foregoing discussion that the heterogeneity of leukemias defies a rational classification that is scientifically accurate as well as clinically useful. In the ensuing discussion we therefore follow the traditional, but admittedly imperfect, practice of segregating the acute and chronic leukemias from the chronic myeloproliferative disorders such as polycythemia vera and myeloid metaplasia.

Our discussion focuses initially on the distinctive pathophysiologic and clinical features of different forms of leukemias; this is followed by the description of morphologic changes that are common to most leukemias, and, finally, a discussion of the cause and pathogenesis of leukemias and lymphomas.

Acute Leukemias

As with all leukemias, the acute ones have their origin in transformation of hematopoietic stem cells. Acute leukemias are characterized by a paucity of mature cells and an accumulation of leukocyte precursors (leukemic blasts).

PATHOPHYSIOLOGY. Morphologic and cell kinetic studies have indicated that in acute leukemias there is a block in differentiation of leukemic stem cells and that the leukemic blasts have a prolonged rather than shortened generation time. *Thus the accumulation of leukemic blasts in acute leukemia results from clonal expansion of the transformed stem cells as well as a failure of maturation of the progeny into functional end cells.* In some cases failure of maturation may be more important than rapid proliferation of the neoplastic cells. As the leukemic blasts accumulate in the marrow, they suppress normal hematopoietic stem cells by mysterious mechanisms. A simple hypothesis based on "crowding out" by the malignant cells seems unlikely. Suppression of normal hematopoietic stem cells in acute leukemia has two important clinical implications: (1) the major manifestations result from the paucity of normal red cells, white cells, and platelets, and (2) therapeutically the aim is to reduce the population of the leukemic clone enough to allow recovery of the few remaining normal stem cells.

CLASSIFICATION. Leukemic transformation may affect any stage during the differentiation of pluripotent hematopoietic stem cells. Involvement of the lymphoid series gives rise to ALL, whereas neoplastic transformation of myeloid progenitor cells is expressed in various forms of AML. Each of these two major subtypes is considered separately after discussion of clinical and laboratory features common to all acute leukemias.

CLINICAL FEATURES. The acute leukemias have the following characteristics:

- *Abrupt stormy onset:* Most patients present within three months of the onset of symptoms.
- *Symptoms related to depression of normal marrow function:* fatigue due mainly to anemia; fever, reflecting an infection due to absence of mature leukocytes; bleeding (petechiae, ecchymoses, epistaxis, gum bleeding) secondary to thrombocytopenia.
- *Bone pain and tenderness,* resulting from marrow expansion with infiltration of the subperiosteum.
- *Generalized lymphadenopathy, splenomegaly,* and *hepatomegaly,* reflecting dissemination of the leuke-

mic cells; this occurs in all acute leukemias, but more commonly in ALL.

- *Central nervous system manifestations* such as headache, vomiting, and nerve palsies resulting from meningeal spread; these features are more common in children than in adults, and more common in ALL than in AML.

LABORATORY FINDINGS. Anemia is almost always present. The white blood cell count is variably elevated, sometimes to more than 100,000 cells per microliter, but in about 50% of the patients is less than 10,000 cells per microliter. Much more important is the identification of immature white cells, including blast forms, in the circulating blood and the bone marrow, where they make up 60 to 100% of all the cells. The platelet count is usually depressed to less than 100,000 per microliter. Uncommonly, there is pancytopenia with few blast cells in the blood (aleukemic leukemia), but the bone marrow is nonetheless flooded with blasts, ruling out aplastic anemia. With this review we can turn to specific forms of acute leukemia.

ACUTE LYMPHOBLASTIC LEUKEMIA

ALL is primarily a disease of children and young adults. It accounts for 80% of childhood acute leukemias and the peak incidence is at approximately four years of age.

MORPHOLOGY. The nuclei of leukemic blasts in Wright-Giemsa–stained preparations have somewhat coarse and clumped chromatin and one or two nucleoli. In contrast to the blasts of AML, the cytoplasm of ALL blasts does not contain azurophilic granules but contains large aggregates of periodic acid–Schiff (PAS)-positive material. Terminal deoxytransferase (TdT), a DNA polymerase, is a useful marker because it is present in 95% of cases of ALL and only 5% of AMLs.

IMMUNOLOGIC SUBTYPES. Five subtypes, based on the origin of the leukemic lymphoblasts and stage of differentiation, are recognized. Because immunophenotyping has prognostic implications it is detailed in Table 12–11. It will be noted that the vast majority of ALLs are of B-cell origin, mainly of the early B

precursor type. All B-cell ALLs, regardless of their level of maturity, express the pan–B cell marker CD19. T-cell ALLs are akin to lymphoblastic lymphoma and are associated with prominent mediastinal masses.

KARYOTYPIC CHANGES. More than two thirds of patients with ALL have nonrandom karyotypic abnormalities. Most common is hyperdiploidy (51 to 60 chromosomes) in early precursor B-cell ALL. The Philadelphia chromosome (p. 369) is present in about 5 to 10% of patients and may be associated with any of the phenotypic subtypes of ALL; it carries a very poor prognosis, as does a t(8;14) translocation characteristic of ALL with a mature B-cell phenotype.

PROGNOSIS. Dramatic advances have been made in the treatment of ALL. The favorable prognostic groups were pointed out in Table 12–11. Overall, 90% of children with ALL achieve complete remission with chemotherapy, and more than 60% can be considered cured. Adults and those with translocations fare less well.

ACUTE MYELOBLASTIC LEUKEMIA

AML primarily affects adults between ages 15 and 39 years. It is an extremely heterogeneous disorder as will be discussed below.

MORPHOLOGY. In most cases myeloblasts can be readily distinguished from lymphoblasts in the usual Wright-Giemsa stain. They reveal delicate nuclear chromatin, three to five nucleoli, and fine, azurophilic, myeloperoxidase-positive granules in the cytoplasm (Fig. 12–22). Distinctive red-staining rod-like structures (Auer rods) are present in some cases, more often in the promyelocytic variant. Monocytic differentiation is associated with staining for lysosomal nonspecific esterases TdT is present in less than 5% of cases.

CLASSIFICATION. AMLs (also called acute nonlymphocytic leukemias) are of diverse origin. Some arise from transformation of multipotent stem cells, even though myeloblasts dominate the picture. In others the common monocyte-granulocyte precursor is involved, giving rise to myclomonocytic leukemia. Based on the line of differentiation and the maturity of cells, AMLs

TABLE 12–11. MAJOR IMMUNOLOGIC SUBTYPES OF ACUTE LYMPHOBLASTIC LEUKEMIA AND ASSOCIATED PROGNOSIS

Subtype	Phenotype	Approximate Frequency (%)	Prognosis
Early B-precursor			Very good
CALLA (CD10) negative	SIg⁻, Cμ⁻, CD19⁺, CD10⁻	5–10	
CALLA positive	SIg⁻, Cμ⁻, CD19⁺, CD10⁺	55–60	
Pre-B	SIg⁻, Cμ⁺, CD19⁺, CD10⁺	20	Intermediate
Mature B	SIg⁺, Cμ⁻, CD19⁺, CD10±	1–2	Poor
Immature T	SIg⁻, CD19⁻, CD10⁻, T⁺	15	Intermediate

Key: SIg, surface Ig; Cμ, cytoplasmic μ chains; T, antigens associated with T cells, e.g., CD2, CD5, CD7.

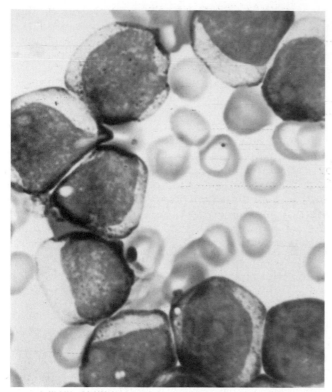

Figure 12–22. Acute myelocytic leukemia (M1). Myeloblasts flood the peripheral blood. (Courtesy of Dr. Robert W. McKenna, Department of Pathology, Southwestern Medical School, Dallas, Texas.)

are divided into seven groups in the widely used French-American-British (FAB) classification. These are listed in Table 12–12, along with their relative frequency and special features. Several cytogenetic changes have been noted in AML; some that are correlated with particular FAB groups and influence prognosis are also indicated in Table 12–12.

PROGNOSIS. AML is a devastating disease. Although the majority of patients achieve remission with intensive chemotherapy, most suffer relapse, and only 10 to 15% enjoy long-term disease-free survival. An increasing number of patients with AML are being treated with bone marrow transplantation, and for certain ones (e.g., younger patients in first remission) this treatment is proving quite effective.

Myelodysplastic Syndromes

In this group of related disorders the bone marrow is partly or wholly replaced by a clone of stem cells that retain the capacity to differentiate but in a manner that is both ineffective and disordered. Thus the myelodysplastic marrow is cellular but is populated by aberrant cells such as megaloblastoid erythroid precursors, bizarre-looking blasts, and agranular megakaryocytes. Since normal cell maturation does not occur, many patients present with pancytopenia. Cytogenetic studies reveal that up to 60% of the patients have a chromosomally abnormal clone of cells in the marrow. Some common karyotypic abnormalities include a loss of chromosomes 5 or 7, or deletions of their long arms. About a third of these patients develop AML; the remainder are constantly threatened by infections, anemia, and hemorrhages due to lack of differentiated myeloid cells. In this respect, these diseases resemble aplastic anemias, from which they must be distinguished by an examination of bone marrow.

Most patients are older males between 50 and 70 years of age. They present with weakness, infections, and hemorrhages. The majority of cases are idiopathic, but some develop the syndrome after chemotherapy with alkylating agents, with or without radiation therapy. The prognosis is variable; median survival time varies from one to five years.

TABLE 12–12. FAB CLASSIFICATION OF ACUTE MYELOBLASTIC (MYELOCYTIC) LEUKEMIAS

Class		Morphology	Comments
M1	Acute myelocytic leukemia without differentiation	Myeloblasts predominate; distinct nucleoli; few granules or Auer rods	20% of AML; presence of Ph¹ chromosome in some cases worsens prognosis
M2	Acute myelocytic leukemia with differentiation	Myeloblasts and promyelocytes predominate; Auer rods may be present	30% of AML; presence of t(8;21) translocation associated with good prognosis
M3	Acute promyelocytic leukemia	Hypergranular promyelocytes; often with many Auer rods per cell; may have reniform or bilobed nuclei	5% of AML; disseminated intravascular coagulation common; presence of t(15;17) translocation is characteristic
M4	Acute myelomonocytic leukemia	Myelocytic and monocytic differentiation evident; myeloid elements resemble M2; peripheral monocytosis	30% of AML; presence of inv 16 or del 16q associated with better prognosis
M5	Acute monocytic leukemia	Promonocytes or undifferentiated blasts	10% of AML; usually in children and young adults; gum infiltration common
M6	Acute erythroleukemia	Bizarre, multinucleated, megaloblastoid erythroblasts predominate; myeloblasts also present	5% of AML; high blood counts and organ infiltration are rare
M7	Acute megakaryocytic leukemia	Pleomorphic undifferentiated blasts; react with antiplatelet antibodies; myelofibrosis or increased bone marrow reticulin	—

Chronic Myeloid Leukemia

Chronic myeloid leukemia (CML) principally affects adults between 25 and 60 years of age and accounts for 15 to 20% of all cases of leukemia. The peak incidence is in the fourth and fifth decades of life.

PATHOPHYSIOLOGY. As mentioned earlier, CML is one of the four chronic myeloproliferative disorders. Unlike other myeloproliferative disorders, however, CML is associated with the presence of a unique chromosomal abnormality, the Ph¹ (Philadelphia) chromosome. *In approximately 90% of patients with CML, the Ph¹ chromosome, usually representing a reciprocal translocation from the long arm of chromosome 22 to another chromosome (usually the long arm of chromosome 9), can be identified in all the dividing progeny of multipotent myeloid stem cells (i.e., granulocytic, erythroid, and megakaryocytic precursors). This finding is firm evidence for the clonal origin of CML from the myeloid stem cells.* There is some evidence that the transformation may occur at an even earlier stage in differentiation, affecting the pluripotent stem cells. For example, in some cases the Ph¹ chromosome can be seen in B cells, and during the terminal phase (blast crisis) of CML, leukemic blasts of B-cell origin may be seen. It will be recalled that the *translocation responsible for the appearance of Ph¹ chromosome gives rise to a bcr-c-abl fusion gene that may be critical for neoplastic transformation* (p. 189). Indeed most patients who appear to be Ph¹ negative by cytogenetic studies, reveal rearrangement of the *bcr* gene at the molecular level.

Although CML originates in the pluripotent stem cells, granulocyte precursors constitute the dominant cell line. *In contrast to acute leukemias, there is no block in the maturation of leukemic stem cells,* as evidenced by the vast number of granulocytes in the peripheral blood. The basis of the increased myeloid stem cell mass in CML seems to lie in a failure of stem cells to respond to physiologic signals that regulate their proliferation.

CLINICAL FEATURES. The onset of CML is usually slow, and the initial symptoms may be nonspecific

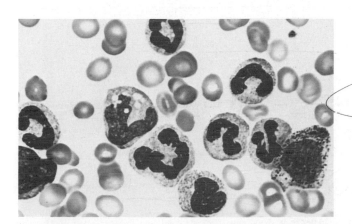

Figure 12–23. Chronic myeloid leukemia. Peripheral blood smear shows many mature neutrophils, some metamyelocytes, and a myelocyte. (Courtesy of Dr. Robert W. McKenna, Department of Pathology, Southwestern Medical School, Dallas, Texas.)

(e.g., easy fatigability, weakness, and weight loss). Sometimes the first symptom is a dragging sensation in the abdomen caused by the extreme splenomegaly that is characteristic of this condition. The laboratory findings are extremely important in making the diagnosis. Usually, there is marked elevation of the leukocyte count, commonly exceeding 100,000 cells per microliter. The circulating cells are predominantly neutrophils and metamyelocytes (Fig. 12–23), but basophils and eosinophils may also be prominent. A small proportion of myeloblasts, usually less than 10%, can be detected in the peripheral blood. Since CML originates from the myeloid stem cell, it is not surprising that as many as 50% of patients have thrombocytosis. *A characteristic finding in CML is the almost total lack of alkaline phosphatase in granulocytes.* This helps to distinguish CML from a leukemoid reaction, which is also associated with a striking elevation of the granulocyte count in response to infection, stress, chronic inflammation, and certain neoplasms. *More important for differentiating leukemoid reactions from CML is the presence of Ph¹ chromosome* and increased numbers of basophils in the peripheral blood, both of which are quite typical of CML. The course of CML is one of slow progression, and even without treatment permits survival of two to three years. After a variable (and unpredictable) period, approximately 50% of patients enter an "accelerated phase," during which there is gradual failure of response to treatment, increasing anemia and thrombocytopenia, acquisition of additional cytogenetic abnormalities, and, finally, transformation into a picture resembling AML (blast crisis). In the remaining 50%, blast crises occur abruptly without an intermediate accelerated phase. It is of interest to note that in 30% of patients, the blasts contain the enzyme TdT, a marker of primitive lymphoid cells. The lymphoblasts belong to the B-cell lineage, as evidenced by the presence of immunoglobulin gene rearrangements and expression of B-lineage markers (CD10, CD19). The treatment of CML is unsatisfactory. Although it is possible to induce remissions with chemotherapy, the median survival time (three to four years) remains unchanged. Recent results of bone marrow transplantation are encouraging. Fifty to seventy per cent of younger patients who receive transplants during the first year of the chronic phase of their disease can be cured by this form of treatment.

Chronic Lymphocytic Leukemia

Chronic lymphocytic leukemia (CLL), the most indolent of all leukemias, accounts for 30% of leukemias in Western countries. It is quite uncommon in Asia. CLL typically affects persons older than 50 years and shows considerable overlap with small lymphocytic lymphoma.

PATHOPHYSIOLOGY. In more than 95% of cases CLL is a neoplasm of B cells. The leukemic cells bear markers of mature B cells (e.g., IgM, IgD, and either λ or κ light chains), indicating monoclonality. Like all B cells they also express CD19 and CD20 antigens, but unlike the vast majority of peripheral B cells they express the T-cell–associated antigen CD5 (a feature shared with small lymphocytic lymphoma). The leukemic B cells fail to respond to antigenic stimulation, hence these patients have hypogammaglobulinemia. Paradoxically, approximately 15% of patients have antibodies against autologous red cells, giving rise to a hemolytic anemia. It is interesting to note that the CD5+ subset of B cells has been incriminated as the source of autoantibodies in diseases such as lupus erythematosus. Presumably in some cases neoplastic CD5+ B cells retain the ability to secrete autoantibodies. To summarize, CLL *is characterized by the accumulation of long-lived, nonfunctional B lymphocytes that infiltrate the bone marrow, blood, lymph nodes, and other tissues.*

CLINICAL FEATURES. CLL is often asymptomatic. When symptoms are present, they are nonspecific and include easy fatigability, loss of weight, and anorexia. Because of hypogammaglobulinemia there is increased susceptibility to bacterial infections. Autoimmune hemolytic anemia may be present. Generalized lymphadenopathy and hepatosplenomegaly are present in 50 to 60% of the cases. Total leukocyte count may be increased only slightly or may reach 200,000 per microliter. In all cases there is absolute lymphocytosis of small, mature-looking lymphocytes. Only a small fraction of lymphocytes are large ones with indented nuclei and nucleoli. Smudge cells (crushed nuclei of lymphocytes) are commonly seen in peripheral smears. The course and prognosis of CLL are extremely variable. Many patients live more than ten years after diagnosis and die of unrelated causes. The median survival is four to six years. Unlike CML, transformation to acute leukemia with blast crisis is rare.

Hairy Cell Leukemia

This uncommon form of chronic B-cell leukemia is distinguished by the presence of leukemic cells that have fine, hair-like cytoplasmic projections, best recognized under the phase contrast microscope but also visible in routine blood smears. A cytochemical feature that is quite characteristic of hairy cells is the presence of tartrate-resistant acid phosphatase in neoplastic B cells.

Hairy cell leukemia occurs mainly in older males, and *its manifestations result largely from infiltration of bone marrow and spleen. Splenomegaly,* often massive, is the most common and sometimes the only abnormal physical finding. *Pancytopenia,* resulting from marrow failure and splenic sequestration, is seen in over half the cases. *Hepatomegaly* is less common and not as marked, and lymphadenopathy is distinctly rare. *Leukocytosis* is not a common feature, being present in only 10 to 15% of patients. Hairy cells can be identified in the peripheral blood smear in most cases. The course of this disease is chronic, and the median survival time is four years. Because of pancytopenia, infections can be a major problem. Splenectomy raises the peripheral blood counts and so provides lasting relief from symptoms for approximately two thirds of

the patients. α-Interferon has also proven to be effective in this disease.

MORPHOLOGY OF ALL LEUKEMIAS. There are two aspects of the morphologic feature of leukemias: (1) the specific cytologic details of the leukemic cells seen in peripheral blood smears and bone marrow aspirates and (2) the tissue changes produced by infiltrations of leukemic cells. The cytologic features, specific for each form of leukemia, were discussed earlier. Here we consider the tissue alterations.

The tissue alterations produced by various leukemias are often similar and may be separated into primary changes, attributed directly to the abnormal overgrowth or accumulation of white cells, and secondary changes, caused both by the destructive effects of masses of these cells and by their relative ineffectiveness in protecting against infection.

Although the leukemic cells may infiltrate any tissue or organ of the body, the most striking changes are seen in the bone marrow, spleen, lymph nodes, and liver. In full-blown disease, the **bone marrow** develops a muddy, red-brown to gray-white color as the normal marrow is diffusely replaced by masses of white cells (Fig. 12–24). Sometimes these infiltrates extend into previously fatty marrow and encroach on and erode the cancellous and cortical bone.

Massive **splenomegaly** is characteristic of CML. A spleen weighing 5000 gm or more is not unusual. Such

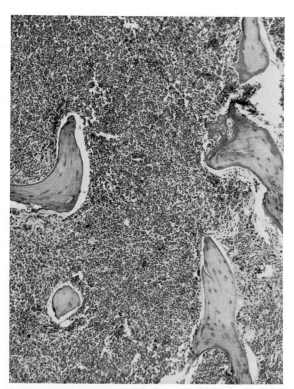

Figure 12–24. Myelogenous leukemia. Low-power view of bone marrow documents the flooding by leukemic cells.

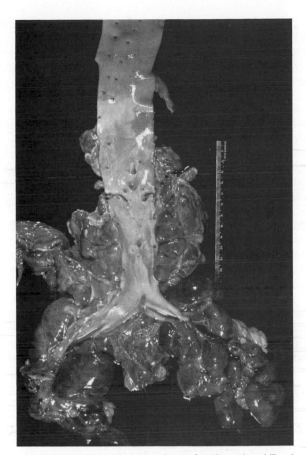

Figure 12–25. Lymphocytic leukemia; periaortic and peri-iliac lymph nodes. The marked lymphadenopathy compresses the vessels.

spleens may virtually fill the abdominal cavity and extend into the pelvis. With CLL, enlargement of the spleen is less striking and the weight of the spleen rarely exceeds 2500 gm. The acute forms of leukemia produce only moderate splenomegaly, usually between 500 and 1000 gm. On sectioning, the parenchyma is firm and muddy gray. When the splenomegaly is massive, as is most characteristic of CML, numerous areas of pale infarction may appear throughout the substance. In minimally enlarged spleens, the histologic appearance may be of focal leukemic infiltrates, with a background of fairly well-preserved normal architecture. In the lymphocytic forms, the white pulp is primarily involved. With more severe involvement the infiltrates become more diffuse. Ultimately, the underlying architecture is obliterated and replaced by a sea of homogeneous leukemic cells.

Whereas splenomegaly is more prominent with myelogenous than with lymphocytic leukemia, extreme **lymph node enlargement** is more characteristic of the lymphocytic forms (Fig. 12–25). Nevertheless, some degree of lymph node involvement is commonly present with all forms of leukemia. The affected nodes remain discrete, rubbery, and homogeneous. On histologic examination, severely involved nodes are seen to be diffusely flooded by the neoplastic cells. The underlying architecture is obliterated, and sometimes the leukemic cells invade the capsule of the node and flood out into the surrounding tissues. With CLL, the histologic picture is identical to that of small lymphocytic lymphoma.

Enlargement of the liver is somewhat more prominent with lymphocytic than with myelogenous leukemia. Histologically, the lymphocytic infiltrates are characteristically confined to the portal areas, whereas infiltrates of myelogenous leukemia are ill-defined and are present within the sinusoids throughout the lobule.

In addition to the principal sites of involvement, other tissues and organs may be affected. Leukemic infiltrates are frequently found in the kidneys, where they begin as small perivascular aggregates that progressively diffuse throughout the stroma. Similar changes may occur in the adrenals, thyroid, myocardium, testes, and, indeed, any tissue. Of particular importance is the infiltration of the central nervous system by leukemic cells. This occurs most commonly in ALL. Protected by the blood-brain barrier from the effects of cytotoxic drugs, cells in the CNS may survive to eventually initiate a relapse unless prophylactic radiation or intrathecal chemotherapy is administered.

The **secondary changes of all forms of leukemia** derive in large part from the loss of mature white cells owing to the inhibition of normal hematopoiesis by leukemic cells. Many times, the bleeding diathesis caused by the thrombocytopenia is the most striking clinical and anatomic feature of acute leukemias. Petechiae and ecchymoses are seen in the skin. Hemorrhages also occur into the serosal linings of the body cavities and into the serosal coverings of the viscera, particularly of the heart and lungs. Mucosal hemorrhages into the gingivae and urinary tract are common. Intraparenchymal hematomas may develop, most frequently in the brain. Disseminated intravascular coagulation, so common in acute promyelocytic leukemia (FAB M3), may also lead to a bleeding disorder.

Infections are a prominent feature, especially in patients with acute leukemias. They are particularly common in the oral cavity, skin, lungs, kidneys, urinary bladder, and colon, and they are often caused by "opportunists" such as fungi, *Pseudomonas* organisms, and commensals.

ETIOLOGY AND PATHOGENESIS OF LEUKEMIAS AND LYMPHOMAS. As with many other forms of cancer, several environmental agents have been implicated in the causation of leukemias and lymphomas. Well-established influences include ionizing radiations and chemicals. Exposure to radiation—occupational, therapeutic, or accidental—increases the incidence of several leukemias (with the curious exception of CLL). The increased risk of leukemias and NHLs following treatment with alkylating agents is also well-established. The risk is even greater if both irradiation and chemotherapy have been used, as for example in the treatment of Hodgkin's disease.

Two viruses, HTLV-1 and EBV, have been associated with acute T-cell leukemia/lymphoma and Burkitt's lymphoma, respectively. Recent studies have implicated HTLV-2 in the causation of mycosis fungoides as well. The possible mechanisms of transformation by these viral agents were discussed earlier (p. 201).

Finally, it should be recalled that with high-resolution banding techniques nonrandom karyotypic abnormalities, most commonly translocations, are noted in more than 60% of all leukemias and lymphomas. In addition to having prognostic implications, study of such abnormalities has provided important insights into the molecular basis of cancer. Several oncogenes located near the breakpoints are dysregulated by the translocations, as was discussed in detail in an earlier chapter (p. 188). In Table 12–13 some common translocations associated with leukemias and lymphomas and the oncogenes located near the breakpoints are presented to emphasize the importance of such changes in the pathogenesis of hematopoietic neoplasms.

Myeloproliferative Disorders

The concept that myeloproliferative disorders result from clonal neoplastic proliferations of the multipotent myeloid stem cells has already been discussed (p. 366). It was mentioned in our earlier presentation that four disorders—CML, polycythemia vera, myeloid metaplasia with myelofibrosis, and essential thrombocythemia—are included in this group. CML was discussed along with other leukemias. Of the remaining three, only polycythemia vera and myeloid metaplasia with myelofibrosis are presented here. Essential thrombocythemia occurs too infrequently to merit further discussion.

POLYCYTHEMIA VERA

As with all myeloproliferative disorders, polycythemia vera is associated with excessive proliferation of erythroid, granulocytic, and megakaryocytic elements, all derived from a single neoplastic stem cell. However, in polycythemia vera the erythroid precursors dominate, so there is an absolute increase in red cell mass. This should be contrasted with relative polycythemia, resulting from hemoconcentration (p. 350). Furthermore, unlike other forms of absolute polycythemia that result from increased secretion of erythropoietin, polycythemia vera is associated with low or virtually undetectable erythropoietin levels. It seems that the neoplastic erythroid stem cells have an intrinsic membrane defect that renders them exquisitely sensitive to low levels of erythropoietin.

MORPHOLOGY. The major anatomic changes stem from the increase in blood volume and viscosity brought about by the erythrocytosis. Plethoric congestion of all tissues and organs is characteristic of polycythemia vera. The liver is enlarged and frequently contains foci of myeloid metaplasia. The spleen is slightly enlarged in about 75% of patients, up to 250 to 300 gm, and is quite firm. The splenic sinuses are packed with red cells, as are all the vessels within the spleen. Occasionally, hematopoiesis can be seen within the red pulp. The major blood vessels are uniformly distended with thick, usually incompletely oxygenated, blood.

Consequent to the increased viscosity and vascular stasis, thromboses and infarctions are common; they affect most often the heart, spleen, and kidneys. Hemorrhages occur in about a third of these patients, probably owing to excessive distention of blood vessels and abnormal platelet function. They usually affect the gastrointestinal tract, oropharynx, or brain. Although these hemorrhages are said on occasion to be spontaneous, more often they follow some minor trauma or surgical procedure. Peptic ulceration has been described in about a fifth of these patients.

The basic changes occur in the bone marrow, which is markedly hypercellular. The fatty marrow is replaced by dark red, succulent, active marrow. Histologically, striking proliferation of all the erythroid forms is seen, particularly the normoblasts. In addition, megakaryocytic and granulocytic hyperplasia (reflecting involvement of myeloid stem cells) is also noted. If the disease changes its course, the marrow reflects the alterations and may become leukemic or fibrotic, as discussed below.

CLINICAL COURSE. Polycythemia vera appears insidiously, usually in late middle age (40 to 60 years). Patients with this disorder classically are plethoric and often somewhat cyanotic. There may be an intense pruritus. Other complaints are referable to the throm-

TABLE 12–13. LEUKEMIAS AND LYMPHOMAS WITH APPARENTLY BALANCED TRANSLOCATIONS AND ASSOCIATED ONCOGENES

Disease	Translocations	Frequency (%)	Oncogene
Leukemias			
CML	t(9;22)(q34;q11)	>90	c-*abl* 9q34
AML (M2)	t(8;21)(q22;q22)	13	c-*mos* 8q22
AML (M3)	t(15;17)(q22;q12)	>90	c-*fes* 15q24
AML (M5)	t(9;11)(p22;q23)	22	None known
ALL	t(9;22)(q34;q11)	18	c-*abl* 9q34
ALL (B cell)	t(8;14)(q24;q32)	>90	c-*myc* 8q24
Lymphomas			
Burkitt's	t(8;14)(q24;q32)	>90	c-*myc* 8q24
Follicular (non-Hodgkin's)	t(14;18)(q32;q21)	>85	*bcl*-2 18q21

botic and hemorrhagic tendencies and to hypertension. Headache, dizziness, gastrointestinal symptoms, hematemesis, and melena are common. Splenic or renal infarction may produce abdominal pain. Hypertension and the increased blood viscosity may lead to heart failure. Owing to the high rate of cell turnover, symptomatic gout is seen in 5 to 10% of cases, although many more patients have hyperuricemia.

The diagnosis is usually made in the laboratory. Red cell counts range from 6 to 10 million per microliter, and the hematocrit may approach 60%. Since there is hyperproliferation of granulocytic precursors as well as megakaryocytes in the bone marrow, the white cell count may be as high as 80,000 per microliter, and platelet count is often greater than 400,000 per microliter. Basophil counts are frequently elevated. About 30% of patients die from some thrombotic complication, affecting usually the brain or heart. An additional 10 to 15% die from some hemorrhagic complication. In patients who receive no treatment, death resulting from these vascular episodes occurs within months after diagnosis; however, if the red cell mass can be maintained near normal by phlebotomies, median survival of 10 years can be achieved.

Prolonged survival with treatment has revealed that the *natural history of polycythemia vera involves a gradual transition to a "spent phase," during which clinical and anatomic features of myeloid metaplasia with myelofibrosis develop*. Approximately 15 to 20% of patients undergo such a transformation after an average interval of 10 years. This transition is brought about by creeping fibrosis in the bone marrow (myelofibrosis) and a shift of hematopoiesis to the spleen, which enlarges markedly. It is ironic that these patients, who may once have had to undergo repeated therapeutic phlebotomies, now require blood transfusions to correct their anemia. This is perhaps the most striking example of conversion of one myeloproliferative disorder to another. As with CML (another myeloproliferative disease), certain patients with polycythemia vera develop a terminal acute myeloblastic leukemia. However, the incidence of this transition is much lower than in CML. It is estimated to be about 2% in patients who are treated with phlebotomy alone and about 15% in those who receive myelosuppressive treatment with chlorambucil or marrow irradiation with radioactive phosphorus. Presumably, the increase is related to the mutagenic effects of these therapeutic agents.

Myeloid Metaplasia with Myelofibrosis

In this chronic myeloproliferative disorder the proliferation of the neoplastic myeloid stem cells occurs principally in the spleen (*myeloid metaplasia*), and in the fully developed syndrome the bone marrow is hypocellular and fibrotic (*myelofibrosis*). Sometimes polycythemia vera (and less often CML) "burns out," as it were, and terminates in a myelofibrotic pattern. In many patients, however, extramedullary hematopoiesis in the spleen and marrow fibrosis arise insidiously without an identifiable preceding syndrome; the term "*agnogenic (idiopathic) myeloid metaplasia*" is sometimes used to describe this condition.

The cause of marrow fibrosis, which is characteristic of myeloid metaplasia, is not clear. Studies with G6PD isoenzymes indicate that the fibroblasts that replace the marrow do not belong to the neoplastic hematopoietic clone. No toxic cause for marrow destruction and subsequent scarring can be demonstrated, a feature that distinguishes this condition from myelophthisic anemias with extramedullary hematopoiesis, in which there are obvious mechanisms of marrow destruction such as metastatic tumors. It has been suggested that *marrow fibroblasts are stimulated to proliferate by platelet-derived growth factor and transforming growth factor-β* released from neoplastic megakaryocytes that undergo intramedullary death. Functional and morphologic abnormalities of platelets are seen in myeloid metaplasia with myelofibrosis, and these two growth factors are known to be mitogenic for fibroblasts. According to this view, the proliferation of neoplastic stem cells begins within the marrow and there is subsequent seeding of the spleen and other organs such as the liver. As the disease progresses, marrow fibrosis occurs secondary to the elaboration of fibroblast growth factors mentioned above. By the time the patient comes to clinical attention, fibroblasts have already taken over the marrow, and the spleen remains the major site of myeloproliferation. This scheme is supported by the occasional finding of hypercellular bone marrow with prominent megakaryocytes early in the course of this disease.

MORPHOLOGY. The principal site of the extramedullary hematopoiesis is the **spleen,** which is usually markedly enlarged, sometimes up to 4000 gm. On section, it is firm, red to gray, and very similar to spleens with myelogenous leukemia. As with CML, multiple subcapsular infarcts may be present. Histologically **there is trilineage proliferation affecting normoblasts, granulocyte precursors, and megakaryocytes; however, megakaryocytes are usually prominent owing to their large size and nuclear morphology.** Sometimes disproportional activity of any one of the three major cell lines is seen. Initially the extramedullary hematopoiesis is confined to the sinusoids, but later it may extend to involve the cords.

The **liver** may be moderately enlarged, with foci of extramedullary hematopoiesis. The **lymph nodes** are only rarely the site of blood cell formation and usually are not enlarged.

The bone marrow in a typical case is hypocellular and shows diffuse fibrosis. However, the marrow is hypercellular in early cases, with equal representation of the three major cell lines. Megakaryocytes are often prominent and may show dysplastic changes.

CLINICAL COURSE. Myeloid metaplasia may begin with a blood picture suggestive of polycythemia vera or myelogenous leukemia, or it may arise as an apparently primary disease. Most patients have moderate to severe anemia. The white cell count may be normal, reduced, or markedly elevated. Early in the course of

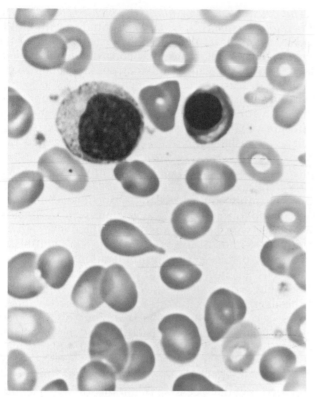

Figure 12-26. Myeloid metaplasia with myelofibrosis. Peripheral blood smear shows a teardrop red cell in the center field. An immature myeloid cell *(left)* and a nucleated red cell *(right)* are seen (Courtesy of Dr. José Hernandez, Department of Pathology, Southwestern Medical School, Dallas, Texas.)

the disease the platelet count is normal or elevated, but eventually patients develop thrombocytopenia. The peripheral blood smear appears markedly abnormal (Fig. 12-26). Red cell abnormalities include the presence of immature forms and bizarre shapes (poikilocytes, teardrop cells). Immature white cells (myelocytes and metamyelocytes) are also seen in the peripheral blood. Platelets are often abnormal in size and shape and defective in function. In some cases, the clinical and blood picture may resemble CML, but the Ph¹ chromosome is absent. Owing to a high rate of cell turnover, hyperuricemia and gout may complicate the picture. The outcome of myeloid metaplasia is variable. There is constant threat of infections, as well as thrombotic and hemorrhagic episodes due to platelet abnormalities. Splenic infarctions are therefore common. As many as 10% of patients eventually suffer a blast crisis resembling AML. The median survival time overall is four to five years.

PLASMA CELL DYSCRASIAS AND RELATED DISORDERS _____

The plasma cell dyscrasias are a group of disorders that have in common the *expansion of a single clone of immunoglobulin-secreting cells and a resultant increase in serum levels of a single homogeneous immu-* noglobulin or its fragments. The homogeneous immunoglobulin identified in the blood is often referred to as an *M component.* Since a common feature of the various plasma cell dyscrasias is the presence in the serum of excessive amounts of immunoglobulins, these disorders have also been called *monoclonal gammopathies, dysproteinemias,* and *paraproteinemias.* In many cases, these dyscrasias behave as malignant diseases, although it should be remembered that M components are also seen in otherwise normal elders (as monoclonal gammopathy of undetermined significance). Collectively, these disorders account for about 15% of deaths from malignant white cell disease; they are most common in middle-aged and elderly persons.

The plasma cell dyscrasias can be divided into six major variants: (1) multiple myeloma, (2) localized plasmacytoma (solitary myeloma), (3) Waldenström's macroglobulinemia, (4) heavy-chain disease, (5) primary or immunocyte-associated amyloidosis, and (6) monoclonal gammopathy of undetermined significance. Each of these disorders will be briefly characterized before the morphologic features of the more common forms are presented.

MULTIPLE MYELOMA. Multiple myeloma is by far the most common of the malignant plasma cell dyscrasias. *It is a clonal proliferation of neoplastic plasma cells in the bone marrow that is usually associated with multifocal lytic lesions throughout the skeletal system.* In approximately 60% of patients the M component is IgG; in 20 to 25%, IgA; and, rarely, IgM, IgD, or IgE. In the remaining 15 to 20% of cases, the plasma cells produce *only* κ or λ light chains, which, because of their low molecular weight, are readily excreted in urine, where they are termed *Bence Jones proteins.* In these patients, Bence Jones proteinuria without serum M component is present (*light-chain disease*). However, in up to 80% of patients the malignant plasma cells synthesize complete immunoglobulin molecules as well as excess light chains, and therefore both Bence Jones proteins and serum M components are present.

LOCALIZED PLASMACYTOMA. This designation refers to the presence of a single lesion in the skeleton or in the soft tissues. Solitary skeletal myeloma tends to occur in the same locations as multiple myeloma, whereas the extraosseous lesions usually form tumorous masses in the upper respiratory tract (sinuses, nasopharynx, larynx). Modest elevations in the levels of M protein are demonstrable in approximately 25% of these patients. Those with solitary skeletal myelomas usually have occult lesions elsewhere. The patients may remain stable for several years, but after a lapse of 10 to 20 years, most develop disseminated disease. Extraosseous (soft tissue) plasmacytomas rarely disseminate. They represent limited disease that can be readily cured by local resection.

WALDENSTRÖM'S MACROGLOBULINEMIA. This disease is best regarded as a hybrid of small lymphocytic lymphoma (SLL) and multiple myeloma. In multiple myeloma, the neoplastic B cells are fully differentiated into immunoglobulin-secreting plasma cells, whereas in SLL the malignant B cells are arrested prior to acquisition of secretory capacity. In between is Waldenström's macroglobulinemia, which involves B cells that are sufficiently differentiated to secrete immunoglobulins but not enough to look like plasma cells. Interestingly, the morphologic and clinical features of Waldenström's macroglobulinemia overlap those of both SLL and myeloma. Like myeloma, there is an M component, which in the great majority of cases is due to the production of monoclonal IgM immunoglobulin. However, unlike myeloma (but resembling lymphoma), the neoplastic B lymphocytes diffusely infiltrate the lymphoid organs, including bone marrow, lymph nodes, and spleen.

HEAVY-CHAIN DISEASE. This is an extremely rare plasma cell dyscrasia in which *only heavy chains are produced.* They may be of the IgG, IgA, or IgM class. Except for the presence of an M component, the disease often mimics a lymphoma-leukemia, and in this respect it resembles Waldenström's macroglobulinemia. However, the precise characteristics depend to some extent on which heavy chain is involved. With IgG heavy-chain disease, there is diffuse lymphadenopathy and hepatosplenomegaly. IgA heavy-chain disease shows a predilection for the lymphoid tissues that are normally the site of IgA synthesis, such as the small intestine and respiratory tract. A small proportion of patients with chronic lymphocytic leukemia secrete IgM heavy chains and hence have concurrent heavy-chain disease.

PRIMARY OR IMMUNOCYTE-ASSOCIATED AMYLOIDOSIS. It may be recalled that monoclonal proliferation of plasma cells, with excessive production of light chains, underlies this form of amyloidosis (p. 166). The amyloid deposits (AL type) consist of partially degraded light chains.

MONOCLONAL GAMMOPATHY OF UNDETERMINED SIGNIFICANCE. M proteins can be detected in the serum of 1 to 3% of asymptomatic, healthy persons over age 50 years. *To this dysproteinosis without any associated disease, the term monoclonal gammopathy of undetermined significance (MGUS) is applied.* This probably is the most common monoclonal gammopathy. Approximately 20% of patients with MGUS develop a well-defined plasma cell dyscrasia (myeloma, Waldenström's macroglobulinemia, or amyloidosis) over a period of 10 to 15 years. The diagnosis of MGUS should be made with caution and after careful exclusion of all other specific forms of monoclonal gammopathies. In general, patients with MGUS have less than 3 gm/dl of monoclonal protein in the serum and no Bence Jones proteinuria.

MORPHOLOGY. Multiple myeloma presents most often as multifocal destructive bone lesions throughout the skeletal system. Although any bone may be affected, the following distribution was found in a large series of cases: vertebral column, 66%; ribs, 44%; skull, 41%; pelvis, 28%; femur, 24%; clavicle, 10%; and scapula, 10%. These focal lesions generally begin in the medullary cavity, erode the cancellous bone, and progressively destroy the cortical bone. The bone resorp-

tion results from the secretion of osteoclast-activating factors (e.g., interleukin 1, tumor necrosis factor–α, lymphotoxin) by myeloma cells. Pathologic fractures are often produced by plasma cell lesions; they are most common in the vertebral column but may affect any of the numerous bones suffering erosion and destruction of their cortical substances. On section, the bony defects are typically filled with soft, red, gelatinous tissue. Most commonly, the lesions appear radiographically as punched-out defects, usually 1 to 4 cm in diameter (Fig. 12–27), but in some of the cases only diffuse demineralization is evident. Microscopic examination of the marrow reveals an increased number of plasma cells, constituting 10 to 90% of all cells in the marrow. The neoplastic plasma cells may resemble normal mature plasma cells, but sometimes more immature forms are found that may even resemble lymphocytes. It may be difficult to identify the neoplastic nature of the well-differentiated plasma cell lesions from the cytologic features of the individual cells; more important is their abnormal aggregation or evidence of their destructive potential in the form of infiltration, invasion, and erosion. With progressive disease, plasma cell infiltrations of soft tissues may be encountered in the spleen, liver, kidneys, lungs, and lymph nodes, or more widely.

Renal involvement, generally called **myeloma nephrosis,** is one of the more distinctive features of multiple myeloma. Grossly, the kidneys may be normal in size or color, slightly enlarged and pale, or shrunken and pale because of interstitial scarring. The most characteristic features are microscopic. Interstitial infiltrates of abnor-

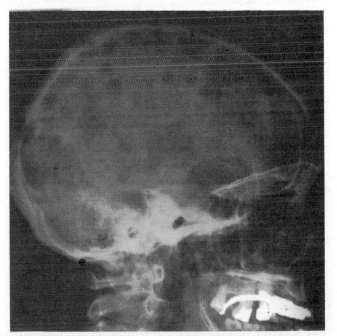

Figure 12–27. Multiple myeloma of the skull (x-ray, lateral view). The sharply punched-out bone defects are most obvious in the calvarium.

mal plasma cells may be encountered. Even in the absence of these, proteinaceous casts are prominent in the distal convoluted tubules and collecting ducts. Most of these casts are made up of Bence Jones proteins, but they may also contain complete immunoglobulins, Tamm-Horsfall protein, and albumin. Some casts have tinctorial properties of amyloid. This is not surprising in view of the fact that AL amyloid is derived from Bence Jones proteins. The casts are usually surrounded by multinucleate giant cells derived from fusion of infiltrating macrophages. Very often the cells lining tubules containing casts become necrotic or atrophic. It is believed that free light chains (Bence Jones proteins), which are filtered by the glomerulus and then reabsorbed by the tubular cells, are toxic to the tubule cells. Metastatic calcification may be encountered within the kidney because of the hypercalcemia that frequently accompanies multiple myeloma. When complicated by amyloidosis, typical glomerular lesions associated with renal amyloidosis are present. Pyelonephritis may occur due to the increased susceptibility of these patients to infections.

In contrast with multiple myeloma, Waldenström's macroglobulinemia and heavy-chain disease are not associated with lytic skeletal lesions. Instead, the neoplastic cells diffusely infiltrate the bone marrow, lymph nodes, spleen, and sometimes the liver. Infiltrations of other organs have also been reported. The cellular infiltrate consists of lymphocytes, plasma cells, lymphocytoid plasma cells, and several other hybrid forms. The remaining forms of plasma cell dyscrasias have either already been described (e.g., primary amyloidosis, p. 166) or are too rare for further description.

CLINICAL COURSE. The clinical manifestations of the plasma cell dyscrasias are varied. _They result from the destructive or otherwise damaging effect of the infiltrating neoplastic cells in various tissues and from the effects of the abnormal immunoglobulins secreted by the tumors._ In multiple myeloma, the pathologic effects of tumorous masses of plasma cells predominate, whereas in Waldenström's macroglobulinemia, most of the signs and symptoms result from the IgM macroglobulins in the serum.

The peak age of incidence of multiple myeloma is between 50 and 60 years. The major clinical features of this disease are as follows:

- _Bone pain,_ resulting from infiltration by neoplastic plasma cells, is extremely common. _Pathologic fractures and_ hypercalcemia occur, with focal bone destruction and diffuse resorption. Hypercalcemia may cause neurologic manifestations such as confusion and lethargy; it also contributes to renal disease. Anemia results from marrow replacement as well as from inhibition of hematopoiesis by tumor cells.
- _Recurrent infections with bacteria_ such as _Staphylococcus aureus, Streptococcus pneumoniae,_ and _Escherichia coli_ are serious clinical problems. They result from severe suppression of normal immunoglobulin

secretion, and from the generation of suppressor T cells with impairment of immunity.

- Excessive production and aggregation of myeloma proteins may lead to the _hyperviscosity syndrome_ (described later).
- As many as 50% of patients suffer _renal insufficiency._ It results from multiple factors, such as recurrent bacterial infections and hypercalcemia, but most importantly from the toxic effects of Bence Jones proteins on tubule cells.
- _Amyloidosis_ develops in 5 to 10% of patients.

The diagnosis of multiple myeloma can be readily made by the characteristic focal, punched-out radiologic defects in the bone, especially when these are present in the vertebrae or calvarium. Electrophoresis of the serum and urine is an important diagnostic tool in suspected cases. _In 99% of cases a monoclonal spike of complete immunoglobulin or immunoglobulin light chain can be detected in the serum or urine, or in both._ In the remaining 1% of cases monoclonal immunoglobulins can be found within the plasma cell masses but not in the serum or urine. Such cases are sometimes called "nonsecretory myelomas."

Waldenström's macroglobulinemia affects somewhat older persons, the peak incidence being between the sixth and seventh decades. Most clinical symptoms of this disease can be traced to the presence of IgM globulins. Because of their size and increased concentration, the macroglobulins form large aggregates that greatly increase the viscosity of blood, giving rise to the _hyperviscosity syndrome._ This is characterized by the following features:

- _Visual impairment_ related to the striking tortuosity and distention of retinal veins; retinal hemorrhages and exudates may also contribute to the visual problems.
- _Neurologic problems_ such as headaches, dizziness, deafness, and stupor, stemming from sluggish blood flow and sludging.
- _Bleeding_ related to the formation of complexes between macroglobulins and clotting factors as well as interference with platelet functions.
- _Cryoglobulinemia_ related to precipitation of macroglobulins at low temperatures produces symptoms such as Raynaud's phenomenon and cold urticaria.

Multiple myeloma and Waldenström's macroglobulinemia are progressive diseases with median survival in the range of two to four years.

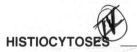

HISTIOCYTOSES _____

The term "histiocytosis" is an umbrella designation for a variety of proliferative disorders of histiocytes or macrophages. Some, such as the rare histiocytic lymphomas mentioned earlier, are clearly malignant. Others, such as the reactive histiocytic proliferations in lymph nodes, are clearly benign. Between these two extremes is a small cluster of conditions characterized by proliferation of a special type of histiocyte called

Langerhans' cells (p. 119). These disorders, called Langerhans' cell histiocytoses, are associated with tumor-like proliferations, but there is insufficient evidence to consider them truly neoplastic. It is to these disorders that our attention is now directed, but briefly because of their relative rarity.

Langerhans' Cell Histiocytosis

In the past these disorders were referred to as histiocytosis X and subdivided into three categories: Letterer-Siwe syndrome, Hand-Schüller-Christian disease, and eosinophilic granuloma. These three conditions are now believed to represent different expressions of the same basic disorder. The proliferating cell in all forms is the Langerhans' cell of marrow origin that is normally found in the epidermis. These cells, believed to be a part of the mononuclear phagocyte system, are HLA-DR positive and express the CD1 antigen. They have abundant, often vacuolated cytoplasm, with vesicular oval or indented nuclei. *Characteristic is the presence of HX bodies (Birbeck granules) in the cytoplasm. Under the electron microscope these are seen to have a pentalaminar, rod-like, tubular structure, with characteristic periodicity and sometimes a dilated terminal end (tennis-racket appearance).*

Langerhans' cell histiocytosis presents as three clinicopathologic entities:

Acute disseminated Langerhans' cell histiocytosis (Letterer-Siwe disease) mostly occurs before two years of age but occasionally may involve adults. The dominant clinical feature is the development of cutaneous lesions that resemble a seborrheic eruption secondary to infiltrations of Langerhans' histiocytes over the front and back of the trunk, and the scalp. Most of those affected have concurrent hepatosplenomegaly, lymphadenopathy, pulmonary lesions, and, eventually, destructive osteolytic bone lesions. Extensive infiltration of the marrow often leads to anemia, thrombocytopenia, and predisposition to recurrent infections such as otitis media and mastoiditis. The course of untreated disease is rapidly fatal. With intensive chemotherapy 50% of patients survive five years.

Unifocal and multifocal Langerhans' cell histiocytosis (unifocal and multifocal eosinophilic granuloma). Both of these variants are characterized by expanding, erosive accumulations of Langerhans' cells, usually within the medullary cavities of bones. Histiocytes are variably admixed with eosinophils, lymphocytes, plasma cells, and neutrophils. The eosinophilic component ranges from scattered mature cells to sheetlike masses of cells.

Virtually any bone in the skeletal system may be involved, most commonly the calvarium, ribs, and femur. Similar lesions may be found in the skin, lungs, or stomach, either as unifocal lesions or as components of the multifocal disease.

Unifocal lesions usually affect the skeletal system. They may be asymptomatic or may cause pain and tenderness, and in some instances pathologic fractures. This is an indolent disorder that may heal spontaneously or be cured by local excision or irradiation.

Multifocal Langerhans' cell histiocytosis usually affects children, who present with fever; diffuse eruptions, particularly on the scalp and in the ear canals; and frequent bouts of otitis media, mastoiditis, and upper respiratory tract infections. An infiltrate of Langerhans' cells may lead to mild lymphadenopathy, hepatomegaly, and splenomegaly. In about 50% of patients, involvement of the posterior pituitary stalk of the hypothalamus leads to diabetes insipidus. The combination of calvarial bone defects, diabetes insipidus, and exophthalmos is referred to as the Hand-Schüller-Christian triad. Many patients experience spontaneous regression; others can be treated with chemotherapy.

Bleeding Disorders

These disorders are characterized by spontaneous bleeding or excessive bleeding following trauma. Such abnormal hemorrhage may have as its cause (1) increased fragility of the vessels or (2) inadequacy of hemostatic responses, in the form of either platelet deficiency or dysfunction or derangement in the clotting mechanism.

Increased fragility of the vessels is associated with severe *vitamin C deficiency (scurvy)* (p. 255), as well as with a large number of infectious and hypersensitivity *vasculitides.* These include meningococcemia, infective endocarditis, the rickettsial diseases, typhoid, and Henoch-Schönlein purpura. Some of these conditions are discussed in other chapters; others are beyond the scope of this book. *A hemorrhagic diathesis that is purely the result of vascular fragility is characterized by (1) the apparently spontaneous appearance of petechiae and ecchymoses in the skin and mucous membranes (probably owing to minor trauma), (2) a normal platelet count and coagulation time, and (3) a bleeding time that is usually normal.*

Deficiencies of platelets (thrombocytopenia) are important causes of hemorrhagic disorders. They may occur in a variety of clinical settings, which are discussed later. Here we would like to point out that there are disorders in which platelet function is impaired, *despite a normal platelet count.* Such qualitative defects are seen in uremia, after aspirin ingestion, in von Willebrand's disease, and in a variety of rare inherited disorders. *Thrombocytopenia and platelet dysfunction are similar to increased vascular fragility in that petechiae and ecchymoses are present, as well as easy bruising, nosebleeds, excessive bleeding from minor trauma, and menorrhagia. Similarly, the coagulation time is normal; although, in contrast to the vascular disorders, the bleeding time is always prolonged.*

A bleeding diathesis based purely on a *derangement in the intricate clotting mechanism* differs in several respects from those resulting from defects in the vessel walls or in platelets. The coagulation time and activated partial thromboplastin time are usually prolonged, whereas the bleeding time is normal. *Petechiae and ecchymoses, as well as other evidence of bleeding from very minor surface trauma, are usually absent.* However, massive hemorrhage may follow operative or dental procedures or severe trauma. Moreover, hemorrhages into areas of the body subject to trauma, such as the joints of the lower extremities, are characteristic. In this category is a group of *congenital coagulation disorders.*

One of the most complex of the bleeding diatheses, *disseminated intravascular coagulation* (DIC, below), involves consumption of both platelets and the clotting factors, so it presents laboratory and clinical features of both thrombocytopenia and a coagulation disorder. *von Willebrand's disease* also involves derangements in both modalities.

In this section the following hemorrhagic disorders are discussed in this order: (1) DIC—consumption of fibrinogen and platelets; (2) thrombocytopenia—deficiency of platelets; (3) coagulation disorders—deficiency in clotting factors.

DISSEMINATED INTRAVASCULAR COAGULATION ____

DIC is an acute, subacute, or chronic thrombohemorrhagic disorder that occurs as a secondary complication in a variety of diseases. *It is characterized by activation of the coagulation sequence that leads to formation of thrombi throughout the microcirculation. As a consequence of the widespread thromboses, there is consumption of platelets and coagulation factors and, secondarily, activation of fibrinolysis.* Thus DIC may give rise either to tissue hypoxia and microinfarcts caused by myriad microthrombi or to a bleeding disorder related to pathologic activation of fibrinolysis and depletion of the elements required for hemostasis (hence the term *consumption coagulopathy*), or to both derangements. This entity is probably a more important cause of bleeding than all the congenital coagulation disorders, which will be discussed later.

ETIOLOGY AND PATHOGENESIS. Before presenting the specific disorders associated with DIC, we shall discuss in a general way the pathogenetic mechanisms by which intravascular clotting can occur. Reference to the earlier comments on normal blood coagulation (p. 67) may be helpful at this point. It suffices here to recall that clotting may be initiated by either of two pathways: the *extrinsic pathway,* which is triggered by

the release of tissue factor ("tissue thromboplastin"), or the *intrinsic pathway,* which involves the activation within the blood of factor XII by surface contact, collagen, or other negatively charged substances. Both pathways lead to the generation of thrombin. *Clot-inhibiting influences* include the rapid clearance of activated clotting factors (factors Xa and XIa) by the reticuloendothelial system or by the liver; activation of endogenous anticoagulants (e.g., protein C); and activation of fibrinolysis.

Two major mechanisms may trigger DIC: (1) release of tissue factor or thromboplastic substances into the circulation and (2) widespread injury to endothelial cells (Fig. 12-28).

The tissue thromboplastic substances released into the circulation may be derived from a variety of sources, for example from the placenta in obstetric complications, from the cytoplasmic granules in the leukemic cells of acute promyelocytic leukemia, or from neoplastic cells in mucin-secreting adenocarcinomas. Carcinomas may also release other thromboplastic substances such as proteolytic enzymes, mucin, and other undefined tumor products. In gram-negative sepsis (an important cause of DIC) endotoxins cause increased synthesis, membrane exposure, and release of tissue factor from monocytes. Furthermore, activated monocytes release IL-1 and TNF-α, both of which increase the expression of tissue factor on endothelial cell membranes and simultaneously decrease the expression of thrombomodulin. The latter, you may recall, activates protein C, an anticoagulant. The result is both activation of the extrinsic clotting system and inhibition of coagulation control.

Endothelial cell injury can initiate DIC by causing release of tissue factor and by promoting platelet aggregation and activation of the intrinsic coagulation cascade as a result of the exposure of subendothelial collagen (p. 66). Even subtle damage to the endothelium can unleash procoagulant activity by enhancing membrane expression of tissue factor. Widespread endothelial injury may be produced by deposition of antigen-antibody complexes (e.g., in systemic lupus erythematosus), temperature extremes (e.g., in heat stroke or burns), or by microorganisms (e.g., meningococci and rickettsiae). As discussed in Chapter 4 (Fig. 4-17, p. 79), endothelial injury is an important consequence of endotoxemia, and, not surprisingly, DIC is a frequent complication of gram-negative sepsis.

Several additional disorders associated with DIC are listed in Table 12-14. Of these, DIC is most likely to follow *sepsis, obstetric complications, malignancy,* and *major trauma.* The initiating factors in these conditions are multiple and often interrelated. For example, in obstetric conditions, tissue factor derived from the placenta, retained dead fetus, or amniotic fluid may enter the circulation; however, shock, hypoxia, and acidosis often coexist and may cause widespread endothelial injury. Supervening infections may complicate the problem further.

Whatever the pathogenetic mechanism, DIC has two consequences. First, there is widespread fibrin deposition within the microcirculation. This leads to ische-

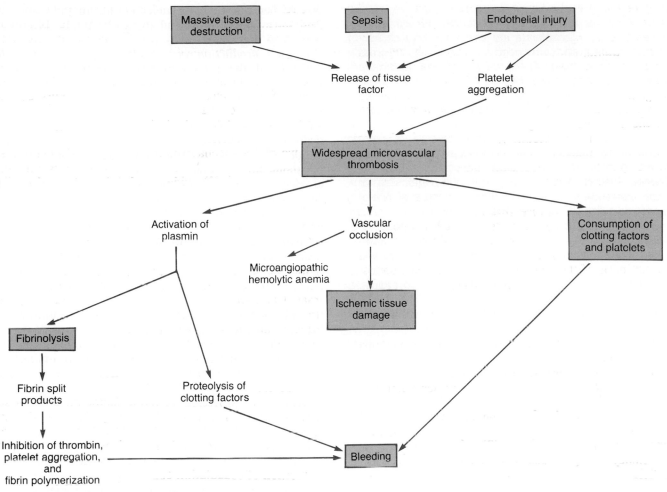

Figure 12–28. Pathophysiology of DIC.

mia in the more severely affected or more vulnerable organs and to hemolysis as the red blood cells are traumatized while passing through the fibrin strands (*microangiopathic hemolytic anemia*). Second, a bleeding diathesis ensues as the platelets and clotting factors are consumed and there is secondary release of plasminogen activators. Plasmin can not only cleave fibrin (fibrinolysis) but also digest factors V and VIII, thereby reducing their concentration further. In addition, fibrinolysis leads to the formation of fibrin degradation products, which themselves have an inhibitory effect on platelet aggregation, have antithrombin activity, and impair fibrin polymerization, all of which contribute to the hemostatic failure (Fig. 12–28).

TABLE 12–14. CLINICAL DISORDERS ASSOCIATED WITH DIC

Obstetric Complications
  Abruptio placentae
  Retained dead fetus
  Septic abortion
  Amniotic fluid embolism
  Toxemia
Infections
  Gram-negative sepsis
  Meningococcemia
  Malaria
Neoplasms
  Carcinomas of pancreas, prostate, lung, and stomach
  Acute promyelocytic leukemia
Massive Tissue Injury
  Trauma
  Burns
  Extensive surgery
Miscellaneous
  Intravascular hemolysis due to incompatible blood transfusion, shock, vasculitis, liver disease

MORPHOLOGY. The anatomic changes of DIC are related, on the one hand, to the widespread fibrin deposition and, on the other, to hemorrhage.

The microthrombi are found principally in the arterioles and capillaries of the kidneys, adrenals, brain, and heart, but no organ is spared, and the lungs, liver, and gastrointestinal mucosa may also be prominently involved. The glomeruli contain small fibrin thrombi, which may evoke only a reactive swelling of the endothelial cells or may be surrounded by a florid focal glomerulitis. The resultant ischemia leads to microinfarcts in the renal cortex. In severe cases, the ischemia may even extend to destroy the entire cortex (**bilateral renal cortical necrosis**—see p. 458). Involvement of the adrenal glands reproduces the picture of the **Waterhouse-Friderichsen syndrome** (see p. 673). Microinfarcts are also commonly encountered in the brain, surrounded by microscopic or gross foci of hemorrhage. These may give rise to bizarre neurologic signs. Similar changes are seen in the heart and often in the anterior pituitary. It has been suggested that DIC may contribute to **Sheehan's postpartum pituitary necrosis** (see p. 647).

When the underlying disorder is toxemia of pregnancy, the placenta is the site of capillary thromboses and, occasionally, florid degeneration of the vessel walls. Such changes are in all likelihood responsible for the premature loss of cytotrophoblasts and syncytiotrophoblasts that characterizes this condition.

The bleeding tendency associated with DIC is manifested not only by larger than expected hemorrhages near foci of infarction but also by diffuse petechiae and ecchymoses, which may be found on the skin, serosal linings of the body cavities, epicardium, endocardium, lungs, and the mucosal lining of the urinary tract.

CLINICAL COURSE. The clinical picture is an apparent paradox, with a bleeding tendency in the face of evidence of widespread coagulation. It is almost impossible to detail all the potential clinical manifestations. In general, *acute DIC (for example, that associated with obstetric complications) is dominated by a bleeding diathesis, whereas chronic DIC (such as may occur in a patient with cancer) tends to present with thrombotic complications.* Typically, the abnormal clotting occurs only in the microcirculation, although large vessels are involved occasionally. The manifestations may be minimal, or there may be shock with acute renal failure, dyspnea, cyanosis, convulsions, and coma. Hypotension is characteristic. Most often, attention is called to the presence of a bleeding diathesis by prolonged and copious postpartum bleeding or by the presence of petechiae and ecchymoses on the skin. These may be the only manifestations, or there may be severe hemorrhage into the gut or urinary tract.

The prognosis with DIC is highly variable and depends on the underlying disorder as well as on the degree of intravascular clotting, the activity of the mononuclear phagocyte system, and the amount of fibrinolysis. In some cases, it can be life threatening; in others, it can be treated with anticoagulants such as heparin or coagulants contained in fresh-frozen plasma. The underlying disorder must be treated simultaneously to prevent the progressive derangement of hemostasis.

THROMBOCYTOPENIA _____

Thrombocytopenia is characterized by spontaneous bleeding, a prolonged bleeding time, and a normal coagulation time. A platelet count of 100,000 per microliter or less is generally considered to constitute thrombocytopenia, although spontaneous bleeding does not become evident until the count falls below 20,000 per microliter. Platelet counts in the range of 20,000 to 50,000 may lead to posttraumatic bleeding. *The drop in platelets may occur because of either (1) decreased production or (2) excessive destruction.* A decrease in the production of platelets is associated with various forms of marrow failure or injury; these include idiopathic aplastic anemias, drug-induced marrow failure, and marrow infiltration by tumors. In all of these settings the cytopenia is associated with a decrease in marrow megakaryocytes. On the other hand, excessive destruction or peripheral consumption of platelets is characterized by a normal or an increased number of megakaryocytes in the marrow. Accelerated destruction of platelets is often immunologically mediated, resulting from formation of antiplatelet antibodies or adsorption of immune complexes formed in the circulation. Antibody-mediated destruction of platelets may be associated with well-known autoimmune diseases such as SLE, or it may appear as an apparently isolated derangement *(idiopathic thrombocytopenic purpura, ITP).* Some of the drug-induced thrombocytopenias are also suspected to be immunologically mediated. *Thrombocytopenia is one of the most common hematologic manifestations of AIDS. It may occur early in the course of human immunodeficiency virus (HIV) infection and is believed to result from immune complex–mediated injury of platelets and HIV-mediated suppression of megakaryocytes.* Excessive destruction of platelets is in some cases mediated by nonimmunologic means. As mentioned earlier, excessive utilization of platelets occurs in DIC. Other nonimmunologic causes include prosthetic heart valves and the rare disorder called *thrombotic thrombocytopenic purpura* (TTP), to be described later.

Whatever its pathogenetic mechanism, thrombocytopenia is associated with bleeding from small blood vessels. Petechiae or, sometimes, large ecchymoses are commonly found in the skin and mucous membranes of the gastrointestinal and urinary tracts, but no site is immune. Bleeding into the central nervous system constitutes a major hazard in patients whose platelet count is markedly depressed.

IDIOPATHIC THROMBOCYTOPENIC PURPURA ____

A disorder of autoimmune origin, idiopathic thrombocytopenic purpura (ITP) most often occurs as an apparently isolated derangement but sometimes as a first manifestation of systemic lupus erythematosus. Although an acute form has been described in children, most of the patients are adult females between ages 20 and 40 years.

Antiplatelet immunoglobulins directed against platelet membrane glycoproteins IIb/IIIa complex or Ib have been identified in the majority of patients with ITP. In some patients, such autoantibodies may bind to megakaryocytes and impair platelet production as well. In most cases megakaryocyte injury is not significant enough to deplete their numbers. The spleen plays an important role in the pathogenesis of this disorder. It is the major site of production of the antiplatelet antibodies and destruction of the IgG-coated platelets. In more than two thirds of patients, splenectomy is followed by return of normal platelet counts and complete remission of the disease. The spleen usually appears remarkably normal, with only minimal, if any, enlargement. Such splenomegaly as may be present is attributable to congestion of the sinusoids and enlargement of the lymphoid follicles, which have prominent germinal centers. Histologically, the marrow may appear normal but usually reveals increased numbers of megakaryocytes, some of which have only a single nucleus and are thought to be young. A similar marrow picture is noted in most forms of thrombocytopenia that result from accelerated platelet destruction. The importance of marrow examination is to rule out thrombocytopenia resulting from marrow failure. Indeed, significant findings are confined mostly to the secondary hemorrhages. Hemorrhages may be seen dispersed throughout the body, particularly in the serosal and mucosal linings.

THROMBOTIC THROMBOCYTOPENIC PURPURA

Thrombotic thrombocytopenic purpura (TTP) is a rare disorder of obscure origin. It is characterized by widespread microthrombi in the arterioles, capillaries, and venules of all organs; thrombocytopenia; and hemolytic anemia. The microthrombi are composed primarily of dense aggregates of platelets that become consolidated and are eventually replaced by fibrin. The clinical manifestations result largely from the ischemia of various organs, particularly the central nervous system (transient neurologic deficits) and the kidneys. In addition, the microcirculatory lesions cause microangiopathic hemolytic anemia because of fragmentation of red cells (p. 344). The cause of TTP is not known; it could be the result of immunologically mediated endothelial injury, but firm evidence is lacking. Alternatively, it has been proposed that the primary defect is formation of platelet aggregates in the circulation that then lodge in the microvasculature. Despite similarities with DIC, the two conditions are thought to be separate and distinct. Unlike DIC, activation of the clotting system is not of primary importance.

COAGULATION DISORDERS

These disorders result from either congenital or acquired deficiencies of the clotting factors. The latter, which are much more common and relatively straightforward, are considered first.

Acquired coagulation disorders are usually associated with deficiencies of multiple clotting factors. As discussed in an earlier chapter (p. 252), vitamin K deficiency may be associated with a severe coagulation defect, since this nutrient is essential for the synthesis of prothrombin and clotting factors VII, IX, and X. The liver is the site of synthesis of several coagulation factors; thus, parenchymal diseases of the liver are among the commonest causes of hemorrhagic diath-

eses. In addition, several liver diseases are associated with complex derangements of platelet function and fibrinogen metabolism, all of which contribute to the coagulopathy in liver disease.

Hereditary deficiencies have been identified for each of the coagulation factors that characteristically occur singly. Hemophilia A, resulting from deficiency of factor VIII, and hemophilia B (Christmas disease), resulting from deficiency of factor IX, are transmitted as X-linked recessive disorders, whereas most others are autosomal disorders. Most of these conditions are rare; only von Willebrand's disease, hemophilia A, and hemophilia B are common enough to warrant further consideration.

DEFICIENCIES OF FACTOR VIII–VON WILLEBRAND'S FACTOR COMPLEX

Hemophilia A and von Willebrand's disease, two of the most common inherited disorders of bleeding, are caused by qualitative or quantitative defects involving factor VIII–von Willebrand's factor (vWF) complex. Before we can discuss these disorders it is essential to review the structure and function of these proteins.

Plasma factor VIII–vWF is a complex made up of two separate proteins that can be distinguished by functional, biochemical, and immunologic criteria. One component, which is required for the activation of factor X in the intrinsic coagulation pathway, is called *factor VIII procoagulant protein, or factor VIII* (Fig. 12–29). Deficiency of factor VIII gives rise to hemophilia. Through noncovalent bonds, factor VIII is linked to a much larger protein, *von Willebrand's factor.* The latter, which forms approximately 99% of the factor VIII–vWF complex, is not a discrete protein but exists in the form of a series of multimers that range in size from 4×10^5 to 20×10^6 daltons. vWF can bind to collagen as well as to platelet membrane glycoprotein Ib, and can therefore "glue" these structures together (Fig. 12–29). *Indeed, the most important function of vWF in vivo is to facilitate the adhesion of platelets to subendothelial collagen.* Thus vWF is crucial to the normal process of hemostasis (p. 66), and its absence in von Willebrand's disease leads to a bleeding diathesis. In addition to its function in platelet adhesion, vWF also serves as a carrier for factor VIII. Von Willebrand's factor can be assayed by immunologic techniques or by the so-called *ristocetin aggregation test.* Ristocetin (once used as an antibiotic) binds to platelets in vitro and activates vWF receptors on their surface. This leads to platelet aggregation if vWF is available to "bridge" the platelets (see Fig. 12–29). Thus ristocetin-induced platelet aggregation can be used as a bioassay for vWF.

The two components of the factor VIII–vWF complex are coded by separate genes and are synthesized by different cells. Although vWF is produced by both endothelial cells and megakaryocytes, the former cells are the major source of plasma vWF. Factor VIII can be synthesized by several tissues, but liver is the major source of this protein. To summarize, *the two compo-*

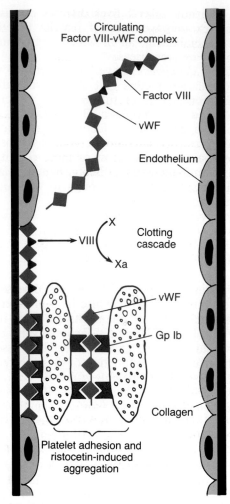

Figure 12–29. Structure and function of factor VIII–von Willebrand factor (vWF) complex. Factor VIII is synthesized by the liver and vWF in the endothelial cells. The two circulate as a complex in the circulation. Factor VIII takes part in the coagulation cascade by activating factor X. vWF causes adhesion of platelets to subendothelial collagen via Gp Ib platelet receptor. Ristocetin activates Gp Ib receptors in vitro and causes platelet aggregation if vWF is present.

nents of factor VIII–vWF complex, synthesized separately, come together and circulate in the plasma as a unit that serves to promote clotting as well as platelet–vessel wall interactions necessary to ensure hemostasis. With this background we can turn to the discussion of diseases resulting from deficiencies of factor VIII–vWF complex.

Von Willebrand's Disease

Von Willebrand's disease is characterized clinically by spontaneous bleeding from mucous membranes, excessive bleeding from wounds, menorrhagia, and a prolonged bleeding time in the presence of *a normal platelet count.* In most cases it is transmitted as an autosomal dominant disorder, but several rare autosomal recessive variants have been identified. Its precise incidence is difficult to estimate because in many instances the clinical manifestations are mild and the diagnosis requires sophisticated tests; it may well be the most common inherited bleeding disorder.

Without delving into great complexities, we can state that the *classic and most common variant (type I) of von Willebrand's disease is characterized by a reduced quantity of circulating vWF.* Because vWF stabilizes factor VIII by binding to it, a deficiency of vWF is associated with a secondary decrease in the levels of factor VIII. *To summarize, patients with von Willebrand's disease have a compound defect involving platelet function and the coagulation pathway.* However, except in the most severely affected (e.g., homozygous patients), effects of factor VIII deficiency that characterize hemophilia, such as bleeding into the joints, are uncommon.

Factor VIII Deficiency (Hemophilia A, Classic Hemophilia)

Hemophilia A is the most common hereditary disease associated with serious bleeding. It is caused by a reduced amount or activity of factor VIII. As an X-linked recessive trait it occurs in males or in homozygous females. However, excessive bleeding has been described in heterozygous females, presumably owing to extremely unfavorable lyonization (inactivation of the normal X chromosome in most of the cells). Approximately 30% of cases are due to new mutations and hence do not have a family history. Overt clinical symptoms develop only in the presence of severe deficiency (less than 1% factor VIII activity; normal 50 to 200%). Mild (more than 5% activity) or moderate (1 to 5% activity) degrees of deficiency are usually asymptomatic, although posttraumatic bleeding may be somewhat excessive. The variable degrees of deficiency in the level of factor VIII procoagulant are related to the type of mutation in the factor VIII gene. As with thalassemia, several genetic lesions (e.g., deletions, slice junction mutations, nonsense mutations) have been identified. To add to the complexities, in about 10% of patients levels of factor VIII appear normal by immunoassay, but the coagulant activity detected by bioassay is low. In these patients a mutation causes the synthesis of an antigenically normal but functionally abnormal protein. In any event, in all symptomatic cases there is a tendency toward massive hemorrhage following trauma or operative procedures. In addition, "spontaneous" hemorrhages are frequently encountered in regions of the body normally subject to trauma, particularly the joints, where they are known as *hemarthroses*. Recurrent bleeding into the joints leads to progressive deformities that may be crippling. *Petechiae and ecchymoses are characteristically absent.* Typically patients with hemophilia A have normal bleeding time and platelet counts, with prolonged partial thromboplastin time. Factor VIII assays are required for diagnosis.

Treatment of hemophilia A involves infusion of factor VIII derived from human plasma. Replacement therapy, however, is not an unalloyed blessing. It carries with it the risk of transmission of viral diseases.

As discussed in Chapter 6, prior to 1985 thousands of hemophiliacs received factor VIII preparations contaminated with HIV. Subsequently many became seropositive and developed AIDS. However, with current practices of blood banking, the risk of HIV transmission has been virtually eliminated but the threat of other undetected infections remains. Ultimately the only safe factor VIII will be one derived from the cloned human gene. Clinical trials with recombinant factor VIII are in progress.

FACTOR IX DEFICIENCY (HEMOPHILIA B, CHRISTMAS DISEASE)

Severe factor IX deficiency is a disorder that is clinically indistinguishable from hemophilia A. Moreover, it is also inherited as an X-linked recessive trait and may occur asymptomatically or with associated hemorrhage. It is much less common than hemophilia A. In about 14% of these patients, factor IX is present but nonfunctional. *The partial thromboplastin time is prolonged; bleeding time is normal.* Identification of Christmas disease (named after the first patient with this condition and not the holy day) is possible only by assay of the factor levels.

DISORDERS THAT AFFECT THE SPLEEN

The spleen is frequently involved in a wide variety of systemic diseases. In virtually all cases, the splenic changes are secondary to disease that is primary elsewhere, and in almost all instances the presentation of the splenic lesion is enlargement. Excessive destruction by the spleen of red cells, leukocytes, and platelets may ensue. Evaluation of splenomegaly is a common clinical problem, aided considerably by a knowledge of the usual limits of splenic enlargement caused by the disorders being considered. Obviously, it would be erroneous to attribute enlargement of the spleen into the pelvis to vitamin B_{12} deficiency and equally erroneous to accept as classic a case of chronic myeloid leukemia unless there is significant splenomegaly. As an aid to diagnosis, then, we present the following list of disorders, classified according to the degree of splenomegaly characteristically produced:

A. Massive splenomegaly (over 1000 gm)
1. Chronic myeloproliferative disorders (chronic myeloid leukemia, myeloid metaplasia with myelofibrosis)
2. Chronic lymphocytic leukemia (less massive)
3. Hairy cell leukemia
4. Lymphomas
5. Malaria
6. Gaucher's disease
7. Primary tumors of the spleen (rare)
B. Moderate splenomegaly (500 to 1000 gm)
1. Chronic congestive splenomegaly (portal hypertension or splenic vein obstruction)
2. Acute leukemias (inconstant)
3. Hereditary spherocytosis
4. Thalassemia major
5. Autoimmune hemolytic anemia
6. Amyloidosis
7. Niemann-Pick disease
8. Langerhans' histiocytosis
9. Chronic splenitis (especially with infective endocarditis)
10. Tuberculosis, sarcoidosis, typhoid
11. Metastatic carcinoma or sarcoma
C. Mild splenomegaly (under 500 gm)
1. Acute splenitis
2. Acute splenic congestion
3. Infectious mononucleosis
4. Miscellaneous acute febrile disorders, including septicemia, systemic lupus erythematosus, and intraabdominal infections

The microscopic changes associated with most of the previously mentioned diseases need not be described here since they have been discussed in the relevant sections of this and other chapters.

An enlarged spleen may remove excessive amounts of one or more of the formed elements of blood, resulting in anemia, leukopenia, or thrombocytopenia. This is referred to as *hypersplenism* and may be associated with many of the diseases of the spleen listed previously. In some cases, however, hypersplenism is associated with an apparently normal spleen, without any known cause for splenic hyperfunction. These cases are labeled *primary hypersplenism.*

Bibliography

Anastasi, J., Bitter, M. A., Vardiman, J. W.: The histopathologic diagnosis and subclassification of Hodgkin's disease. Hematol. Oncol. Clin. North Am. 3:187, 1989. (A modern discussion of the morphologic subtypes of Hodgkin's disease.)

Beutler, E.: The common anemias. JAMA 259:2433, 1988. (A brief commonsense approach to the understanding of thalassemias, iron-deficiency anemia, and anemia of chronic disease.)

Borowitz, M. J.: Immunologic markers in childhood acute lymphoblastic leukemia. Hematol. Oncol. Clin. North Am. 4:743, 1990. (A detailed discussion of immunophenotyping of ALL and its clinical relevance.)

Bussel, J. B.: Autoimmune thrombocytopenic purpura. Hematol. Oncol. Clin. North Am. 4:179, 1990. (An excellent discussion of the immunopathogenesis and clinical features of autoimmune thrombocytopenia.)

Dehner, L. P.: Morphologic findings in the histiocytic syndromes. Semin. Oncol. 18:8, 1991. (A modern perspective on the Langerhans' cell histiocytosis.)

Diehl, V., et al.: The cell of origin in Hodgkin's disease. Semin. Oncol. 17:660, 1990. (An update on the origin of Reed-Sternberg cells.)

Foon, K. A., Rai, K. R., Gale, R. P.: Chronic lymphocytic leukemia: New insights into biology and therapy. Ann. Intern Med. 113:525, 1990. (An excellent discussion of etiology, immunology, and clinical features of CLL.)

Giller, R. H., Grose, C.: Epstein-Barr virus: The hematologic and oncologic consequences of virus-host interaction. Crit. Rev. Oncol. Hematol. 9:149, 1989. (A detailed discussion of virology of EBV and the clinical manifestations of EBV infection: infectious mononucleosis, Burkitt's lymphoma, and nasopharyngeal carcinoma.)

Heerema, N. A.: Cytogenetic abnormalities and molecular markers of acute lymphoblastic leukemia. Hematol. Oncol. Clin. North Am.

4:795, 1990. (A detailed review of the chromosomal abnormalities in ALL and their impact on prognosis.)

Jaffe, E. S.: The role of immunophenotypic markers in the classification of non-Hodgkin's lymphoma. Semin. Oncol. *17:*11, 1990. (A short discussion of an immunologic classification of non-Hodgkin's lymphomas.)

Kazazian, H. J. Jr.: The thalassemia syndromes: Molecular basis and prenatal diagnosis in 1990. Semin. Hematol. *27:*209, 1990. (Clinical and molecular features of thalassemias; emphasis is on molecular pathology.)

Miller, J. L.: von Willebrand's Disease. Hematol. Oncol. Clin. North Am. *4:*107, 1990. (A review of the structure and function of von Willebrand's factor and consequences of inherited deficiencies.)

Moake, J. L.: Hypercoagulable states. Adv. Intern. Med. *35:*235, 1990. (A good general discussion of inherited and acquired states of hypercoagulability, including the pathogenesis of DIC.)

Silver, R. T.: Chronic myeloid leukemia. A perspective of the clinical and biologic issues of the chronic phase. Hematol. Oncol. Clin. North Am. *4:*319, 1990. (A good overview of chronic myeloid leukemia.)

Urba, W. J., Longo, D. L.: Lymphocytic lymphomas: Epidemiology, etiology, pathology and staging. In Moossa, A. R., et al. (eds.): Comprehensive Textbook of Oncology. 2nd ed. 1991. Williams & Wilkins, Baltimore, pp. 1268, 1277. (Two clinically oriented chapters that deal with non-Hodgkin's lymphoma, including classification and pathology.)

THIRTEEN

The Respiratory System

MARY F. LIPSCOMB, M.D.

ATELECTASIS

PEDIATRIC LUNG DISEASES
  Respiratory Distress Syndrome of the
    Newborn
  Sudden Infant Death Syndrome

OBSTRUCTIVE AND RESTRICTIVE LUNG
DISEASES

OBSTRUCTIVE LUNG DISEASES
  Asthma
  Chronic Obstructive Lung Diseases
    Emphysema
    Chronic Bronchitis
  Bronchiectasis

RESTRICTIVE LUNG DISEASES
  Acute Restrictive Lung Diseases
    Adult Respiratory Distress Syndrome –
      Diffuse Alveolar Damage
  Chronic Restrictive Lung Diseases
    Idiopathic Pulmonary Fibrosis
    Sarcoidosis
    Hypersensitivity Pneumonitis
    Diffuse Pulmonary Hemorrhage
      Syndromes

VASCULAR LUNG DISEASES
  Pulmonary Thromboembolism, Hemorrhage,
    and Infarction
  Pulmonary Hypertension and Vascular
    Sclerosis

PULMONARY INFECTIONS
  Acute Bacterial Pneumonias
  Primary Atypical Pneumonias
  Actinomycosis and Nocardiosis
  Tuberculosis
    Primary Tuberculosis
    Secondary Tuberculosis (Reactivation
      Tuberculosis)
  Fungal Infections
    Histoplasmosis
    Coccidioidomycosis
    Candidiasis
    Other Fungal Infections

Lung Abscess
Cytomegalovirus Infections
Pneumocystis Pneumonia

LUNG TUMORS
  Bronchogenic Carcinoma
  Bronchial Carcinoid
  Malignant Mesothelioma

BENIGN PLEURAL LESIONS
  Pleural Effusion and Pleuritis
  Pneumothorax, Hemothorax, and Chylothorax

LESIONS OF THE UPPER RESPIRATORY TRACT
  Acute Infections
  Nasopharyngeal Carcinoma
  Laryngeal Tumors
    Benign Tumors
    Carcinoma of the Larynx

The major function of the lung is to excrete carbon dioxide from blood and replenish oxygen. The chest wall and diaphragm act as bellows to move air in and out of the lungs, allowing gas exchange across the alveolar-capillary membrane. Obviously, opportunities for disease in this important organ system are legion. A common approach in the study of lung pathology, and one that provides the framework for this chapter, is to organize lung diseases into those affecting (1) the airways, (2) the interstitium, and (3) the pulmonary vascular system. This division into discrete compartments is, of course, deceptively neat. In reality, disease in one compartment is generally accompanied by alterations of morphology and function in another.

The respiratory system includes, in addition to the lungs, (1) the diaphragm and muscles of the chest wall, (2) the regulatory neural circuits, (3) the pleural spaces, and (4) the upper respiratory tract (nasopharynx and trachea, including the larynx). Diseases affecting the first two will not be discussed but those affecting the pleura and upper respiratory tract will be considered after a discussion of the diseases of lung. We begin our discussion with atelectasis since it can complicate many primary lung disorders.

ATELECTASIS

Atelectasis is loss of lung volume due to inadequate *expansion of air spaces*. It is associated with shunting of inadequately oxygenated blood from pulmonary arteries into veins, thus giving rise to a ventilation-perfusion imbalance and hypoxia. On the basis of the underlying mechanism or the distribution of alveolar collapse, atelectasis is divided into the following categories (Fig. 13–1).

Resorption Atelectasis. *Resorption atelectasis* occurs when an obstruction prevents air from reaching distal airways. The air already present gradually becomes absorbed and alveolar collapse follows. It is important to note that bronchial obstruction does not inevitably lead to atelectasis because there is extensive collateral air flow in the lungs. Depending on the level of airway obstruction, an entire lung, a complete lobe, or a patchy segment may be involved. The most frequent cause of resorption collapse is obstruction of a bronchus by a mucous or mucopurulent plug. This frequently occurs postoperatively but may also complicate bronchial asthma, bronchiectasis, or acute or chronic bronchitis. Sometimes obstruction is caused by the aspiration of foreign bodies, particularly in children, or blood clots during oral surgery or anesthesia. Airways may also be obstructed by tumors (especially bronchogenic carcinoma), by enlarged lymph nodes (as from tuberculosis), and, rarely, by vascular aneurysms.

Compression Atelectasis. *Compression atelectasis* (sometimes called passive or relaxation atelectasis) is usually associated with accumulations of fluid, blood, or air within the pleural cavity, which mechanically collapse the adjacent lung. This is a frequent occurrence with pleural effusions, caused most commonly by congestive heart failure. Leakage of air into the pleural cavity (pneumothorax) also leads to compression atelectasis. Basal atelectasis resulting from the elevated position of the diaphragm commonly occurs in bedridden patients, in patients with ascites, and in surgical patients during and after the operation.

Microatelectasis. *Microatelectasis* (or nonobstructive atelectasis) is a generalized loss of lung expansion due to a complex set of events, the most important of which is loss of surfactant. Microatelectasis is present in both adult and neonatal respiratory distress syndromes and in several lung diseases associated with interstitial inflammation. It is also believed to be an important component of postsurgical atelectasis.

Contraction Atelectasis. *Contraction* (or cicatrization) *atelectasis* occurs when either local or generalized fibrotic changes in the lung or pleura hamper expansion and increase elastic recoil during expiration.

> With massive pulmonary parenchymal collapse, or with a large pneumothorax, the entire lung may be folded against the mediastinum, although the collapse is usually not complete. Compression atelectasis, whether related to pleural effusions or elevated diaphragms, is usually basal and bilateral. The collapsed lung parenchyma is shrunken below the level of the surrounding lung substance and is purple, rubbery, and subcrepitant, with a wrinkled overlying pleura. Histologically, the collapsed alveoli are slit-like. Congestion and dilatation of the septal vasculature are usually present. Edema fluid is often present in the alveolar spaces, and in later stages foamy alveolar macrophages may accumulate. Compensatory overinflation of unaffected lung tissue usually occurs. In long-standing cases, fibrosis and chronic inflammation may develop.

Atelectasis (except that caused by contraction) is potentially reversible and should be treated promptly to prevent hypoxemia and superimposed infection of the collapsed lung.

PEDIATRIC LUNG DISEASES

RESPIRATORY DISTRESS SYNDROME OF THE NEWBORN

There are many causes of respiratory distress in the newborn, including excessive sedation of the mother,

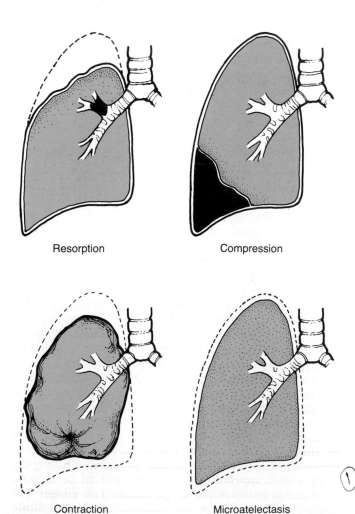

Resorption

Compression

Contraction

Microatelectasis

Figure 13–1. Various forms of atelectasis in adults.

fetal head injury during delivery, aspiration of blood or amniotic fluid, and intrauterine hypoxia due to coiling of the umbilical cord about the neck. However, the most common cause is respiratory distress syndrome (RDS), also known as *hyaline membrane disease* because of the formation of "membranes" in the peripheral air spaces of infants who succumb to this condition. Although with the other causes of respiratory distress the newborn may be apneic or hypoxic from the moment of birth, infants with RDS usually appear normal at birth but within minutes to a few hours develop a labored, grunting respiration that progressively worsens and, unless controlled by therapy, causes death. Indeed, RDS is the major cause of death in the neonatal period.

RDS is basically a disease of premature infants. It affects 15 to 20% of those born between 32 and 36 weeks' gestation and the prevalence increases to 60% for infants delivered before 28 weeks. Other contributing influences are diabetes in the mother, caesarian section before the onset of labor, and prenatal asphyxia. Males are at greater risk than females.

PATHOGENESIS. The fundamental defect in RDS is the inability of immature lung to synthesize sufficient surfactant. Surfactant is a complex of surface-active lipids, principally dipalmitoyl phosphatidyl choline (lecithin) and at least two proteins thought to be essential to the normal function and metabolism of the lipid. It is synthesized by type II pneumocytes and, with the healthy newborn's first breath, rapidly coats the surface of alveoli, reducing surface tension and thus decreasing the pressure required to keep alveoli open. In a lung deficient in surfactant, alveoli tend to collapse and a relatively greater inspiratory effort is required with each breath to open the alveoli. The infant rapidly tires of breathing, and generalized atelectasis sets in. The resulting hypoxia sets into motion a sequence of events that lead to epithelial and endothelial damage and eventually to the formation of hyaline membranes (Fig. 13–2).

Surfactant synthesis is regulated by hormones. Corticosteroids stimulate the formation of surfactant lipids and associated apoproteins. Thyroxine acts synergistically with corticosteroids, but insulin antagonizes this effect. Uncontrolled diabetes in a pregnant woman gives rise to compensatory hyperinsulinism in the fetus, which in turn can suppress surfactant synthesis. This may explain the higher risk of RDS in infants born to diabetic mothers.

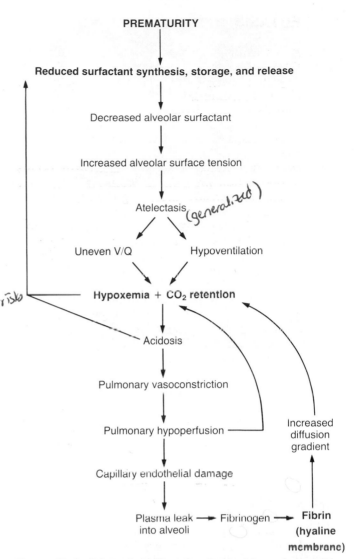

Figure 13–2. Schematic outline of pathophysiology of respiratory distress syndrome. (V/Q, ventilation-perfusion ratio.) (From Oh, W., Stern, L.: Respiratory diseases of the newborn. *In* Stern, L., Vert, P. (eds.): Neonatal Medicine. New York, Masson Publishing USA, 1987, p. 396.)

MORPHOLOGY. The lungs in RDS are of normal size but are heavy and relatively airless. They have a mottled purple color and microscopically the tissue appears solid, with poorly developed, generally collapsed (atelectatic) alveoli. If the infant dies within the first several hours of life, only necrotic cellular debris is present in the terminal bronchioles and alveolar ducts. Later in the course hyaline membranes line the respiratory bronchioles, alveolar ducts, and random alveoli (Fig. 13–3). These "membranes," produced by increased capillary permeability, consist mainly of fibrinogen and fibrin admixed with necrotic epithelial cells. In addition to the formation of membranes, there is intense vascular congestion. If the infant dies after several days, evidence of reparative changes, including proliferation of alveolar lining cells and interstitial fibrosis, is seen.

Treatment is designed to support ventilation until the infant is able to breathe on its own, which in milder cases can be expected by the third or fourth day of life. In some centers use of aerosolized human, animal, or synthetic surfactants produces a gratifying reduction in mortality, so that now overall 85 to 90% of these infants survive to go home. The greater the birth weight the better the outlook. Death and morbidity may result not only from hypoxemia but also

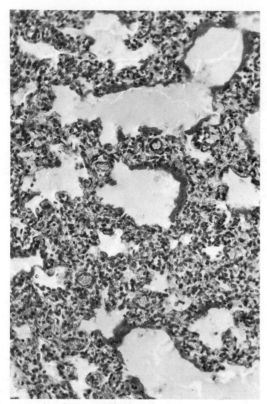

Figure 13-3. Hyaline membrane disease. There is atelectasis of alveoli and dilatation of alveolar ducts, which are filled with fluid and lined by thick hyaline membranes.

from (1) intraventricular hemorrhage, to which the immature brain is particularly vulnerable during hypoxemia, (2) heart failure secondary to patent ductus arteriosus, and (3) necrotizing enterocolitis.

A minority of the infants who survive suffer long-term sequelae related to neurodevelopmental defects and chronic lung disease. The neurologic abnormalities result from the effects of hypoxia on neurons or from intracerebral hemorrhage. The chronic lung disease manifested as *bronchopulmonary dysplasia* is multifactorial. It results from the primary anoxic injury as well as exposure to high concentrations of oxygen and positive pressure ventilation required for the treatment of these severely ill infants. Pathologic findings in bronchopulmonary dysplasia include metaplasia of bronchial epithelium, peribronchial fibrosis, hypertrophy of bronchial smooth muscle, fibrotic obliteration of bronchioles, and overdistended alveoli. In some of these patients abnormal radiographic findings and pulmonary function persist into adulthood.

The most effective method of reducing the morbidity and mortality from RDS is prevention—notably prevention of premature delivery until the maturing lung is capable of adequate surfactant synthesis. Reasonably reliable estimates of fetal pulmonary maturity can be achieved by measuring the concentration of surfactant in amniotic fluid obtained by amniocentesis. The most common test is the lecithin-sphingomyelin ratio (L/S). The lecithin level rises sharply at 34 to 36 weeks' gestation, whereas the level of sphingomyelin

either falls or does not change. An L/S ratio of 2 indicates fetal pulmonary maturity, 1.2 indicates a possible risk of RDS, and less than 1 a definite risk. When the test indicates pulmonary immaturity, efforts are made to delay delivery until the lung matures. If early delivery is unavoidable, administration of corticosteroids to the mother may decrease the risk of RDS by increasing surfactant synthesis.

SUDDEN INFANT DEATH SYNDROME

The current definition of sudden infant death syndrome (SIDS) is: *the sudden and unexpected death of an infant under one year of age whose death remains unexplained after the performance of an adequate autopsy, examination of the scene of death, and review of the case history.* SIDS, sometimes referred to as "crib death," is discussed here because most evidence favors some form of respiratory dysfunction as the primary cause in most cases. Often these infants have had prior irregularities of the respiratory rhythm with apneic spells, sometimes prolonged (near SIDS), which either resolved spontaneously or required resuscitation. Thus abnormal breathing patterns predict a high risk for SIDS. Usually death occurs during sleep and without apparent struggle. SIDS is not a rare event, accounting for approximately 7000 deaths annually in the United States. It is the single most common cause of death in infants younger than one year once they are out of the immediate neonatal period. Even higher rates are encountered in many developing countries. Many factors relating to both mother and infant are associated with an increased risk of SIDS (Table 13-1).

Anatomic studies of victims have yielded a variety of findings, although these are usually subtle, of uncertain significance, and not present in all cases. But by definition an overt cause of death such as bronchopneumonia or a lethal malformation is lacking. In about two thirds of cases, subtle alterations have been identified in the structures that control respiratory and cardiac rhythm (brain stem, carotid bodies, vagus nerves) and in tissues sensitive to chronic hypoxemia (brain, lungs, periadrenal brown fat). These changes

TABLE 13-1. FACTORS ASSOCIATED WITH SIDS

Maternal	Infant
Youth (less than 20 years of age)	Prematurity
	Low birth weight
Unmarried	Male sex
Short intergestational intervals	Product of a multiple birth
	Not the first sibling
Low socioeconomic group	SIDS in a prior sibling
Smoking	
Drug abuse	
African-American (? socioeconomic)	

could well lead to or be secondary to chronic hypoxia, so the possibility exists that they are not, of themselves, the basic defects. Airway blockage has been implicated, such as might occur with a particularly large tongue that might recess during sleep, a hypermobile mandible that might prolapse during deep sleep, or laryngeal mucous gland hyperplasia that could contribute to excessive secretions. The inconstancy of these findings is not surprising, because many different mechanisms could all lead to sudden death.

In about a third of SIDS cases mechanisms other than those relating to the cardiopulmonary systems have been implicated. Principal among these is infection. Most deaths occur during the winter months and therefore upper respiratory viral infections are suspected. Furthermore, attention has been drawn to unsuspected intestinal infections by *Clostridium botulinum* as a potential cause of death. Defective control of body temperature, leading to acute and lethal development of hyperthermia (malignant hyperthermia) has also been incriminated. This is difficult to document, however, because the infants have often been dead for several hours when discovered. Suffice it to say that the cause of SIDS is unknown; and unfortunately only when the cause is known will there be hope of preventing these tragic deaths.

OBSTRUCTIVE AND RESTRICTIVE LUNG DISEASES

Diffuse pulmonary diseases can be classified in two categories: (1) *obstructive disease* (airway disease), characterized by an increase in resistance to air flow due to partial or complete obstruction at any level and (2) *restrictive disease*, characterized by reduced expansion of lung parenchyma accompanied by decreased total lung capacity.

The *major obstructive disorders* (excluding tumor or inhalation of a foreign body) are *asthma, emphysema, chronic bronchitis, bronchiectasis, cystic fibrosis, and bronchiolitis*. In patients with these diseases, total lung capacity (TLC) is either normal or increased but the hallmark is a decreased expiratory flow rate. Expiratory obstruction may result either from anatomic airway narrowing, classically observed in asthma, or from loss of elastic recoil, characteristic of emphysema.

In contrast, in *restrictive diseases*, TLC is reduced and the expiratory flow rate is normal. The restrictive defect occurs in two general conditions: (1) *extrapulmonary disorders* that affect the ability of the chest wall to act as a bellows (e.g., severe obesity, kyphoscoliosis, and neuromuscular disorders such as the Guillain-Barré syndrome, p. 734, that affect the respiratory muscles) and (2) *acute or chronic interstitial lung diseases*. The classic acute restrictive disease is adult respiratory distress syndrome (ARDS). *Chronic* restrictive diseases include the pneumoconioses (p. 220), sarcoidosis, and idiopathic pulmonary fibrosis.

OBSTRUCTIVE LUNG DISEASES

ASTHMA

Asthma is characterized by episodic, reversible bronchoconstriction resulting from increased responsiveness of the tracheobronchial tree to various stimuli. The basis of bronchial hyperreactivity is not entirely clear, but accumulating evidence suggests that persistent bronchial inflammation plays an important role. Clinically, asthma is manifested by dyspnea, cough, and wheezing (a soft whistling sound during expiration). This common disease affects about 5% of adults and 7 to 10% of children.

Because asthma is a heterogeneous disease triggered by a variety of inciting agents there is no universally accepted simple classification. Nevertheless, it is customary to classify asthma into two major categories based on the presence or absence of an underlying immune disorder:

(1) *Extrinsic asthma*, in which the asthmatic episode is initiated by a type I hypersensitivity reaction induced by exposure to an extrinsic antigen (p. 122). Three types of extrinsic asthma are recognized: *atopic asthma, occupational asthma* (many forms), and *allergic bronchopulmonary aspergillosis* (bronchial colonization with *Aspergillus* organisms followed by development of immunoglobulin E [IgE] antibodies). *Atopic asthma is the most common type of asthma; its onset is usually in the first two decades of life, and it is commonly associated with other allergic manifestations in the patient as well as in other family members.*

(2) *Intrinsic asthma*, in which the triggering mechanisms are nonimmune. In this form, a number of stimuli can initiate bronchospasm, including (a) aspirin, (b) pulmonary infections, especially those caused by viruses, (c) cold, (d) psychological stress, (e) exercise, and (f) inhaled irritants such as sulfur dioxide. *It must be emphasized, however, that, because of inherent tracheobronchial hyperreactivity, a person who has extrinsic asthma is also susceptible to developing an asthmatic attack when exposed to one of the mentioned agents. Thus, in many cases a neat distinction between intrinsic and extrinsic asthma is not possible.*

PATHOGENESIS. As emphasized at the outset, the common denominator underlying all forms of asthma is increased airway reactivity to a variety of stimuli. Bronchial hyperresponsiveness can be readily demonstrated in the form of increased sensitivity to bronchoconstrictive agents such as histamine or methacholine (a cholinergic agonist). It seems that persons with an "asthmatic diathesis" are primed to develop acute episodes of bronchospasm when they encounter any one of the inciting agents (extrinsic or intrinsic) mentioned earlier.

Although the importance of airway hyperirritability is established, the basis of the abnormal bronchial response is not fully understood. *Most current evidence suggests that bronchial inflammation is the substrate for hyperresponsiveness.* Persistent inflammation of bronchi, manifested by the presence of inflammatory cells (particularly eosinophils, lymphocytes, mast cells) and by damage to the bronchial epithelium, is a constant feature of bronchial asthma, rendering the airways hyperresponsive to various stimuli.

What causes the bronchial inflammation? In the allergic or atopic asthma, it is readily explained by type I hypersensitivity reactions but the cause is much less clear in those with so-called intrinsic asthma. Because the basis of bronchial inflammation is better understood in allergic (atopic) asthma, this will be considered first. The details of type I hypersensitivity were discussed in an earlier chapter (p. 122), so only a brief capsule with emphasis on mechanisms that are of particular importance in the pathogenesis of asthma

will be reviewed (Fig. 13–4). Like all type I hypersensitivity reactions, attacks of atopic asthma often demonstrate two phases, an early phase, beginning between 30 and 60 minutes after antigen exposure and then remitting, followed 4 to 8 hours later by a more protracted late phase. As might be expected, the initial triggering of mast cells occurs on the mucosal surface; the resultant mediator release opens mucosal intercellular junctions, allowing penetration of the antigen to more numerous submucosal mast cells. In addition, direct stimulation of subepithelial vagal (parasympathetic) receptors provokes reflex bronchoconstriction. As detailed on page 123, mast cell activation leads to

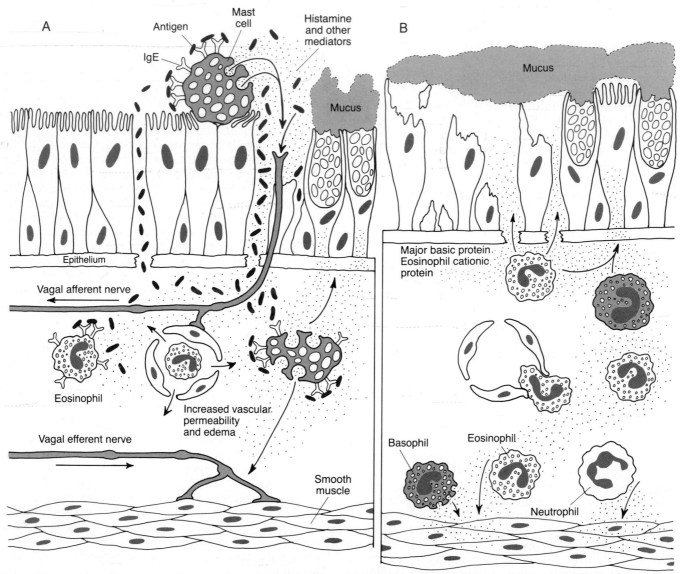

Figure 13–4. A model for immediate and late stages of allergic asthma. *A,* The immediate reaction is triggered by Ag-induced cross-linking of IgE bound to IgE receptors (FcRε) on mast cells (and possibly FcRε-expressing eosinophils and macrophages) in the airways. These cells release preformed mediators that open tight junctions between epithelial cells. Antigen can then enter the mucosa to activate mucosal mast cells and eosinophils, which in turn release additional mediators. Collectively the mediators, either directly or via neuronal reflexes, induce bronchospasm, increased vascular permeability, and mucus production as well as recruit additional mediator-releasing cells from the blood. *B,* The arrival of recruited cells signals the initiation of the late stage of asthma, in which residual antigen binding to IgE (not shown) may trigger a fresh round of mediator release. Factors, particularly from eosinophils, may also stimulate release of mediators from other inflammatory cells and cause damage to the epithelium. (Modified from Lichtenstein, L.: The nasal late phase response—an in vivo model. Hosp. Pract. *23:*121, 1988).

the release of a variety of primary and secondary mediators. Those considered important in the pathogenesis of asthma include:

- Leukotrienes C4, D4, and E4; these are extremely potent mediators that cause prolonged bronchoconstriction, increase vascular permeability, and increase mucin secretion.
- Prostaglandin D_2 (PGD_2), which elicits bronchoconstriction and vasodilatation.
- Eosinophilic and neutrophilic chemotactic factors, and leukotriene B4, which recruit and activate eosinophils and neutrophils.
- Platelet-activating factor (PAF), which causes aggregation of platelets and release of histamine from their granules; *more important, PAF causes sustained recruitment of eosinophils into the lungs.*

Together these mediators induce bronchoconstriction, edema, and mucus secretion; these initial reactions are followed by the late phase, which is dominated by additional recruitment of leukocytes —basophils, neutrophils, and eosinophils. Not only do these cells release additional waves of mediators and thus intensify the initial response, they also cause epithelial cell damage. *Eosinophils* are particularly important in this phase. Their armamentarium of mediators is as extensive as that of mast cells and in addition they produce major basic protein (MBP) and eosinophil cationic protein (ECP), which are toxic to the epithelial cells. Activated eosinophils also produce leukotriene C4 and PAF and directly activate mast cells to release mediators. Thus eosinophils can amplify and sustain the inflammatory response without additional exposure to the triggering antigen.

The mechanism of bronchial inflammation and hyperresponsiveness is much less clear in patients with intrinsic (nonatopic) asthma. Incriminated in such cases are *viral infections of the respiratory tract and inhaled air pollutants such as sulfur dioxide, ozone, and nitrogen dioxide.* In some of these patients bronchial hyperresponsiveness is superimposed on clinically manifest chronic bronchitis—referred to as chronic asthmatic bronchitis (p. 396). In such patients the distinction between chronic bronchitis and asthma may be quite hazy.

In closing it should be mentioned that bronchial hyperresponsiveness has also been ascribed to some fundamental defect in autonomic regulation. Perhaps there is a hereditary or acquired overactivity of the cholinergic (constrictor) response or reduced activity of the β-adrenergic (bronchodilator) pathway; however, the possible existence and importance of an underlying abnormality in the autonomic control of bronchial constriction is still unproved.

MORPHOLOGY. The morphologic changes in asthma have been described principally in patients who die of prolonged severe attacks, but it appears that in nonfatal cases the pathologic process is similar albeit less pronounced. Grossly, the lungs are overdistended because of overinflation, and there may be small areas of atelectasis. **The most striking macroscopic finding is occlusion of bronchi and bronchioles by thick, tenacious mucus plugs.** Histologically, the mucus plugs contain whorls of shed epithelium (Curschmann's spirals). Numerous eosinophils and Charcot-Leyden crystals (collections of crystalloids made up of eosinophil proteins) are also present. The other characteristic histologic findings in asthma include: (1) patchy necrosis of epithelial cells; (2) an increase in fibrous tissue immediately beneath the basement membrane, giving the appearance of a thickened basement membrane; (3) edema and an inflammatory infiltrate in the bronchial walls, with prominent eosinophils, which may constitute 5 to 50% of the cellular infiltrate; also present are mast cells and basophils, macrophages, lymphocytes, and plasma cells, and some neutrophils; (4) an increase in size of the submucosal mucous glands (or increased numbers of goblet cells in bronchiolar epithelium); and (5) hypertrophy of the bronchial wall muscle, a reflection of prolonged vasoconstriction.

CLINICAL COURSE. An asthma attack is characterized by severe dyspnea with wheezing; the chief difficulty is in expiration. The victim labors to get air into the lungs and then cannot get it out, so that there is progressive hyperinflation of the lungs with air trapped distal to the bronchi, which are constricted and filled with mucus and debris. In the usual case, attacks last from one to several hours and subside either spontaneously or with therapy, usually bronchodilators and corticosteroids. Intervals between attacks are characteristically free from respiratory difficulty, but persistent, subtle respiratory deficits can be detected by spirometric methods. Occasionally, a severe paroxysm occurs that does not respond to therapy and persists for days and even weeks *(status asthmaticus).* The associated hypercarbia, acidosis, and severe hypoxia may be fatal, although in most cases the disease is more disabling than lethal. Many children "outgrow" asthma, although in those with the most hyperreactive airways the vulnerability to recurrent attacks persists into adulthood. The frequency with which chronic obstructive pulmonary disease (COPD) develops later is not known, but the risk is thought to be small unless the patient takes up cigarette smoking.

CHRONIC OBSTRUCTIVE LUNG DISEASES

Despite the wide use of the designation chronic obstructive pulmonary disease, or COPD, there is no general agreement on its precise definition. According to some, it is defined strictly on the basis of pulmonary function tests and is said to exist when there is objective evidence of persisting (and irreversible) air flow obstruction. Others use the term more broadly to include two common conditions: chronic bronchitis and emphysema, recognizing that in some cases either of these conditions can exist without air flow obstruction. Despite these uncertainties, one thing is clear: *by the time patients with chronic bronchitis or emphysema develop sufficient dyspnea (breathlessness) to seek medical attention, airway obstruction can be readily demonstrated.* Furthermore, as will be emphasized again, these two conditions often coexist, so on practical clinical grounds the grouping of chronic bronchitis and emphysema under the rubric of COPD is justified.

Emphysema

Emphysema is characterized by *permanent enlargement of the air spaces* distal to the terminal bronchioles accompanied by *destruction of their walls.* There are several conditions in which enlargement of air spaces is not accompanied by destruction; this is more correctly called *overinflation.* For example, the distention of air spaces in the opposite lung following unilateral pneumonectomy is compensatory overinflation rather than emphysema.

The relationship between chronic bronchitis and emphysema is complicated, but the use of precise definitions has helped bring some order to what was once chaos. At the outset it should be emphasized that the definition of emphysema is a morphologic one, whereas chronic bronchitis (defined later, p. 396) is characterized in clinical terms by the presence of chronic and recurrent cough with excess mucus secretion. Although chronic bronchitis may exist without demonstrable emphysema and almost pure emphy-

sema may occur (particularly in patients with inherited α_1-antitrypsin deficiency), the two diseases usually coexist, because the major pathogenic mechanism, cigarette smoking, is common to both. Predictably, when the two entities coexist, the clinical and physiologic features overlap.

TYPES OF EMPHYSEMA. Emphysema is not only defined in terms of the anatomic nature of the lesion but it is further classified according to its distribution in the lobule and acinus. Recall that an acinus is the part of lung distal to the terminal bronchiole and a cluster of three to five acini is referred to as a lobule. There are three types of emphysema: (1) centriacinar, (2) panacinar, and (3) distal acinar. The first two are more important but their differentiation is often difficult in advanced disease and so they are briefly diagrammed (Fig. 13–5) and described below.

Centriacinar (Centrilobular) Emphysema. The distinctive feature of this type of emphysema is the pattern of involvement of the lobules: the central or proximal parts of the acini, formed by respiratory bronchioles, are affected, while distal alveoli are spared. Thus, both emphysematous and normal air spaces exist within the same acinus and lobule (Fig. 13–6A). The lesions are more common and severe in the upper lobes, particularly in the apical segments. In severe centriacinar emphysema the distal acinus also becomes involved, and so, as noted, the differentiation from panacinar emphysema becomes difficult.

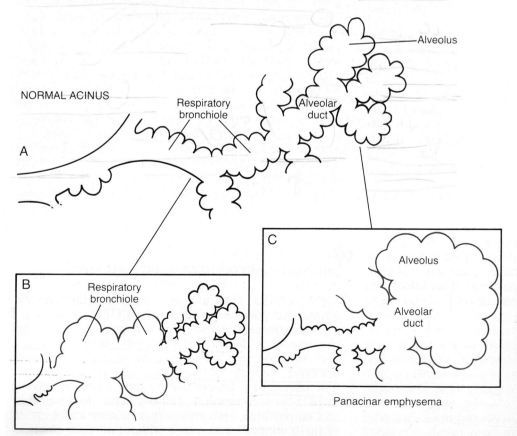

NORMAL ACINUS

Alveolus

Respiratory bronchiole

Alveolar duct

A

B

Respiratory bronchiole

Centrilobular emphysema

C

Alveolus

Alveolar duct

Panacinar emphysema

Figure 13–5. *A,* Diagram of normal structures within the acinus, the fundamental unit of the lung. A terminal bronchiole (not shown) is immediately proximal to the respiratory bronchiole. *B,* Centrilobular emphysema with dilatation that initially affects the respiratory bronchioles. *C,* Panacinar emphysema with initial distention of the peripheral structures (i.e., alveolus and alveolar duct); the disease later extends to affect the respiratory bronchioles. (RB, respiratory bronchiole; AD, alveolar duct; AS, alveolus.)

Figure 13–6. *A,* Centrilobular emphysema (magnification ×5). The pulmonary arteries contain injected barium. The emphysematous foci (E) abut the arteries but normal alveolar spaces are adjacent to the septa (S). *B,* Panacinar emphysema (×5) demonstrates a more generalized distribution of the permanently enlarged emphysematous foci. Compare with *A.* (From Bates, D. V., et al.: Respiratory Function in Disease. 2nd ed. Philadelphia, W. B. Saunders, 1971.)

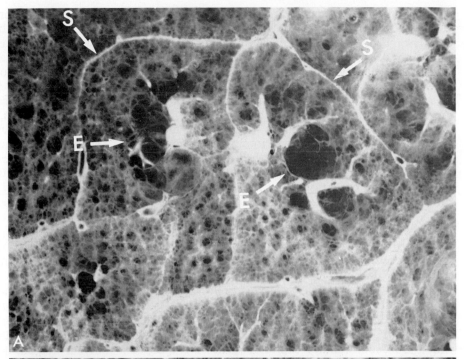

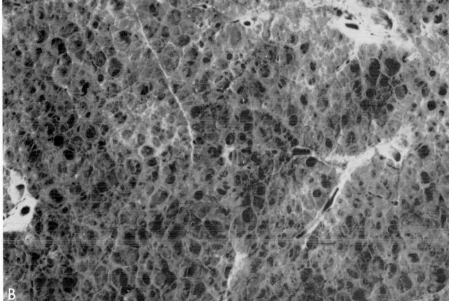

Panacinar (Panlobular) Emphysema. In this type of emphysema the acini are uniformly enlarged from the level of the respiratory bronchiole to the terminal blind alveoli (Fig. 13–6B). In contrast to centriacinar emphysema, panacinar emphysema tends to occur more commonly in the lower lung zones and is the type of emphysema that occurs in α_1-antitrypsin deficiency.

Distal Acinar (Paraseptal) Emphysema. In this form the proximal portion of the acinus is normal but the distal part is dominantly involved. The emphysema is more striking adjacent to the pleura, along the lobular connective tissue septa, and at the margins of the lobules. It occurs adjacent to areas of fibrosis, scarring, or atelectasis and is usually more severe in the upper half of the lungs. The characteristic findings are of multiple, contiguous, enlarged air spaces that range in diameter from less than 0.5 mm to more than 2.0 cm, sometimes forming cyst-like structures that with progressive enlargement are referred to as bullae. This type of emphysema probably underlies many of the cases of spontaneous pneumothorax in young adults.

INCIDENCE. Emphysema is a common disease, but its precise incidence is difficult to estimate because a definite diagnosis, which is based on morphology, can be made only by examination of the lungs at autopsy. In one autopsy series, it was present in 65% of adult men and 25% of adult women. Most were asymptomatic. Emphysema, especially centriacinar, is much more common and more severe in men than in women. *There is a clear association between heavy* _cigarette smoking and emphysema,_ and the most severe type occurs in those who smoke heavily. Although emphysema does not become disabling until the fifth to eighth decade of life, ventilatory deficits may become clinically evident decades earlier. Indeed, emphysematous changes were found in the lungs of teenagers who died of accidental causes and who had been exposed to environmental air pollution.

PATHOGENESIS. The genesis of the two common forms of emphysema—centriacinar and panacinar—is unsettled. The most plausible hypothesis to explain alveolar wall destruction and air space enlargement _invokes excess protease or elastase activity unopposed by appropriate antiprotease regulation_ (Fig. 13–7).

This hypothesis is based on the observation that patients with a genetic deficiency of the antiprotease α_1-antitrypsin have a markedly enhanced tendency to develop pulmonary emphysema, which is compounded by smoking. About 2% of all patients with emphysema have this defect. α_1-Antitrypsin, normally present in serum, tissue fluids, and macrophages, is a major inhibitor of proteases (particularly elastase) secreted by neutrophils during inflammation. This enzyme is encoded by codominantly expressed genes on the proteinase inhibitor (Pi) locus on chromosome 14. The Pi locus is extremely polymorphic, with approximately 80 different alleles. Most common is the normal (M) allele and the corresponding PiMM phenotype. Approximately 0.012% of the United States population is homozygous for the Z allele (PiZZ), associated with markedly decreased serum levels of α_1-antitrypsin. Many of these persons develop symptomatic emphysema.

The following sequence is postulated: (1) Neutrophils (the principal source of cellular elastase) are normally sequestered in peripheral capillaries, including those in the lung, and a few gain access to the alveolar spaces. (2) Any stimulus that increases either the number of leukocytes (neutrophils and macrophages) in the lung or the release of their elastase-containing granules will increase elastolytic activity. (3) With low levels of serum α_1-antitrypsin, elastic tissue destruction is unchecked and emphysema results. _Thus, emphysema is seen to result from the destructive effect of high protease activity in subjects with low antiprotease activity._ This hypothesis is strongly supported by studies in experimental animals in which intratracheal instillation of the proteolytic enzymes

papain and, more important, human neutrophil elastase, results in the degradation of elastin accompanied by the development of emphysema.

The protease-antiprotease hypothesis also helps explain the effect of cigarette smoking in the production of emphysema, particularly the centriacinar form in subjects with normal α_1-antitrypsin levels.

- Smokers have greater numbers of neutrophils and macrophages in their alveoli.
- Smoking stimulates release of elastase from neutrophils.
- Smoking enhances elastase activity in macrophages; macrophage elastase is not inhibited by α_1-antitrypsin, and indeed can proteolytically digest this antiprotease.
- Oxidants in cigarette smoke and oxygen free radicals secreted by neutrophils inhibit α_1-antitrypsin and thus decrease net anti-elastase activity in smokers.

In summary, it is likely that impaction of smoke particles predominantly at the bifurcation of respiratory bronchioles results in the influx of neutrophils and macrophages, both of which secrete elastase. An increase in the elastase activity localized in the centriacinar region, together with the smoke-induced decrease of α_1-antitrypsin activity, causes the centriacinar pattern of emphysema seen in smokers. This schema also explains the additive influence of smoking and α_1-antitrypsin deficiency in inducing serious obstructive airway disease.

MORPHOLOGY. The diagnosis and classification of emphysema depend largely on the macroscopic appearance of lung. Panacinar emphysema, when well developed, produces pale, voluminous lungs, which often obscure the heart when the anterior chest wall is removed at autopsy. The macroscopic features of centriacinar emphysema are less impressive. The lungs are a deeper pink and less voluminous unless the disease is well advanced. Generally in centriacinar emphysema the upper two thirds of the lungs is more severely affected than the lower lungs and may demonstrate bullae.

Histologically, there is thinning and destruction of alveolar walls. With advanced disease, adjacent alveoli become confluent, creating large air spaces. Terminal and respiratory bronchioles may be deformed because of the loss of septa that help tether these structures in

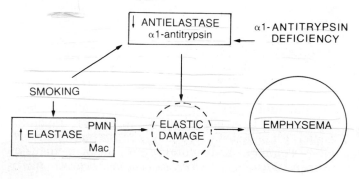

Figure 13–7. Protease-antiprotease mechanism of emphysema. Smoking inhibits antielastase and favors the recruitment of leukocytes and release of elastase. (PMN, polymorphonuclear leukocytes; Mac, alveolar macrophages.)

the parenchyma. With the loss of elastic tissue in the surrounding alveolar septa, there is reduced radial traction on the small airways. As a result they tend to collapse during expiration—an important cause of chronic air flow obstruction in severe emphysema. In addition to alveolar loss, the number of alveolar capillaries is diminished. There may be evidence of accompanying bronchitis and bronchiolitis.

CLINICAL COURSE. The clinical manifestations of emphysema do not appear until at least one third of the pulmonary parenchyma is affected. Dyspnea is usually the first symptom; it begins insidiously but is steadily progressive. In patients with underlying chronic bronchitis or chronic asthmatic bronchitis, cough and wheezing are initial complaints. Weight loss is common and may be so severe as to suggest a hidden malignant tumor.

The classical presentation in patients who have no "bronchitic" component is one in which the patient is barrel-chested and dyspneic, with obviously prolonged expiration, sitting forward in a hunched-over position, attempting to squeeze the air out of the lungs with each expiratory effort. In these patients overdistention is severe and diffusing capacity is low. Dyspnea and hyperventilation are prominent, so that until very late in the disease gas exchange is adequate and blood gas values are relatively normal. Because of prominent dyspnea and adequate oxygenation of hemoglobin these patients are sometimes called "pink puffers."

On the other extreme are patients with emphysema who also have pronounced chronic bronchitis and a history of recurrent infections and purulent sputum. They usually have less prominent dyspnea and respiratory drive, so they retain carbon dioxide, become hypoxic, and are often cyanotic. For reasons not entirely clear, they tend to be obese. Often they seek medical help after the onset of congestive heart failure (cor pulmonale, p. 315) and associated edema. Patients with this clinical picture are sometimes unflatteringly called "blue bloaters."

Most patients with emphysema and COPD fall somewhere between these two classic extremes. For all of them a hazard is that hypoxemia can lead to pulmonary vascular spasm, pulmonary hypertension, and cor pulmonale. Death from emphysema is related to (1) pulmonary failure with respiratory acidosis, hypoxia, and coma or (2) right-sided heart failure.

CONDITIONS RELATED TO EMPHYSEMA. Several conditions resemble emphysema or are inappropriately referred to as emphysema.

Compensatory emphysema is a term used to designate the compensatory dilatation of alveoli in response to loss of lung substance elsewhere, such as occurs in residual lung parenchyma following surgical removal of a diseased lung or lobe. Usually there is no destruction of septal walls.

Senile emphysema refers to the overdistended lungs of elders, which result from age-related alterations of the internal geometry of the lung (e.g. larger alveolar ducts and smaller alveoli). There is no significant tissue destruction and a better designation for such aging lungs would be **senile hyperinflation.**

Obstructive overinflation refers to the condition in which the lung expands because air is trapped within it. A common cause is subtotal obstruction by a tumor or foreign object. Overinflation in obstructive lesions occurs either (1) because of a ball-valve action of the obstructive agent, so that air enters on inspiration but cannot leave on expiration or (2) because the bronchus may be totally obstructed but ventilation through "collaterals" brings in air from behind the obstruction. Obstructive overinflation can be a life-threatening emergency if the affected portion extends sufficiently to compress the remaining normal lung.

Bullous emphysema refers to any form of emphysema that produces large bullae (spaces more than 1 cm in diameter in the distended state, Fig. 13–8). These

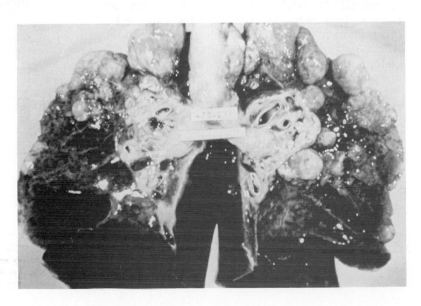

Figure 13-8. Bullous emphysema with large apical and subpleural bullae.

represent localized accentuations of emphysema and are most often subpleural, near the apex. Bullae assume clinical importance if they compress adjacent normal lung to compromise normal ventilatory function or if they rupture to cause pneumothorax (p. 433).

Mediastinal (interstitial) emphysema designates the entrance of air into the connective tissue stroma of the lung, mediastinum, and subcutaneous tissue. This may occur spontaneously with a sudden increase in intraalveolar pressure (as with vomiting or violent coughing) that causes a tear, with dissection of air into the interstitium. Sometimes it occurs in children with whooping cough. It is particularly apt to occur in patients on respirators who have partial bronchiolar obstruction, or in persons who suffer a perforating injury, (e.g., fractured rib). When the interstitial air enters the subcutaneous tissue, the patient may literally blow up like a balloon, with marked swelling of the head and neck and crackling crepitation all over the chest. In most instances the air is resorbed spontaneously when the site of entry is sealed.

Chronic Bronchitis

Chronic bronchitis is common among cigarette smokers and urban dwellers in smog-ridden cities; some studies of men in the 40- to 65-year age group indicate that 20 to 25% have the disease. The diagnosis of chronic bronchitis is made on clinical grounds: *it is defined as a persistent productive cough for at least three consecutive months in at least two consecutive years.* It can occur in several forms. Most patients have *simple chronic bronchitis:* the productive cough raises mucoid sputum, but air flow is not obstructed. If the sputum contains pus, presumably because of secondary infections, the patient is said to have "*chronic mucopurulent bronchitis.*" Some patients with chronic bronchitis may demonstrate hyperresponsive airways and intermittent episodes of asthma. This condition, termed "*chronic asthmatic bronchitis,*" is often difficult to distinguish from atopic asthma. A small subpopulation of bronchitic patients develops chronic outflow obstruction as measured by pulmonary function tests. These patients almost always have evidence of associated emphysema (i.e., permanent enlargement of the air spaces distal to the terminal bronchioles). Thus, it is generally believed (at least in Western countries) that chronic bronchitis is associated with significant outflow obstruction only when it is complicated by emphysema. Between 5 and 15% of smokers develop physiologic evidence of COPD and many of these present initially with chronic bronchitis. At present, it is not possible to determine which cigarette smokers, including those with chronic bronchitis, will develop COPD, with its potentially dire consequences.

PATHOGENESIS. The distinctive feature of chronic bronchitis is hypersecretion of mucus that starts in the large airways. Although the single most important causative factor is cigarette smoking, other air pollutants, such as sulfur dioxide and nitrogen dioxide, may contribute. These irritants, directly or through neurohumoral pathways, induce *hypersecretion of the bronchial mucous glands, cause hypertrophy of mucous glands, and lead to metaplastic formation of mucin-secreting goblet cells in the surface epithelium of bronchi.* Microbial infection is often present, but it plays a secondary role, mainly by maintaining the inflammation and exacerbating symptoms. In addition to the changes in the bronchi, small airway disease affecting bronchioles is also induced by airborne pollutants, as described in greater detail under morphology.

MORPHOLOGY. Grossly, the mucosal lining of the larger airways is usually hyperemic and swollen by edema fluid. Frequently it is covered by a layer of mucinous or mucopurulent secretions. The smaller bronchi and bronchioles may also be filled with similar secretions. Histologically, the diagnostic feature of chronic bronchitis in the trachea and larger bronchi is enlargement of the mucus-secreting glands (Fig. 13–9). The magnitude of the increase in size is assessed by the Reid index, the ratio of the thickness of the submucosal gland layer to that of the bronchial wall. Normally the index is 1:3; with clinically significant chronic bronchitis the ratio usually exceeds 1:2. There is often an increased number of goblet cells in the lining epithelium with concomitant loss of ciliated epithelial cells. Squamous metaplasia frequently develops, followed by dys-

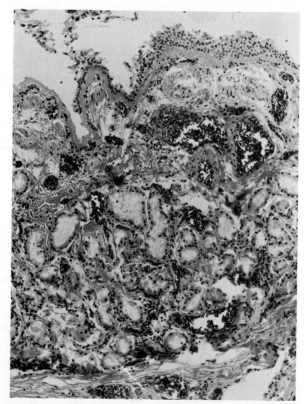

Figure 13–9. Chronic bronchitis. Lumen of bronchus is above. Note slight desquamation of mucosal epithelial cells and marked thickening of mucous gland layer (approximately twice normal). Vascular congestion is evident.

plastic changes in the lining epithelial cells, a sequence of events that may lead to the evolution of bronchogenic carcinoma. A variable density of inflammatory cells, largely mononuclear but sometimes admixed with neutrophils, is frequently present in the bronchial mucosa. **Chronic bronchiolitis,** characterized by goblet cell metaplasia (normally the number of goblet cells is small in peripheral airways), inflammation, fibrosis in the walls, and smooth muscle hyperplasia may also be present. It has been suggested that chronic bronchiolitis may be a morphologic correlate of so-called small airway disease, the forerunner of significant airway obstruction in COPD. The current consensus, however, is that while inflammation of small airways can contribute to mild to moderate airway obstruction, it is the destructive lesions of emphysema with resultant distortion of the small airways that is the most important contributor to expiratory air flow resistance.

CLINICAL COURSE. In patients with chronic bronchitis, a prominent cough and the production of sputum may persist indefinitely without ventilatory dysfunction; however, as alluded to earlier, some patients develop significant COPD with outflow obstruction. This is accompanied by hypercapnia, hypoxemia, and, in severe cases, cyanosis. Differentiation of this form of COPD from that caused by emphysema can be made in the classic case, but as mentioned many patients have both conditions. With progression, chronic bronchitis is complicated by cardiac failure (cor pulmonale, p. 315). Recurrent infections and respiratory failure are constant threats.

BRONCHIECTASIS

Bronchiectasis is the permanent dilatation of bronchi and bronchioles due to destruction of the muscle and elastic supporting tissue, resulting from or associated with chronic necrotizing infections. It is not a primary disease but rather is secondary to persisting infection or obstruction caused by a variety of conditions. Once developed it gives rise to a characteristic symptom complex dominated by cough and expectoration of copious amounts of purulent sputum. Diagnosis depends on an appropriate history along with radiographic demonstration of bronchial dilatation. The conditions that most commonly predispose to bronchiectasis include the following:

1. *Bronchial obstruction.* Common causes are tumors, foreign bodies, and, occasionally, mucus impaction. Under these conditions, the bronchiectasis is localized to the obstructed lung segment. Bronchiectasis can also complicate atopic asthma and chronic bronchitis.
2. *Congenital or hereditary conditions.* Only a few are cited:
   - In cystic fibrosis, widespread severe bronchiectasis is a reflection of the generalized defects in exocrine

gland secretion and is an important and serious complication (p. 89).
   - In immunodeficiency states, particularly immunoglobulin deficiencies, bronchiectasis is prone to develop because of an increased susceptibility to repeated bacterial infections; localized or diffuse bronchiectasis can occur.
   - Kartagener's syndrome, an autosomal recessive disorder, is frequently associated with bronchiectasis and sterility in males. Structural abnormalities of the cilia impair mucociliary clearance in the airways, leading to persistent infections, and reduce the mobility of spermatozoa.
3. *Necrotizing, or suppurative, pneumonia* may predispose to bronchiectasis. In the past it was sometimes a sequel to childhood pneumonias complicating measles, whooping cough, and influenza. Although this form of postinfective bronchiectasis is no longer common in the United States, it continues to be an important problem in underdeveloped countries.

PATHOGENESIS. Two processes are critical in the pathogenesis of bronchiectasis: (1) obstruction or abnormal dilatation of bronchi and (2) chronic persistent infection. Either of these two processes may come first: normal clearance mechanisms are hampered by obstruction or dilatation of bronchi so secondary infection soon follows; conversely, chronic infection will in time cause damage to bronchial walls, leading to weakening and dilatation. For example, obstruction due to a bronchogenic carcinoma or a foreign body impairs clearance of secretions. As air is resorbed from dependent lung parenchyma, the loss of support for occluded airways allows the bronchi to dilate. Although these changes are initially reversible, superimposed infection damages the wall and the accumulating exudate further distends the airways, leading to irreversible dilatation. Conversely, a persistent necrotizing inflammation in the bronchi or bronchioles may cause obstructive secretions, inflammation throughout the wall (with peribronchial fibrosis and scarring traction on the walls), and, eventually, the train of events already described.

In the usual case a mixed flora can be cultured from the involved bronchi, including staphylococci, streptococci, pneumococci, enteric organisms, anaerobic and microaerophilic bacteria, and, particularly in children, *Haemophilus influenzae* and *Pseudomonas aeruginosa.*

MORPHOLOGY. Bronchiectatic involvement of the lungs usually affects the lower lobes bilaterally, particularly those air passages that are most vertical. When tumors or aspiration of foreign bodies lead to bronchiectasis, involvement may be sharply localized to a single segment of the lungs. Usually the most severe involvement is found in the more distal bronchi and bronchioles. The airways may be dilated as much as four times their usual diameter and on gross examination of the lung can be followed nearly to the pleural surfaces (Fig. 13–10). (By contrast, in normal lungs the bronchioles cannot be followed by ordinary gross examination

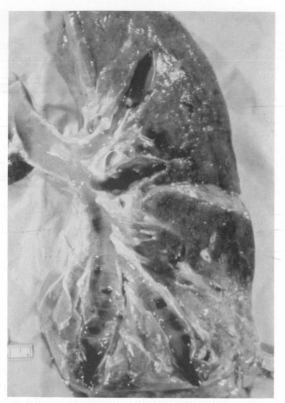

Figure 13–10. Bronchiectasis. Dilated bronchi extend almost to the pleura in the left lower lung lobe.

beyond a point 2 to 3 cm from the pleural surfaces.) In severe involvement the dilatation may produce a cystic pattern on the cut surface of the lung. Varying degrees of emphysema and atelectasis are frequently present together.

The histologic findings vary with the activity and chronicity of the disease. In the full-blown, active case, there is an intense acute and chronic inflammatory exudate within the walls of the bronchi and bronchioles and desquamation of lining epithelium, leaving extensive areas of ulcerated epithelium. There may be pseudo-stratification of the columnar cells or squamous metaplasia of the remaining epithelium. In some instances, **the necrosis destroys the bronchial or bronchiolar walls and forms a lung abscess.** Fibrosis of the bronchial and bronchiolar walls and peribronchiolar fibrosis develop in the more chronic cases. When healing occurs, there may be complete regeneration of the lining epithelium; however, usually so much injury has occurred that abnormal dilatation and scarring persist.

CLINICAL COURSE. The clinical manifestations consist of severe, persistent cough with expectoration of mucopurulent, sometimes fetid sputum. The sputum may contain flecks of blood; frank hemoptysis can occur. Symptoms are often episodic and are precipitated by upper respiratory tract infections or the introduction of new pathogenic agents. Clubbing of the fingers may develop. In cases of severe, widespread

bronchiectasis, significant obstructive ventilatory defects develop, with hypoxemia, hypercarbia, pulmonary hypertension and, rarely, cor pulmonale. Metastatic brain abscesses and reactive amyloidosis are other less frequent complications of bronchiectasis.

RESTRICTIVE LUNG DISEASES _____

Restrictive lung diseases are characterized by reduced compliance (i.e., more pressure is required to expand the lungs because they are stiff). Although chest wall abnormalities, some mentioned earlier (p. 389), can also cause restrictive disease, this discussion will concentrate on parenchymal causes.

Before we discuss the individual disorders it will be useful to consider two general features of restrictive pulmonary diseases, beginning with a brief review of the microanatomy of the septal wall.

- As noted in Figure 13–11, only a thin basement membrane, scant pericapillary interstitial tissue, and the cytoplasm of two very flat cells, endothelium and alveolar epithelium, are interposed between air and blood. The initiating injury in these diseases usually affects either of these two cell types, although with chronicity changes in the interstitium tend to

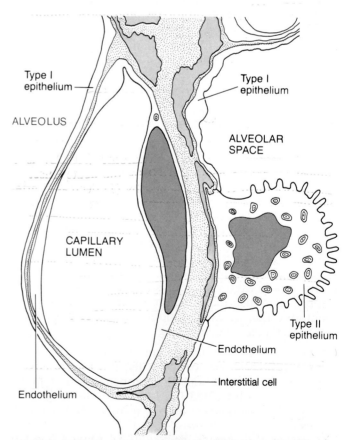

Figure 13–11. Microscopic structure of alveolar wall. Note that the basement membrane (stippled red) is thin on one side and widened where it is continuous with the interstitial space. Portions of interstitial cells are shown.

dominate the picture. Because of prominent changes in the interstitium, these disorders are often referred to as "interstitial lung disease." It should be evident from Figure 13–11, however, that because of their intimate relationship changes in the interstitium can affect both alveoli and capillaries.

- The important signs and symptoms of restrictive lung disease can be inferred from the morphologic changes. Interstitial fluid or fibrosis produces a "stiff lung," which in turn necessitates increased effort of breathing (dyspnea). Furthermore, damage to the alveolar epithelium and interstitial vasculature produces abnormalities in the ventilation-perfusion ratio that lead to hypoxia. For example, damaged or underventilated air units (alveoli) may still be perfused, and, conversely, with damage to the capillaries, underperfusion of ventilated air spaces occurs. With progression, patients develop severe hypoxia, respiratory failure, often in association with pulmonary hypertension, and cor pulmonale (p. 315).

Restrictive lung disease can be either (1) acute, associated with an abrupt decrement in respiratory function and demonstrable pulmonary edema, often with accompanying inflammation, or (2) chronic, associated with insidious development of respiratory dysfunction. Chronic restrictive lung disorders demonstrate variable amounts of chronic inflammation and fibrosis, although some demonstrate unique features described later. In the discussion that follows, we first consider ARDS, the prototypic and most important acute restrictive lung disease, and then several examples of chronic interstitial disorders.

ACUTE RESTRICTIVE LUNG DISEASES _____

Adult Respiratory Distress Syndrome – Diffuse Alveolar Damage _____

Adult respiratory distress syndrome (ARDS) is a clinical syndrome characterized by the acute onset of respiratory distress accompanied by (1) decreased arterial oxygen pressure, (2) decreased lung compliance, and (3) the development of diffuse pulmonary infiltrates on radiographs, without evidence of primary left-sided heart failure. *Diffuse alveolar damage (DAD) is the morphologic counterpart of ARDS*. It is associated with diffuse alveolar endothelial and epithelial injury and, usually, pulmonary edema. DAD occurs in a multitude of clinical settings (Table 13–2), all characterized by a cascade of events that lead to a common pattern of acute injury of the alveolar-capillary membrane.

PATHOGENESIS. Some conditions that lead to ARDS primarily damage the alveolar epithelium; in others the endothelium is the primary target, but ultimately both are involved. In some clinical settings the toxins responsible for the damage can be identified. For example, ARDS following exposure to high oxygen concentrations results from injurious oxygen-derived free radicals; however, in many instances including some common conditions (see Table 13–2), the specific

TABLE 13–2. CONDITIONS ASSOCIATED WITH DEVELOPMENT OF *ARDS*

Infection	Inhaled irritants
*Sepsis	Oxygen toxicity
*Diffuse pulmonary infections: Viral, mycoplasma, and *Pneumocystis* pneumonia; miliary tuberculosis	Smoke
	Irritant gases and chemicals
	Chemical injury
	Heroin or methadone overdose
*Gastric aspiration	Acetylsalicylic acid
Physical injury	Barbiturate overdose
*Mechanical trauma, including head injuries	Paraquat
Pulmonary contusions	**Hematologic conditions**
Near drowning	Multiple transfusions
Fractures with fat embolism	DIC
Burns	**Pancreatitis**
Ionizing radiation	**Uremia**
	Cardiopulmonary bypass

*More than 50% of cases of ARDS are associated with these four conditions.
DIC = disseminated intravascular coagulation.

toxic agent has not been identified. *Nevertheless, there is compelling evidence that neutrophils—and most likely macrophages—are involved in mediating the injury in most cases.* The postulated sequence of events in gram-negative sepsis, an important cause of ARDS, is illustrated in Figure 13–12. Endotoxin (1) triggers the release of tumor necrosis factor alpha (TNF-α, p. 78) from monocytes and alveolar macrophages, and (2) activates the alternate pathway of complement to generate C5a. This complement component up-regulates the expression of adhesion molecules on neutrophils (p. 28), whereas TNF-α activates endothelial cells to up-regulate adhesion molecules (ELAM-1, ICAM-1) and to produce cytokines. TNF-α can also cause endothelial cell necrosis. This sequence of changes leads to sequestration of neutrophils in lung capillaries, which are then activated by TNF-α and complement to secrete preformed proteases and generate damaging oxygen-derived free radicals. Additional mediators that may play roles include (1) the eicosanoids, some of which increase vascular permeability; thromboxane A$_2$, which can cause vascular constriction and platelet aggregation; and LTB4, which is a chemotaxin; (2) interleukin 8 (IL-8), a potent neutrophil chemotaxin, which is made not only by macrophages but also by stimulated epithelial and endothelial cells; and (3) tissue thromboplastin, which can be released by endothelial cells to trigger coagulation. *Collectively the consequences of all these mediators and reactions are edema formation, necrosis of cells, and digestion of lung matrix.* Although early in the course of ARDS there is little evidence of generalized thrombosis, within 72 hours this process becomes evident and complicates the clinical picture.

MORPHOLOGY. The anatomic changes in DAD are remarkably consistent, whatever the precipitating condition. On gross examination early in the disease, the lungs resemble the liver; they are dark red, firm, airless,

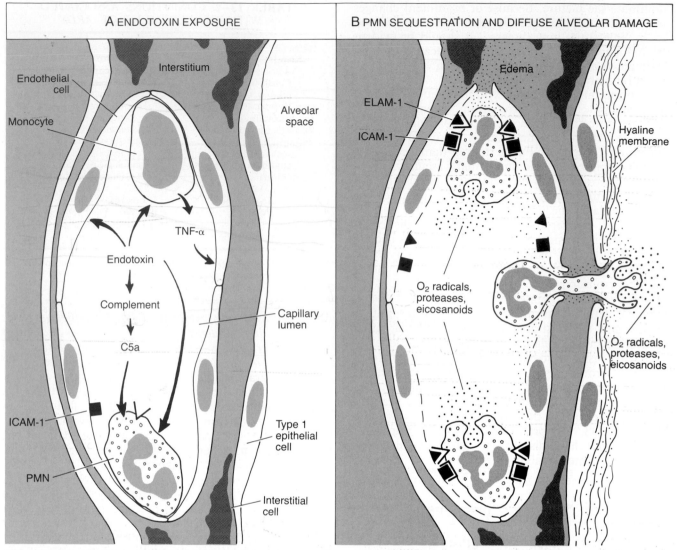

Figure 13–12. A simplified model for DAD in endotoxemia. *A,* Endotoxin associated with gram-negative organisms acts on multiple targets. It induces monocytes and lung macrophages to release mediators, including TNF-α and chemotactic peptides (e.g., LTB4, IL-8). Endotoxin-induced activation of complement via the alternate pathway releases C5a, which together with bacterial lipopolysaccharide and TNF-α activates PMN. *B,* Endotoxin activates endothelial cells to upregulate adhesion molecules (ICAM-1 and ELAM-1) that facilitate binding neutrophils. Activation of PMN results in the up-regulation of adhesion molecules and the release of oxidants, proteases, and eicosanoids. The net result is the sequestration of PMN in pulmonary capillaries, damaged endothelial and epithelial cells, and the development of interstitial edema and alveolar hyaline membranes.

and heavy. If the patient dies after the first week, the lungs are still solid but not as beefy red. Late in the course, with deposition of collagen, they become diffusely gray and glistening. Microscopically, the process may be divided into exudative, proliferative (or repair), and fibrotic phases. In the exudative phase there is capillary congestion, interstitial and intraalveolar edema and hemorrhage, necrosis of alveolar epithelial cells, and, particularly with sepsis, collections of neutrophils in capillaries. The alveolar ducts are dilated and alveoli tend to collapse, in all likelihood owing to a secondary impairment of surfactant synthesis (microatelectasis). Endothelial damage may be evident by light microscopy, or may be subtle and visible only under the electron

microscope. Fibrin thrombi may be present in capillaries and large vessels. **The most characteristic finding, however, is hyaline membranes, particularly lining the distended alveolar ducts.** Such membranes consist of protein-rich edema fluid admixed with remnants of necrotic epithelial cells. Overall, the picture is remarkably similar to that seen in RDS in the newborn (see Fig. 13–3). In the proliferative phase, beginning as early as three or four days, but readily appreciated by day 10, there is proliferation of type II pneumocytes and interstitial fibroblasts. The latter also invade the exudates that have accumulated in the air spaces. Finally the progressive fibrosis involving the alveolar space may result in marked distortion of lung parenchyma. In some areas there is alveolar collapse and obliteration of the normal alveolar capillary unit, but in others there is dilatation of alveoli and alveolar ducts. After several weeks, a picture of diffuse interstitial fibrosis interspersed with dilated distorted air spaces (honeycomb lung) develops.

CLINICAL COURSE. The prognosis of ARDS is grim and has not improved in recent years despite better understanding of the pathophysiology. About 50% of patients die during the acute phase. The more severe the initial permeability leak in alveolar-capillary membranes, the poorer the prognosis. Patients who develop associated hypoxic multisystem failure (especially cardiac, renal, or hepatic) generally have an especially poor outcome. A confounding clinical problem is that the high levels of oxygen, sometimes used to treat hypoxemia, may lead to additional alveolar damage owing to oxygen toxicity.

The alveolar exudates also provide a rich culture medium for microorganisms, and secondary infections are common. At autopsy it is often difficult to distinguish changes due to the initial injury from secondary infection and the effects of oxygen. Should the patient survive the acute stage, diffuse interstitial fibrosis may occur and continue to compromise respiratory function. However, in most patients who survive the acute insult and are spared the chronic sequelae, normal respiratory function returns within four to six months.

CHRONIC RESTRICTIVE LUNG DISEASES ____

The chronic restrictive (interstitial) diseases of the lung parenchyma are a heterogeneous group with little uniformity regarding terminology and classification. Many entities are of unknown cause and pathogenesis; some have an intraalveolar as well as an interstitial component; and there is frequent overlap in histologic features among the different conditions. Nevertheless, the presence of similar clinical signs, symptoms, radiographic alterations, and pathophysiologic changes justify their consideration as a group.

Chronic restrictive lung disorders account for about 15% of noninfectious diseases seen by pulmonary physicians. They can be divided into two broad categories (Table 13–3), those with known causes and those of unknown cause, and further divided on the basis of the presence or absence of granulomas. This distinction is of some utility when diagnosis is made from biopsy tissue. The most common conditions are those caused by specific environmental agents (24%), sarcoidosis (20%), idiopathic pulmonary fibrosis (15%), and the collagen-vascular diseases (8%). The remainder have more than 150 different causes and associations in addition to those listed here.

The chronic interstitial diseases probably evolve over time from low-grade inflammation that may resemble a more limited form of ARDS. Indeed, there are a few agents that in large doses can cause ARDS and in smaller doses and following repeated exposure can lead

TABLE 13–3. MAJOR CATEGORIES OF CHRONIC INTERSTITIAL LUNG DISEASE WITH SELECTED EXAMPLES*

Known Etiology	Unknown Etiology
A. Lung response: Alveolitis, interstitial inflammation, and diffuse fibrosis	
†Environmental agents: Asbestos, fumes, gases Ionizing radiation Following ARDS Drugs: Bulsulfan, bleomycin	†Collagen-vascular diseases: Scleroderma, rheumatoid arthritis, systemic lupus erythematosus, dermatomyositis, mixed connective tissue disease †Idiopathic pulmonary fibrosis (IPF) Goodpasture's syndrome Idiopathic pulmonary hemosiderosis
B. Lung response: As in A but with granulomas	
Beryllium Hypersensitivity pneumonitis	†Sarcoidosis Eosinophilic granuloma Wegener's granulomatosis

*Adapted from Reynolds, H. Y.: Interstitial lung diseases. *In* Wilson, J. E., et al. (eds.): Harrison's Principles of Internal Medicine. 12th edition. New York, McGraw-Hill, 1991, p. 1083).
†Most common causes.

to interstitial fibrosis and restrictive lung disease (e.g., radiation injury and bleomycin toxicity). Some of the more common and prototypic forms of chronic restrictive diseases are described next.

Idiopathic Pulmonary Fibrosis ____

Idiopathic pulmonary fibrosis (IPF) refers to a poorly understood pulmonary disorder of unknown cause characterized histologically by diffuse interstitial fibrosis, which in advanced cases results in severe hypoxemia and cyanosis. There are at least 20 synonyms for this entity (e.g., chronic interstitial pneumonitis, Hamman-Rich syndrome, diffuse or cryptogenic fibrosing alveolitis). Males are affected more often than females, and most patients are between 30 and 50 years old when the condition is diagnosed. It should be stressed that similar clinical and pathologic findings may occur with well-defined entities such as asbestosis, the connective tissue diseases, and a number of other conditions (see Table 13–3). Therefore known causes must be ruled out before the appellate "idiopathic" is used.

The proposed sequence of events in IPF begins with some form of alveolar wall injury, which results in interstitial edema and accumulation of inflammatory cells (alveolitis). Fibroblasts then proliferate, and progressive fibrosis of both the alveolar septa and the alveolar exudate results in obliteration of normal pulmonary architecture. Immune mechanisms are suspected to trigger this sequence of events. There are often circulating immune complexes or cryoimmunoglobulins in the serum of patients with IPF, particularly in cases in which the biopsy shows significant cellular infiltration rather than interstitial fibrosis. Granular deposits of IgG have been detected in alveolar walls, suggesting again that immune complexes may play a pathogenetic role, but the nature of the antigens in the complexes is unknown. Figure 13–13 outlines the possible sequence of events in immune-mediated IPF. Macrophages are probably the key players that orchestrate the tissue injury and ensuing fibrosis. Immune complexes might bind to the Fc receptors of alveolar macrophages to stimulate the release of factors that recruit neutrophils. The soluble mediators released from macrophages and recruited neutrophils injure cells and degrade connective tissue. Alveolar macrophages from patients with IPF secrete increased amounts of fibronectin and platelet-derived growth factor (PDGF), which can both attract fibroblasts and stimulate their proliferation. Insulin-like growth factor and IL-1 are yet other macrophage cytokines that drive fibroblastic proliferation.

MORPHOLOGY. The morphologic changes vary according to the stage of the disease. In early cases, the lungs are firm; microscopically they show pulmonary edema, intraalveolar exudate, hyaline membranes, and infiltration of the alveolar septa with mononuclear cells. Type I pneumocytes are particularly susceptible to injury. Subsequently there is hyperplasia of type II pneumocytes, which appear as cuboidal or even columnar cells lining the alveolar spaces. With advancing disease, there is organization of the intraalveolar exudate by fibrous tissue, as well as thickening of the alveolar septa owing to fibrosis and variable amounts of inflammation. At this stage the lungs demonstrate alternating areas of fibrosis and normal tissue. In the end, the lung consists of spaces lined by cuboidal or columnar epithelium separated by inflammatory fibrous tissue, an appearance referred to as honeycomb lung (Fig. 13–14). There is also intimal thickening of the pulmonary arteries and lymphoid infiltration in the fibrotic interstitium.

Although most patients with IPF exhibit the morphologic changes just described, there are instances in which the interstitial pneumonitis is accompanied by the accumulation of large numbers of pulmonary alveolar macrophages within the air spaces. When first described, this variant was called desquamative interstitial pneumonitis (DIP), but according to current thinking, DIP is probably one variant of an early phase of IPF. Thus the more typical pattern of IPF, which lacks the desquamative component, is sometimes termed usual interstitial pneumonitis (UIP). DIP is more likely to respond to steroid therapy, perhaps because it represents an earlier stage, whereas UIP, with its more marked fibrosis, responds very poorly to this intervention.

Clinically, patients exhibit respiratory difficulty and, in advanced cases, hypoxemia and cyanosis. The septal fibrosis constitutes a significant alveolocapillary block. Cor pulmonale and cardiac failure may result. The progression in individual cases is unpredictable. In some patients the disease remits spontaneously. In a

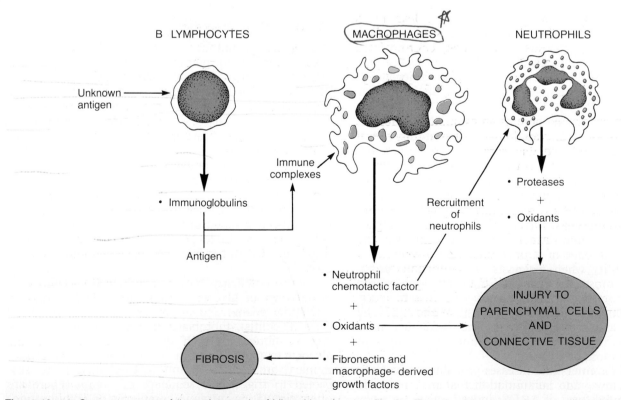

Figure 13–13. Current concepts of the pathogenesis of idiopathic pulmonary fibrosis. The role of the macrophage is pivotal in the induction of interstitial fibrosis, the most important component of IPF. (Modified from Crystal, R. G., et al.: Interstitial lung disease of unknown cause. Disorders characterized by chronic inflammation of the lower respiratory tree. N. Engl. J. Med. *310:*161, 1984.)

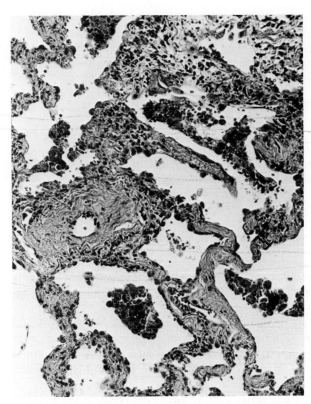

Figure 13–14. Idiopathic pulmonary fibrosis. The alveolar walls are thickened by fibrosis. In addition there is an increase in interstitial lymphocytes and increased numbers of type II pneumocytes lining the distended air spaces. Capillaries are noticeably decreased in number.

few the process progresses very rapidly, leading to fibrosis in a matter of weeks, whereas in others it develops over many years. The median course of the disease is about five years.

Sarcoidosis

Although considered here as an example of a restrictive lung disease with granulomatous tissue response, it should be remembered that *sarcoidosis is a multisystem disease of unknown cause characterized by noncaseating granulomas* in many tissues and organs (p. 42). Other diseases, including mycobacterial or fungal infections and berylliosis, sometimes also produce noncaseating granulomas; *therefore, the histologic diagnosis of sarcoidosis is one of exclusion.* Although the multisystem involvement of sarcoidosis can present in many clinical guises, bilateral hilar lymphadenopathy or lung involvement, visible on chest radiographs, are the major presenting manifestations in 90% of cases. Eye and skin involvement each occur in about 25% of cases, and may occasionally be the presenting feature of the disease.

Sarcoidosis occurs worldwide, but the frequency varies in different populations. In the United States it occurs in one to four per 10,000 and is ten times more prevalent in blacks.

ETIOLOGY AND PATHOGENESIS. The distinctive granulomatous tissue response seen in sarcoidosis suggests that the disease represents a cell-mediated immune response to an unidentified antigen. Many causal agents have been proposed as the immunogen (atypical mycobacteria, pine pollen, and so forth) but none has been proved. Several features support a role for a deranged immune response to one or more still unidentified agents in the pathogenesis of sarcoidosis.

- Most patients manifest cutaneous anergy to common skin test antigens (e.g., *Candida,* mumps, purified protein derivative [PPD]) to which normal persons have been exposed and sensitized.
- The number of peripheral blood T lymphocytes is often decreased, resulting in an absolute lymphopenia, and the CD4 to CD8 ratio may be reduced to less than 0.8 (normal 0.9 to 2.5).
- Bronchoalveolar lavage fluids from patients with active sarcoid lung lesions demonstrate an increased number of T lymphocytes with a CD4 to CD8 T-cell ratio of up to 10:1. CD4+ T cells demonstrate cell surface activation markers, including the interleukin-2 (IL-2) receptor (IL-2R), and lavage fluids contain detectable levels of secreted IL-2 and IL-2R.
- Circulating B cells are normal in number but the serum contains excess polyclonal immunoglobulins, secreted by B cells in lymphoid tissues.

All these findings are consistent with a cell-mediated immune response (type IV hypersensitivity reaction) to an unidentified antigen. Still unexplained is the distribution of lesions. The depletion of CD4+ T cells in the peripheral blood and cutaneous anergy is most likely due to the recruitment of the CD4+ T cells into the lesions.

MORPHOLOGY. Virtually any organ may be affected; the most common morphologic changes will be described.

Lymph nodes are involved in almost all cases, commonly the hilar and paratracheal ones, but any node in the body may be involved, particularly those in the head and neck. The tonsils are affected in about a quarter to a third of cases. The nodes are characteristically enlarged and discrete, and sometimes lobulated (when viewed on chest radiographs, the bilateral hilar lymphadenopathy is referred to as "potato nodes"). Histologically, all involved nodes show classic noncaseating granulomas (Fig. 13–15). These are made up of aggregates of tightly clustered epithelioid cells, often with Langhans' or foreign body-type giant cells. The granulomas are surrounded by a rim of lymphocytes, mostly CD4+, helper T cells. Rarely, central necrosis is present. In chronic disease, the granulomas may become enclosed within fibrous rims or eventually be replaced by hyaline fibrous scars. Two other microscopic features are often present in the granulomas: (1) Schaumann bodies, laminated concretions composed of calcium and proteins, and (2) asteroid bodies, stellate inclusions enclosed within giant cells (Fig. 13–16). The latter are found in approximately 60% of sarcoid granulomas but may occur in granulomas of other origins.

The lungs are a common site of involvement. Typi-

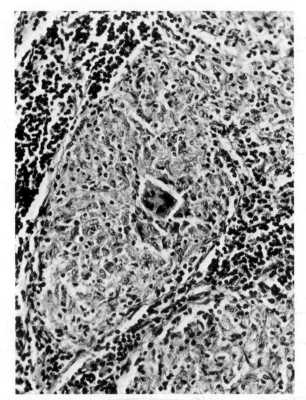

Figure 13-15. Sarcoidosis. The characteristic noncaseating granuloma contains a central multinucleate giant cell.

cally, grossly detectable lesions are absent; however, microscopic lesions are distributed throughout the parenchyma, usually bilaterally, with some tendency to localize in the walls of peribronchiolar and perivenular lymphatics. The granulomas may be cellular with collections of macrophages surrounded by lymphocytic infiltrates, or they may exhibit variable amounts of fibrosis. In a minority of patients the granulomas are eventually replaced by diffuse interstitial fibrosis accompanied by pulmonary artery sclerosis and cor pulmonale.

Skin lesions are encountered in a third to a half of the cases. Sarcoidosis of the skin assumes a variety of macroscopic appearances (e.g., discrete subcutaneous nodules; focal, slightly elevated, erythematous plaques; flat lesions that are slightly reddened and scaling and resemble those of lupus erythematosus or erythema nodosum on the anterior tibia). Lesions may also appear on the mucous membranes of the oral cavity and upper respiratory tract. In all instances, these lesions reveal noncaseating granulomas.

Involvement of the eye, lacrimal glands, and salivary glands occurs in about one fifth to one half of the cases. The ocular involvement takes the form of iritis or iridocyclitis and may be unilateral or bilateral. As a consequence corneal opacities, glaucoma, and, less commonly, total loss of vision may develop. The posterior uveal tract is also affected with resultant choroiditis, retinitis, and optic nerve involvement. These ocular lesions are frequently accompanied by inflammation in the

lacrimal glands with suppression of lacrimation. When bilateral sarcoidosis of the parotid, submaxillary, and sublingual glands occurs the combined uveoparotid involvement is designated as **Mikulicz's syndrome.**

The spleen may appear unaffected grossly but in about three quarters of the cases it contains granulomas. In 18% it becomes enlarged.

The liver demonstrates microscopic granulomatous lesions, usually in portal triads, about as often as the spleen but only about a third of the patients demonstrate hepatomegaly or abnormal liver function.

Less frequently affected organs include kidneys, bones, joints, muscles, and endocrine glands. Bone lesions, usually involving the short bones of hands and feet, can be identified in 3 to 5% of patients. Sometimes there is hypercalcemia and hypercalciuria. This is not related to bone destruction but is rather due to increased calcium absorption secondary to production of active vitamin D by the mononuclear phagocytes in the granulomas.

CLINICAL COURSE. The clinical presentation of sarcoidosis is variable. In many patients the disease is entirely asymptomatic, discovered on routine chest films as bilateral hilar adenopathy or as an incidental finding at autopsy. Peripheral lymphadenopathy, cutaneous lesions, eye involvement, splenomegaly, or hepatomegaly may be presenting manifestations. In about two thirds of symptomatic cases, patients seek medical attention because of the insidious onset of respiratory symptoms (shortness of breath, cough, or vague sub-

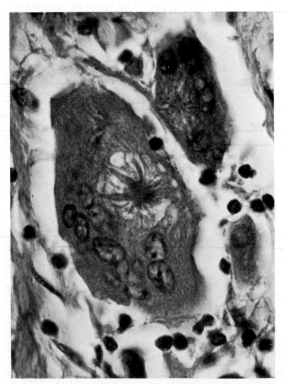

Figure 13-16. Characteristic asteroid body within a giant cell.

sternal discomfort) or with constitutional signs and symptoms (fever, fatigue, weight loss, anorexia, night sweats). Occasionally the presentation is as a systemic hypersensitivity reaction with fever, erythema nodosum, and polyarthritis associated with bilateral hilar adenopathy or, alternatively, eye and salivary gland involvement (Mikulicz's syndrome). Because of the variable and nondiagnostic clinical features, resort is frequently made to lung or lymph node biopsy. Although other sites such as liver and bone marrow may be sampled, these tissues are less useful. The presence of noncaseating granulomas is suggestive of sarcoidosis, but other identifiable causes of granulomatous inflammation must be excluded.

Sarcoidosis follows an unpredictable course characterized by either progressive chronicity or periods of activity interspersed with remissions. The remissions may be spontaneous or initiated by steroid therapy and are often permanent. Overall, 65 to 70% of affected patients recover with minimal or no residual manifestations. Twenty per cent develop permanent lung dysfunction or visual impairment. Of the remaining 10%, most succumb to progressive pulmonary fibrosis and cor pulmonale.

Hypersensitivity Pneumonitis

This is an immune-mediated inflammatory lung disease that primarily affects the alveoli and is therefore often called "allergic alveolitis." Most often it is an occupational disease that results from heightened sensitivity to inhaled antigens in the form of organic dusts such as moldy hay (Table 13–4). Unlike bronchial asthma, in which bronchi are the focus of immune-mediated injury, the damage in hypersensitivity pneumonitis occurs at the level of alveoli. Hence it presents

TABLE 13–4. SELECTED CAUSES OF HYPERSENSITIVITY PNEUMONITIS

Syndrome	Exposure	Antigens
Microbes Contaminating Vegetable Matter or Water		
Farmer's lung	Moldy hay	Various actinomycetes, *Aspergillus* spp.
Bagassosis	Moldy pressed sugar cane (bagasse)	Thermophilic actinomycetes
Maple bark disease	Maple bark	*Cryptostroma corticale*
Humidifier lung	Cool-mist humidifier	Thermophilic actinomycetes, *Aureobasidium pullulans*, protozoal proteins
Animal Products		
Pigeon breeder's lung	Pigeons	Pigeon serum proteins in droppings
Chemicals		
Trimellatic anhydride pneumonia	Chemical industry	Haptenated protein

as a predominantly restrictive lung disease with decreased diffusing capacity, lung compliance, and total lung volume. The occupational exposures are diverse but each syndrome shares common clinical and pathologic findings, and likely very similar pathophysiology.

Hypersensitivity pneumonitis may present either as an *acute reaction* with fever, cough, dyspnea, and constitutional complaints 4 to 8 hours following exposure or as a *chronic disease* with insidious onset of cough, dyspnea, malaise, and weight loss. In all probability, acute syndromes result from the combination of (1) a direct irritant effect, (2) activation of the alternate complement pathway (perhaps because the inhaled material is contaminated by endotoxin), and (3) immune complex– and T cell–mediated injury. The chronic form of the disease is mediated almost entirely by delayed hypersensitivity reactions.

MORPHOLOGY. The histopathology of both acute and chronic forms of hypersensitivity pneumonitis demonstrates mononuclear cell infiltrates in the alveoli and alveolar walls and around terminal bronchioles. Lymphocytes predominate, but plasma cells and large foamy macrophages are also present. In acute forms of the disease variable numbers of neutrophils may also be seen. Interstitial noncaseating granulomas reflecting type IV hypersensitivity reaction are present in more than two thirds of cases. In advanced chronic cases diffuse interstitial fibrosis occurs.

The clinical course is variable. If antigenic exposure is terminated following acute attacks of the disease, fever and cough usually last a few days and constitutional complaints clear in several weeks. The chronic form of the disease resolves more slowly and most patients continue to experience mild to moderate symptoms. In a small number of cases (about 5%) respiratory failure and death may occur.

Diffuse Pulmonary Hemorrhage Syndromes

Hemorrhage in the lung is a dramatic complication of some interstitial and vascular lung disorders. These so-called pulmonary hemorrhage syndromes include (1) Goodpasture's syndrome, (2) idiopathic pulmonary hemosiderosis, and (3) vasculitis-associated hemorrhage.

Goodpasture's syndrome is an uncommon but intriguing condition characterized by a proliferative, usually rapidly progressive glomerulonephritis (p. 450), and hemorrhagic interstitial pneumonitis. Both the renal and pulmonary lesions are caused by antibodies to antigens common to glomerular and pulmonary basement membranes. The immunopathogenesis of Goodpasture's syndrome and the changes in the glomeruli are discussed on page 441. It suffices to say that most cases begin clinically with respiratory symptoms, principally hemoptysis, and with radiographic evidence of bilateral fluffy infiltrates.

> Microscopic examination of the lungs demonstrates focal necrosis of alveolar walls associated with intraalveolar hemorrhages, fibrous thickening of the septa, and hypertrophy of septal lining cells. The once dismal prognosis for this disease has been markedly improved by immunosuppressive therapy either with or without plasma exchange. With severe renal disease, renal transplantation is eventually required.

Idiopathic pulmonary hemosiderosis is an uncommon pulmonary disease of uncertain cause that usually presents with insidious onset of productive cough, hemoptysis, anemia, and weight loss, and with pulmonary infiltrates on x-ray. Microscopically, the lung reveals intraalveolar hemorrhage with hemosiderin-filled macrophages. There is mild to moderate interstitial fibrosis. The pulmonary manifestations are similar to those of Goodpasture's syndrome, but there is no associated renal disease or circulating anti–basement membrane antibody. Clinically, the course is usually mild to moderate, with periods of activity followed by prolonged remissions—and often spontaneous remission.

Vasculitis-associated hemorrhage is infrequent but can occur in some conditions, most commonly in systemic lupus erythematosus (p. 139), Wegener's granulomatosis (p. 289), and *microscopic* polyarteritis (p. 288). In this group there is necrotizing inflammation of the pulmonary capillaries. Although pulmonary manifestations in lupus are common, pulmonary hemorrhage occurs in only 2%. In Wegener's granulomatosis mild intra-alveolar hemorrhage is present in up to 50% of cases but massive hemorrhage is much less frequent. Alveolar hemorrhage occurs in about a third of patients with microscopic polyarteritis.

VASCULAR LUNG DISEASES _____

PULMONARY THROMBOEMBOLISM, HEMORRHAGE, AND INFARCTION _____

The embolization of venous and right-sided cardiac thrombi to the lungs is an extremely important clinical problem. Indeed, pulmonary thromboembolism is the most common preventable cause of death in hospitalized patients. In total, thromboembolism causes approximately 50,000 deaths per year in the United States. Even when not directly fatal, it can complicate the course of other diseases. The true incidence of nonfatal pulmonary embolism is not known. Some undoubtedly occur outside the hospital in ambulatory patients and are small and clinically silent. Even among hospitalized patients, not more than a third are diagnosed before death. Moreover, when the diagnosis of a fatal pulmonary embolism is made clinically, postmortem examination fails to document the presence of emboli in approximately 50% of cases. Unfortunately, autopsy data on the incidence of pulmonary emboli vary widely, ranging from less than 1% to the extreme of 64%. If only fatal pulmonary emboli are considered, they are detected at postmortem in about 0.3% of hospitalized patients who have medical diseases, 1% of patients who have undergone surgery, and 5 to 8% of patients with hip fractures.

More than 95% of all pulmonary emboli arise from thrombi within the large deep veins of the lower legs. Thromboemboli do not commonly arise from superficial or smaller leg veins. It should be noted that even when a patient has a well-documented pulmonary embolus, deep vein thrombosis can be identified clinically in only 20 to 70% of instances; this variation reflects whether or not invasive procedures such as venography were used.

The influences that predispose to venous thrombosis in the legs were discussed on p. 69, but the following risk factors should be emphasized: (1) prolonged bed rest (particularly with immobilization of the legs), (2) surgery on the legs (as following knee surgery), (3) severe trauma (including burns or multiple fractures), (4) congestive heart failure, (5) women in the period around parturition or who take birth control pills with high estrogen content, and (6) disseminated cancer.

The pathophysiologic consequences of thromboembolism in the lung depend largely on the size of the embolus, which in turn dictates the size of the occluded pulmonary artery, and on the cardiopulmonary status of the patient. There are two important consequences of embolic pulmonary arterial occlusion: (1) an increase in pulmonary artery pressure due to blockage of flow and, possibly, vasospasm caused by neurogenic mechanisms and/or release of mediators (e.g., TXA_2 and serotonin) and (2) ischemia of the downstream pulmonary parenchyma. Thus, occlusion of a *major vessel* results in a sudden increase in pulmonary artery pressure, a diminished cardiac output, right-sided heart failure (cor pulmonale), or even death. Usually hypoxemia develops, due to multiple mechanisms: (1) *perfusion of lung zones that have become atelectatic;* the alveolar collapse occurs in the ischemic areas due to a reduction in surfactant production, and because pain associated with embolism leads to reduced movement of the chest wall; in addition some of the pulmonary blood flow is redirected through areas of the lung that are normally hypoventilated. You may recall that under physiologic conditions the vessels that supply such zones are constricted and hence little perfusion occurs. With embolism, the associated increase in pulmonary vascular pressure may cause these channels to open, thus perfusing poorly ventilated parts of the lung; (2) the decrease in cardiac output causes a *widening of the difference in arterial-venous oxygen saturation;* and (3) *right-to-left shunting* of blood may occur in some patients through a patent foramen ovale, present in 30% of normal persons. If *smaller vessels* are occluded, the result is less catastrophic and the event may even be clinically silent. Recall that lung is oxygenated not only by the pulmonary arteries but also by bronchial arteries and directly from air in the alveoli. If the bronchial circulation is normal and adequate ventilation is maintained then the resultant decrease in blood flow does not cause tissue necrosis. Indeed, ischemic necrosis (infarction) resulting from pulmonary thromboembolism is the exception rather than the rule, occurring in only about 10% of cases. It occurs only if there is compromise in cardiac function or bronchial circulation or if the region of the lung at risk is underventilated owing to underlying pulmonary disease.

MORPHOLOGY. The morphologic consequences of pulmonary embolism, as noted, depend on the size of the embolic mass and the general state of the circulation. Large emboli impact in the main pulmonary artery or its major branches or lodge astride the bifurcation as a saddle embolus (Fig. 13–17). Death usually follows so suddenly from hypoxia or acute failure of the right side of the heart (acute cor pulmonale) that there is no time for morphologic alterations in the lung.

Smaller emboli become impacted in medium-sized and small pulmonary arteries. With adequate cardiovascular circulation and bronchial arterial flow, the vitality of the lung parenchyma is maintained but the alveolar spaces often fill with blood to produce **pulmonary hemorrhage** as a result of ischemic damage to the endothelial cells.

With compromised cardiovascular status, as may occur with congestive heart failure, **infarction** results. The more peripheral the embolic occlusion, the more likely is infarction. About three fourths of all infarcts affect the lower lobes, and more than half are multiple. They vary in size from lesions barely visible to involvement of large parts of a lobe. Characteristically, they are wedge shaped with their base at the pleural surface and the apex pointing toward the hilus of the lung. As discussed earlier (p. 76) pulmonary infarcts are typically hemorrhagic and appear as raised, red-blue areas in the early stages (Fig. 13–18). The adjacent pleural surface is often covered by a fibrinous exudate. If the occluded vessel can be identified it is usually found near the apex of the infarcted area. The red cells begin to lyse within 48 hours and the infarct pales, eventually becoming red-brown as hemosiderin is produced. In time, fibrous replacement begins at the margins as a gray-white peripheral zone and eventually converts the infarct into a scar that is contracted below the level of the lung substance. Histologically, the hallmark of fresh infarcts is coagulative necrosis of the lung parenchyma in the area of hemorrhage. If it is caused by the infected embolus, the infarct is modified by a more intense neutrophilic inflammatory reaction. Such lesions are referred to as septic infarcts and some convert to abscesses. If an infarct occurs in an area of underlying pneumonia a similar outcome occurs.

CLINICAL COURSE. The clinical consequences of pulmonary thromboembolism are summarized here and in Figure 13–19.

- Most pulmonary emboli (60 to 80%) are clinically silent because they are small; the embolic mass is rapidly removed by fibrinolytic activity and the bronchial circulation sustains the viability of the affected lung parenchyma until this is accomplished.
- Embolic obstruction of middle-sized arteries (10 to 15% of cases) that are not end-arteries is usually not associated with pulmonary infarction but instead results in more centrally located pulmonary hemorrhage. Patients with hemorrhage usually manifest dyspnea or hemoptysis, but rarely pleuritic chest pain because the central hemorrhage does not in-

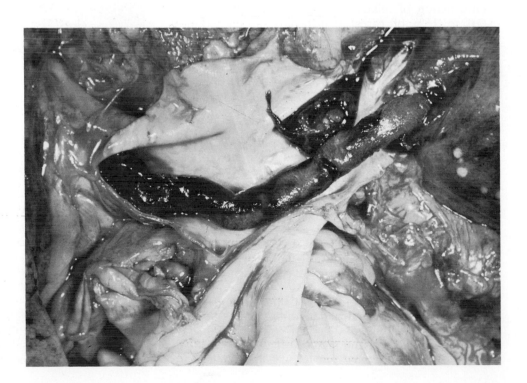

Figure 13–17. Large saddle embolus from femoral vein lying astride main left and right pulmonary arteries.

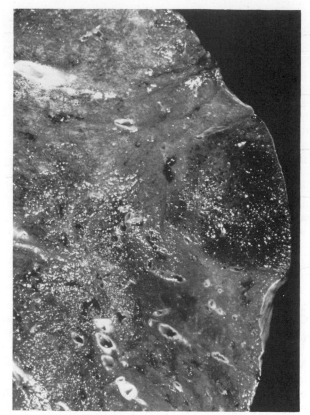

Figure 13-18. A relatively recent, small, roughly wedge-shaped hemorrhagic pulmonary infarct *(right).*

volve the pleura. If an infiltrate appears on the chest radiograph, it clears in a few days because there is no tissue necrosis or subsequent scarring as with an infarct.

● Obstruction of relatively small pulmonary branches (10 to 15% of cases) that behave as end-arteries usually causes pulmonary infarction, especially when some element of circulatory insufficiency is present. Typically, patients who sustain an infarct manifest dyspnea, the basis of which is not fully understood.

● In 5% of cases sudden death, acute right-sided heart failure (acute cor pulmonale), or cardiovascular collapse (shock) may occur when more than 60% of the total pulmonary vasculature is obstructed by a large embolus or multiple, simultaneous, small emboli. Massive pulmonary embolism is one of the few causes of literally instantaneous death, even before the patient experiences chest pain or dyspnea.

● In a small but significant subset of patients (less than 3%) recurrent multiple emboli lead to pulmonary hypertension, chronic right-sided heart strain (chronic cor pulmonale), and, in time, pulmonary vascular sclerosis with progressively worsening dyspnea.

Emboli usually resolve after the initial acute insult. They contract, and endogenous fibrinolytic activity may cause total lysis of the clot. However, in the presence of an underlying predisposing factor, a small innocuous embolus may presage a larger one, and

patients who have experienced one pulmonary embolus have a 30% chance of developing a second. Thus, recognition and appropriate preventive treatment are essential. Prophylactic therapy includes early ambulation for postoperative and postpartum patients, elastic stockings, and isometric leg exercises for bedridden patients. Anticoagulation for persons at high risk is warranted. It is sometimes necessary to insert a screen (or umbrella) into the inferior vena cava—or even to ligate it, if anticoagulation is not feasible—in order to prevent repeat thromboembolism.

PULMONARY HYPERTENSION AND VASCULAR SCLEROSIS _____

Pulmonary hypertension is most often caused by a decrease in the cross-sectional area of the pulmonary vascular bed but it may also result from increased pulmonary vascular blood flow. It is most frequently *secondary* to (1) chronic obstructive or interstitial lung disease, (2) recurrent pulmonary emboli, or (3) heart disease in which there is a left-to-right shunt. Rarely (less than 5% of cases), pulmonary hypertension exists even though all known causes of increased pulmonary pressure can be excluded; this is referred to as primary, or *idiopathic, pulmonary hypertension.* Distinction of primary hypertension from that caused by recurrent thromboembolism may be particularly difficult, but angiography and radioisotope scanning may be helpful. Table 13-5 provides an overview of causes of pulmonary hypertension.

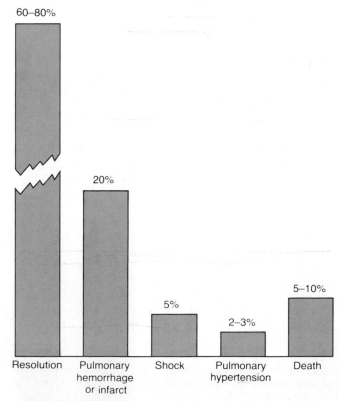

Figure 13-19. Clinical outcome of pulmonary thromboembolism.

TABLE 13–5. CAUSES OF PULMONARY HYPERTENSION AND VASCULAR SCLEROSIS

Secondary Pulmonary Hypertension

Cardiac disease: Left-to-right shunts: septal defects; mechanical obstructions: atrial myxoma, mitral stenosis
Inflammatory vascular disease: Scleroderma and other connective tissue diseases; other forms of vasculitis
Lung disease: Chronic hypoxia: high-altitude hypoxia, extraparenchymal restrictive lung diseases (obesity); chronic hypoxia with destruction of vascular bed: COPD, chronic interstitial fibrosing diseases, pneumoconiosis
Recurrent thromboembolism*

Primary Pulmonary Hypertension

Plexiform pulmonary arteriopathy (30–70% of cases)
Thrombotic pulmonary arteriopathy (20–50% of cases)*
Pulmonary venoocclusive disease (~10% of cases)

*These two diseases are difficult to distinguish clinically or morphologically.

hypertrophy, and reduplication of the internal and external elastic membranes. In these vessels the wall thickness may exceed the diameter of the lumen, which is sometimes narrowed to the point of near obliteration. In patients with severe, long-standing primary pulmonary hypertension, additional changes take the form of "plexiform" lesions and necrotizing arteritis with fibrinoid necrosis and thrombosis. The plexiform lesions consist of a multichanneled outpouching of the pulmonary arterial wall. These may represent aneurysmal dilatation of the vessel wall or reparative lesions in areas of previous fibrinoid necrosis. When there is prominent thrombosis and recanalization of arteries without plexiform lesions the disease has been referred to as thrombotic pulmonary arteriopathy. This pattern of primary pulmonary hypertension is difficult to distinguish from secondary disease resulting from recurrent thromboembolism.

Because many of the diseases that give rise to secondary pulmonary vascular hypertension have already been discussed, only primary pulmonary hypertension is considered here. It should be stated at the outset that the mechanism of primary pulmonary hypertension is not known. According to current thinking, chronic vasoconstriction resulting from vascular hyperreactivity gives rise to pulmonary hypertension and, in time, its morphologic counterpart, intimal and medial vascular hypertrophy. The importance of vascular hyperreactivity is supported by the fact that about 10% of patients with primary pulmonary hypertension often suffer from vasospastic disorders such as Raynaud's phenomenon (p. 153). In addition, pulmonary vascular resistance can sometimes be rapidly decreased with vasodilators. The hyperreactivity is believed to be secondary to an acquired defect in endothelial regulation of smooth muscle relaxation. Several mechanisms have been postulated to explain such dysfunction. One notion is that it is immune-mediated, because both Raynaud's phenomenon and pulmonary hypertension also occur in the immune-mediated connective disease diseases (scleroderma, systemic lupus erythematosus, rheumatoid arthritis). A connection with the connective tissue diseases is also in keeping with the prevalence of the disease in young women and its occasional occurrence in families.

CLINICAL COURSE. *Secondary pulmonary vascular sclerosis* may develop at any age. The clinical features reflect the underlying disease, usually pulmonary or cardiac, with accentuation of respiratory insufficiency and right-sided heart strain. *Primary pulmonary vascular sclerosis,* on the other hand, is almost always encountered in young persons, more commonly women, and is marked by fatigue, syncope (particularly on exercise), dyspnea on exertion, and sometimes chest pain. These patients eventually develop severe respiratory insufficiency and sometimes cyanosis. In patients with primary pulmonary hypertension death usually results from right-sided heart failure within a few years of the diagnosis. Some amelioration of the respiratory distress can be achieved by vasodilators, but without lung transplantation the prognosis is grim.

PULMONARY INFECTIONS

Pulmonary infections in the form of pneumonia are responsible for one sixth of all deaths in the United States. This is not surprising because (1) the epithelial surfaces of the lung are constantly exposed to liters of variously contaminated air; (2) nasopharyngeal flora is regularly aspirated during sleep, even by normally healthy persons; and (3) other common lung diseases render the lung parenchyma vulnerable to virulent organisms. It is therefore a small miracle that the normal lung parenchyma remains sterile. This attests to the efficiency of a series of pulmonary defense mechanisms. We will briefly review these to facilitate an understanding of lung infections.

Pulmonary defenses can be divided into those that involve the upper airways (from the nasopharynx to the level of the terminal bronchioles) and the lower airways (the respiratory bronchioles and distal air spaces). They can be further categorized into those that are immune and those that are not. Nonimmune defense mechanisms are important not only in protecting against microbes but also in removing other particulates. Microorganisms in the air drawn through

MORPHOLOGY. Vascular alterations in all forms of pulmonary sclerosis (primary and secondary) involve the entire arterial tree, but the nature of the vascular change tends to vary with the size of the vessel. The various arterial lesions are as follows: (1) The main elastic arteries develop atheromas similar to those in systemic atherosclerosis but rarely as severe. (2) In medium-sized muscular arteries, proliferation of myointimal cells and smooth muscle causes thickening of the intima and media with narrowing of the lumens. (3) Smaller arteries and arterioles also develop changes: thickening, medial

the nose may be filtered out by vibrissae lining the mucosa. A mucous blanket coats the ciliated epithelium lining the upper respiratory tract and traps microorganisms; the coordinated beating of the cilia propels the debris-laden mucus layer to the pharynx, where it can be swallowed or expectorated. Coughing enhances the function of this mucociliary elevator.

In the air-exchanging spaces of the lung comprising the lower respiratory tract, mucous and ciliated cells are absent so resident alveolar macrophages serve as the primary defense mechanism. If this vigilant cell is overwhelmed, it secretes mediators that increase vascular permeability and local levels of complement and recruit neutrophils. If the host is immune to the microorganism because of previous exposure, immune defenses amplify the nonspecific mechanisms. A primary immune response is initiated in the regional lymph nodes. A humoral response gives rise to IgA that finds its way to the surface of the trachea, bronchi, and bronchioles. This immunoglobulin effectively

blocks epithelial attachment of a number of pathogenic microorganisms, including mycoplasmas and viruses. Serum immunoglobulins of all classes enter the alveolar lining fluid, particularly when there is local inflammation. Induction of cell-mediated immunity generates sensitized T cells that accumulate in the interstitium and alveolar spaces. These mechanisms are summarized in Figure 13–20. From this review it can be predicted that abnormalities that affect either nonimmune or immune defense mechanisms predispose to lung infections. A partial list of common conditions associated with an increased risk for developing lung infections follows:

- Injury to the mucociliary elevator from tobacco smoke, toxic fumes, viral infections, or genetic defects in cilia.
- Loss of the gag or cough reflex as a result of anesthesia, drugs, coma, or neuromuscular disorder; voluntary suppression of cough because of chest pain.

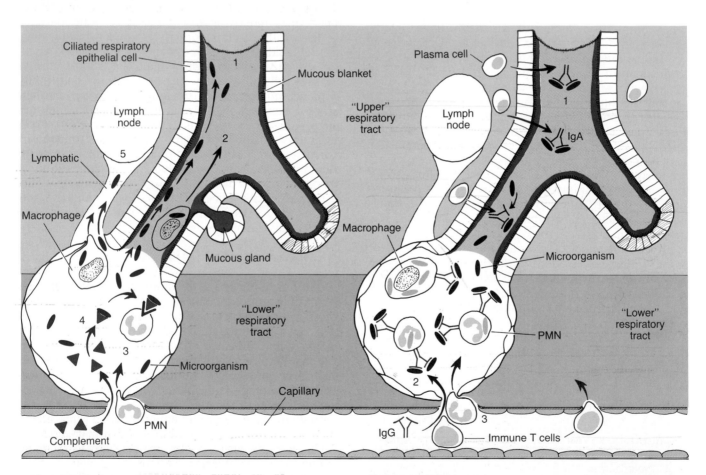

A NONIMMUNE LUNG   B IMMUNE LUNG

Figure 13–20. Lung defense mechanisms. *A,* In the nonimmune lung, removal of microbial organisms depends upon (1) entrapment in the mucous blanket and removal via the mucociliary elevator, (2) phagocytosis by alveolar macrophages that can kill and degrade organisms and remove them from the air spaces by migrating onto the mucociliary elevator, or (3) phagocytosis and killing by neutrophils recruited by macrophage factors. (4) Serum complement may enter the alveoli and be activated by the alternate pathway to provide the opsonin C3b that enhances phagocytosis. (5) Organisms including those ingested by phagocytes may reach the draining lymph nodes to initiate immune responses. *B,* Additional mechanisms operate in the immune lung. (1) Secreted IgA can block attachment of the microorganism to epithelium in the upper respiratory tract. (2) In the lower respiratory tract, serum antibodies (IgM, IgG) are present in the alveolar lining fluid. They activate complement more efficiently by the classical pathway, yielding C3b (not shown). In addition, IgG is also opsonic. (3) The accumulation of immune T cells is important in controlling infections by viruses and other intracellular microorganisms.

- Abnormal phagocytic function either secondary to viral infections, smoking, inhaled toxins, or antiinflammatory therapy, or as a primary genetic defect (e.g., chronic granulomatous disease). Pulmonary edema resulting from congestive heart failure in all likelihood interferes with normal phagocyte recruitment and function.
- Immune deficiency states, particularly secondary to immunosuppressive therapy or human immunodeficiency virus (HIV) infection.

Defects in nonimmune defenses (including neutrophil and complement defects) and humoral immunodeficiency typically lead to an increased incidence of infections with pyogenic bacteria. On the other hand, cell-mediated immune defects lead to increased infections with intracellular microbes such as mycobacteria and herpesviruses as well as with microorganisms of very low virulence such as *Pneumocystis carinii*. Several of these infectious agents will be discussed after a general review of pneumonias.

Pneumonia can be very broadly defined as any infection in the lung (Table 13–6). It may present as acute, fulminant clinical disease or as chronic disease with a more protracted course. A given pathogen

TABLE 13–6. LUNG INFECTIONS

Acute Bacterial Pneumonias
 Community-acquired, often following influenza: *Streptococcus pneumoniae* (single most common cause), *Haemophilus influenzae, Staphylococcus aureus, Klebsiella pneumoniae* and other gram-negative rods, *Legionella pneumophila,* aspiration pneumoniae with mixed aerobes and anaerobes, *Branhamella catarrhalis*
 Hospital-acquired (nosocomial): *Pseudomonas* spp., other gram-negative bacilli, *Staphylococcus aureus,* commonly penicillin resistant
"Atypical" Pneumonias
 Mycoplasma pneumoniae
 Viruses: Children: respiratory syncytial virus, parainfluenza virus; adults: influenza A and B, adenovirus (in military recruits)
 Chlamydia (*C. psittici, C. trachomatis,* and *C. pneumoniae*)
 Rickettsiae *(Coxiella burneti, Rickettsia rickettsiae)*
Chronic Pneumonias
 Nocardia spp.
 Actinomyces spp.
 Granulomatous: *Mycobacterium tuberculosis* and atypical mycobacteria, *Histoplasma capsulatum, Coccidioides immitis, Blastomyces dermatitidis, Paracoccidioides brasiliensis*
Lung Abscesses
 Mixed anaerobes, with or without accompanying aerobes (particularly *Streptococcus* spp.)
 Aerobes, uncommonly isolated alone: *Staphylococcus aureus, Streptococcus* spp., *Klebsiella pneumonia, Nocardia* spp.
*Pneumonias Largely Limited to Neutropenic or Immunosuppressed Persons**
 CMV
 Pneumocystis carinii (particularly in AIDS)
 Mycobacterium avium–Intracellulare
 Invasive aspergillosis
 Invasive candidiasis

*These patients are also at increased risk for the development of pneumonias caused by most of the other agents in this listing, particularly gram-negative bacilli.

usually causes only one of these forms of pneumonia (Table 13–6). *Acute pneumonias* may be caused by pyogenic bacteria that induce primarily neutrophilic exudates in alveoli, bronchioles, and bronchi or by a miscellaneous group of microorganisms that induce predominantly peribronchiolar and interstitial mononuclear inflammation. As commonly used the term "pneumonia" usually refers to the acute bacterial pneumonias, whereas the term "pneumonitis" is reserved for inflammatory conditions that primarily affect the interstitium and present clinically as "atypical" pneumonias (p. 415). In contrast to these two forms of acute pneumonias, the *chronic pneumonias* are usually caused by fungi, parasites, and intracellular bacteria as well as by the filamentous bacteria, *Nocardia* and *Actinomyces* species. Some of the chronic pneumonias may demonstrate a neutrophilic inflammatory component, but, as expected, chronic inflammation predominates, often with a striking granulomatous component. With this background we can discuss pulmonary infections by individual bacterial, viral, and fungal agents. This presentation follows the general sequence outlined in Table 13–6.

ACUTE BACTERIAL PNEUMONIAS ———

Bacterial pneumonias are typically associated with intraalveolar exudation resulting in *consolidation* (solidification) of lung parenchyma. They tend to conform to one of two anatomic and radiographic patterns, referred to as *lobar pneumonia* and *bronchopneumonia.* In lobar pneumonia the contiguous air spaces of part or all of a lobe are homogeneously filled with an exudate that can be visualized on radiographs as a lobar or segmental consolidation and is thus sometimes referred to as "air space" pneumonia (Fig. 13–21A). In contrast, bronchopneumonia implies a patchy distribution of inflammation that generally involves more than one lobe (Fig. 13–21B). This pattern results from an initial infection of the bronchi and bronchioles with extension into the adjacent alveoli. Certain organisms tend to cause bronchopneumonia, whereas others such as *Streptococcus pneumoniae* tend to produce a lobar pattern. More than 90% of lobar pneumonias are caused by *S. pneumoniae,* sometimes referred to as "pneumococcus," so this pattern is usually predictive of this specific pathogen. It should be noted, however, that the causal associations are not clear cut. For example, less commonly other bacteria such as *Klebsiella* can produce a lobar consolidation. Even mycoplasmas, which typically cause interstitial rather than intraalveolar inflammation, may give the appearance of lobar consolidation on chest radiographs. Furthermore, as will be discussed, one organism may produce bronchopneumonia on one occasion and lobar pneumonia in other hosts. Sometimes bronchopneumonia can become confluent and induce almost total lobar consolidation, or lobar pneumonia may not involve an entire lobe. *Ultimately, the terms "bronchopneumonia" and "lobar pneumonia" merely give some indication of the anatomic distribution of the*

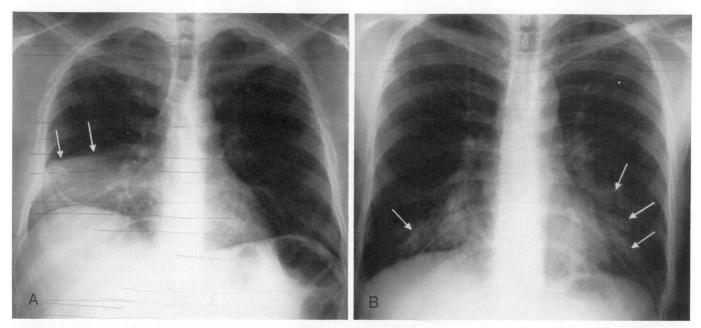

Figure 13–21. *A,* Chest radiograph of lobar pneumonia involving the right lower lobes. Arrows demonstrate the interlobar fissure. *B,* Radiograph of bronchopneumonia illustrating the patchy distribution of the infiltrates. The arrows demonstrate patches in the right and left lower lobes. (Courtesy of Dr. Michael Landay, Department of Radiology, Southwestern Medical School, Dallas, TX.)

infection and the likely causative agent, but there is much overlap. More significant is the total amount of involvement and, especially, the identity of the specific invader and its vulnerability to particular antibiotics. Therefore in the ensuing discussion bacterial pneumonias are categorized on the basis of the causative agent.

S. pneumoniae is the most common bacterial cause of acute community-acquired bacterial pneumonia, producing so-called *pneumococcal pneumonia.* This is described first and is followed by a discussion of pneumonias caused by other organisms.

Pneumococcal pneumonia occurs in all age groups, but elders and infants are particularly vulnerable. Those with underlying congestive heart failure, chronic obstructive lung disease, diabetes, or alcoholism are especially prone. Typically, the infection follows a viral upper respiratory tract infection. The onset is abrupt, with high fever and an episode of a severe shaking chill accompanied by pleuritic chest pain and a cough productive of rusty-colored purulent sputum.

MORPHOLOGY. With pneumococcal lung infection both patterns of pneumonia, lobar and bronchopneumonia, may occur; the latter is much more prevalent at the extremes of age. Regardless of the distribution of the pneumonia, because pneumococcal lung infections usually originate by aspiration of pharyngeal flora (20% of adults harbor *S. pneumoniae* in their throats), the lower lobes or the right middle lobe is most frequently involved.

In the preantibiotic era, pneumococcal pneumonia involved whole or almost whole lobes and evolved through four stages: congestion, red hepatization, gray hepatization, and resolution. Early antibiotic therapy alters or halts this typical progression so that at autopsy the anatomic changes may not conform to the classic stages.

During the first stage, that of congestion, the affected lobe(s) is heavy, red, and boggy, and histologically there is vascular congestion with proteinaceous fluid, scattered neutrophils, and many bacteria in the alveoli. Within a few days the stage of red hepatization ensues, in which the lung lobe is liver-like in consistency, the alveolar spaces are packed with neutrophils, red cells, and fibrin, and the pleura usually demonstrates a fibrinous or fibrinopurulent exudate. In the next stage, gray hepatization, the lung is dry, gray, and firm, and the fibrinous exudate persists within the alveoli but is relatively depleted of red cells (Fig. 13–22). Resolution follows in uncomplicated cases as exudates within the alveoli are enzymatically digested and either resorbed or expectorated leaving the basic architecture intact. The pleural reaction may similarly resolve or undergo organization, leaving fibrous thickening or permanent adhesions.

In the bronchopneumonic pattern, foci of inflammatory consolidation are distributed in patches throughout one or several lobes, most frequently bilateral and basal. Well-developed lesions up to 3 or 4 cm in diameter are slightly elevated, dry, granular, gray-red to yellow, and poorly delimited at their margins (Fig. 13–22). Confluence of these foci may occur in severe cases, producing the appearance of a lobar consolidation. The lung substance immediately surrounding areas of consolidation is usually hyperemic and edematous, but the large intervening areas are generally normal. Pleural involvement is less common than in lobar pneumonia. Histologically, the reaction consists of a suppurative

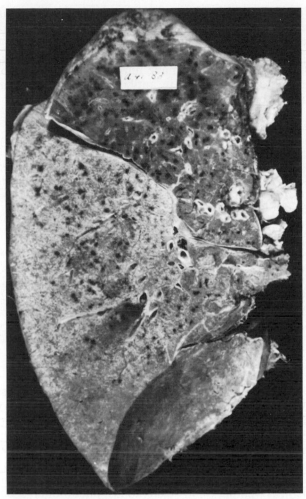

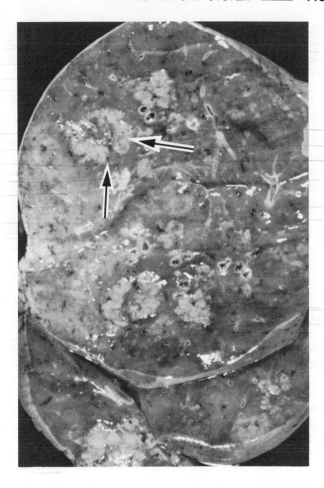

Figure 13–22. *Left,* Lobar pneumonia. The lower lobe is uniformly consolidated, whereas the upper lobe is relatively unaffected. Note the "plaster-cast" impression of the dome of the diaphragm, preserved in the bottom of the lower lobe, and the fibrinous exudate (pleuritis) layering this diaphragmatic surface. *Right,* Bronchopneumonia. A gross section of lung showing patches of gray purulent consolidation *(arrows).*

exudate that fills the bronchi, bronchioles, and adjacent alveolar spaces.

With appropriate therapy, complete restitution of the lung is the rule for both forms of pneumococcal pneumonia, but in occasional cases complications may occur: (1) tissue destruction and necrosis may lead to **abscess** formation; (2) suppurative material may accumulate in the pleural cavity, producing an **empyema**; (3) organization of the intraalveolar exudate may convert areas of the lung into solid fibrous tissue; and (4) bacteremic dissemination may lead to **meningitis**, **arthritis**, or **infective endocarditis**. Complications are much more likely with serotype 3 pneumococci.

Examination of Gram-stained sputum is an important step in the diagnosis of acute pneumonia. The presence of numerous neutrophils containing the typical gram-positive, lancet-shaped diplococci is good evidence of pneumococcal pneumonia, but it must be remembered that *S. pneumoniae* is a part of the endogenous flora and therefore false positive results may

be obtained by this method. Isolation of pneumococci from blood cultures is more specific. During early phases of illness blood cultures may be positive in 20 to 30% of patients.

Pneumococcal pneumonias respond readily to penicillin treatment but there is an increasing awareness that penicillin-resistant strains of pneumococci occur, so whenever possible antibiotic sensitivity should be determined.

Haemophilus influenzae, a small, gram-negative coccobacillus long known to be the most frequent cause of meningitis in children, is increasingly recognized as an important lung pathogen. Encapsulated *H. influenzae type b* is also an important cause of epiglottitis in children. Both unencapsulated and encapsulated forms are important in the causation of bronchopneumonias following viral infections, and in patients with chronic pulmonary diseases such as cystic fibrosis, chronic bronchitis, and bronchiectasis. The morphologic changes are indistinguishable from those of other bacterial bronchopneumonias. *H. influenzae* pneumonia is typically milder than other forms of pneumonia, has a more insidious onset, and in adults rarely results in abscess formation or empyema. Children are more likely to develop empyema and extrapulmonary complications such as otitis media, epiglottitis, arthritis, pericarditis, or meningitis.

Staphylococcus aureus is also an important cause of secondary bacterial pneumonia in children and healthy adults following viral respiratory illnesses: measles in children and influenza in both children and adults. _S. aureus_ may also cause a primary pneumonia in persons with chronic pulmonary disease, a particularly serious problem in hospitalized patients who are intubated or suffer aspiration. Hospital-acquired infections are of particular concern because the causative strains are frequently penicillin resistant and a significant minority (5%) are unresponsive to most antibiotics. Staphylococcal pneumonia occurring in association with right-sided staphylococcal endocarditis is a serious complication of intravenous drug abuse. Most often _S. aureus_ causes a bronchopneumonia with formation of multiple abscesses, but occasionally it can produce a lobar pattern of consolidation.

Klebsiella pneumoniae is the most common cause of gram-negative bacillary pneumonia, most frequently among debilitated and malnourished persons, particularly chronic alcoholics. The onset is abrupt and prostrating, similar to that of pneumococcal pneumonia, and it may be even more severe. Thick and gelatinous sputum is quite characteristic because the organism produces an abundant viscid capsular polysaccharide and the patient may have difficulty coughing it up. The pattern of pneumonia is frequently lobar and there is a propensity for distention of the lobes, seen as bulging of the interlobar fissures on radiographs. Even with treatment, this type of pneumonia has a considerably greater mortality rate than does pneumococcal pneumonia. If the patient survives, complete resolution is less frequent, and abscesses, fibrosis, and bronchiectasis may remain.

Legionella pneumophila, the agent of Legionnaires' disease, received its colorful name by being recognized first after an epidemic of frequently fatal pneumonia among delegates to the 1976 American Legion convention in Philadelphia. The spread of infection was traced to a contaminated water-cooled air-conditioning system in the convention hotel. It soon became evident, however, that Legionnaires' disease occurs endemically and sporadically and is a common cause of severe pneumonia requiring hospitalization. _L. pneumophila_ is also frequently involved in hospital-acquired respiratory infections. Other species of _Legionella_ are also pathogenic.

Legionella species are gram-negative rods that are ubiquitous in water, particularly standing tepid or warm water. Inhalation of airborne contaminated droplets is the likely mode of spread. _Legionella_ pneumonia is unusual in children and is more common in elders and persons with some predisposing condition such as cardiac, renal, immunologic, or hematologic disease. The clinical presentation does not distinguish this pneumonia from pneumonias caused by other bacteria. Unfortunately, the organism is difficult to identify and culture in sputum, and diagnosis usually depends on direct identification of the bacteria by fluorescent antibody techniques in samples obtained by transtracheal aspiration or bronchoalveolar lavage. Often the diagnosis is made retrospectively by demonstrating a fourfold rise in antibody titer in acute- and convalescent-phase sera.

> The lung changes may take the form of patchy bronchopneumonia or sometimes complete consolidation of one or more lobes. Microscopically, the alveolar spaces in the consolidated areas are filled with an inflammatory exudate composed of neutrophils and more macrophages than is usual in other bacterial pneumonias. Often there are areas of necrosis of the native architecture that create small abscesses. Organisms cannot be visualized by the usual bacterial stains but can be identified both within phagocytes and extracellularly using immunochemical stains or by using the Dieterle silver stain.

Pseudomonas aeruginosa, a common cause of nosocomial _(hospital-acquired)_ pneumonia, occurs almost exclusively in persons who have some defect in natural defenses. It is particularly prone to occur in patients rendered neutropenic, usually by chemotherapy for hematopoietic malignancies; in patients with extensive burns or cystic fibrosis; and in patients requiring mechanical ventilation. _Pseudomonas_ pneumonia occurs with or without bacteremia. Nonbacteremic _Pseudomonas_ pneumonia presents as a diffuse bronchopneumonia with abscess formation and a high incidence of empyema reminiscent of staphylococcal pneumonia. Bacteremic _Pseudomonas_ pneumonia is a progressive necrotizing pneumonia in which there is prominent blood vessel invasion and consequent extrapulmonary manifestations. Both forms of pneumonia are associated with a high mortality rate.

Aspiration bronchopneumonia occurs in markedly debilitated patients or those who aspirate gastric contents either while unconscious or during repeated vomiting. The resultant pneumonia is partly chemical, owing to the extremely irritating effects of the gastric acid, and partly bacterial. The bacterial component is a mixture of anaerobic and microaerophilic organisms normally present in the oral cavity. This type of pneumonia is often necrotizing, pursues a fulminant clinical course, and is a frequent cause of death in patients predisposed to aspiration. In those that survive, abscess formation is a common complication.

Branhamella catarrhalis was once considered a harmless commensal in the nasopharynx. It is now implicated in invasive infectious diseases, including pneumonia, in adults who have an underlying chronic obstructive lung disease. The pneumonia resembles that caused by _H. influenzae_.

PRIMARY ATYPICAL PNEUMONIAS _____

The concept of primary atypical pneumonia was set forth in 1938 with the description of eight cases in which pharyngitis and systemic flu-like symptoms evolved into laryngitis and finally tracheobronchitis and pneumonia. Unlike "typical" acute pneumonias, sputum production was modest, there were no physical findings of consolidation, the white cell count was only moderately elevated, and bacteria and influenza A viruses could not be isolated. In retrospect these cases were probably caused by *Mycoplasma pneumoniae.* This agent is the *most common cause of atypical pneumonias*, particularly at times when influenza A epidemics are not present in the community. A similar syndrome may occur with a number of other agents, including viruses, chlamydia, and rickettsiae. Nearly all these agents can also cause a primarily upper respiratory tract infection with coryza (inflammation with diffuse discharge from the nasal mucosa), pharyngitis, laryngitis, and tracheobronchitis. The common pathogenetic mechanism is attachment of the organisms to the respiratory epithelium followed by necrosis of the cells and an inflammatory response. When the process extends to alveoli there is usually *interstitial* inflammation, but there may also be some outpouring of fluid into alveolar spaces so that on chest films the changes may mimic bacterial pneumonia. Damage to and denudation of the respiratory epithelium inhibits mucociliary clearance and predisposes to secondary bacterial infections. Viral infections of the respiratory tract are well known for this complication.

Mycoplasma infections are particularly common among children and young adults. They occur sporadically or as local epidemics in closed communities (schools, military camps, prisons). Viral lower respiratory tract infections may occur at any age, and in adults they are most often caused by influenza viruses A and B (see Table 13–6). Less common offenders are *parainfluenza and respiratory syncytial viruses,* the latter especially in infants and children. *Adenovirus pneumonias* are particularly common in young army recruits. A number of other viruses are sometimes implicated, including those that cause measles and chickenpox. Much depends on the resistance of the host, so atypical pneumonias range from mild to severe. More serious lower respiratory tract infection is favored by infancy, old age, malnourishment, alcoholism, and immunosuppression. Not surprisingly, viruses and mycoplasmas are frequently involved in outbreaks of infection in hospitals.

MORPHOLOGY. Regardless of cause, the morphologic patterns in atypical pneumonias are similar. The process may be patchy, or it may involve whole lobes bilaterally or unilaterally. Macroscopically, the affected areas are red-blue, congested, and subcrepitant. The weight of the lungs is moderately increased. Because much of the reaction is interstitial, little inflammatory exudate escapes on sectioning of the lung, although there may be slight oozing of red, frothy fluid. Histologically, the inflammatory reaction is largely confined within the walls of the alveoli (Fig. 13–23). The septa are widened and edematous; they usually contain a mononuclear inflammatory infiltrate of lymphocytes, histiocytes, and occasionally plasma cells. In very acute cases, neutrophils may also be present. In contrast to bacterial pneumonias alveolar spaces are remarkably free of cellular exudate but may contain a proteinaceous fluid and occasional mononuclear cells. In severe cases full-blown **diffuse alveolar damage with hyaline membranes may develop.** Fibrin thrombi may be seen within the alveolar capillaries in areas of necrosis of the alveolar walls. In less severe, uncomplicated cases subsidence of the disease is followed by reconstitution of the native architecture. Superimposed bacterial infection, as expected, results in a mixed histologic picture.

CLINICAL COURSE. The clinical course of primary atypical pneumonia is extremely varied, even among cases caused by a single pathogen. Often, primary atypical pneumonia masquerades as a severe upper respiratory infection or "chest cold," and presumably many of these go undiagnosed. In contrast, in some patients, particularly those with underlying immunodeficiency, the course is fulminant and death may

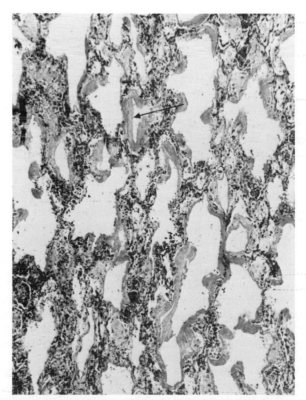

Figure 13–23. Viral pneumonia. The thickened alveolar walls are heavily infiltrated with mononuclear leukocytes. Coagulation of protein-rich intraalveolar exudate has formed hyaline membranes *(arrow).*

occur within a few days. More typically, the onset is that of an acute, nonspecific febrile illness characterized by fever, headache, and malaise. Only later do localizing symptoms appear. Chest radiographs usually reveal transient, ill-defined patches, mainly in the lower lobes. Physical findings are characteristically minimal, indistinguishable from bronchopneumonia, although, particularly with mycoplasma, lobar consolidations may occur. Because the edema and exudation are both in a strategic position to cause an alveolocapillary block there may be respiratory distress seemingly out of proportion to the physical and radiographic findings.

Identifying the causative agent is difficult. Indeed, in most cases the pathogen remains undetermined. Culture of the organism is possible but is often difficult. Rising titers of specific antibodies point to the diagnosis but these results are usually obtained after the patient has begun to recover. Elevations in the titers of cold agglutinins occur in mycoplasma infection, but this is present in only 50% of cases. Because this test is not specific, it is not widely utilized. As a practical matter, patients with community-acquired pneumonia, for which a bacterial agent seems unlikely, are often treated with an antibiotic (erythromycin) effective against _Mycoplasma_ organisms because they are the most common treatable cause.

The prognosis for uncomplicated cases is good; generally, complete recovery is the rule. The most serious infections, caused by influenza viruses in infirm and elderly persons, are often complicated by bacterial superinfection.

ACTINOMYCOSIS AND NOCARDIOSIS _____

The agents that most commonly cause actinomycosis (_Actinomyces israelii_) and nocardiosis (_Nocardia asteroides_) are bacteria belonging to the order Actinomycetales, but because of their filamentous morphology and slow growth they were originally considered fungi. These organisms produce chronic infections that are more indolent than those caused by pyogenic bacteria.

A. israelii is a normal anaerobic inhabitant of the oral cavity. There are three classic patterns of actinomycosis: (1) _cervicofacial_ (involving the jaw extending into the neck), (2) _thoracic,_ and (3) _abdominal and pelvic._ _A. israelii,_ an anaerobe, becomes pathogenic whenever there is devitalization of tissues and reduced oxygen tension. Thus actinomycosis may develop in the jaw and neck following an intraoral infection or dental surgery or in the lung or gastrointestinal tract, superimposed on an antecedent disorder (e.g., lung abscess, ulceroinflammatory disease of the gut) that provides a favorable environment for its growth.

Nocardia organisms are aerobic and are not usually normal inhabitants of the oral cavity. They are weakly acid fast (as compared to the mycobacteria), which distinguishes them from other actinomycetes. _Nocardia_ infections usually take the form of an acute bronchopneumonia with abscess formation, although they may

occasionally simulate tuberculosis. Sometimes there is an associated empyema. Nocardia has a propensity to disseminate, and in a third of cases it may infect the brain, where it typically causes abscesses.

MORPHOLOGY. The gross appearance of the lesions caused by both actinomycetes is essentially intense suppuration with abscess formation. Within the suppurative exudate, _A. israelii_ **grows in colony formation with a tangled mass of filaments surrounded by radiating, sometimes terminally clubbed, organisms.** These colonies are grossly visible as yellow to gray "sulfur granules." The branching filaments of nocardia rarely form colonies. Typical of both organisms is great chronicity, burrowing spread of the infection, and, sometimes, the development of penetrating sinus tracts. Thus lesions in the lung produced both by _A. israelii_ and _Nocardia_ resemble bronchopneumonia with abscess formation. In time, the abscesses are enclosed by a fibroblastic reaction, but sometimes fistulous sinus tracts penetrate to the pleural cavities or even through the chest wall. The fibroblast response is much more pronounced in actinomycosis. A similar sequence occurs wherever the organisms become implanted.

The diagnosis must be suspected whenever there is persistent suppurative chronic infection with abscess formation. It can be confirmed by identification of sulfur granules within the inflammatory exudate (actinomycosis) or the characteristic acid-fast forms in smears of exudate (nocardiosis) or culture of the causative agents.

TUBERCULOSIS _____

Tuberculosis (TB) is a communicable chronic _granulomatous disease_ caused by _Mycobacterium tuberculosis._ It usually involves the lungs but may affect any organ or tissue in the body. Typically, _the centers of tubercular granulomas undergo caseous necrosis._ Among medically and economically deprived persons throughout the world, TB remains a leading cause of death. It is estimated that 1 billion individuals are infected worldwide, with 8 million new cases and 3 million deaths per year. In the Western world deaths due to TB peaked in 1800 and steadily declined throughout the 1800s and early 1900s. With the development of streptomycin, an effective anti-TB drug, in the 1940s, the incidence of TB declined even more precipitously, but in 1984 the decline in new cases stopped abruptly, a change that resulted from the increased incidence of tuberculosis in HIV-infected persons.

It is important that _infection_ be differentiated from _disease._ Infection implies seeding of some focus with organisms, which may or may not cause clinically significant tissue damage (i.e., disease). Although other routes may be involved, most infections are acquired by direct person-to-person transmission of airborne droplets of organisms from an active case to a susceptible host. *In most persons an asymptomatic focus of pulmonary infection appears that is self-limited, although, uncommonly, primary tuberculosis may result in the development of fever and pleural effusion.* Generally, the only evidence of infection, if any remains, is a tiny, telltale fibrocalcific nodule at the site of the infection. Viable organisms may remain dormant in such loci for decades—and possibly for the life of the host. Such persons are infected, but do not have active disease and so cannot transmit organisms to others. Yet when their defenses are lowered, the infection may "reactivate" to produce communicable and potentially life-threatening disease.

Infection, whether active or inactive, can be detected by the tuberculin (Mantoux) test, which reveals the development of skin sensitivity to tuberculoprotein. About 2 to 4 weeks after the infection has begun, intracutaneous injection of 0.1 ml of purified protein derivative (PPD) induces a visible and palpable induration (at least 5 mm in diameter) that peaks in 48 to 72 hours. Sometimes, more PPD is required to elicit the reaction, and unfortunately, in some responders, the standard dose may produce a large, necrotizing lesion. A positive tuberculin test result signifies the presence of cell-mediated hypersensitivity to tubercular antigens. It does not differentiate between infection and disease. The possibility has been raised, but not proven, that a positive reaction requires that viable organisms persist in the latent focus of infection. It is well recognized that *false negative reactions (or skin test anergy) may be produced by certain viral infections, sarcoidosis, malnutrition, Hodgkin's disease, immunosuppression, and, notably, overwhelming active tuberculous disease.* False positive reactions may also result from infection by atypical mycobacteria.

About 80% of the population of South India (and many other Asian and African countries) are tuberculin positive. By contrast, in 1980 in the United States, 5 to 10% of the population reacted positively to tuberculin, indicating the marked difference in rates of exposure to the tubercle bacillus. Of the approximately 15 million persons exposed to tubercle bacilli in the United States, only 23,000 developed active disease in 1986. Thus, only a small fraction of those who contract an infection develop active disease.

Tuberculosis flourishes wherever there is poverty, crowding, and chronic debilitating illness. Similarly, elders, with their weakened defenses, are vulnerable. In the United States, American blacks, native Americans, the Inuit, and Hispanics have higher attack rates than other segments of the population. Whether this disparity can be ascribed entirely to socioeconomic factors or is in part genetic in origin is not known. Certain diseases also increase the risk: diabetes mellitus, Hodgkin's disease, chronic lung disease (particularly silicosis), malnutrition, alcoholism, and immunosuppression. In areas of the world where HIV infection is prevalent, this infection has become the single most important risk factor for development of tuberculosis. All these predisposing conditions are most likely related to a decrease in the capacity to develop and maintain T cell–mediated immunity against the infectious agent.

ETIOLOGY. Mycobacteria are slender rods and acid fast (i.e., they have a high content of complex lipids that readily bind the Ziehl-Neelsen [carbol fuchsin] stain and subsequently stubbornly resist decolorization). *M. tuberculosis hominis* is responsible for most cases of tuberculosis; the reservoir of infection is usually humans with active pulmonary disease. Transmission is usually direct, by inhalation of airborne organisms in aerosols generated by expectoration or by exposure to contaminated patient secretions. Oropharyngeal and intestinal tuberculosis contracted by drinking milk contaminated with *Mycobacterium bovis* is now rare in developed nations but still prevalent in countries that have tuberculous dairy cows and unpasteurized milk. Both *M. hominis* and *M. bovis* species are obligate aerobes whose slow growth is retarded by a pH lower than 6.5 and by long-chain fatty acids, hence the difficulty of finding tubercle bacilli in the centers of large caseating lesions where anaerobiosis, low pH, and increased levels of fatty acids are present.

PATHOGENESIS. There are three important considerations in understanding the pathogenesis of tuberculosis: (1) the basis of virulence of the organism, (2) the relationship of hypersensitivity (as expressed by a positive skin test result) to immunity against the infection, and (3) the pathogenesis of the caseation necrosis.

The virulence of the tubercle bacillus is not related to any known endotoxin. The ability of *M. tuberculosis* to induce disease in experimental animals appears to be related to mycosides (covalently linked complex lipids and carbohydrates) in the lipid fraction of the bacterium. One mycoside derivative, called "cord factor" (because it is responsible for the serpentine, cord-like growth of *M. tuberculosis* in vitro), is highly toxic to mice. Components of the cell wall of the bacillus, notably wax D (a glycolipid) and muramyl dipeptide, are powerful adjuvants (i.e., when injected with an antigen they induce a heightened immune response to it). The adjuvant effect is probably important in both the development of delayed hypersensitivity skin reactions and the granulomatous inflammation at sites of infection.

The development of cell-mediated, or type IV, hypersensitivity to the tubercle bacillus probably explains the organism's destructiveness in tissues and also the emergence of resistance to the organisms. On the initial exposure to the organism, the inflammatory response is nonspecific, resembling the reaction to any form of bacterial invasion. Within two or three weeks, coincident with the appearance of a positive skin reaction, the reaction becomes granulomatous and the centers of granulomas become caseous, forming typical "soft tubercles." The sequence of events following an initial lung infection is outlined in Figure 13–24 and summarized here:

- Antigen from the tubercle bacillus reaches draining lymph nodes and is presented to T cells. T cells are sensitized and recirculate to the site of infection.
- T cells release cytokines when exposed to antigen at the site of infection.

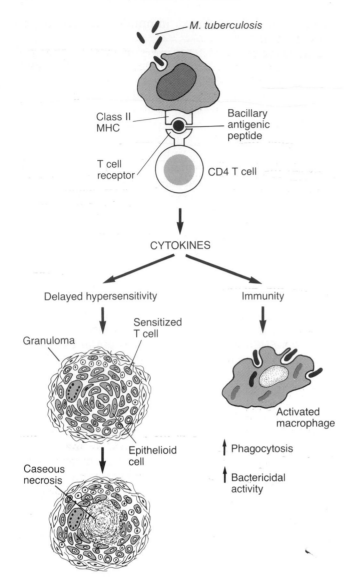

Figure 13-24. Tuberculosis: the dual consequences of the emergence of macrophage activation and sensitization.

- Monocytes are recruited and activated (particularly by γ-interferon from the T cells) to kill or inhibit the growth of the organism.
- In response to cytokines and possibly the constituents of the cell wall of the bacillus, some of the activated macrophages form granulomas, which may subsequently entrap the residual microorganisms.

Thus, it is apparent, *the development of hypersensitivity is requisite for granuloma formation and for enhanced resistance to the organisms.* Whether hypersensitivity and resistance are separate but concurrent functions or are interdependent is uncertain. In experimental animals T cells reactive with the antigens of tubercle bacilli can be cloned. Upon infusion into nonimmune animals some sensitized T-cell clones confer resistance to the infection but fail to transfer delayed type hypersensitivity; others do the opposite, and still other clones transfer both properties. Thus there is some evidence that hypersensitivity and resistance can be dissociated.

As mentioned, *typical granulomas in tuberculosis have central caseation (soft tubercles), although sometimes there is no caseation (hard tubercles).* What induces the caseation remains a mystery. The epithelioid cells that form the granuloma have characteristics of secretory rather than phagocytic cells, and it is likely that their products are responsible for the necrosis.

In summary, the appearance of hypersensitivity signals the acquisition of immunity and resistance to the organism. But at the same time, hypersensitivity is accompanied by the caseating destructive response to the tubercle bacillus. Thus, the sensitized host more rapidly mobilizes a defensive reaction but suffers enhanced necrosis of tissue. Whether the protective or destructive response predominates determines whether the primary focus of infection remains localized and disseminated organisms are destroyed or disabling disease appears.

Primary Tuberculosis

Primary tuberculosis is the form of disease that develops in a previously unexposed, and therefore unsensitized, person. Elders and profoundly immunosuppressed persons may lose their sensitivity to the tubercle bacillus and so may develop primary tuberculosis more than once. With primary tuberculosis, the source of the organism is exogenous. About 5% of those newly infected develop significant disease.

MORPHOLOGY. In countries where bovine tuberculosis and infected milk have largely disappeared, primary tuberculosis almost always begins in the lungs. Typically, the inhaled bacilli implant in the distal air spaces of the lower part of the upper lobe or the upper part of the lower lobe, usually close to the pleura. As sensitization develops, a 1- to 1.5-cm area of gray-white inflammatory consolidation emerges, **the Ghon focus.** In most cases the center of this focus undergoes caseation necrosis. Tubercle bacilli, either free or within phagocytes, drain to the regional nodes to initiate gray-white foci of consolidation, which also often caseate. **This combination of parenchymal lesion and nodal involvement is referred to as the Ghon complex** (Fig. 13-25). In most cases the pulmonary and nodal involvement is unilateral, but rarely bilateral or multiple Ghon foci or complexes are encountered. In most cases, the Ghon complex in time undergoes progressive fibrosis, often followed by calcification.

Histologically, **sites of active involvement are marked by a characteristic granulomatous inflammatory reaction that forms both caseating and noncaseating tubercles** (Fig. 13-26). Individual tubercles are microscopic; it is only when multiple granulomas coalesce that they become macroscopically visible. The granulomas are usually enclosed within a fibroblastic rim punctuated by lymphocytes. Multinucleate giant cells (typically Langhans' type) are present in the granulomas. In the more vulnerable host, the fibroblastic rim is poorly

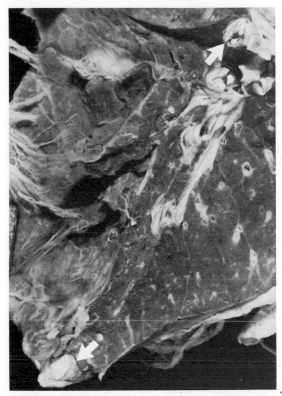

Figure 13–25. Primary pulmonary tuberculosis—Ghon complex. The parenchymal focus is present in the lower left subpleural location *(arrow)*. Lymph nodes with caseation are visible in the upper right *(arrow)*.

developed and the lymphocytic infiltrate sparse. To establish a diagnosis of tuberculosis **at autopsy or in a biopsy specimen the organisms must be identified by special stains or culture because the granulomatous reaction may occur in other diseases as well (p. 42).**

The chief implications of primary tuberculosis are that (1) it induces hypersensitivity and increased resistance; (2) the foci of scarring may harbor viable bacilli for years, perhaps for life, and thus be the nidus for reactivation at a later time when host defenses are compromised; and (3) uncommonly, the disease may develop without interruption into so-called progressive primary tuberculosis or disseminated disease. In progressive primary tuberculosis, the primary focus enlarges, caseates, and cavitates, sometimes spreading through the airways or lymphatics to multiple sites within the lung or perhaps causing multiple patchy white areas of cheesy consolidation that may cavitate. Blood-borne dissemination may give rise to miliary tuberculosis. These consequences also occur in secondary tuberculosis and so are described later.

Secondary Tuberculosis (Reactivation Tuberculosis)

Secondary tuberculosis is the pattern of disease that arises in a previously sensitized host. It may follow shortly after primary tuberculosis but more commonly it arises from reactivation of dormant primary lesions many decades after initial infection, particularly in those with weakened host resistance. Occasionally it results from exogenous reinfection because of waning of the protection afforded by the primary disease or

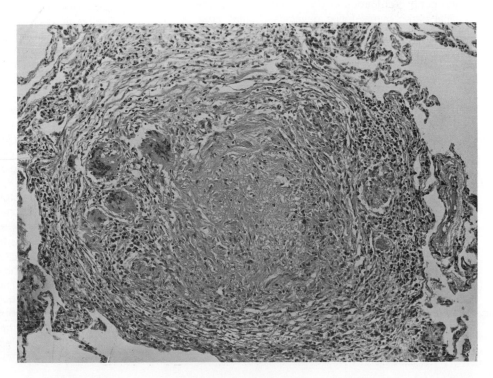

Figure 13–26. A characteristic tubercle in detail illustrates central caseation and both epithelioid and giant cells.

because of a large inoculum of virulent bacilli. Whatever the source of the organism, only a few patients (fewer than 5%) with primary disease subsequently develop secondary tuberculosis.

Secondary pulmonary tuberculosis is <u>classically localized to the apex of one or both upper lobes.</u> The reason is obscure, but it may relate to high oxygen tension in the apices. Because of the preexistence of hypersensitivity, the bacilli excite a prompt and marked tissue response that tends to wall off the focus. As a result of this localization, the regional lymph nodes are less prominently involved early in the developing disease than they are in primary tuberculosis. On the other hand, cavitation occurs readily in the secondary form, resulting in bronchogenic dissemination. Indeed, cavitation is almost inevitable in neglected secondary tuberculosis and erosion into an airway becomes an important source of infectivity because the patient now raises sputum containing bacilli. *It is noteworthy that in patients with HIV infection who are known to have been previously exposed to tuberculosis, reactivation disease does not usually present with apical lesions; cavitation is distinctly uncommon and mediastinal lymphadenopathy usually occurs.* Thus, in these markedly immunodeficient persons, the pattern of reactivation tuberculosis is more like that of primary tuberculosis. Because of impaired T-cell immunity in acquired immunodeficiency syndrome (AIDS) dissemination of tuberculosis occurs in about 50% of cases.

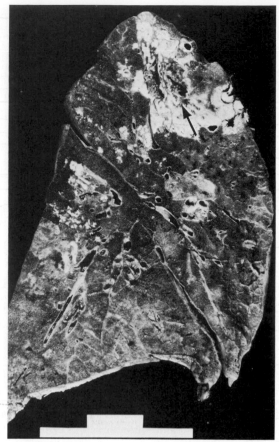

Figure 13–27. Secondary pulmonary tuberculosis. The cut section of the lung discloses massive caseation and cavitation *(arrow)* in the apex. Scattered foci of caseation as well as areas of pneumonic consolidation are present in both lobes.

MORPHOLOGY. The initial lesion is usually a small focus of consolidation, less than 2 cm in diameter, located within 1 to 2 cm of the apical pleura. Such foci are sharply circumscribed, firm, gray-white to yellow areas that have a variable amount of central caseation and peripheral fibrous induration. In favorable cases, the initial parenchymal focus develops a small area of caseation necrosis that does not cavitate because it fails to communicate with a bronchus or bronchiole. The subsequent course may be one of progressive fibrous encapsulation, leaving only fibrocalcific scars that depress and pucker the pleural surface and cause focal pleural adhesions. Histologically, the active lesions show characteristic coalescent tubercles with central caseation. Although tubercle bacilli can be demonstrated by appropriate methods in early exudative and caseous phases of granuloma formation, it is usually impossible to find them in the late, fibrocalcific, stages. Localized, apical, secondary pulmonary tuberculosis may undergo fibrocalcific arrest either spontaneously or following therapy, or the disease may progress and extend along several different pathways:

(1) **Progressive pulmonary tuberculosis** may ensue. The primary apical lesion enlarges with expansion of the area of caseation. Erosion into a bronchus evacuates the caseous center, creating a ragged, **irregular cavity lined by caseous material** that is poorly walled off by fibrous tissue (Fig. 13–27). Erosion of blood vessels may result in hemoptysis. The infection may spread by direct expansion, by dissemination through airways and lymphatic channels, or by miliary dissemination through the vascular system to other parts of the lungs alone or throughout the body. **Miliary pulmonary disease** occurs when organisms drain through lymphatics into the lymphatic ducts, which empty into the venous return to the right side of the heart and thence into the pulmonary arteries. Individual lesions are either microscopic or small, visible (2-mm) foci of yellow-white consolidation scattered through the lung parenchyma. Miliary lesions may expand and coalesce to yield almost total consolidation of large regions or even whole lobes of the lung (pneumonia alba). With chronicity, secondary scarring may markedly distort the pulmonary architecture. With progressive pulmonary tuberculosis, the pleural cavity is invariably involved, and serous **pleural effusions, tuberculous empyema**, or **obliterative fibrous pleuritis** may develop.

(2) **Endobronchial, endotracheal, and laryngeal tuberculosis** may develop when infective material is spread either through lymphatic channels or from expectorated infectious material. The mucosal lining may be studded with minute granulomatous lesions, sometimes apparent only on microscopic examination.

(3) **Systemic miliary tuberculosis** ensues when infective foci in the lungs seed the pulmonary venous return to the heart; the infection subsequently disseminates through the systemic arterial system. Almost every organ in the body may be seeded. Lesions resemble those in the lung. Miliary tuberculosis is most prominent in the liver, bone marrow, spleen, adrenals, meninges, kidneys, fallopian tubes, and epididymis.

(4) **Isolated-organ tuberculosis** may appear in any one of the organs or tissues affected by miliary dissemination. Organs typically involved include the meninges (tuberculous meningitis), kidneys (renal tuberculosis), adrenals (formerly an important cause of Addison's disease), bones (osteomyelitis), and fallopian tubes (salpingitis). When the vertebrae are affected, the disease is referred to as Pott's disease.

(5) In years past, **intestinal tuberculosis** contracted by drinking contaminated milk was fairly common as the primary focus of tuberculosis. It was often preceded by tuberculous involvement of the oropharyngeal lymphoid tissue with spread to the lymph nodes in the neck (scrofula). In developed countries today intestinal tuberculosis is more often a complication of protracted advanced secondary tuberculosis, secondary to swallowing coughed-up infective material. Typically, the organisms are trapped in mucosal lymphoid aggregations of the small and large bowel, which then undergo inflammatory enlargement with ulceration of the overlying mucosa, particularly in the ileum.

The many patterns of tuberculosis are depicted in Figure 13–28.

CLINICAL COURSE. Secondary tuberculosis, when localized, may be asymptomatic. When manifestations appear they are usually insidious in onset; there is gradual development of both systemic and localizing symptoms. Systemic symptoms are probably related to cytokines released by activated macrophages (e.g., TNF-α and IL-1). They often appear early in the course and include malaise, anorexia, weight loss, and fever. Commonly the fever is low grade and remittent (appearing late each afternoon and then subsiding), and night sweats occur. With progressive pulmonary involvement, localizing symptoms appear. One of the earliest is cough that gradually becomes more distressing and yields increasing amounts of sputum, at first mucoid and later purulent. When cavitation is present, the sputum contains tubercle bacilli. Some degree of hemoptysis is present in about half of all cases of pulmonary tuberculosis. Pleuritic pain may also be the first manifestation of the disease, resulting either from spontaneous pneumothorax or from extension of the infection to the pleural surfaces. The diagnosis is based in part on the history and on the physical and radiographic findings of consolidation or cavitation in the apices of the lungs. Ultimately, however, tubercle bacilli must be identified. Acid-fast smears and cultures of the sputum of patients suspected of having tuberculosis should be performed. Because cultures may take up to 10 weeks to become positive, there is much interest in the new DNA-based diagnostic techniques. In some recent studies, rapid diagnosis of tuberculosis has been accomplished by amplification of mycobacterial DNA in clinical samples. Miliary tuberculosis is difficult to diagnose, often presenting, particularly in elders and patients with AIDS, as a fever of unknown

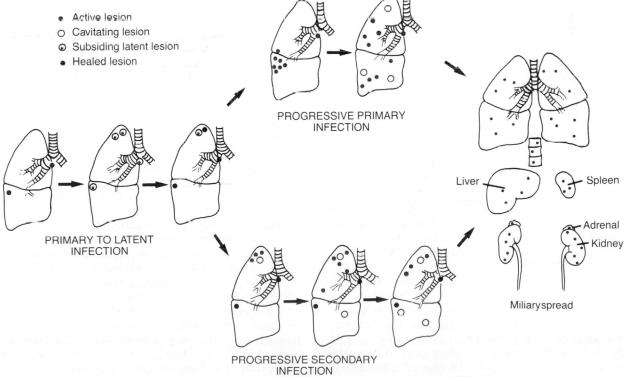

- Active lesion
- Cavitating lesion
- Subsiding latent lesion
- Healed lesion

PROGRESSIVE PRIMARY INFECTION

PRIMARY TO LATENT INFECTION

Liver

Spleen

Adrenal

Kidney

Miliary spread

PROGRESSIVE SECONDARY INFECTION

Figure 13–28. Potential progressions of pulmonary tuberculosis.

origin in the absence of apparent active pulmonary disease. The diagnosis may depend on identifying tubercles containing acid-fast bacilli in bone marrow or liver tissue.

The prognosis is generally good when infections are localized to the lungs, except when they are caused by drug-resistant strains or occur in aged, debilitated, or immunosuppressed persons, who are at high risk for developing miliary tuberculosis. Amyloidosis may appear in persistent cases.

FUNGAL INFECTIONS

Many pathogenic fungi (e.g., the dermatophytes) limit their activities to the skin, producing superficial mycoses. Those that cause systemic infections (deep mycoses) are, of course, of greater medical concern. The *dimorphic fungi: Histoplasma capsulatum, Coccidioides immitis,* and *Blastomyces dermatitidis,* all cause pulmonary disease in ostensibly normal hosts following inhalation of the infective stage of the organism. As would be expected, the infections are likely to be more severe in the immunosuppressed. The *nonseptate hyphal fungi* belonging to the order Mucorales, and the mold-like fungus, *Aspergillus,* are strictly opportunistic infectious agents. They are particularly aggressive in patients with decreased numbers or functions of phagocytes. The *yeast-like fungi, Candida* species and *Cryptococcus neoformans,* can cause disease in otherwise healthy hosts, but they are best considered opportunistic infectious agents because they clearly cause more serious infection in immunocompromised patients. All systemic fungi can infect the lung, although extrapulmonary disease may be more frequent and clinically more important with some fungi.

Histoplasmosis

Infection caused by *H. capsulatum* mimics tuberculosis in many ways. It typically begins with a primary pulmonary infection that is localized and asymptomatic in 90% of cases. It may progress to more extensive pulmonary involvement, sometimes cavitary, and in predisposed persons may disseminate in a miliary pattern. Histoplasmosis, one of the most common systemic fungal infection in the U.S., is endemic in the Ohio and central Mississippi River Valleys and along the Appalachian Mountains in the southeastern United States. Warm, moist soil, enriched by droppings from bats and birds, provides the optimal medium for the growth of the mycelial form, which produces infectious spores. When airborne and inhaled, the spores germinate into the parasitic yeast form in the lungs. In most normal adults in endemic areas the infection is asymptomatic and takes the form of a peripheral pulmonary lesion associated with hilar lymphadenopathy, recapitulating the Ghon complex of tuberculosis. Unlike tuberculosis, however, the initial lesions of histoplasmosis are often multiple. Exposed persons develop a positive histoplasmin skin reaction (analogous to the tuberculin test). The primary infection may undergo fibrosis and calcification and be discovered only by radiography in a person with a positive histoplasmin skin test result who is tuberculin negative. In children or adults with lowered resistance or defective immune responses, this primary complex may be followed by pulmonary infection, leading in some instances to lymphohematogenous dissemination and extrapulmonary disease.

> **MORPHOLOGY. The round to oval histoplasma yeast forms, 2- to 5-μm in diameter, infect and multiply within mononuclear phagocytes.** The primary pulmonary nodules, composed of aggregates of macrophages stuffed with organisms, are usually located in a lower lobe and are associated with similar lesions in the regional lymph nodes. These lesions develop into small granulomas complete with Langhans' giant cells and may develop central necrosis and later fibrosis and calcification. The similarity to tuberculosis is striking, and differentiation requires identification of the yeast forms (best seen with periodic acid-Schiff [PAS] or silver stains). In the vulnerable host upper lobe chronic cavitary disease develops, resembling the secondary form of tuberculosis. Histologically, the margins of the cavity exhibit coalescent granulomas with central necrosis. In infants or immunocompromised adults, particularly those with HIV infection, histoplasmosis develops into disseminated disease (analogous to miliary tuberculosis). Under these circumstances, when T cell–mediated immunity is markedly impaired, there is no granuloma formation. Instead focal collections of phagocytes stuffed with yeast forms expand the tissue spaces and cause enlargement of the organs comprising the mononuclear phagocyte system, including the liver, spleen, lymph nodes, lymphoid tissue of the gastrointestinal tract, and bone marrow. The adrenals and meninges may also be involved, and in about 25% of cases ulcers form in the nose and mouth, on the tongue, or in the larynx.

CLINICAL COURSE. The clinical manifestations of histoplasmosis are almost indistinguishable from those of tuberculosis. The infection may be asymptomatic, or it may cause only vague manifestations such as fever, malaise, and myalgias and be readily mistaken for "flu." With more extensive pulmonary involvement, cough, hemoptysis, and even dyspnea and chest pain may appear. Disseminated disease is a hectic, febrile illness that may be accompanied by hepatosplenomegaly, anemia, leukopenia, or thrombocytopenia, as well as manifestations relating to principal sites of localization. Although the histoplasmin skin test and elevated serum antibody titers reveal exposure to the organism, they do not distinguish present from past disease. The diagnosis of active infection is best made by direct visualization of the organism in the lesion and by culture of sputum or material from bone marrow or liver biopsy.

Coccidioidomycosis

Coccidioidomycosis, or "cocci," as some call it, is caused by *C. immitis*. It results from inhalation of infective arthrospores and is endemic in the Southwest and far West of the United States, particularly in the San Joaquin Valley, where it is known as valley fever. There, almost 80% of the population are coccidioidin skin test positive (analogous to the tuberculin test). Coccidioidomycosis, like histoplasmosis and tuberculosis, takes the forms of (1) *an asymptomatic pulmonary infection (about 60% of exposed persons)*, (2) *progressive pulmonary disease*, or (3) *miliary disease*.

MORPHOLOGY. The primary pulmonary form consists of a small focus of consolidation in the middle or lower lung field. Spread to the hilar lymph nodes simulates the Ghon complex of tuberculosis. The sites of infection are usually marked by granulomas, which often have central caseation and giant cells. **Fungi appearing as thick-walled, nonbudding spherules, 20 to 60 μm in diameter (often filled with small endospores, Fig. 13–29),** can be visualized around the necrotic debris, or sometimes within macrophages or giant cells. In most instances the lesions heal by progressive fibrosis and calcification and the infection is asymptomatic. In about 40% of patients, the disease produces symptoms such as fever, chills, cough, and pleuritic chest pain, mimicking a pneumonia caused by a mycoplasma or virus. Often such persons have hypersensitivity reactions, such as erythema nodosum or erythema multiforme, polyarthritis, pleuritis, and pericarditis. In these cases, the histologic reaction may be granulomatous but may take the form of suppuration in which fungal spherules can be seen. Progressive disease is marked by more disseminated involvement of the lungs and coalescent areas of consolidation. In fewer than 10%, miliary dissemination follows with spread to the skin, bones, adrenals, lymph nodes, spleen, liver, and meninges. Systemic spread is more likely to occur in blacks, Asians, or Filipinos than in Caucasians, unless they have underlying AIDS. Suppuration, rather than granuloma formation, is the rule in disseminated disease and likely reflects loss of cell-mediated immunity.

The clinical diagnosis can be suspected with a positive coccidioidin skin test, which develops within ten days to three weeks of infection, and is further supported by elevated IgM antibody titers, which develop within the first month of infection. Diagnosis is confirmed by culture of the organism.

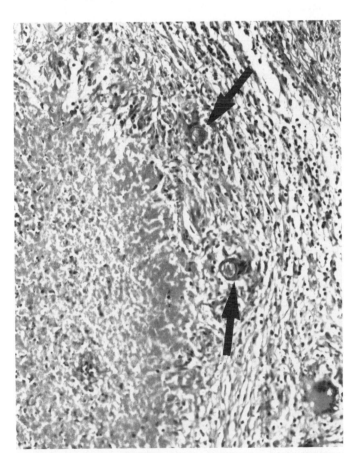

Figure 13–29. Coccidioides spherules *(arrows)* in a caseating granuloma from a patient with pulmonary coccidioidomycosis.

Candidiasis

Candida albicans is the most frequent disease-causing fungus. It is a normal inhabitant of the oral cavity, gastrointestinal tract, and vagina in many individuals. The spectrum of candidiasis is broad. *C. albicans* most frequently causes superficial, bothersome infections of the mouth, nails, genital tract (vaginitis in females), and perianal area of infants (diaper rash), but in immunosuppressed persons it can cause widespread mucocutaneous involvement or become systemic, producing abscesses in many organs. The source of infection in fungemic states is often contaminated indwelling intravenous lines, surgical drains, or urinary tract catheters. In many cases in which *Candida* is consistently isolated from the blood, the patient improves when the infecting source is simply removed, particularly if the patient is not severely immunosuppressed.

The most common pattern of candidiasis takes the form of a superficial infection on mucosal surfaces of the oral cavity (thrush) or vagina. Florid proliferation of the fungi creates gray-white, dirty-looking superficial membranes composed of matted organisms and inflammatory debris. Deep to the surface there is mucosal hyperemia and a superficial inflammation. This form of candidiasis is seen in newborns, diabetics, debilitated patients, or persons receiving broad-spectrum antibiotics that destroy competing normal bacterial flora. However, vaginal candidiasis may develop in otherwise healthy women; it is particularly common in pregnant women and in those who take oral contraceptives. A more erosive chronic mucocutaneous candidiasis occurs, particularly in the esophagus, in the mortally ill or in association with any hematologic or

T-cell derangement that markedly impairs the inflammatory-immune response. *Oral thrush, often accompanied by esophageal candidiasis, is extremely common in patients with AIDS.*

Invasive candidiasis implies blood-borne dissemination of organisms to various tissues or organs. Common patterns are: (1) renal abscesses, (2) myocardial abscesses and endocarditis, (3) brain involvement (most commonly meningitis, but parenchymal microabscesses occur), (4) endophthalmitis (virtually any eye structure can be involved), (5) hepatic abscesses, and (6) pulmonary lesions (manifest as irregular or cannonball abscesses of varying sizes, which are sometimes hemorrhagic owing to vascular invasion).

Blood-borne dissemination and miliary abscess formation is likely to occur when there is extensive tissue trauma or neutrophil defects. Patients receiving chemotherapy for acute lymphoblastic leukemia are particularly susceptible because of neutropenia associated with bone marrow suppression. In patients who have valvular heart disease or a prosthetic heart valve, or who are heroin addicts, candidemia is particularly prone to cause *Candida* endocarditis, which then serves as a continuing source of seeding via the bloodstream.

Other Fungal Infections

Blastomycosis, caused by *B. dermatitidis,* is most easily remembered as being similar to histoplasmosis and coccidioidomycosis. *It may take the form of an asymptomatic primary pulmonary infection, progressive pulmonary disease, or (rarely) disseminated miliary disease.*

Similarly, the histologic changes are most often granulomatous but may be suppurative in particularly vulnerable hosts. "Blasto," however, has the following differences from "cocci":

- The pathogen is smaller (5 to 25 μm diameter), round to oval, thick walled, and reproduces by budding rather than endosporulation.
- The endemic area is confined in the United States to areas overlapping with those where histoplasmosis is found.
- There is no reliable skin test and serologic tests are relatively insensitive.
- Dissemination frequently involves the skin in the form of indolent papules or enlarging fungating ulcers.
- Cutaneous infections frequently induce striking pseudoepitheliomatous hyperplasia, which is easily mistaken for squamous cell carcinoma.

Cryptococcosis, caused by *C. neoformans,* rarely occurs in otherwise healthy persons. It almost always represents an opportunistic infection in immunocompromised hosts, particularly those with AIDS, leukemia, lymphoma, or Hodgkin's disease. The fungus, a 5- to 10-μm yeast, has a thick, gelatinous capsule and reproduces by budding. Like the previously described systemic fungi, the infective form is most likely present in the soil and is acquired by inhalation. The fungus initially localizes in the lungs and then disseminates to other sites, particularly the meninges. *Sites of involvement are marked by a variable tissue response, which ranges from florid proliferation of gelatinous organisms with a minimal or absent inflammatory cell infiltrate (in immunodeficient hosts) to a granulomatous reaction (in the more reactive host).* Patients with cryptococcal meningitis present with headache and fever. The cerebrospinal fluid contains an elevated concentration of protein and demonstrates moderate lymphocytosis, although both of these changes may be minimal in profoundly immunodeficient patients, such as those with AIDS. Diagnosis can be made in about 70% of cases by adding India ink to a drop of centrifuged spinal fluid to demonstrate the yeast cell body surrounded by the halo of the polysaccharide capsule. However, the most sensitive test is based on detection of cryptococcal antigen by utilizing antibodies to cryptococcal polysaccharide attached to latex particles. Results of the latex agglutination test are positive in more than 95% of cases and should be confirmed by culture.

Mucormycosis and *invasive aspergillosis* are uncommon infections limited to immunocompromised hosts, particularly those with diabetes or leukemia-associated neutrophil defects and those receiving steroid treatment. *Both diseases are caused by fungi that assume mycelial forms in lesions.* In mucormycosis, the hyphae are nonseptate and branch at right angles; and in aspergillosis the hyphae are septate and branch at more acute angles. In mucormycosis, the organisms preferentially localize in the nose (from which they may rapidly spread to the sinuses and brain), lungs, and gastrointestinal tract. *Aspergillus* species favor the lungs, from whence they may disseminate. Both agents cause a nondistinctive, suppurative, sometimes granulomatous, reaction with a predilection for invading blood vessel walls, causing vascular necrosis and infarction.

In addition to the invasive aspergillosis seen in severely compromised patients, two other forms of pulmonary aspergillosis may occur: (1) colonization of pulmonary cavities (e.g., ectatic bronchi or lung cysts), to create fungus balls; these may act as ball valves, occluding the cavity and thus predisposing to infection and hemoptysis; (2) allergic bronchopulmonary aspergillosis; in this form patients with asthma develop an exacerbation of symptoms due to development of type I hypersensitivity against the fungus growing in the bronchi.

LUNG ABSCESS

Lung abscess refers to a localized area of suppurative necrosis within the pulmonary parenchyma. The causative organism may be introduced into the lung by any of the following mechanisms:

- *Aspiration of infective material* from carious teeth or infected sinuses or tonsils, particularly likely during oral surgery, anesthesia, coma, or alcoholic intoxication, and in debilitated patients with depressed cough reflexes.

- *Aspiration of gastric contents,* usually accompanied by infectious organisms.
- As a *complication of acute bacterial pneumonia,* particularly that caused by *S. aureus, K. pneumoniae, Pseudomonas* species, and, occasionally, type 3 pneumococci. Mycotic infections and bronchiectasis may also lead to lung abscesses.
- *Bronchial obstruction,* particularly with bronchogenic carcinoma obstructing a bronchus or bronchiole. Impaired drainage, distal atelectasis, and aspiration of blood and tumor fragments all contribute to the development of abscesses. An abscess may also form within an excavated necrotic portion of a tumor.
- *Septic embolism,* from septic thrombophlebitis or from infective endocarditis of the right side of the heart.

In addition, lung abscesses may result from hematogenous spread of bacteria in disseminated pyogenic infection. When all of the above pathogenetic pathways are excluded, there are still a large number of cases of mysterious origin, referred to as "primary cryptogenic lung abscesses."

Anaerobic bacteria are present in almost all lung abscesses, sometimes in vast numbers, and they are the exclusive isolates in a third to two thirds of cases. The most frequently encountered anaerobes are commensals normally found in the oral cavity, principally species of *Bacteroides, Fusobacterium, Peptococcus,* and microaerophilic streptococci. Often there is a mixed anaerobic-aerobic infection; the most commonly isolated aerobic organisms are *S. aureus,* β-hemolytic streptococci, *Nocardia,* and many different gram-negative organisms.

> **MORPHOLOGY.** Abscesses vary in diameter from a few millimeters to large cavities of 5 to 6 cm. The localization and number of abscesses depend on their mode of development. Pulmonary abscesses resulting from aspiration of infective material are much more common on the right side (more vertical airways) than on the left, and most are single. On the right side they tend to occur in the subapical and axillary portions of the upper lobe and in the apical portion of the lower lobe, because these locations reflect the likely course of aspirated material when the patient is recumbent. Abscesses that develop in the course of pneumonia or bronchiectasis are commonly multiple, basal, and diffusely scattered. Septic emboli and abscesses arising from hematogenous seeding or from empyemas are commonly multiple and may affect any region of the lungs.
>
> As the focus of suppuration enlarges, it almost inevitably ruptures into airways. Thus, the contained exudate may be partially drained, producing an air-fluid level on radiographic examination. The proteolytic digestion of the exudate favors the growth of organisms, including saprophytes; thus a lung abscess may rapidly become a multilocular cavity with poor margination. The expanding mass may infringe on the blood supply, leading to **gangrene** of the lung. Occasionally, abscesses rupture into the pleural cavity and produce bronchopleural fistu-

> las, the consequence of which is pneumothorax or empyema. Histologically, as expected with any abscess, there is suppuration surrounded by variable amounts of fibrous scarring and mononuclear infiltration (lymphocytes, plasma cells, macrophages), depending on the chronicity of the lesion.

CLINICAL COURSE. The manifestations of a lung abscess are much like those of bronchiectasis and include a prominent cough that usually yields copious amounts of foul-smelling, purulent, or sanguineous sputum; occasionally hemoptysis occurs. If there is no avenue for drainage of the abscess cavity, sputum may be minimal. Spiking fever and malaise are common, and there may be pleuritic pain. Clubbing of the fingers, weight loss, and anemia may all occur. Infective abscesses occur in 10 to 15% of patients with bronchogenic carcinoma; thus, when a lung abscess is suspected in an older patient underlying carcinoma must be considered. When discovered early the vast majority of abscesses are eliminated by appropriate antibiotic therapy. Surgical resection or drainage may be necessary in some cases. Secondary amyloidosis develops infrequently in chronic cases. Overall, the mortality rate is in the range of 10%.

CYTOMEGALOVIRUS INFECTIONS ————

Cytomegalovirus (CMV), a member of the herpesvirus family, may produce a variety of disease manifestations, depending partly on the age of the infected host but even more on the host's immune status. *Cells infected by the virus exhibit gigantism of both the entire cell and its nucleus. Within the nucleus is an enlarged inclusion, which gives the name to the classic form of symptomatic disease that occurs in neonates, cytomegalic inclusion disease* (CID). Although classic CID is a multisystem disease, CMV infections are discussed here because in immunosuppressed adults, particularly AIDS patients and transplant recipients, CMV pneumonitis is a serious problem. Transmission of CMV occurs at three peak periods:

- Transplacentally from a newly acquired or chronic asymptomatic infection in the mother
- During the first year of life, by transmission of the virus through cervical or vaginal secretions at birth, or later, through breast milk from a mother who has active infection
- After 15 years of age from respiratory secretions, via the fecal-oral route, from blood transfusions or organ grafts, or by venereal routes

In healthy young children and adults the disease is nearly always asymptomatic. In surveys around the world, 50 to 100% of adults demonstrate serum antibody titers, indicating exposure. About 5% of healthy blood donors possess demonstrable CMV-infected leukocytes. Occasionally some immunocompetent patients develop an infectious mononucleosis–like illness, with fever, atypical lymphocytosis, lymphadenopathy, and hepatomegaly accompanied by abnormal liver function tests suggesting mild hepatitis.

Infection acquired in utero may take many forms. In approximately 90% of cases it is asymptomatic, but in some, mainly those who acquire the virus from a mother with primary infection, classic CID develops. Affected infants may be profoundly ill and manifest jaundice, hepatosplenomegaly, anemia, and bleeding due to thrombocytopenia. Such findings mimic erythroblastosis fetalis (p. 343). Those infants who survive usually bear permanent residual effects, including mental retardation and various neurologic impairments. The congenital infection is not always devastating, however, and may take the form of an interstitial pneumonitis, hepatitis, encephalitis, or a hematologic disorder. Most infants with this milder form of CID recover, although a few may later be mentally retarded. Rarely, a totally asymptomatic infection may be followed months to years later by neurologic sequelae, including delayed-onset mental retardation, hearing deficits, and cerebral calcifications.

Immunosuppression can predispose children and adults to serious CMV infections that primarily affect the lungs, gastrointestinal tract, or retina; the central nervous system is usually spared. As mentioned, immunosuppressed transplant recipients and patients with AIDS are particularly vulnerable. In the pulmonary infection, an interstitial mononuclear infiltrate with foci of necrosis develops, accompanied by typical enlarged cells with inclusions. The pneumonitis can progress to full blown ARDS. Intestinal necrosis and ulceration can develop and be extensive, leading to debilitating diarrhea. CMV chorioretinitis can occur either alone or in combination with involvement of the lungs and intestinal tract. An overview of the many outcomes of infection is offered in Figure 13–30.

In classic severe neonatal disease (CID) the organs most often affected, in order of frequency, are the salivary glands, kidneys, liver, lungs, pancreas, thyroid, adrenal, and brain. Grossly, anatomic changes are minimal, consisting chiefly of slight enlargement of the involved organs, particularly liver and spleen. The brain is often smaller than normal (microcephaly) and may show foci of calcification. Histologically, the characteristic enlargement of cells can be appreciated. In the glandular organs, the parenchymal epithelial cells are affected; in the brain, the neurons; in the lungs, the alveolar macrophages and epithelial and endothelial cells; and in the kidneys, the tubular epithelial and glomerular endothelial cells. Random cells are involved and are strikingly enlarged, often to a diameter of 40 μm, and show cellular and nuclear polymorphism. Prominent intranuclear basophilic inclusions spanning half the nuclear diameter are usually set off from the nuclear membrane by a clear halo (Fig. 13–31). Within the cytoplasm of these cells, smaller basophilic inclusions may also be seen. Interstitial pneumonitis may be present, as well as focal necrosis within the liver and adrenals. Focal necrosis with ulcerations occurs in the small and large intestines. The affected ganglion cells within the brain are often surrounded by a glial reaction, sometimes with calcification. There is a tendency for the brain lesions to center around the third ventricle, aqueduct, and fourth ventricle.

PNEUMOCYSTIS PNEUMONIA ——————

P. carinii is an opportunistic infectious agent of uncertain classification. Although the terminology applied to protozoa is used to describe the various stages

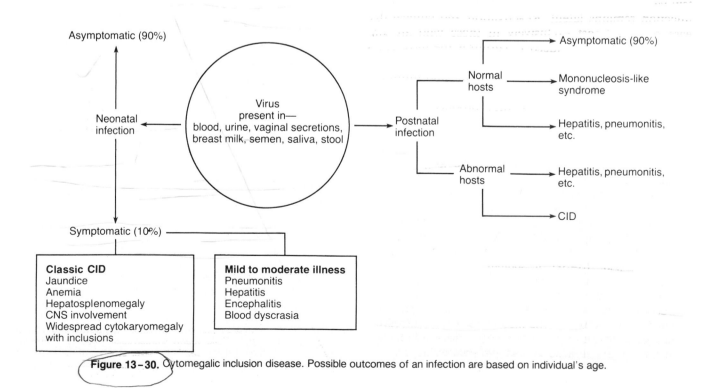

Figure 13–30. Cytomegalic inclusion disease. Possible outcomes of an infection are based on individual's age.

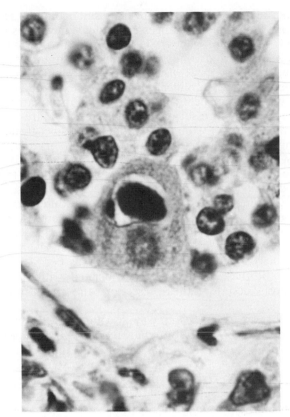

Figure 13–31. Cytomegalic inclusion disease. The markedly enlarged cell in the pancreatic islet has a prominent nuclear inclusion surrounded by a cleared halo. There are basophilic cytoplasmic inclusions as well.

of its life cycle, genetic analysis links it most closely to fungi. Serologic evidence indicates that virtually all persons are exposed to pneumocystis during the first few years of life, but in the overwhelming majority the infection remains latent. Reactivation and clinical disease occurs almost exclusively in those who are immunocompromised. Indeed *P. carinii* is the most common cause of infection in patients with AIDS and may also infect severely malnourished infants and immunosuppressed persons. Pneumocystis infections are largely confined to the lung, where they produce interstitial pneumonitis.

Microscopically, involved areas of the lung demonstrate intraalveolar foamy, pink-staining exudate (with hematoxylin and eosin), and the septa are thickened by edema and a minimal mononuclear infiltrate. Special stains are required to visualize the organism in either the trophozoite or encysted form. Silver stains of tissue sections reveal cup-shaped cyst walls in the alveolar exudates (Fig. 13–32). If sputum production can be successfully induced in the patient, Giemsa or methylene blue stains can demonstrate the trophozoite forms of organism (about 6 μm in diameter with long filopodia) in about 50% of patients. The most sensitive and effective method of diagnosis is to identify the organism in bronchoalveolar lavage fluids or in a transbronchial biopsy.

Fever, dry cough, and dyspnea occur in 90 to 95% of patients, who typically demonstrate bilateral perihilar and basilar infiltrates. Hypoxia is frequent; pulmonary function studies show a restrictive lung defect, and carbon monoxide diffusing capacity is invariably low. If treatment is initiated before widespread involvement, the outlook for recovery is good; however, because residual organisms are likely to remain, particularly in patients with AIDS, relapses are common unless the underlying immunosuppression is reversed.

LUNG TUMORS

Although lungs are frequently the site of metastases from cancers in extrathoracic organs, primary lung cancer is also a common disease. Ninety-five per cent of primary lung tumors arise from the bronchial epithelium (bronchogenic carcinomas), and the remaining 5% are a miscellaneous group that includes bronchial carcinoids, mesotheliomas, bronchial gland neoplasms, mesenchymal malignancies (e.g., fibrosarcomas, leiomyomas), lymphomas, and a few benign lesions. The

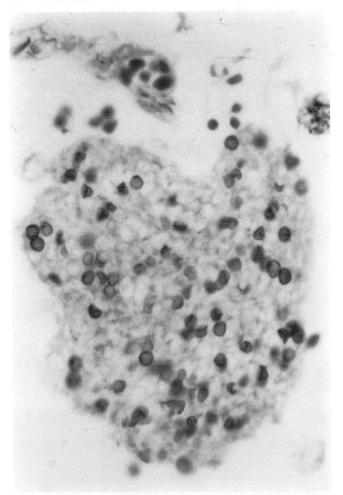

Figure 13–32. *Pneumocystis* pneumonia. A high-power photomicrograph of the characteristic foamy intraalveolar exudate containing cysts of the organism made visible by silver staining of the cyst wall. Note some of the cysts demonstrate a cup shape.

most common benign lesions are spherical, small (3- to 4-cm), discrete hamartomas that often show up as "coin" lesions on chest radiographs. They consist mainly of mature cartilage but often are admixed with fat, fibrous tissue, and blood vessels in varying proportions.

BRONCHOGENIC CARCINOMA

Bronchogenic carcinoma is without doubt the number one cause of cancer-related deaths in industrialized countries. It has long held this position among males in the United States, accounting for about a third of their cancer deaths, and it has become the leading cause of cancer deaths in women. In 1991, lung cancer was expected to cause 142,000 deaths in the United States alone. The rate of increase among males is slowing down, but it continues to accelerate among females. These statistics are undoubtedly related to the causal relationship of cigarette smoking and bronchogenic carcinoma. The peak incidence of lung cancer occurs between ages 40 and 70 years; currently, the male to female ratio is about 2:1. Male cigarette smokers are about 10 times more likely to die of bronchogenic carcinoma than are nonsmokers.

There are four major histologic types of bronchogenic carcinomas: squamous cell carcinoma, adenocarcinoma, large cell undifferentiated carcinoma, and small cell carcinoma. It has become apparent that for most therapeutic decisions, the first three can be lumped into a category termed non–small cell lung carcinoma (NSCLC) to distinguish them from small cell lung cancer (SCLC). In some cases there is a combination of histologic patterns. This classification is summarized in Table 13–7.

ETIOLOGY AND PATHOGENESIS. The evidence is now overwhelming that all forms of cancer result from genetic damage (p. 184). The relevant issues with bronchogenic carcinoma, as with all cancers, relate to the nature of genetic changes that result in malignant transformation of bronchial epithelium and the factors that induce these changes. Both of these issues are discussed at length in the general discussion of carcinogenesis in Chapter 7. Only those aspects that are pertinent to carcinomas of the lung are reiterated here briefly.

TABLE 13–7. HISTOLOGIC CLASSIFICATION OF BRONCHOGENIC CARCINOMA AND APPROXIMATE INCIDENCE

I. Non–Small Cell Lung Carcinoma (NSCLC) (70–75%)
1. Squamous cell (epidermoid) carcinoma (25–30%)
2. Adenocarcinoma, including bronchioloalveolar carcinoma (30–35%)
3. Large cell carcinoma (10–15%)
II. Small Cell Lung Carcinoma (SCLC) (20–25%)
III. Combined patterns (5–10%)
Most frequently
Mixed squamous cell and adenocarcinoma
Mixed squamous cell and SCLC

Like all cancers, lung cancers result from an accumulation of genetic changes that affect oncogenes and tumor suppressor genes. SCLCs are characterized by changes in several oncogenes, including amplification of the *myc* family (L-*myc*, N-*myc*) and mutations of *raf* gene. L-*myc* amplification is associated with particularly aggressive behavior. Mutational inactivation of the tumor suppressor genes p53 and *Rb* are quite common in SCLC and the latter may be the first change during neoplastic transformation. In addition, all SCLCs have a deletion of the short arm of chromosome 3, where a cancer suppressor gene is likely to be found. The genetic alterations in NSCLC are somewhat different. Many with squamous differentation over-express epidermal growth factor receptors, suggesting a role for this polypeptide in the growth of these cancers. Mutations of the K-*ras* oncogene are particularly relevant in adenocarcinomas because activation of these oncogenes is associated with a poor prognosis despite radical resection and small tumor load.

With regard to carcinogenic influences, there is strong evidence that smoking, and, to a much lesser extent, other environmental insults, are the main culprits responsible for the genetic changes that give rise to lung cancers. First, the evidence relating to cigarette smoking will be given, followed by a few brief comments on the less important factors.

An impressive body of evidence—statistical, clinical, and experimental—incriminates cigarette smoking. Statistically there is a nearly linear correlation between the frequency of lung cancer and pack-years of cigarette smoking. The increased risk becomes 20 times greater among habitual heavy smokers (40 or more cigarettes a day for a span of years) as compared with nonsmokers. About 80% of lung cancers occur in active smokers or those who stopped recently. Cessation of cigarette smoking for at least 15 years brings the risk down nearly to control levels. Passive smoking (proximity to cigarette smokers) increases the risk, but less than twice that of nonsmokers. Smoking pipes and cigars also increases the risk, but only modestly. The use of filter cigarettes reduces the risk somewhat, but only for those who have used them exclusively for the last 5 to 10 years.

The *clinical evidence* is largely composed of the documentation of progressive alterations in the lining epithelium of the respiratory tract in habitual cigarette smokers. In essence, there is a linear correlation between the intensity of exposure to cigarette smoke and the appearance of ever more worrisome epithelial changes, beginning with atypical squamous metaplasia, then dysplasia, and ultimately abnormalities approaching carcinoma in situ, followed in most instances by the bad news.

The *experimental evidence,* although it mounts with each passing year, lacks one important link: it has not been possible to date to produce lung cancer in an experimental animal by exposing it to cigarette smoke. Nonetheless, cigarette smoke condensate is a witch's brew of tumorigenic delicacies, such as polycyclic hydrocarbons and other potent mutagens and carcinogens. Despite the lack of an experimental model, the chain of evidence linking cigarette smoking to lung cancer grows ever stronger.

Other influences may act in concert with smoking or may by themselves be responsible for some lung cancers. Environmental and occupational air pollutants undoubtedly can contribute; witness the increased incidence of this form of neoplasia in miners of radioactive ores, asbestos workers (particularly when coupled with smoking), and workers exposed to dusts containing arsenic, chromium, uranium, nickel, vinyl chloride, and mustard gas. Heavy smokers exposed to asbestos have an approximately 55 times greater risk of lung cancer than do nonsmokers not exposed to asbestos. Radiation exposure (in miners of radioactive ores, those who construct atomic bombs) has yielded an increased incidence of lung cancer.

Despite the fact that environmental factors are paramount in the causation of lung cancer, it is well known that all persons exposed to similar quantities of tobacco smoke or other environmental carcinogens do not develop cancer. Perhaps the mutagenic effect of carcinogens is conditioned by hereditary (genetic) factors. Recall that many chemicals (procarcinogens) require metabolic activation via the P-450 monooxygenase enzyme system for conversion into ultimate carcinogens (p. 199). There is evidence that exposure of this enzyme system is under genetic control, and conceivably persons who rapidly metabolize the procarcinogens incur the greatest exposure. Indeed, such individuals have a greater risk of developing lung cancer.

MORPHOLOGY. Bronchogenic carcinomas in the various histologic categories share several features:

- They arise in the lining epithelium of major bronchi, usually close to the hilus of the lung.
- All patterns are associated with cigarette smoking; the strongest association is with squamous cell and small cell carcinomas.
- All are aggressive, locally invasive, widely metastasizing neoplasms (particularly SCLC) with a propensity for spread to the liver, adrenals, brain, and bones, although almost every organ in the body can be affected.
- All varieties, especially SCLC, have the capacity to synthesize bioactive products, producing paraneoplastic syndromes.

These tumors begin as small mucosal lesions, usually firm and gray-white, that may follow one of several patterns of growth. They may form intraluminal masses; they may invade the bronchial mucosa, infiltrating longitudinally in the peribronchial connective tissue; or they may form large bulky masses pushing into adjacent lung parenchyma. Some large masses undergo cavitation due to central necrosis or develop focal areas of hemorrhage. Finally, these tumors may extend to the pleura, invade the pleural cavity and chest wall, and spread to adjacent intrathoracic structures. More distant spread can occur via lymphatics or the hematogenous route.

Squamous cell carcinomas are more common in men than in women; they tend to arise centrally in major bronchi and eventually spread to local hilar nodes, but they disseminate outside the thorax later than do other histologic types. More is known about the natural history of squamous cell carcinomas than of other variants. Squamous cell carcinomas are often preceded for years by atypical metaplasia or dysplasia in the bronchial epithelium, which then transforms to carcinoma in situ, a phase that may last for several years. A small area (1 to 2 cm in diameter) of thickened, irregularly nodular mucosa gradually develops. By this time, atypical cells may be identified in cytologic smears of sputum or in bronchial lavage fluids or brushings, although the lesion is asymptomatic and undetectable on radiographs. Eventually the small neoplasm reaches a symptomatic stage, when a well-defined tumor mass begins to obstruct the lumen of a major bronchus, often producing distal atelectasis and infection. Simultaneously, the lesion invades surrounding pulmonary substance (Fig. 13–33).

Histologically, these tumors range from well-differentiated squamous cell neoplasms showing keratin pearls and intercellular bridges to poorly differentiated neoplasms having only minimal residual squamous cell features (Fig. 13–34). Squamous cell carcinomas have a slightly better prognosis than other histologic types because they tend to develop into large, bulky, centrally obstructing symptomatic masses before they metastasize and are, therefore, more often surgically resectable.

Adenocarcinomas are almost equally common in men and women, and the association with cigarette smoking is weaker than for squamous cell carcinoma. They may occur as central lesions like the squamous cell variant but are usually more peripherally located, many arising in relation to peripheral lung scars. In general, these tumors grow slowly and form smaller masses than do the other subtypes, but they tend to metastasize widely at an early stage. Histologically, the neoplastic cells are generally cuboidal to columnar, frequently secrete mucin, and typically form tubular, acinar, or papillary structures.

Bronchioloalveolar carcinoma (BAC), a special category of adenocarcinoma, occurs as two variants. Less than half of BAC are multifocal mucinous masses that sometimes are discrete but at other times coalescent (simulating pneumonic consolidation). Most often they are confined to a single lobe, but they sometimes involve multiple lobes and may even be bilateral. Histologically, these masses consist of tall columnar cells, regularly arrayed along preserved alveolar septa, having abundant intra- and extracellular mucin and basally located small nuclei. The cytologic appearance is deceptively benign and mitoses are rare. The other variant is a single, localized gray-white nodule that may be up to 10 cm in diameter and is most often located near the periphery in an upper lobe. In contrast to the multifocal variant, the neoplastic cells usually do not elaborate mucin, are low columnar or cuboidal, and are somewhat irregularly aligned along the tumor's fibrovascular stroma rather than the alveolar septa; papillary configurations

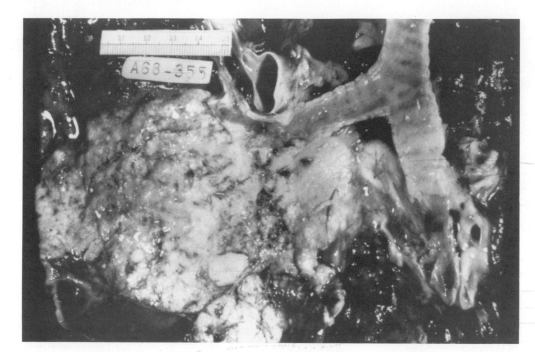

Figure 13–33. Bronchogenic carcinoma. The gray-white tumor tissue is seen infiltrating the lung substance. Histologically, this large tumor mass was identified as a squamous cell carcinoma.

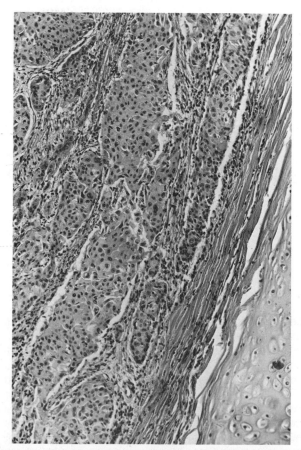

Figure 13–34. Bronchogenic carcinoma, squamous cell type. The bronchial cartilage is seen at the lower right. The neoplasm has replaced the mucosa and is growing into the lumen.

are prominent. The nuclei are large, centrally placed, and hyperchromatic and may reveal mitoses. BAC has a better prognosis than other bronchogenic carcinomas: the multifocal variant has a 20 to 25% five-year survival rate, and the localized single mass has a 50 to 70% five-year rate.

Large cell carcinomas constitute a group of neoplasms that lack cytologic differentiation and probably represent squamous cell or glandular neoplasms that are too undifferentiated to permit categorization. The cells are usually anaplastic and have large vesicular nuclei. Sometimes a tumor is composed of wildly anaplastic giant cells; others may have clear cells or spindle-shaped cells. These neoplasms are generally bulky and are more often peripheral than central. They have a poor prognosis because of their tendency to spread to distant sites early in their course. More than half involve the central nervous system at the time of diagnosis, and the five-year survival rate is 2 to 3%.

Small cell lung carcinomas are more common in men, than in women and are strongly associated with cigarette smoking. They generally appear as pale gray, centrally located masses with extension into the lung parenchyma and early involvement of the hilar and mediastinal nodes. These cancers are composed of small, dark, round-to-oval, lymphocyte-like cells (albeit larger than lymphocytes) that have scant cytoplasm and hyperchromatic nuclei, among which mitoses are numerous (Fig. 13–35). This is the classic "oat" cell. In some cases the tumor cells are spindle-shaped or fusiform. Penetration of submucosal vessels is often seen.

SCLCs are rapidly growing lesions that tend to infiltrate widely and disseminate early in their course and so are rarely resectable. They are therefore almost always treated by combined radiotherapy and chemotherapy,

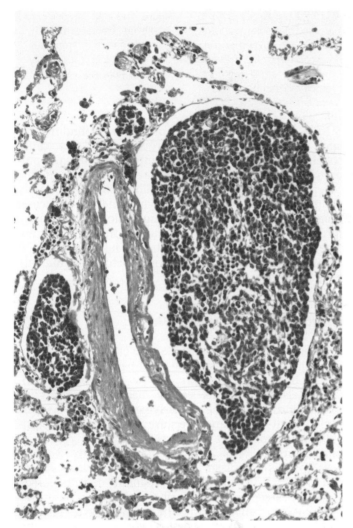

Figure 13–35. Small cell lung carcinoma. The cells are small round, oval, or spindle-shaped with deep, basophilic nuclei. Note, the large and small nests of tumor cells in perivascular lymphatics.

but even with these modalities, the two-year survival rate is only 5 to 8%; newer protocols have improved the outlook somewhat. The histogenesis of these neoplasms is still unclear. On the one hand, SCLCs exhibit neuroendocrine properties: expression of neuron-specific enolase, presence of neurosecretory granules (detected by electron microscopy), presence of neurofilaments, and the ability to secrete a host of polypeptide hormones including ACTH, calcitonin, gastrin-releasing peptide, and chromogranin A. On the other hand these neoplasms may contain areas of squamous cell and adenocarcinomatous differentiation, suggesting that the cells of origin are the same as those that give rise to all other histologic variants.

Combined patterns require no further comment, but it should be noted that a significant minority of bronchogenic carcinomas reveal more than one line of differentiation, sometimes several (see Table 13–7).

For all these neoplasms one can trace involvement of successive chains of nodes about the carina, in the mediastinum, and in the neck (scalene nodes) and clavicular regions, and, sooner or later, distant metastases. Involvement of the supraclavicular node (Virchow's node) is particularly characteristic and sometimes calls attention to an occult primary tumor. These cancers, when advanced, often extend into the pericardial or pleural spaces, leading to inflammation and effusions. They may compress or infiltrate the superior vena cava to cause venous congestion or the full-blown vena caval syndrome. Apical neoplasms may invade the brachial or cervical sympathetic plexus to cause severe pain in the distribution of the ulnar nerve or to produce Horner's syndrome (ipsilateral enophthalmos, ptosis, meiosis, and anhidrosis). Such apical neoplasms are sometimes called Pancoast's tumors, and the combination of clinical findings Pancoast's syndrome. A Pancoast's tumor is often accompanied by destruction of the first and second ribs and sometimes thoracic vertebrae.

STAGING. As with other cancers, tumor-node-metastases (TNM) categories (p. 208) have been established to indicate the size and spread of the primary neoplasm. Although the details of staging are beyond our scope, some concept of the system can be derived from the following abbreviated version:

Occult: No clinical or radiographic evidence of the primary tumor or of spread, but bronchopulmonary secretions contain malignant cells (TX N0 M0).

Stage I: A tumor smaller than 3 cm in greatest diameter distal to the origin of a lobar bronchus, with (T1 N1 M0) or without (T1 N0 M0) metastasis to ipsilateral regional nodes, or a larger tumor distal to the carina that invades the visceral pleura but does not have nodal or distant metastases (T2 N0 M0).

Stage II: A tumor of any size, distal to the carina, that invades the visceral pleura and extends only to the nodes in the ipsilateral hilar region (T2 N1 M0).

Stage III: Any tumor that is more extensive locally or shows metastasis beyond the ipsilateral lymph nodes (e.g., contralateral nodes, mediastinum, liver, brain).

CLINICAL COURSE. Bronchogenic carcinomas are silent, insidious lesions that more often than not have spread so as to be unresectable before they produce symptoms. Cure by surgical resection is largely limited to the 10 to 15% of neoplasms discovered by chance on radiographs or by cytologic examination. In some instances, chronic cough, expectoration, dyspnea, and wheezing call attention to still localized, resectable disease. When hoarseness, chest pain, superior vena caval syndrome, pericardial or pleural effusion, or persistent segmental atelectasis or pneumonitis make their appearance the prognosis is grim. Too often the tumor presents with symptoms emanating from metastatic spread to the brain (mental or neurologic changes), liver (hepatomegaly), or bones (pain). Although the adrenals may be nearly obliterated by metastatic disease, adrenal insufficiency (Addison's disease) is uncommon because islands of cortical cells sufficient to maintain adrenal function usually persist.

Because of the prevalence and mortality associated

with lung carcinomas, intensive efforts have been made to discover these tumors at an early stage. Periodic chest radiography and cytologic screening of sputum or investigation of mysteriously appearing paraneoplastic syndromes (p. 207) sometimes leads to the discovery of occult lesions. It is variously estimated that about 3 to 10% of all lung cancer patients develop clinically overt paraneoplastic syndromes. These include (1) *hypercalcemia* (due to secretion of a parathormone-like peptide or occasionally to osteolytic lesions); (2) *Cushing's syndrome* (from increased production of ACTH); (3) *diabetes insipidus* (inappropriate secretion of antidiuretic hormone); (4) *neuromuscular syndromes* including a myasthenic syndrome, peripheral neuropathy, and polymyositis; (5) *clubbing of the fingers* and hypertrophic pulmonary osteoarthropathy; and (6) *hematologic manifestations,* including migratory thrombophlebitis, nonbacterial endocarditis, and disseminated intravascular coagulation (DIC). Secretion of calcitonin and other ectopic hormones has also been documented by assays, but these products usually do not provoke distinctive syndromes. *Hypercalcemia is most often encountered with squamous cell neoplasms; the hematologic syndromes with adenocarcinomas; the remaining syndromes are much more frequent with small cell neoplasms, but exceptions abound.*

The outlook for persons with particular histologic variants of bronchogenic carcinoma differs, as previously noted, but overall the five-year survival rate is in the range of 5 to 10%.

BRONCHIAL CARCINOID

Bronchial carcinoids show the neuroendocrine differentiation of Kulchitsky cells in the bronchial mucosa and resemble intestinal carcinoids (p. 517). The cells contain dense core neurosecretory granules in their cytoplasm and rarely may secrete hormonally active polypeptides. They occasionally occur as part of multiple endocrine neoplasia (p. 679). Bronchial carcinoids appear at an early age (mean 40 years) and represent about 5% of all pulmonary neoplasms. In happy contrast to bronchogenic carcinomas, they are often resectable and curable.

Most bronchial carcinoids originate in main stem bronchi and grow in one of two patterns: (1) an obstructing polypoid, spherical, intraluminal mass or (2) a mucosal plaque penetrating the bronchial wall to fan out in the peribronchial tissue—the so-called collar-button lesion. Even these penetrating lesions push into the lung substance along a broad front and are therefore reasonably well-demarcated. About 30% of these tumors metastasize to hilar nodes, and a few to more distant sites such as liver. Histologically, these neoplasms, like their counterparts in the intestinal tract, are composed of uniform cuboidal cells that have regular round nuclei with few mitoses and little or no anaplasia. Occasional tumors are less well-differentiated. The cells are disposed in nests, cords, glandular patterns, or small masses separated by a delicate stroma and may therefore resemble small cell carcinomas. In these cases differentiating the highly malignant small cell cancer from the much more indolent carcinoid can be difficult.

Most bronchial carcinoids present with findings related to their intraluminal growth (i.e., they cause cough, hemoptysis, and recurrent bronchial and pulmonary infections). Some are asymptomatic and discovered by chance on chest radiographs. Only rarely do they induce the carcinoid syndrome. In any case, because they are slow growing lesions that rarely spread beyond the local hilar nodes, these tumors are amenable to conservative resection. The reported 5- to 10-year survival rate ranges from 50 to 95%, but late recurrences sometimes develop.

MALIGNANT MESOTHELIOMA

Malignant mesothelioma is a rare cancer of mesothelial cells, usually arising in the parietal or visceral pleura but less commonly in the peritoneum, and, rarely, elsewhere. This cancer has a propensity to spread and encase the underlying organs. It has assumed great importance because it is related to occupational exposure to asbestos in the air (p. 223). Indeed, up to 8% of *heavily exposed* asbestos workers develop this neoplasm, usually after a long latent period of 35 to 50 years. Malignant mesotheliomas have appeared in persons whose only exposure was living in proximity to an asbestos factory or being a family member of an asbestos worker; however, approximately 20% of persons with mesothelioma have no history of exposure. The combination of cigarette smoking and asbestos does not increase the risk as it does for bronchogenic carcinoma.

The basis for the carcinogenicity of asbestos is still a mystery. Clearly the physical form of the asbestos is critical; very nearly all cases are related to exposure to amphibole asbestos, which has long, straight fibers, and not to serpentine chrysotile. Asbestosis of the lungs occurs concurrently in only 20% of cases.

MORPHOLOGY. In the pleural cavity, malignant mesotheliomas presumably begin in a localized area, provoke an effusion, and in the course of time spread widely either by contiguous growth or seeding of the effusion and opposing pleural surfaces. At autopsy, the affected lung is typically ensheathed by a yellow-white, firm, sometimes gelatinous layer of tumor that obliterates the pleural space. The neoplasm may directly invade the thoracic wall or the subpleural lung tissue; often it extends into interlobar fissures and sometimes into hilar nodes. Histologically, mesotheliomas conform to one of three patterns: (1) sarcomatoid, in which spindled and sometimes fibroblastic-appearing cells grow in nondistinctive sheets; (2) epithelial, in which cuboidal cells line tubular and microcystic spaces, into which small papillary buds project (resembling an adenocarcinoma); and (3) biphasic, the most common pattern, having both sarcomatoid and epithelioid areas. It is evident that the sarcomatoid variant may be difficult to differentiate from other forms of sarcoma, and the epithelial variant from primary or metastatic adenocarcinomas. Special stains and electron microscopy are essential adjuncts when the diagnosis is in doubt. Under the electron microscope mesotheliomas reveal long, slender microvilli and abundant tonofilaments.

Pleural mesotheliomas tend to remain confined to the thorax but sometimes spread to the liver and other distant sites. Although metastatic spread is detected at autopsy, it is often not clinically significant.

CLINICAL COURSE. Symptoms of malignant mesothelioma include chest or shoulder pain and recurrent effusions with few manifestations of respiratory dysfunction, although in time, cough, dyspnea, weight loss, and sometimes finger clubbing and pulmonary osteoarthropathy develop. The diagnosis can usually be suggested by computed tomography (CT), but open lung biopsy is almost always required to confirm the diagnosis. The prognosis is dismal: few patients survive longer than a year after the diagnosis.

BENIGN PLEURAL LESIONS _____

PLEURAL EFFUSION AND PLEURITIS _____

Pleural effusion, the presence of fluid in the pleural space, can be either a transudate or an exudate. A pleural effusion that is a transudate is termed *hydrothorax.* Hydrothorax from congestive heart failure is probably the most common cause of fluid in the pleural cavity. An exudate, characterized by a specific gravity greater than 1.020 and, often, inflammatory cells, implies pleuritis. The four principal causes of pleural exudate are (1) microbial invasion via either direct extension of a pulmonary infection or bloodborne seeding; (2) cancer (bronchogenic carcinoma), metastatic neoplasms to the lung or pleural surface, mesothelioma; (3) pulmonary infarction; and (4) viral pleuritis. There are other less common causes of exudative pleural effusions, such as systemic lupus erythematosus, rheumatoid arthritis, uremia, and following thoracic surgery. Tuberculosis has become a much less common cause of pleural effusion than it once was, but it still must be considered when there is no other obvious underlying cause. Pleuritis without effusion may be encountered in a host of conditions, including any of the causes of pleural exudate listed earlier. There are a number of causes of pleuritis, however, in which effusions are decidedly unusual, such as the pneumoconioses.

Cancer should be suspected as the underlying cause of an exudative effusion in any patient over age 40 years, particularly when there is no febrile illness, no pain, and a negative tuberculin test result. These effusions characteristically are large and frequently are serosanguineous. Cytologic examination may reveal malignant and inflammatory cells.

Whatever the cause, transudates and serous exudates are usually resorbed without residual effects if the inciting cause is controlled or remits. In contrast, fibrinous, hemorrhagic, and suppurative exudates may lead to fibrous organization, yielding adhesions or fibrous pleural thickening, and sometimes minimal to massive calcifications.

PNEUMOTHORAX, HEMOTHORAX, AND CHYLOTHORAX _____

Pneumothorax refers to air or other gas in the pleural sac. It may occur in the absence of known pulmonary disease (simple or spontaneous pneumothorax), or as a result of some thoracic or lung disorder (secondary pneumothorax), such as emphysema or a fractured rib. Secondary pneumothorax occurs with rupture of any pulmonary lesion situated close to the pleural surface that allows inspired air to gain access to the pleural cavity. Such pulmonary lesions include emphysema, lung abscess, tuberculosis, carcinoma, and many other, less common processes. Because these lung diseases are most prevalent after age 40 years, it is apparent that secondary pneumothorax tends to occur in the older age group. Mechanical ventilatory support with high pressure may also trigger secondary pneumothorax. In contrast, simple pneumothorax characteristically occurs in young, otherwise healthy adults, usually men. The cause is unknown; rarely, latent tuberculosis is present.

There are several possible complications of pneumothorax. A ball-valve leak may create a tension pneumothorax that shifts the mediastinum. Compromise of the pulmonary circulation may follow and may even be fatal. If the leak seals and the lung is not reexpanded within a few weeks (either spontaneously or through medical or surgical intervention), enough scarring may occur so that it can never be fully reexpanded. In these cases, serous fluid collects in the pleural cavity and creates hydropneumothorax. With prolonged collapse, the lung becomes vulnerable to infection, as does the pleural cavity when communication between it and the lung persists. Empyema is thus an important complication of pneumothorax. Finally, pneumothorax tends to be recurrent. This is understandable when it complicates other pulmonary disease, because the predisposing condition remains. What is less readily understood is that simple pneumothorax is also recurrent.

Hemothorax refers to the collection of whole blood (in contrast to bloody effusion) in the pleural cavity, and is almost always a fatal complication of a ruptured intrathoracic aortic aneurysm. With hemothorax, in contrast to bloody pleural effusions, the blood clots within the pleural cavity.

Chylothorax is a pleural collection of a milky lymphatic fluid containing microglobules of lipid. The total volume of fluid may not be large, but chylothorax is always significant because it implies obstruction of the major lymph ducts, usually by an intrathoracic cancer (e.g., a primary or secondary mediastinal neoplasm, such as a lymphoma).

LESIONS OF THE UPPER RESPIRATORY TRACT

ACUTE INFECTIONS

Acute infections of the upper respiratory tract are among the most common afflictions of man, most commonly presenting as the common cold. The clinical features are well known to all: nasal congestion accompanied by watery discharge; sneezing; scratchy, dry sore throat; and a slight increase in temperature that is more pronounced in young children. The most common pathogens are rhinoviruses, but coronaviruses, respiratory syncytial viruses, parainfluenza and influenza viruses, adenoviruses, enteroviruses, and even group A β-hemolytic streptococci have also been implicated. In a significant number of cases (around 40%) the cause cannot be determined; perhaps new viruses will be discovered. Most of these infections occur in the fall and winter and are self-limiting (usually lasting for a week or less). In a minority of cases, colds may be complicated by the development of bacterial otitis media or sinusitis.

In addition to the common cold, infections of the upper respiratory tract may present with signs and symptoms that are localized to the pharynx, epiglottis, or larynx. *Acute pharyngitis,* manifesting as a sore throat, may be caused by a host of agents. Mild pharyngitis with minimal physical findings frequently accompanies a cold and is the most frequent form of pharyngitis. More severe forms with tonsillitis, associated with marked hyperemia and exudates, occur with β-hemolytic streptococci and adenovirus infections. In the latter infection the conjunctiva may be inflamed to produce the complex referred to as pharyngoconjunctival fever. Herpes simplex and coxsackievirus A may produce pharyngeal vesicles and ulcers. Pharyngitis is also an important component of infectious mononucleosis caused by Epstein-Barr virus (EBV).

Acute *bacterial epiglottitis* is a syndrome predominantly of young children who have an infection of the epiglottis by *H. influenzae* in which pain and airway obstruction are the major findings. The onset is abrupt. Failure to appreciate the need to maintain an open airway for a child with this condition can be fatal.

Acute laryngitis can be the result of irritant or allergic insults, but a significant number of cases are due to the same agents that produce the common cold and usually involve the pharynx and nasal passages as well as the larynx. Brief mention should be made of two uncommon but important forms of laryngitis: *tuberculous* and *diphtheritic.* The former is almost always a consequence of protracted active tuberculosis,

during which infective sputum is coughed up. Rarely, this laryngeal involvement may be an expression of miliary tuberculosis. Diphtheritic membranous laryngitis is often accompanied by inflammation that begins in the pharynx and extends distally into the trachea, but this has fortunately become uncommon because of the widespread immunization of young children against diphtheria toxin. After it is inhaled, *Corynebacterium diphtheriae* implants at any location on the mucosa of the upper airways and elaborates a powerful exotoxin that causes necrosis of the mucosal epithelium accompanied by a dense fibrinopurulent exudate that creates the classic superficial, dirty gray membrane of diphtheria. The major hazards of this infection are sloughing and aspiration of the membrane (causing obstruction of major airways), and absorption of bacterial exotoxins (producing myocarditis, peripheral neuropathy, or other tissue injury).

In children, influenza A and B viruses and respiratory syncytial virus are important causes of laryngotracheobronchitis, more commonly known as *croup.* Although self-limited, croup may cause disturbing inspiratory stridor and harsh persistent cough. In occasional cases the laryngeal inflammatory reaction may narrow the airway sufficiently to cause respiratory failure. Anatomic changes described in fatal cases of croup consist of marked edema and infiltration of mononuclear inflammatory cells into the mucosa. Viral infections in the upper respiratory tract predispose the patient to secondary bacterial infection, particularly by staphylococci, streptococci, and *H. influenzae.*

NASOPHARYNGEAL CARCINOMA

This rare neoplasm merits comment because of (1) the strong epidemiologic links to the EBV and (2) the high frequency of this form of cancer in Chinese people, which raises the possibility of viral oncogenesis on the background of genetic susceptibility. EBV infects the host by first replicating in the nasopharyngeal epithelium (and then infecting nearby tonsillar lymphocytes). In some persons this leads to transformation of the epithelial cells. Unlike the case in Burkitt's lymphoma (p. 202), another EBV-associated tumor, the EBV genome is found in virtually all nasopharyngeal carcinomas, including those that occur outside the endemic areas in Asia.

There are three histologic variants: squamous cell carcinoma, nonkeratinizing carcinoma, and undifferentiated carcinoma; the last mentioned is the most common and the one most closely linked with the EBV. The undifferentiated neoplasm is characterized by a syncytial pattern of large epithelial cells resembling the transitional epithelial cells of the urinary bladder, having indistinct cell borders and prominent nuclei. It should be recalled that in infectious mononucleosis, EBV directly infects B lymphocytes, after which a marked proliferation of reactive T lymphocytes causes atypical lymphocytosis, seen in the peripheral blood, and enlarged lymph nodes (p. 352).

Similarly, in nasopharyngeal carcinomas there is often a striking influx of mature lymphocytes. These neoplasms are therefore referred to as "lymphoepitheliomas," a true misnomer because the lymphocytes are not part of the neoplastic process, nor is the tumor benign. Nasopharyngeal carcinomas invade locally, spread to cervical lymph nodes, and then metastasize to distant sites. They tend to be radiosensitive and five-year survival rates of 50% are reported for even advanced cancers.

LARYNGEAL TUMORS

A variety of benign and malignant neoplasms of squamous epithelial and mesenchymal origin may arise in the larynx, but only vocal cord nodules, papillomas, and squamous cell carcinomas are sufficiently common to merit comment. In all of these conditions, the most common presenting feature is hoarseness.

Benign Tumors

Vocal cord nodules ("polyps") are smooth, hemispheric protrusions (usually less than 0.5 cm in diameter) located, most often, on the true vocal cords. They are composed of fibrous tissue and covered by stratified squamous mucosa that is usually intact but can be ulcerated by contact trauma with the other vocal cord. These lesions occur chiefly in heavy smokers or singers (singer's nodes), suggesting that they are the result of chronic irritation or abuse. The occasional presence of mononuclear white cells within the fibrous stroma and prominent vascularization also support the notion of an inflammatory origin.

Laryngeal papilloma is a benign neoplasm, usually located on the true vocal cords, that forms a soft raspberry-like excrescence rarely more than 1 cm in diameter. Histologically it consists of multiple, slender, finger-like projections supported by central fibrovascular cores and covered by an orderly, typical, stratified squamous epithelium. When the papilloma is located on the free edge of the vocal cord, trauma may lead to ulceration that can be accompanied by hemoptysis and exuberant regenerative epithelial activity; the gross appearance of the resultant lesion may mimic squamous cell carcinoma. Indeed, instances of carcinomas arising in preexisting papillomas have been reported.

Papillomas are usually single in adults, but often multiple in children, where they are referred to as *juvenile laryngeal papillomatosis*. The latter (and perhaps also the former) are caused by the human papillomavirus type 6 and 11; do not become malignant; and often spontaneously regress at puberty. Nevertheless, if extensive they cause obstruction. This may necessitate a permanent tracheostomy, because they are difficult to treat and tend to recur.

Carcinoma of the Larynx

Carcinoma of the larynx represents only 2% of all cancers. It most commonly occurs after age 40 years and is more common in males (7:1) than in females. Environmental influences are very important in its causation; nearly all cases occur in smokers, and alcohol and asbestos exposure may also play roles.

About 95% of laryngeal carcinomas are typical squamous cell lesions. Rarely, adenocarcinomas are seen, presumably arising from mucous glands. The tumor usually develops directly on the vocal cords, but it may arise above or below the cords, on the epiglottis or aryepiglottic folds, or in the piriform sinuses. Those confined within the larynx proper are termed "intrinsic," whereas those that arise or extend outside the larynx are called "extrinsic." Squamous cell carcinomas of the larynx follow the growth pattern of all squamous cell carcinomas (p. 210). They begin as in situ lesions that later appear as pearly gray, wrinkled plaques on the mucosal surface, ultimately ulcerating and fungating (Fig. 13–36). The degree of anaplasia of these laryngeal tumors is highly variable. Sometimes massive tumor giant cells and multiple bizarre mitotic figures are seen. As expected with lesions arising from recurrent expo-

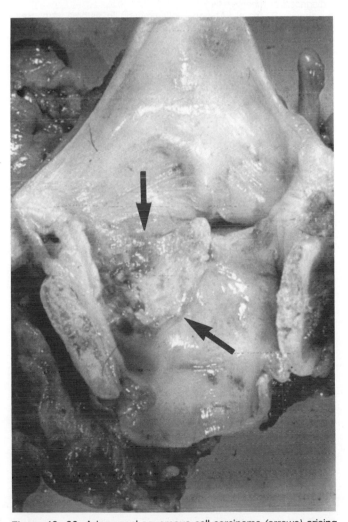

Figure 13–36. A laryngeal squamous cell carcinoma *(arrows)* arising on the true vocal cord.

sure to environmental carcinogens, adjacent mucosa may demonstrate squamous cell hyperplasia with foci of dysplasia, or even carcinoma in situ.

Carcinoma of the larynx manifests itself clinically by persistent hoarseness. At presentation about 60% of these cancers are confined to the larynx; as a result the prognosis is better than for those that have spread into adjacent structures. Later, laryngeal tumors may produce pain, dysphagia, and hemoptysis. Patients with this condition are extremely vulnerable to secondary infection of the ulcerating lesion. With surgery, radiation, or combined therapeutic treatments many patients can be cured, but about a third die of their disease. The usual cause of death is infection of the distal respiratory passages or widespread metastases and cachexia.

Bibliography

American Thoracic Society: Diagnostic standards and classification of tuberculosis. Am. Rev. Respir. Dis. *142:*725, 1990. (A summary of the etiology, pathogenesis, clinical features, and, especially, diagnosis of tuberculosis.)

Djukanovic, R., et al.: Mucosal inflammation in asthma. Am. Rev. Respir. Dis. *142:*434, 1990. (A review of the cells and mediators involved in asthma, with an extensive bibliography.)

Katzenstein, A. A., Askin, F. B.: Surgical Pathology of Nonneoplastic Lung Disease. Philadelphia, W. B. Saunders, 1982. (An overview of the pathology of several important lung diseases, including diffuse alveolar damage, the chronic interstitial fibrosing diseases, and vascular lung diseases.)

Mandel, G. L., Douglas, R. G., Bennett, J. E.: Principles and Practice of Infectious Diseases. 3rd ed. Edinburgh, Churchill Livingstone, 1990. (A virtual treasure trove of scholarly information on infectious diseases. Especially useful for understanding pulmonary infections are chapters on Acute Pneumonia by J. R. Donowitz and G. L. Mandel, Lung Abscess by Sydney M. Finegold, Chronic Pneumonia by W. E. Dismarkes, *Mycobacterium tuberculosis* by R. M. DesPrez and C. R. Heim, Cytomegalovirus by M. Ho, and *Pneumocystis carinii* by P. D. Walzer.)

Murray, J. F.: The white plague: Down and out, or up and coming? Am. Rev. Respir. Dis. *140:*1788, 1989. (An interesting discussion of the changing face of tuberculosis.)

Murray, J. F., Nadel, J. A. (eds.): Textbook of Respiratory Medicine. Philadelphia, W. B. Saunders, 1988. (An excellent, well-written two-volume overview of pulmonary diseases, including in depth analyses of pathogenetic mechanisms.)

Thurlbeck, W. M.: Pathophysiology of chronic obstructive pulmonary disease. Clin. Chest Med. *11:*389, 1990. (A review of the relationship of pathologic findings in COPD, with clinical and physiologic abnormalities, citing important autopsy studies.)

Valdes-Dapena, M.: A pathologist's perspective on the Sudden Infant Death Syndrome—1991. Pathol Ann. 27(Part 1):133, 1992. (A comprehensive and up-to-date review by a leader in this field.)

Wernberger, S. E., Drazen, J. M.: Disturbances of respiratory function. *In* Wilson, J. D., et al. (eds.): Harrison's Principles of Internal Medicine. 12th ed. New York, McGraw-Hill, 1991. (A succinct overview of pulmonary function in relation to lung pathology.)

Wiedeman, H. P., Matthay, R. A.: Adult respiratory distress syndrome. Clin. Chest Med. Vol 2, 1990. (A collection of articles on ARDS by experts in the field, includes pathophysiology and histopathology.)

Willey, J. C., Harris, C. C.: Cellular and molecular biological aspects of human bronchogenic carcinogenesis. Crit. Rev. Oncol. Hematol. *10:*181, 1990. (A clearly written review of the subject, beginning with a general overview of the principles of carcinogenesis, with special attention to those of likely importance in the lung, and a summary of phenotypic and genotypic changes found in lung cancer cells.)

FOURTEEN

The Kidney and Its Collecting System

CLINICAL MANIFESTATIONS OF RENAL DISEASES
GLOMERULAR DISEASES
   Pathogenesis of Primary Glomerular Diseases
      Circulating Immune Complex Nephritis
      Immune Complex Nephritis In Situ
      Cytotoxic Antibodies
      Cell-Mediated Immune Glomerulonephritis
      Mediators of Immune Injury
      Other Mechanisms of Glomerular Injury
   Glomerular Syndromes and Disorders
      The Nephrotic Syndrome
         Minimal Change Disease (Lipoid Nephrosis)
         Membranous Glomerulonephritis (Membranous Nephropathy)
         Focal Segmental Glomerulosclerosis
         Membranoproliferative Glomerulonephritis
      The Nephritic Syndrome
         Acute Proliferative (Poststreptococcal, Postinfectious) Glomerulonephritis
         Rapidly Progressive (Crescentic) Glomerulonephritis
         Focal (Proliferative) Glomerulonephritis
         IgA Nephropathy (Berger's Disease)
         Hereditary Nephritis
         Chronic Glomerulonephritis
DISEASES AFFECTING TUBULES AND INTERSTITIUM
   Tubulointerstitial Nephritis
      Acute Pyelonephritis
      Chronic Pyelonephritis and Reflux Nephropathy
      Drug-Induced Interstitial Nephritis
   Acute Tubular Necrosis
   Diffuse Cortical Necrosis

DISEASES INVOLVING BLOOD VESSELS
   Hypertension
      Mechanisms of Secondary Hypertension
      Mechanisms of Essential Hypertension
      Benign Nephrosclerosis
      Malignant Hypertension and Malignant Nephrosclerosis
CYSTIC DISEASES OF THE KIDNEY
   Simple Cysts
   Autosomal Dominant Polycystic Kidney Disease
   Autosomal Recessive Polycystic Kidney Disease
URINARY OUTFLOW OBSTRUCTION
   Renal Stones
   Hydronephrosis
TUMORS
   Renal Cell Carcinoma
   Wilms' Tumor
   Tumors of the Urinary Collecting System (Renal Calyces, Pelvis, Ureter, Bladder, and Urethra)

The kidney is a structurally complex organ that has evolved to subserve a number of important functions: excretion of the waste products of metabolism, regulation of body water and salt, maintenance of appropriate acid balance, and secretion of a variety of hormones and autocoids. Diseases of the kidney are as complex as its structure, but their study is facilitated by dividing them into those that affect the four basic morphologic components: glomeruli, tubules, interstitium, and blood vessels. This traditional approach is useful because the early manifestations of diseases that affect each of these components tend to be distinctive. Further, some components appear to be more vulnerable to specific forms of renal injury; for example, *glomerular diseases are most often immunologically mediated whereas tubular and interstitial disorders are more likely to be caused by toxic or infectious agents.* Nevertheless, some disorders affect more than one structure. In addition, the anatomic interdependence of structures in the kidney implies that damage to one almost always secondarily affects the others. Thus, severe glomerular damage impairs the flow through the peritubular vascular system; conversely, tubular destruction, by increasing intraglomerular pressure, may induce glomerular atrophy. Thus, whatever the origin, there is a tendency for all forms of chronic renal disease ultimately to destroy all four components of the kidney, culminating in chronic renal failure and what has been called end-stage contracted kidneys. The functional reserve of the kidney is large, and much damage may occur before functional impairment is evident. For these reasons, the early signs and symptoms are particularly important to the clinician, and these are referred to in the discussion of individual diseases.

CLINICAL MANIFESTATIONS OF RENAL DISEASES

The clinical manifestations of renal disease can be grouped into reasonably well-defined syndromes. Some are peculiar to glomerular diseases; others are present in diseases that affect any one of the components. Before we list the syndromes a few terms must be clarified.

Azotemia is a biochemical abnormality that refers to an elevation of the blood urea nitrogen (BUN) and creatinine levels and is largely related to a decreased glomerular filtration rate (GFR). Azotemia is produced by many renal disorders, but it also arises from extrarenal disorders. *Prerenal azotemia* is encountered when there is hypoperfusion of the kidneys, which impairs renal function *in the absence of parenchymal damage.* Similarly, *postrenal azotemia* is seen whenever urine flow is obstructed below the level of the kidney. Relief of the obstruction is followed by prompt correction of the azotemia.

When azotemia becomes associated with a constellation of clinical signs and symptoms and biochemical abnormalities, it is termed uremia. Uremia is characterized not only by failure of renal excretory function but also by a host of metabolic and endocrine alterations incident to renal damage. There is, in addition, secondary gastrointestinal (e.g., uremic gastroenteritis), neuromuscular (e.g., peripheral neuropathy), and cardiovascular (e.g., uremic fibrinous pericarditis) involvement, which are usually necessary for the diagnosis of uremia.

We can now turn to a brief description of the major renal syndromes:

1. *Acute nephritic syndrome* is a glomerular syndrome dominated by the acute onset of usually grossly visible hematuria (red blood cells in urine), mild to moderate proteinuria, and hypertension; it is the classic presentation of acute poststreptococcal glomerulonephritis (GN).
2. The *nephrotic syndrome* is characterized by heavy proteinuria (more than 3.5 gm per day), hypoalbu-

minemia, severe edema, hyperlipidemia, and lipiduria (lipid in the urine).
3. *Asymptomatic hematuria or proteinuria,* or a combination of these two, is usually a manifestation of subtle or mild glomerular abnormalities.
4. *Acute renal failure* (ARF) is dominated by oliguria or anuria (no urine flow), with recent onset of azotemia. It can result from glomerular injury (such as crescentic GN), interstitial injury, or acute tubular necrosis.
5. *Chronic renal failure,* characterized by prolonged symptoms and signs of uremia, is the end result of all chronic renal diseases.
6. *Urinary tract infection* (UTI) is characterized by bacteriuria and pyuria (bacteria and leukocytes in the urine). The infection may be *symptomatic* or *asymptomatic,* and it may affect the kidney *(pyelonephritis [PN])* or the bladder *(cystitis)* only.
7. *Nephrolithiasis* (renal stones) is manifested by renal colic, hematuria, and recurrent stone formation (p. 465).

In addition to these renal syndromes, *urinary tract obstruction* (p. 465) and *renal tumors* (p. 467) represent specific anatomic lesions that often have varied manifestations.

GLOMERULAR DISEASES

The glomerulus is the prima ballerina of the kidney, and glomerular diseases constitute some of the major problems encountered in nephrology; indeed, chronic GN is the most common cause of chronic renal failure in humans. Recall that the glomerulus consists of an anastomosing network of capillaries invested by two layers of epithelium. The visceral epithelium is incorporated into and becomes an intrinsic part of the capillary wall, whereas the parietal epithelium lines Bowman's space, the cavity in which plasma filtrate first collects. The glomerular capillary wall is the filtering membrane and consists of the following structures (Figs. 14–1, 14–2):

1. A thin layer of fenestrated *endothelial cells,* each fenestrum being about 70 to 100 nm in diameter.
2. A *glomerular basement membrane* (GBM) with a thick, electron-dense central layer, the *lamina densa,* and thinner, electron-lucent peripheral layers, the *lamina rara interna* and *lamina rara externa.* The GBM consists of collagen, mostly type IV, laminin, polyanionic proteoglycans, fibronectin, and several other glycoproteins.
3. The *visceral epithelial cells* (podocytes), structurally complex cells that possess interdigitating processes embedded in and adherent to the lamina rara externa of the basement membrane. Adjacent *foot processes* (pedicels) are separated by 20- to 30 nm wide *filtration slits,* which are bridged by a thin diaphragm.
4. The entire glomerular tuft is supported by *mesangial cells* lying between the capillaries. Basement membrane–like mesangial matrix forms a mesh-

Figure 14-1. Schematic representation of a glomerular lobe.

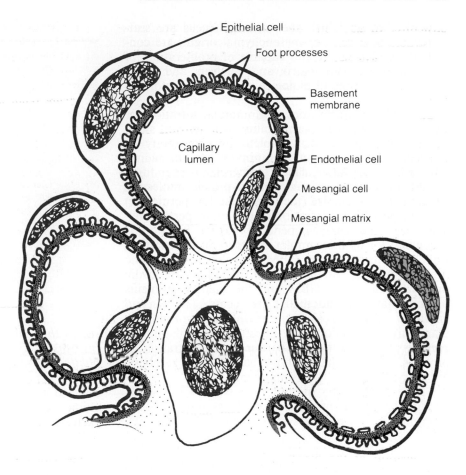

Epithelial cell

Foot processes

Basement membrane

Capillary lumen

Endothelial cell

Mesangial cell

Mesangial matrix

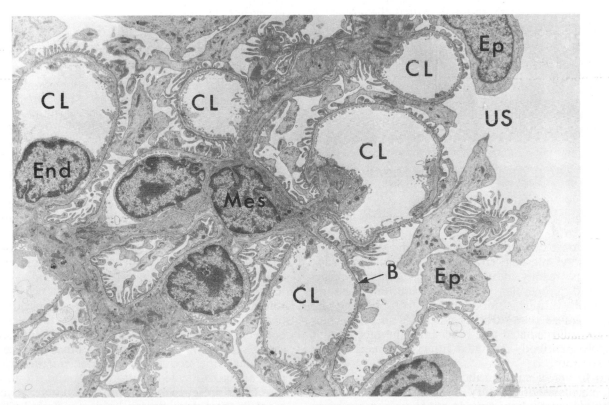

Figure 14-2. Low-power electron micrograph of rat glomerulus. (CL, capillary lumen; End, endothelium; Mes, mesangium; B, basement membrane; Ep, visceral epithelial cells with foot processes; US, urinary space.)

work through which the mesangial cells are scattered. These cells, of mesenchymal origin, are contractile, phagocytic, and capable of proliferation, of laying down both matrix and collagen, and of secreting a number of biologically active mediators, as we shall see.

The major characteristics of glomerular filtration are an extraordinary high permeability to water and small solutes and an almost complete impermeability to molecules of the size of albumin (+ 3.6 nm radius; 70,000 kd). The latter, called glomerular barrier function, discriminates among various protein molecules depending on their size (the larger, the less permeable) and charge (the more cationic, the more permeable). This size- and charge-dependent barrier function is accounted for by the complex structure of the capillary wall, the integrity of the GBM, and the many anionic moieties present within the wall, including the acidic proteoglycans of the GBM and the sialoglycoproteins of epithelial and endothelial cell coats. The *visceral epithelial cell* is critical to the maintenance of glomerular barrier function: its filtration slit diaphragm presents a distal diffusion barrier to the filtration of proteins, and it is the cell type that is largely responsible for synthesis of GBM components.

Glomeruli may be injured by a variety of factors and in the course of a number of systemic diseases. Immune diseases such as systemic lupus erythematosus (SLE), vascular disorders such as hypertension and polyarteritis nodosa, metabolic diseases such as diabetes mellitus, and some purely hereditary conditions such as Fabry's disease often affect the glomerulus. These are termed secondary glomerular diseases to differentiate them from those in which the kidney is the only or predominant organ involved. The latter constitute the various types of *primary GN* or *glomerulopathy.* Here we shall discuss the various types of primary GN. The glomerular alterations in systemic diseases are covered in other parts of this book.

Table 14–1 lists the most common forms of GN that have reasonably well-defined morphologic and clinical manifestations.

PATHOGENESIS OF PRIMARY GLOMERULAR DISEASES

Although we know little of etiologic agents or triggering events, it is clear that immune mechanisms underlie most cases of primary GN and many of the secondary glomerular involvements. Experimentally, GN can be readily induced by antigen-antibody reactions, and glomerular deposits of immunoglobulins, often with various components of complement, are found in more than 70% of patients with GN. Thus, although cell-mediated and other immune mechanisms play roles, antibody-mediated injury has received the most attention.

Two forms of such antibody-associated injury have been established: (1) injury resulting from deposition of *soluble circulating antigen-antibody complexes* in the glomerulus and (2) injury by *antibodies reacting in*

TABLE 14–1. GLOMERULAR DISEASES

Primary Glomerulonephritis
Acute diffuse proliferative glomerulonephritis (GN)
Rapidly progressive (crescentic) GN
Membranous GN
Lipoid nephrosis (minimal change disease)
Focal segmental glomerulosclerosis
Membranoproliferative GN
IgA nephropathy
Chronic GN
Secondary (Systemic) Diseases
Systemic lupus erythematosus
Diabetes mellitus
Amyloidosis
Goodpasture's syndrome
Polyarteritis nodosa
Wegener's granulomatosis
Henoch-Schönlein purpura
Bacterial endocarditis
Hereditary Disorders
Alport's syndrome, Fabry's disease

situ within the glomerulus, either with insoluble fixed (instrinsic) glomerular antigens or with molecules planted within the glomerulus (Fig. 14–3). In addition there is experimental evidence that *cytotoxic antibodies* directed against glomerular cell components may cause glomerular injury. These pathways are not mutually exclusive, and in humans all may contribute to injury.

Circulating Immune Complex Nephritis

The pathogenesis of immune complex diseases (type III hypersensitivity reactions) was discussed in detail in an earlier chapter (p. 127). Here we shall briefly review the salient features that relate to glomerular injury. *With circulating immune complex disease, the glomerulus may be considered an "innocent bystander" because it does not incite the reaction. The antigen is not of glomerular origin.* It may be endogenous as in the glomerulopathy associated with SLE, or it may be exogenous, as is likely in the glomerulonephritis that follows certain bacterial (streptococcal), viral (hepatitis B), parasitic (*plasmodium falciparum* malaria), and spirochetal *(Treponema pallidum)* infections. Sometimes the inciting antigen is unknown. Whatever the antigen may be, antigen-antibody complexes are formed in the circulation and are then trapped in the glomeruli, where they produce injury, in large part through the binding of complement, although complement-independent injury may also occur (see later). The glomerular lesions usually consist of leukocytic infiltration in glomeruli and proliferation of endothelial, mesangial, and parietal epithelial cells. Electron microscopy reveals the complexes as electron-dense deposits or clumps that lie either in the mesangium, between the endothelial cells and the GBM *(subendothelial deposits),* or between the outer surface of the GBM and the podocytes *(subepithelial deposits).* Deposits may be located at more than one site in a given case. The presence of immunoglobulins and complement in these deposits can be demonstrated by immunofluorescence microscopy. When *fluoresceinated anti-*

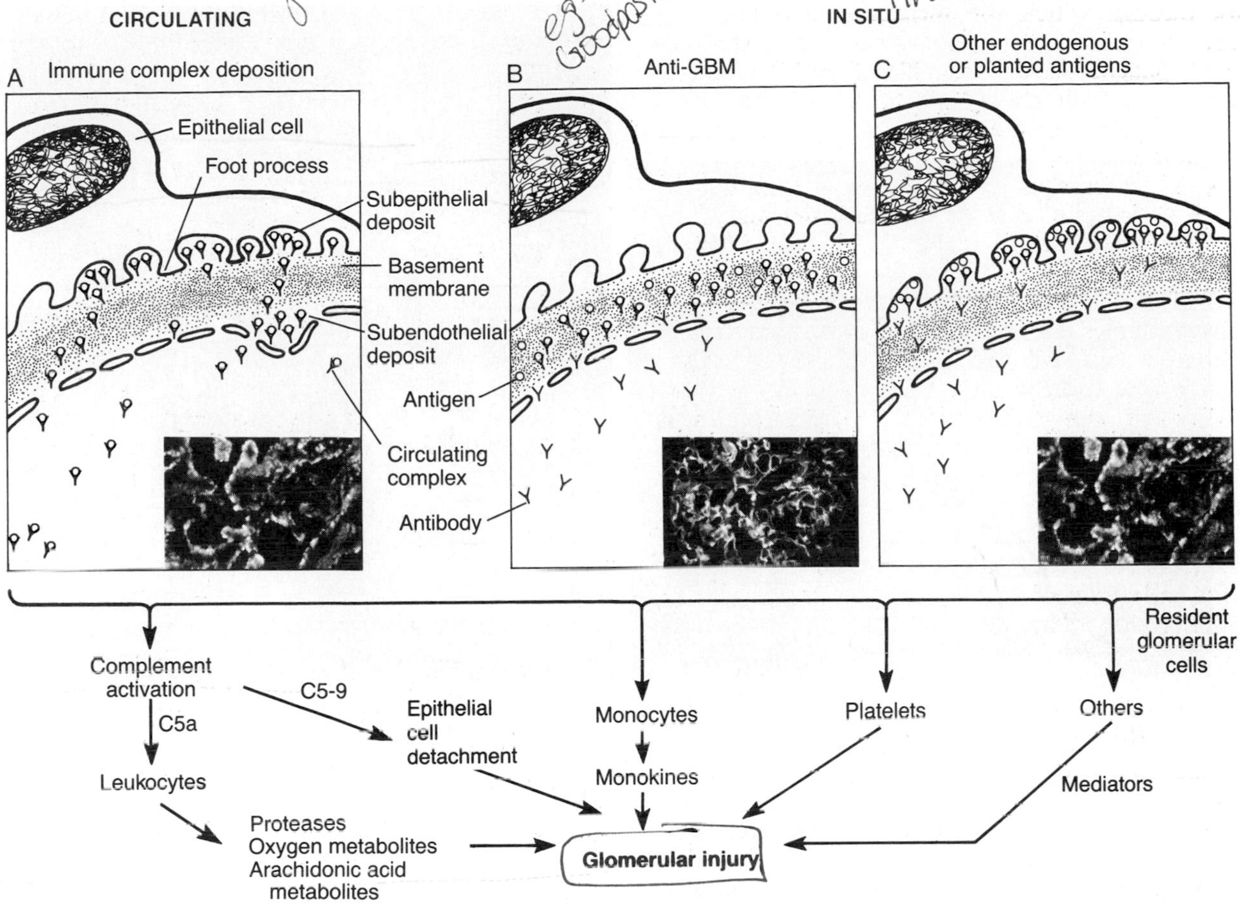

Figure 14-3. Antibody-mediated glomerular injury can result either from the deposition of circulating immune complexes *(left panel)* or from formation in situ of complexes *(middle and right panels)*. Anti-GBM disease *(middle panel)* is characterized by *linear* immunofluorescence patterns, whereas circulating and other lesions induced in situ develop *granular* patterns. The glomerular injury *(bottom)* results from mediators and toxic products derived from complement, neutrophils, monocytes, platelets, and other factors.

Immunoglobulin or anticomplement antibodies are used, the immune complexes are seen as granular deposits in the glomerulus. (Fig. 14-4A). Once deposited in the kidney, immune complexes may eventually be degraded, mostly by infiltrating monocytes and phagocytic mesangial cells, and the inflammatory changes may then subside. Such a course occurs when the exposure to the inciting antigen is short lived and limited, as in most cases of poststreptococcal GN. However, if a continuous shower of antigens is provided, repeated cycles of immune complex formation, deposition, and injury may occur, leading to chronic GN. In some cases the source of chronic antigenic exposure is clear, such as in SLE, in which autoimmune injury to the tissues constantly releases nuclear and cytoplasmic antigens. In many cases, however, the antigen is unknown.

Immune Complex Nephritis in Situ

As noted, antibodies in this form of injury react directly with fixed or planted antigens in the glomerulus.

ANTI-GLOMERULAR BASEMENT MEMBRANE. The best-established model is so-called classic anti-GBM nephritis (Fig. 14-3, middle panel). *In this type of injury antibodies are directed against fixed antigens in the glomerular basement membrane and reveal a linear pattern of localization by immunofluorescence microscopy.* It has its experimental counterpart in the nephritis of rabbits called *Masugi nephritis* or *nephrotoxic serum nephritis*. This is produced by injecting rats with anti-GBM antibodies produced by immunization of rabbits with rat kidney. Although in the experimental model anti-GBM antibodies are produced by injecting "foreign" kidney antigens into an animal, *spontaneous anti-GBM nephritis in humans results from the formation of autoantibodies directed against GBM.* The antibodies directly bind along the GBM to create a "linear pattern," as seen with immunofluorescent techniques, in contrast to the granular pattern described for other forms of antibody-mediated nephritis (Fig. 14-4B). Often the anti-GBM antibodies cross-react with other basement membranes, especially those in the lung alveoli, resulting in simultaneous lung and kidney lesions *(Goodpasture's syndrome)*. It must be clear that this form of GN is an autoimmune disease, so any one of the several mechanisms discussed earlier (p. 138) in relation to autoimmunity may be involved in triggering the disease. Anti-GBM nephritis accounts for less

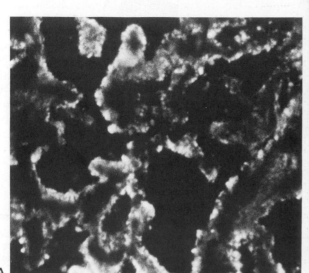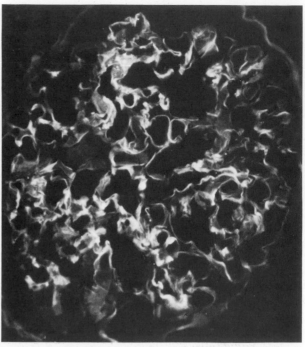

Figure 14-4. Two patterns of deposition of immune complexes as seen by immunofluorescence microscopy. *A, Granular,* characteristic of circulating and in situ immune complex nephritis; *B, linear,* characteristic of classical anti-GBM disease.

than 5% of human GN. It is solidly established as the cause of injury in Goodpasture's syndrome (p. 450). Most instances of anti-GBM nephritis are characterized by very severe glomerular damage and the development of rapidly progressive renal failure. The basement membrane antigen responsible for classic anti-GBM nephritis of Goodpasture's syndrome is a component of the noncollagenous domain of the α_3 chain of collagen type IV.

HEYMANN NEPHRITIS. Although classic anti-GBM disease is the one extablished form of injury to a glomerular antigen, other fixed antigens have been identified experimentally that initiate immune deposition in situ. Some of these are distributed in a *discontinuous* pattern along the visceral epithelial cell foot processes; thus, the resultant pattern of immune deposition in the glomerulus is *granular* (see Fig. 14-3, *right*) rather than diffuse and linear. One of these is the so-called *Heymann* antigen. The Heymann model of rat GN is induced by immunizing animals with preparations of proximal tubular brush border in Freund's adjuvant. The rats develop antibodies to brush border antigens and a membranous GN (p. 445) that closely resembles human membranous GN. This is characterized on immunofluorescence by the deposition of immunoglobulins and complement in a granular (rather than linear) pattern along the GBM. Although it was once thought to be due to trapping of circulating immune complexes, it is now clear that the GN results from the reaction of the anti–brush border antibody with a fixed but discontinuously distributed 330-kd glycoprotein (GP330) present on the base of visceral epithelial cells and cross-reactive with brush

border antigen. Heymann nephritis most resembles human membranous GN, in which the epithelial cell antigen appears to be a homologue of GP330.

Antibodies may also react in situ with previously "planted" nonglomerular antigens, which may localize in the kidney by interacting with various intrinsic components of the glomerulus. Planted antigens include cationic molecules that bind to glomerular capillary anionic sites; DNA, which has an affinity for GBM components; bacterial products, such as endostreptosin, a protein of group A streptococci; large aggregated proteins (e.g., aggregated IgG), which deposit in the mesangium because of their size; and immune complexes themselves, since they continue to have reactive sites for further interactions with free antibody, free antigen, or complement. Most of these planted antigens induce a granular and variable pattern of immunoglobulin deposition by fluorescence microscopy.

Factors that affect glomerular localization of antigen, antibody, or complexes are legion. The molecular charge and size of these reactants are clearly important. The pattern of localization is also affected by changes in glomerular hemodynamics, mesangial function, and integrity of the charge-selective barrier in the glomerulus. These influences may well explain the variable pattern of immune reactant deposition and histologic change in glomerulonephritis. Studies in experimental models have shown that complexes deposited in the proximal zones of the GBM (endothelium or subendothelium) elicit an inflammatory reaction in the glomerulus with infiltration of leukocytes. In contrast, antibodies directed to distal zones of the GBM (epithelium and subepithelium) are largely noninflammatory and elicit lesions similar to those of Heymann or membranous GN.

Cytotoxic Antibodies

In addition to producing immune deposits, antibodies directed to glomerular cell antigens may cause direct cell injury, often without deposits. Antibodies to mesangial cell antigens, for example, cause mesangiolysis followed by mesangial cell proliferation; antibodies to endothelial cell surface proteins cause endothelial injury; and antibodies to certain visceral epithelial cell glycoproteins cause proteinuria in experimental animals. These mechanisms may well play a role in human immune disorders that are not associated with immune deposits.

To conclude the discussion of antibody-mediated injury, it must be stated that *antigen-antibody deposition in the glomerulus is a major pathway of glomerular injury; and that immune reactions in situ, trapping of circulating complexes, interactions between these two events, and local hemodynamic and structural determinants in the glomerulus all contribute to the morphologic and functional alterations in GN.*

Cell-Mediated Immune Glomerulonephritis

There is increasing evidence that sensitized T cells, as a reflection of a cell-mediated immune reaction, can cause glomerular injury. The idea is an attractive one, as it may account for the many instances of GN in which either there are no immune deposits or the deposits do not correlate with the severity of damage. Clues to its occurrence include the presence of macrophages and T lymphocytes in the glomerulus in some forms of human and experimental GN, evidence in vitro of lymphocyte reactivity on exposure to altered GBM antigen in progressive human GN, and an increasing number of experimental models of cell-mediated injury in the glomerulus.

Mediators of Immune Injury

Once immune reactants are localized in the glomerulus, how does glomerular damage ensue? *Glomerular damage is reflected physiologically by loss of glomerular barrier function manifested by proteinuria, and in some instances by reductions in GFR.* One well-established pathway is the *complement-leukocyte–mediated mechanism* (see Fig. 14–3). Activation of complement initiates the generation of chemotactic agents (mainly C5a) and the recruitment of neutrophils and monocytes. Neutrophils release proteases, which cause GBM degradation; oxygen-derived free radicals, which cause cell damage; and arachidonic acid metabolites, which contribute to the reductions in GFR. However, this mechanism applies only to some types of GN, since many types show few neutrophils in the damaged glomeruli. Some models suggest complement- but not neutrophil-dependent injury, owing to an effect of the C5-C9 lytic component (membrane attack complex) of

complement, which causes epithelial cell detachment and stimulates mesangial and epithelial cells to secrete damaging chemical mediators. Other mediators of glomerular damage include (1) *monocytes and macrophages,* which infiltrate the glomerulus in antibody- and cell-mediated reactions, and, when activated release a vast number of biologically active molecules (p. 40); (2) *platelets,* which aggregate in the glomerulus during immune-mediated injury and release prostaglandins and growth factors; (3) *resident glomerular cells*—epithelial, mesangial, and endothelial—which can be stimulated to secrete mediators such as cytokines (interleukin-1), arachidonic acid metabolites, growth factors, nitric oxide, and endothelin; and (4) *fibrin-related products,* which cause leukocyte infiltration and glomerular cell proliferation.

Other Mechanisms of Glomerular Injury

Other mechanisms may contribute to glomerular damage in certain primary renal disorders. Three that deserve special mention are epithelial cell injury, renal ablation glomerulopathy, and interstitial inflammation.

EPITHELIAL CELL INJURY: This can be induced by antibodies to visceral epithelial cell antigens; by toxins, as in an experimental model of proteinuria induced by puromycin aminonucleoside; conceivably by certain cytokines; or by unknown factors, as is the case in lipoid nephrosis (p. 445). Such injury is reflected by morphologic changes in the visceral epithelial cells, which include loss of foot processes, vacuolization, retraction and *detachment* of cells from the GBM, and functionally by proteinuria. It is hypothesized that the detachment of visceral epithelial cells is caused by loss of its adhesive interactions with the basement membrane, and that this detachment leads to protein leakage (Fig. 14–5).

RENAL ABLATION GLOMERULOPATHY. It has been documented that once any renal disease, glomerular or

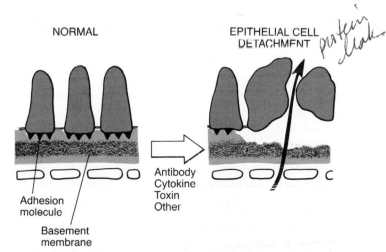

Figure 14–5. Epithelial cell injury. The postulated sequence is a consequence of antibodies to epithelial cell antigens, or toxins, or cytokines or other factors causing injury and detachment of epithelial cells, and protein leakage through defective GBM and filtration slits. (Adapted from Couser W. G.: Mediation of immune glomerular injury. Am. Soc. Nephrol. 1:13, 1990.)

otherwise, destroys sufficient functioning nephrons to reduce the GFR to about 30 to 50% of normal, progression to end-stage renal failure proceeds inexorably although the rate varies. Such patients develop proteinuria and their kidneys show widespread *glomerulosclerosis*. Recent studies suggest that progressive sclerosis may be initiated by the adaptive changes that occur in the relatively unaffected glomeruli of diseased kidneys. Such a mechanism is suggested by experiments in rats subjected to ablation of renal mass by subtotal nephrectomy. Compensatory hypertrophy of the remaining glomeruli serves to maintain renal function in these animals, but proteinuria and focal glomerulosclerosis soon develop, leading eventually to total glomerular obsolescence and uremia. The glomerular hypertrophy is associated with hemodynamic changes, including increases in single-nephron GFR, blood flow, and transcapillary pressure (capillary hypertension). The sequence of events (Fig. 14–6) leading to sclerosis entails endothelial and epithelial cell injury, increased glomerular permeability to proteins, accumulation of proteins in the mesangial matrix, and fibrin deposition. This is followed by proliferation of mesangial cells, increased deposition of mesangial matrix, and sclerosis of glomeruli. The latter results in further reductions in nephron mass and a vicious cycle of continuing glomerulosclerosis.

INTERSTITIAL INFLAMMATION IN GN. It has long been known that many human and experimental models of GN are associated with the presence of inflammatory cells—lymphocytes and macrophages—*in the interstitium*. In some instances, as in anti-GBM disease, the infiltrate may be related to cross-reacting antibodies with tubular basement membranes. In others, the nature of the infiltrate suggests an interstitial delayed hypersensitivity reaction. Recent evidence *suggests* that this intersitital reaction plays a role in both the acute and the progressive renal dysfunction in some forms of immune GN; however, the precise mechanisms of inflammatory cell accumulation and the manner by which such inflammation affects glomerular function are still unclear.

We now turn to a consideration of specific types of GN and the glomerular syndromes they produce.

GLOMERULAR SYNDROMES AND DISORDERS _____

The Nephrotic Syndrome _____

The nephrotic syndrome refers to a clinical complex comprised of the following: (1) massive proteinuria, with the daily loss in the urine of 3.5 gm or more of protein; (2) generalized edema, the most obvious clinical manifestation; (3) hypoalbuminemia, with plasma albumin levels less than 3 gm per 100 ml; and (4) hyperlipidemia and lipiduria. At the onset there is little or no azotemia, hematuria, or hypertension. The components of the nephrotic syndrome bear a logical relationship to one another. The initial event is a derangement in the capillary walls of the glomeruli, resulting in increased permeability to the plasma proteins. It will be remembered from the previous discussion of the normal kidney that the glomerular capillary wall, with its endothelium, GBM, and visceral epithelial cells, acts as a barrier through which the glomerular filtrate must pass. Any increased permeability resulting from either structural or physicochemical alterations allows protein to escape from the plasma into the glomerular filtrate. Massive proteinuria may result. With longstanding or extremely heavy proteinuria, the serum albumin tends to become depleted, resulting in hypoalbuminemia and a reversed albumin-globulin ratio. The generalized edema of the nephrotic syndrome is in turn largely a consequence of the drop in osmotic pressure produced by hypoalbuminemia. As fluid escapes from the vascular tree into the tissues, there is a concomitant drop in plasma volume, with diminished glomerular filtration. Compensatory secretion of aldosterone, along with the reduced GFR, promotes retention of salt and water by the kidneys, thus further aggravating the edema. By repetition of this chain of events, massive amounts of edema (termed *anasarca*) may accumulate. The genesis of the hyperlipidemia is more obscure. Presumably hypoalbu-

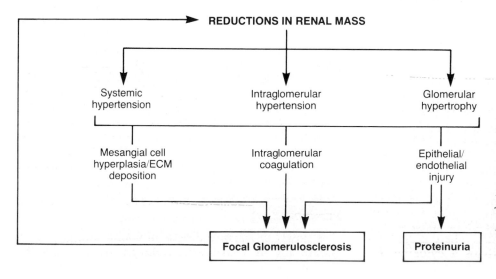

Figure 14–6. Nonimmune mechanisms in progressive glomerulosclerosis caused by reductions in renal mass. The adaptive changes in glomeruli (hypertrophy and glomerular capillary hypertension), as well as systemic hypertension, cause epithelial and endothelial injury and resultant proteinuria. The mesangial response, involving mesangial cell proliferation and extracellular matrix (ECM) production together with intraglomerular coagulation, causes the glomerulosclerosis. This results in further loss of functioning nephrons and a vicious circle of progressive glomerulosclerosis.

TABLE 14–2. CAUSES OF NEPHROTIC SYNDROME

	Children %	Adults %
Primary glomerular diseases	95	60
Minimal change disease (lipoid nephrosis) aka min. disease	61	9
Focal sclerosis	10	9
Membranous GN	5	25
Membranoproliferative GN	9	4
Other proliferative GN (e.g., focal, pure mesangial, diffuse)	10	13
Associated with systemic disease (most commonly diabetes, SLE, amyloidosis)	5	40

minemia triggers increased synthesis of all forms of plasma proteins, including lipoproteins. Peripheral breakdown of lipoproteins may also be impaired. The lipiduria in turn simply reflects the hyperlipoproteinemia and increased GBM permeability.

The relative frequencies of the several causes of the nephrotic syndrome vary according to age. In children younger than age 15 years, for example, the nephrotic syndrome is almost always caused by a lesion primary to the kidney, whereas among adults it may often be associated with a systemic disease. Table 14–2 represents a composite derived from several studies of the causes of the nephrotic syndrome and is therefore only approximate. As the table indicates, the most frequent *systemic* causes of the nephrotic syndrome are SLE, diabetes, and amyloidosis. The renal lesions produced by these disorders are described elsewhere in this text. The most important of the *primary* glomerular lesions that characteristically lead to the nephrotic syndrome are *lipoid nephrosis (minimal change disease)* and *membranous GN.* The former is most important in children; the latter in adults. Two other primary lesions, *focal glomerulosclerosis* and *membranoproliferative GN,* also produce the nephrotic syndrome. These four lesions are discussed individually below. The fifth possible primary cause of this syndrome, *proliferative GN,* is not considered in this section because this lesion frequently presents with the nephritic syndrome.

LIPOID NEPHROSIS (MINIMAL CHANGE DISEASE)

This relatively benign disorder is the most frequent cause of the nephrotic syndrome in children. *It is characterized by glomeruli that have a normal appearance under the light microscope but disclose diffuse loss of visceral epithelial foot processes when viewed with the electron microscope.* Although it may develop at any age, it is most common between ages two and three years.

The pathogenesis of lipoid nephrosis is shrouded in mystery. *There is no evidence for either an immune complex or an anti-GBM mechanism, but the ultrastructural changes in glomerular epithelial cells clearly point to primary epithelial cell injury.* There is *speculation* that a circulating toxin, perhaps a cytokine, se-

creted by immune lymphocyte or macrophage activation, might be the culprit in causing such injury. Certain studies invoke loss of glomerular polyanionic molecules as a result of epithelial injury as one possible cause of the proteinuria. It is currently thought that the charge on the GBM imparted by glomerular polyanions is an important factor in its barrier function (p. 440). The negatively charged GBM allows greater penetration of neutral and cationic molecules than it does of anionic molecules of the same size. In lipoid nephrosis, reduction in negative charges due to loss of glomerular polyanions permits transmembrane passage of anionic serum albumin, resulting in albuminuria. Detachment of epithelial cells (Fig. 14–5) as a result of loss of adhesion to the GBM may also contribute to the protein loss.

MORPHOLOGY. With the light microscope the glomeruli appear nearly normal (Fig. 14–7A). The cells of the proximal convoluted tubules are often heavily laden with lipids, but this is secondary to tubular reabsorption of the lipoproteins passing through the diseased glomeruli. This appearance of the proximal convoluted tubules is the basis for the older term for this disorder, **"lipoid nephrosis."** Even with the electron microscope, the GBM appears normal. The only obvious glomerular abnormality is the uniform and diffuse loss of the foot processes of the podocytes (Fig. 14–7C). The cytoplasm of the podocytes thus appears smeared over the external aspect of the GBM, obliterating the network of arcades between the podocytes and the GBM. There are also epithelial cell vacuolization, microvillus formation, and occasional focal detachments. The changes in the podocytes are completely reversible after remission of the proteinuria.

CLINICAL COURSE. The disease manifests itself by the insidious development of the nephrotic syndrome in an otherwise healthy person. There is no hypertension, and renal function is preserved in most patients. The protein loss is usually confined to the smaller serum proteins, chiefly albumin (selective proteinuria). The prognosis in children with this disorder is good. More than 90% of the cases respond to a short course of steroid therapy; however, proteinuria recurs in more than two thirds of the initial responders, some of whom become steroid dependent. A few develop progressive deterioration of renal function. In one large study of biopsy-proved cases followed for up to 10 years, 71% were in complete remission, 22% had persistent disease, and the remaining 7% had died of renal failure. Because of its responsiveness to therapy in children, lipoid nephrosis must be differentiated from the other causes of the nephrotic syndrome in nonresponders. Adults also respond to steroid therapy but relapses are more common.

MEMBRANOUS GLOMERULONEPHRITIS (MEMBRANOUS NEPHROPATHY)

This slowly progressive disease of young adulthood and middle age is *characterized morphologically by the*

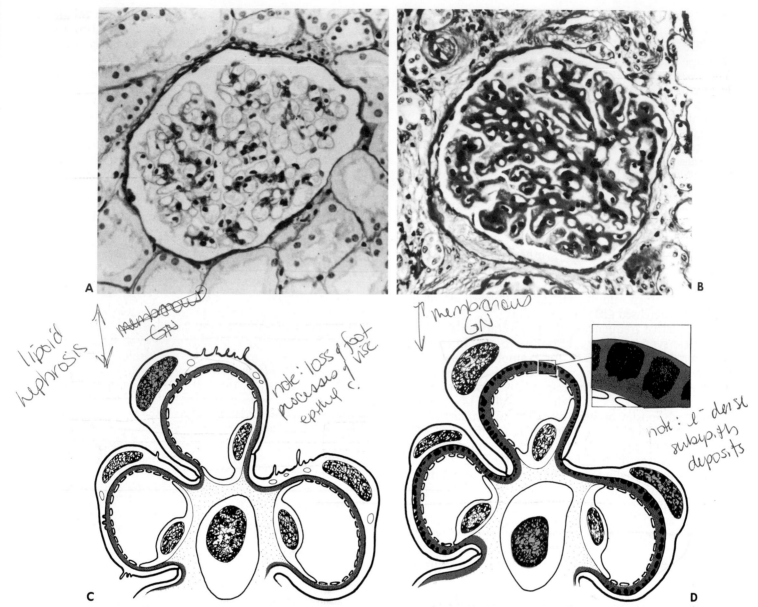

Handwritten annotations: lipoid nephrosis ↕; membranous GN; note: loss of foot processes of visc epithel c.; ↑ membranous GN ↓; note: e-dense subep.th deposits

Figure 14–7. Lipoid nephrosis, *A, C,* and membranous glomerulonephritis, *B, D.* Note that under the light microscope the glomerulus appears normal, with a thin basement membrane, in lipoid nephrosis, *A.* Compare this with the diffuse thickening of the basement membrane in membranous glomerulonephritis, *B.* On electron microscopy, lipoid nephrosis exhibits diffuse loss of foot processes of visceral epithelial cells, *C,* whereas membranous glomerulonephritis, *D,* is characterized by electron-dense subepithelial deposits.

presence of subepithelial immunoglobulin-containing deposits along the glomerular capillary wall. Early in the disease, the glomeruli may appear normal by light microscopy, but well-developed cases show *diffuse thickening of the capillary wall.*

Membranous GN (MGN) may occur in association with known disorders or agents (secondary MGN): (1) malignant epithelial tumors, particularly carcinoma of the lung and colon and melanoma; (2) SLE; (3) exposure to inorganic salts (gold, mercury); (4) drugs (penicillamine, captopril); (5) infections (chronic hepatitis B, syphilis, schistosomiasis, malaria); and (6) metabolic disorders (diabetes mellitus, thyroiditis). In about 85% of cases; the condition is truly idiopathic (primary).

MGN is a form of chronic immune complex ne-

phritis. Although circulating complexes of known exogenous (e.g., hepatitis B) or endogenous (DNA in SLE) antigen can cause MGN, it is now thought that most idiopathic forms are induced by antibodies reacting in situ to endogenous or planted glomerular antigens.

Genetic susceptibility is suggested by the increased prevalence of HLA-DR3 in European and HLA-DR2 in Japanese patients with MGN. This points to possible defects in immune regulation, and indeed an imbalance in helper and suppressor T-lymphocyte function has been reported in these patients.

The lesions bear a striking resemblance to those of experimental Heymann nephritis, which, as you recall, is induced by antibodies to an intrinsic tissue antigen

(GP330) present in visceral epithelial cells. Susceptibility to Heymann nephritis in rats and MGN in humans is linked to the HLA locus, which influences the ability to elaborate antibodies to the *nephritogenic* antigen. The possibility thus exists that idiopathic MGN, like Heymann nephritis, is an autoimmune disease linked to susceptibility genes and caused by antibodies to a renal antigen similar to GP330.

Begging the question of the nature of the immune deposits, how does the glomerular capillary wall become leaky? In the absence of neutrophils, monocytes, or platelets and the virtually uniform presence of complement, current work points to a direct action of C5b-9, the membrane-attack complex of complement, as described previously (p. 443).

MORPHOLOGY. Seen by light microscopy, the basic change appears to be diffuse thickening of the GBM (see Fig. 14–7B). By electron microscopy, it can be seen that the apparent thickening is caused in part by subepithelial deposits that nestle against the GBM and are separated from each other by small spike-like protrusions of GBM matrix ("spike and dome" pattern; (see Fig. 14–7D). As the disease progresses, these spikes close over the deposits, incorporating them into the GBM. In addition, the podocytes lose their foot processes. The consequent close apposition of the podocytes to the GBM contributes to the appearance of GBM thickening on light microscopy. Later in the disease, the incorporated deposits are catabolized and eventually disappear, leaving for a time cavities within the GBM. These are later filled in with progressive deposition of GBM matrix. With further progression, the glomeruli become sclerosed and finally become completely hyalinized. Fluorescence microscopy shows typical granular deposition of immunoglobulins and complement along the GBM (see Fig. 14–4A).

CLINICAL COURSE. The onset is characterized by the insidious development of the nephrotic syndrome, usually without antecedent illness; however, proteinuria may be present without the full-blown nephrotic syndrome. In contrast to minimal change disease, the proteinuria is usually nonselective and does not usually respond to corticosteroid therapy. Globulins are lost in the urine, as are the smaller albumin molecules. MGN follows a notoriously variable and often indolent course. Overall, about 50% of patients suffer progressive disease terminating in renal failure after 2 to 20 years. An additional 10 to 30% have a more benign course with partial or complete remission of proteinuria, and the others have persistent proteinuria.

FOCAL SEGMENTAL GLOMERULOSCLEROSIS

Focal segmental glomerulosclerosis (FSG) is characterized by sclerosis affecting some but not all glomeruli and involving only segments of each glomerulus. It can occur as a secondary event in a variety of glomerular (*IgA nephropathy*) and tubulointerstitial diseases (*reflux nephropathy*) or may be primary. Primary (or idio-

pathic) FSG accounts for approximately 10% of all cases of the nephrotic syndrome. In children it is important to distinguish this cause of the nephrotic syndrome from lipoid nephrosis because the clinical course is markedly different. Unlike the case with lipoid nephrosis, patients with this lesion have a higher incidence of hematuria and hypertension, their proteinuria is nonselective, and in general their response to corticosteroid therapy is poor. In one series that included both children and adults, 50% of the patients died within 10 years of diagnosis; of the survivors, most (90%) had persistent urinary abnormalities. Adults in general fare less well than children.

MORPHOLOGY. The disease first affects only some of the glomeruli (thus the term *focal*) and initially only the juxtamedullary glomeruli (Fig. 14–8). With progression, eventually all levels of the cortex are affected. Histologically, focal glomerulosclerosis is characterized by sclerosis and hyalinization of some tufts within a glomerulus and sparing of the others. Thus, the involvement is both focal and segmental. Occasionally glomeruli are completely sclerosed (global sclerosis). In affected glomeruli, immunofluorescent microscopy reveals deposits of immunoglobulins, usually IgM, and complement in the mesangium. Electron microscopy shows increased mesangial matrix in affected glomeruli, along with electron-dense granular deposits in the mesangium. The visceral epithelial cells exhibit loss of foot processes, as in lipoid nephrosis, but also a **greater degree of epithelial cell detachment** with denudation of underlying GBM.

In time progression of the disease leads to total sclerosis of the glomeruli with pronounced tubular atrophy and interstitial fibrosis. This advanced picture would be difficult to differentiate from other forms of chronic GN (p. 452).

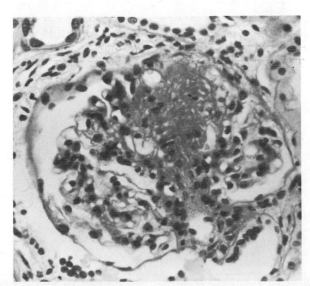

Figure 14–8. Focal segmental sclerosis, high-power view. Only one portion of the glomerulus shows an area of sclerosis. There is slight mesangial hyperplasia in the rest of the glomerulus.

The pathogenesis of primary focal glomerulosclerosis is unknown. Some investigators have suggested that focal glomerulosclerosis is a variant, albeit an aggressive one, of lipoid nephrosis. Others believe it to be a distinct clinicopathologic entity. In any case, *the characteristic disruption of visceral epithelial cells is thought to represent the hallmark of FSG.* The hyalinosis and sclerosis represent entrapment of plasma proteins in hyperpermeable foci and mesangial cell reaction to such proteins and to fibrin deposits. The recurrence of proteinuria in patients with focal sclerosis who receive renal allografts, sometimes within 24 hours of transplantation, suggests a circulating toxin (cytokine?) as the cause of the epithelial damage.

There is little tendency for spontaneous remission of idiopathic FSG, and responses to corticosteroid therapy are poor. Progression to renal failure occurs at varying rates and about 50% of patients suffer renal failure after 10 years.

MEMBRANOPROLIFERATIVE GLOMERULONEPHRITIS

Membranoproliferative GN (MPGN) is characterized histologically by alterations in the basement membrane and proliferation of glomerular cells. It accounts for 5 to 10% of cases of idiopathic nephrotic syndrome in children and adults. Some patients present only with hematuria or proteinuria in the nonnephrotic range and others have a combined nephrotic-nephritic picture. Two types of MPGN (I and II) are recognized on the basis of distinct ultrastructural, immunofluorescent, and probably pathogenic, findings.

By light microscopy both types are similar. The glomeruli are large and show proliferation of mesangial cells as well as infiltrating leukocytes (Fig. 14–9A). They have a "lobular" appearance. The GBM is thickened, and the glomerular capillary wall often shows a double-contour or "tramtrack" appearance, especially evident in silver or periodic acid–schiff stains. This is caused by "splitting" of the basement membrane because of the inclusion within it of processes of mesangial cells extending into the peripheral capillary loops, so-called mesangial interposition.

Types I and II have different ultrastructural and immunofluorescent features (Fig. 14–19B). Type I MPGN (two thirds of cases) is characterized by the presence of subendothelial electron-dense deposits. By immunofluorescence, C3 is deposited in a granular pattern, and IgG and early complement components (C1q and C4) are often also present, suggesting an immune complex pathogenesis.

In type II lesions, the lamina densa of the GBM is transformed into an irregular, ribbon-like, extremely electron-dense structure, owing to the deposition of dense material of unknown composition in the GBM proper, giving rise to the term **dense-deposit disease.** C3 is present in irregular granular-linear foci in the basement membranes and mesangium in characteristic circular aggregates (mesangial rings). IgG is usually absent, as are the early-acting complement components (C1q and C4).

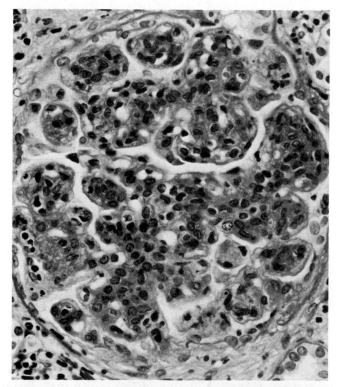

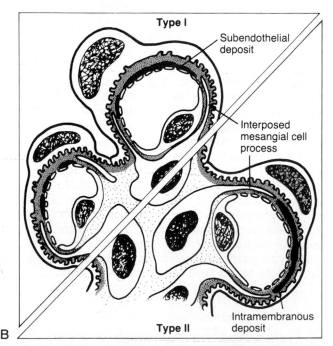

A

B

Figure 14–9. *A,* Membranoproliferative GN, showing mesangial cell proliferation, basement membrane thickening, leukocyte infiltration, and accentuation of lobular architecture. *B,* Schematic representation of patterns in the two types of membranoproliferative glomerulonephritis as seen by electron microscopy. In type I there are *subendothelial deposits;* type II is characterized by *intramembranous dense deposits* (dense deposit disease). In both, mesangial interposition gives the appearance of split basement membranes when viewed in the light microscope.

Although there is considerable overlap, different pathogenic mechanisms are involved in the evolution of type I and type II disease. Most cases of type I MPGN appear to be caused by a chronic immune complex reaction, but the inciting antigen is not known. The pathogenesis of type II MPGN is less clear. The serum of patients with type II MPGN has a factor called "C3 nephritic factor" (C_3NeF), which can activate the alternate complement pathway. This factor is an immunoglobulin that reacts with C3 convertase of the alternate complement pathway (p. 34) and serves to stabilize it, thus activating the pathway and resulting in the elaboration of biologically active complement fragments. C_3NeF is thus an autoantibody and as in other autoimmune diseases there is a genetic predisposition to developing MPGN. The hypocomplementemia, more marked in type II, is contributed in part by the excessive consumption of C3 and in part by reduced synthesis of C3 by the liver. It is still not clear how the complement abnormality induces the glomerular changes.

CLINICAL COURSE. The principal mode of presentation is the nephrotic syndrome, although MPGN may begin as acute nephritis or more insidiously as mild proteinuria. The prognosis of MPGN is uniformly poor. In one study, none of 60 patients followed for one to 20 years showed complete remission. Forty per cent progressed to end-stage renal failure, 30% had variable degrees of renal insufficiency, and the remaining 30% had persistent nephrotic syndrome without renal failure. Type II disease has a worse prognosis, and it tends to recur in transplant recipients.

The Nephritic Syndrome

Nephritic syndrome is a clinical complex, usually of acute onset, characterized by (1) hematuria with red cell and hemoglobin casts in the urine, (2) some degree of oliguria and azotemia, and (3) hypertension. Although there may also be some proteinuria and even edema these are usually not sufficiently marked to cause the nephrotic syndrome. The lesions that cause this syndrome have in common proliferation of the cells within the glomeruli, often accompanied by a leukocytic infiltrate. This inflammatory reaction injures the capillary walls, permitting escape of red cells into the urine, and induces hemodynamic changes that lead to a reduction in the GFR. The reduced GFR is manifested clinically by oliguria, reciprocal fluid retention, and azotemia. Hypertension is probably a result of both the fluid retention and some augmented renin release from the ischemic kidneys.

The acute nephritic syndrome may be produced by systemic disorders such as SLE or may be the result of primary glomerular disease. The latter, which is more common, is exemplified by acute diffuse proliferative GN, discussed below.

ACUTE PROLIFERATIVE (POSTSTREPTOCOCCAL, POSTINFECTIOUS) GLOMERULONEPHRITIS

Diffuse proliferative GN (PGN), one of the more frequent of the glomerular disorders, typically is caused by immune complexes. The inciting antigen may be either exogenous or endogenous. The prototype *exogenous pattern* is postinfectious GN, whereas that produced by an *endogenous* antigen is *lupus nephritis,* seen in SLE (p. 143). Infections by organisms other than the streptococci may also be associated with diffuse PGN. These include certain staphylococcal infections as well as a number of common viral diseases such as mumps, measles, chickenpox, and hepatitis B.

The classic case of poststreptococcal GN develops in a child one to four weeks after the patient recovers from a group A streptococcal infection. Only certain "nephritogenic" strains of the β-hemolytic streptococci are capable of evoking glomerular disease. In most cases the initial infection is pharyngitis or a skin infection. It is generally agreed that acute poststreptococcal GN is mediated by deposition of immune complexes. *Typical features of immune complex disease, such as hypocomplementemia and granular deposits of IgG and complement on the GBM, are seen.* Nevertheless, the nature of the pathogenic antigen remains mysterious and it is not clear whether circulating or formed complexes in situ are the predominant forms. Streptococcal antigens, altered GBM, and altered forms of IgG have been implicated at one time or another.

MORPHOLOGY. In the rare fatal cases the kidneys are grossly smooth and show fine, punctate petechiae scattered over the cortical surface. Under the light microscope, the most characteristic change is a fairly uniformly increased cellularity of the glomerular tufts affecting nearly all glomeruli, hence the term **diffuse.** The increased cellularity is caused both by proliferation and swelling of endothelial and mesangial cells and by a neutrophilic and monocytic infiltrate. Sometimes there are thrombi within the capillary lumens and necrosis of the capillary walls. In a few cases there may also be "crescents" (p. 450) inside Bowman's capsule. In general, these are an ominous finding. When they involve most of the glomeruli, the pattern merges with that of rapidly progressive GN, to be discussed. In the early stages of the disease, the electron microscope shows the immune complexes arrayed as subendothelial, intramembranous, or most often subepithelial "humps" nestled against the GBM (Fig. 14-10). Immunofluorescence studies reveal IgG and complement within the deposits. These deposits are usually cleared over a period of about two months.

CLINICAL COURSE. The onset of the kidney disease tends to be abrupt, heralded by malaise, a slight fever, nausea, and the nephritic syndrome. In the usual case, oliguria, azotemia, and hypertension are only mild to moderate. Characteristically, there is gross hematuria, the urine appearing smoky brown rather than bright red. Some proteinuria is a constant feature of the disease and, as mentioned earlier, it may occasionally be severe enough to produce the nephrotic syndrome.

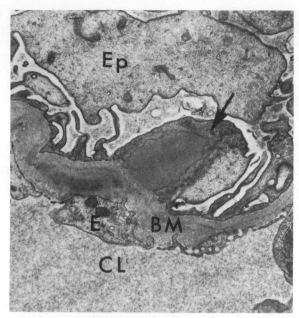

Figure 14–10. Poststreptococcal GN. Electron micrograph shows a hump-shaped, electron-dense deposit *(arrow)* on epithelial side of basement membrane (BM). There is also a dense deposit within BM. (CL, capillary lumen; E, endothelium; Ep, epithelium.)

Serum complement levels are low and serum anti-streptolysin O titers elevated in poststreptococcal cases.

Complete recovery occurs in most children in epidemic cases. A very few children (1%) develop rapidly progressive GN or chronic renal disease. The prognosis in sporadic cases is less clear. In adults, 15 to 50% of cases become chronic depending on the clinical and histologic severity. In contrast, the prevalence of chronicity after sporadic cases of acute GN in children is much lower.

RAPIDLY PROGRESSIVE GLOMERULONEPHRITIS (RPGN; CRESCENTIC GLOMERULONEPHRITIS)

Rapidly progressive glomerulonephritis (RPGN) is a clinicopathologic syndrome and not a specific etiologic form of glomerulonephritis. Clinically it is characterized by rapid and progressive loss of renal function associated with severe oliguria and (if untreated) death from renal failure within weeks to months. Regardless of the cause, *the histologic picture is characterized by the presence of crescents in most of the glomeruli (crescentic GN).* These are produced in part by proliferation of the parietal epithelial cells of Bowman's capsule and in part by infiltration of monocytes and macrophages.

The conditions in which the syndrome of RPGN may occur can be grouped into three categories: (1) postinfectious (poststreptococcal RPGN), (2) GN associated with systemic diseases, and (3) idiopathic RPGN (also called primary or isolated RPGN). As might be expected from the list of associated conditions (Table 14–3) no single pathogenic mechanism can explain all cases. There is little doubt, however, that in most cases the glomerular injury is immunologically mediated. In SLE, and in poststreptococcal settings, RPGN is me-

diated by immune complexes. RPGN associated with Goodpasture's syndrome is a classic example of anti-GBM nephritis (p. 441). In this condition, circulating anti-GBM antibodies can be detected in more than 95% of cases by radioimmunoassay. These antibodies cross-react with pulmonary alveolar basement membranes to produce the clinical picture of pulmonary hemorrhages associated with renal failure. Linear deposits of IgG, and in many cases C3, can be visualized by immunofluorescence along both the glomerular and alveolar basement membranes. What triggers the formation of anti–basement membrane antibodies is not clear. It should be emphasized that Goodpasture's syndrome is not a common disorder but (if untreated) is frequently fatal; patients die of renal failure or of pulmonary complications.

Idiopathic RPGN accounts for about half of all cases. In a fourth of these, linear glomerular deposits are found (as in Goodpasture's syndrome) but there is no pulmonary involvement. In another fourth, granular glomerular deposits are present, related to the deposition of immune complexes. But in about half the patients there are minimal immune deposits or none *(pauci-immune crescentic GN)*. Antineutrophil cytoplasmic antibodies (ANCA), which as we have seen (p. 288) play a role in some forms of vasculitis, are virtually always present in pauci-immune GN. Thus idiopathic *crescentic* GN can be caused by different pathogenic mechanisms, inducing severe glomerular injury.

MORPHOLOGY. The kidneys are enlarged and pale, often with petechial hemorrhages on the cortical surfaces. Depending on the underlying cause, the glomeruli may show focal necrosis (Goodpasture's syndrome), diffuse or focal endothelial proliferation, and mesangial proliferation. However, the histologic picture is dominated by the formation of distinctive crescents (Fig. 14–11). Crescents are formed by proliferation of parietal cells and by migration of monocytes into Bowman's space. The crescents eventually obliterate Bowman's space and compress the glomeruli. Fibrin strands are prominent between the cellular layers in the crescents,

---

TABLE 14–3. RAPIDLY PROGRESSIVE GLOMERULONEPHRITIS (RPGN)

1. Postinfectious RPGN
   Poststreptococcal
2. Associated with systemic diseases
   SLE
   Polyarteritis
   Goodpasture's syndrome
   Wegener's granulomatosis
   Henoch-Schönlein purpura
3. Idiopathic
   Immune complex
   Anti-GBM
   Pauci-immune

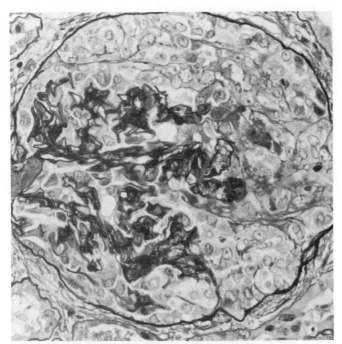

Figure 14-11. Crescentic glomerulonephritis; PAS stain. Note the collapsed glomerular tuft and the mass of proliferating cells internal to Bowman's capsule. (Courtesy of Helmut Rennke, M.D., Brigham and Women's Hospital, Boston.)

and some believe that it is the escape of fibrin into Bowman's space that incites crescent formation. Electron microscopy may, as expected, disclose subepithelial deposits in some cases but in all cases shows distinct ruptures in the GBM. In time, most crescents undergo sclerosis.

CLINICAL COURSE. The onset of RPGN is much like that of the nephritic syndrome except that the oliguria and azotemia are more pronounced. Ninety per cent of these patients become anephric and require long-term dialysis or transplantation. The prognosis can be roughly related to the number of crescents: patients with crescents in fewer than 80% of the glomeruli have a slightly better prognosis than those with higher percentages of crescents. Plasma exchange benefits some patients, particularly those with Goodpasture's syndrome.

FOCAL (PROLIFERATIVE) GLOMERULONEPHRITIS

Focal GN is a histologic diagnosis based on the presence of proliferative changes that affect only some of the glomeruli (*focal involvement*) and only isolated tufts within the glomerulus (*segmental involvement*). Depending on the underlying cause, the clinical picture is variable, and except in the case of one pattern known as *Berger's disease,* discussed below, there is no typical clinical syndrome associated with focal GN. Many cases of focal GN are secondary to one of a number of systemic diseases. The most frequent of these systemic diseases are *Henoch-Schönlein purpura*

in children, SLE, and occasional cases of polyarteritis nodosa in adults. Other causes are infective endocarditis, Wegener's granulomatosis, and the early stages of Goodpasture's syndrome. Like diffuse PGN, this is usually an immune complex disease but differs in that the immune complexes are largely localized to the mesangium of glomeruli.

IgA NEPHROPATHY (BERGER'S DISEASE)

This condition usually affects children and young adults and begins as an episode of gross hematuria occuring within a day or two of a nonspecific upper respiratory tract infection. Typically, the hematuria lasts several days then subsides, only to recur every few months. IgA nephropathy is one of the most common causes of recurrent microscopic or gross hematuria. It is often associated with loin pain.

Although the cause of Berger's disease is unknown, the pathogenic hallmark is the deposition of IgA in the mesangium. Some have considered Berger's disease to be a variant of Henoch-Schönlein purpura, often characterized by IgA deposition in the mesangium. In contrast to Berger's disease, which is purely a renal disorder, Henoch-Schönlein purpura is a systemic syndrome involving the skin (purpuric rash), gastrointestinal tract (abdominal pain), joints (arthritis), and kidneys.

Histologically, the lesions vary considerably. The glomeruli may be normal or may show mesangial widening and segmental proliferation confined to some glomeruli (focal GN); diffuse mesangial proliferation (mesangioproliferative); or rarely, overt crescentic GN. The characteristic immunofluorescent picture is of mesangial deposition of IgA, often with C3 and properdin and smaller amounts of IgG or IgM. Early complement components are usually absent. Electron microscopy confirms the presence of electron-dense deposits in the mesangium.

The pathogenesis is unknown, although there are several clues. Taken together, these clues suggest a primary (probably genetic) abnormality in regulation of IgA production and increased IgA synthesis in response to some environmental agent (? viruses, food proteins). IgA aggregates or complexes are then entrapped in the mesangium, where they activate the alternate complement pathway.

Clinically, IgA nephropathy is a heterogeneous disease. Although most children have a benign course, the disease appears to be slowly progressive in adults. It is estimated that chronic renal failure develops in more than 50% of cases over a period of 20 years.

HEREDITARY NEPHRITIS

Hereditary nephritis refers to a group of hereditary familial renal diseases associated primarily with glomerular injury. The best-studied entity is *Alport's syndrome, in which nephritis is accompanied by nerve deafness and various eye disorders, including lens dislocation, posterior cataracts, and corneal dystrophy.* Males tend to be affected more frequently and more severely than females and are more likely to progress to renal failure. The patients present at age 5 to 20 years with gross or microscopic hematuria and proteinuria, and overt renal failure occurs between ages 20 and 50 years. The inheritance is heterogeneous, being either X-linked or autosomal dominant in most pedigrees.

Histologically, there is segmental glomerular proliferation or sclerosis, or both, and an increase in mesangial matrix. In some kidneys, glomerular or tubular epithelial cells take on a foamy appearance owing to accumulation of neutral fats and mucopolysaccharides **(foam cells).** With progression, there is increasing glomerulosclerosis, vascular narrowing, tubular atrophy, and interstitial fibrosis. With the electron microscope, the basement membrane of glomeruli and tubules shows irregular foci of thickening or attenuation, with pronounced splitting and lamination of the lamina densa.

The basement membrane defect has been traced, in some kindreds, to a disturbance in the synthesis of a GBM component that is a novel chain ($\alpha 5$) of collagen type IV. How loss of this molecule causes the glomerular lesions is unclear.

CHRONIC GLOMERULONEPHRITIS

Having discussed various forms of glomerular disease, we should now turn to one of their unfortunate outcomes, chronic GN. It is the most common cause of end-stage renal disease presenting as chronic renal failure. Approximately 60% of all patients who require chronic hemodialysis or renal transplantation have the diagnosis of chronic GN.

By the time chronic GN is discovered, the glomerular changes are so far advanced that it is difficult to discern the nature of the original lesion. It probably represents the end stage of a variety of entities, prominent among which are focal glomerulosclerosis, membranous, and membranoproliferative GN. It has been estimated that perhaps 20% arise with no history of symptomatic renal disease. Although chronic GN may develop at any age, it is usually first noted in young and middle-aged adults.

MORPHOLOGY. Classically, the kidneys are symmetrically contracted and their surfaces are red-brown and diffusely granular, closely resembling kidneys in advanced benign nephrosclerosis (p. 462).

Microscopically, the feature common to all cases is advanced scarring of the glomeruli and Bowman's spaces, sometimes to the point of complete replacement or "hyalinization" of the glomeruli (Fig. 14–12). This obliteration of the glomeruli is the end point of all cases, and it is impossible to ascertain from such kidneys the nature of the earlier lesion.

The obstruction to blood flow between afferent and efferent arterioles secondary to glomerular damage must of necessity have an impact on the other elements of the kidney. There is, then, marked interstitial fibrosis,

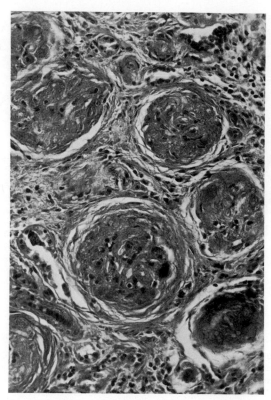

Figure 14–12. Chronic glomerulonephritis. The glomeruli are totally replaced by hyaline connective tissue.

associated with atrophy and replacement of many of the tubules in the cortex. The small and medium-sized arteries are frequently thick walled, with narrowed lumens, secondary to hypertension. Lymphocytic (and, rarely, plasma cell) infiltrates are present in the interstitial tissue. As damage to all structures progresses it may become difficult to ascertain whether the primary lesion was glomerular, vascular, or interstitial. Such markedly damaged kidneys are thus designated "end-stage kidneys."

CLINICAL COURSE. Most often chronic GN develops insidiously and is discovered only late in its course, after the onset of renal insufficiency. Very frequently, renal disease is first suspected with the discovery of proteinuria, hypertension, or azotemia on routine medical examination. In some patients the course is punctuated by transient episodes of either the nephritic or the nephrotic syndrome. Some of these may seek medical attention for their edema. As the glomeruli become obliterated, the avenue for protein loss is progressively closed and the nephrotic syndrome thus becomes less common with more advanced disease. Some proteinuria, however, is constant in all cases. Hypertension is very common and its effects may dominate the clinical picture. Although microscopic hematuria is usually present, grossly bloody urine is infrequent.

Without treatment, the prognosis is poor; relentless progression to uremia and death is the rule. The rate

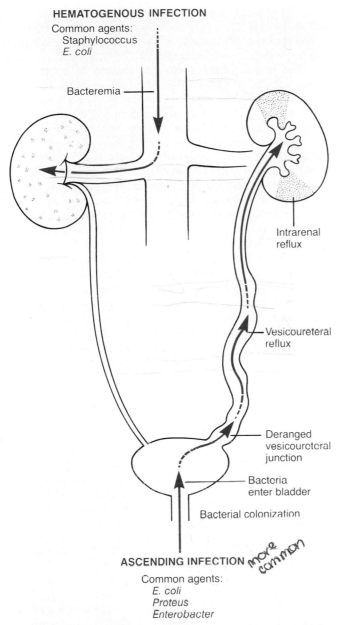

HEMATOGENOUS INFECTION
Common agents:
Staphylococcus
E. coli

Bacteremia

Intrarenal
reflux

Vesicoureteral
reflux

Deranged
vesicoureteral
junction

Bacteria
enter bladder

Bacterial colonization

ASCENDING INFECTION *more common*

Common agents:
E. coli
Proteus
Enterobacter

Figure 14–13. Schematic representation of pathways of renal infection. *Hematogenous* infection results from bacteremic spread. More common is *ascending infection,* which results from a combination of urinary bladder infection, vesicoureteral reflux, and intrarenal reflux.

of progression is extremely variable, however, and 10 years or more may elape between onset of the first symptoms and death. Renal dialysis, of course, alters this course and allows long-term survival.

DISEASES AFFECTING TUBULES AND INTERSTITIUM

Most forms of tubular injury also involve the interstitium, so the two are discussed together. Under this heading we present diseases characterized by (1) inflammatory involvement of the tubules and interstitium *(interstitial nephritis),* and (2) ischemic or toxic

tubular injury, leading to *acute tubular necrosis* and acute renal failure. Although *diffuse cortical necrosis* involves all elements of the renal cortex, it is also presented in this section, because its cause and clinical manifestations overlap with those of acute tubular necrosis.

TUBULOINTERSTITIAL NEPHRITIS _____

Tubulointerstitial nephritis (TIN) refers to a group of inflammatory diseases of the kidneys that primarily involve the interstitium and tubules. The glomeruli may be spared altogether or affected only late in the course. In most cases of TIN caused by bacterial infection the renal pelvis is prominently involved, hence the more descriptive term *pyelonephritis (pyelo,* pelvis). The term *interstitial nephritis* is generally reserved for cases that are noninfectious in origin. These include tubular injury resulting from drugs, metabolic disorders such as hypokalemia, physical injury such as irradiation, and immune reactions. On the basis of clinical features and the character of the inflammatory exudate, TIN, regardless of the etiologic agent, can be divided into acute and chronic categories. In the following section we present pyelonephritis first, followed by other noninfectious forms of interstitial nephritis.

Acute Pyelonephritis _____

Acute pyelonephritis, a common suppurative inflammation of the kidney and the renal pelvis, is caused by bacterial infection. It is an important manifestation of urinary tract infection (UTI), which implies involvement of the lower (cystitis, prostatitis, urethritis) or the upper (pyelonephritis) urinary tract, or both. As we shall see, pyelonephritis almost always is associated with infection of the lower urinary tract. The latter, however, may remain localized without extending to involve the kidney. UTIs are extremely common clinical problems.

ETIOLOGY AND PATHOGENESIS. The principal causative organisms are the enteric gram-negative rods. *Escherichia coli* is by far the most common one. Other important organisms are species of *Proteus, Klebsiella, Enterobacter,* and *Pseudomonas;* these are usually associated with recurrent infections, especially in patients who undergo urinary tract manipulations. Staphylococci and *Streptococcus fecalis* may also cause pyelonephritis, but only uncommonly.

There are two routes by which bacteria can reach the kidneys: through the bloodstream (hematogenous) and from the lower urinary tract (ascending infection). Although *hematogenous spread* is the far less common of the two, acute pyelonephritis may result from seeding of the kidneys by bacteria in the course of septicemia or infective endocarditis (Fig. 14–13). *Ascending infection* from the lower urinary tract is the most important route by which the bacteria reach the kidney. The first step in the pathogenesis of ascending infection appears to be colonization of the distal urethra (and the introitus in females) by gram-negative coliform bacteria. From here the organisms must gain access to the bladder, moving against the flow of urine. This may occur during urethral instrumentation, including catheterization and cystoscopy, which are important predisposing factors in the pathogenesis of UTIs. In the absence of instrumentation, UTI most commonly affects females, whose short urethra, and perhaps trauma to the urethra during sexual intercourse, facilitate the entry of bacteria into the urinary bladder. Ordinarily, bladder urine is sterile and remains so owing to antimicrobial properties of the bladder mucosa and owing to the flushing action associated with periodic voiding of urine. With outflow obstruction or bladder dysfunction, however, the natural defense mechanisms of the bladder are overwhelmed, setting the stage for UTI. Obstruction at the level of the urinary bladder results in incomplete emptying and increased residual volume of urine. In the presence of stasis, bacteria introduced into the bladder (as by catheterization) can multiply undisturbed, without being unceremoniously flushed out or destroyed by the bladder wall. From the contaminated bladder urine, the bacteria ascend along the ureters to infect the renal pelvis and parenchyma. Accordingly, UTI is particularly frequent among patients with urinary tract obstruction, as may occur with benign prostatic hypertrophy and uterine prolapse.

Although obstruction is an important predisposing factor in the pathogenesis of ascending infection, *it is incompetence of the vesicoureteral orifice* that allows bacteria to ascend the ureter into the pelvis. The normal ureteral insertion into the bladder is a competent one-way valve that prevents retrograde flow of urine, especially during micturition, when the intravesical pressure rises. An incompetent vesicoureteral orifice allows the reflux of bladder urine into the ureters (vesicoureteral reflux, VUR). The effect of VUR is similar to that of an obstruction in that after voiding there is residual urine in the urinary tract, which favors bacterial growth. Furthermore, VUR affords a ready mechanism by which the infected bladder urine can be propelled up to the renal pelves and further into the renal parenchyma through open ducts at the tips of the papillae (intrarenal reflux). Reflux can be demonstrated radiographically by a voiding cystourethrogram: the bladder is filled with a radiopaque dye and films are taken during micturition. VUR can be demonstrated in about 50% of infants and children with urinary tract infection.

Besides the various predisposing factors already discussed (obstruction, VUR, pregnancy, and instrumentation of the urinary tract), diabetes tends to increase the risk of serious complications of pyelonephritis, including septicemia, necrotizing papillitis, and recurrence of infection.

MORPHOLOGY. One or both kidneys may be involved. The affected kidney may be normal in size or enlarged. **Characteristically, discrete, yellowish, raised abscesses are grossly apparent on the renal surface**

(Fig. 14–14). They may be widely scattered or limited to one region of the kidney, or they may coalesce to form a single large area of suppuration.

The characteristic histologic feature of acute pyelonephritis is suppurative necrosis or abscess formation within the renal substance. In the early stages, the suppurative infiltrate is limited to the interstitial tissue, but later, abscesses rupture into tubules. Large masses of neutrophils frequently extend within involved nephrons into the collecting ducts, giving rise to the characteristic white cell casts found in the urine. Typically, the glomeruli appear to be resistant to the infection.

When the element of obstruction is prominent, the suppurative exudate may be unable to drain and thus fills the renal pelvis, calyces, and ureter, producing **pyonephrosis.**

A second (and, fortunately, infrequent) form of pyelonephritis is necrosis of the renal papillae, known as **necrotizing papillitis** or **papillary necrosis.** This is particularly common among diabetics who develop acute pyelonephritis and may also complicate acute pyelonephritis when there is significant urinary tract obstruction. It is also seen with the chronic interstitial nephritis asso-

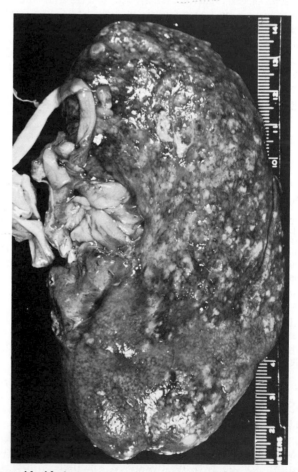

Figure 14–14. Acute pyelonephritis. The cortical surface is studded with focal pale abscesses, more numerous in the upper pole and midregion of the kidney; the lower pole is relatively unaffected. Between the abscesses there is dark congestion of the renal surface.

ciated with analgesic abuse (p. 456). This lesion consists of a combination of ischemic and suppurative necrosis of the tips of the renal pyramids (renal papillae). **The pathognomonic gross feature of necrotizing papillitis is sharply defined gray-white to yellow necrosis of the apical two thirds of the pyramids.** One, several, or all papillae may be affected. Microscopically, the papillary tips show characteristic coagulative necrosis, with surrounding neutrophilic infiltrate.

When the bladder is involved in a urinary tract infection, as it often is, **acute** or **chronic cystitis** results. In long-standing cases associated with obstruction, the bladder may be grossly hypertrophic, with trabeculation of its walls, or it may be thinned and markedly distended from retention of urine.

CLINICAL COURSE. When uncomplicated acute pyelonephritis is clinically apparent, the onset is usually sudden, with pain at the costovertebral angle and systemic evidence of infection, such as chills, fever, and malaise. Urinary findings include pyuria and bacteriuria. In addition, there are usually indications of bladder and urethral irritation (i.e., dysuria, frequency, urgency). Even without antibiotic treatment, the disease tends to be benign and self-limited. The symptomatic phase of the disease usually lasts no longer than a week, although bacteriuria may persist much longer. In cases involving predisposing influences, the disease may become recurrent or chronic. The development of necrotizing papillitis is associated with a much poorer prognosis. These patients have evidence of overwhelming sepsis—and often renal failure. Bilateral necrotizing papillitis is usually but not invariably fatal.

Chronic Pyelonephritis and Reflux Nephropathy _____

Chronic pyelonephritis (CPN) is defined here *as a morphologic entity in which predominantly interstitial inflammation and scarring of the renal parenchyma is associated with grossly visible scarring and deformity of the pelvicalyceal system.* CPN, an important cause of chronic renal failure, accounts for up to 20% of patients requiring dialyis or transplantation. CPN can be divided into two forms: chronic obstructive and chronic reflux-associated.

CHRONIC OBSTRUCTIVE PYELONEPHRITIS

We have seen that obstruction predisposes the kidney to infection. Recurrent infections superimposed on diffuse or localized obstructive lesions lead to recurrent bouts of renal inflammation and scarring, which eventually cause CPN. The disease can be bilateral, as with congenital anomalies of the urethra (posterior urethral valves), and result in fatal renal insufficiency unless the anomaly is corrected, or unilateral, such as occurs with calculi and unilateral obstructive anomalies of the ureter.

REFLUX NEPHROPATHY (CHRONIC REFLUX-ASSOCIATED PYELONEPHRITIS)

This is by far the more common form of chronic pyelonephritic scarring, and results from superimposition of a UTI on congenital VUR and intrarenal reflux. Reflux may be unilateral or bilateral; thus, the resultant renal damage either may cause scarring and atrophy of one kidney or may involve both and lead to chronic renal insufficiency. Whether VUR causes renal damage in the absence of infection (sterile reflux) is uncertain, because it is difficult clinically to rule out remote infection in a patient first seen with pyelonephritic scarring.

MORPHOLOGY. One or both kidneys may be involved, either diffusely or patchily. **Even when involvement is bilateral, the kidneys are not equally damaged and therefore are not equally contracted. This uneven scarring is useful in differentiating chronic PN from the more symmetrically contracted kidneys caused by benign nephrosclerosis (p. 462) and chronic GN. The hallmark of CPN is scarring involving the pelvis or calyces, or both, leading to papillary blunting and marked calyceal deformities** (Fig. 14–15).

The microscopic changes are largely nonspecific, and similar alterations may be seen with other tubulointersti-

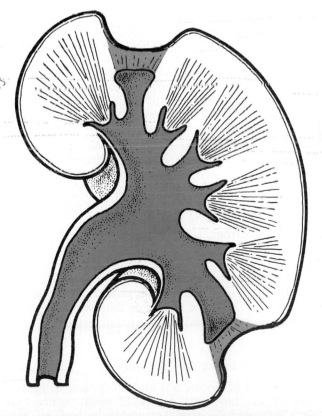

Figure 14–15. Typical coarse scars of chronic pyelonephritis associated with vesicoureteral reflux. The scars are usually polar and are associated with underlying blunted calyces.

tial disorders, such as analgesic nephropathy. The parenchyma shows the following features:

- Uneven interstitial fibrosis and an inflammatory infiltrate of lymphocytes, plasma cells, and occasionally neutrophils.
- Dilatation or contraction of tubules, with atrophy of the lining epithelium: Many of the dilated tubules contain pink to blue glassy-appearing casts known as colloid casts, which suggest the appearance of thyroid tissue, hence the descroptive term "throidization" of the kidney. Often neutrophils are seen within tubules.
- Concentric fibrosis about the parietal layer of Bowman's capsule, termed periglomerular fibrosis: Glomeruli may appear normal in early cases but eventually undergo hyalinization.
- In some cases, glomerular lesions, which are indistinguishable morphologically and by immunofluorescence from those present in idiopathic focal glomerulosclerosis, are seen. Such cases are often associated with heavy proteinuria, and it is believed that glomerular lesions contribute significantly to the progression of renal failure associated with reflux nephropathy.
- Chronic inflammatory infiltration and fibrosis involving the calyceal mucosa and wall.
- Vascular changes similar to those of hyaline or proliferative arteriolosclerosis caused by the frequent association with hypertension.

CLINICAL COURSE. Many patients with CPN come to medical attention relatively late in the course of their disease because of the gradual onset of renal insufficiency or because signs of kidney disease are noticed on routine laboratory tests. Often the renal disease is heralded by the development of hypertension. Pyelograms are characteristic and therefore are important in confirming the diagnosis; they show the affected kidney to be asymmetrically contracted, with some degree of blunting and deformity of the calyceal system (caliectasis). The presence or absence of significant bacteriuria is not particularly helpful diagnostically. Its absence certainly should not rule out CPN. If the disease is bilateral and progressive, tubular dysfunction occurs with loss of concentrating ability, manifested by polyuria and nocturia.

As noted earlier, some patients with CPN or reflux nephropathy ultimately develop glomerular lesions of *focal segmental glomerulosclerosis.* These are associated with proteinuria and eventually lead to progressive chronic renal failure. Such glomerular lesions may be caused by adaptive responses that occur in glomeruli as a result of reductions of renal mass (p. 443).

Drug-Induced Interstitial Nephritis

In this era of antibiotics and analgesics, drugs have emerged as important causes of renal injury. Two forms of tubulointerstitial nephritis caused by drugs are recognized.

ACUTE DRUG-INDUCED INTERSTITIAL NEPHRITIS

This is an adverse hypersensitivity reaction to an increasing number of drugs, particularly synthetic penicillins (methicillin), diuretics, and nonsteroidal antiinflammatory agents. The reactions begin about 15 days after exposure to the drug and consist of fever, eosinophilia, rash, hematuria, mild proteinuria, and eosinophils in the urine. Moderate to severe renal dysfunction may develop but usually abates promptly or slowly with discontinuation of the drug.

Renal biopsy reveals interstitial edema, a mononuclear peritubular infiltrate, and tubular necrosis. Neutrophils and eosinophils may also be seen in the interstitial infiltrate (Fig. 14–16). The presence of (1) eosinophilia, (2) a mononuclear infiltrate, (3) deposits of IgG along tubular basement membranes (seen in some patients), (4) the reported elevation of serum IgE levels, and (5) the latent period all support an immune-mediated basis for the renal injury. It is thought that the drugs act as haptens, which during secretion by tubules bind to tubular components, rendering them antigenic, with resultant antibody or cell-mediated tubule injury.

It is important to recognize this type of acute drug-induced renal reaction, as it is becoming a relatively common cause of acute but reversible renal dysfunction.

CHRONIC ANALGESIC NEPHRITIS

Patients who consume large quantities of analgesics may develop chronic interstitial nephritis, often asso-

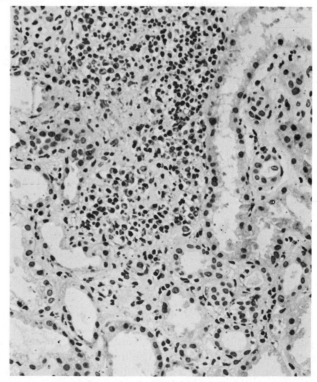

Figure 14–16. Acute drug-induced interstitial nephritis. Note interstitial inflammation and edema.

ciated with renal papillary necrosis. Although the renal damage was initially ascribed to phenacetin, most patients who develop this nephropathy consume mixtures containing some combination of phenacetin, aspirin, and acetaminophen. For interstitial nephritis to develop, prolonged exposure to excessive amounts of analgesics is necessary. It has been estimated that consumption of a least 2 to 3 kg of analgesics over a two- to three-year period is essential for renal damage to occur. Although phenacetin, aspirin, and acetaminophen each produce lesions experimentally, a mixture of aspirin and phenacetin produces papillary necrosis much more readily and at smaller doses. The pathogenesis of the renal lesions is not entirely clear. It seems that papillary necrosis is the initial event, and the interstitial nephritis in the overlying renal parenchyma is a secondary phenomenon. Acetaminophen, a phenacetin metabolite, injures cells by both *covalent binding* and *oxidative damage*. The ability of aspirin to inhibit prostaglandin synthesis suggests that this drug may induce its potentiating effect by inhibiting the vasodilatory effects of prostaglandin, and predisposing the papilla to ischemia. Thus, the papillary damage may be due to a combination of direct toxic effects of phenacetin metabolites as well as ischemic injury to both tubule cells and vessels.

The necrotic papillae appear yellowish-brown, owing to the accumulation of breakdown products of phenacetin and other lipofuscin-like pigments. Later on, the papillae may shrivel, be sloughed off, and drop into the pelvis. Microscopically the papillae show coagulative necrosis associated with loss of cellular detail but preservation of tubular outlines. Foci of dystrophic calcification may occur in the necrotic areas. The cortex drained by the necrotic papillae shows tubular atrophy, interstitial scarring, and inflammation. The small vessels in the papillae and urinary tract submucosa exhibit characteristic PAS-positive basement membrane thickening (analgesic microangiopathy).

Common clinical features of analgesic nephropathy include chronic renal failure, hypertension, and anemia. The latter results in part from damage to red cells by phenacetin metabolites. Cessation of analgesic intake may stabilize or even improve renal function. Another complication of analgesic abuse is the increased incidence of transitional cell carcinoma of the renal pelvis in patients who survive the renal failure.

ACUTE TUBULAR NECROSIS

Acute tubular necrosis (ATN) is a clinicopathologic entity characterized morphologically by destruction of tubular epithelial cells and clinically by acute suppression of renal function. It is the most common cause of acute renal failure (ARF). ARF signifies an acute suppression of renal function and urine flow, falling, within 24 hours, to less than 400 ml (oliguria). There are other causes of ARF: (1) severe glomerular diseases such as RPGN, (2) diffuse renal vessel diseases such as polyarteritis nodosa and malignant hypertension, (3) acute papillary necrosis associated with acute pyelonephritis, (4) acute drug-induced interstitial nephritis, and (5) diffuse cortical necrosis. Here we discuss ATN; diffuse cortical necrosis follows in the next section. The other causes of ARF are discussed elsewhere in this chapter.

ATN is a reversible renal lesion that arises in a variety of clinical settings. Most of these, ranging from severe trauma to acute pancreatitis to septicemia, have in common a period of inadequate blood flow to the peripheral organs, usually accompanied by marked hypotension and shock. The pattern of ATN associated with shock is called *ischemic ATN*. Mismatched blood transfusions and other hemolytic crises also produce a picture resembling ischemic ATN. The second pattern, called *nephrotoxic ATN*, is caused by a variety of poisons, including heavy metals (e.g., mercury), organic solvents (e.g., carbon tetrachloride), and a multitude of drugs such as gentamicin, other antibiotics, and radiographic contrast agents. Because of the many precipitating factors, ATN occurs quite frequently. Moreover, its reversibility adds to its clinical importance because proper management means the difference between full recovery and certain death.

PATHOGENESIS. The critical event in both ischemic and nephrotoxic ATN is believed to be *tubular damage* (Fig. 14–17). Tubular epithelial cells are particularly sensitive to anoxia, and they are also vulnerable to toxins. Several factors predispose the tubules to toxic injury, including a vast electrically charged surface for tubular reabsorption, active transport systems for ions and organic acids, and the capability for effective concentration. Ischemia causes numerous structural alterations in epithelial cells; loss of cell polarity appears to be a functionally important early event. Once tubular injury has occurred, the progression to ARF may follow one of several hypothetic pathways. Tubular damage has been postulated to trigger vasoconstriction of preglomerular arterioles, resulting in reduced GFR due to glomerulotubular feedback. The *vasoconstriction* has been ascribed to activation of the renin-angiotensin system, but other vasoconstrictive agents such as renin, adenosine, thromboxanes, and endothelin have also been implicated. Alternatively, loss of vasodilator effects (prostaglandin, nitric oxide/endothelium-derived relaxation factor) may be involved. Damage to the tubules can itself result in oliguria, because tubular debris could block urine outflow and eventually increase intratubular pressure, thereby decreasing the GFR. Additionally, fluid from the damaged tubules could leak into the interstitium, resulting in increased interstitial pressure and collapse of the tubule. Finally, there is some evidence of a direct effect of toxins on the ultrafiltration coefficient of the glomerular capillary wall. Which one of these mechanisms is most important in the onset of the oliguria is controversial. Most investigators

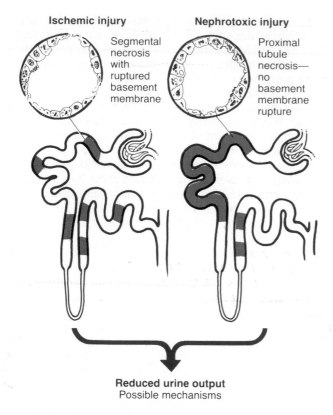

Ischemic injury

Segmental necrosis with ruptured basement membrane

Nephrotoxic injury

Proximal tubule necrosis— no basement membrane rupture

Reduced urine output
Possible mechanisms

1. Arteriolar vasoconstriction
2. Blockage of tubules ⟶ ↑intratubular pressure
3. Leakage from tubules ⟶ ↑interstitial pressure collapse of tubules
4. Direct effect on glomerular capillaries

Figure 14–17. Ischemic and nephrotoxic patterns of tubular injury in acute tubular necrosis (see text).

agree, however, that a combination of these events may result in renal failure.

MORPHOLOGY. Ischemic ATN is characterized by necrosis of short segments of the tubules. Most of the lesions are seen in the straight portions of the proximal tubule and the ascending thick limbs, but no segment of the proximal or distal tubules is spared. Tubular necrosis is often subtle, requiring careful histologic examination; it is usually associated with the difficult-to-discern rupture of the basement membrane **(tubulorrhexis).** A striking additional finding is the presence of proteinaceous casts in the distal tubules and collecting ducts. They consist of Tamm-Horsfall protein (secreted normally by tubular epithelium) along with hemoglobin and other plasma proteins. When crush injuries have produced ATN, the casts are composed of myoglobin. The interstitium usually discloses generalized edema along with an inflammatory infiltrate consisting of polymorphonuclear leukocytes, lymphocytes, and plasma cells. The histologic picture in **toxic ATN** is basically similar, with some differences. Necrosis is most prominent in the proximal tubule, and the tubular basement membranes are generally spared.

If the patient survives for a week, epithelial regeneration becomes apparent in the form of mitotic activity in the persisting tubular epithelial cells. Except where the basement membrane is destroyed, regeneration is total and complete.

CLINICAL COURSE. The clinical course of ATN may be divided into *initiating, maintenance,* and *recovery* stages. The initial phase, lasting for about 36 hours, is usually dominated by the inciting medical, surgical, or obstetric event in the ischemic form of ATN. The only indication of renal involvement is a slight decline in urine output with a rise in BUN. At this point, oliguria could be explained on the basis of a transient decrease in blood flow to the kidneys.

The *maintenance* phase begins anywhere from the second to the sixth day. Urine output falls dramatically, usually to between 50 and 400 ml per day. Sometimes it declines to only a few milliliters per day, but complete anuria is rare. Oliguria may last only a few days, or it may persist as long as three weeks. The clinical picture is dominated by the signs and symptoms of uremia and fluid overload. In the absence of careful supportive treatment or dialysis, most patients die during this phase. With good care, however, survival is the rule.

The *recovery* is ushered in by a steady increase in urine volume, reaching up to about 3 liters per day over the course of a few days. Because tubular function is still deranged, serious electrolyte imbalances may occur during this phase. There also appears to be an increased vulnerability to infection. For these reasons, about 25% of deaths from ATN occur during this phase.

During the final phase, there is a progressive return of the patient's well-being. Urine volume returns to normal; however, subtle functional impairment of the kidneys, particularly of the tubules, may persist for months. With modern methods of care, patients who do not succumb to the underlying precipitating problem have a 90 to 95% chance of recovering from ATN.

DIFFUSE CORTICAL NECROSIS

This is an infrequent lesion that in about 50% of cases follows the obstetric emergency of premature separation of the placenta (abruptio placentae). Another 30% of cases occur as a complication of septic shock. At one time this condition was thought to be invariably fatal, but recently it has been appreciated that patchy involvement of the cortices may occur, and this is compatible with survival.

PATHOGENESIS. The morphologic alterations in the kidney suggest that diffuse cortical necrosis results from severe and widespread cortical ischemia. In many instances, renal ischemia is simply the result of generalized hypotension. In addition, however, disseminated intravascular coagulation (DIC) within the interlobular and afferent arterioles is a common antecedent of cortical necrosis. This is most marked when the underlying disorder is an obstetric complication. Local vasoconstriction and intrarenal shunting of blood from the cortex to medulla may also contribute to cortical ischemia. Conceivably, many of these pathogenic pathways are operative when cortical necrosis follows premature separation of the placenta, or sepsis.

> **MORPHOLOGY.** The gross alterations of massive yellowish white infarction necrosis of the parenchyma are sharply limited to the cortex. The histologic appearance is that of acute ischemic infarction. Rarely, there may be areas of apparently better-preserved cortex. At the deeper levels, the areas in contact with the preserved medulla have usually a massive leukocytic infiltration. Intravascular thromboses may be prominent, and occasionally acute necroses of small arterioles and capillaries are present. Hemorrhages occur into the glomeruli, together with precipitation of fibrin.

CLINICAL COURSE. The onset of cortical necrosis is similar to that of ATN. Urine output falls, reaching oliguric levels within a day or two. In contrast to ATN cortical necrosis frequently is characterized by complete anuria; however, more often urine output is in the range of 50 to 100 ml daily. The clinical picture is that of uremia, and unless dialysis is performed, death occurs within days. Occasionally, when the involvement is patchy, renal function returns and the patient survives. In these cases, the kidney is scarred, with areas of necrosis visible on radiographs as spotty calcifications.

DISEASES INVOLVING BLOOD VESSELS

Nearly all diseases of the kidney involve the renal blood vessels secondarily. Systemic vascular disease, such as various forms of arteritis, also involves renal blood vessels, and often their effects on the kidney are clinically important. These were considered in an earlier chapter (p. 277). We will discuss in this chapter hypertension and its effects on renal blood vessels. Although the effects of hypertension are systemic, we have chosen to discuss this entity here, owing to the intimate relationship between the kidney and blood pressure.

HYPERTENSION

Elevated blood pressure is a staggering health problem for three reasons: it is very common, its effects are sometimes devastating, and it remains asymptomatic until late in its course. Its effects are widespread, and no organ is spared. Hypertension has been identified as one of the most important risk factor in both coronary

heart disease (p. 307) and cerebrovascular accidents (p. 713); it may also lead directly to congestive heart failure (hypertensive heart disease, p. 314) and to renal failure. There is no magic threshold of blood pressure above which an individual is considered hypertensive and below which he or she is safe. Rather, the detrimental effects of blood pressure increase continuously as the pressure increases. Hypertension, then, must be defined somewhat arbitrarily. Most would agree that a sustained diastolic pressure greater than 90 mm Hg is an essential feature. A sustained systolic pressure in excess of 140 mm Hg also constitutes hypertension, but its clinical consequences differ somewhat from those of diastolic hypertension. By means of these criteria, the percentage of hypertensive persons in the general population in screening programs is 25%. However, most surveys use systolic and diastolic pressures of 160/95 as the dividing line for adults. Even with these values, the prevalence was an alarming 18% in the study already mentioned. The prevalence increases with age, although when present in young adults it tends to be more severe. Blacks are affected about twice as often as whites and apparently are more vulnerable to its complications. Although females are hypertensive more often than males, this sex preponderance is limited to the older age groups, in which the disease is likely to be relatively benign. Before 50 years hypertension is more common in males.

About 90% of hypertension is idiopathic and apparently primary (essential hypertension). Of the remaining 10%, most is secondary to renal disease or, less often, to narrowing of the renal artery, usually by an atheromatous plaque (renovascular hypertension). Only relatively infrequently is secondary hypertension the result of adrenal disorders, such as primary aldosteronism, Cushing's syndrome, and pheochromocytoma. *Both essential and secondary hypertension may be either benign or malignant, according to the clinical course.* In most cases hypertension remains fairly stable over years to decades and, unless a myocardial infarction or cerebrovascular accident supervenes is compatible with a long life. This form of the disorder, termed *benign hypertension,* produces a renal lesion known as *benign nephrosclerosis.* Although a benign course is most characteristic of idiopathic or essential hypertension it may also be seen with the secondary disorder. About 5% of hypertensive persons show a rapidly rising blood pressure, which, untreated, leads to death within a year or two. Appropriately enough, this is called *accelerated* or *malignant hypertension,* and the corresponding renal lesion *malignant nephrosclerosis.* The full-blown clinical syndrome of malignant hypertension includes severe hypertension (a diastolic pressure over 120 mm Hg), renal failure, and bilateral retinal hemorrhages and exudates, with or without papilledema. This form of hypertension may develop in previously normotensive persons or it may be superimposed on preexisting benign hypertension, either essential or secondary. In its pure form, malignant hypertension usually affects younger persons than does benign hypertension. Typically, it develops in the fourth decade.

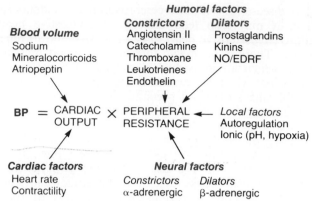

Figure 14–18. Blood pressure regulation. NO/EDRF denotes nitric oxide–endothelium-derived growth factor.

The morphology and clinical course of the two renal lesions, benign and malignant nephrosclerosis, will be considered separately later (p. 462). First we shall discuss what is known of the cause and pathogenesis of hypertension in general.

REGULATION OF NORMAL BLOOD PRESSURE. Although the cause of most cases of hypertension is unknown, speculations abound and the subject is a source of lively controversy. For our consideration, a reasonable starting point is the well-known observation that arterial pressure is a product of cardiac output and peripheral resistance. These two are in turn affected by a variety of factors, depicted schematicaly in Figure 14–18. These factors are shown as affecting either vascular resistance or cardiac output, but only to avoid a maze of crisscrossing lines. In reality, most of these factors act at several points; for example, angiotensin not only causes vasoconstriction but also stimulates aldosterone secretion, which in turn affects salt retention and fluid volume. Analogously, salt retention not only increases cardiac output but may also increase peripheral resistance by altering the sensitivity of the vascular smooth muscle to vasoactive stimuli. Such interactions are too numerous to detail, but several examples have been cited to emphasize that in most hypertensive persons elevation of blood pressure results from an interaction of multiple factors.

MECHANISMS OF RENAL HYPERTENSION. The kidneys play an important role in blood pressure regulation by at least three mechanisms:

1. *Renin-Angiotensin system* (Fig. 14–19). Through the elaboration of renin, the kidney eventually forms *angiotensin II* (AII), which alters blood pressure by increasing both peripheral resistance and blood volume. The former effect is achieved largely by its ability to cause vasoconstriction through direct action on vascular smooth muscle, the latter by stimulation of aldosterone secretion, which increases distal tubular reabsorption of sodium, and thus of water.

2. *Sodium Homeostasis.* The kidney is intimately involved in the complex process of sodium homeostasis. One mechanism already discussed is the renin-angiotensin system, which affects distal tubular reabsorption of sodium through the mediation of aldosterone secretion. Two other renal factors have important bearing on sodium homeostasis: the *GFR* and *GFR-independent natriuretic factors.* When

RENIN-ANGIOTENSIN SYSTEM

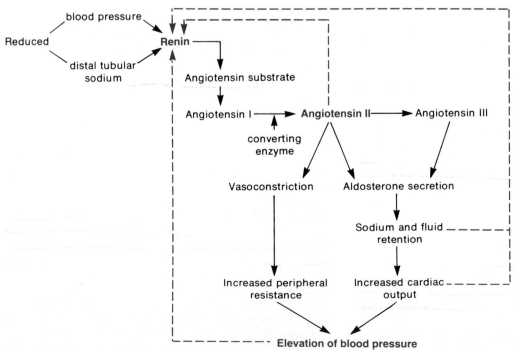

Figure 14–19. Role of renin-angiotensin system in regulation of blood pressure. Solid lines represent positive interactions; broken lines show negative interactions or feedback inhibition.

Figure 14–20. Hypothetical scheme for pathogenesis of essential hypertension implicating genetic defects in renal sodium excretion, or in sodium/calcium transport, or causing increased neurohormonal release—coupled with excess salt intake. Increased cardiac output and increased total peripheral resistance contribute to the hypertension.

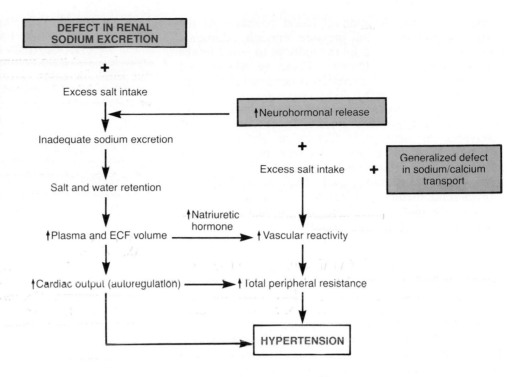

blood volume is reduced, the GFR falls; this in turn leads to increased reabsorption of sodium by proximal tubules in an attempt to conserve sodium and expand blood volume. Such GFR-independent factors include atrial natriuretic factor or atriopeptin, a group of peptides secreted by heart atria in response to volume expansion, which inhibit sodium reabsorption at a distal site.

3. *Renal Vasodepressor Substances.* The kidney produces a variety of vasodepressor or antihypertensive substances, which presumably counterbalance the vasopressor effects of angiotensin. The vasodepressor substances include the prostaglandins, a urinary kallikrein-kinin system, platelet-activating factor, and nitric oxide/EDRF (endothelium-derived relaxation factor).

From the point of view of pathogenesis, two categories of renal hypertension can be recognized—those associated with excessive renin secretion (e.g., renovascular hypertension) and those associated with volume excess (e.g., acute GN). In some cases of chronic renal failure, a mixture of both patterns is seen. Experimental models developed by Goldblatt clearly demonstrate these two mechanisms and have greatly helped our understanding of renal hypertension. Renal ischemia, produced by clamping one renal artery (the so-called Goldblatt kidney) leaving the other kidney intact, produces hypertension that is mediated by excessive release of renin. A similar mechanism operates in the hypertension associated with renal artery stenosis, such as may be produced by an atheromatous plaque but which in a few cases is caused by fibromuscular hyperplasia of the renal artery.

Renal hypertension is most likely to respond to drugs that interfere with the renin-angiotensin axis;

however, the treatment of choice in renal arterial hypertension is reconstruction of the artery. When vascular reconstruction is performed or the affected kidney is removed, blood pressure may return to normal, especially if the hypertension is of recent origin. The procedure is less successful in longstanding hypertension, because the contralateral kidney damaged by the hypertension also begins to release excessive amounts of renin and because other less well-understood mechanisms for the perpetuation of hypertension take over.

Activation of the renin-angiotensin system has also been implicated in the pathogenesis of hypertension associated with polyarteritis nodosa, unilateral chronic pyelonephritis, juxtaglomerular cell tumors, malignant hypertension, and chronic renal disease.

MECHANISMS OF ESSENTIAL HYPERTENSION. We come now to the vexing problem of the pathogenesis of essential hypertension. At the outset, it is obvious from the term "essential" that the cause is unknown. At the most elemental level, it must relate to either a primary increase in cardiac output or an increase in peripheral resistance, and the several theories of the origin of hypertension stress one or the other event (Fig. 14–20).

Those who advocate a *primary increase in cardiac output suggest that the basic nonstructural, probably genetic defect is reduced renal sodium excretion in the presence of normal arterial pressure* (defective pressure natriuresis). Decreased sodium excretion would lead to an increase in fluid volume and a rise in cardiac output. In the face of increasing cardiac output, peripheral vasoconstriction occurs to prevent overperfusion of tissues, which would result from an unchecked increase in cardiac output. This process, called autoregulation, leads to increased peripheral resistance and along with it an elevation of blood pressure. At the higher setting of blood pressure enough additional sodium can be excreted by the kidneys to equal intake and prevent fluid retention. Thus, an altered but steady state of sodium excretion is achieved ("resetting of pressure natriuresis").

The second hypothesis implicates vasoconstrictive influences as the primary events. These could be (1) behavioral or neurogenic factors, as shown by the reduction of blood pressure that can be achieved by meditation (the relaxation response); (2) increased release of vasoconstrictor agents (e.g., renin, catecholamines, endothelin); or (3) a primary increased sensitivity of vascular smooth muscle, caused by a genetic defect in cell membrane transport of sodium and calcium, leading to increased intracellular calcium and contraction in the smooth muscle cells.

Both hereditary and environmental factors have been implicated in hypertension. When both parents are hypertensive, the children have a much increased risk of developing hypertension. Studies on twins and familial aggregations support a role for the genetic constitution in the causation of hypertension. If heredity is involved, how is the genetic defect manifested? Defects relating to renal sodium reabsorption or sodium and calcium transport in vascular smooth muscle have been suggested, which could lead to hypertension by the mechanisms described previously. Even if genetic predisposition to hypertension exists, it is likely that environmental factors are also involved in the expression of the genetic abnormalities. The role of environment is illustrated by the lower incidence of hypertension in Chinese people living in their native country as compared with persons of Chinese descent living in the United States. Environmental factors implicated in the causation of hypertension include stress, obesity, smoking, inactivity, and heavy consumption of salt. The evidence linking the level of dietary sodium intake with the prevalence of hypertension in different population groups is impressive. It must be stressed in both of the major hypotheses discussed that heavy sodium intake augments the hypertension.

Essential hypertension is thus a complex disorder that may have more than one cause. It may be initiated by a disturbance in any of the factors that control normal blood pressure, many of which are environmental (stress, salt intake, estrogens) but act in the genetically predisposed individual. In established hypertension, both increased blood volume and increased peripheral resistance contribute to the increased pressure.

Table 14–4 lists the main causes and possible mechanisms of hypertension. We shall now examine some of the renal vascular disorders associated with hypertension.

Benign Nephrosclerosis

Benign nephrosclerosis (BNS), the term used for the kidney of benign hypertension, is always associated with hyaline arteriolosclerosis. Some degree of BNS,

TABLE 14–4. MAIN CAUSES AND POSSIBLE FACTORS IN THE PATHOGENESIS OF HYPERTENSION

Essential hypertension
  Genetic defect in renal sodium excretion
  Genetic defect in sodium/calcium transport in vascular smooth muscle
  Increased vasoconstrictive influences: behavioral, neurogenic, hormonal
Secondary hypertension
  Renal disease: increased renin secretion, sodium and fluid retention, decreased vasodilator (vasodepressor) secretion
  Endocrine causes: aldosteronism, oral contraceptives, pheochromocytoma, thyrotoxicosis
  Vascular causes: coarctation of the aorta, vasculitis
  Neurogenic causes: psychogenic, increased intracranial pressure

albeit mild, is present at autopsy in many persons older than 60 years. The frequency and severity of the lesions are increased in young age groups in association with hypertension and diabetes mellitus.

The kidneys are symmetrically atrophic, each weighing 110 to 130 gm, with a surface of diffuse, fine granularity that resembles grain leather.

Microscopically, the basic anatomic change is hyaline thickening of the walls of the small arteries and arterioles, known as **hyaline arteriolosclerosis.** This appears as a homogeneous, pink hyaline thickening, at the expense of the vessel lumens, with loss of underlying cellular detail. The narrowing of the lumens results in markedly decreased blood flow through the affected vessels and thus produces ischemia in the organ served. All structures of the kidney show ischemic atrophy. The glomeruli develop axial thickening and fibrosis, and sometimes there is fibrotic replacement of Bowman's spaces (Fig. 14–21). In far advanced cases of BNS, the glomerular tufts may become obliterated by this homogeneous hyalinization. Diffuse tubular atrophy and interstitial fibrosis are present. Often there is a scant interstitial lymphocytic infiltrate. The larger blood vessels (i.e., interlobar and arcuate arteries) show reduplication of internal elastic lamina along with fibrous thickening of the media (fibroelastic hyperplasia).

It should be remembered that many renal diseases cause hypertension, which in turn may lead to BNS. Thus, this renal lesion is often seen superimposed on other, primary kidney diseases.

Because this renal lesion alone rarely causes severe damage to the kidney, it very infrequently leads to uremia and death. Nonetheless, there is usually some functional impairment, such as loss of concentrating ability or a variably diminished GFR. A mild degree of proteinuria is a constant finding. Usually these patients die from hypertensive heart disease or from cerebrovascular accidents rather than from renal disease.

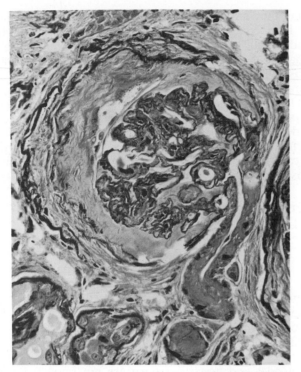

Figure 14–21. Benign nephrosclerosis—microscopic detail of a glomerulus and its afferent arteriole sectioned obliquely. The arteriole has hyaline, thickened walls, and a narrowed lumen. The glomerulus shows diffuse glomerulosclerosis and has marked fibrous thickening of the parietal layer of Bowman's capsule.

Malignant Hypertension and Malignant Nephrosclerosis

Malignant hypertension is far less common than benign hypertension, occurring in only about 5% of patients with elevated blood pressure. It may arise de novo (i.e., without preexisting hypertension) or appear suddenly in a person who had mild hypertension. The basis for this turn for the worse in hypertensive subjects is unclear, but the following sequence of events is suggested. The initial event appears to be some form of vascular damage to the kidneys. This most commonly results from longstanding benign hypertension, with eventual injury to the arteriolar walls, or it may spring from arteritis. In either case, the result is increased permeability of the small vessels to fibrinogen and other plasma proteins, endothelial injury, and platelet deposition. This leads to the appearance of *fibrinoid necrosis* of arterioles and small arteries, and intravascular thrombosis. Mitogenic factors from platelets (e.g., PDGF) and plasma cause intimal smooth hyperplasia of vessels, resulting in the hyperplastic arteriolosclerosis typical of malignant hypertension and further narrowing of the lumens. The kidneys become markedly ischemic. With severe involvement of the renal afferent arterioles, the renin-angiotensin system receives a powerful stimulus, and indeed *patients with malignant hypertension have markedly elevated levels of plasma renin.* This then sets up a self-perpetuating cycle in which angiotensin II causes intrarenal vasoconstriction

and the attendant renal ischemia perpetuates renin secretion. Aldosterone levels are also elevated, and salt retention undoubtedly contributes to the elevation of blood pressure. The consequences of the markedly elevated blood pressure on the blood vessels throughout the body is known as malignant *arteriolosclerosis,* and the renal disorder as *malignant nephrosclerosis* (MNS).

The kidney may be essentially normal in size or slightly shrunken, depending on the duration and severity of the hypertensive disease. Small, pinpoint petechial hemorrhages may appear on the cortical surface from rupture of arterioles or glomerular capillaries, giving the kidney a peculiar flea-bitten appearance.

The microscopic changes reflect the pathogenetic events described earlier. Damage to the small vessels is manifested as **fibrinoid necrosis** of the arterioles. The vessel walls appear to take on a homogeneous, granular eosinophilic appearance masking underlying detail. Also, there is often a sprinkling of inflammatory cells, giving rise to the term **necrotizing arteriolitis**. The inflammation is presumably secondary to vascular damage. A different response is seen in the interlobular arteries and larger arterioles, where the proliferation of intimal cells produces an "onion skin" appearance (Fig. 14–22).

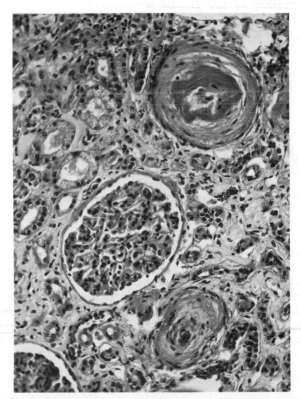

Figure 14–22. Malignant nephrosclerosis. Two markedly thickened vessels are seen above and below the glomerulus. The vessel above contains a heavy deposit of fibrinoid and demonstrates necrotizing arteriolitis.

This name is derived from the concentric arrangement of cells whose origin is believed to be intimal smooth muscle, although this issue is not finally settled. This lesion, called **hyperplastic arteriolosclerosis,** causes marked narrowing of arterioles and small arteries, to the point of total obliteration. Necrotizing arteriolitis may extend to involve the glomeruli (**necrotizing glomerulitis**). Microthrombi may be seen within the glomeruli as well as necrotic arterioles.

The full-blown syndrome of malignant hypertension is characterized by diastolic pressures greater than 120 mm Hg, papilledema, encephalopathy, cardiovascular abnormalities, and renal failure. Most often, the early symptoms are related to increased intracranial pressure and include headaches, nausea, vomiting, and visual impairments, particularly the development of scotomas, or spots before the eyes. At the onset of rapidly mounting blood pressure there is marked proteinuria and microscopic, or sometimes macroscopic, hematuria but no significant alteration in renal function. Soon, however, renal failure makes its appearance. The syndrome is a true medical emergency that requires the prompt institution of aggressive antihypertensive therapy before the irreversible renal lesions develop. About 50% of patients survive at least five years, and further progress is still being made. Ninety per cent of deaths are caused by uremia and others by cerebral hemorrhage or cardiac failure.

CYSTIC DISEASES OF THE KIDNEY _____

Cystic diseases of the kidney are a heterogeneous group comprising hereditary, developmental but non-hereditary, and acquired disorders. As a group, they are important for several reasons: (1) they are reasonably common and often present diagnostic problems for clinicians, radiologists, and pathologists; (2) some forms, such as adult polycystic disease, are major causes of chronic renal failure; (3) they can occasionally be confused with malignant tumors. Here we shall briefly mention simple cysts, the most common form, and discuss in some detail polycystic kidney disease.

SIMPLE CYSTS _____

These generally innocuous lesions occur as multiple or single cystic spaces that vary in diameter within a wide range. Commonly, they are 1 to 5 cm; translucent; lined by a gray, glistening, smooth membrane; and filled with clear fluid. Microscopically, these membranes are composed of a single layer of cuboidal or flattened cuboidal epithelium, which in many instances may be completely atrophic. The cysts are usually confined to the cortex. Rarely, large massive cysts up to 10 cm in diameter are encountered.

Simple *cysts* are a common postmortem finding that has no clinical significance. The main importance of cysts lies in their differentiation from kidney tumors,

when they are discovered either incidentally or because of hemorrhage and pain during life. Radiographic studies show that, in contrast to renal tumors (p. 467), renal cysts have smooth contours, are almost always avascular, and give fluid rather than solid signals on ultrasonography.

Dialysis-associated acquired cysts occur in the kidneys of patients with end-stage renal disease who have undergone prolonged dialysis. They are present in both cortex and medulla and may bleed, causing hematuria. Occasionally, renal adenomas or even adenocarcinomas arise in the wall of these cysts.

AUTOSOMAL DOMINANT (ADULT) POLYCYSTIC KIDNEY DISEASE _____

This is a hereditary disease characterized by multiple expanding cysts of both kidneys that ultimately destroy the intervening parenchyma. It is seen in approximately one in 1000 persons and accounts for 10% of cases of chronic renal failure. Inheritance of this disease is through a dominant autosomal gene of very high penetrance. In most families the defective gene is on the short arm of chromosome 16, but what protein it encodes and how cysts form are not known. Partial intratubular obstruction, loss of tubular basement membrane compliance, and disturbed epithelial cell growth are currently postulated mechanisms of cyst formation.

MORPHOLOGY. The kidneys may achieve enormous size, and weights up to 4 kg for each kidney have been recorded (Fig. 14–23). These very large kidneys are readily palpable abdominally as masses extending into the pelvis. On gross examination, the kidney seems to be composed solely of a mass of cysts of varying sizes up to 3 or 4 cm in diameter with no intervening parenchyma. The cysts are filled with fluid, which may be clear, turbid, or hemorrhagic.

Microscopic examination reveals some normal parenchyma dispersed among the cysts, which may arise at any level of the nephron, from tubules to collecting ducts, and therefore have a variable, often atrophic lining. Occasionally, Bowman's capsules are involved in the cyst formation, and in these cases, glomerular tufts may be seen within the cystic space. The pressure of the expanding cysts leads to ischemic atrophy of the intervening renal substance. Evidence of superimposed hypertension or infection is common.

CLINICAL COURSE. Polycystic kidney disease in adults usually does not produce symptoms until the fourth decade. By this time the kidneys are quite large. The most common complaint of the patient is flank pain or at least a heavy, dragging sensation. Acute distention of a cyst, either by intracystic hemorrhage or by obstruction, may cause excruciating pain. Sometimes attention is first drawn to the lesion by palpation of an abdominal mass. Intermittent gross hematuria commonly occurs. The most important complications,

Figure 14-23. Polycystic kidney disease in an adult. Both kidneys are comprised of masses of cysts with no grossly apparent intervening normal parenchyma. The ureters are also malformed and are abnormally dilated.

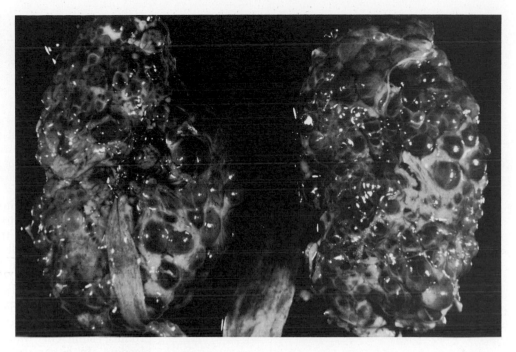

because of their deleterious effect on already marginal renal function, are hypertension and UTI. Hypertension of varying severity develops in about 75% of patients. Berry aneurysms of the circle of Willis are present in 10 to 30% of patients, and these individuals have a high incidence of subarchnoid hemorrhage. Asymptomatic liver cysts occur in one third of patients.

Although the disease is ultimately fatal, the outlook is in general better than with most chronic renal diseases. The condition tends to be relatively stable and progresses only very slowly. End-stage renal failure occurs at about age 50, but there is wide variation in the course of this disorder, and nearly normal life spans are reported. Death usually results from uremia or hypertensive complications.

AUTOSOMAL RECESSIVE (CHILDHOOD) POLYCYSTIC KIDNEY DISEASE _____

This rare developmental anomaly is genetically distinct from adult polycystic kidney disease, having *autosomal recessive* inheritance. Perinatal, neonatal, infantile, and juvenile subcategories have been defined, depending on time of presentation and the presence of associated hepatic lesions. The first two are most common; serious manifestations are usually present at birth, and young infants may succumb rapidly to renal failure. Kidneys exhibit numerous small cysts in the cortex and medulla that give the kidney a sponge-like appearance. Dilated elongated channels at right angles to the cortical surface completely replace the medulla and cortex. The cysts have a uniform lining of cuboidal cells, reflecting their origin from the collecting tubules. The disease is invariably bilateral. *In almost all cases, there are multiple epithelium-lined cysts in the liver as well as proliferation of portal bile ducts.*

Patients who survive infancy develop liver cirrhosis *(congenital hepatic fibrosis).*

URINARY OUTFLOW OBSTRUCTION _____

RENAL STONES _____

Urolithiasis is calculus formation at any level in the urinary collecting system, but most often calculi arise in the kidney. It is a frequent disorder, as evidenced by the finding of stones in about 1% of all autopsies. Symptomatic urolithiasis is most common in males. A familial tendency toward stone formation has long been recognized.

ETIOLOGY AND PATHOGENESIS. About 75% of renal stones are composed of either calcium oxalate or calcium oxalate mixed with calcium phosphate. Another 15% are composed of magnesium ammonium phosphate, and 10% are either uric acid or cystine stones. In all cases, there is an organic matrix of mucoprotein that makes up about 2.5% of the stone by weight (Table 14-5).

The cause of stone formation is often obscure, particularly in the cases of calcium-containing stones. Probably involved is a confluence of predisposing conditions. *The most important is almost certainly increased urine concentration of the stone's constituents.* As shown in Table 14-5, 50% of the patients who develop calcium stones have hypercalciuria that is not associated with hypercalcemia. Most in this group absorb calcium from the gut in excessive amounts and promptly excrete it in the urine, and some have a primary renal defect of calcium reabsorption. *Ten percent* of patients have hypercalcemia (due to hyperparathyroidism, vitamin D intoxication, sarcoidosis) and consequent hypercalciuria. *In 20% of this sub-*

TABLE 14–5. PREVALENCE OF VARIOUS TYPES OF RENAL STONES

Stone	Per Cent of All Stones
Calcium oxalate (phosphate)	75
Idiopathic hypercalciuria (50%)	
Hypercalcemia and hypercalciuria (10%)	
Hyperoxaluria (5%)	
Enteric (4.5%)	
Primary (0.5%)	
Hyperuricosuria (20%)	
No known metabolic abnormality (15–20%)	
Struvite (Mg; NH₃; Ca; PO₄) *mag. alum. phos.*	10–15
Renal infection	
Uric acid	6
Associated with hyperuricemia	
Associated with hyperuricosuria	
Idiopathic (50%)	
Cystine	1–2
Others or unknown	±10

MORPHOLOGY. Stones are unilateral in about 80% of patients. Common sites of formation are renal pelves, calyces, and the bladder. Often many stones are found in one kidney. They tend to be small (average diameter 2 to 3 mm) and may be smooth or jagged. Occasionally, progressive accretion of salts leads to the development of branching structures known as **staghorn calculi,** which create a cast of the renal pelvis and calyceal system. These massive stones are usually composed of magnesium ammonium phosphate.

CLINICAL COURSE. Stones may be present without producing either symptoms or significant renal damage. This is particularly true with large stones lodged in the renal pelvis. Smaller stones may pass into the ureter, producing a typical intense pain known as renal or ureteral colic, characterized by paroxysms of flank pain radiating toward the groin. Often at this time there is gross hematuria. The clinical significance of stones lies in their capacity to obstruct urine flow or to produce sufficient trauma to cause ulceration and bleeding. In either case, they predispose to bacterial infection. Fortunately, in most cases the diagnosis is readily made by radiological means.

group there is excessive excretion of uric acid in the urine, which favors calcium stone formation; presumably the urates provide a nidus for calcium deposition. *In 5% there is hyperoxaluria and in 14 to 20% there is no known metabolic abnormality.*

The causes of the other types of renal stones are better understood. *Magnesium ammonium phosphate (struvite) stones almost always occur in patients with a persistently alkaline urine, owing to urinary tract infections.* In particular, the urea-splitting bacteria, such as *Proteus vulgaris* and the staphylococci, predispose toward urolithiasis. Moreover, bacteria may serve as particulate nidi for the formation of any kind of stone. In avitaminosis A, desquamated squames from the metaplastic epithelium of the collecting system act as nidi.

Gout and diseases involving rapid cell turnover, such as the leukemias, lead to high uric acid levels in the urine and the possibility of *uric acid stones.* About half of the patients with uric acid stones, however, have neither hyperuricemia nor increased urine urate but an unexplained tendency to excrete a persistently acid urine (under pH 5.5) favoring stone formation. *Cystine stones* are almost invariably associated with a genetically determined defect in the renal transport of certain amino acids, including cystine. In contrast to magnesium ammonium phosphate stones, *both uric acid and cystine stones are more likely to form when the urine is relatively acidic.*

Urolithiasis may also conceivably result from the lack of influences that normally inhibit mineral precipitation. Inhibitors of crystal formation in urine include pyrophosphate, mucopolysaccharides, diphosphonates, and a glycoprotein called *nephrocalcin,* but no deficiency of any of these substances has been consistently demonstrated in patients with urolithiasis.

HYDRONEPHROSIS

Hydronephrosis refers to the dilatation of the renal pelvis and calyces, with accompanying atrophy of the parenchyma, caused by obstruction to the outflow of urine. The obstruction may be sudden or insidious, and it may occur at any level of the urinary tract, from the urethra to the renal pelvis. The most common causes are as follows:

A. Congenital: Atresia of the urethra, valve formations in either ureter or urethra, aberrant renal artery compressing the ureter, renal ptosis with torsion, or kinking of ureter.
B. Acquired:
1. Foreign bodies: Calculi, necrotic papillae.
2. Tumors: Benign prostatic hypertrophy (BPH), carcinoma of the prostate, bladder tumors (papilloma and carcinoma), contiguous malignant disease (retroperitoneal lymphoma, carcinoma of the cervix or uterus).
3. Inflammation: Prostatitis, ureteritis, urethritis, retroperitoneal fibrosis.
4. Neurogenic: Spinal cord damage with paralysis of the bladder.
5. Normal pregnancy: Mild and reversible.

Bilateral hydronephrosis occurs only when the obstruction is below the level of the ureters. If blockage is at the ureters or above, the lesion is unilateral. Sometimes obstruction is complete, allowing no urine to pass; usually it is only partial.

Even with complete obstruction, glomerular filtration persists for some time, and the filtrate subsequently diffuses back into the renal interstitium and perirenal spaces, whence it ultimately returns to the lymphatic and venous systems. Because of the continued filtration, the affected calyces and pelvis become dilated, often markedly so. The unusually high pressure thus generated in the renal pelvis, as well as that transmitted back through the collecting ducts, causes compression of the renal vasculature. Both arterial insufficiency and venous stasis result, although the latter is probably more important. The most severe effects are seen in the papillae, because they are subjected to the greatest increases in pressure. Accordingly, the initial functional disturbances are largely tubular, manifested primarily by impaired concentrating ability. Only later does glomerular filtration begin to diminish. Experimental studies indicate that serious irreversible damage occurs in about 3 weeks with complete obstruction and in 3 months with incomplete obstruction.

MORPHOLOGY. Bilateral hydronephrosis (as well as unilateral hydronephrosis when the other kidney is already damaged or absent) leads to renal failure, and the onset of uremia tends to abort the natural course of the lesion. In contrast, **unilateral** involvements display the full range of morphologic changes, which vary with the degree and the speed of obstruction. With subtotal or intermittent obstruction, the kidney may be massively enlarged (lengths in the range of 20 cm) and the organ may consist almost entirely of the greatly distended pelvicalyceal system. The renal parenchyma itself is compressed and atrophied, with obliteration of the papillae and flattening of the pyramids. On the other hand, *when* **obstruction is sudden and complete, glomerular filtration is compromised relatively early, and as a consequence, renal function may cease while dilatation is still comparatively slight.** Depending on the level of the obstruction, one or both ureters may also be dilated **(hydroureter).**

Microscopically, the early lesions show tubular dilatation, followed by atrophy and fibrous replacement of the tubular epithelium with relative sparing of the glomeruli. Eventually, in severe cases the glomeruli also become atrophic and disappear, converting the entire kidney into a thin shell of fibrous tissue. With sudden and complete obstruction, there may be coagulative necrosis of the renal papillae, similar to the changes of necrotizing papillitis (p. 455). In uncomplicated cases, the accompanying inflammatory reaction is minimal. Complicating pyelonephritis, however, is common.

CLINICAL COURSE. *Bilateral* complete obstruction produces anuria, which is soon brought to medical attention. When the obstruction is below the bladder, the dominant symptoms are those of bladder distention. Paradoxically, incomplete bilateral obstruction causes polyuria rather than oliguria, as a result of defects in tubular concentrating mechanisms, and this may obscure the true nature of the disturbance. Un-

fortunately, *unilateral* hydronephrosis may remain completely silent for long periods unless the other kidney is for some reason not functioning. Often the enlarged kidney is discovered on routine physical examination. Sometimes the basic cause of the hydronephrosis, such as renal calculi or an obstructing tumor, produces symptoms that indirectly draw attention to the hydronephrosis. Removal of obstruction within a few weeks usually permits full return of function; however, with time the changes become irreversible.

TUMORS

Many types of benign and malignant tumors occur in the urinary tract. In general, benign tumors such as small (rarely over 2.5 cm in diameter) cortical adenomas or medullary fibromas (interstitial cell tumors) have no clinical significance. The most common malignant tumor of the kidney is the renal cell carcinoma, followed in frequency by Wilms' tumors and by primary tumors of the calyces and pelves. Other types of renal cancer are extremely rare and need not be discussed here. Tumors of the lower urinary tract are about twice as common as renal cell carcinomas, and they are described at the end of this section.

RENAL CELL CARCINOMA

Renal cell carcinoma is the type of neoplasm usually meant by the term "cancer of the kidney." It is an adenocarcinoma arising from tubular epithelial cells and represents 80 to 90% of all malignant tumors of the kidney and 2% of all cancers in adults. The lesions are most common from the fifth to seventh decades, and males are affected twice as often as females. Although no neoplasm has an absolutely predictable course, the renal cell carcinoma distinguishes itself by being especially variable in its behavior. There is a greater frequency in cigarette smokers, and familial forms have been reported. The latter show dominantly inherited aberrations in the short arm of chromosome 3, which have also been detected in some sporadic cases.

MORPHOLOGY. These cancers are usually large by the time they are discovered and appear as spherical masses 3 to 15 cm in diameter. They may arise anywhere in the kidney. The cut surface is yellow-gray-white, with prominent areas of cystic softening or of hemorrhage, either fresh or old (Fig. 14–24). The margins of the tumor are well defined; however, at times small processes project into the surrounding parenchyma and small satellite nodules are found in the surrounding substance, providing clear evidence of the aggressiveness of these lesions. As the tumor enlarges, it may fungate through the walls of the collecting system, extending through the calyces and pelvis as far as

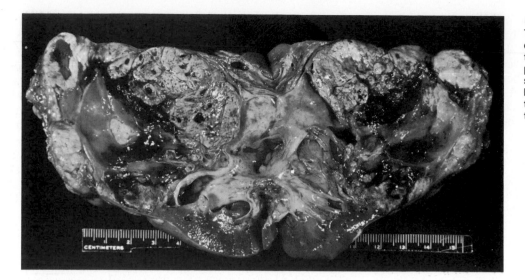

Figure 14-24. Renal cell carcinoma. The kidney has been hemisected to expose the tumor mass, which totally replaces and expands the upper pole of the kidney. Prominently shown are the areas of necrosis, hemorrhage, and cystic softening of the tumor. Only the lower pole of the kidney is recognizable below.

the ureter. Even more frequently, the tumor invades the renal vein and grows as a solid column within this vessel, sometimes extending in serpentine fashion as far as the inferior vena cava and even into the right side of the the heart. Occasionally there is direct invasion into the perinephric fat and adrenal gland.

Depending on the amount of lipid and glycogen present, the tumor cells may appear almost totally vacuolated or they may be solid. The classic vacuolated (lipid-laden) or **"clear cells"** are demarcated only by their cell membranes; the nuclei are usually pushed basally and are small (Fig. 14-25). At the other extreme are the granular cells, resembling the tubular epithelium, which have round, small, regular nuclei enclosed within granular pink cytoplasm. These cells may show great regularity of cytologic detail. Some tumors exhibit marked degrees of anaplasia, with numerous mitotic figures, and giant cells. Between the extremes of clear cells and solid cells, all intergradations may be found. The cellular arrangement, too, varies widely; the cells may form abortive tubules or papillary patterns, or they may cluster in cords or disorganized masses. The stroma is usually scant but highly vascularized.

CLINICAL COURSE. Renal cell carcinomas have several peculiar clinical characteristics that create especially difficult but challenging diagnostic problems. The symptoms vary, but the _most frequent presenting manifestation is hematuria, occurring in more than 50% of cases_. Macroscopic hematuria tends to be intermittent and fleeting, superimposed on a steady microscopic hematuria. In other patients, the tumor may declare itself simply by virtue of its size, when it has grown large enough to produce flank pain and a palpable mass. Extrarenal effects are fever and polycythemia, both of which may be associated with a renal cell carcinoma but which, because they are nonspecific, may be misinterpreted for some time before their true significance is appreciated. Polycythemia affects 5

to 10% of patients with this disease. It is assumed that the polycythemia results from elaboration of erythropoietin by the renal tumor. Uncommonly, these tumors produce a variety of hormone-like substances, resulting in hypercalcemia, hypertension, Cushing's syndrome, or feminization or masculinization. In many patients, the primary tumor remains silent and is discovered only after its metastases have produced symptoms. The prevalent locations for metastases are the lungs and the bones. It must be apparent that renal cell carcinoma presents in many fashions, some quite

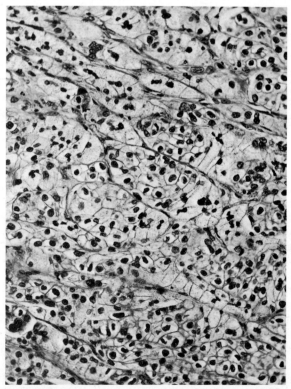

Figure 14-25. A high-power detail of the "clear cell" pattern of renal cell carcinoma.

devious, but *the triad of painless hematuria, long-standing fever, and dull flank pain is characteristic.*

WILMS' TUMOR

Although Wilms' tumor occurs infrequently in adults, it is the third most common organ cancer in children under the age of 10 years. It is therefore one of the major cancers of children. These tumors contain a variety of cell and tissue components, all derived from the mesoderm. *Wilms' tumor, like retinoblastoma, may arise sporadically or be familial with the susceptibility to tumorigenesis inherited as an autosomal dominant trait. Many tumors are associated with deletions in the short arm of chromosome 11 (11p13) and loss of the cancer suppressor gene WT-1* (p. 189). *Recent studies suggest that, unlike childhood retinoblastoma, Wilms' tumor is genetically heterogeneous, and in some cases loci other than 11p13 are involved.*

Grossly, these tumors are generally large, expansile, spherical masses that totally dwarf the kidney. In certain cases, they may grow so large as to produce distention of the abdomen and a readily observable mass on casual inspection. They are usually unilateral but, in familial cases, bilateral tumors are encountered. Grossly, myxomatous, soft; fish-flesh areas; solid gray, hyaline cartilaginous tissue; and areas of hemorrhagic necrosis are the common components. They often invade the capsule and perirenal tissues.

Histologically, the tumor consists of nests and sheets of primitive blastema with intervening mesenchyme. Abortive tubules are frequently seen with surrounding spindle cell stroma often having a sarcomatoid pattern. Abortive glomeruli may also be present. In addition, striated muscle, smooth muscle, collagenous fibrous tissue, cartilage, bone, fat cells, and areas of necrotic tissue containing cholesterol crystals and lipid macrophages may be seen. The degree of anaplasia in the stromal component generally correlates with the prognosis.

CLINICAL COURSE. Patients' complaints are usually referable to the tumor's enormous size. Commonly there is a readily palpable abdominal mass, which may extend across the midline and down into the pelvis. Less often, the patient presents with fever and abdominal pain, with hematuria, or, occasionally, with intestinal obstruction as a result of pressure from the tumor. The outlook for patients with Wilms' tumor is generally very good. Excellent results are obtained with a combination of radiotherapy, nephrectomy, and chemotherapy. Two-year survival rates are as high as 90%, and survival for two years usually implies a cure. These results are all the more remarkable because in many of these patients, pulmonary metastases, present at diagnosis, may disappear under the therapeutic regimen.

TUMORS OF THE URINARY COLLECTING SYSTEM (RENAL CALYCES, PELVIS, URETER, BLADDER, AND URETHRA)

The entire urinary collecting system from renal pelvis to urethra is lined with transitional epithelium, so its epithelial tumors assume similar morphologic patterns. Tumors in the collecting system above the bladder are relatively uncommon; those in the bladder, however, are an even more frequent cause of death than are kidney tumors. Nevertheless, in the individual case, a small lesion in the ureter, for example, may cause urinary outflow obstruction and have greater clinical significance than a much larger mass in the capacious bladder. We shall consider first the range of anatomic patterns, principally as they occur in the urinary bladder, followed by their clinical implications.

MORPHOLOGY. Tumors arising in the urinary bladder range from small benign papillomas to large invasive cancers (Fig. 14-26). The rare benign **papillomas** are small (0.2 to 1.0 cm), frond-like structures, having a delicate fibrovascular axial core covered by multilayered, well-differentiated transitional epithelium. In some of these lesions, the covering epithelium appears as normal as the mucosal surface whence these tumors arise; such lesions are almost invariably noninvasive and benign and do not recur once removed.

Transitional cell carcinomas (TCC) range from papillary to flat, noninvasive to invasive, and from extremely well-differentiated (grade I, Fig. 14-27) to highly anaplastic aggressive cancers (grade III). Grade I carcinomas are rarely invasive but may recur after removal. Whether the regrowth is a true recurrence or a second primary growth is uncertain. Progressive degrees of cellular atypia and anaplasia are encountered in papillary exophytic growths, accompanied by increase in size of the lesion and evidence of invasion of the submucosal or muscular layers. These tumors are unequivocally transitional cell carcinomas, grade II or grade III. As

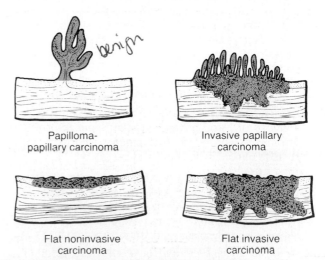

Figure 14-26. Four morphologic patterns of bladder tumors.

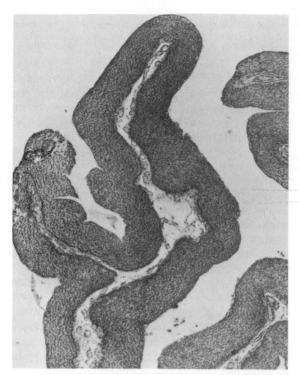

Figure 14–27. A Grade I papillary transitional cell carcinoma of the bladder. The delicate papilla is covered by orderly transitional epithelium.

these cancers approach the grade III pattern they tend to be flatter than the less aggressive forms, to cover larger areas of the mucosal surface, to invade deeper, and to have a shaggier necrotic surface. Occasionally these cancers show foci of squamous cell differentiation, but only 5% of bladder cancers are true **squamous cell carcinomas.** Carcinomas of grades II and III infiltrate surrounding structures, spread to regional nodes, and on occasion metastasize widely. Recently the suggestion has been made to divide all transitional cell tumors into two grades:

1. **Low-grade TCCs** are papillary tumors with normal to slightly atypical appearing transitional epithelium. These tumors retain blood group antigens, normal chromosomes, and have normal proliferative indexes. Patients may have multiple tumors, and almost none are invasive.
2. **High-grade TCCs** may have a papillary component but are usually flat with downward growth. They are comprised of pleomorphic cells with abnormal ploidy and loss of blood group antigens. Some 85 to 95% of patients who die of TCC present with high-grade invasive tumors as the first, and usually only, tumor.

In addition to overt carcinoma, an **in situ stage of bladder carcinoma can be recognized,** most frequently in patients with previous or simultaneous papillary or invasive tumors. Indeed, wide areas of atypical hyperplasia and dysplasia are often present. It is now thought that these epithelial changes and lesions in situ

are caused by the generalized influence of a putative carcinogen on urothelium and that they may be the precursors of invasive carcinomas in some patients. The extent of the "restless epithelium" provides a plausible source for multiple and recurrent lesions. The staging of bladder cancer is complex and beyond our scope.

CLINICAL COURSE. Painless hematuria is the dominant clinical presentation of all these tumors. Because most arise in the bladder we shall consider these first. They affect men about twice as frequently as women and usually develop between the ages of 50 and 70 years. Although most occur in persons who have no known history of exposure to industrial solvents, bladder tumors are 50 times more frequent in those exposed to β-naphthylamine. Cigarette smoking, chronic cystitis, schistosomiasis of the bladder, and certain drugs (cyclophosphamide) are also believed to induce higher attack rates.

The clinical significance of bladder tumors depends on several factors: obviously on their benign or malignant nature, on their location within the bladder, and —most important— on the depth of invasion of the lesion. Except for the clearly benign papillomas, all tend stubbornly to recur after removal and tend to kill by infiltrative obstruction of ureters rather than by metastasis. Lesions that invade the ureteral or urethral orifices cause urinary tract obstruction. In general, with shallow lesions, the prognosis after removal is good, but when deep penetration of the bladder wall has occurred, whatever the histologic pattern, the five-year survival rate is less than 20%. Overall five-year survival is 57%.

Although papillary and cancerous neoplasms of the lining epithelium of the collecting system occur much less frequently in the renal pelvis than in the bladder, they nonetheless make up 5 to 10% of primary renal tumors. Painless hematuria is the most characteristic feature of these lesions, but in their critical location they produce pain in the costovertebral angle as hydronephrosis develops. Infiltration of the walls of the pelvis, calyces, and renal vein worsens the prognosis. Despite removal of the tumor by nephrectomy, fewer than 50% of patients survive for five years. Cancer of the ureter is, fortunately, the rarest of the tumors of the collecting system. The five-year survival rate is less than 10%.

Bibliography

Andres, G., et al.: Biology of disease. Formation of immune deposits and disease. Lab. Invest. *55:*519, 1989. (A review of how immune deposits are formed in the glomerulus.)

Atkins, R. C.: Pathogenesis of Glomerulonephritis. Nephrology, Vol. I. Tokyo, Springer-Verlag, 1991.

Bane, B., et al.: Renal Cell Carcinoma. Review and Update. In Advances in Pathology, Vol. V Chicago, Mosby-Year Book, 1992.

Cotran, R. S.: Tubulointerstitial Nephropathies. New York, Churchill Livingstone, 1986. (A review of tubulointerstitial diseases, including reflux nephropathy, obstructive uropathy, and drug-induced interstitial diseases.)

Couser, W. G.: Mediation of immune glomerular injury. J. Am. Soc. Nephrol. *1:*13, 1990. (An up-to-date review.)

Gardner, K. D., and Bernstein J. (eds.): The Cystic Kidney. Dordrecht, The Netherlands, Kluwer Academic Publ., 1990. (A treatise on cystic kidney diseases.)

Gabow, P. A.: Polycystic kidney disease: Clues to pathogenesis. Kidney Int. *40:*989, 1991. (A summary of fascinating recent work on the genetics and possible mechanisms of cystogenesis).

Heptinstall, R. H.: Pathology of the Kidney. 4th Ed. Boston, Little Brown, 1992. (Classic illustrated written text of renal pathology.)

Hill, G. (ed.): Uropathology. New York, Churchill Livingstone, 1989. (A multiauthor book dealing with pathology of the lower urinary tract.)

Laragh, J. H. et al.: Hypertension: Pathophysiology, Diagnosis and Management. New York, Raven Press, 1990.

Molitoris, B. A.: New insights into the cell biology of ischemic acute renal failure. J. Am. Soc. Nephrol. *1:*1263, 1991. (A review of current work on cell polarity in ischemic renal failure.)

Murphy, W. (ed.): Urologic Pathology. Philadelphia, W. B. Saunders, 1989. (A comprehensive review of lesions of the lower urinary tract.)

Neilson, E. G. (ed.): Cell biology of the tubulointerstitium. Kidney Int. *39:*370. 1991.

Rennke, H. G., and Klein, P. S.: Pathogenesis and significance of nonprimary focal and segmental glomerulosclerosis. Am. J. Kid. Dis. *12:*443, 1989.

Striker, L. J., Olson, J. L., and Striker, G. E.: The Renal Biopsy. Philadelphia, W. B. Saunders, 1990. (A concise description of renal biopsy findings in glomerulonephritis.)

Tisher, C., and Brenner, B. M.: Renal Pathology, with Clinical and Pathological Correlations. Philadelphia, J. B. Lippincott, 1990. (A multiauthor renal pathology reference work.)

FIFTEEN

The Gastrointestinal Tract

ORAL CAVITY p473
ULCERATIVE AND INFLAMMATORY LESIONS
LEUKOPLAKIA
CANCER OF THE ORAL CAVITY (INCLUDING TONGUE)
SALIVARY GLAND DISEASES
   Sialadenitis
   Tumors
ESOPHAGUS p478
MOTOR DISORDERS
   Achalasia
   Other Motor Disorders
MISCELLANEOUS LESIONS
REFLUX ESOPHAGITIS
ESOPHAGEAL CARCINOMA
STOMACH p484
PYLORIC STENOSIS
GASTRITIS
   Acute (Erosive or Hemorrhagic) Gastritis
   Chronic (Nonerosive) Gastritis
STRESS ULCERS
PEPTIC ULCERS
TUMORS
   Gastric Polyps
   Gastric Carcinoma
   Gastrointestinal Lymphomas
SMALL AND LARGE INTESTINE p494
DEVELOPMENTAL ANOMALIES
   Megacolon

DIVERTICULA
VASCULAR DISORDERS
   Ischemic Bowel Disease
   Angiodysplasia
   Hemorrhoids
INFLAMMATORY DISEASES
   Crohn's Disease
   Ulcerative Colitis
INFECTIOUS ENTEROCOLITIS
   Enterotoxin-Induced Diarrhea
   Enteroinvasive Organisms
MALABSORPTION SYNDROMES
   Disaccharidase Deficiency
   Celiac Sprue
   Postinfectious (Tropical) Sprue
   Whipple's Disease
NEOPLASMS OF SMALL AND LARGE INTESTINE
   Polyps (Adenomas)
      Nonneoplastic Polyps
      Sporadic Adenomatous Polyps
      Hereditary Familial Polyposis
   Colorectal Carcinoma
   Carcinoid Tumors (Argentaffinomas)
OBSTRUCTIVE LESIONS
APPENDIX p519
APPENDICITIS
TUMORS

Oral Cavity

Only the more common conditions affecting the soft tissues will be considered. Excluded are the too painful to mention dental disorders as well as the basically extraoral diseases that sometimes involve the mouth and pharynx, such as diphtheria, lichen planus, and leukemia, some of which are considered elsewhere.

ULCERATIVE AND INFLAMMATORY LESIONS

Although several ulcerative and inflammatory conditions are discussed below, it is well to remember that mechanical trauma and cancer may also produce ulcerations in the oral cavity that must be considered in the differential diagnosis.

Aphthous ulcers (canker sores) are extremely common, small (usually less than 5 mm in diameter), painful, shallow ulcers. Characteristically, they take the form of rounded, superficial erosions, often covered with a gray-white exudate, having an erythematous rim. They appear singly or in crops on the nonkeratinized oral mucosa, particularly the soft palate, buccal-labial mucosa, floor of the mouth, and lateral borders of the tongue. They are more common in the first two decades of life and are often apparently triggered by stress, fever, ingestion of certain foods, and activation of inflammatory bowel disease. Although the cause remains unknown, an autoimmune basis is suspected. Self-limited, they usually resolve within a few weeks but may recur in the same location or a different one.

Herpetic stomatitis is an extremely common infection caused by herpes simplex virus type 1 (HSV-1). The pathogen is transmitted from person to person, most often by kissing; by middle life over three quarters of the population have been infected. In most adults, the primary infection is asymptomatic but the virus persists in a dormant state within ganglia about the mouth (e.g., trigeminal). With reactivation (fever, sun or cold exposure, respiratory tract infection, trauma), solitary or multiple, small (less than 5 mm in diameter) vesicles containing clear fluid appear, most often on the lips or about the nasal orifices—the well-known "cold sores" or "fever blisters." They soon rupture, leaving shallow, painful ulcers that heal within a few weeks, but recurrences are common. Histologically, the vesicles begin as an intraepithelial focus of inter- and intracellular edema. The infected cells become ballooned and develop intranuclear acidophilic viral inclusions. Sometimes adjacent cells fuse to form _giant cells_ or _polykaryons_. Necrosis of the infected cells and the focal collections of edema fluid account for the intraepithelial vesicles seen clinically. Identification of the inclusion-bearing cells or polykaryons in smears of blister fluid constitutes the diagnostic _Tzanck test_ for HSV infection.

When the primary infection occurs in a prepubescent child or immunocompromised adult, a more virulent disseminated eruption is likely to occur, marked by multiple vesicles throughout the oral cavity including the pharynx _(herpetic gingivostomatitis)_. In passing, we should note that HSV-I may localize in many other sites including the conjunctivae (keratoconjunctivitis), and in children and vulnerable adults, may spread to the esophagus when a nasogastric tube is introduced through an infected oral cavity, or worse a viremia may seed the brain (encephalitis) or produce visceral and disseminated lesions. HSV-2 (the agent of herpes genitalis), on the other hand, is transmitted sexually and produces vesicles on the genital mucous membranes and external genitalia that have the same histologic characteristics as those that occur about the mouth.

Oral candidiasis (thrush, moniliasis) is a common fungal infection among predisposed persons rendered vulnerable by diabetes mellitus, anemia, antibiotic or glucocorticoid therapy, some form of immunodeficiency, or debilitating illnesses such as disseminated cancer. _Candida albicans_ is a normal inhabitant of the oral cavity found in 30 to 40% of the population; it causes disease only when there is some impairment of the usual protective mechanisms. Typically, oral candidiasis takes the form of a superficial, white, curd-like, circumscribed membrane of myriad organisms sitting on the mucosa anywhere in the oral cavity. The membrane can be scraped off to reveal an underlying granular erythematous inflammatory base; in milder infections there is minimal ulceration, but in particularly vulnerable persons the mucosa may be denuded. The fungi can be identified within these membranes as boxcar-like chains of tubular cells producing pseudohyphae from which bud 2- to 4-μm, typically ovoid yeast forms. In the particularly vulnerable host, the infection may spread into the esophagus, especially when a nasogastric tube has been introduced, or may produce visceral lesions when the fungus gains entry into the bloodstream. For poorly understood reasons, similar monilial lesions may appear in the vagina, not only in predisposed persons but also in apparently healthy young women, particularly ones who are pregnant or using oral contraceptives.

Acquired immunodeficiency syndrome (AIDS) and less advanced forms of HIV infection are often associated with lesions in the oral cavity. They may take the form of candidiasis, herpetic vesicles, or some other microbial infection (e.g., gingivitis, glossitis). Of particular interest are the intraoral lesions of _Kaposi's sarcoma (KS)_ and _hairy leukoplakia (HL)_. KS, as described on page 302, is a multifocal, systemic disease that eventually evolves into highly vascular tumorous aggregates. Although KS may occur in the absence of the AIDS virus, it affects about 20% of AIDS patients, particularly homosexual or bisexual males. More than 50% of those afflicted develop intraoral purpuric discolorations or violaceous, raised, nodular masses, and sometimes this involvement constitutes the presenting manifestation of KS.

Hairy leukoplakia (HL) is an uncommon lesion seen virtually only in persons infected with human immunodeficiency virus (HIV). It constitutes white confluent patches, anywhere on the oral mucosa, that have a "hairy" or corrugated surface resulting from marked epithelial thickening (acanthosis), hyperkeratosis, and sometimes koilocytosis. In addition to HIV, human papillomavirus (HPV) and Epstein-Barr virus (EBV) can sometimes be identified by in situ hybridization in these lesions and may play roles in inducing the epithelial proliferation. Occasionally, the development of HL calls attention to the existence of the underlying HIV infection.

LEUKOPLAKIA

As generally used, _the term "leukoplakia" refers to a whitish, well-defined, mucosal patch or plaque caused by epidermal thickening or hyperkeratosis not attributable to any physical or chemical agent save possibly_ *the use of tobacco.* The term generally is not applied to other white lesions, such as those caused by candidiasis, lichen planus, or white sponge nevus among many others.

The plaques are more frequent among older men and are most frequently located on the vermilion border of the lower lip, buccal mucosa, and the hard and soft palates, and less frequently on the floor of the mouth and other intraoral sites. *They appear as localized, sometimes multifocal or even diffuse, smooth or roughened, leathery, white, discrete areas of mucosal thickening that on microscopic evaluation vary from banal hyperkeratosis without underlying epithelial dysplasia to mild to severe dysplasia bordering on carcinoma in situ* (Fig. 15–1). Only histologic evaluation distinguishes among these changes. The lesions are of unknown cause save that there is a strong association with the use of tobacco, particularly pipe smoking and smokeless tobacco (pouches, snuff, chewing). Less strongly implicated are chronic friction as may be produced by ill-fitting dentures or jagged teeth, alcohol abuse, and irritant foods (so, pizza freaks, relax). More recently, HPV antigen has been identified in some tobacco-related lesions, raising the possibility that the virus and tobacco act in concert in the induction of these lesions.

Oral leukoplakia is an important finding because about 5 to 15% (depending somewhat on location) undergo transformation to squamous cell carcinoma and it is virtually impossible to distinguish the innocent from the ominous. The transformation rate is greatest with lip and tongue lesions and lowest with those on the floor of the mouth.

Two somewhat related lesions must be differentiated from oral leukoplakia. Hairy leukoplakia, described above and seen only in patients with AIDS, has a corrugated or "hairy" surface rather than the white, opaque thickening of oral leukoplakia, and moreover has not been related to the development of oral cancer. *Erythroplasia* refers to red, velvety, often granular, circumscribed areas, having poorly defined, irregular boundaries, that may or may not be elevated. Sometimes these lesions are speckled or have whitish areas *(erythroleukoplakia).* Histologically, erythroplasia almost invariably reveals marked epithelial dysplasia (the malignant transformation rate is more than 50%), so recognition of this lesion becomes even more important than identification of oral leukoplakia.

CANCERS OF THE ORAL CAVITY (AND TONGUE)

The overwhelming preponderance of oral cavity cancers are squamous cell carcinomas. They are relatively uncommon, representing about 3% of all cancers in the United States, but they are disproportionately important because although almost all are readily accessible to biopsy and early identification, about half kill within five years and indeed may have already metastasized by the time the primary lesion is discovered. Significantly, the five-year survival rate with nodal involvement is 30%, and 70% with node-negative disease. These cancers tend to occur later in life and are rare before age 40 years. In the past there was

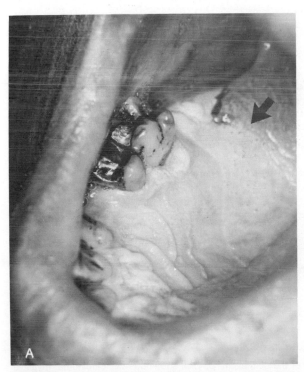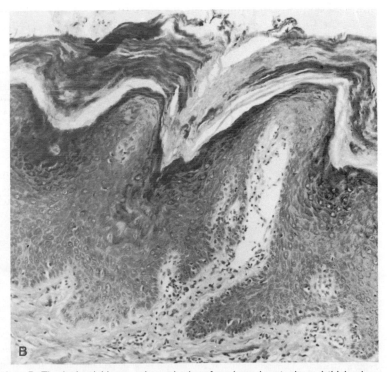

Figure 15–1. *A,* Leukoplakia of floor of mouth *(arrow)* in a smoker. *B,* The leukoplakia reveals marked surface hyperkeratosis and thickening of the mucosa but no dysplasia. (*A,* Courtesy of Dr. Gerald Shklar, Harvard Dental School, Boston, MA.)

a strong male preponderance, but currently the ratio is about 2:1.

ETIOLOGY AND PATHOGENESIS. The various influences thought to be important in development of these cancers are summarized in Table 15-1.

MORPHOLOGY. Despite reported differences, the three predominant sites of origin of oral cavity carcinomas are (in order of frequency) (1) vermilion border of the lateral margins of the lower lip, (2) floor of the mouth, and (3) lateral borders of the mobile tongue. Early lesions appear as pearly white to gray, circumscribed thickenings of the mucosa closely resembling leukoplakic patches. They then may grow in an exophytic fashion to produce

readily visible and palpable nodular and eventually fungating lesions, or they may assume an endophytic, invasive pattern with central necrosis to create a cancerous ulcer. The squamous cell carcinomas are usually moderately to well differentiated keratinizing tumors, but uncommonly are very anaplastic and undifferentiated. Before the lesions become advanced it may be possible to identify epithelial atypicality, dysplasia, or carcinoma in situ in the margins, suggesting origin from leukoplakia or erythroplasia (Fig. 15-2). Spread to regional nodes is present at the time of initial diagnosis only rarely with lip cancer, in about 50% of cases of tongue cancer, and in more than 60% of those with cancer of the floor of the mouth. More remote spread to tissues or organs in the thorax or abdomen is less common than extensive regional spread.

TABLE 15-1. IMPORTANT PATHOGENIC INFLUENCES ON ORAL CANCER

Factor	Comments
Leukoplakia, erythroplasia	See discussion on p. 475
Tobacco use	Best-established influence, particularly pipe smoking and smokeless tobacco
Alcohol abuse	Less strong influence than tobacco
Human papillomavirus types 16, 18, 11	Identified by molecular probes in some (not all) cases
Protracted irritation	Weakly associated
Plummer-Vinson syndrome	Association questionable

see p346, 479

CLINICAL COURSE. These lesions may cause local pain or difficulty in chewing, but many are relatively asymptomatic and so the lesion (very familiar to the exploring tongue) is ignored. It is tragic that so many are not discovered until beyond cure. The five-year survival rates, despite surgery and radiation, vary from 91% for lip cancer to about 30% for cancers of the base of the tongue, pharynx, and floor of the mouth.

SALIVARY GLAND DISEASES

Although diseases primary in the major salivary glands are in general uncommon, the parotids bear the

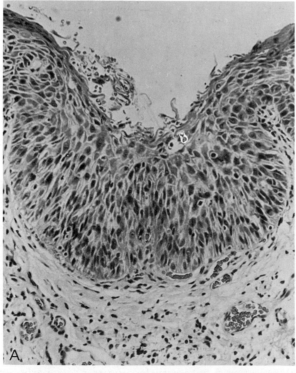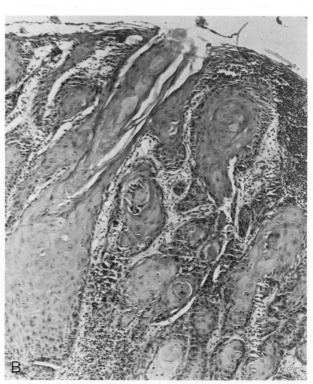

Figure 15-2. *A,* Oral carcinoma in situ shows nuclear pleomorphism in all strata of the epithelium. *B,* Oral squamous cell carcinoma. Invasive tumor islands show formation of keratin pearls. (Courtesy of Dr. L. R. Eversole, Professor and Chairman, Department of Oral Diagnostic Sciences, College of Dentistry, University of Florida, Gainesville, FL.)

brunt of these involvements. Among the many possible disorders, attention will be restricted to sialadenitis and salivary gland tumors.

SIALADENITIS

Inflammation of the major salivary glands may be of viral, bacterial, or autoimmune origin. Dominant among these causations is the infectious viral disease mumps, which may produce enlargement of all the major salivary glands but predominantly the parotids. Uncommonly, the parotitis is unilateral or affects the other major salivary glands as well. The paramyxovirus produces usually a diffuse, interstitial inflammation marked by edema and a mononuclear cell infiltration. Occasionally there are focal areas of parenchymal necrosis, apparently produced by marked inflammatory swelling of the encapsulated glands to the point of compression of the vascular supply. Although self-limited in childhood rarely leaving residua, in adults mumps may be accompanied by pancreatitis or orchitis; the latter sometimes causes permanent sterility.

Presumed *autoimmune sialadenitis,* almost invariably bilateral, is seen in Sjogren's syndrome discussed on page 149. All of the salivary glands, major and minor, as well as the lacrimal glands may be affected in this disorder, which induces dry mouth *(xerostomia)* and dry eyes *(keratoconjunctivitis sicca).* The combination of salivary and lacrimal gland inflammatory enlargement, usually painless, and xerostomia, whatever the cause, is sometimes referred to by the generic term *Mikulicz syndrome,* embracing sarcoidosis, leukemia, lymphoma, and idiopathic lymphoepithelial hyperplasia.

Bacterial sialadenitis most often occurs secondary to some obstructive process in the major excretory ducts such as stone formation *(sialolithiasis)* or inspissated secretions in xerostomia or fibrocystic disease of the pancreas. Rarely, bacterial inflammation appears in the absence of ductal obstruction, usually for completely obscure reasons, mostly in elderly persons following a major surgical procedure elsewhere in the body. Depending on the pathogen, the sialadenitis may be largely interstitial or cause focal areas of suppurative necrosis or even abscess formation.

TUMORS

The salivary glands give rise to a surprising diversity of tumors, about 80% of which occur within the parotid glands and most of the others in the submandibular. Males and females are affected about equally, usually in the sixth or seventh decade of life. In the parotids 70 to 80% are benign, whereas in the submaxillary glands only half are benign. Thus it is evident that a neoplasm in the submaxillary glands is more ominous than one in the parotids. The dominant tumor arising in the parotids is the benign, pleomorphic adenoma, sometimes called mixed tumor of salivary gland origin. Much less frequent is the papillary

cystadenoma lymphomatosum (Warthin's tumor). Collectively, these two types account for three quarters of parotid tumors. Whatever the type, they present clinically as a mass causing a swelling at the angle of the jaw. Among the diverse cancers of parotid glands, the two dominant types are malignant mixed tumors arising either de novo or in preexisting, benign, pleomorphic adenomas and mucoepidermoid carcinoma. Only the benign pleomorphic adenoma and Warthin's tumor are sufficiently common to merit description.

The pleomorphic adenoma or benign mixed tumor, as noted above, is the most common tumor of salivary glands. It is a slow growing, well demarcated, apparently encapsulated lesion rarely exceeding 6 cm in greatest dimension. Most often arising in the superficial parotid, they usually cause painless swelling at the angle of the jaw and can be readily palpated as discrete masses, but nonetheless they are often present for years before being brought to medical attention. Histologically, despite the encapsulation, there are often multiple projections of tumor cells penetrating the capsule dictating the need for adequate margins of resection to prevent recurrences. On average, about 10% of excisions are followed by recurrence. The characteristic histologic feature is the heterogeneity implied by the name of this tumor. Basically, there are epithelial elements forming ducts, acini, tubules, strands, or sheets of cells interspersed within a loose often myxoid connective tissue stroma sometimes bearing islands of apparent chondroid or, rarely, bone. In some tumors, the epithelial structures dominate whereas in others the stroma dominates (Fig. 15–3). The epithelial cells are small, dark, and range from cuboidal to spindle forms, depending on their organization. Immunohistochemical evidence suggests that all of the diverse cell types within these tumors, including those within the stroma, are of myoepithelial derivation. When primary or recurrent benign tumors are present for many years (10 to 20 years), malignant transformation may occur, referred to then as a malignant mixed salivary gland tumor. Whether such cancers were occult from inception and restricted to a hidden focus that was left behind in the previous surgical excision or whether there was indeed malignant transformation of a benign lesion remains a persistent question. Equally uncertain is the role of previous surgery in precipitating malignant transformation, but clearly this occurs in the absence of previous treatment.

Papillary cystadenoma lymphomatosum or Warthin's tumor occurs infrequently and virtually only in the parotid gland of either sex. These curious benign neoplasms are generally small, well-encapsulated, round to ovoid masses that on transection often reveal mucin-containing, cleft-like or cystic spaces within a soft, gray background. Microscopically, they are very characteristic, composed basically of an epithelial element lining the branching, cystic or cleft-like spaces based on an immediately subjacent, well-developed lymphoid tissue sometimes forming germinal centers. The epithelium is double tiered with a surface layer of regularly arrayed, tall, slender epithelial cells underlaid by inconspicuous, cuboidal to polygonal, apparent myoepithelial cells.

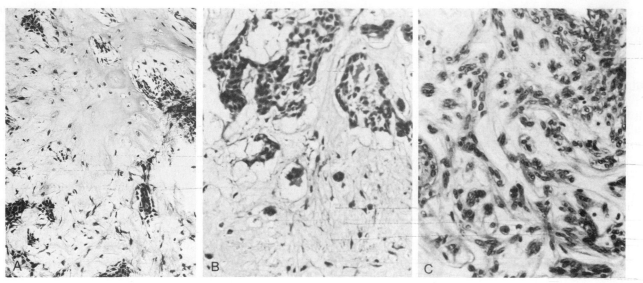

Figure 15–3. *A,* Low-power view of a pleomorphic adenoma showing abundant myxoid stroma with areas of chondroid and osteoid cells and interspersed islands of epithelial cells. *B,* The epithelial acinar formations scattered through a loose myxoid stroma. *C,* Islands and strands of myoepithelial cells with small, dark-staining nuclei.

The luminal columnar cells are often deeply acidophilic and have many of the features of oncocytes (i.e., densely packed mitochondria). A recurrence rate of about 10% is attributed to incomplete excision, multicentricity, or a second primary; malignant transformation is rare and controversial.

Esophagus

The many widely differing esophageal lesions evoke a remarkably limited range of symptoms, rendering diagnosis difficult. Most cause dysphagia (difficulty in swallowing) or "heartburn" (retrosternal pain), sometimes both. Less commonly, esophageal varices and lacerations cause significant, sometimes severe, bleeding with vomiting of blood (hematemesis) or blood in the stools (melena). With upper gastrointestinal bleeding, the critical issue arises of whether it is esophageal or gastric in origin, because its management depends much on its source.

MOTOR DISORDERS

The selection of the conditions to be discussed under this heading is admittedly arbitrary, because certain disorders not included here, such as esophageal cancer, also produce disordered esophageal motility. In some measure the selection reflects the lack of a better banner under which the following conditions might march.

ACHALASIA

The term achalasia means "failure to relax," and in the present context applies to incomplete relaxation of the lower esophageal sphincter (LES) in response to swallowing, thus, in effect producing a functional obstruction of the esophagus. There is near consensus that some derangement in the innervation of the LES is at fault rather than a muscle disorder, but the nature of the neural defect is still uncertain. Equally ardently proposed are the following mechanisms:

- A reduction in the number of ganglion cells in the esophageal myenteric plexus, though some contend that the reduction is most marked in patients who have long-standing disease and so is likely to be secondary rather than primary.
- Primary degenerative changes in the vagal branches to the esophagus in the form of loss of myelin sheaths and disruption of axonal membranes, leading in time to loss of post-synaptic ganglion cells.
- Degeneration of the cells of the central vagal nuclei, accounting for the changes in the terminal vagal branches.
- Decreased neural formation of the inhibitory vasoactive intestinal polypeptide that induces the relaxation of the circular smooth muscle of the sphincter.

Among these several proposals, most weight is accorded the reduction in the number of ganglion cells, but whichever view obtains, what is the cause of the change? Viral infection has been suggested but without proof.

In only one situation is the cause of achalasia

known—Chagas' disease caused by *Trypanosoma cruzi*. In this infection, the organisms directly invade and destroy the ganglion cells within the myenteric plexus, sometimes throughout the gastrointestinal tract and urinary tract, inducing among other derangements, achalasia. With this exception, the cause and pathogenesis of achalasia are unknown.

> The body of the esophagus above the level of the lower esophageal sphincter is generally flaccid and often distended (megaesophagus). The wall may be of normal thickness, thickened by hypertrophy, or thinned by dilatation. The myenteric ganglion cells are reduced in number within the esophageal wall, particularly in the lower esophagus. There may also be degeneration of the myelin sheaths and breaks in the axonal membranes of the intraesophageal ramifications of the vagus nerves, and in a few cases reduction in the number of ganglion cells in central vagal nuclei. Secondary changes may appear incident to stasis of food, such as chronic esophagitis sometimes accompanied by leukoplakia and mucosal dysplasia most severe proximal to the lower esophageal functional obstruction. Superimposed carcinoma sometimes develops.

Dysphagia, sometimes accompanied by retrosternal chest pain and vomiting, is the predominant clinical manifestation of achalasia. Weight loss may be associated with long-standing disease. Of greater importance is the predisposition to carcinoma, appearing in 2 to 7% of patients with long-standing disease. Still unexplained is the persistence of the increased predisposition to cancer even after seemingly successful control of the motor dysfunction.

OTHER MOTOR DISORDERS

Congenital Atresia and Stenosis

Congenital atresia and stenosis are both serious defects in newborns that require prompt intervention. *Atresia* implies failure of development of a segment of the esophagus, creating discontinuous, blind upper and lower pouches. Most blind lower pouches communicate through a fistulous tract with the trachea or a main stem bronchus, but seldom does an upper pouch communicate with the airways. In addition to causing reflux vomiting, atresia leads to aspiration of food or refluxed gastric contents causing severe, potentially fatal respiratory difficulty. Early correction is therefore mandatory.

Stenosis, on the other hand, implying marked narrowing of the esophageal lumen, may occur as a developmental defect or may be acquired secondary to: (1) chronic esophagitis with inflammatory fibrosis, (2) neoplastic narrowing, (3) collagenization of the esophageal wall as with systemic scleroderma, or (4) extrinsic

compression by some expansile mediastinal tumor or aneurysm. Whatever the basis, stenosis causes marked dysphagia, vomiting, and feeding difficulties requiring dilatation or another form of intervention.

Diverticula

Outpouchings of the esophageal wall tend to occur in three locations but may be located elsewhere: (1) at the pharyngoesophageal junction where defects in the posterior pharyngeal wall create loci of weakness (*Zenker's diverticulum*); (2) near the midpoint of the esophagus where the tracheal bifurcation may cause slight narrowing of the esophageal lumen; and (3) immediately above the lower esophageal sphincter, typically in patients with motility disorders. At all locations, the saccular outpouchings tend to be small (1 to 3 cm in diameter) and to have large mouths, and they are lined by normal esophageal mucosa but have thinned muscularis or sometimes none. Although those in the midportion of the esophagus are sometimes referred to as traction diverticula, it is likely that all are related to some combination of defective muscle support, narrowing or functional obstruction of the lumen, and increased intraluminal peristaltic pressure, producing what is in effect a saccular "aneurysm of the esophagus."

These lesions are generally of little clinical significance save that when distended with food they may compress the esophagus or may develop ulceroinflammatory changes, causing dysphagia and retrosternal pain.

Rings and Webs

These two terms are used interchangeably, but sometimes rings and webs are differentiated on the basis of location within the esophagus and the presence or absence of muscularis within the constriction, or each term is used to mean whatever the author intends it to mean, to paraphrase Alice of "Wonderland" fame. The lesions are ring-like, concentric constrictions of the esophagus, some comprising only thin mucosal folds, others being thicker and containing submucosa as well as muscularis. Those in the lower esophagus are often referred to as *Schatzki's rings* in token of the radiologist who first described them. Upper esophageal rings, more often referred to as webs are sometimes accompanied by atrophic glossitis and iron deficiency anemia, typically in elderly women. The complex of web-induced dysphagia, glossitis, and iron deficiency anemia has come to be known as the *Plummer-Vinson or Paterson-Brown-Kelly syndrome*. The causal relationship of these various features is obscure and may well be coincidental. Not surprisingly, these lesions, if sufficiently obstructive, hamper the passage of food, cause intermittent dysphagia, and sometimes produce sudden regurgitation of solid lumps such as a piece of meat, which may then be aspirated (the "steak house syndrome").

MISCELLANEOUS LESIONS ————————

HIATAL HERNIA ————————————————

In this disorder a dilated segment of the stomach protrudes above the diaphragm. Two patterns are distinguished: (1) sliding esophageal hiatal hernia and (2) paraesophageal hiatal hernia (Fig. 15–4).

In the much more common *sliding hiatal hernia* the esophagogastric junction is displaced cephalad, resulting in a dilated, bell-shaped segment of the stomach lying above the diaphragm. The basis for this derangement is obscure and has been variously attributed to an abnormally short esophagus, gastric reflux leading to esophageal spasm and traction on the stomach, repeated episodes of increased intraabdominal pressure produced by vomiting that displace the stomach upward, and other equally unconvincing explanations. The importance of the sliding hernia is its association with reflux esophagitis in some patients. Most patients with a sliding hernia, however, do not have reflux, but most patients with severe reflux esophagitis do have a sliding hiatal hernia.

Paraesophageal hiatal hernias account for only 10% of hiatal hernias. Here a defect or weakening of the diaphragmatic esophageal hiatus permits a portion of the gastric fundus to balloon into the thorax. The sac tends to roll up alongside of the esophagus, hence the synonym *"rolling hiatus hernia."* In most cases, the sac is relatively small (3 to 6 cm in greatest dimension), but occasionally the diaphragmatic defect is sufficiently large or expanded to permit other abdominal viscera to accompany the herniated stomach. These hernias are not necessarily associated with reflux esophagitis or other symptoms, but occasionally dysphagia is noted, or vague substernal discomfort.

LACERATIONS (MALLORY-WEISS SYNDROME) ——

Linear tears in the gastroesophageal wall are uncommon lesions encountered most frequently in chronic alcoholics after a bout of retching or vomiting. Occasionally they are seen without documented prior vomiting or with no history of alcohol abuse. These tears, oriented in the long axis of the esophagus, stomach, or both, are usually not perforating and extend through mucosa and submucosa, rarely through the muscularis, and on average are 2 to 3 cm long. They may be located in the terminal esophagus, astride the esophagogastric junction, or in the proximate gastric mucosa. Some experts believe that there is always accompanying relaxation of the diaphragmatic support of the terminal esophagus or a concurrent sliding hernia.

The presumed pathogenesis is a wave of strong antiperistalsis overwhelming the lower esophageal sphincter with massive stretching and tearing of the esophagogastric junction. The tears account for about 5 to 10% of all instances of massive hematemesis, but generally the bleeding is not profuse and subsides spontaneously with medical therapy. Sometimes such measures as balloon tamponade, embolization of the left gastric artery, or surgery are required. A rare complication is infection followed by perforation, but most often these lesions heal spontaneously, leaving no residua.

VARICES ————————————————————

When sufficiently severe and prolonged, portal hypertension, of whatever cause, induces the formation of bypass channels between the portal vein and superior vena cava. The causes of portal hypertension

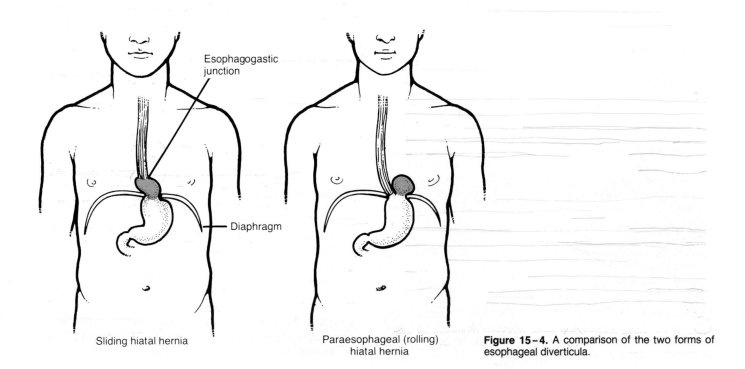

Sliding hiatal hernia

Paraesophageal (rolling) hiatal hernia

Esophagogastric junction

Diaphragm

Figure 15–4. A comparison of the two forms of esophageal diverticula.

(principally cirrhosis) and the genesis of these venous bypasses are considered on page 545. Here it suffices that with an increase in pressure in the portal vein, flow is diverted through the coronary veins of the stomach into the submucosal plexus of the lower esophagus, thus permitting drainage through the azygos vein into the superior vena cava. With prolonged increased pressure, the veins in the lower esophageal plexus and sometimes those in the gastric mucosa in the region of the gastroesophageal junction dilate and eventually become variceal. They are difficult to visualize after death with loss of the distending pressure, but under appropriate conditions they appear as longitudinal, tortuous, dilated veins that protrude directly beneath the mucosa of the lower esophagus, gastroesophageal junction, or proximate cardiac region (Fig. 15–5). When unruptured the overlying mucosa may be normal, but often it is eroded and inflamed, further weakening the tissue support of the dilated veins. Rupture with massive bleeding is at least alarming and at worst fatal. The mechanism of rupture appears to be increased tension on the wall of the veins (a function of the diameter of the vessel) as they progressively dilate. Episodes of vomiting with increased intraabdominal pressure further raise the level of the portal hypertension and predispose to rupture.

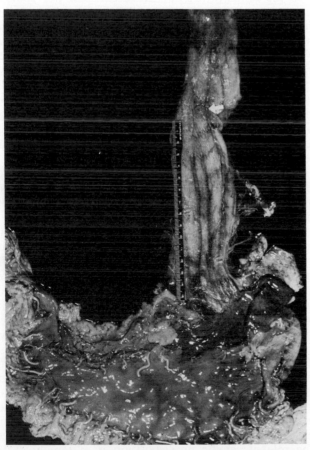

Figure 15–5. Three submucosal veins, rendered prominent by their marked variceal dilatation, are seen in the lower half of the esophagus. The arrow points to one of them.

Varices develop in approximately two thirds of all cirrhosis patients and are most often associated with alcoholic cirrhosis. With variceal rupture, the mortality rate from massive hematemesis is at least 30% during the initial hospitalization, and even with survival a 50% likelihood of rebleeding at some subsequent date exists with all of its attendant risk. In contrast to lacerations, emergency intervention is frequently necessary, such as balloon tamponade, embolization, endoscopic sclerotherapy, or direct surgical ligation of the bleeding focus. Before such therapy can be used, the critical question of the source of the bleeding must be resolved, because massive upper gastrointestinal bleeding has many origins in the general population, principally (1) peptic ulcer (2) hemorrhagic gastritis (3) esophageal varices, and (4) esophageal lacerations, in descending order of frequency. However, in cirrhosis patients, varices vie with peptic ulcers for first place.

REFLUX ESOPHAGITIS

Injury to the esophageal wall with subsequent inflammation is a common condition worldwide. In northern Iran the prevalence of esophagitis is over 80%. There is also an extremely high incidence of esophagitis in regions of China. The basis for this prevalence is unknown. In the United States and other western countries it is thought to be present in 10 to 20% of the general population. Here it may have many origins—prolonged gastric intubation, uremia, ingestion of corrosive or irritant substances, radiation, and graft-versus-host disease, but most important is chronic esophageal reflux. Heavy smoking and alcohol consumption are important cofactors. It should be noted, however, that in Iran religious prohibitions exclude both of these contributors. Whether excessive consumption of very hot liquids in the high-incidence locales plays a role remains uncertain. *Notwithstanding these enigmas, the overwhelming preponderance of cases in the western world constitute reflux esophagitis. Much less often direct microbial invasion, usually by viruses or fungi, is implicated in immunodeficient and debilitated patients* such as those with leukemia and terminal cancer. These unfortunates are vulnerable to the development of candidal or herpes simplex esophagitis when there are oral infections and gastric intubation has been introduced through the infected territory. Less common microbial causes include cytomegalovirus, aspergillus, and sundry bacteria. With these few comments on other patterns of esophagitis, our attention can now be directed to the "big banana," reflux esophagitis.

PATHOGENESIS. Many factors are involved in the causation of reflux esophagitis:

- Impairment of the efficacy of the lower esophageal antireflux mechanism that prevents acid peptic secretions from inundating the lower esophagus. Reflux is known to occur in normal asymptomatic subjects, but in those with symptomatic esophagitis the frequency and quantity of reflux are greater.
- A sliding hiatal hernia significantly predisposes. As

noted, most patients with moderate to severe esophagitis have a sliding hiatal hernia.

- Increased gastric volume, whatever its basis, contributes to the volume of reflux.
- The levels of acid and of pepsin in the gastric secretion determine the injury-producing potential of the refluxate.
- Inadequate or slowed esophageal clearance of refluxate is an important contributing influence. Not only is clearance of the fluid involved but also restoration of the normal esophageal pH, mainly by swallowing of saliva.
- The reparative capacity of the esophageal mucosa is itself reduced by protracted exposure to gastric reflux. Although the normal stratified squamous esophageal mucosa is impermeable to hydrogen ions and to peptic digestion, with prolonged exposure the mucosa becomes permeable, potentiating cell injury and ultimately epithelial desquamation and erosion.

Any one of these influences may assume primacy in the individual case, but more than one is likely to be involved in most instances.

MORPHOLOGY. Grossly, depending on the severity and duration of the esophagitis, there may be only minimal hyperemia and superficial spotty erosions, or with more severe disease, thickening of the wall owing to edema or fibrosis along with confluent epithelial erosions or total ulceration of the mucosa. These changes are most marked in the distal esophagus but in severe cases may extend into more proximal levels. The granular, red, ulcerated surface may be covered by a gray-white inflammatory membrane (pseudomembrane), as is typical of candidiasis.

The histologic features of well-developed reflux esophagitis are: mucosal erosion or deeper ulceration accompanied by an acute and chronic inflammatory cell infiltrate. Earlier, less severe changes include basal cell hyperplasia and submucosal papillae extending into the superficial third of the epithelium with scattered intraepithelial eosinophils and "polys." Sometimes present are dysplastic changes in the squamous epithelial cells or mural fibrosis with long-standing chronic disease. As will be emphasized later, chronic esophagitis is a fertile soil for the development of carcinoma.

Barrett's esophagus may appear as a reparative response in patients with long-standing reflux esophagitis. It is characterized by replacement in the distal esophagus of the normal stratified squamous mucosa by a metaplastic columnar-type epithelium having both gastric and intestinal type glands. In instances with severe reflux esophagitis the lower third or even half of the esophagus may undergo such transformation. Rarely, peptic ulceration (p. 487) occurs within the transformed mucosa. In some instances, the columnar epithelium undergoes dysplastic change and indeed sometimes becomes cancerous.

CLINICAL CORRELATION. The dominant manifestation of reflux disease is heartburn, sometimes accompanied by regurgitation of a sour brash. Rarely these chronic symptoms are punctuated by attacks of severe chest pain mimicking a "heart attack." Although largely limited to adults over age 40, uncommonly reflux esophagitis is seen in infants and children. The potential consequences: of prolonged, severe reflux esophagitis are development of a cancer, stricture, bleeding, and possibly Barrett's esophagus with its attendant risks of peptic ulceration and esophageal adenocarcinoma (generally cited as a 10% risk).

ESOPHAGEAL CARCINOMA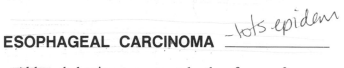

Although benign tumors and other forms of cancer may arise in the esophagus, collectively they are totally overshadowed by esophageal carcinoma, more than 95% of which are squamous cell tumors and the remainder adenocarcinomas. In the United States, most occur in adults over the age of 50 with a male-female ratio of 3:1 and they account for 1 to 2% of all cancer deaths. There are, however, striking and puzzling differences in the incidence of this form of cancer around the world and even within a single country. Whereas the prevalence in the United States is in the range of six new cases per year per 100,000 males, in the "Asian esophageal cancer belt" extending from the northern provinces of China to the Caspian littoral in Iran, the prevalence is well over 100 per 100,000, females being affected more often than males. In Sri Lanka, esophageal carcinoma is the most common carcinoma of the gastrointestinal tract. Equally puzzling is the three- to fourfold higher incidence of this form of malignancy among black Americans than among whites. These epidemiologic contrasts must contain causative clues, but to date they have not been deciphered.

ETIOLOGY AND PATHOGENESIS. A large number of clinical, environmental, and genetic predisposing influences have been identified, some better established than others (Table 15–2).

Common to most of the predisposing clinical conditions is retardation of the passage of food through the esophagus, exposing the mucosa longer to potential carcinogenic influences. Tobacco use and alcohol abuse rank high among these putative dangers. Not surprisingly, therefore, there is a well-defined predisposing role for chronic esophagitis, itself associated with abuse of alcohol and tobacco. Together these two hazards, when sufficiently excessive, increase the risk of cancer about fortyfold. However, these influences cannot underlie the very high incidence of this tumor among the orthodox Moslems of Iran, who neither drink nor smoke. Here is where some of the other questionable environmental factors mentioned are invoked, but without much direct causal evidence. The role of genetic predisposition is extremely ill-defined, but its possible contribution cannot be dis-

TABLE 15-2. PREDISPOSING INFLUENCES TO ESOPHAGEAL CANCER

Established	Questionable
Clinical	
Achalasia	
Hiatal hernia	
Reflux esophagitis	
Barrett's esophagus	
Plummer-Vinson syndrome	
Caustic-induced strictures	
Environmental	
Alcohol abuse	Aflatoxins
Tobacco use	Nitrosamines
	Nutritional deficiencies (e.g., vitamins A, C, riboflavin)
	Some trace chemical excess or deficiency (e.g., zinc)
Genetic	
One rare autosomal condition with 100% risk; tylosis	

missed; witness the 100% risk of esophageal cancer in tylosis.

MORPHOLOGY. Periodic cytologic screenings in high-risk locales have revealed that a long prodrome of mucosal epithelial dysplasia, atypical dysplasia, and finally carcinoma in situ precedes the appearance of overt tumors. In the United States and most other low-risk regions, the tumors are not identified until they are relatively advanced. They then typically take one of three forms: (1) polypoid fungating masses that protrude into the lumen, (2) necrotizing cancerous ulcerations that extend deeply and sometimes (about 10%) erode into the respiratory tree, aorta, or elsewhere, or (3) diffuse infiltrative neoplasms that cause thickening and rigidity of the wall with narrowing of the lumen (Fig. 15-6). Whichever the pattern, about 20% arise in the cervical and upper thoracic esophagus, 50% in the middle third, and 30% in the lower third. As noted earlier, at least 95% are squamous cell carcinomas, ranging from well-differentiated keratinizing lesions to very anaplastic undifferentiated patterns. Characteristically these cancers tend to extend locally rather than metastasizing early. Complete excision is therefore uncommon, and indeed obvious residual neoplasm is perforce left behind in more than a third of resected cases. Eventually they spread to lymph nodes, lungs, and liver in the majority of cases.

The remaining 5% of malignant neoplasms of the esophagus are mostly **adenocarcinomas arising in a Barrett's esophagus;** however, some distal adenocarcinomas are of gastric origin and directly invade the esophagus. On gross inspection, these neoplasms cannot be distinguished from squamous cell carcinomas,

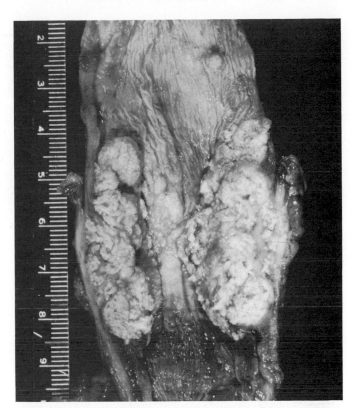

Figure 15-6. Esophageal carcinoma just above the gastroesophageal junction. The fungating mass has been transected anteriorly.

but histologically they reveal usually intestinal type cancerous glands or in a few instances an adenosquamous pattern, representing an admixture of adenocarcinoma and squamous cell carcinoma, either of which may predominate. The patterns of regional and systemic spread are similar to those of squamous cell lesions.

CLINICAL COURSE. Although dysphagia is usually the first manifestation of esophageal carcinoma, it appears late in the course, when the disease is already well-advanced. Weight loss, anorexia, fatigue, and weakness soon appear and are followed by pain, sometimes severe, usually related to swallowing. The diagnosis is usually made by imaging techniques and endoscopic biopsy. Regrettably, even after all modalities of therapy currently available have been employed, only about 3% of patients survive two years. Thus, there is emphasis on routine screening procedures, particularly in those with manifestations of chronic esophagitis and Barrett's esophagus. Repeated endoscopic biopsies are recommended to detect the appearance of dysplasia in the mucosal epithelium in the hope of discovering cancerous transformation at a stage when it is still resectable.

Stomach

Gastric lesions are frequent causes of clinical disease. They range from transient attacks of acute gastritis to anything but transient gastric carcinomas. Between these extremes fall the very common peptic ulcer and a few other lesions.

PYLORIC STENOSIS

This condition appears in two settings:
- In infants within the first month of life as an apparent polygenic familial disorder that affects males three to four times more often than females.
- Rarely in adults, possibly secondary to local disease such as a pyloric ulcer, prolonged pyloric spasm, or underlying pyloric carcinoma, but sometimes in the absence of any antecedent condition raising the possibility of the delayed appearance of the childhood pattern.

In both settings there is marked muscular hypertrophy of the pylorus with thickening of the wall creating a sausage-shaped mass that is readily palpable in the infant. Mucosal edema with submucosal lymphocytic infiltration further narrows the pyloric canal.

These changes typically produce persistent, projectile, nonbilious vomiting in infants and similar but less striking manifestations in adults. Surgical muscle splitting is curative.

GASTRITIS

This diagnosis is both overused and often missed; overused when it is applied loosely to any transient upper abdominal complaint in the absence of any validating clinical or anatomic evidence, and often missed because most patients with chronic gastritis are asymptomatic. Although there are numerous clinical subvarieties of gastritis, here they are simply divided into acute (erosive or hemorrhagic) and chronic (nonerosive) gastritis. There are in addition a few uncommon specific patterns, one of which will be mentioned later. These subsets of gastritis and some common associations are cited in Table 15–3.

ACUTE (EROSIVE OR HEMORRHAGIC) GASTRITIS

This diagnosis can be firmly established only by a combination of endoscopic observations and histologic evaluation of biopsy specimens. Although mucosal erosions and hemorrhages are frequently visible to the endoscopist, acute gastritis may exist in an earlier or milder nonerosive form with merely mucosal congestion and edema and histologic evidence of inflammation. The early changes are transient and completely

TABLE 15–3. TYPES OF GASTRITIS AND THEIR MAJOR ASSOCIATIONS*

Acute (erosive/hemorrhagic) gastritis
  NSAIDs esp. aspirin
  Alcohol abuse
  Low-flow states (shock)
  Stress, including illness, trauma, emotional problems
  Cigarette smoking
  Uremia
  Toxic substances (e.g., staphylococcal food poisoning, suicidal agents such as acids, alkalis)
  Radiation
  ?Helicobacter (formerly Campylobacter) pylori
Chronic (nonerosive)
  Aging
  H. pylori
  Autoantibodies (pernicious anemia)
  Idiopathic
  ?Peptic ulcer
Specific forms of gastritis
  Menetrier's disease
  Crohn's disease
  Others

* From Weinstein, W.M.: Gastritis. In Sleisenger, M.H., Fordtran, J.S. (eds.): Gastrointestinal Disease; Pathophysiology, Diagnosis, Management. 4th ed. Philadelphia, W.B. Saunders, 1989, p. 793.

reversible within a few days, but the development of erosions and hemorrhages is more serious and sometimes causes major upper gastrointestinal bleeding or leads to stress ulcerations (described later) or even death.

PATHOGENESIS. The following factors are important to the development of erosive or hemorrhagic gastritis:
- Luminal acid and pepsin are requisite.
- Increased mucosal tissue acidosis with subsequent decreased secretion of bicarbonate (the alkaline "tide")
- Reduced mucosal blood flow, whatever its basis (shock, drugs, stress), causing hypoxic injury and impairing the secretion of bicarbonate
- Disruption of the so-called mucosal barrier (i.e., the intact layer of surface mucosal epithelial cells), permitting back-diffusion of hydrogen ions and, in turn, increased shedding of surface cells. In this manner deeper layers are exposed with the potential of ulceration.

How the various associations mentioned in the previous table interact with these pathogenic influences is not always clear. Long-term use of nonsteroidal antiinflammatory drugs (NSAIDs), particularly aspirin, may damage cell junctions, permitting back-diffusion of hydrogen ions and increasing surface shedding. At the same time, aspirin and other NSAIDs inhibit cyclooxygenase and could reduce mucosal secretion of various prostaglandins thought to have "cytoprotective" effects. In experimental models, alcohol causes injury to the mucosal microvessels, thereby producing hemorrhage and potential ischemic injury. Stress may induce autonomic vasoconstriction of the mucosal blood supply. Analogously, the nicotine in cigarette smoke may lead to acute gastritis by vasoconstrictive actions. *Helicobacter pylori* is strongly associated with certain forms of chronic gastritis. Whether this organism has a causal role in acute gastritis remains unknown, but it has been shown that two healthy volunteers developed acute gastritis soon after ingesting *H. pylori* (Fig. 15-7). Much is speculative or unknown, hence the numerous cases of so-called idiopathic or incidental acute gastritis.

MORPHOLOGY. There is a spectrum of severity ranging from localized (most often involving the acid-secreting mucosa of the fundus and body) to diffuse, and from superficial inflammation not associated with significant hemorrhage or erosions to transmural involvement frequently accompanied by focal erosions and hemorrhages. All variants are marked by mucosal and sometimes submucosal hyperemia, edema, and an inflammatory infiltrate of lymphocytes, macrophages, and occasionally neutrophils. The acute erosive lesions are but one step removed from stress ulcers, to be described. Between the erosions there may be regeneration in the form of basophilic, flattened, cuboidal epithelium devoid of mucus secretion. Indeed, acute gastritis under appropriate circumstances may disappear within days with complete restitution of the normal mucosa.

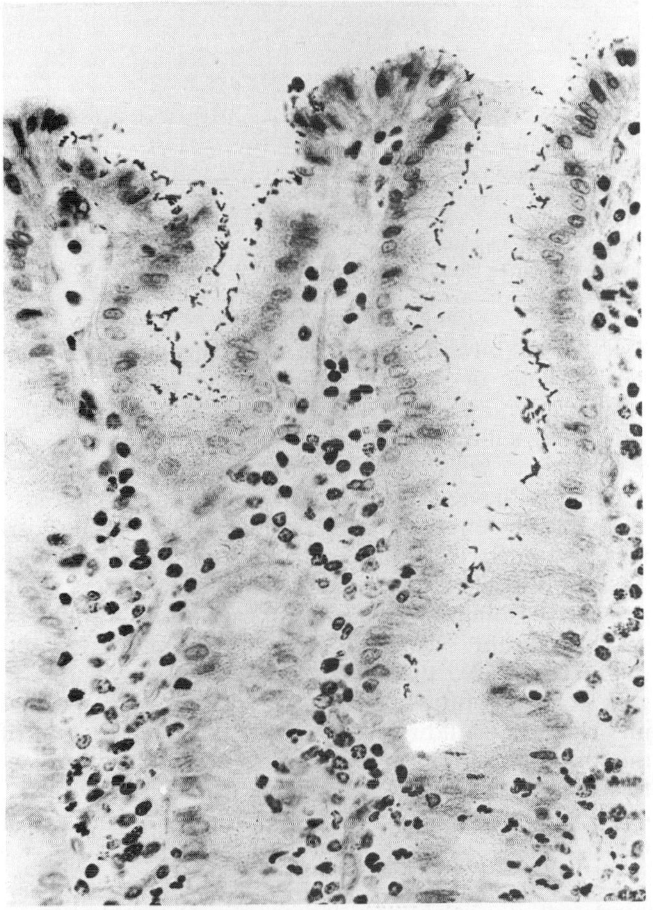

CLINICAL COURSE. Depending on the severity of the anatomic changes, acute gastritis may be entirely asymptomatic, may cause variable epigastric pain, nausea, and vomiting, or with overt hemorrhagic erosive changes may be responsible for massive hematemesis and potentially fatal blood loss. Overall it is one of the major causes of massive hematemesis. In particular settings, the condition is quite common. As many as 25% of persons who take regular aspirin daily for rheumatoid arthritis developed acute gastritis, many with bleeding.

CHRONIC (NONEROSIVE) GASTRITIS _____

Chronic gastritis is characterized by the absence of grossly visible mucosal erosions and by chronic inflammatory changes leading eventually to mucosal (gastric) atrophy and possibly atypical metaplasia. The epithelial changes may become dysplastic and possibly be transformed into carcinoma. Although usually asymptomatic, chronic gastritis has many important associations, mainly pernicious anemia, gastric and duodenal ulcer, as well as gastric carcinoma. Each of these conditions relates to a particular variant of chronic gastritis:

- Type A gastritis, related to pernicious anemia, involves mainly the fundus and body of the stomach and is an autoimmune disease.
- Type B gastritis (much more common than type A) is of nonimmune origin and has been further subdivided:

(1) "Hypersecretory" antral gastritis, with its elevated levels of gastric acid and pepsin, is related to duodenal ulcer disease. About 90% of persons with a duodenal ulcer have antral gastritis.

(2) "Environmental" gastritis, which is multifocal (type AB) and often involves multiple regions of the stomach, is associated with gastric ulcer, atypical metaplasia, and carcinoma. About 75% of persons with a gastric ulcer have this pattern of gastritis.

PATHOGENESIS. The fundal (type A) variant associated with pernicious anemia is clearly autoimmune in origin, as is discussed on page 348. The type B gastritis, sometimes involving only the antrum or in other instances being more generalized, is likely to be of multifactorial origin, but many experts accord *H. pylori* the major role. Colonization with *H. pylori* is common in the general population, and its increasing prevalence with age could explain the increased prevalence of chronic gastritis in the elderly. *H. pylori* organisms are present in about 90% of cases of chronic

Figure 15-7. *Helicobacter* gastritis. A Warthin-Starry stain showing large numbers of *Helicobacter* organisms along the luminal surface of the gastric epithelial cells. Note that no tissue invasion is present. (Courtesy of Drs. Yogeshwar Dayal and Ronald DeLellis, New England Medical Center, Boston, MA.)

gastritis. They are restricted to the surface mucus layer secreted by the mucosal epithelial cells and do not invade cells or tissue. They thrive best at pH levels considerably above those encountered in the gastric lumen but are presumably partially protected from the high levels of gastric acid by being buried within the mucus layer, and by their elaboration of an enzyme urease with the release of ammonia, which buffers the acidity in their microenvironment. In a study of asymptomatic persons, all those who had *H. pylori* infection had gastritis. Type AB, so-called environmental gastritis, probably has much the same origins as type B. Very likely it is multifactorial in origin, aging and *H. pylori* providing a "substrate" on which other pathogenic influences may act, such as chronic alcohol abuse, cigarette smoking, reflux of biliary secretions into the stomach (particularly associated with the postgastrectomy state), and the chronic use of NSAIDs. Recurrent attacks of acute gastritis are *not* accorded any causal importance.

> **MORPHOLOGY.** Regardless of the regional distribution of the chronic gastritis, the chronic inflammatory changes may be limited to the superficial zone or may extend throughout the mucosa. With more severe involvements, the inflammation is accompanied by variable gland loss and mucosal atrophy **(atrophic gastritis).** In the fundic type A autoimmune variant, there is particularly prominent loss of parietal cells, owing to antibodies targeted on these cells and intrinsic factor. Notably, there are no erosions in any form of chronic gastritis, but the surface epithelium may undergo intestinal metaplasia and in some instances atypical metaplasia, accounting presumably for the increased incidence of gastric carcinoma among these persons.

CLINICAL COURSE. Chronic (nonerosive) gastritis usually causes few symptoms related directly to the gastric changes, (i.e., nausea, vomiting, and upper abdominal discomfort are uncommon). However, the loss of parietal cells and their production of intrinsic factor blocks the absorption of vitamin B_{12}, inducing pernicious anemia (p. 348). Most important is the relationship of chronic gastritis to the development of peptic ulcer and gastric carcinoma. It suffices here that most patients with a peptic ulcer, whether duodenal or gastric, have gastritis that persists after the ulcer heals, suggesting that the gastritis is primary. The long-term risk of gastric carcinoma for persons with gastric atrophy is in the range of 2 to 4%.

STRESS ULCERS ——————————

About 10 to 20% of patients admitted to hospital intensive care units acutely develop superficial gastric mucosal erosions, referred to as stress ulcers. They are more likely to appear in the following settings.

- Severe trauma including major surgical procedures, serious sepsis, or grave illness of any type

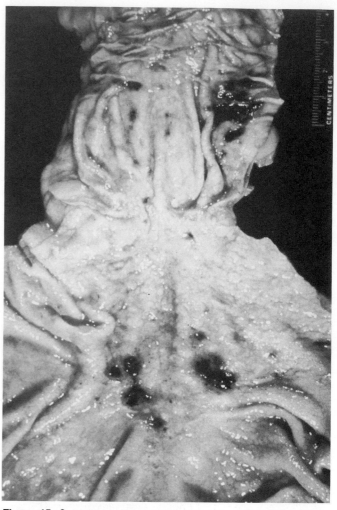

Figure 15-8. Multiple stress ulcers of the stomach, highlighted by the dark digested blood in their bases.

- Extensive burns (referred to as Curling's ulcers)
- Traumatic or surgical injury to the central nervous system or an intracerebral hemorrhage (also called Cushing's ulcers)
- Long-term use of gastric irritant drugs, the worst offenders being aspirin, NSAIDs, and corticosteroids.

The pathogenesis of these mucosal lesions is uncertain and may well vary with the setting. Only with Cushing's ulcers is there hypersecretion of gastric acid-pepsin, so some contend that these lesions should be set apart from "stress ulcers." In the remaining settings, the favored theory is splanchnic vasoconstriction with reduced mucosal perfusion causing mucosal injury directly or indirectly by impairing the secretion of the protective mucus layer or so-called "cytoprotective" prostaglandins (PGs, see page 484). Many of the implicated drugs may act by blocking the synthesis of PGs.

> Typically, stress ulcers are small, round to ovoid, sometimes irregular, mucosal defects that initially involve only the proximal portion of the gastric mucosa but then may

extend throughout the entire stomach. **They rarely exceed 2.5 cm in diameter, usually have a brown base of digested blood, and only exceptionally penetrate more deeply than the muscularis mucosa** (Fig. 15–8). Histologically, the lesions appear to result from enzymatic digestion with only a mild to moderate inflammatory infiltration. In some cases, particularly in association with burns and head lesions, stress ulcers may extend into the duodenum and in this location are more likely to be deep or penetrating.

Most often stress ulcers are totally silent and come to clinical attention only when they cause bleeding, which is sometimes massive and then carries more than a 50% risk of death. Much attention, therefore, has been directed at preventing their development in patients at risk, by such means as the administration of antacids and hydrogen receptor antagonists.

PEPTIC ULCER

Put most simply, *a peptic ulcer can be defined as a "hole in the mucosa" of any portion of the gastrointestinal tract exposed to acid-pepsin secretion*. Both the acid and the pepsin are critical. The definition should be further qualified as noted in Table 15–4.

At least 98% of peptic ulcers are located either in the first portion of the duodenum or in the stomach in a ratio of about 4:1. Although the great majority of individuals have a single ulcer, occasionally, particularly in certain families and in the Zollinger-Ellison syndrome, there are concurrent ulcers in the stomach and duodenum. Despite a remarkably uniform morphology, gastric ulcers (GU) and duodenal ulcers (DU) may well constitute different diseases, as will become apparent.

EPIDEMIOLOGY. It is difficult to provide accurate data on the frequency of peptic ulcers because they are remitting, relapsing lesions that generally first appear in middle to later life, usually heal with or without

TABLE 15–4. DISTINCTIVE FEATURES OF PEPTIC ULCER

Usually a single lesion
Tends to be a small mucosal defect (less than 4 cm diameter)
Almost always penetrates the muscularis mucosa and may perforate the wall
Is frequently recurrent (although may heal)
Is located in the following sites, in descending order of frequency:
 1. Duodenum, first portion
 2. Stomach, usually antrum
 3. Within a Barrett's esophagus (p. 482)
 4. In the margins of a gastroenterostomy (stomal ulcer)
 5. In the duodenum, stomach, or jejunum in patients with Zollinger-Ellison syndrome (p. 580)
 6. Within a Meckel's diverticulum that contains ectopic gastric mucosa

therapy, and frequently recur at some later date (once an ulcer patient, always an ulcer patient). Best estimates suggest that in the American population about 2% of males and 1.5% of females have peptic ulcers. In terms of a lifetime, American males have about a 10% chance of having a peptic ulcer, and females about a 5% chance. For unknown reasons, there has been a significant decrease in the prevalence of DUs over the past decades but little change in the prevalence of GUs. No significant racial differences have been identified.

There are hints of genetic susceptibility to DU but not to GU. Twenty to forty per cent of DU patients have a positive family history, and there is a 50% concordance in monozygotic twins as compared to 14% in dizygotic twins. There are in addition rare familial syndromes associated with DU, such as the autosomal dominant hyperpepsinogenemia I. Persons with blood group O have a 30% greater risk for DU than those who have other blood groups. The capacity to secrete mucopolysaccharide blood group substances into salivary and gastrointestinal secretions is an inherited trait. Nonsecreters are 50% more prone to DUs than are secreters. None of these influences relates to GU.

Acquired disease may also predispose to DU: alcoholic cirrhosis, chronic obstructive pulmonary disease, chronic renal failure, hyperparathyroidism. The only basis for these associations relates to hyperparathyroidism; hypercalcemia, whatever its cause, stimulates gastrin secretion and therefore acid secretion.

PATHOGENESIS. The more writing about a problem, the less is understood. Reams are devoted to the pathogenesis of peptic ulceration, but we are left only with the generalization that *peptic ulcers must be produced by some imbalance between the gastroduodenal mucosal defensive and aggressive forces, cited in Table 15–5*. It is more remarkable that the stomach does not entirely digest itself; consider what happens to a swallowed piece of meat.

Incorporation of the many countervailing influences into a unifying theory is impossible because pieces are still missing from the puzzle. Moreover, there may be subsets of peptic ulcers and many pathways may be involved. Certainly there are differences between DU and GU.

Gastric acid and pepsin are requisite for all peptic ulcerations. The importance of the acid is evidenced by the Zollinger-Ellison syndrome (p. 580) with its multiple peptic ulcerations owing to excess gastrin and acid production. Nonetheless, as indicated earlier, only a minority of patients with DU have hyperacidity and only very few with GU. The basis for the hyperacidity, when present, is not always clear, but possible causes are increased parietal cell mass, increased sensitivity to secretory stimuli, increased basal acid secretory drive, or impaired inhibition of stimulatory mechanisms such as gastrin release. In some patients with DU there is too rapid gastric emptying, exposing the duodenal mucosa to an excessive acid load.

In addition to the clear-cut erosiveness of acid and pepsin, *H. pylori is strongly suspected of playing some*

TABLE 15–5. MAJOR FACTORS IN THE PATHOGENESIS OF PEPTIC ULCERS

Defensive Forces	Aggressive Forces
• Secretion of a surface mucus layer by epithelial cells	• Acid secretion, but only about a third of patients with DU secrete excess acid and hyperacidity is not a feature of GU; nonetheless, "No acid—no ulcer."
• Secretion of bicarbonate into the mucus layer, thus producing a pH gradient from the highly acidic gastric lumen to the almost neutral mucosal surface	• Peptic activity derived from pepsinogen is critical to ulcer production, but hypersecretion is not requisite.
• The specialized apical surface of the gastric mucosal cells that protects against diffusion of H$^+$ ions into the mucosa	• *Helicobacter* (formerly *Campylobacter*) *pylori* infection of the gastric antrum is generally viewed as important (but there are doubters).
• A remarkable regenerative capacity of mucosal epithelial cells for rapid repair of injuries	• NSAIDs may be ulcerogenic. The risk has been estimated to be about 2 to 4% per patient-year. Aspirin (time-dose dependent) is the worst offender, but a variety of other NSAIDs have also been implicated.
• Mucosal elaboration of prostaglandins having "cytoprotective" activity, possibly by maintaining adequate mucosal blood flow and by stimulating secretion of mucus and bicarbonate	• Impaired inhibition of stimulatory mechanisms such as gastrin release

role. The organisms remain attached to the mucus layer and do not penetrate mucosal epithelial cells and no cytodestructive toxins have been identified. Nonetheless, *H. pylori* has been identified in the antrum of more than 90% of patients with DU and some lesser number of those with GU. In most instances there is an associated antral—or sometimes more diffuse—gastritis. The gastritis persists after the peptic ulcers have healed, implying that it is the primary lesion. Could the organism be responsible for the gastritis predisposing the inflamed mucosa to other ulcerogenic influences? The minority of patients who do not have *H. pylori* infection often are habitual users of aspirin or other NSAIDs.

Impaired mucosal defense must be invoked to explain why some persons with normal levels of gastric acid and pepsin and no *H. pylori* infection develop an ulcer; however, no specific defects such as impaired secretion of mucus or bicarbonate or reduced mucosal blood flow can be clearly identified in ulcer subjects. Only with the use of NSAIDs and suppression of prostaglandin synthesis can a finger be pointed with some assurance. Yet one of the effective modalities of treating peptic ulcers enhances mucus secretion, emphasizing the importance of defensive mechanisms.

Other possible ulcerogenic influences require mention. *Cigarette smoking* impairs healing and favors recurrence and so is suspected of being ulcerogenic. *Alcohol* has not been proved to directly cause peptic ulceration, but it certainly is responsible for alcoholic

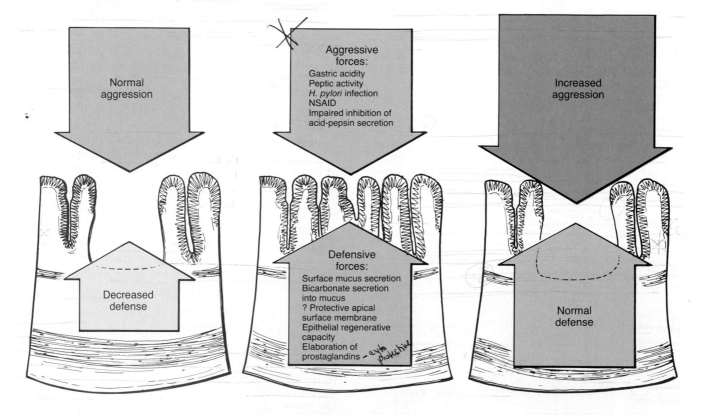

Figure 15–9. Peptic ulcer. A schematic representation of the imbalance in the defensive and aggressive forces thought to underlie the genesis of these lesions.

cirrhosis, in turn associated with an increased incidence of ulcer disease. *Corticosteroids* in high dose and with protracted use have been reported to increase the risk of ulcerogenesis, but the evidence is open to challenge. Finally, there is a widespread belief that *psychologic stress* is an important contributing factor: while it may activate or enhance symptoms, hard data on cause and effect are lacking. It is clear that there is still great uncertainty about the origins of peptic ulcers (Fig. 15–9).

MORPHOLOGY. All peptic ulcers, whether gastric or duodenal, have a basically identical gross and microscopic appearance. **They are usually round, sharply punched out defects in the mucosa that penetrate at least into the submucosa, usually into the muscularis and sometimes more deeply.** Most are 2 to 4 cm in diameter; those in the duodenum tend to be smaller, and occasional gastric lesions significantly larger. Favored sites are the anterior and posterior walls of the first portion of the duodenum and the lesser curvature of the stomach. The location within the stomach is dictated by the extent of the associated gastritis. Usually it involves the entire antrum with the ulcer crater in the margin of the affected area close to the adjacent acid-secreting fundic mucosa, but it may be more proximal or distal. Occasional gastric ulcers occur on the greater curvature or anterior or posterior walls of the

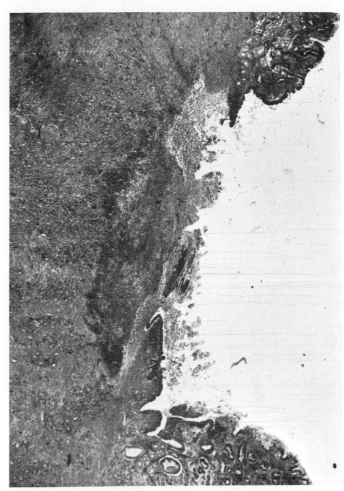

Figure 15–11. A low-power view of a peptic ulcer, illustrating the depth of the lesion.

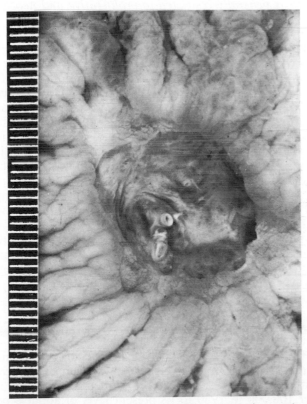

Figure 15–10. A gastric peptic ulcer. The crater has a maximum diameter of about 2 cm, is sharply punched out and has a deceptively clean base and an eroded, almost transected artery protruding from it. Note the radiating mucosal folds.

stomach, the very same locations of most ulcerative cancers.

Classically, **the margins of the crater are perpendicular and there is some mild edema of the immediately adjacent mucosa, but no significant elevation or beading of the edges (features of ulcerative cancer; (Fig. 15–10).** The surrounding mucosal folds tend to radiate as wheel spokes. The base of the crater appears remarkably clean owing to peptic digestion of the inflammatory exudate and necrotic tissue. Infrequently, an eroded artery is visible in the ulcer (usually associated with a history of significant bleeding); the crater penetrates through the duodenal or gastric wall to produce a localized or generalized peritonitis; or the perforation is sealed by some structure such as adherent omentum, liver, or pancreas.

The histologic appearance varies with the activity, chronicity, and degree of healing. During the active phase, four zones can be distinguished: (1) the base and margins have a thin layer of necrotic fibrinoid debris underlain by (2) a zone of active nonspecific inflammatory infiltration with neutrophils predominating, underlain by (3) active granulation tissue, deep to which is (4) fibrous, collagenous scar that fans out widely from the margins of the ulcer (Fig. 15–11). Vessels trapped within the scarred area are characteristically thickened and occasionally thrombosed, but in some instances they are widely patent. In GU the surrounding mucosa typically shows chronic atrophic gastritis, and often there is intestinal metaplasia of the glands.

Both gastric and duodenal ulcers may heal. First the crater fills with granulation tissue, followed by reepithelialization from the margins and eventually more or less restoration of the normal architecture. Extensive fibrous scarring hampers the reparative process.

CLINICAL COURSE. The great majority of peptic ulcers cause epigastric gnawing, burning, or boring pain, but a significant minority first come to light with complications such as hemorrhage or perforation. The pain tends to be worse at night and occurs usually one to three hours after meals during the day. Classically, the pain is relieved by alkalis or food, but there are many exceptions. Nausea, vomiting, bloating, belching, and significant weight loss (raising the specter of some hidden malignancy) are additional manifestations. Occasionally with penetrating ulcers the pain is referred to the back, the left upper quadrant, or chest, and it may be misinterpreted as being of cardiac origin.

The diagnosis rests ultimately on various imaging techniques and endoscopy. Collectively these methods can accurately detect and diagnose more than 98% of peptic ulcers. Gastric analyses for acidity, endoscopic biopsy, and cytologic examinations of gastric aspirate or brushings may be necessary in rare instances to differentiate a benign gastric peptic ulcer from an ulcerative gastric carcinoma.

The complications of peptic ulcer disease are shown in Table 15–6. Malignant transformation is unknown with duodenal ulcers and is extremely rare with gastric ulcers and always open to the possibility that the seemingly benign lesion was from the outset a deceptive, ulcerative, gastric carcinoma.

Peptic ulcers are notably chronic recurring lesions. They more often impair the quality of life than shorten it; however, with present-day effective therapies aimed at neutralization of gastric acid, promotion of mucus secretion, and inhibition of acid secretion (H_2 receptor antagonists and parietal cells' ATPase inhibitors) most ulcer victims escape the surgeon's knife and die of unrelated conditions with their entrails intact.

TUMORS

A wide variety of mesenchymal neoplasms, such as stromal cell tumors, leiomyomas, leiomyoblastomas, neurofibromas, and lipomas as well as their malignant counterparts may arise in the stomach but are all too rare for inclusion here. Also, carcinoids are sometimes primary tumors in the stomach. Because these neoplasms are identical to those in the intestines, where they are more frequent, they are described in a later section (p. 517). Only polyps, gastric carcinoma, and gastrointestinal lymphomas remain for our present consideration.

GASTRIC POLYPS

The term "polyp" is applied to any nodule or mass that projects above the level of the surrounding mucosa. Occasionally, a lipoma or leiomyoma arising in the wall of the stomach may protrude beneath the mucosa to produce an apparent polypoid lesion. However, *the use of the term "polyp" in the gastrointestinal tract is generally restricted to proliferative and neoplastic lesions arising in the mucosal epithelium*. Gastric polyps are uncommon and are found in 0.4% of routine autopsies, as compared with colonic polyps, which are seen in 25 to 50% of older persons. *In the stomach, these lesions can be divided into: (1) hyperplastic polyps (80%) and (2) adenomatous polyps (20%).* They are most frequent in elders and are associated with achlorhydria and atrophic gastritis; therefore, they are reported in 5% of all patients with pernicious anemia. The essential features of these lesions are given in Table 15–7. From the clinical viewpoint, the likelihood of carcinoma in an adenomatous polyp is correlated with its size and irregularity of contour. Often the stomach harboring a polyp contains a separate carcinoma that may have arisen from a polyp or from an area of chronic atrophic gastritis, which is commonly found in these cases. Multiple polyps are seen in familial adenomatous polyposis and Peutz-Jeghers and Gardner's syndromes (p. 513).

GASTRIC CARCINOMA

This form of neoplasia is a challenge on many scores. For no apparent reason the incidence of gastric carcinoma has declined in the United States from 33 per 100,000 in 1930 to its present level of about 6 per 100,000. Yet it remains among the leading killer cancers, in some large part because the overall five-year survival rate is less than 10%, a rate that has not

TABLE 15–6. COMPLICATIONS OF PEPTIC ULCER DISEASE

Bleeding
  Occurs in 25 to 33% of patients
  Most frequent complication; may be massive
  Accounts for about 25% of ulcer deaths
  May be first indication of presence of ulcer
Perforation
  Occurs in only 5% of patients
  Accounts for two thirds of all ulcer deaths
  Rarely, is first indication of ulcer
Obstruction from edema or scarring of pyloric canal or duodenum
  Causes incapacitating, crampy abdominal pain
  Rarely, may lead to total obstruction with intractable vomiting
Intractable pain

TABLE 15-7. COMPARISON OF HYPERPLASTIC AND ADENOMATOUS GASTRIC POLYPS

Hyperplastic (80%)	Adenomatous (20%)
May be single, often multiple	Usually single, but sometimes multiple
Soft, pink, nipple-shaped	Have raspberry-like head or appear verrucose and corrugated; may be sessile or pedunculated
Usually less than 1 cm in diameter; rarely exceed 2 cm in diameter	May be small, but often exceed 4 cm in diameter
Composed of hyperplastic, sometimes cystic, glands lined by normal epithelium resembling that found in surrounding normal gastric pits	Epithelium ranges from well-differentiated, benign-appearing neoplastic cells to poorly differentiated cells with hyperchromatic, overly large nuclei; frequent mitotic figures
Intervening stroma usually contains a chronic inflammatory infiltrate	Wide reported range (average 40%) malignant transformation
Low (0.5%) malignant potential	

TABLE 15-8. MAJOR FEATURES OF LAURENS' CLASSIFICATION OF ADVANCED GASTRIC CARCINOMA*

Feature	Intestinal	Diffuse
Major gross configurations	Polypoid; fungating	Ulcerative; infiltrating
Microscopic features		
Differentiation	Well-differentiated: papillary or solid	Poorly differentiated: signet ring cells
Mucin production	Limited; confined to gland lumens	Extensive: frequently prominent in stroma around glands ("colloid" carcinoma)
Growth pattern	Expansile: inflammation often prominent	Noncohesive
Associated intestinal metaplasia	Almost universal	Less frequent
Clinical features		
Mean age (years)	55	48
Sex ratio (M:F)	2:1	~1:1
Associated with decreasing incidence in Western countries	Yes	No
Three-year survival rate (cases operated upon for potential cure)	43%	35%

*From Antonioli, D.A.: Gastric carcinoma and its precursors. Monogr. Pathol. 31:144, 1990.

changed over the past 50 years. Moreover, there are puzzling geographic differences in this tumor. It is much more common in such countries as Colombia, Costa Rica, Hungary, and Japan than in the United States. In 1981 it became the leading cause of cancer death in Japan. Even more puzzling is that the incidence of certain patterns of gastric carcinoma have declined while others have not.

Some time ago this form of neoplasia was divided by Laurens into intestinal and diffuse morphologic types (Table 15-8). The intestinal variant is thought to arise from gastric mucous cells that have undergone metaplasia into intestinal type cells. This pattern of cancer tends to be better differentiated, is the more common type in high-risk populations, and is the pattern that is progressively diminishing in frequency in the United States. In contrast, the diffuse variant is thought to arise de novo from native gastric mucous cells, tends to be poorly differentiated, and is becoming comparatively more common in the United States. Whereas the intestinal type carcinoma occurs primarily after age 50 years in 2:1 male predominance, the diffuse lesion occurs at an earlier age with no male predominance. It would almost appear that there are two quite disparate forms of gastric cancer.

PATHOGENESIS. The major factors thought to affect the genesis of this form of cancer are summarized in Table 15-9.

Environmental influences are thought to be most important. When families migrate from high-risk to low-risk areas (or the reverse), successive generations acquire the level of risk that prevails in the new locales. The diet is suspected to be the likely offender, and particularly the potential for the formation of

TABLE 15-9. FACTORS THAT MAY AFFECT THE DEVELOPMENT OF GASTRIC CARCINOMA

Diet
Nitrites derived from nitrates (found in food, drinking water, and used as preservatives in prepared meats) may undergo nitrosation to form nitrosamines and nitrosamides known to be carcinogenic in laboratory animals.
Smoked foods and pickled vegetables are associated with an increased incidence.
Fresh vegetables, citrus fruits (vitamin C) decrease the risk, possibly by inhibiting nitrosation.

Genetic Influences
Blood group A slightly increases risk.
Close relatives (e.g., siblings of a patient) have an above average attack rate.

Predisposing Conditions
Chronic atrophic gastritis is often associated with intestinal metaplasia and dysplasia with increased risk. The attendant hypochlorhydria favors gastric colonization by nitrite-forming bacteria permitting increased formation of nitrosamines.
Pernicious anemia, because of its associated chronic atrophic gastritis.
Gastric adenomatous polyps substantially increase the risk (p. 490).

nitroso compounds (lack of refrigeration, common use of nitrite preservatives, contaminated water with a high nitrate content, and lack of fresh fruit and vegetables). Significantly, the altered risk results from a change in the incidence of the intestinal type of gastric carcinoma that is often referred to as the environmental form.

MORPHOLOGY. Strenuous efforts by Japanese endoscopists to discover gastric carcinomas at a more curable stage has led to the identification of so-called **early gastric carcinoma (EGC). EGC constitutes a lesion confined to the mucosa and submucosa, regardless of the presence or absence of perigastric lymph node metastases.** EGC is not synonymous with carcinoma in situ. Despite the possible presence of nodal metastasis, the mean five-year survival rate for EGC after surgery is over 90%. In Japan roughly a third of gastric carcinomas are classified as EGC. They occur anywhere in the stomach, vary greatly in size, may exceed 10 cm in diameter, and range from exophytic lesions that protrude into the gastric lumen to slightly elevated, flat or depressed lesions, to shallow ulcerative craters with slightly heaped-up margins. They display the same histologic patterns found in the more advanced tumors. Whether EGC is merely an early stage of advanced gastric carcinoma or a special subset is still uncertain, but present evidence favors the former.

Advanced gastric carcinoma (AGC) is a neoplasm that has extended below the submucosa, into the muscularis, and has perhaps spread more widely. In the United States and most Western countries most lesions are, unfortunately, AGC. Most arise in the gastric antrum, but some more proximally, notably in the cardia close to the esophageal junction (about 30 to 40%). They have been variously subclassified, but **the two most important variants, as noted earlier, are the intestinal type and the diffuse type.** The former usually appear exophytic, fungating, or sometimes polypoid. The latter tend to be ulcerative tumors with irregular craters and heaped-up, beaded margins (Fig. 15–12) or they diffusely infiltrate, smooth out, and flatten the mucosa and cause indurative thickening of the wall **(linitis plastica, leather-bottle stomach).** The cancerous craters can often be differentiated from peptic ulcers by their heaped-up, beaded margins and shaggy, necrotic bases, and generally the underlying overt neoplastic tissue extending into the surrounding wall (Fig. 15–13). Histologically, **the intestinal variant of AGC is composed of characteristic neoplastic glands resembling those of colonic carcinoma, that permeate the wall but grow along broad cohesive fronts and so have also been categorized as having an "expanding growth pattern."** By contrast, the "diffuse" variant derived from gastric mucous cells is not marked by glandular formations but rather by permeation of the wall by scattered individual cells or small clusters (an infiltrative pattern). Mucus secretion often expands the

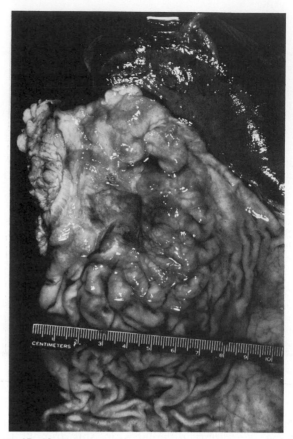

Figure 15–12. Gastric carcinoma, ulcerative pattern. The irregular ulcer crater is situated high in the fundus and has penetrated into the adjacent spleen, which can be seen above it. Note the beaded margins of the ulcer crater and the irregular base.

cells and pushes the nucleus to the periphery, creating signet ring conformations. Often the tumor evokes a strong desmoplastic reaction in which the scattered cells are embedded.

Whatever the variant, all gastric carcinomas eventually penetrate the wall to involve the serosa and then may spread to regional and more distant lymph nodes and elsewhere, notably the liver. Two patterns of spread are particularly distinctive. For obscure reasons, gastric carcinomas frequently metastasize to the supraclavicular sentinel (Virchow's) node as the first clinical manifestation of an occult neoplasm. More uncommonly, these cancers metastasize to one or both ovaries to cause solid tumorous enlargements called Krukenberg tumors (p. 628).

CLINICAL COURSE. EGC is generally asymptomatic and can be discovered only by repeated endoscopic examination of persons at high risk, as is the practice in Japan. Advanced carcinoma may also be asymptomatic, but often first comes to light because of abdominal discomfort or weight loss. Uncommonly, these neoplasms may cause dysphagia when they are located

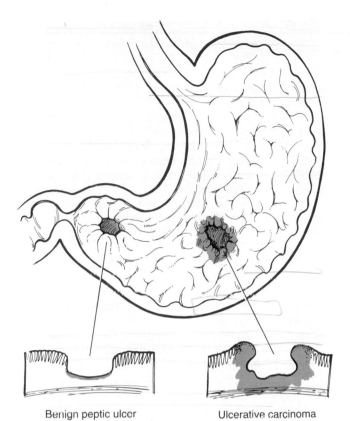

Benign peptic ulcer   Ulcerative carcinoma

Figure 15–13. A schematic comparison of the gross appearance of benign and malignant gastric ulcers. The margins of the benign ulcer are modestly elevated and the mucosal folds radiate spoke-like. The margins of the ulcerative cancer are elevated and beaded, and the crater is enclosed within cancerous tissue.

in the cardia or obstructive symptoms when they arise in the pyloric canal.

The diagnosis is based largely on barium x-ray studies or computed tomography (CT), results of which can be deceptively negative with EGC unless specialized radiographic procedures disclose the mucosal relief. Cytologic methods may be useful but only with positive diagnoses, since negative results do not rule out cancer. Most accurate is gastric endoscopy and adequate biopsy of suspected lesions. EGC yields highly commendable 90% five- and 75% ten-year survival rates, in striking contrast to the dismal outlook (about 10% five-year survival) for advanced lesions.

GASTROINTESTINAL LYMPHOMAS ——————

Unlike Hodgkin's disease, which is almost exclusively a nodal disease, non-Hodgkin's lymphoma (NHL) may sometimes be primary outside of nodes, almost half of which arise in the gastrointestinal tract. Nonetheless, they represent only 1 to 4% of all gastrointestinal neoplasms. More frequently (in more than 50% of patients) systemic nodal NHL in time involves the gastrointestinal tract, but usually such involvement

is multifocal and often primarily affects the mesenteric lymph nodes with extension into the gut. *For lymphomas to qualify as* primary in the gastrointestinal tract *there must be no involvement of nonregional lymph nodes, liver, and spleen, nor radiographic or hematologic evidence of extraintestinal disease.* The peak incidence is in the sixth decade with a much smaller peak in the first decade. The male-female ratio is about 2:1.

In Western countries, the stomach is the primary site (50 to 60%) more often than the small bowel (about 30%), followed by the ileocecal segment and the colon. Wherever they arise they take one of three forms: (1) polypoid masses projecting into the lumen, (2) large elevated plaques often having shaggy necrotic ulcerated craters, or (3) infiltrative neoplasms producing irregular thickening of the wall of the gut. Any one of these three patterns may occur in a single focus, but often they are multicentric, usually in one segment of the gut. The infiltrative pattern in the stomach may cause massive thickening of the rugal folds that closely resembles infiltrative diffuse carcinoma or the rare hypertrophic Menetrier's gastritis (gastropathy).

Histologically, they recapitulate the patterns of NHL arising in lymph nodes described on page 354. More than 80% are B-cell neoplasms and 10% or less are of T-cell origin (p. 000). Over half represent histologically aggressive subgroups, principally diffuse large cell and immunoblastic lymphomas. Most of the remainder include small cleaved cell, mixed large and small cell, and follicular patterns, and a distinctive gut-associated lymphoid tumor lying intermediate between lymphoid reactive hyperplasia and usual lymphoma.

The risk of developing a primary NHL, principally in the small intestine, is significantly increased in patients with a malabsorption disorder (notably celiac disease, regional enteritis) or depressed immune function. Those associated with celiac sprue are most often T-cell lymphomas. AIDS has come to be the major immunodeficiency state associated with the development of NHL, most often primary in the gastrointestinal tract. In the Middle East and many Third World countries, a distinctive form of *immunoproliferative small intestinal disease* (IPSD) occurs particularly in young patients with protracted bacterial and parasitic enteric infections. Whether IPSD is itself malignant or in some cases converts to Mediterranean lymphoma is uncertain, but in either case these lesions tend to have a mixed population of lymphocytes, plasma cells, and plasmacytoid cells, and many are associated with α–heavy chain paraproteinemia.

Recognition of primary gastrointestinal lymphomas is important because combinations of surgery, chemotherapy, and radiotherapy yield in all but AIDS cases 35 to 80% cure rates, depending on the stage at the time of diagnosis and the histologic subtype of the disease.

Small and Large Intestine

Many conditions such as infections, vascular insufficiency, and Crohn's disease affect both levels of the intestines, so it seems prudent and more efficient to consider together the disorders of both the small and large intestine. Collectively these conditions account for a large fraction of gastrointestinal disease.

DEVELOPMENTAL ANOMALIES

On the whole these deviations from the norm are uncommon sources of clinical disease.

In the *small intestine* the major anomalies are as follows:

* *Atresia or stenosis,* the former being complete failure of development of the intestinal lumen and the latter representing only narrowing. Both defects usually involve only a segment of bowel.
* *Duplication* usually takes the form of saccular to long, tubular, cystic structures, which may or may not communicate with the lumen of the small intestine.
* *Meckel's diverticulum* is the most common of the anomalies. It results from failure of complete obliteration of the omphalomesenteric duct, leaving a persistent tubular diverticulum up to 5 to 6 cm long with a variable diameter sometimes approximating that of the small intestine itself. Such diverticula are usually located in the ileum within 85 cm of the cecum and are composed of all layers of the normal small intestine. Rarely, pancreatic rests are found in a Meckel's diverticulum, and in about half of the cases there are heterotopic islands of functioning gastric mucosa. Peptic ulceration in the adjacent intestinal mucosa sometimes is responsible for mysterious intestinal bleeding or symptoms resembling acute appendicitis. Other complications include diverticulitis, perforation with peritonitis, intestinal obstruction secondary to intussusception (p. 519), or diverticular adhesions (Fig. 15–14).
* *Omphalocele* is herniation of intestines into a sac created by a congenital defect in the umbilical region of the abdominal wall.

In the *large intestine* the major anomalies are the following ones:

* *Malrotation* so that the cecum fails to achieve its normal position in the right-side lower quadrant and may be found anywhere back to the splenic flexure. This may predispose to volvulus (p. 519) or to confusing clinical syndromes when acute appendicitis presents with left side upper quadrant pain.
* *Congenital aganglionosis*—Hirschsprung's disease —leading to congenital megacolon (discussed next).

MEGACOLON

Distention of the colon to greater than 6 or 7 cm in diameter (megacolon) occurs as a congenital and as an acquired disorder.

Congenital megacolon (Hirschsprung's disease) results when during development, the caudad migration of cells from the neural crest destined to become the intramural plexuses of the colon arrest at some point before reaching the anus. Hence *an aganglionic segment remains that lacks both Meissner's submucosal and Auerbach's myenteric plexuses, causing in effect functional obstruction and progressive distension of the colon proximal to it.* In most instances, only the rectum and sigmoid are aganglionic, but in about a fifth of cases longer segments, and rarely the entire colon, are affected.

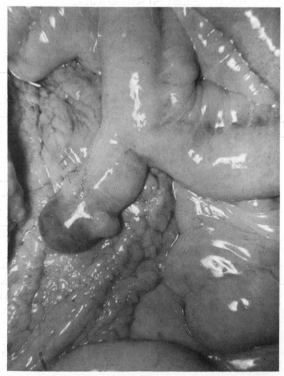

Figure 15–14. Meckel's diverticulitis. The tip of the diverticulum is reddened because of peptic ulceration near a contained rest of gastric epithelium.

Morphologically, the colon may be massively distended, sometimes achieving a diameter of 15 to 20 cm. The wall may be thinned by distension or in some cases be thickened by muscle hypertrophy. The critical lesion is the lack of ganglion cells in the plexuses but this is sometimes accompanied by thickened and hypertrophic nerve fibers highlighted by specific stains for acetylcholinesterase (Fig. 15–15). To be noted, the ganglia are present in the distended colon. The mucosal lining of the distended portion may be intact or have shallow, so-called **stercoral ulcers** produced by impacted, inspissated feces.

Figure 15–15. Megacolon. To the left is seen the congenital form (Hirschsprung's) with its distal aganglionic functional obstruction. On the right the acquired form is depicted with normal innervation; there are various causes for obstruction, most often an intraluminal mass.

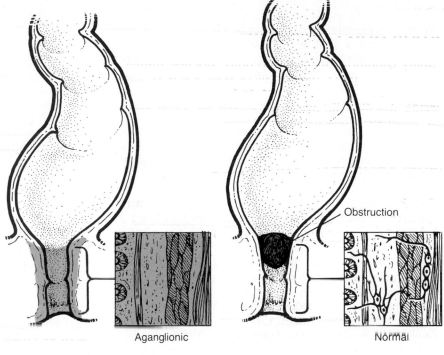

Congenital (Hirschsprung's) megacolon

Acquired megacolon

The precise genetics of this condition have not been worked out but there are some indications of a familial distribution: siblings have a greater incidence of the same condition than controls. There is a high level of concordance in monozygotic but not dizygotic twins. Congenital megacolon is much more frequent in those with Down's syndrome as well as other congenital anomalies such as hydrocephalus, ventricular septal defect, and Meckel's diverticulum.

Clinically, in most cases there is delay in the initial passage of meconium, which is followed by vomiting in 48 to 72 hours. When a very short distal segment of the rectum alone is involved, the obstruction may not be complete and may not produce manifestations until later in infancy, in the form of alternating periods of obstruction and passage of diarrheal stools. The principal threat to life is superimposed enterocolitis with fluid and electrolyte disturbances. More rarely the distended colon perforates, usually in the cecum. The diagnosis is established by the absence of ganglion cells in a biopsy of the mucosa and submucosa of the nondistended bowel, and if necessary a full-thickness biopsy at least 3 cm proximal to the pectinate line. Acquired megacolon may result from: (1) Chagas' disease, in which the trypanosomes directly invade the bowel wall to destroy the plexuses, (2) organic obstruction of the bowel as by a neoplasm or inflammatory stricture, (3) toxic megacolon complicating ulcerative colitis or Crohn's disease, or (4) a functional psychosomatic disorder. Save for the trypanosomal Chagas' disease, where the inflammatory involvement of the ganglia is evident, the remaining forms of megacolon are not associated with any deficiency of mural ganglia.

DIVERTICULA

Diverticula in the small intestine are uncommon save for the Meckel's variety described earlier (p. 494). They generally are small (2 to 3 cm diameter) saccular outpouchings, but when present are asymptomatic save when they permit bacterial overgrowth that depletes vitamin B_{12}, producing a syndrome similar to pernicious anemia. Whether the saccules are of congenital origin or develop slowly over the course of years through points of congenital bowel weakness remains unknown.

Diverticular disease of the colon by contrast is increasingly common with advancing age in Western countries, reaching a frequency of over 50% in the eighth and ninth decades of life. Significantly, this condition is relatively infrequent in native populations of Third World countries. This disparity is attributed to the more refined, low-fiber diet of privileged societies resulting in reduced stool bulk with increased difficulty in passage of intestinal contents. Exaggerated spastic contractions of the colon isolate segments of the colon (segmentation) in which the intraluminal pressure becomes markedly elevated with consequent herniation of the bowel wall through points of weakness, particularly alongside penetrating vessels. The important role of foci of weakness is borne out by the early development of diverticula in individuals with such connective tissue disorders as Marfan's and Ehlers-Danlos syndrome. Thus, two factors are thought to be important in the genesis of these protrusions: (1) foci of muscle weakness in the colonic wall and (2) exaggerated peristaltic contractions with abnormal elevation of intraluminal pressure.

In the past, much was made of the separation of *diverticulosis* from *diverticulitis*. The former term was applied to the presence of diverticula free of inflammatory changes that were assumed to be asymptomatic. Clinical manifestations such as lower abdominal pain were thought to arise only when inflammation developed in and about the diverticula. Although diverticulitis is more likely to be symptomatic and associated with fever and leukocytosis, it may also be silent, and conversely diverticulosis with its increased peristaltic contractions may cause abdominal complaints. Hence the preferred designation today is *diverticular disease* to encompass all forms.

In approximately 95% of patients the diverticula are limited to the sigmoid colon. Infrequently more proximal levels are affected and sometimes the entire colon. The exaggerated peristalsis often induces hypertrophy of the musculature of affected segments. The taenia coli and circular muscle bundles are unusually prominent, and most saccules are found penetrating between the bundles of circular muscle fibers between the mesenteric and lateral taeniae at points where the entering arterioles branch out into the submucosa. They comprise small, flask-like or spherical outpouchings usually 0.5 to 1 cm in diameter that frequently dissect into the appendices epiploicae and may therefore be inapparent on casual inspection (Fig. 15–16). In the uninflamed state the walls are usually very thin, made up largely of mucosa and submucosa enclosed within fat or an intact peritoneal covering (Fig. 15–17). Inflammatory changes may supervene to produce both diverticulitis and peridi-

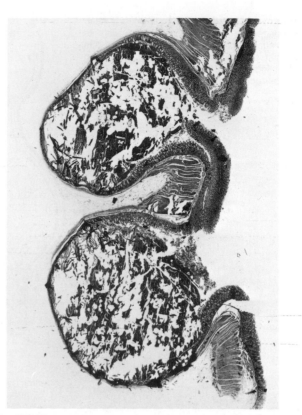

Figure 15–17. Diverticulosis of the colon. A low-power micrograph of two diverticula shows their thin walls and absence of muscular coats. There is no evidence of inflammation, but they are stuffed with fecal matter.

verticulitis, and indeed sometimes perforation leads to localized peritonitis. When multiple closely adjacent diverticula become inflamed, the bowel wall may be enclosed by fibrous tissue with narrowing of the lumen producing a remarkable resemblance to a cancerous stricture.

In the great majority of persons, diverticular disease is asymptomatic and is discovered only at autopsy or by chance during a laparoscopy or barium enema for some other problem. In about only a fifth of the cases does intermittent cramping or sometimes continuous left-side lower quadrant pain or discomfort appear with a sensation of never being able to completely empty the rectum. Superimposed diverticulitis accentuates the symptoms and produces left-side lower quadrant tenderness along with fever. Superimposed complications are uncommon and take the forms of minimal, chronic, or intermittent bleeding or rarely (5 to 10%) brisk hemorrhage, perforation with pericolic abscess, or fistula formation.

The treatment of this condition merits brief mention because it bears on its pathogenesis. Currently a high-fiber diet is recommended on the theory that the increased stool bulk reduces the exaggerated peristalsis as the source of discomfort. Coarse wheat bran is recommended in part because it is extremely effective

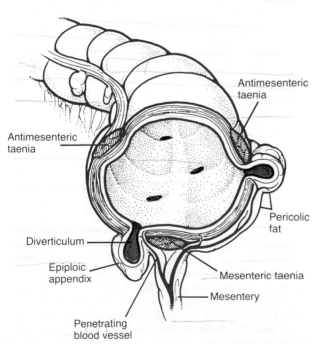

Figure 15–16. Diverticulosis of the colon. The favored locations for the diverticula (beside the taeniae) and the penetrating mesenteric vessels are shown.

in holding fluid and increasing stool bulk, but in greater part because most patients claim to be cured of their disease to avoid being faced with a daily ration of "sawdust."

VASCULAR DISORDERS

ISCHEMIC BOWEL DISEASE

Ischemic lesions may be restricted to the small intestine or to the large intestine or may affect both, depending on the particular vessel(s) affected. The severity of the injury ranges from outright transmural infarction of the gut to ischemic injury of only the most vulnerable mucosa and sometimes also the submucosa, sparing the deep muscularis and serosa. *Almost always, transmural infarction implies embolism or thrombosis of one of the major arteries or veins of the intestines, whereas partial-thickness injury may result from hypoperfusion.*

The three major supply trunks—celiac, superior, and inferior mesenteric arteries—are richly interconnected by arcades. Loss of one may be without effect, so outright infarction almost always requires occlusion of at least two of the major vessels either by thrombosis or embolism, or occlusion of one with marked atherosclerotic narrowing of another. In most large analyses of ischemic bowel disease, thrombosis or embolism of the superior mesenteric artery accounts for about 30% of the cases, venous thrombosis about 10%, nonocclusive hypoperfusion about 30%, and the remainder (usually instances of transmural infarction) remain unexplained either because the occlusive lesion fragmented and was driven out into the periphery or because by the time of exploration it had undergone lysis.

The various predisposing clinical conditions are as follows:

- *Arterial embolism.* Myocardial infarction with mural thrombosis, cardiac vegetations, atrial fibrillation and thrombosis, angiographic procedures, and atheroembolism.
- *Arterial thrombosis.* Severe atherosclerosis usually at the origin of the vessel, systemic vasculitis, dissecting aneurysm, angiographic procedures, aortic reconstructive surgery, hypercoagulable states, and oral contraceptives.
- *Venous thrombosis.* Hypercoagulable states, oral contraceptives, antithrombin III deficiency, intraperitoneal sepsis, invasive neoplasms, and abdominal trauma.
- *Nonocclusive ischemia.* Cardiac failure, shock, dehydration, vasoconstrictor drugs (e.g., digitalis, vasopressin, propranolol).
- *Miscellaneous.* Bowel resection, volvulus, and stricture or hernia.

Transmural intestinal Infarction, also called **gangrene of the bowel, mesenteric thrombosis,** and **ischemic**

enterocolitis, may involve a short or long segment depending on the particular vessel affected and the patency of the anastomotic supply. Whether the occlusion is arterial or venous, the infarction always appears hemorrhagic because of reflow of blood into the damaged area, and within 18 to 24 hours there is obvious subserosal hemorrhage and a thin, fibrinous exudate over the serosa (Fig. 15–18). The ischemic injury usually begins in the mucosa and extends outward. With arterial occlusion the demarcation from adjacent normal bowel is fairly sharply defined but with venous occlusion the margins are less distinct. Histologically, the changes are those that would be anticipated with marked edema, interstitial hemorrhage, and sloughing necrosis of the mucosa. The ischemic necrosis and inflammatory necrosis are seldom fully developed because surgical intervention or death intercedes. Within 24 hours intestinal bacteria produce outright gangrene and sometimes perforation of the bowel.

Mucosal and mural infarction, often called **"acute hemorrhagic enteropathy,"** characteristically is marked by multifocal lesions interspersed with spared areas. Depending on preexisting atherosclerotic narrowing of the arterial supply of the gut, the lesions may be largely confined to the small or the large intestine, but often

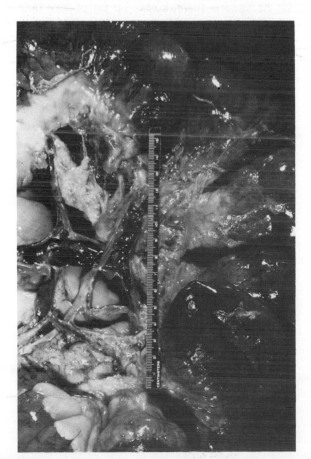

Figure 15–18. The mesenteric veins contain a dark thrombus, and the involved loops of small intestine are darkened by the venous infarction.

involve both. Affected foci may or may not be visible from the serosal surface because by definition the entire thickness of the bowel and serosal layer is not affected. When the bowel is opened there is hemorrhagic edematous thickening of the mucosa, sometimes with superficial ulcerations. The histologic changes range from marked vascular congestion with surrounding edema to hemorrhagic suffusion to outright necrosis of the mucosa and submucosa (Fig. 15–19). Sometimes an inflammatory membrane (pseudomembrane) coats the affected mucosa, usually secondary to bacterial superinfection. With the passage of time, a nonspecific inflammatory infiltrate becomes evident at the margins of the lesions.

CLINICAL COURSE. Ischemic bowel injury is most common in the later years of life. The clinical manifestations depend on the severity and suddenness of the occlusion, the distribution of the lesions, and whether outright infarction has occurred or only mucosal or mural infarction. With the transmural lesions, there is the sudden onset of abdominal pain, often out of proportion to the physical signs. Sometimes the pain is accompanied by bloody diarrhea or is soon followed by vascular collapse. The onset of pain tends to be more sudden with mesenteric embolism than with arterial or venous thrombosis. To be of any help the diagnosis must be made promptly, and making it requires a high index of suspicion in the appropriate setting (e.g., recent myocardial infarct, atrial fibrilla-

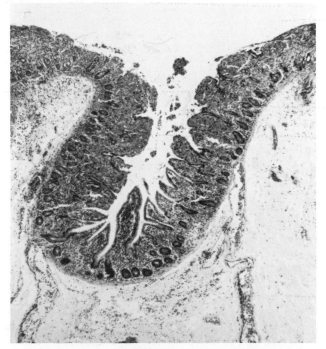

Figure 15–19. Mucosal infarction of small intestine with hemorrhagic suffusion of the lamina propria and superficial sloughing of the surface at upper left. There is marked edema but no hemorrhage in the noninfarcted submucosa.

tion, or manifestations suggestive of some form of vegetative endocarditis).

In contrast, nonocclusive ischemia may appear only as unexplained abdominal distention or gastrointestinal bleeding, but sometimes it is accompanied by the gradual onset of abdominal pain or discomfort. Helpful in establishing this diagnosis is a background favoring hypoperfusion of the bowel such as an episode of severe cardiac decompensation or shock.

The mortality rate with infarction of the bowel approaches 90%, largely because the window of time between onset of symptoms and perforation is so small. Mucosal and mural infarction, on the other hand, is not by and of itself fatal, and indeed if the cause of the hypoperfusion can be corrected the lesions are reversible.

ANGIODYSPLASIA

Angiodysplasia is the term applied to a focus of markedly dilated tortuous submucosal veins, usually directly beneath the mucosa most often located in the cecum or right colon. These vascular ectasias may occur as isolated lesions in the gut but are sometimes part of a systemic disorder such as hereditary hemorrhagic telangiectasia (Osler-Weber-Rendu syndrome) or the CREST syndrome (calcinosis, Reynaud's phenomenon, esophageal dysmotility, sclerodactyly, telangiectasia). They are prone to rupture and may cause massive gastrointestinal bleeding the origin of which is difficult to identify because of their small size and their tendency to collapse once ruptured. Angiography is almost always required to establish the diagnosis.

The pathogenesis of the isolated dilatations is uncertain, but it is speculated that they develop over the span of decades and thus become manifest relatively late in life. As penetrating veins pass through the muscularis they are subject to intermittent occlusion during peristaltic contractions, but the thicker-walled arteries remain patent, to thus produce venous distension and ectasia. The capacious cecum and right colon are favored locations, because according to physical laws, the greater the diameter of a cylinder, the greater the wall tension at any given intraluminal pressure.

HEMORRHOIDS

These are variceal dilatations of the hemorrhoidal venous plexuses. They are extremely common after age 50 years as a consequence of chronic constipation over the span of years and straining at stool. Other predisposing influences are repeated pregnancies with pelvic venous stasis and, least often but most important, portal hypertension usually related to cirrhosis of the liver. Those that arise as varicosities of the superior and middle hemorrhoidal veins appear above the anorectal line and are covered by rectal mucosa (internal hemorrhoids). In contrast those that appear below the anorectal line represent dilatations of the inferior hemorrhoidal plexus and are covered by anal mucosa *(external hemorrhoids).* They are thin-walled, dilated typical varices that may become thrombosed, particularly when subject to trauma. Internal hemorrhoids may *prolapse* during straining at stool and then become trapped by the compressive anal sphincter leading to sudden, extremely painful, edematous hemorrhagic enlargement or *strangulation.* They commonly bleed, sometimes masking far more serious bleeding from higher origins.

INFLAMMATORY DISEASES

Included under this heading are two important disorders of unknown cause, Crohn's disease (CD) and ulcerative colitis. The two entities have many overlaps and so are often referred to collectively as inflammatory bowel disease (IBD). There are in addition a number of specific enteric infections caused by viruses, bacteria, or larger parasites. They range clinically from the more annoying than serious *Escherichia coli*-induced traveler's diarrhea to the potentially lethal cholera. Certain of these microbial agents tend to affect the small intestine more than the colon and others the reverse, but in many instances both levels of the gut are affected. Before a diagnosis of IBD can be made in a patient with abdominal cramps and diarrhea the known microbial causes must be first ruled out.

CROHN'S DISEASE

This chronic, relapsing, inflammatory disorder of obscure origin may affect any portion of the gastrointestinal tract from esophagus to anus but most often involves the small intestine and colon. Early descriptions emphasized the sharply segmental transmural fibrosis and thickening of the terminal ileum accounting for the designation "terminal ileitis," but to encompass other localizations the name "regional enteritis" was applied. Now the eponymic Crohn's disease is preferred. The small bowel alone (particularly the terminal ileum) is affected in about 30% of cases, the small bowel and colon together in 50% of cases, and the colon alone in approximately 20% of cases. The colonic involvement is referred to as Crohn's colitis to distinguish it from ulcerative colitis (UC, discussed later). In about 40 to 60% of cases of CD granulomas are present in the inflammatory reaction, and when they are present Crohn's colitis can be readily differentiated from the nongranulomatous UC. When granulomas are lacking, however, the diagnosis of "indeterminate colitis" may be necessary. Although principally a disorder of the alimentary tract, the lesions of Crohn's disease have been identified in the mouth, larynx, esophagus, stomach, skin, and elsewhere. Moreover, active cases of CD are often accompanied by extraintestinal complications (probably of immune origin) such as iritis, ankylosing spondylitis, erythema nodosum, pericholangitis, sclerosing cholangitis, and various renal disorders, including nephrolithiasis and a predisposition to urinary tract infections. It is evident that CD is a systemic disease with mainly GI involvement.

EPIDEMIOLOGY. Worldwide in distribution, CD is much more prevalent in the United States, Great Britain, and Scandinavia than in Central Europe and is rare in Asia and Africa. Some of these differences may be spurious. In the United States, the incidence is about 3 to 10 cases per 100,000 population. There is evidence of an increasing incidence over the past few decades not attributable to improved case finding. Whites are more frequently affected than nonwhites and Jews more than non-Jews. There is a slight female preponderance, and although the disease may first become manifest at any age, the major peak occurs in the second and third decades with a smaller peak in the sixth and seventh decades. Genetic predisposition exists. Familial aggregations have been repeatedly observed; there is a 15 to 40% risk for first-degree relatives and an increased concordance in identical twins. Some studies point to an association with HLA-A2 not confirmed by other studies but HLA-B27 is common among those who also have ankylosing spondylitis.

ETIOLOGY AND PATHOGENESIS. The search for the cause(s) of CD and UC has revealed many parallels, not the least of which is that both remain idiopathic. Indeed, there are so many parallels that both conditions are often regarded as IBD. So it is reasonable to consider here such evidence as has been accumulated for both conditions.

Virtually every known microbial agent has at one time or another been incriminated and then discounted, all manner of immune and autoimmune abnormalities identified and queried, dietary factors suspected, and psychosomatic derangements examined, but no smoking pistol has been found. Recourse has therefore been made to more complex formulations, the favored one today being that *both CD and UC result from some genetically conditioned, abnormal reaction (immune?) to a microbial antigen or autoantigen.* Regrettably the evidence supporting this view is not much more substantial than other proposals, so the discussion of all can be brief.

- *Infectious causes.* Among the many potential offenders investigated, current favorites include diverse mycobacteria, uncharacterized RNA viruses, certain subspecies of *E. coli,* and cell wall–defective enteric bacteria.
- *Abnormal reactivity.* A constitutional susceptibility to a microbial or intestinal autoantigen, or more likely an abnormal immune reaction to it, could explain many of the accumulated findings, a few of which will be cited. Indicative of immune activation in IBD is increased production of IL-1, IL-2, and IL-6, but these findings may be epiphenomena. Patients with UC (but not CD) have an increased frequency of other autoimmune diseases. Some patients with IBD have circulating cytotoxic antibodies to colon epithelial cells. Colonic tissue–bound antibody has been identified in both UC and CD. Peripheral blood lymphocytes (presumably in the form of natural killer [NK] cells) have been reported

that are cytotoxic in vitro to colonic epithelial cells. Although the granulomatous reaction of CD points to cell-mediated immunity, no consistent T-cell abnormalities have been found save a reduced number in the circulation. Finally, the fact that marked clinical improvement follows immunosuppressive therapy such as corticosteroids might support an immune-mediated pathogenesis, but the beneficial effect may merely reflect nonspecific damping of epiphenomena.

- *Dietary factors.* Since both conditions are more common in industrialized countries and appear to be increasing in prevalence, some component of refined diets has been suspected. Perhaps certain dietary antigens are inappropriately absorbed because of some defect in mucosal cell permeability. Unfortunately, convincing experimental evidence is lacking.
- *Psychosomatic influences.* When all else fails, the psyche can be accused of attacking the soma. Repeated studies have called attention to the relationship between emotional events and the onset, or more often recurrence, of IBD. While a possible contributory role cannot be ruled out, it is difficult to explain sharply segmental involvement in CD or partial colon involvement in UC on these grounds.

We must leave it that the origins of both forms of IBD are obscure.

MORPHOLOGY. As noted before, **any level of the GI tract may be affected in CD, but wherever the involvement, it is segmental and sharply demarcated from adjacent normal bowel.** Occasionally several involved segments are separated by normal bowel; this condition is called "skip lesions." The earliest observable gross alteration is hyperemia, edema, and bogginess of the wall, followed in time by small, shallow, "aphthoid" mucosal ulcers. These coalesce to form irregular serpentine ulcers in the long axis of the bowel,

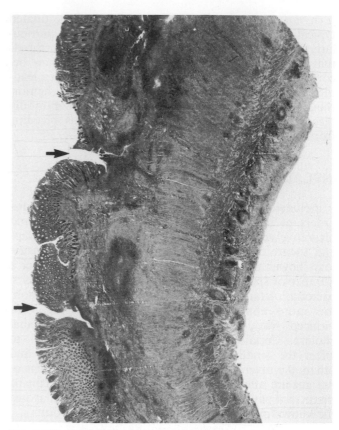

Figure 15-21. Crohn's disease. A low-power cross section of the markedly thickened wall. The narrow serpentine ulcerations are seen on cross section *(arrows).* The dark areas are masses of inflammatory cells, most numerous in the submucosa, subserosa, and margins of the ulcers.

creating deep fissures separated by nodular mucosal thickenings giving a "cobblestone" appearance. The subsequent fibrosis throughout the wall thickens it and produces the characteristic rubber hose rigidity of involved segments. The lumen is markedly narrowed and so permits passage of only a thin stream of barium, creating the radiographic string sign (Fig. 15-20). The mesentery simultaneously becomes thickened and fibrotic and sometimes appears to creep over the bowel serosa. Penetration of the ulcers may produce adhesion to adjacent loops of bowel, fistulous communications, or localized, walled-off abscesses. The mural thickening and narrowing of the lumen in Crohn's colitis are rarely seen in ulcerative colitis.

Microscopic examination characteristically reveals a marked, chronic transmural inflammatory reaction with a prominent infiltration of lymphocytes, histiocytes, and plasma cells, but the margins of the ulcers retain a neutrophilic infiltrate (Fig. 15-21). The fibrosis permeates all layers but is particularly evident in the submucosal and subserosal layers. Distinctive of CD, but present in only 40 to 60% of cases, are the noncaseating granulomas most numerous in the inflammatory foci of the submucosa and subserosa. Similar granulomas may be present in the chronic reactive regional lymph nodes.

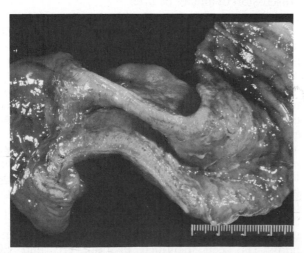

Figure 15-20. Crohn's disease involving a segment of the terminal ileum. Note the sharp borders of the lesion, the markedly thickened wall, and the narrowed lumen.

Granulomas are not present in UC. Vasculitis sometimes develops in the mural vessels trapped in areas of active inflammation.

Particularly important with long-standing chronic disease are the dysplastic changes appearing in the mucosal epithelial cells. These may be focal or widespread, tend to become more marked with time, and are thought to be related to the increased risk of carcinoma. In those with colitis there is a two- to threefold increased risk of colon cancer. Rarely the tumor occurs in the small bowel with Crohn's enteritis.

The essential morphologic similarities and contrasts between UC and CD are given in Table 15–10.

CLINICAL COURSE. The presentation of Crohn's disease is highly variable and ultimately unpredictable. The dominant manifestations are recurrent episodes of diarrhea, crampy abdominal pain, and fever lasting days to weeks. These manifestations usually begin insidiously, but in some instances, particularly in young persons, the onset of the pain is so abrupt and the diarrhea so mild that abdominal exploration is performed with a diagnosis of appendicitis. Some melena is present in about 50% of cases with colon involvement, usually mild but sometimes massive. Weight loss may become marked in some patients. In most patients, after an initial attack, the manifestations remit either spontaneously or with therapy, but characteristically they are followed by relapses and intervals between successive attacks grow shorter. For about 10 to 20% of patients the symptom-free interval after the initial attack may last for decades, and for very fortunate ones the first attack is the last.

Superimposed on this course are the potential development of perianal or perirectal fissures, fistulas, or abscesses, manifestations of malabsorption, and some of the extraintestinal manifestations mentioned earlier.

The feared consequences of Crohn's disease include: (1) intestinal narrowing of a degree that surgical intervention is required, (2) perforation of a deep fissure with peritonitis or fistula formation, (3) massive bleeding usually from a colonic focus, (4) toxic dilatation of the colon, (5) systemic amyloidosis, and (6) carcinoma of the colon or small intestine, the risk depending on the duration of the disease. Significant as the increased risk is, it is substantially less than that associated with UC.

ULCERATIVE COLITIS _____

UC is a common, chronic, recurrent diarrheal disease of unknown cause characterized by severe ulcerations that begin in the rectum but may extend proximally, sometimes to involve the entire colon. The diagnosis of UC clinically requires that other forms of colitis of known cause, such as those caused by *Yersinia* and *Campylobacter,* be ruled out first. There are, as we pointed out on p. 499, many similarities between UC and CD, and hence both are sometimes referred to as "inflammatory bowel disease" (IBD). In CD the colon is frequently affected, sometimes without small intestinal involvement. There is a familial predisposition to both diseases, a higher concordance in monozygotic than in dizygotic twins, an increased incidence among Jews (except those in Israel), and an association with many systemic complications such as ankylosing spondylitis, sacroiliitis, erythema nodosum, sclerosing cholangitis, and iritis. As with CD, 90% of patients who have UC and ankylosing spondylitis also have HLA-B27. There are, however, differences between the two conditions:

- UC is restricted to the colon, except possibly for some "backwash ileitis" when there is total colon involvement. Beginning in the rectum, it spreads proximally. Skip lesions are not seen in UC as they are in CD.
- The ulceroinflammatory process in UC is nonspecific, whereas many cases of CD have a granulomatous reaction.
- CD is characterized by transmural inflammation and fibrosis, but in UC the colon ulcers rarely extend below the submucosa and there is a surprisingly minimal fibrosing reaction.
- Patients with UC are at greater risk of developing colorectal cancer than those with CD.

UC is somewhat more common than CD in the United States and other Western countries, with an incidence of 5 to 15 cases per 100,000 population, but it is infrequent in Asia, Africa, and South America. Unlike that of CD there is no evidence that the incidence is rising. The disease begins most often in the second or third decade of life, is more common than CD in the first decade, and has a small peak in the seventh decade. There is no significant sex predominance, and whites are affected more often than nonwhites. For obscure reasons, smokers are less often affected than nonsmokers.

ETIOLOGY AND PATHOGENESIS. The current state of uncertainty about the cause or causes of IBD (and therefore of UC) was detailed earlier (p. 499). You may recall that the search has focused on the following lines of investigation.

- A possible microbial invader.
- Abnormal (immune?) reactivity to an exogenous (dietary?, microbial?) antigen or possibly an autoimmune reaction to an endogenous (colonic) antigen. In UC particular attention has been devoted to a failure of the mucosal immunoglobulin A (IgA) system.
- Genetic predisposition to particular challenges.
- A psychosomatic basis.

Most widely held is the view that, in genetically predisposed persons, some form of autoimmune reaction underlies UC, perhaps initiated by one of many relatively innocuous dietary or microbial colonic antigens.

MORPHOLOGY. As noted, UC begins in the rectum and spreads proximally in continuity. Involvement of only the rectum or rectosigmoid accounts for about 80% of cases. In about 10% of cases the entire colon is affected.

In the acute stage, the mucosa is hyperemic, edematous, and friable. With progression, small aphthoid ulcers appear underlain by foci of suppuration. Coalescence of these lesions leads to irregular, broad-based ulcers ranging up to many centimeters in longest dimension. They rarely extend below the submucosa, but coalescence of adjacent ulcerations may literally denude large tracts of the colon. Typically the ulcerations are separated by narrow strands of residual mucosa that are sometimes undermined to leave tenuous bridges (Fig. 15–22). Small islands of edematous hyperemic mucosa may persist as **"pseudopolyps."** Usually there is minimal fibrous induration. Uncommonly the ulcerations penetrate more deeply, sometimes to perforate and produce pericolic abscesses, fistulas, or perianal or ischiorectal abscesses. Also infrequently in extremely acute cases there is toxic dilatation of the colorectum. With chronicity, cases with deep mural penetration may develop fibrous thickening of the bowel wall.

The histologic changes are essentially those of nonspecific acute and chronic ulcerative inflammation. The initial lesions comprise minute crypt abscesses with suppurative necrosis of the surrounding epithelium. Enlargement of these and coalescence eventually produce the larger ulcers described. In chronic cases, the neutrophilic infiltration in the margins of the ulcerative lesions is underlain by numerous lymphocytes, macrophages, and plasma cells. An acute vasculitis may appear in this inflammatory zone. With remission of the activity, granulation tissue fills the ulcer craters, followed by regeneration of the mucosal epithelium. The electron microscopic changes are those that would be anticipated in any inflammatory reaction and are not significantly contributory.

The most serious complication of UC is the development of colon carcinoma. Two factors govern the risk: duration of the disease and its extent. Although the reported data vary greatly, there is an overall consensus that the frequency of carcinoma has been overstated in the past. Currently it is believed that at 10 years with disease limited to the left colon the risk is minimal, at 20 years the risk is of the order of 2% with left-sided disease and about 10% with total colon involvement, rising at 30 years to about 3 to 4% and 15 to 25%, respectively. Long before these cancers appear there is an important sequential development of at first mucosal inflammatory metaplasia in areas of involvement eventually transforming into ever more marked dysplasia eventuating in neoplasia.

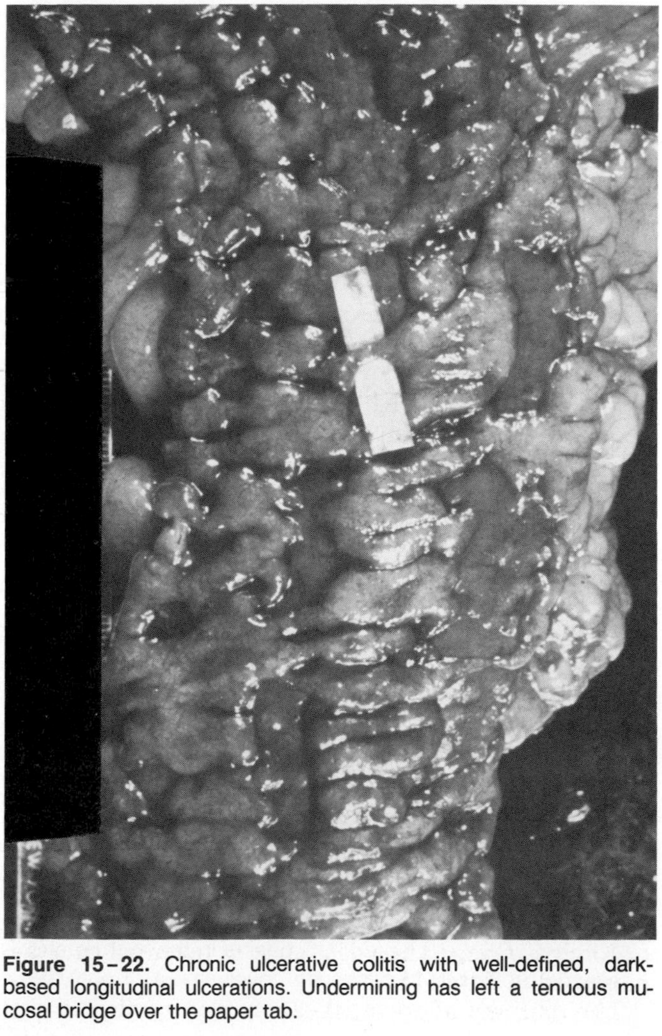

Some of the comparative features of CD and UC are given in Table 15–10 and shown in Figure 15–23.

CLINICAL COURSE. Most commonly UC appears insidiously with cramps and discomfort progressing to diarrhea that is often bloody with mucus and flecks of feces; the tenesmus and colicky lower abdominal pain

Figure 15–22. Chronic ulcerative colitis with well-defined, dark-based longitudinal ulcerations. Undermining has left a tenuous mucosal bridge over the paper tab.

TABLE 15–10. RELATIVE FREQUENCY OF MORPHOLOGIC FINDINGS IN ULCERATIVE COLITIS (UC) VS. CROHN'S DISEASE OF COLON (CD)*

Features	UC	CD
Gross		
Total colonic involvement	+++	+
Distal predominance	++++	+
Small intestinal involvement	0	+++
"Skip" lesions	0	+++
Broad-based ulcers	+++	+
Serpentine fissures	+	++++
Transmural fibrous thickening	+	++++
Pseudopolyps	+++	0
Microscopic		
Granulomas	0	+++
Nonspecific acute and chronic inflammation	++++	++
Crypt abscesses	++++	+
Transmural inflammation	+	+++

* Modified from Yardley, J.H., Donowitz, M.: Colorectal biopsy in inflammatory bowel disease. *In* Yardley, J.H., et al. (eds.): The Gastrointestinal Tract. Baltimore, Williams & Wilkins Co., 1977, p. 50.

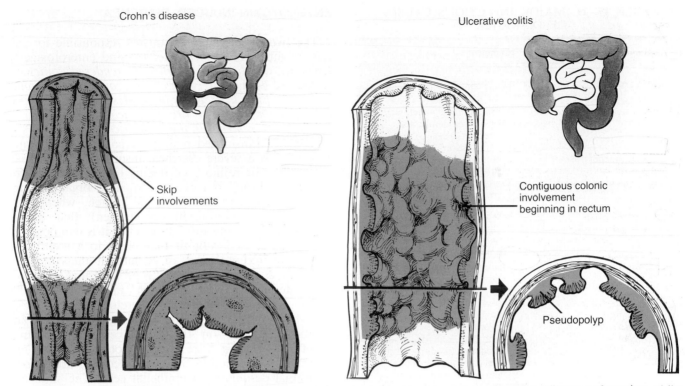

Figure 15–23. The distribution patterns of Crohn's disease and ulcerative colitis are compared as well as the different conformations of the ulcers and wall thickenings.

are relieved by defecation. Some patients manifest fever and weight loss. Grossly bloody stools are far more common with UC than with CD, and the blood loss may be considerable. Extragastrointestinal complications are also more common with UC than with CD. Arthritis is commonest but also encountered are spondylitis, skin lesions, hepatic lesions (e.g., fatty change, hepatitis, pericholangitis, and sclerosing cholangitis), eye changes, finger clubbing, and amyloidosis.

The course is variable. Most patients' disease follows a chronic relapsing, remitting course, with exacerbations often triggered by emotional or physical stress. During severe attacks or when the onset is acute the colon may become markedly distended: *toxic dilatation* or *toxic megacolon* requires emergency measures. Other life-threatening complications include massive hemorrhage and perforation with peritonitis. Inflammatory strictures of the colorectum, while uncommon, must be differentiated from cancer.

The diagnosis can usually be made by endoscopic examination and biopsy. Specific infectious causes must always be ruled out. The prognosis varies with the clinical activity of the disease. The outlook for recovery from the first attack is excellent, but about 5% of patients whose onset of disease is severe and unremitting die within a year of peritonitis, sepsis, hemorrhage, or fluid and electrolyte disturbances. The darkest cloud on the horizon is the development of colon cancer. These cancers may be difficult to detect because they are often infiltrative and easily mistaken for inflammatory stenoses; moreover, several may arise concurrently. The sequential mucosal changes from

dysplasia to neoplasia provide the rationale for surveillance programs of repeated colonoscopies and multiple biopsies aimed at detecting "premalignant" changes.

INFECTIOUS ENTEROCOLITIS _____

This heading refers to a group of diseases of microbial origin marked principally by clinically significant diarrhea and sometimes ulceroinflammatory changes in the small or large intestine, or sometimes both. Frequently (in 40 to 50% of cases) the specific cause cannot be isolated but there are convincing features of an infection (i.e., more or less acute onset, limited duration, rising antibody titers to a particular pathogen, and frequently response to antibiotic therapy).

These conditions constitute a global problem of staggering proportions, causing more than 10,000 deaths per day among children in the developing countries. Although far less prevalent in industrialized nations, these infections still have attack rates of one to two illnesses per person per year. A large number of causative agents including viruses, bacteria, and protozoa are responsible; the major offenders vary with the age, nutrition, immune status of the host, and the environment (living conditions, public health measures, and such special predispositions as hospitalization, immunodeficiency [AIDS], wartime dislocation, or foreign travel). The wide range of potential causes is presented in Table 15–11.

The diversity of potential causes requires that further

TABLE 15–11. MAJOR INFECTIOUS CAUSES OF DIARRHEA

Organism	Comment
Viruses	
Rotaviruses	Principally in children under age six. Sporadic—from contaminated water, may become epidemic; also direct fecal-oral transmission
Enteric adenoviruses	Common in infants and children, mostly sporadic
Norwalk virus	Young and old, mainly epidemic; fecal-oral
Bacteria	
Enterotoxigenic *Escherichia coli*	Major cause of traveler's diarrhea, food- and water-borne, previously unencountered strains
Campylobacter jejuni	Major global cause, any age, mainly children, transmission by contaminated water and food
Yersinia enterocolitica	Similar to above
Shigella	Major global offender, children and adults, fecal-oral direct transmission and contaminated water and food, endemic and epidemic
Enteropathogenic *E. coli*	Children and nursery outbreaks
Salmonella spp.	Large number serotypes with range of clinical syndromes, children and adults, food- and water-borne, human and animal reservoirs
Clostridium difficile	Antibiotic-associated, hospital-acquired, mainly in predisposed adults
Vibrio cholerae, Aeromonas, others	
Parasites	
Giardia lamblia	Carrier state common, major cause of traveler's diarrhea, contaminated drinking water, high infection rate in Russia, Northwestern United States, other locales; may become epidemic
Entamoeba histolytica	Large reservoir of asymptomatic carriers in developed countries and endemic in developing areas, fecal-oral, sexual transmission particularly among homosexuals, and from contaminated water and food

comments of necessity be limited largely to pathophysiologic categories.

There are several mechanisms by which the various intestinal pathogens cause illness, mainly diarrhea, and the major offenders will be discussed in pathophysiologic categories.

ENTEROTOXIN-INDUCED DIARRHEA

The two prototypical organisms responsible for this type of illness are *Vibrio cholerae* and enterotoxigenic *Escherichia coli*. The diarrhea is rendered somewhat distinctive because it is purely an "overflow phenomenon," resulting from toxin-induced secretion in excess of absorption, so there are no mucosal ulcerations or white cells or red cells in the fecal discharge.

Cholera (transmitted mainly by contaminated water and food) is a severe diarrheal disorder that has been responsible for millions of deaths in the past and for epidemics throughout the world. The organisms remain restricted to the intestinal lumen, where they elaborate an enterotoxin (choleragen) that affects mainly the small intestine. In essence it is composed of two subunits, a B subunit that binds to a membrane ganglioside receptor and an A subunit that probably binds to a transmembrane G protein that activates adenylate cyclase, resulting in raised intracellular cAMP levels and increased secretory activity (Fig. 15–24). Simultaneously the choleragen exerts an antiabsorptive effect on the villus cells. Thus comes about the copious "rice water" stools devoid of inflammatory cells and bearing only flecks of mucus and occasional desquamated epithelial cells. The small intestinal mucosa is basically normal. With this understanding of the pathophysiology of cholera, the mortality rate has been dramatically reduced by the simple expedient of fluid and electrolyte repletion.

E. coli may cause disease by one of several plasmid-transmitted virulence factors, which produce strains that are enterotoxigenic or enteropathogenic or both, and still others that are enteroinvasive or have other attributes.

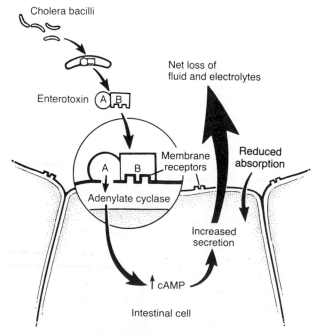

Figure 15–24. A schema of the mechanisms of action of the cholera enterotoxin in its induction of excessive mucosal secretory activity.

The *enterotoxigenic strains (ETEC)* elaborate two types of enterotoxins. The heat-labile toxin (LT) acts on small intestinal epithelium exactly as the cholera toxin binding to membrane receptors and ultimately activating adenylate cyclase. Facilitating its pathogenicity are pili or fimbriae that permit adherence of the organisms to the epithelial cells. The second heat-stable toxin (ST) has no similarity to the cholera toxin and produces excessive fluid secretion by activation of guanylate cyclase. Certain ETEC strains can elaborate both LT and ST.

ENTEROINVASIVE ORGANISMS

The major pathogens to be considered here are enteropathogenic *Shigella*, enteropathogenic *E. coli*, *Salmonella*, *Clostridium difficile*, and *Entamoeba histolytica*, with a few concluding remarks about *Yersinia* and *Campylobacter*. All have the capacity to invade intestinal mucosa and produce ulceroinflammatory lesions in the small intestine, large intestine, or both. As a consequence, the stool generally contains white cells and red cells, which differentiates it from that of enterotoxigenic diarrhea.

Four *Shigella species*, *Shigella dysenteriae*, *-flexneri*, *-boydii*, and *-sonnei*, produce potentially serious diarrhea called generically "*bacillary dysentery*," a designation implying diarrheal stools containing inflammatory white cells and red cells. All strains are pathogenic; Shiga bacillus produces the severest disease, but *S. sonnei* is now the major cause of bacillary dysentery in the United States. Disease caused by these organisms becomes particularly prevalent with population dislocations such as wars, but there is a constant low level of endemicity in tropical countries. Transmission is mainly fecal-oral, but in underdeveloped countries contaminated food and water have produced epidemics. The precise mechanism of production of the diarrhea is poorly understood but it appears to relate to a Shiga toxin that acts on the small intestine as well as a cytotoxic toxin that permits invasion of the colonic epithelium. The Shiga toxin has a B subunit that binds to specific membrane receptors and an A subunit that is internalized and appears to inhibit peptide chain elongation. Whether this action underlies its secretory effect is not clear.

The major locus of attack is the colon; the organisms invade the lamina propria and are carried to the intestinal lymph nodes but do not produce bacteremia. *The mucosal invasion yields a nonspecific fibrinosuppurative exudate in the form of a dirty gray pseudomembrane that in time leads to increased friability of the underlying mucosa, intramucosal suppuration, and the eventual development of ulcerations.* Large tracts of the colonic mucosa may be sloughed. Impaired colonic absorption may contribute to the dysentery.

Enteropathogenic E. coli is responsible for serious outbreaks, principally in children. These serotypes, different from enterotoxigenic strains, have adherence factors as well as the capacity to invade and destroy cells and to produce toxins some of which are Shiga-like (p. 266). Thus the resultant diarrhea is the consequence of direct mucosal injury and toxin-induced oversecretion.

Salmonella species, of which there are more than 1500 serotypes, produce a range of clinical syndromes: (1) typhoid fever caused by *Salmonella typhi*, (2) enteric fever (a milder form of typhoid fever), (3) gastroenteritis, (4) bacteremia, (5) localized abscesses anywhere in the body including bones and arterial walls, and (6) an asymptomatic chronic carrier state. All of the nontyphoidal syndromes may be caused by *Salmonella cholerae-suis* or any one of the hundreds of serotypes of *Salmonella enteritidis*. Only typhoid fever as the archetypal salmonellosis and the gastroenteritis will be characterized.

Typhoid fever is an acute serious systemic infection characterized at the outset by intestinal colonization leading rapidly to bacteremia and daily spiking fevers, yet a slow pulse; abdominal manifestations such as crampy pain and diarrhea sometimes alternating with constipation; and toward the end of the first week a characteristic, mainly central macular rash of "rose spots." Thereafter a steady febrile state ensues with mental disturbances (delirium) and severe diarrhea. After about four weeks, in the absence of serious complications, there is slow progressive improvement. The causative agent, *S. typhi*, is almost always food or water borne, from infected humans including carriers. There are no natural animal reservoirs. Following ingestion, the organisms penetrate the small bowel mucosa, soon drain through lymphatics, and induce the bacteremia. *Activation of the mononuclear-phagocyte system leads to inflammatory enlargement of lymph nodes, hepatomegaly, splenomegaly, and enlargement of lymphoid follicles in the gut such as Peyer's patches.* The macrophages form small nodular aggregates of plump phagocytic cells, often containing red cells (erythrophagocytosis) and nuclear debris. With progressive enlargement of the Peyer's patches the overlying mucosa ulcerates, producing an oval mucosal defect with the long dimension in the axis of the bowel. *The shallow ulceration surmounting an enlarged plateau of lymphoid tissue with striking hyperplasia of erythrophagocytic macrophages is virtually diagnostic of typhoid fever.* The major threats to life are fluid and electrolyte disturbances, intestinal hemorrhage, and perforation, but additional complications derive from the blood-borne dissemination of the bacillus with its localization in any site (e.g., pneumonia, pyelonephritis, osteomyelitis, arthritis, and cholecystitis [the latter may induce an asymptomatic chronic carrier state]).

Gastroenteritis may be caused by any one of the salmonellae save *S. typhi*. They lack enterotoxins; their pathogenicity is related to flagellar (H), somatic (O), and especially coat (V_1) antigens. The organisms may be transmitted from infected humans, but other major sources of infection are animals and their products, including poultry, meat, eggs, and dairy foods. Community suppers and barbecues are notorious for *Salmonella* outbreaks. Following ingestion of the bacilli there is within hours to days onset of nausea and vomiting, followed by abdominal cramps and diarrhea.

The organisms mainly attack the ileum and to a lesser extent the colon. The anatomic changes have not been well documented, but biopsies have revealed crypt abscesses and shallow ulcers with hyperemia and friability of the intervening mucosa. Save for the predominance of macrophages and mononuclear cells in the inflammatory reaction about the ulcers (reminiscent of typhoid fever) the changes closely mimic those of ulcerative colitis.

C. difficile is an important cause of diarrhea, seen mainly in hospitalized, usually elderly, patients taking broad-spectrum antibiotics. Rarely it appears in the absence of antibiotic therapy in persons predisposed by surgery, trauma, cancer, or other serious illness. Although a large number of antibiotics have at one time or another been implicated, the major offenders today are ampicillin, amoxicillin, clindamycin, and cephalosporins. Approximately 20% of patients who are confined to the hospital for longer than a few days acquire C. difficile as a nosocomial infection. In most the infection remains asymptomatic, but when antibiotic therapy destroys the normal gut microflora C. difficile proliferate and elaborate two toxins, designated A and B. A is less cytotoxic than B, but it impairs the cytoskeletal structure of mucosal epithelial cells and loosens their tight junctions, facilitating increased fluid secretion and diarrhea. Toxin B is highly cytotoxic. These toxins achieve their highest intraluminal level in the colon and there cause initially hyperemia and crypt abscesses. In time, the suppuration extends into the lamina propria and at the same time erupts to the surface of the mucosa in "volcano-like" fashion, yielding focal gray-white coagula of inflammatory cells, mucosal cell debris, plasma proteins, and mucus. Coalescence of these coagula eventually produces the classic _yellow-gray, loosely attached pseudomembrane that may be focal and patchy in some areas but elsewhere may cover significant segments of the colonic mucosa_ (Fig. 15–25). Although the pseudomembrane is characteristic of C. difficile infection it may be mimicked by a large number of other organisms such as Candida, staphylococci, and Yersinia, to mention only a few, particularly when the gut is predisposed by hypoperfusion as in cardiac failure. The appropriate diagnosis is best made by C. difficile toxin assays.

Amebiasis caused by _Entamoeba histolytica_ is a major global problem. Spread is by contaminated water and food or direct fecal-oral contact facilitated by the ability of the parasite to encyst and survive in most environments for weeks to months. In developing areas, the prevalence of infection (not necessarily disease) may be as high as 50%. In the United States, it is estimated to be about 4% generally and much greater among mentally retarded persons, promiscuous homosexual males, those with immunodeficiency (e.g., AIDS), and malnourished persons. Fortunately in the

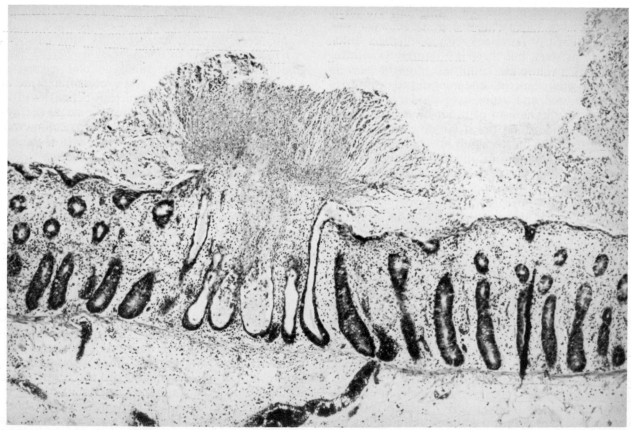

Figure 15–25. Pseudomembranous colitis. A focal area of mucosal inflammation has erupted in volcano-like fashion producing a surface layer of exudate.

United States up to 99% of infected individuals remain asymptomatic and often eliminate the parasite from the gut within a year. Whether asymptomatic "cyst passers" have avirulent strains remains uncertain. Prevalence figures are often spuriously high because there are other nonpathogenic amebae that inhabit the gut of humans, such as *E. hartmanni, E. nana,* and *E. coli.* Pathogenic *E. histolytica* can be most certainly identified as a uninuclear trophozoite actively engulfing red cells. Nonpathogenic and nonvirulent strains are nonphagocytic. The cysts by contrast are quadrinucleate. Transmission is fecal-oral, usually from asymptomatic persons who harbor only cysts.

The major clinical syndrome of active infection is acute or chronic invasive colitis with scattered discrete mucosal ulcerations interspersed by normal-looking mucosa. Once excysted, the amebae invade the crypts at the level of the muscularis mucosa and fan out to produce classic flask-shaped ulcers. As the undermined mucosa sloughs, larger craters are produced, but generally there are intervening areas of relatively normal-looking mucosa. The ulcers may be restricted to the mucosa and submucosa but in more severe cases may penetrate deeply and perforate. There is surprisingly little inflammatory suppuration in the margins of the ulcers, but typically destructive trophozoites can be found in the advancing edges.

The pathogenicity of invasive amebiasis has now been partially unravelled, revealing that *E. histolytica* adheres to colonic epithelial cells by virtue of galactose-containing lectins for which intestinal mucins have a high affinity. Following binding they kill target cells on direct contact. There is some evidence that they generate a surface "amebopore protein" that punches holes in the host cell membranes, permitting the unregulated influx and efflux of solutes. Whatever the method, amebae may penetrate the colon, produce peritonitis or pericolic amebomas, or drain into the portal venous system to produce, in up to 40% of patients, hepatic abscesses (discrete, often solitary cavities filled with brown pastelike debris) and potentially thereafter lung and brain abscesses.

The diagnosis depends on identification of cysts or trophozoites in the stools, requiring optimally an experienced observer.

Two other intestinal pathogens merit brief characterization. *Campylobacter jejuni* is transmitted to humans from animals or animal products by the consumption of improperly cooked food, or rarely of contaminated water. It produces an acute, usually short-lived colitis that has many of the clinical and pathologic features of idiopathic ulcerative colitis. Generally the lesions are confined to the rectosigmoid, and only isolation of the offender in the stool or visualization of the curved motile rods in dark-field or phase-contrast microscopy permits recognition of this form of colitis. *Yersinia enterocolitica,* on the other hand, typically involves the terminal ileum and colon and often produces manifestations characterized as "pseudoappendicitis." The organism is widely prevalent in a variety of animals and animal products, and most human infections result from ingestion of contaminated food and water. The

relatively nondistinctive shallow mucosal ulcerations are scattered mainly through the terminal ileum but sometimes extend into the colon. The gross and microscopic lesions are not distinctive and the causative agent can be identified only by stool culture or serologic methods. Virulent strains are capable of invading and destroying epithelial cells and penetrating the mucosa. Drainage of the agent to the regional lymph nodes and bacteremic spread may then follow with focal infections anywhere throughout the body. In addition, postinfective complications may appear, including arthritis and erythema nodosum.

MALABSORPTION SYNDROMES _____

The normal digestion and absorption of foods involves three sequential stages:

1. An *intraluminal stage,* in which proteins and fats are broken down into assimilable forms and fats are solubilized by bile salts. Within the lumen iron and vitamin B_{12} are converted into forms capable of being absorbed or bound to appropriate cofactors necessary for their absorption (for example, intrinsic factor with vitamin B_{12}).
2. An *intestinal stage* which involves the further hydrolysis of carbohydrates by disaccharidases in the brush border of the small intestine, and the mucosal cell uptake and transport of hydrolyzed products derived from foods as well as the formation of chylomicrons from triglycerides and cholesterol.
3. *Transport across the epithelial cells* to lymphatics or blood vessels is the final stage in the normal handling of foodstuffs.

A host of disorders interrupt or disrupt some necessary step in the sequence described (Table 15–12).

Only a few prototypes of the three stages of digestion will be described briefly. Other syndromes—pernicious anemia (p. 347), pancreatitis (p. 581)—are discussed elsewhere.

DISACCHARIDASE DEFICIENCY _____

A deficiency of lactase in the brush border of the small intestinal epithelial cells impairs the breakdown of the unabsorbable disaccharide, lactose, into its absorbable components glucose and galactose. The low levels of lactase may represent an acquired deficiency seen in any disease that damages the small intestinal mucosa, such as celiac sprue, postinfectious sprue, radiation injury, and extensive Crohn's disease. On the other hand, lactase deficiency may represent a congenital disorder of great consequence because in infants it produces milk intolerance, leading to diarrhea, weight loss, and failure to thrive. The diagnosis is most readily made by measurement of the breath hydrogen level, a reflection of bacterial overgrowth in the excess intraluminal carbohydrate.

TABLE 15–12. SOME MAJOR FORMS OF MALABSORPTION*

Deranged Stage	Clinical Syndrome	Pathophysiology
Intraluminal Stage		
Digestion of fats, proteins	Pancreatic damage: pancreatitis (p. 581), cystic fibrosis (p. 89), carcinoma (p. 585)	Decreased production of pancreatic enzymes
	Zollinger-Ellison syndrome (p. 580)	Inactivation of pancreatic enzymes by excess gastric acid
Solubilization of fat	Biliary tract obstruction (p. 526), cholestatic liver disease (p. 526)	Inadequate delivery of bile to the duodenum or disruption of the enterohepatic circulation
	Terminal ileal resection or disease	Disruption of the enterohepatic circulation
Preabsorption, modification of particular nutrients	Pernicious anemia (p. 347)	Deficiency of intrinsic factor required for vitamin B$_{12}$ absorption
	Blind loop syndrome, tapeworm infection	Competitive uptake of vitamin B$_{12}$ by bacteria or worms
	Iron deficiency from impaired absorption (p. 345)	Gastric hypochlorhydria; inadequate dietary ascorbic acid, citric acid; phylates, tannates, in the diet
Intestinal Stage		
Mucosal cell digestion	Lactase deficiency	Inability to hydrolyze the disaccharide lactose into absorbable monosaccharides
Mucosal uptake and transport	Crohn's disease (p. 499), celiac sprue, postinfectious (tropical) sprue, ileal resection, Whipple's disease	Reduction of absorptive surface area, mucosal cell injury
Transport Stage		
Lymphatic transport	Lymphoma (p. 493), tuberculosis, Whipple's disease	Obstruction to intestinal lacteals or ducts

* From Wright, T.L., Heyworth, M.F.: Maldigestion and malabsorption. *In* Sleisenger, M.H., Fordtran, J.S. (eds.): Gastrointestinal Disease, Pathophysiology, Diagnosis, Management. 4th ed. Philadelphia, W.B. Saunders, 1989, p. 263.

CELIAC SPRUE

This malabsorption syndrome is neither common nor rare but is important to recognize because an appropriate diet produces remarkable benefits. The malabsorption is related to immune-mediated damage to the small intestinal mucosa following dietary exposure to gluten-containing grains, principally wheat, rye, oats, and barley. It is the gliadin in the gluten that is the culprit.

The morphologic alterations are limited to the small intestinal mucosa, tending to be more marked in the more proximal levels but sometimes involving all of it. On exposure to gluten, there is progressive loss of the normal villus structure with elongation of the crypts. Thus, there is flattening of the mucosal surface. Histologically the surface epithelial cells are quite atypical, cuboidal, or even squamoid with loss of the microvilli, often vacuolated, and sometimes infiltrated by inflammatory cells. The increased number of mitoses in the crypts suggests excessive proliferative activity. The numbers of lymphocytes and plasma cells in the lamina propria are moderately increased; some of them may appear immunoblastoid or plasmacytoid. Most observers contend that there is a disproportionate number of CD4 helper cells relative to the CD8 suppressor-cytotoxic cells. Although the loss of villi is striking, as will be seen, it may also be encountered in postinfectious sprue as well as other conditions.

Several sets of influences underlie the intolerance to gluten gliadin, (1) genetic, (2) immune, and (3) toxic. Evidence of the role of genetics is the greater incidence of the disease in first-degree relatives of patients and the high concordance rate (over 70%) for monozygotic twins. In addition there is a strong association with HLA-B8, HLA-DR3, HLA-DR7, and/or HLA-DQw2. Recall that the class II major histocompatibility complex plays an important role in determining the cell-mediated response to particular antigens. Yet not all patients with these histocompatibility antigens develop celiac sprue, nor do all affected persons bear these antigens.

The immunologic evidence is abundant but inconclusive. The great majority of patients with celiac sprue have elevated levels of antigliadin antibodies, most of which are IgA. Whether they directly contribute to the damage remains unestablished and so attention has turned to a cell-mediated immune response. As noted, most of the lymphocytes bear markers of suppressor cytotoxic lymphocytes. There is, however, no formal evidence that these T cells directly injure mucosal epithelium. Alternatively, elaboration of toxic lymphokines has been postulated, but again not proven.

Direct toxic injury has not been excluded. Certain polypeptide fractions derived from gluten are directly toxic to mucosal cells in vitro and disrupt the normal mucosal intercellular tight junctions.

Whatever the cause, the mucosal changes are accompanied by an increased net efflux (shedding) of surface cells, which leads to a strikingly increased proliferative reaction in the crypts with inadequate maturation of the newly formed cells, which are incapable of synthesizing disaccharidases, peptidases, and other enzymes important in digestion. Absorption is therefore deficient in these patients. *The malabsorption in celiac sprue, then, is multifactorial, arising from both reduction in the absorptive area of the small intestine and deficient intraluminal digestion.* Remarkably, all these derangements and the small intestinal mucosal changes revert in most cases to normal within a few weeks of rigid exclusion of gluten from the diet. Regrettably, a few patients are refractory to gluten-free diets or revert following a period of benefit.

Long-standing disease, in addition to impairing growth and development in the growing child or adult, leads to an approximately 10% incidence of some form of malignant disease, principally lymphomas of the intestines but also carcinomas of the esophagus and small intestine.

POSTINFECTIOUS SPRUE (TROPICAL SPRUE)

Although the small intestinal mucosal changes in this condition are identical to those in celiac sprue the two conditions appear to be totally unrelated. The best evidence suggests that tropical sprue is caused by an antecedent enteric infection; principally implicated are *E. coli, Klebsiella,* and *Enterobacter* species. Puzzling is the geographic distribution of this condition. Worldwide, it is particularly prevalent in the Caribbean, but it has not been reported in Jamaica. It is also endemic in North and South America but rare in Central America and Mexico. Another large pocket is India and Southeast Asia. The malabsorption usually becomes apparent within days or a few weeks of an acute diarrheal enteric infection in visitors to endemic locales; natives are almost never affected. The condition is rarely encountered in persons who have never visited or lived in these locales. Administration of antibiotics such as tetracycline corrects the malabsorption. If untreated, it can persist and be responsible for weight loss and in particular depletion of folates leading to megaloblastic anemia. Lymphoma of the small intestine does not appear to be a hazard, as it is following celiac sprue.

WHIPPLE'S DISEASE

Whipple's disease is quite uncommon, but it is so intriguing and frustrating that it invites brief characterization. A systemic condition, it may involve any organ of the body but principally manifests itself in intestinal derangements, central nervous system involvement, and arthritis. The wall of the small intestine is thickened largely by edema of the mucosa; sometimes expansion of the villi creates a shaggy, bearskin-rug appearance. Much of this thickening is related to masses of macrophages stuffed with bacilli creating large PAS-positive granules (Fig. 15–26). Some bacilli are extracellular in the lamina propria. Bacilli-laden macrophages can also be found in the synovial membranes of affected joints, the brain, cardiac valves, and elsewhere. Simultaneously, mucosal

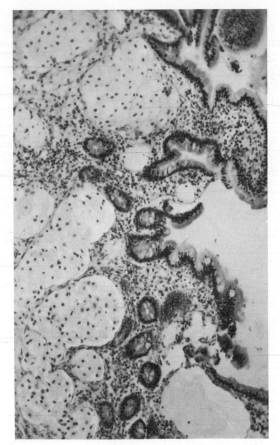

Figure 15–26. Whipple's disease with clusters of distended macrophages lying within the lamina propria of the intestinal mucosa.

and submucosal lymphatics are dilated, presumably because of obstruction, and filled with fat droplets, which may also be found in the lymphatics and lymph nodes of drainage. Rupture of these lymphatics may yield lipogranulomas. Underlying these changes and central to the mystery are innumerable tiny bacilli (visible only by electron microscopy) within the cells, in the underlying lamina propria, and within distended macrophages. Yet they cannot be isolated by culture methods, cannot be transmitted, are uniform in appearance from one case to the next (which implies that they are more than coincidental), and disappear soon after appropriate antibiotic therapy in association with prompt and dramatic clinical improvement.

NEOPLASMS OF SMALL AND LARGE INTESTINES

Despite "the miles" of small intestine, neoplasms in this segment of the gastrointestinal tract are rare relative to the number in the much shorter large intestine. The most frequent benign tumors in the small intestine are adenomas (polyps), stromal cell tumors (mostly leiomyomas), and lipomas, followed, down the line, by various neurogenic, vascular, and hamartomatous lesions. All more or less resemble their counterparts in other locations. They tend to be small, polypoid, or intramural masses, are distributed throughout the small intestine with a tendency to be more numerous closer to the ileum, and seldom produce clinical manifestations, mainly obstructive symptoms or intussusception (p. 519). Despite their rarity, benign tumors are more common than cancers.

Cancers of the small intestine represent about 1% of all gastrointestinal malignancies. In most analyses adenocarcinomas are the commonest, followed in order by carcinoids, lymphomas, and sarcomas. In contrast to the distribution of benign tumors, adenocarcinomas tend to occur in the proximal levels (duodenum and upper jejunum, more than half close to the ampulla of Vater), carcinoids anywhere in the small intestine though somewhat more often in the ileum, and sarcomas and lymphomas more often distally. The adenocarcinomas tend to produce encircling "napkin ring" lesions resembling left-sided colonic carcinomas. Like all malignancies they eventually spread to regional lymph nodes, liver, and sometimes elsewhere. The carcinoid tumors are described in a separate section later (p. 517). The sarcomas may be derived from any of the mesenchymal elements in the bowel wall (e.g., smooth muscle cells, fibroblasts, and fatty, vascular, and neural elements). Whatever the histology they may become large, bulky neoplasms by the time they are discovered, tending to extend centrifugally and thus not produce intestinal obstruction. Despite their large size, they often remain localized but eventually may spread through the bloodstream, and rarely the lymphatics. Lymphomas of the small intestine were described previously along with those of the stomach.

The large intestine is the unfortunate host to more primary neoplasms than any other organ in the body. If all ages are included, adenomas (polyps) of the colon occur in 30 to 50% of the population (the frequency increasing with age), and the incidence of colorectal cancer is exceeded only by that of bronchogenic carcinoma among visceral malignant neoplasms. The other forms of neoplasia mentioned in the small intestine (e.g., benign mesenchymal tumors, carcinoids, sarcomas, and lymphomas) may also arise in the colon. With this brief overview we can turn to the predominant forms of intestinal neoplasia: polyps, adenomas, and carcinomas of the colorectum.

POLYPS (ADENOMAS)

Almost all adenomas of the large bowel protrude into the lumen and so are referred to as polyps. Although an expanding submucosal lipoma or intramural leiomyoma may appear as a polyp, unless qualified, the term "polyp" as used here implies a mucosal epithelial lesion. *Colorectal polyps can be divided into (1) nonneoplastic, (2) sporadic adenomatous polyps of which there are three variants, tubular, tubulovillous, and villous, and (3) heredofamilial polyposis syndromes.* An additional form of sporadic neoplastic lesion about which nothing further will be said is the

nonpolypoid "flat adenoma." Nonneoplastic polyps are best viewed as benign, controlled proliferations. In contrast, adenomatous polyps are neoplasms that range from small, benign, often pedunculated lesions usually composed of tubular glands to large, villous neoplasms that are usually sessile and often have overt cellular atypia, and frequently areas of carcinoma (Fig. 15–27). *There is strong evidence that most, perhaps all, colorectal carcinomas arise in preexisting adenomatous polyps.* Thus, a spectrum of neoplastic proliferation is proposed in which loss of growth controls in the cells lining one or several mucosal crypts leads to an expanding mass of epithelium recognized as an adenoma that may in time become more uncontrolled, eventuating in a carcinoma, the so-called *adenoma-carcinoma sequence.*

The reported frequency of the different types of colonic polyps varies greatly, but nonetheless there is agreement that nonneoplastic polyps represent about 90% of all epithelial polyps in the large intestine. Among the adenomatous lesions the great majority are

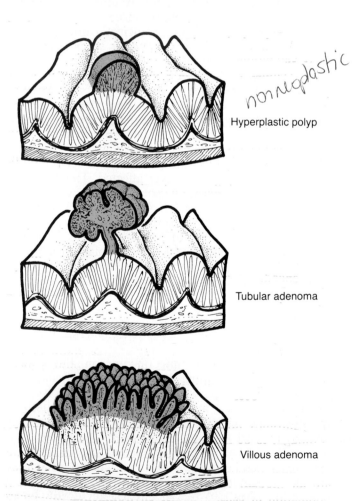

nonneoplastic

Hyperplastic polyp

Tubular adenoma

Villous adenoma

Figure 15–27. A diagrammatic representation of the three principal forms of colonic polyps. The hyperplastic polyp *(above)* sits as a hemispheric dome on top of the mucosal fold. The tubular (pedunculated) adenoma *(middle)* has a slender stalk and a knobby, raspberry-like head. The sessile villous adenoma *(below)* has a broad base and myriad delicate papillae protruding into the lumen.

tubular, about 5 to 10% tubulovillous, and only 1% villous. The frequency of all polyps increases with age, and thus nonneoplastic polyps are found in more than half of all persons age 60 years and older. Similarly, the prevalence of adenomatous polyps is about 20 to 30% before age 40, rising to 40 to 50% after age 60. Males and females are affected equally. There is a well-defined familial predisposition to sporadic adenomatous lesions, accounting for about a fourfold greater risk of similar lesions in first-degree relatives, and also a fourfold greater risk of colorectal carcinoma.

PATHOGENESIS. A large number of genetic alterations have been uncovered in the epithelial cells of colon adenomas. They are of two forms, activation of protooncogenes and loss of cancer suppressor genes. K-*ras*, the protooncogene frequently involved, is located at 12p, whereas the relevant cancer suppressor genes have been mapped to 5q21, 17p, and 18q. Located at 5q21 is the APC gene (about which more is said later); 17p harbors the well-known p53 tumor suppressor gene; and at 18q resides the *Deleted in Colon Carcinoma* (DCC) gene (p. 190). It is important to emphasize that small adenomas with little cellular dysplasia generally have none of these alterations; they tend to be associated with larger lesions characterized by severe dysplasia and often cancer in situ or foci of overt carcinoma. Moreover, even the adenomas with severe cellular changes have only one or two of these genotypic changes. There is therefore a correlation between the level of dysplasia in an adenoma and the number of genomic alterations in the cells. Later it will be seen colorectal cancers have the same types of mutations but more of them, so the development of a cancer appears to result from the cumulative effects of many mutations.

What do all of these molecular deviations mean in the evolution of adenomas, and ultimately carcinomas? Only speculation is possible, but according to one view the process starts in the basal crypt epithelium (the normal locus of cell division in the colonic mucosa) with activation of one or more protooncogenes. These may encode as growth promoters. Indeed a protein kinase, PP60^{c-src}, which is the cellular homologue of a retroviral-coded transforming protein, has been identified in the polypoid epithelium, the level being highest in those polyps with the greatest malignant potential. Thereafter it is speculated that one or more of the deletions may constitute loss of one or more cancer suppressor genes, contributing to the tumor progression (this process has been well documented with the retinoblastoma, p. 190). Except in the familial polyposis syndromes, none of the genetic alterations described is thought to be inherited because they are not present in small, clearly benign adenomas and indeed are sometimes missing from larger adenomas. Rather they are all thought to be acquired in a rapidly dividing population of cells. Whether environmental influences contribute to the neoplastic progression remains uncertain, but the question arises because dietary factors are thought to play a role in the genesis of colorectal cancer, as will be discussed presently. We can now turn to the various subsets of polyps.

Nonneoplastic Polyps

The two major patterns of nonneoplastic polyps are hyperplastic and juvenile.

Hyperplastic polyps are small (less than 5 mm in diameter), nipple-like, hemispheric, smooth, moist protrusions of the mucosa, usually positioned on the tops of mucosal folds. They may occur singly but are more often multiple. Although they may be located anywhere in the colon, well over half are found in the rectosigmoid. Histologically, they are composed of well-differentiated glands and crypts separated by connective tissue lamina propria. Rarely, large hyperplastic polyps develop foci of adenomatous change, and even more rarely they become dysplastic or even carcinomatous. Nonetheless, the generalization obtains: *the usual small, hyperplastic polyp has virtually no malignant potential.*

Juvenile polyps are essentially hamartomatous proliferations, mainly of the lamina propria, enclosing widely spaced, dilated cystic glands. Macroscopically, they are large (1 to 3 cm in diameter), rounded, smooth or slightly lobulated lesions, some with a stalk, sometimes 2 cm long. Almost always they appear in children younger than five years, usually in the rectum, although rarely they may be scattered throughout the colon. In general they occur singly, and being hamartomatous lesions have no malignant potential. They may, however, be the source of rectal bleeding and in some instances become twisted on their stalks to undergo painful infarction. In a rare, autosomal dominant, familial condition, the *juvenile polyposis syndrome*, multiple juvenile polyps appear throughout the colon.

Sporadic Adenomatous Polyps

The segregation of these polyps into three subsets is based on histologic architecture. Tubular adenomas are marked by a network of branching glands lined by more or less undifferentiated columnar cells or mucin-secreting cells. In villous adenomas the test tube–straight glands penetrate from the surface of the lesion to the center, creating myriad finger-like projections. Sometimes there is a mixture of both the tubular and villous patterns, creating tubulovillous adenoma. The epithelium in all is neoplastic and therefore to some extent abnormal, which classically is subdivided into three grades—mild, moderate, and severe dysplasia.

It is impossible from gross inspection of a polyp to accurately determine its clinical significance, but although there are exceptions, the following generalizations are frequently valid:

- *Most tubular adenomas are small and pedunculated; conversely most pedunculated polyps are tubular.*
- *Villous adenomas tend to be large and sessile, and conversely villous features should be suspected in any sessile polyp.*
- *The period required for an adenoma to double in size is about ten years. Thus, they are slow growing and must certainly have been present for many years.*
- *The malignant risk with an adenomatous polyp is*

correlated with three interactive features: polyp size, histologic architecture, and severity of epithelial dysplasia as follows:

- Cancer is rare in polyps smaller than 1 cm in diameter.
- The risk of cancer is high (approaching 40%) in villous sessile adenomas more than 4 cm in diameter.
- Dysplasia when present is likely to be found in villous areas, whatever the type of polyp.

We turn now to a few details about each of the patterns.

Tubular adenomas may arise anywhere in the large intestine, but about half are found in the rectosigmoid, the proportion increasing with age. In about half of the instances they occur singly, but in the remainder two or more lesions are distributed at random. Most have slender stalks 1 to 2 cm long and raspberry-like heads. They only uncommonly exceed 2.5 cm in diameter (Fig. 15–28A). Histologically, the stalk is covered by normal colonic mucosa but the head is composed of neoplastic epithelium forming branching glands lined by tall, hyperchromatic, somewhat disorderly cells, which may or may not show mucin secretion (Fig. 15–28B). In some instances there are foci of villous architecture, but by convention the lesion is still considered a tubular adenoma if no more than 20 to 25% of it is villous. In the clearly benign lesion, the branching glands are well separated by lamina propria and the level of dysplasia or cytologic atypia is slight. However, all degrees of dysplasia may be encountered, usually in the larger tubular adenomas ranging up to carcinoma in situ or overt

cancer confined to the mucosa or possibly with invasion below the muscularis mucosa into the stalk of the lesion. As long as the cancerous change is entirely intramucosal, even if there is microscopic invasion of the lamina propria, there is little if any metastatic potential and such lesions can be locally excised with cure. However, with penetration below the muscularis mucosa the lesion acquires the potential to spread to regional nodes or more widely. Histologic features suggestive of such aggressive behavior are vascular invasion, severe cytologic atypia, penetration of the stalk and possibly extension into the base of the lesion.

Tubular adenomas may be asymptomatic, but many are discovered in the course of investigation of bleeding, usually occult, or anemia.

Villous adenomas are the largest and the most ominous of the epithelial polyps. They tend to occur in older persons, preponderantly in the rectum and rectosigmoid, but may be located elsewhere. They are generally sessile, up to 10 cm in diameter, velvety or cauliflower-like masses projecting about 1 to 3 cm above the surrounding normal mucosa. The histology is that of test tube–like glands separated by scant connective tissue. The resultant finger-like papillae are covered by dysplastic, sometimes very disorderly, sometimes piled-up, columnar epithelium showing considerable hyperchromasia

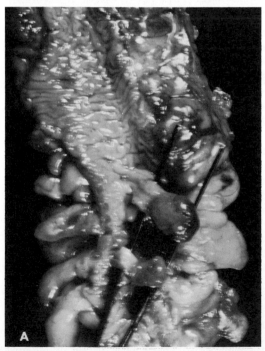

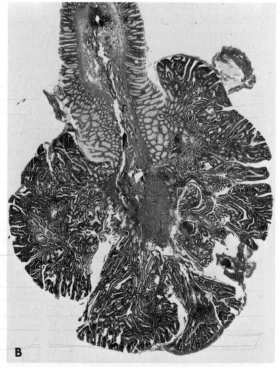

Figure 15–28. *A,* Two pedunculated adenomas of the colon, displayed on top of the forceps. The berry-like heads are attached on elongated, slender stalks. *B,* Low-power view of one of these lesions, showing the normal mucosa covering the stalk and the polypoid hyperplasia of the epithelium in the head of the polyp.

and variation in nuclear size (Fig. 15-29). To be categorized as a villous adenoma at least 50% of the lesion should present the histologic picture described. All degrees of dysplasia up to frank anaplasia may be encountered. Invasive carcinoma is found in up to 40% of these lesions, the frequency being correlated as noted earlier with the size of the polyp and the level of dysplasia.

Villous adenomas are much more frequently symptomatic than the other patterns and often are discovered because of overt or occult rectal bleeding. They may also hypersecrete copious amounts of mucoid material rich in protein and potassium, leading possibly to either hypoproteinemia or hypokalemia. When cancerous changes are present the lesions have the capacity to spread to regional nodes, liver, and elsewhere. On discovery, these polyps are to be considered malignant or potentially malignant and so in practical terms require prompt and adequate excision.

Tubulovillous adenomas are by definition composed of 25 to 50% villous areas, the remainder being tubular. They are intermediate between the tubular and the villous lesions in terms of their frequency of having a stalk or being sessile, their size, the general level of dysplasia found in such lesions, and the risk of harboring in situ or invasive carcinoma.

CLINICAL SIGNIFICANCE. Most important is the relationship of the various types of adenomas to the possible development of carcinoma, traditionally referred to as the adenoma-carcinoma sequence. *Presently, it is generally accepted that most if not all colorectal cancers arise within adenomatous polyps,* as the following observations strongly suggest.

- Populations that have a high prevalence of adenomas have a high prevalence of colorectal cancer and vice versa.
- The distribution of adenomas within the colorectum is more or less comparable to that of colorectal cancer.
- The peak incidence of adenomatous polyps antedates by some years the peak for colorectal cancer.
- Tiny foci of cancer are relatively common within adenomatous polyps but are extraordinarily rare as lesions arising directly from the nonpolypoid mucosa.
- The risk of cancer is directly related to the number of adenomas and hence is virtually 100% for patients who have familial multipolyposis syndromes with myriad adenomas.
- Programs that assiduously follow up patients for the development of adenomas and remove all that are suspicious have substantially reduced the incidence of colorectal cancer.
- Finally, at the genetic level evidence accumulates that adenomas and cancers have similar types of mutations with a strong suggestion that the superimposition of additional genomic alterations onto those found in adenomas results in the progression to cancer (Fig. 15-30).

All these observations underscore the clinical importance of the appropriate management of colorectal polyps.

Hereditary Familial Polyposis Syndromes

These uncommon syndromes fall into two major categories, one in which the polyps are adenomatous and have a very high frequency of giving rise to a carcinoma, and the other in which the polyps are hamartomatous and only occasionally are associated

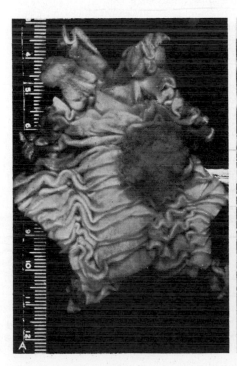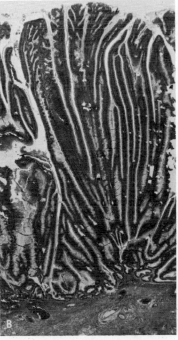

Figure 15-29. *A,* Villous adenoma of the colon, seen grossly. *B,* High-power detail of the long, villous glandular fronds. There is no evidence of cellular atypicality or of carcinoma in the view given.

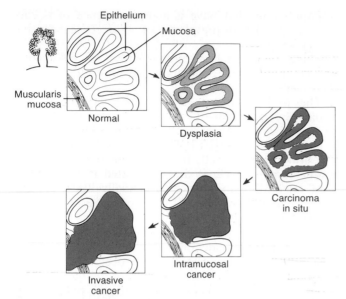

Figure 15–30. A schematic diagram of the potential progression of epithelial changes over time in an adenomatous polyp *(left)*. The initial focus of dysplasia converts in time into carcinoma in situ, which sometime later breaks through the basement membrane to become an intramucosal (still curable) carcinoma, but eventually an invasive cancer.

with cancer, frequently in extragastrointestinal sites. Both the adenomatous and hamartomatous familial syndromes are mostly autosomal dominant conditions. The essential features of the major disorders are presented in Table 15–13, followed by brief characterization of two prototypes.

Familial adenomatous polyposis (FAP) is the archetype of the adenomatous polyposis syndromes. It has many similarities to Gardner's syndrome, as is evident in Table 15–13, and indeed both syndromes may be variants of a single condition. Both, as noted, are autosomal dominant conditions. The genetic defect underlying FAP has been localized to 5q21, the site of the putative APC (*A*denomatous *P*olyposis *C*oli) suppressor gene. (Immediately adjacent to the APC gene lies another suppressor, the *M*utated in *C*olon *C*arcinoma [MCC] gene, which is affected in colon cancers, but not in familial polyps.) Both FAP and Gardner's syndrome are marked by innumerable 1- to 3-cm adenomatous polyps that carpet the gastrointestinal tract. The major target in both conditions is the colon, but in Gardner's syndrome there are frequently extraintestinal lesions (Table 15–13). Both conditions are associated with an excessively high gastrointestinal cancer rate. The average age of onset of the polyps in FAP is about 25 years, followed in virtually 100% of cases by cancer in 10 to 15 years unless surgical resections interrupt the natural progress of this condition.

Peutz-Jeghers (PJ) syndrome, also autosomal dominant, is characterized mainly by mucocutaneous pigmentations and gastrointestinal hamartomatous polyps. Although the polyps may be numerous, they rarely achieve the numbers found in FPC and sometimes

TABLE 15–13. FAMILIAL POLYPOSIS SYNDROMES*

Syndrome	Location of Polyps	Associated Lesions
Adenomatous Polyps		
FAP	Mostly colorectal; fewer in small intestine and stomach; lymphoid polyps of terminal ileum	Osteomas of the mandible fairly common; occasionally dental abnormalities
Gardner's syndrome	Same distribution of adenomatous polyps as in FAC	Osteomas of the mandible, skull, long bones; exostoses; epidermoid cysts; dental abnormalities; desmoids (in about 20% of patients)
Turcot's syndrome	Colonic adenomas	Brain tumors, mostly gliomas
Hamartomatous Polyps		
Peutz-Jeghers syndrome	Hamartomatous polyps singly or multiply throughout entire GI tract; most abundant in small intestine	Mucosal and cutaneous melanotic pigmentations around the lips, oral mucosa, face, genitalia, and palmar surfaces of the hands; occasional skin and visceral cancers

(handwritten annotations: "AD", "dolon", "Onset 25 yrs", "AD", "colon & extraintestinal lesions", "high ca. incid.", "low potential malig transf; but ↑ risk dev - S, L intest ca.")

* Modified from Boland, C.R., Itzkowitz, S.H., Kim, Y.S.: Colonic polyps and the gastrointestinal polyposis syndromes. *In* Sleisinger, M.H., Fordtran, J.S. (eds.): Gastrointestinal Disease, Pathophysiology, Diagnosis, and Management. 4th ed. Philadelphia, W.B. Saunders, 1989, p. 1501.

only a few are present. The mucosal and cutaneous pigmentations are brown-black, macular, and by their distribution (cited in Table 15–13) are quite distinctive of this syndrome. Despite the fact that hamartomatous polyps have a low potential for malignant transformation, patients with the PJ syndrome have a modestly increased risk of developing carcinomas of the small or large intestine (possibly from concomitant adenomatous polyps or mixed lesions) as well as carcinomas of the stomach, pancreas, breast, lung, ovary, and uterus. The risk of cancer is of a different order of magnitude from that accompanying FAP or Gardner's syndrome.

COLORECTAL CARCINOMA

In the United States, colorectal carcinoma is second only to cancer of the lung among the cancer killers. Every one of the 145,000 annual deaths represents in some measure a preventable tragedy because the modalities for discovering these cancers at an early stage are widely available: rectal digital examination, sigmoidoscopy, colonoscopy, radiography, CT, magnetic resonance studies, and biopsy. There is a remarkable variation in the frequency of this form of neoplasm among various countries. The incidence rates are highest in the United States, Canada, Australia, New Zealand, and other affluent countries and substantially lower in the native populations of Asia (notably Japan), South America, and Africa. The extent of the difference is remarkable: sixtyfold between the highest and lowest rates. Some of these striking contrasts must reflect environmental factors, because families who migrate from low-risk locales to high-risk locales over the course of several decades "acquire" the attack rate prevailing in the new environment. The converse is equally true. Changes in the diet are thought to be responsible. The peak incidence of colorectal carcinoma is 60 to 70 years; fewer than 20% of cases occur before age 50 years. When colorectal carcinoma is found in a young person, preexisting ulcerative colitis or one of the FAP syndromes must be suspected. With lesions in the rectum, the male-female ratio is 2:1; for more proximal tumors there is no gender difference.

PATHOGENESIS. There is little doubt now that most, perhaps all, colorectal carcinomas arise in preexisting adenomatous polyps. The great majority of these polyps are sporadic, but it is estimated that about 2 or 3% of all colorectal cancers begin in FAP syndromes. In the previous discussion of these precursor lesions it was pointed out that mutations affecting K-*ras*, as well as deletions or mutations at 5q21, 17p, and 18q, are present in some adenomas, the number of mutations being proportional to the size and level of dysplasia, and hence malignant potential, of the lesion. The 5q21 locus is of particular interest because it harbors two tumor suppressor genes: (1) the APC gene, inactivated in familial polyposis coli, and (2) the MCC gene, mutated in many colon cancers. The adenoma-carcinoma progression is thus viewed as a multiple-hit, multi-step phenomenon involving the additive effects of sequential genetic alterations. Compatible with this thesis are the larger number and greater frequency of genetic changes in carcinomas than in adenomas (p. 193).

Despite all the genetic changes thought to be involved in carcinogenesis, the epidemiologic data cited earlier point to environmental factors as well, and indeed both sets of influences may work in concert. Most attention has centered on (1) the dietary fat intake, (2) the refined carbohydrate intake, (3) the level of fiber intake, and (4) the adequacy of such protective micronutrients as vitamins A, C, and E in the diet. Correlations have been drawn between the amount of fat in the diet and the attack rate of colorectal cancer. It is theorized that high fat intake enhances the synthesis of cholesterol and bile acids by the liver, which may be converted into potential carcinogens by the bacterial flora of the large intestine. *Bacteroides* organisms in particular are suspected; their proliferation in the colon is favored by a high dietary level of refined sugars. There is some laboratory evidence supporting this concept, but no clear documentation of fat-derived fecal carcinogens in humans.

Dietary fiber is thought to play a protective role that accounts for the higher incidence of colorectal cancer in affluent Western societies that live on more refined, low-fiber diets than are characteristic of the lower socioeconomic populations in Asia, Africa, and elsewhere, where simpler natural foods with a higher fiber content are the rule. The fiber is thought to increase the stool bulk and thereby dilute the concentration of putative carcinogens and at the same time speed the transit through the large intestine, thereby decreasing the mucosal exposure to the possible offenders. In addition, some fiber components may serve to bind toxic compounds, adding yet another line of protection. Intriguing as these dietary speculations may be, they remain speculations.

MORPHOLOGY. The distribution of the cancers in the colorectum appears to be undergoing change in the United States: there is a well-defined shift toward the right colon, particularly in elders. Currently about 25% of the cancers are located in the cecum or ascending colon and a similar proportion in the rectum and distal sigmoid. An additional 25% are located in the descending colon and proximal sigmoid; the remainder scattered elsewhere. No longer are more than half of colorectal cancers readily detectable by digital or proctosigmoidoscopic examination. Most often single, infrequently multiple carcinomas are present, particularly in patients with familial polyposis syndrome, numerous sporadic adenomas, or ulcerative colitis. As mentioned earlier, it is extremely rare to find a minute carcinoma arising de novo from apparently normal mucosa. It is equally rare to find recognizable remnants of the preexisting adenoma, because as these neoplasms enlarge they obliterate their origins. **On the left side most colorectal** **cancers are annular, napkin-ring lesions** which generally markedly narrow the lumen and sometimes cause distension of the proximal bowel (Fig. 15–31). The margins of the napkin ring are classically heaped up, beaded, and firm, and the midcircumference ulcerated. These neoplasms directly penetrate the bowel wall over the course of time (probably years), and may appear as subserosal and serosal, firm, white nodules. Spread occurs particularly to the regional lymph nodes and liver but eventually elsewhere.

Cancers in the right colon typically have a polypoid fungating appearance protruding into the lumen as cauliflower-like masses (Fig. 15–32). Plaque-like or ulcerative lesions are much less common. Whatever their gross morphology, the tumors eventually penetrate the wall and extend to the mesentery and regional lymph nodes. More distant dissemination to the liver and other sites may follow. Because these neoplasms arise in the more capacious cecum and ascending colon where the fecal stream is more fluid, they rarely cause obstruction and so remain silent clinically for long periods, save possibly for causing occult bleeding.

Uncommonly, but particularly in association with ulcerative colitis, colorectal cancers are insidiously infiltrative and difficult to identify radiographically and macroscopi-

crampy left lower quadrant discomfort with lesions in the left colon. Right-sided cancers are frequently found in the investigation of fatigue or weakness of obscure origin or an unexplained iron deficiency anemia. It is a clinical maxim that this type of anemia in a male means gastrointestinal cancer, usually in the right colon unless other obvious causes such as malnutrition or chronic inflammatory bowel disease are present. In females the situation is less clear because menstrual losses, multiple pregnancies, or abnormal uterine bleeding might well underlie such an anemia. Systemic manifestations such as weakness, malaise, and weight loss appear only when the neoplasm has already spread to the liver and possibly elsewhere. Indeed, these lesions are so often clinically silent that about one third of patients already have hematogenous spread before coming to clinical attention.

The diagnosis of these neoplasms relies on a variety of methods, including barium enema, sigmoidoscopy, colonoscopy, computed tomography (CT), and biopsy. Elevated blood levels of carcinoembryonic antigen (CEA) are of little diagnostic value because they reach significant levels only after the tumor has achieved a considerable size and has very likely spread; only about 25% of early, so-called favorable, cases have diagnostic levels. Moreover, "positive" CEA levels may be produced by carcinomas of the lung, breast, ovary, urinary bladder, and prostate as well as such nonneoplastic disorders as alcoholic cirrhosis, pancreatitis, and ulcerative colitis. This marker has its greatest value in

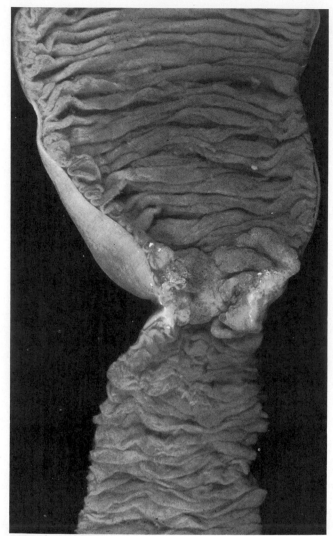

Figure 15-31. Carcinoma of the rectosigmoid. The constricting annular lesion has caused obstructive dilatation of the proximal colon above.

cally. Such lesions tend to be exceedingly aggressive, infiltrative, and spread at an early stage in their evolution.

Unlike the macroscopic differences between right- and left-sided tumors, **histologically 95% of all carcinomas of the colorectum are adenocarcinomas, many of which produce mucin.** Frequently the mucin is secreted extracellularly either within the neoplastic gland lumens or within the interstitium of the gut, dissecting the layers of the wall and facilitating invasion and spread. Tumors arising close to the anus often have foci of squamous cell differentiation and so are called **adenosquamous carcinomas.** Another infrequent variant is the small cell undifferentiated carcinoma, which presumably arises from neuroendocrine cells and therefore has the potential to produce various paraneoplastic syndromes by the elaboration of hormones or other bioactive products.

CLINICAL COURSE. Colorectal cancers remain asymptomatic for years and come to attention by producing occult bleeding, changes in bowel habit, or

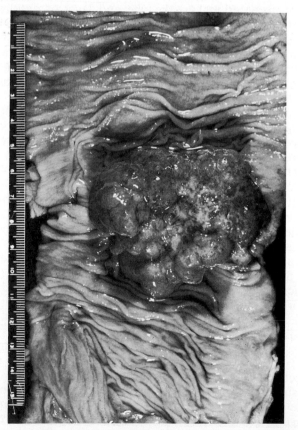

Figure 15-32. Carcinoma of the right colon. The polypoid cancer projects into the lumen but has not caused obstruction.

monitoring possible recurrence of the neoplasm following resection of the primary tumor. If total removal has been accomplished, the CEA disappears. Return of positivity is an indicator of recurrence.

The prognosis for patients is directly dependent on the extent of the tumor, and accordingly numerous staging systems have been devised. Perhaps simplest and most widely used is the modified Dukes' classification presented in Table 15–14 and diagrammed in Figure 15–33.

This staging system can be applied only after the neoplasm has been resected and the extent of spread determined by surgical exploration and anatomic examination. Thus the patient with a Dukes' A lesion has a 70 to 100% chance for five-year survival following resection, falling to 65% with a B1 lesion, 43% with a B2 lesion, and 15% with a C2 lesion. It is evident that the challenge is to discover these neoplasms when curative resection is possible, preferably when they have not yet evolved from preexisting adenomatous polyps. Much can be said, therefore, in favor of screening programs for colon polyps in persons at high risk for this form of cancer.

CARCINOID TUMORS (ARGENTAFFINOMAS) _____

The prolonged survival of patients with these tumors despite their local invasiveness and sometimes metastases made early observers consider them carcinoma-like, hence the designation "carcinoid." They arise from neuroendocrine cells (also called enterochromaffin or Kulchitsky cells) dispersed throughout the gastrointestinal tract and also present in many other organs such as lung, biliary tract, pancreas, and elsewhere. The great preponderance of these tumors arise in the gastrointestinal tract: about 75% in the midgut (ileum, right colon, appendix), 10 to 20% in the hindgut (left colon, rectum), and the small residuum in the foregut (esophagus, stomach, upper small intestine). The peak incidence of these neoplasms is in the sixth decade, but they may appear at any age.

The cells in carcinoids have an affinity for soluble silver salts hence the designation "argentaffinoma." In

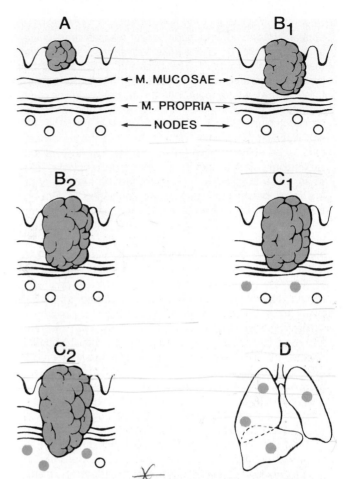

Figure 15–33. Pathologic staging of colorectal cancer. This Astor-Coller modification of Dukes' classification for grading colorectal cancer is based on the extent of local spread of the tumor (stages A through C) and the presence of distant visceral metastases (stage D). This scheme of staging has significant prognostic implications in that the five-year mortality figures progressively increase with the stage of the tumor.

some neoplasms the cells can directly deposit the silver salt and are termed *argentaffin* positive. In others the deposition requires a reducing agent, and such cells are termed *argyrophil* positive. These versatile cells also have the capacity to synthesize and secrete a variety of bioactive and hormonal products, most notably serotonin (5-hydroxytryptamine), histamine, gastrin, adrenocorticotropic hormone (ACTH), calcitonin, insulin, and others. Hence, as will be seen, some of these neoplasms (not all are secretory) are associated with striking systemic syndromes.

TABLE 15–14. MODIFIED DUKES' CLASSIFICATION OF CARCINOMA OF THE COLON*

Dukes' Type	Stage of Neoplasm
A	Limited to mucosa
B1	Extending into muscularis propria but not penetrating through it with uninvolved nodes
B2	Through entire wall with uninvolved nodes
C1	Limited to the wall with involved nodes
C2	Through all layers of the wall with involved nodes
D	With distant metastatic spread

* From Astler, V.B., Coller, F.A.: The prognostic significance of direct extension of carcinoma of the colon and rectum. Ann. Surg. *139*:846, 1954.

MORPHOLOGY. The sites of origin of gastrointestinal carcinoid are (1) appendix (35 to 45%), (2) small bowel, chiefly ileum (25 to 50%), (3) stomach (5 to 10%), (4) colon (5 to 10%), and (5) rectum (approximately 5%). In the appendix they appear as bulbous swellings of the tip, which on transection reveal obliteration of the lumen by solid, gray-yellow neoplasm. Only rarely are the serosa or the regional lymph nodes involved. In the gut they appear as intramural or submucosal masses that create small, polypoid or plateau-like elevations rarely more than 3 cm in diameter. The overlying mucosa may be intact or ulcerated and on transection the tumor constitutes a gray-white to yellow-tan infiltrative lesion that permeates the submucosa and sometimes the muscularis into the mesentery. Those that arise in the stomach and ileum are frequently multicentric, but the remainder tend to be solitary lesions (Fig. 15–34). The tumors are exceedingly firm owing to a striking desmoplasia, and when these fibrosing lesions penetrate the mesentery of the small bowel they may cause angulation or kinking that can sometimes be obstructive. A high proportion of ileal, gastric, and colonic carcinoids have already metastasized to regional nodes by the time they are detected, and many to the liver and elsewhere. Visceral metastases are usually small, dispersed nodules and rarely achieve the number or size seen with typical gastrointestinal carcinomas. By contrast, **rectal and appendiceal carcinoids almost never metastasize.**

Histologically, the neoplastic cells may form discrete islands, trabeculae, strands, glands, or undifferentiated sheets, but whatever their organization the tumor cells are monotonously similar, have a scant pink granular cytoplasm, and a round to oval stippled nucleus. Classically there is minimal variation in cell and nuclear size and mitoses are infrequent or absent (Fig. 15–34). In the unusual case there may be more significant anaplasia and sometimes mucin secretion within the cells and gland formations. By electron microscopy the cells in most tumors contain cytoplasmic, well-formed, membrane-bounded, secretory granules in keeping with their neuroendocrine origin.

The definitive identification of these tumors requires various histochemical procedures. In most midgut carcinomas the secretory granules are argentaffin and argyrophil positive. Foregut lesions are frequently argentaffin negative but argyrophil positive and hindgut tumors are almost always argentaffin negative and only sometimes argyrophil positive. In addition the secretory granules in most neoplasms can be shown to contain chromogranin A, which is sometimes also present in elevated levels in the plasma. Neuron-specific enolase is also found in these cells as it is in many other cells of neuroendocrine origin. In individual lesions appropriate antibodies and immunoperoxidase methods may disclose other bioactive or hormonal secretory products.

CLINICAL COURSE. Gastrointestinal carcinoids are frequently asymptomatic as are virtually all appendiceal primaries. Only rarely do they produce local symptoms owing to angulation or obstruction of the small intestine; however, the secretory products of carcinoids may produce a variety of syndromes or endocrinopathies such as the carcinoid syndrome (to be described), the Zollinger-Ellison syndrome related to excessive elaboration of gastrin, Cushing's syndrome associated with ACTH secretion, hyperinsulinism, and others. Only 1% of all patients with carcinoids, 10% of those with gastrointestinal tumors, and 20% of those

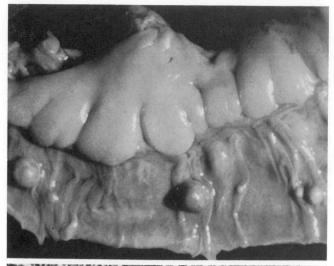
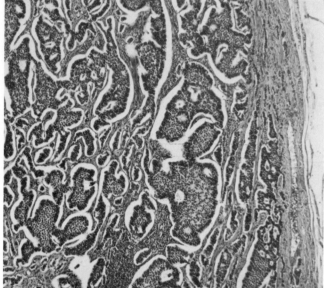
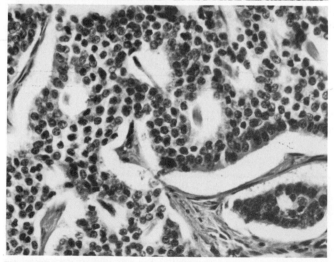

Figure 15–34. Multiple protruding ileal carcinoids *(top).* Middle panel reveals nests of cells invading the submucosa. The uniformity of the cells is evident below.

Know XS 5HT elaboration?

TABLE 15–15. CLINICAL FEATURES OF THE CARCINOID SYNDROME

Vasomotor disturbances
  Cutaneous flushes and apparent cyanosis (in almost all patients)
Intestinal hypermotility
  Diarrhea, cramps, nausea, vomiting (in almost all patients)
Asthmatic bronchoconstrictive attacks
  Cough, wheezing, dyspnea (in about a third of cases)
Cardiac involvement
  Thickening and stenoses of the pulmonic valve leaflets and endocardial fibrosis, principally in right ventricle (in about one half of cases); bronchial carcinoids affect the left side of the heart
Hepatomegaly
  Sometimes nodular; related to hepatic metastases (clinically apparent only in some cases)

with widespread metastases develop any manifestations of a carcinoid syndrome; the full-blown syndrome is even more unusual. Its essential features are detailed in Table 15–15.

Still uncertain is the precise origin of the manifestations, but most are thought to arise from excess elaboration of serotonin (5-hydroxytryptamine—5-HT). Elevated levels of 5-HT and its metabolite, 5-hydroxyindoleacetic acid (5-HIAA) are present in the blood and urine of most patients with the classic syndrome. 5-HT is degraded in the liver to functionally inactive HIAA. Thus with gastrointestinal carcinoids hepatic metastases must be present for the development of the syndrome. In contrast, hepatic metastases are not required for extraintestinal carcinoids such as those in the lungs or ovaries, since their venous drainage bypasses the liver. The possibility that other secretory products of carcinoids such as histamine, bradykinin, kallikrein, and prostaglandins contribute to the manifestations of the carcinoid syndrome has not been excluded. The fibrosing reaction seen throughout the body in some instances of the carcinoid syndrome is particularly striking. Not only is there thickening of the pulmonic valve and the right ventricular endocardium by the deposition of a dense layer of collagen on top of the endocardium, but there may also be in unusual cases similar changes on the left side of the heart, extensive retroperitoneal and pelvic fibrosis, collagenous thickenings overlying metastases in the liver, dense collagenous intimal aortic plaques, and collagenous pleural plaques. The basis for these changes is mysterious. The overall five-year survival rate is approximately 90%; even with small bowel tumors and hepatic metastases it is better than 50%.

OBSTRUCTIVE LESIONS

The major causes of intestinal obstruction are listed in Table 15–16. Surprisingly tumors and infarction account for a relatively small proportion. Four entities —hernias, intestinal adhesions, intussusception, and volvulus—account for at least 80%.

A hernia is a weakness or defect in the wall of the peritoneal cavity that permits a serosa-lined sac to pouch out, into which the gut or other viscera may protrude. The commonest hernias are located in the inguinal and femoral canals, at the umbilicus, and in surgical scars. Rarely they may occur in retroperitoneal locations (e.g., about the ligament of Treitz). They are important because segments of the small bowel, for example, may become trapped within the sac *(incarcerated)* and sometimes compromise their blood supply leading to infarction or gangrene of the trapped segments *(strangulation)*.

Intussusception (which is nearly impossible to spell) denotes telescoping of a proximal segment of bowel into the immediately distal segment. In children, this phenomenon sometimes occurs without apparent anatomic basis, perhaps related to excessive peristaltic activity, but in adults intussusception often points to an intraluminal mass (e.g., tumor) that becomes trapped by a peristaltic wave and pulls its point of attachment along with it into the distal segment. Not only does intestinal obstruction ensue but the vascular supply may be compromised, with infarction of the trapped segment.

Volvulus refers to twisting of a loop of bowel or other structure (e.g., ovary) about its base of attachment, constricting the venous outflow and sometimes the arterial supply as well. Volvulus affects the small bowel most often and rarely the redundant sigmoid. Intestinal obstruction and infarction may follow.

TABLE 15–16. MAJOR CAUSES OF INTESTINAL OBSTRUCTION

Mechanical obstruction
  Strictures, congenital and acquired; atresias
  Meconium in mucoviscidosis
  Imperforate anus
  Obstructive gallstones, fecaliths, foreign bodies
  Adhesive bands or kinks
  Hernias
  Volvulus
  Intussusception
  Neurogenic paralytic ileus
  Tumors
Vascular obstruction
  Bowel infarction

Appendix

The appendix is the most lucrative organ in the abdomen; it alone is responsible for about 10% of all emergency abdominal surgery. The reason for almost all of the "openings" is appendicitis, which will be considered here along with tumors, including mucocele.

APPENDICITIS _____

Surveys indicate that approximately 10% of persons in the United States and other Western countries develop appendicitis at some time. No age is immune, but the peak incidence is in the second and third decades, although lately a second smaller peak is appearing among elders. Males are affected more often than females in a ratio of 1.5:1.

PATHOGENESIS. Despite the frequency of appendicitis, its pathogenesis remains uncertain. Traditionally it has been attributed to luminal obstruction leading to distension of the obstructed segment as mucinous secretions accumulate, followed by vascular compromise of the wall and secondary bacterial invasion by enteric organisms. Unfortunately luminal obstruction can be identified in only about half the cases, usually by a fecalith and uncommonly by angulation or kinking, a tangled mass of pinworms or other foreign body, or exuberant enlargement of the mucosal lymphoid follicles (e.g., in measles or other viral infection). Fruit devotees will be relieved to learn that neither grape seeds nor peach pits have been implicated. Other pathogenic mechanisms must exist to account for all of the cases in which an identifiable obstruction is lacking.

> **MORPHOLOGY. Appendicitis is classically divided into acute, suppurative, and gangrenous stages.** Initially the acute reaction is marked by neutrophilic exudation **throughout** the thickness of the wall. The lumen may be filled with pus. The subserosal vessels are congested and often there is a fibrinous exudate covering the serosa, accounting for the reddened, granular appearance of the "acute appendix." With progression the neutrophilic exudate becomes more marked and foci of suppurative necrosis may appear within the wall as well as within the mucosa, producing sometimes sloughing necrosis. Now the serosal reaction is more marked, with purulent exudate layering the serosa. Often the suppuration extends onto contiguous structures such as the enveloping omentum (Fig. 15–35). At this stage the changes comprise **acute suppurative appendicitis.** If the process continues, edema compromises the blood supply, greatly augmenting the inflammatory process and resulting in large areas of greenish hemorrhagic ulceration of the mucosa and green-black foci of necrosis extending throughout the wall to the serosa. This stage of **acute gangrenous appendicitis** immediately preceeds rupture of the appendix. Now the periappendiceal reaction is more marked, with the possible development of either a localized periappendiceal abscess or possibly generalized peritonitis. To be noted, suppurative exudate within the lumen in the absence of well-defined acute inflammation in the wall cannot be construed as acute appendicitis, since it may merely reflect drainage from a more proximal inflammatory lesion. Contrariwise, fibrous obliteration of the lumen does not signify previous inflammation because it may simply be developmental in origin. True chronic inflammation of the appendix, in the absence of Crohn's disease, is vanishingly rare.

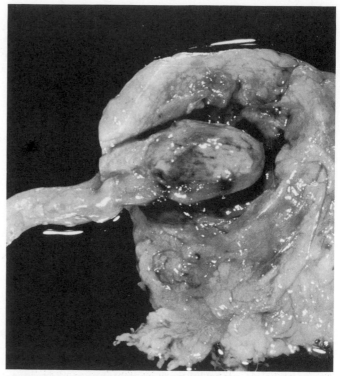

Figure 15–35. Acute suppurative appendicitis involving mainly the tip which is partially enclosed within an omental bed. The appendiceal serosa is layered with exudate as is the adjacent omental bed.

CLINICAL COURSE. Acute appendicitis is the easiest and most difficult of abdominal diagnoses. The classic case is marked by (1) mild periumbilical discomfort, followed by (2) anorexia, nausea, and vomiting, soon associated with (3) right lower quadrant tenderness, which in the course of hours is transformed into (4) a deep constant ache or pain in the right lower quadrant. Fever and leukocytosis appear early in the course. Regrettably, a large number of cases are not classic and the condition can be remarkably silent, particularly in elders, or can fail to reveal localizing right-side lower quadrant signs, particularly when the appendix is retrocecal or there is malrotation of the colon. Moreover, the following disorders may present many of the clinical features of acute appendicitis: (1) mesenteric lymphadenitis following a viral systemic infection, (2) gastroenteritis with mesenteric adenitis, (3) pelvic inflammatory disease with tuboovarian involvement, (4) rupture of an ovarian follicle at the time of ovulation, (5) ectopic pregnancy, (6) Meckel's diverticulitis, and other conditions as well. Thus, as many as 40% of patients with a preoperative diagnosis of acute appendicitis do not have the condition when they undergo surgical exploration. However, it is generally conceded that it is better to have a substantial negative diagnostic error than to suffer the consequences of failing to operate when acute appendicitis is indeed present, permitting perforation and localized or generalized peritoneal infection. The operative mortality rate of uncomplicated acute appendicitis is generally 0 to 0.3%, but after perforation it ranges from 1 to 15%, depending on the age of the patient.

TUMORS

Carcinoids (p. 517) are the commonest form of neoplasia in the appendix. The only other tumorous involvement worthy of mention is mucocele of the appendix and its possible associated pseudomyxoma peritonei.

Mucocele refers to dilatation of the lumen of the appendix by mucinous secretion. It may be caused by (1) nonneoplastic obstruction of the lumen or (2) neoplastic mucinous secretions produced by cystadenomas or cystadenocarcinomas of the appendiceal mucosa.

Obstructive mucocele is usually associated with a fecalith in the lumen, permitting the slow accumulation of mucinous secretions without triggering bacterial invasion. Eventually the distension, which is usually mild to moderate, reaches the point of inducing atrophy of the mucin-secreting mucosal cells and the distended appendix stops enlarging. This pattern is usually asymptomatic and is discovered as an incidental finding at laparotomy.

Neoplastic mucocele may result from a *mucinous cystadenoma* of the appendix. The benign tumorous proliferation of mucosal mucin-secreting epithelium distends the lumen with mucin. The cystadenoma is histologically identical to analogous tumors in the ovary (p. 623). Not only is the distension (2 to 3 cm) greater than that encountered in obstructive mucocele, but appendiceal perforation occurs in about 20% of such cases with spillage of the secretions into the localized periappendiceal region. Rarely pockets of mucin may be found elsewhere in the peritoneal cavity, but significantly *the collections reveal no neoplastic cells or tumorous peritoneal implants.* Much less frequently, the mucin-secreting neoplasms are malignant *(cystadenocarcinomas),* and in such instances rupture of the appendix or penetration of the wall by the cancer cells is followed by implantation of cancer cells throughout the peritoneal cavity, which becomes filled with mucin *(pseudomyxoma peritonei).* Characteristic of this condition are the neoplastic implants throughout the peritoneum as well as islands of neoplastic epithelium sometimes floating free in the mucinous secretions. An identical form of pseudomyxoma peritonei may be produced by ovarian mucinous cystadenocarcinomas.

BIBLIOGRAPHY

ORAL CAVITY

Greenspan, D., Greenspan, J. S.: Oral mucosal manifestations of AIDS. Dermatol. Clin. 5:733, 1987. (An important review because of the prevalence of oral lesions in the AIDS population.)

Hogewind, W. F., et al.: Oral leukoplakia, with emphasis on malignant transformation. A follow-up study of 46 patients. J. Cranial Maxillofacial Surg. 17:128, 1989. (A detailed analysis with good morphologic and etiologic details.)

Illes, R. W., Brian, M. B.: A review of the tumors of the salivary gland. Surg. Gynecol. Obstet. 163:399, 1986. (An excellent brief survey of the range of salivary gland tumors with essential clinical and morphologic details.)

Oral hairy leucoplakia. Lancet 2:1194, 1989. (A brief discussion with emphasis on pathogenesis.)

Randle, H. W.: White lesions of the mouth. Dermatol. Clin. 5:641, 1987. (A detailed discussion of oral leukoplakia and look-alike lesions. Good for morphologic details.)

Rich, A. M., Radden, B. G.: Squamous cell carcinoma of the oral mucosa: A review of 244 cases in Australia. J. Oral Pathol. 13:459, 1984. (A balanced review of the possible causative influences.)

Stead, R. H., et al.: An immunohistochemical study of pleomorphic adenomas of the salivary gland: Glial fibrillary acidic protein-like immunoreactivity identifies a major myoepithelial component. Hum. Pathol. 19:32, 1988. (A study that aids in the characterization of the diverse cells comprising these tumors.)

ESOPHAGUS

Ansari, A.: Mallory-Weiss syndrome. Experience in a community hospital. Postgrad. Med. 76:189, 1984. (An abbreviated consideration of this fortunately infrequent condition.)

Goff, J. S.: Infectious causes of esophagitis. Ann. Rev. Med. 39:163, 1988. (A clear and concise discussion of the more important causes of microbial-induced esophagitis.)

Hamilton, S. R.: Reflux esophagitis and Barrett esophagus. Monogr. Pathol. 31:11, 1990. (A detailed definitive discussion of all aspects of reflux esophagitis and Barrett esophagus.)

Reynolds, J. C., Parkman, H. P.: Achalasia. Gastroenterol. Clin. North Am. 18:223, 1989. (A comprehensive excellent review.)

Sons, H. U.: Etiologic and epidemiologic factors of carcinoma of the esophagus. Surg. Gynecol. Obstet. 165:100, 1987. (A comprehensive analysis of these intriguing aspects of this form of cancer.)

Stair, J. M., Brian, J. E.: The spectrum of esophageal carcinoma. J. Arkansas Med. Soc. 82:107, 1985. (An excellent overview of the etiology, pathogenesis, morphology, and clinical aspects of this form of cancer.)

STOMACH

Antonioli, D. A.: Gastric carcinoma and its precursors. Monogr. Pathol. 31:144, 1990. (An authoritative discussion of early gastric carcinoma, gastric polyps, and intestinal metaplasia as precursors of gastric carcinoma.)

Blaser, M. J.: Epidemiology and pathophysiology of *Campylobacter pylori* infections. Rev. Infect. Dis. 12(suppl 1):899, 1990. (An up-to-date consideration of this challenging but still controversial causation of chronic gastritis.)

Friedman, G.: Peptic ulcer disease. Clin. Symp. 40:2, 1988. (A detailed, but simplified, consideration of all major facets of peptic ulcer disease, very well illustrated.)

Haber, D. A., Mayer, R. J.: Primary gastrointestinal lymphoma. Semin. Oncol. 15:154, 1988. (A fine summary of the patterns found in Western countries, with good histologic, diagnostic, and therapeutic details.)

MacLellan, D. G.: Stress ulceration: The enigma continues. Dig. Dis. 7:159, 1989. (A general overview of the origins, appearance, and significance of these lesions.)

Ohta, H., et al.: Early gastric carcinoma with special reference to macroscopic classification. Cancer 60:1099, 1987. (A detailed analysis with excellent clinicopathologic details of these interesting lesions.)

Peterson, W. L.: *Helicobacter pylori* and peptic ulcer disease. N. Engl. J. Med. 324:1043, 1991. (A balanced presentation of the possible role of this organism in peptic ulcer and nonulcer diseases of the stomach.)

Silen, W.: Pathogenetic factors in erosive gastritis. Am. J. Med. 79:45, 1985. (A clear, succinct presentation of the factors important in the pathogenesis of acute erosive gastritis.)

Soll, A. H.: Pathogenesis of peptic ulcer and implications for therapy. N. Engl. J. Med. 322:909, 1990. (Excellent for pathogenesis and treatment. Presents no morphology.)

Talley, N. J.: Chronic (nonerosive) gastritis: Pathogenesis and management. Digest. Dis. 7:61, 1989. (A very helpful brief review of classification and the pathogenesis of the major categories.)

SMALL AND LARGE INTESTINE

Albert, M. B., Nochomovitz, L. E.: Dysplasia and cancer surveillance in inflammatory bowel disease. Gastroenterol. Clin. North Am. 18:83, 1989. (A very well illustrated presentation of the dysplasia-carcinoma sequence in these disorders.)

Black, R. E.: Epidemiology of traveler's diarrhea and relative importance of various pathogens. Rev. Infect. Dis. *12*(suppl 1):S73, 1990. (Good update on this problem.)

Cartwright, C. A., et al.: Activation of the pp60$^{c\text{-}src}$ protein kinase is an early event in colonic carcinogenesis. Proc. Natl. Acad. Sci. USA *87*:558, 1990. (An up-to-date analysis of the possible steps involved in colon carcinogenesis.)

Editorial: Molecular secrets of colorectal cancer. Lancet *338*:1363, 1991. (Further analysis of this rapidly evolving area.)

Ekbom, A., et al.: Increased risk of large-bowel cancer in Crohn's disease with colonic involvement. Lancet *336*:357, 1990. (A study of a large cohort.)

Guerrant, R. L., et al.: Diarrhea in developed and developing countries: Magnitude, special settings, and etiologies. Rev. Infect. Dis. *12*(suppl 1):S41, 1990. (An excellent analysis of the various etiologies and their prevalence.)

Hunter, G. C., Guernsey, J. M.: Mesenteric ischemia. Med. Clin. North Am. *72*:1091, 1988. (A concise but thorough overview of the many patterns of ischemic gut injury.)

Levison, D. A., et al.: The gut-associated lymphoid tissue and its tumours. Curr. Top. Pathol. *81*:133, 1990. (An authoritative presentation with excellent morphologic details.)

Manousos, O. N.: Diverticular disease of the colon. Digest. Dis. *7*:86, 1989. (Thorough review with good discussion of pathogenesis and clinical features.)

Nishisho, I., et al.: Mutations of chromosome 5q21 genes in FAP and colorectal cancer patients. Science *253*:665, 1991. (Further progress in the genetic mutations underlying familial polyposis and colorectal cancer.)

Podolsky, D. K.: Inflammatory bowel disease, N. Engl. J. Med. *325*:929, 1008, 1991. (An excellent summary of both Crohn's disease and ulcerative colitis, highlighting the similarities and contrasts.)

Ravdin, J. I.: *Entameoba histolytica:* From adherence to enteropathy. J. Infect. Dis. *159*:420, 1989. (An authoritative review with excellent pathogenic details.)

Sjoblom, S.-M.: Clinical presentation and prognosis of gastrointestinal carcinoid tumours. Scand. J. Gastroenterol. *23*:779, 1988. (A brief review of the morphology and functional activity of these neoplasms.)

Tanaka, M., Riddell, R. H.: The pathological diagnosis and differential diagnosis of Crohn's disease. Hepatogastroenterology *37*:18, 1990. (A detailed presentation of morphology and helpful comparison of Crohn's disease and ulcerative colitis.)

Willet, W. C., et al.: Relation of meat, fat, and fiber intake to the risk of colon cancer in a prospective study among women. N. Engl. J. Med. *323*:1664, 1990. (A large-scale authoritative study implicating high animal fat intake in the causation of colon cancer.)

Willson, J. K. V.: Biology of large bowel cancer. Hematol. Oncol. Clin. North Am. *3*:19, 1989. (An excellent overview of the origins of this form of cancer.)

Wilson, J. L.: Diverticular disease of the colon. Gastrointest. Dis. *15*:111, 1988. (An overall perspective of this condition with consideration of its epidemiology, pathogenesis, and clinical presentation.)

SIXTEEN

The Liver and the Biliary Tract

MARY F. LIPSCOMB, M.D.

THE LIVER

JAUNDICE AND HEREDITARY DISORDERS OF BILIRUBIN METABOLISM
- Unconjugated Hyperbilirubinemia
- Conjugated Hyperbilirubinemia
- Hereditary Disorders of Bilirubin Metabolism

HEPATIC FAILURE

PEDIATRIC LIVER DISEASE
- Neonatal Hepatitis
- Extrahepatic Biliary Atresia
- Reye's Syndrome

CIRCULATORY DISORDERS

VIRAL HEPATITIS
- Etiologic Agents
- Pathogenesis
- Clinical Syndromes
    - Acute Viral Hepatitis
    - Fulminant Viral Hepatitis
    - The Carrier State
    - Chronic Hepatitis

AUTOIMMUNE CHRONIC HEPATITIS

DRUG- AND TOXIN-INDUCED LIVER DISEASE

CIRRHOSIS
- Portal Hypertension
- Alcoholic Liver Disease and Cirrhosis

Postnecrotic Cirrhosis
Biliary Cirrhosis
Hemochromatosis — Pigment Cirrhosis
Wilson's Disease
α_1-Antitrypsin Deficiency

TUMORS
- Primary Carcinoma

THE BILIARY TRACT

CHOLANGITIS AND LIVER ABSCESS

CHOLELITHIASIS

CHOLECYSTITIS

CARCINOMA OF THE GALLBLADDER

CARCINOMA OF EXTRAHEPATIC BILE DUCTS, INCLUDING AMPULLA OF VATER

The liver and biliary tract are included together in this chapter because of their anatomic proximity and interrelated functions, and because of the similarity of symptoms and signs that arise when they are diseased. Thus, pain in the upper abdomen or jaundice may result from disorders in any of these organs, and a common clinical problem is to identify the specific culprit. The liver dominates our discussion, because it plays a central role in metabolic homeostasis and because a wide variety of diseases afflict it.

The Liver

The number of metabolic functions performed by the liver is enormous; it is not surprising therefore that this important organ has a tremendous reserve capacity. Indeed, up to 75% can be removed without loss of life, and compensatory hyperplasia rapidly restores normal or nearly normal function. Metabolic functions of the liver include synthesis and degradation of carbohydrates and proteins as well as regulation of lipid metabolism. Regulation of blood levels of glucose and amino acids depends on a normally functioning liver, as does maintenance of normal levels of several other metabolites, including hemoglobin breakdown products (e.g., bilirubin), coagulation proteins, albumin, cholesterol, hormones, and ammonia. When the liver is injured, a number of extrahepatic organs may be affected secondarily by alterations in the levels of these compounds. Measurement of blood levels of several such components (e.g., albumin and bilirubin) helps determine the nature and extent of the liver injury. Two of the most frequent clinical presentations in patients with a wide variety of liver diseases are jaundice and hepatic failure; these syndromes are discussed before we embark on a description of specific liver diseases.

JAUNDICE AND HEREDITARY DISORDERS OF BILIRUBIN METABOLISM

Jaundice (icterus) is the yellow discoloration of skin and sclerae that occurs when bilirubin is elevated in the blood (a normal value is less than 1.2 mg/dl) and is deposited in tissues. Jaundice becomes evident when bilirubin levels rise above 2.0 to 2.5 mg/dl. As might be expected, jaundice is more difficult to appreciate in dark-skinned people, although examination of the sclera should reveal the discoloration.

A brief review of bilirubin metabolism will serve to illustrate the mechanisms of jaundice and its significance in the diagnosis of liver disease (Fig. 16–1). The majority of bilirubin (about 70%) is derived from the breakdown of effete red blood cells. Heme pigment is oxidized to biliverdin by heme oxygenase, then reduced to bilirubin by biliverdin reductase. This conversion occurs within the cells of the mononuclear phagocyte system, principally in the spleen. Most of the remaining bilirubin (30%) is derived from breakdown of nonhemoglobin heme proteins in the liver (e.g., cytochrome P-450), but a small fraction is produced by the lysis of immature red cells in the bone marrow. This latter pathway becomes particularly important in hematologic disorders associated with excessive intramedullary hemolysis of abnormal red cells ("ineffective erythropoiesis," p. 339).

Whatever its origin, bilirubin formed outside the liver is bound principally to albumin and is transported via the blood to the liver. Its further metabolism can be divided into four steps: (1) transfer into liver cells from hepatic sinusoidal blood, (2) intracellular binding to a specific cytosolic protein, presumably ligandin, for transport into endoplasmic reticulum, (3) conjugation to one or two molecules of glucuronic acid, and (4) transport of conjugated bilirubin into bile canaliculi. The mechanisms involved in the uptake of bilirubin from the blood to its eventual excretion into the bile canaliculi are complex and still poorly understood. A number of hereditary diseases of bilirubin metabolism, to be briefly described later in this section, have offered some insight into these complexities.

Once in the canaliculus, the bilirubin participates in bile flow and eventually reaches the intestines, where the glucuronides are split and the bilirubin converted by bacterial action into urobilinogens, most of which are excreted in the feces. Approximately 20% of the urobilinogens formed are reabsorbed in the ileum and colon, returned to the liver, and again promptly excreted into the bile. A small amount that escapes this enterohepatic circulation reaches the kidneys and is excreted with urine.

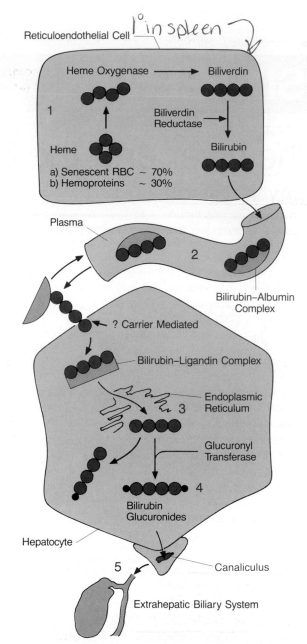

Figure 16–1. Schematic of bilirubin metabolism indicates types of derangements that lead to jaundice: (1) excessive release of heme pigment (hemolytic anemia); (2) reduced hepatic uptake; (3) impaired conjugation of bilirubin; (4) deranged intrahepatic bilirubin excretion; (5) extrahepatic biliary tract obstruction.

There are important pathophysiologic differences between unconjugated bilirubin and the conjugated form. *Unconjugated bilirubin is soluble in lipids, toxic, and tightly complexed to albumin, a form that cannot be excreted in the urine even when blood levels are high.* Normally, a very small amount of unconjugated bilirubin is present as an albumin-free diffusible anion in plasma. High blood levels of diffusible unconjugated bilirubin may enter the tissues, particularly the brain in infants, and produce toxic injury. This is of particular concern in hemolytic disease of the newborn (erythroblastosis fetalis) in which the accumulation of unconjugated bilirubin in the brain can lead to severe neurologic damage, referred to as *kernicterus.* In contrast, *conjugated bilirubin is water soluble, nontoxic, and only loosely bound to albumin. Because of its solubility and weak association with albumin, conjugated bilirubin, when present in excess in plasma (as in obstructive jaundice), is excreted in the urine.*

Having reviewed bilirubin metabolism, we can turn now to the pathophysiologic mechanisms that cause jaundice. Normal serum bilirubin levels vary between 0.3 and 1.2 mg/dl and are maintained within this range because the rate of bilirubin production is equal to rates of hepatic uptake, conjugation, and biliary excretion. Jaundice occurs when the equilibrium between bilirubin production and clearance is disturbed by one or more of the following mechanisms: *(1) excessive production of bilirubin; (2) reduced liver cell uptake; (3) impaired conjugation; (4) decreased intrahepatic excretion of bilirubin; and (5) impaired extrahepatic biliary excretion.* The first three mechanisms produce unconjugated hyperbilirubinemia, the last two conjugated hyperbilirubinemia (cholestatic jaundice).

More than one mechanism may operate to produce jaundice in some diseases, but in general in a given disease state, one mechanism predominates. Therefore, when a patient presents with jaundice, a knowledge of the predominant form of plasma bilirubin (i.e., conjugated or unconjugated) is of great clinical value in arriving at the possible cause of hyperbilirubinemia. For example, unconjugated hyperbilirubinemia often indicates excessive production of bilirubin, as occurs in hemolytic anemia, whereas the presence of conjugated bilirubin points to a disorder "distal" to the hepatic conjugating enzyme systems. An example of the latter is biliary tract obstruction, which leads to regurgitation of conjugated bilirubin into the blood. As expected, in conjugated hyperbilirubinemias, bilirubin is present in the urine, whereas in unconjugated hyperbilirubinemias it is not. With this general discussion, we can now illustrate some specific examples of jaundice with respect to the type of accumulated bilirubin and the mechanism of hyperbilirubinemia (Table 16–1).

UNCONJUGATED HYPERBILIRUBINEMIA

In unconjugated hyperbilirubinemia 80% or more of the serum bilirubin is unconjugated. It is caused by three major mechanisms:

1. *Overproduction of bilirubin.* Hemolytic disease is the most common cause of excessive bilirubin production. The hyperbilirubinemia rarely exceeds 5 mg/dl even when the rate of hemolysis is high, because the normal liver is capable of handling most of the overload. On occasion, patients with pulmonary hemorrhage or infarcts or massive hemorrhage into other tissues may become icteric, presumably as a result of resorption of heme pigment from destroyed red cells.

2. *Reduced hepatic uptake of bilirubin.* This is a very uncommon mechanism of unconjugated hyperbilirubinemia. It is encountered in some cases of the genetic disorder called Gilbert's syndrome (discussed later) and after administration of certain drugs such as rifampin.

3. *Impaired conjugation of bilirubin.* Bilirubin is conjugated in the smooth endoplasmic reticulum of the hepatocytes through the action of glucuronyl transferase. The activity of glucuronyl transferase is low at birth and does not reach normal levels until about two weeks after birth. Thus almost every newborn develops transient and mild unconjugated hyperbilirubinemia (often called *neonatal jaundice* or *physiologic jaundice of the newborn*). Of greater clinical impact are several conditions caused by a genetic or acquired lack of the conjugating enzyme. Gilbert's syndrome and Crigler-Najjar syndrome (see Table 16–2) are characterized by hereditary glucuronyl transferase deficiency. Acquired deficiency may result from any cause of diffuse hepatocellular damage; however, because hepatic parenchymal diseases are often associated with impaired secretion of bile into the canaliculi as well, conjugated bilirubin also accumulates. Indeed, transport of bile into the canaliculi is the rate-limiting step in bilirubin excretion and, therefore, the hyperbilirubinemia of hepatocellular diseases is predominantly of the conjugated type.

TABLE 16–1. PATHOPHYSIOLOGIC CLASSIFICATION OF JAUNDICE, WITH EXAMPLES

I. **Predominantly unconjugated hyperbilirubinemia**
  A. Excess production of bilirubin
    1. Hemolytic anemias
    2. Resorption of blood from large internal hemorrhages
    3. Ineffective erythropoiesis
  B. Reduced hepatic uptake
    1. Drugs
    *2. Possibly some cases of Gilbert's syndrome
  C. Impaired bilirubin conjugation
    *1. Gilbert's syndrome
    *2. Crigler-Najjar syndromes I and II
    3. Physiologic jaundice of the newborn
    4. Diffuse hepatocellular disease (e.g., hepatitis, cirrhosis)

II. **Predominantly conjugated hyperbilirubinemia (cholestatic jaundice)**
  A. Decreased intrahepatic excretion of bilirubin
    *1. Dubin-Johnson syndrome
    *2. Rotor's syndrome
    3. Drug-induced (e.g., oral contraceptives)
    4. Hepatocellular disease (e.g., viral hepatitis)
    5. Primary biliary cirrhosis
    6. Sclerosing cholangitis
  B. Extrahepatic biliary obstruction
    1. Gallstones
    2. Carcinomas of head of pancreas, extrahepatic bile ducts, ampulla of Vater
    3. Extrahepatic biliary atresia

* Hereditary forms of hyperbilirubinemia (see also Table 16–2).

CONJUGATED HYPERBILIRUBINEMIA

In conjugated hyperbilirubinemia more than half of the serum bilirubin is conjugated. This occurs when the secretion or excretion of conjugated bilirubin is impaired at the level of the liver cell membrane, within the bile canaliculi, or at any level within the excretory duct system (cholestasis). *Depending on the level of the derangement, disorders of bilirubin secretion or excretion are usually divided into intrahepatic and extrahepatic causes of cholestasis.*

Intrahepatic cholestasis occurs in two hereditary disorders, the *Dubin-Johnson* and *Rotor's syndrome*, in which the defect appears to reside in the transfer of bilirubin and other organic anions across the hepatocyte membrane into the canaliculi. Various *drugs* (p. 542) may also cause intrahepatic cholestasis. Acute viral infection of the liver *(viral hepatitis)* and cirrhosis may act at several levels to produce hyperbilirubinemia. Thus damage to liver cells may impair conjugating or secretory mechanisms; and swelling and disorganization of liver cells can compress and block the canaliculi or cholangioles.

Extrahepatic cholestasis results from obstruction of the extrahepatic bile ducts. Frequent causes include *gallstones* impacted in the common or main hepatic ducts, and *carcinoma* of the extrahepatic bile ducts, ampulla of Vater, or head of the pancreas (which may impinge on the distal common bile duct). Less common causes of extrahepatic obstruction include (1) acute infection of the biliary tree, filling the lumens with pus (cholangitis), (2) congenital atresia of the extrahepatic ducts, and (3) tumors or inflammatory lesions (e.g., in lymph nodes) causing extrinsic pressure on the bile ducts at any site.

When bile duct obstruction is complete, bile disappears from the stools altogether. Stools lose their characteristic brown color and become gray and putty-like. Obviously, urinary urobilinogen also disappears. However, the urine contains bilirubin, because conjugated bilirubin is water soluble and hence readily filtered by the kidney. Since bile is necessary for the absorption of fats from the small intestine, malabsorption of fats and fat-soluble vitamins appears. With the impaired absorption of vitamin K hypoprothrombinemia occurs, predisposing to hemorrhage, a particular threat to persons who may require surgery, for example to relieve biliary obstruction. In all forms of obstructive jaundice, whether intrahepatic or extrahepatic, bile salts as well as bilirubin may be regurgitated into the blood. Accumulated bile salts produce intense itching, a particularly distressing symptom to patients with obstructive lesions. Cholestasis is also associated with significant elevations of plasma cholesterol levels, and, indeed, these patients may develop localized accumulations of macrophages laden with cholesterol in the skin (xanthomas). Another very important feature of cholestatic jaundice is the elevation of the serum alkaline phosphatase value. The increased enzyme levels result from increased synthesis rather than decreased excretion. It should be noted, however, that alkaline phosphatase is really a family of related enzymes derived from a variety of sources (bones, kidneys, white cells, intestines, and the placenta), and elevated serum levels may also be encountered in nonhepatic disorders. If conditions that affect other tissues rich in alkaline phosphatase can be excluded, notably bone disease and pregnancy, an increase in the level of this enzyme is a very sensitive marker of impaired biliary excretion. Indeed, in partial or early obstructive disease an elevated alkaline phosphatase level may suggest the diagnosis before the bilirubin level increases.

A recapitulation of some of these patterns of jaundice is provided in Table 16–1. *Overall, the most frequent causes of jaundice in adults are viral hepatitis, cirrhosis, extrahepatic biliary obstruction, and drug reactions.*

HEREDITARY DISORDERS OF BILIRUBIN METABOLISM

A number of conditions, most quite rare, are characterized by hyperbilirubinemia related to an inherited defect in the metabolism of bilirubin. Most are innocuous and make the patient "more yellow than sick," but one disorder, the Crigler-Najjar syndrome, may be lethal. The importance of these disorders is that they provide insight into the dynamics of bilirubin metabolism and most, while innocuous, biochemically mimic some of the more ominous acquired hepatobiliary disorders. They should be kept in mind when dealing with the differential diagnosis of jaundice. The clinical and pathologic features of several hereditary disorders are summarized in Table 16–2. Only Gilbert's syndrome is common enough to warrant additional comments.

Affecting up to 7% of the population, *Gilbert's syndrome* is associated with mild unconjugated hyperbilirubinemia and impaired bilirubin clearance in the absence of abnormal liver morphology or any other functional derangements. The hyperbilirubinemia may go undiscovered for many years. If it becomes apparent, it is not until adolescence and then usually in association with stress such as an intercurrent illness, fasting, or strenuous exercise. Mild hemolytic anemia has been described as part of the syndrome, but it is not intrinsic to this condition. More likely, the hemolysis is unrelated and merely elevates the bilirubin level sufficiently for jaundice to become apparent. The mode of inheritance and the precise defect are not certain but family studies suggest an autosomal dominant disorder with incomplete penetrance. Virtually all patients have decreased levels of glucuronyl transferase, but there is evidence for a defect in hepatic uptake of bilirubin as well. It is important to recognize this disease to allay the anxiety that a jaundiced sufferer might justifiably experience with this otherwise innocuous condition.

HEPATIC FAILURE

The ultimate consequence of many liver diseases is hepatic failure. This may come about by slow, cell-by-cell, insidious erosion of the enormous functional reserve of the liver, by repetitive discrete waves of parenchymal damage, or in some cases by sudden or

TABLE 16-2. THE HEREDITARY HYPERBILIRUBINEMIAS

Disorder	Inheritance	Defects in Bilirubin Metabolism	Liver Pathology	Clinical Course
Unconjugated Hyperbilirubinemia:				
Crigler-Najjar syndrome type I	Autosomal recessive	Absent glucuronyl transferase activity	Canalicular cholestasis	Fatal in neonatal period
Crigler-Najjar syndrome type II	Autosomal dominant with variable penetrance	Decreased glucuronyl transferase activity	Normal	Generally mild, occasional kernicterus
Gilbert's syndrome	? Autosomal dominant	Decreased glucuronyl transferase activity, with decreased conjugation, ? decreased hepatic uptake	None	Innocuous
Conjugated Hyperbilirubinemia:				
Dubin-Johnson syndrome	Autosomal recessive	Impaired biliary secretion (? canalicular membrane-carrier defect)	"Melanin-like" pigment in hepatocyte cytoplasm	Innocuous
Rotor syndrome	Autosomal recessive	? Decreased hepatic uptake and storage ? Decreased biliary secretion	Normal	Innocuous

relatively sudden massive hepatic destruction. Whatever the sequence, the hepatic damage must ultimately be widespread because focal lesions, such as primary or metastatic tumors, focal infections, or trauma, rarely deplete the functional reserve. In some instances, diffuse liver injury is compatible with marginal compensation, but intercurrent disease (as, for example, severe infection or massive hemorrhage) tips the balance and leads to hepatic failure.

The morphologic disorders that cause liver failure can be divided into three categories: (1) *ultrastructural lesions that do not necessarily produce obvious liver cell necrosis,* (2) *chronic liver disease,* and (3) *massive hepatic necrosis.* The major conditions, many of which will be cited in greater detail later, that fall within these categories are as follows:

1. *Without apparent significant liver cell necrosis.* These disorders are Reye's syndrome in children, tetracycline toxicity, and acute fatty liver of pregnancy.

2. *Chronic liver disease.* The commonest disorders in this category are chronic active hepatitis (usually of viral origin, but also associated with drugs or autoimmunity) and the many types of cirrhosis, all to be described later.

3. *Widespread massive necrosis.* Destruction of virtually the entire liver is most often caused by fulminant viral hepatitis. In addition, massive necrosis may follow exposure to drugs and chemicals such as acetaminophen, the anesthetic halothane, monoamine oxidase inhibitors used as antidepressants, certain agents employed in the treatment of tuberculosis (e.g., rifampin), and industrial chemicals such as phosphorus and carbon tetrachloride.

Whatever the basis, liver failure manifests itself in a host of clinical dysfunctions. Disturbance of any one of the hundreds of liver functions may dominate the symptom complex. Certain features are, however, usual.

Jaundice is an almost invariable finding. With hepatocellular failure, all steps of bilirubin metabolism are affected to some degree. Since the rate-limiting step is excretion of conjugated bilirubin, most often conjugated hyperbilirubinemia predominates.

Fetor hepaticus, a characteristic odor variously described as "musty" or "sweet and sour," occurs in some but not all instances. It is related to the formation of mercaptans by the action of gastrointestinal bacteria on the sulfur-containing amino acid methionine and shunting from the portal into the systemic circulation (portosystemic shunting).

Neuropsychiatric abnormalities, also called *hepatic encephalopathy,* frequently appear in hepatic failure. They may manifest as disturbances in consciousness, ranging from subtle behavioral abnormalities to marked confusion and stupor to deep coma. Other findings include fluctuating neurologic signs such as rigidity, hyperreflexia, and, rarely, seizures. Particularly characteristic is a peculiar flapping tremor of the outstretched hands (asterixis). The genesis of this encephalopathy is uncertain but is quite likely due to more than one factor. It has been attributed to elevated blood levels of ammonia, short-chain fatty acids, and other toxic substances, or depletion of normal neurotransmitters such as noradrenaline and dopamine, with corresponding elevations of false neurotransmitters (such as phenylethanolamine and octopamine). Whatever the precise agent inducing the encephalopathy, two factors appear to be important: (1) shunting of blood around the liver, as occurs from spontaneous portosystemic connections that develop in the course of intrahepatic disease or as a consequence of surgical shunts to relieve portal hypertension; and (2) severe loss of hepatocellular function, as may occur in fulminant hepatic necrosis. In either case, potentially neurotoxic substances present in the portal blood reach the systemic circulation. One important agent appears to be of nitrogenous origin, derived from the action of gastrointestinal bacteria on the contents of the gut, because coma can be worsened by increased dietary protein or gastrointestinal bleeding and ameliorated by antibiotics that destroy the flora of the gut.

How any or all of these toxins produce generalized central nervous system depression is poorly understood. There is increasing evidence that some disturbance in neurotransmission involving γ-aminobutyric acid (GABA) is important. Increased GABA neurotransmission results in altered consciousness and motor control. In hepatic encephalopathy, GABA neurotransmission might be stimulated by benzodiazepine-type compounds that can be derived from food and accumulate in the brain. This schema is supported by the recent finding that administration of benzodiazepine antagonists reversed hepatic encephalopathy in some patients.

Renal failure may occur in patients with extensive liver disease. It may, of course, be caused by some toxic agent, such as carbon tetrachloride or mycotoxins, which simultaneously damages kidney and renal parenchyma. Analogously, hepatic and renal disease is seen in Wilson's disease due to copper toxicity. Mysteriously, however, hepatic failure alone may cause renal failure, referred to as the *hepatorenal syndrome,* or *hepatic nephropathy.* This syndrome may also follow surgical procedures for obstructive jaundice. Few terms in medicine have caused more confusion than "hepatorenal syndrome." Present consensus restricts the term to patients with combined hepatic (or biliary obstructive) disease whose *renal failure is not associated with visible morphologic changes in the kidneys.* Indeed, kidneys from such patients have been successfully used for transplantation and have functioned normally in their new hosts. The cause of the renal failure is still uncertain, but increasingly the evidence points to reduction of renal blood flow due to generalized renal vasoconstriction, particularly marked in the cortex. The mechanisms of this vasoconstriction are not known, but it may be caused by (1) gut-derived bacterial endotoxins that escape normal clearance by the liver, (2) increased production of thromboxane A_2 by activated platelets, and (3) increased renin and aldosterone secretion secondary to reduced circulating blood volume (from loss of fluid into ascites).

A host of *other abnormalities* may be encountered in hepatic failure secondary to altered hepatic metabolism. Useful diagnostically is evidence of *hypogonadism and gynecomastia* secondary to impaired degradation of estrogens. *Palmar erythema* (a reflection of local vasodilatation) and telangiectasias of the skin ("spider angiomas") are also attributed to hyperestrinism but with little proof. Each angioma is a central, pulsating, dilated arteriole from which small vessels radiate. *Ascites* is particularly prominent in chronic liver failure associated with the combination of portal hypertension and hypoalbuminemia and will be dis-

cussed in more detail later (p. 544). *Weight loss, muscle wasting, hypoglycemia, prolongation of the prothrombin time,* and a *bleeding tendency* (because of impaired synthesis of blood clotting factors II, VII, IX, and X) are also frequent.

As might be expected, laboratory tests that reflect deranged liver metabolism are useful for confirming the presence of serious liver injury. In particular, blood levels of liver enzymes, bilirubin, albumin, and coagulation factors are useful. The outlook of full-blown hepatic failure is grave; a rapid downhill course is usual, with death occurring within weeks to a few months in about 80%. In selected cases liver transplantation may save the patient. A fortunate few can be tided over an episode of acute necrosis until regeneration restores adequate hepatic function.

PEDIATRIC LIVER DISEASE ————

Jaundice in the neonate is a common and often difficult diagnostic problem. Most commonly, it results from immaturity of the glucuronyl transferase system and is therefore associated with unconjugated hyperbilirubinemia. Understandably, preterm infants are more likely to be affected. In some cases there is an associated mild-to-moderate red cell hemolysis. Less common causes of hyperbilirubinemia are hereditary defects in bilirubin metabolism. Also uncommon is neonatal jaundice associated with cholestasis and conjugated hyperbilirubinemia. This may result from (1) hepatic parenchymal cell injury (e.g., "neonatal hepatitis") in about 80% of cases and (2) *extrahepatic biliary atresia* (EHBA) in about 20% of cases. Sometimes these two conditions have been called collectively "*infantile obstructive cholangiopathy*" because they share some laboratory and morphologic similarities. Nevertheless they must be distinguished because without early surgical intervention the prognosis of EHBA is grim, whereas in neonatal hepatitis the treatment is medical and the outlook in most cases is better.

NEONATAL HEPATITIS ————

A number of hepatic parenchymal disorders result in *neonatal hepatitis,* but in about 60% of cases it is idiopathic. The remaining 40% of cases are caused by a wide array of agents, including viruses (e.g., CMV), bacteria (e.g., *Treponema pallidum*), and genetic or metabolic disorders such as α_1-antitrypsin deficiency, galactosemia, and total parenteral nutrition. It is evident that some of the causes are not inflammatory, so "hepatitis" is a misnomer, as are an unfortunately large number of other medical terms the student must endure.

Neonatal hepatitis is associated with disarray of the orderly arrangement of hepatocytes within the lobule, prominent hepatocytic giant cells, mononuclear infiltrates in the portal areas, increased number and size of Kupffer cells, and presence of bile in ductules and canaliculi. Depending on the cause, specific changes may be identified, including intracytoplasmic inclusions in α_1-antitrypsin deficiency, intranuclear inclusions in CMV, or fatty change or cirrhosis in metabolic disorders such as tyrosinemia or galactosemia. In some cases changes mimic EHBA with cholangiolar proliferation and portal fibrosis.

Most patients with neonatal hepatitis are male and have a low birth weight; nearly a third have other congenital abnormalities. In the idiopathic and viral disorders, the disease is usually self-limited.

EXTRAHEPATIC BILIARY ATRESIA _____

EHBA is complete obstruction of at least some of the hepatic ducts or common bile duct in the absence of trauma. It is an uncommon condition encountered most often in normal-weight, full-term, female infants. The laboratory studies are those anticipated with an obstructive jaundice and do not differentiate the condition from intrahepatic cholestasis.

Salient histologic features of EHBA include (1) inflammation and fibrosing stricture of the hepatic or common bile ducts; (2) periductular inflammation of intrahepatic ductules and cholangioles; (3) proliferation of smaller bile ducts, with possibly some disappearance of larger interlobular ducts; and (4) periportal fibrosis and cirrhosis after several months. Cholestasis is evident and in some cases there are changes in the hepatic parenchyma resembling those of "neonatal hepatitis."

Clinically, infants with EHBA develop progressive jaundice. Laboratory findings do not distinguish between atresia and neonatal hepatitis, but a biopsy establishes the diagnosis in 90% of cases. Surgical procedures can sometimes correct the defect but liver transplantation is being performed in an increasing number of cases. Failure to recognize and treat this condition ultimately leads to cirrhosis and liver failure.

REYE'S SYNDROME _____

Reye's syndrome is a rare disease characterized by fatty change in the liver and encephalopathy that in its most severe forms is often fatal. The mortality rate varies from 10 to 30% in the United States to as high as 50% in the rest of the world. It primarily affects children younger than nine years (most younger than four), although older children and, rarely, adults are afflicted. Typically Reye's syndrome develops following a viral illness, the onset heralded by nausea and vomiting and accompanied by irritability or lethargy. This is followed, in fatal cases, by progressive deterioration of the mental state with delirium, convulsions, and coma.

First described in 1963, the incidence of this disorder is on the wane, with an estimated incidence now of about one or two cases per million. Aspirin given during a preceding viral illness has been strongly linked to development of the syndrome in many studies, notably those from the United States. In contrast, in Australia, where the syndrome was first described, a causal link with drug administration was not found. An association with varicella and influenza A and B infections has also been noted in some cases. In other studies, while a preceding viral illness is the rule, no particular viruses are more common than others. An underlying inborn error of metabolism, particularly affecting fat metabolism (e.g., medium-chain acyl-CoA dehydrogenase deficiency), has been demonstrated in a minority of cases. This suggests that *perhaps more subtle and yet to be identified metabolic disorders predispose a person to Reye's syndrome. A viral infection with or without accompanying drugs then sets into motion a train of events that results in liver failure.*

The major pathologic findings are in the liver and brain. **Liver** changes uniformly consist of fatty change (microvesicular hepatic steatosis, Fig. 16–2). Under the electron microscope mitochondrial injury evidenced by swelling and disruption of cristae and loss of dense bodies is noted. Loss of mitochondrial enzymes that regulate the citric acid cycle and synthesis of urea from ammonia have been detected. This observation partly explains the elevated levels of blood ammonia.

In the **brain** cerebral edema is usually present. Astrocytes are swollen and mitochondrial changes similar to those seen in the liver may develop. Inflammation is notably absent, as is any evidence of viral infection in the central nervous system.

The **kidney** may demonstrate subtle fatty change and muscle cells may demonstrate abnormal mitochondria.

Laboratory findings in Reye's syndrome include elevated serum levels of transaminases, ammonia, fatty acids, and lactic acid (producing a metabolic acidosis) together with a prolonged prothrombin time and hypoglycemia; *jaundice is notably absent.*

CIRCULATORY DISORDERS _____

Hepatic chronic passive congestion (CPC) and central hemorrhagic necrosis (CHN) are two circulatory changes representing essentially a continuum encountered in right-sided heart failure. They are discussed on page 306, and it suffices to state here that CPC of the liver is an extremely common postmortem finding, because some degree of circulatory failure is almost inevitable in the agonal stage of life. CHN, in contrast, is less common, and although it is encountered in severe right-sided heart failure, it may also be caused

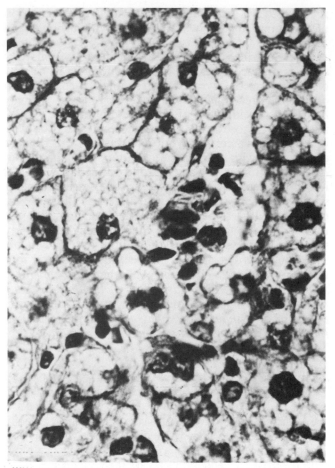

Figure 16–2. Microvesicular hepatic steatosis (fatty change) in a patient with Reye's syndrome.

by disorders that cause arterial hypoperfusion of the liver, such as left-sided heart failure or shock due to other causes. The location of liver injury in CHN is explained by the fact that the perivenular (central) zone of the liver lobule is more susceptible to ischemia than the periportal and middle zones. *Cardiac sclerosis* sometimes follows CHN and, more rarely, long-standing CPC. It is characterized by a delicate fibrosis about the central veins of the liver lobules. Although the fibrotic process and destruction of central hepatocytes may slightly reduce the size of the liver and create a fine pigskin-like granularity to the serosal covering, the criteria required for the diagnosis of cirrhosis detailed on p. 542 are not fulfilled.

That *infarcts* are rare in the liver is not surprising in view of the double blood supply from the hepatic artery and portal vein. Nonetheless, they do occur when an intrahepatic branch of the hepatic artery is occluded, as in polyarteritis nodosa. Even more uncommon are infarcts resulting from embolism or neoplasia- or inflammation-induced thromboses. The typical pale or anemic infarcts are similar to those encountered in other solid parenchymal organs and require no further description.

The *Budd-Chiari syndrome* is thrombosis of the major hepatic veins, and often of the adjacent inferior vena cava. Although highly significant clinically, it is sufficiently rare to warrant only brief consideration. Known causes of the Budd-Chiari syndrome include (1) hematologic disorders with thrombotic tendencies, especially polycythemia vera and paroxysmal nocturnal hemoglobinuria; (2) use of oral contraceptives; (3) tumors, particularly hepatocellular carcinoma and renal cell carcinoma, both of which tend to invade the hepatic vein; (4) intrahepatic infections such as amebic abscesses; and (5) mysterious membranous webs which develop in the venous outflow of the liver or within the inferior vena cava, found mostly in Japanese and other Asians, but relatively uncommon in the U.S. In addition, several cases of hepatic vein thrombosis have been reported during pregnancy or shortly after delivery and may relate to the increased risk of thrombosis in pregnancy. In approximately 30% of the cases, hepatic vein thrombosis appears without apparent cause. Whatever its origins, it is followed by a swollen, tender liver, ascites, portal hypertension (p. 544), and esophageal varices. Unless the obstruction can be bypassed surgically, death follows, usually within months. The anatomic changes are those of severe central passive congestion rapidly progressing to CHN.

Portal vein thrombosis, a less ominous condition than the Budd-Chiari syndrome, results in portal hypertension, ascites, and esophageal varices. Although portal vein thrombosis may occur in the absence of an underlying condition, more commonly it results from (1) abdominal infections resulting in portal vein pylephlebitis, (2) cancer arising in either hepatic or extrahepatic abdominal organs invading the vein, (3) pancreatitis initiating thrombosis in the splenic vein followed by propagation of the thrombus, (4) abdominal surgical trauma, or (5) cirrhosis.

Two extremely rare conditions of the liver vasculature are important to note because of their causal link to various commonly used drugs. *Venoocclusive disease,* defined as subendothelial sclerosis and obliteration of the smaller and central veins and sublobular veins, is thought to be caused by toxic endothelial injury resulting from (1) drugs (including antineoplastic agents), (2) radiation, and (3) graft-versus-host disease. There is the insidious development of outflow obstruction, which mimics the Budd-Chiari syndrome. *Peliosis hepatis* is gradual generalized dilatation of hepatic sinusoids, giving rise ultimately to grossly visible blood-filled spaces. Historically, the first cases were associated with chronic wasting syndromes, but it is now associated with (1) the use of anabolic steroids and synthetic estrogens, (2) immunosuppressive therapy, and (3) human immunodeficiency virus (HIV) infection and the acquired immunodeficiency syndrome (AIDS). Although the pathogenesis is uncertain, toxic injury to the endothelial cells lining the sinusoids is likely.

VIRAL HEPATITIS

Hepatitis is a term used by the pathologist to describe the presence of inflammation in the liver and by the clinician to describe a syndrome in which the patient demonstrates laboratory evidence of liver cell necrosis, often immediately preceded or accompanied by malaise, fever, and jaundice. It usually presents as an acute, self-limited disease; less commonly, a persisting or recurrent injury causes chronic inflammation, which gives rise to diffuse scarring (cirrhosis), portal hypertension, and liver failure. Hepatitis may be caused by a large number of infectious organisms, therapeutic agents, and toxins, as well as by autoimmune reactions. Only viral hepatitis due to hepatotropic viruses is discussed here. Other infectious agents that cause hepatitis (e.g., tuberculosis, infectious mononucleosis, and cytomegalovirus infection) are usually associated with primary infection of extrahepatic organs and are discussed elsewhere in the text.

Hepatotropic viruses, by definition, infect primarily hepatocytes. Several have been characterized and there is epidemiologic evidence for the existence of more. The known hepatotropic viruses include hepatitis A virus, hepatitis B virus, the hepatitis B–associated delta virus, hepatitis C virus, and hepatitis E virus; these last two were formerly referred to as non-A, non-B hepatitis viruses. Although all cause acute hepatitis, the epidemiology, the spectrum of liver injury, and the incidence of chronicity vary with the pathogen. Therefore, before discussing the features common to most, the epidemiology and biology of the individual agents will be discussed (Table 16–3).

ETIOLOGIC AGENTS

Hepatitis A Virus

Hepatitis A virus (HAV) is a small, nonenveloped RNA virus (a picornavirus) that causes *a benign, acute,* *self-limited disorder that does not lead to chronicity or to a carrier state.* Rarely, it causes massive liver necrosis; the incidence for this dire complication increases after age 40 years. Hepatitis A was formerly referred to as "*infectious hepatitis*" or "*short-incubation hepatitis,*" because the incubation period (relative to hepatitis B and C) is short, from 15 to 45 days (average 15 to 30). The first telltale sign of HAV infection is the presence of the virus in the stools. Fecal shedding (which corresponds to the period of peak infectivity) begins during the final week of the incubation period and continues into the initial (prodromal) phase of illness. A transient viremia begins during the prodrome and rapidly clears with the onset of clinical illness. The virus is not shed in any significant quantities from the saliva, urine, or semen, an important factor in understanding how the disease is transmitted.

HAV provokes the formation of antibodies (anti-HAV), initially of the IgM type, which are followed rapidly by the IgG isotype. As seen in Figure 16–3, the appearance of IgM anti-HAV antibodies coincides roughly with the decline in fecal shedding of the virus. After several weeks to months, the titer of IgM antibodies falls, whereas the IgG antibodies persist for several years and confer long-term immunity. Thus, the identification of IgM anti-HAV is very useful in the diagnosis of acute viral hepatitis, whereas IgG anti-HAV merely documents past exposure.

As expected from a virus shed only in the feces, transmission of HAV occurs almost exclusively by the fecal-oral route, from acutely infected persons, often before they reveal symptoms, or from clinically inapparent (mild) cases. This mode of spread is favored by poor personal hygiene, close contact, and overcrowding. *Hepatitis A may occur as a sporadic or epidemic infection.* It occurs in epidemic proportions among the institutionalized as well as among people of developing

TABLE 16–3. SALIENT FEATURES OF HEPATITIS VIRUS

Virus	Agent	Transmission	Incubation Period (Days)	Fulminant Hepatitis	Carrier State	Chronic Hepatitis	Hepatocellular Carcinoma
HAV	27- 32-nm unenveloped ssRNA (Picornaviridae)	Fecal-oral	15–45	0.1–0.4%	None	None	No
HBV	42-nm enveloped dsDNA (Hepadnaviridae)	Parenteral; close personal contact	30–180	1–4%	0.1–1.0% of blood donors in U.S. and Western world	5–10% of acute infections	Yes
HDV	Enveloped ssRNA; replication defective	Parenteral; close personal contact	30–50 (in superinfection)	?	In U.S., mainly drug addicts and hemophiliacs	<5% coinfection, >70% superinfection	No increase above HBV
HCV	30- 60-nm enveloped ssRNA (? Flaviridae)	Parenteral; close personal contact	20–90	Rare	0.4–1.4% of blood donors in U.S. and Western world	40–60%	Yes
HEV	27- 34-nm unenveloped ssRNA (Caliciviridae)	Water-borne	15–60	0.5–3% (20% in pregnant women)	Unknown	None	Unknown, but unlikely

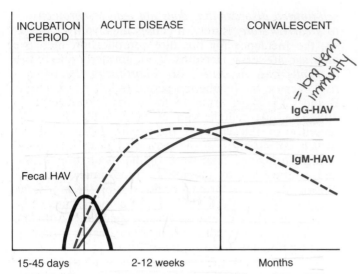

INCUBATION PERIOD	ACUTE DISEASE	CONVALESCENT

= long term immunity

IgG-HAV

IgM-HAV

Fecal HAV

15-45 days | 2-12 weeks | Months

Figure 16–3. The sequence of serologic changes in acute hepatitis A.

countries who live under overcrowded, unsanitary conditions. Such epidemics are often waterborne or related to food handlers. Nonimmune adults are at particular risk when traveling in areas of high endemicity. Promiscuous homosexual males also have a high incidence of infection. The prevalence of this infection in high-endemicity areas can be judged by the fact that more than 80% of blood donors in countries such as Taiwan, Israel, Yugoslavia, and Belgium have anti-HAV anti-

bodies. (In the United States the corresponding rate is about 40%.) Most of these persons were never aware that they had become infected, and probably had only trivial or asymptomatic infection. In developing countries, where the prevalence is high, young children generally show serologic evidence of infection before age five years. In developed countries persons are more likely to develop infection at a later age, and patients are more likely to develop a serious infection. *Sporadic infections* may be contracted by the consumption of raw or steamed shellfish (oysters, mussels, clams), which concentrate the virus from contaminated seawater. The virus can also be transmitted to chimpanzees and marmosets, and infection has occurred in handlers of these primates. *Because the viremia is transient, blood-borne transmission of HAV only rarely occurs and, therefore, blood is not specifically screened for this virus.* This is in contrast to the screening of all blood donors for HBV and HCV.

Hepatitis B Virus

Hepatitis B virus (HBV) hepatitis was formerly known as "*serum hepatitis*" or "*long-incubation hepatitis,*" because it typically occurs 30 days to 6 months (average 1.5 to 2 months) after exposure to infected blood or serum. In passing we might note that HCV also causes a long-incubation type, serum hepatitis. *The clinical spectrum of HBV infection is broader than that of HAV. In addition to acute hepatitis, the infec-*

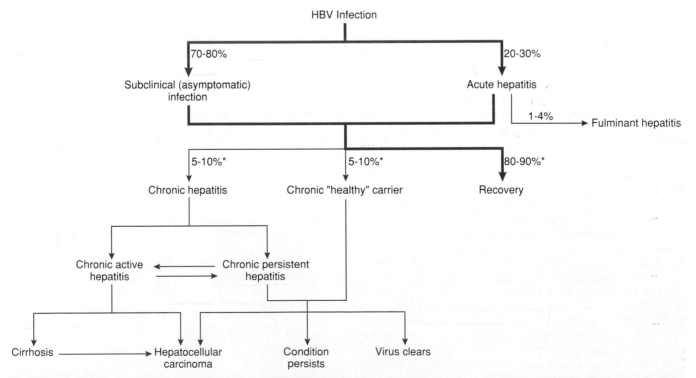

Figure 16–4. Potential outcomes of hepatitis B virus (HBV) infections in adults. Percentages are approximate, and they refer to the proportion of total persons infected with HBV. Frequency of the less common outcomes is not indicated. The thick lines highlight the most common outcomes.

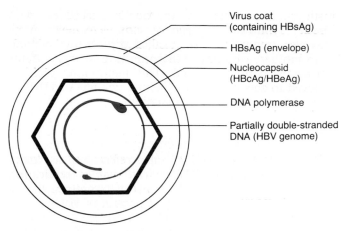

Virus coat
(containing HBsAg)

HBsAg (envelope)

Nucleocapsid
(HBcAg/HBeAg)

DNA polymerase

Partially double-stranded
DNA (HBV genome)

Figure 16–5. Diagrammatic representation of structure and components of hepatitis B. (Drawn from Gerber, M. A., Thung, S. N.: Molecular and cellular pathology of hepatitis B. Lab. Invest. 52:572, 1985.)

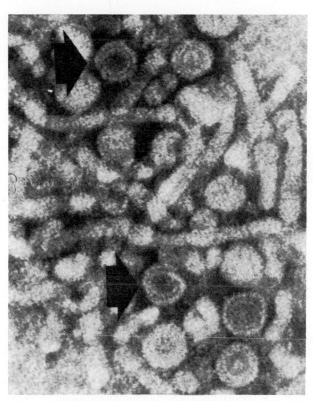

Figure 16–6. Hepatitis B virus. Electron micrograph (× 220,000) of negatively stained pellet prepared from the serum of a patient with chronic hepatitis. Numerous Dane particles *(arrows)* and 22-nm tubules (consisting of HBsAg) are present. (Courtesy of Dr. Michael Gerber, Professor of Pathology, Tulane University School of Medicine, New Orleans.)

tion may result in fulminant hepatitis, a chronic carrier state, chronic hepatitis, or cirrhosis. There is also clearly a link to hepatocellular carcinoma (p. 559). Globally, hepatitis B is an enormous problem. Therefore major efforts are made to avoid transmitting this agent in blood transfusions and to immunize persons who are likely to be exposed. Figure 16–4 diagrams the various outcomes following infection with HBV.

HBV is a hepadnavirus in the form of a 42-nm sphere composed of a central 27-nm nucleocapsid core containing partially double-stranded and partially single-stranded, circular DNA, and an associated DNA polymerase. The nucleocapsid core is enclosed within a lipoprotein coat in which the HBV surface antigen is embedded (Fig. 16–5). Complete virions are sometimes called *Dane particles,* in recognition of the investigator who first described them. During active infection Dane particles can be readily visualized by electron microscopy in infected hepatocytes and less commonly in serum (Fig. 16–6).

Three well-defined antigens are associated with HBV: two (HBcAg and HBeAg) are associated with the virus core, whereas the third, hepatitis B surface antigen (HBsAg), is the major antigenic determinant of the outer surface coat. HBsAg is produced in abundance by infected liver cells and the excess can be visualized within their cytoplasm and in the serum, both as spherical particles 22 nm in diameter and as long, tubular, filamentous forms 22 nm thick (see Fig. 16–6). HBsAg in the past was called *"Australia antigen"* because it was first identified in the serum of an Australian aborigine. Unlike HBsAg, HBcAg is never found free in the circulation because uncoated core particles do not circulate. In contrast, the other core-associated antigen, HBeAg, may be found in the serum as a soluble (nonparticulate) protein. The presence of HBeAg in serum is a marker for active viral replication with shedding of complete virions into the bloodstream and, thus, of high infectivity. HBeAg is not present in the blood in the absence of HBsAg. The antigens

associated with HBV evoke specific antibodies: anti-HBs, anti-HBc, and anti-HBe. These three antibodies, together with viral-specific antigens, are important markers for determining the clinical status of a patient exposed to the virus (Fig. 16–7). HBsAg is first de-

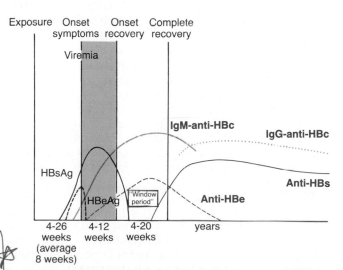

Figure 16–7. Sequence of serologic changes in acute resolving hepatitis B. Note that the color of the labels (e.g., HBeAg) corresponds to the lines that they depict.

tected in blood during the incubation period, in some cases as early as a week after infection. Soon after HBsAg becomes detectable, complete virions and HBeAg also appear in the blood. HBeAg disappears early in the acute illness, usually two to three weeks before the clearance of HBsAg. In a typical case of acute hepatitis B, the HBsAg level begins to decline after the onset of illness and is usually undetectable three months after exposure. Persistence beyond six months usually indicates chronic disease (p. 539). Although core antigen is never found in the serum, antibodies against it (anti-HBc) are the first antiviral antibodies detected after exposure to HBV. Anti-HBc appears toward the end of the incubation period and persists during the acute illness and for several months to years thereafter. The initial anti-HBc response is IgM (a valuable marker for recent exposure), followed six to 18 months later by IgG antibodies. These anti-HBc antibodies are not protective and are detectable in the face of chronic disease. Anti-HBe appears in the serum as the HBeAg begins to disappear, early during the course of acute illness, and its presence signals the onset of resolution of acute hepatitis. Anti-HBs is detected during convalescence (several weeks to months after the disappearance of HBsAg) and usually persists for life; high titers confer immunity. There is a variable interval between the disappearance of HBsAg and the appearance of anti-HBs, called the "window period," during which the presence of anti-HBc may be the only serum marker of hepatitis B infection. The persistence of HBsAg and its relationship to chronic hepatitis B infection are discussed later.

In summary, during the presymptomatic stage of acute hepatitis B, the principal serum markers of the infection are first HBsAg and then HBeAg. As the symptoms appear, IgM anti-HBc becomes detectable, followed after a variable period of weeks to months by anti-HBe and anti-HBs, in that order.

Blood and body fluids of infected persons are the most important reservoirs of infection. HBV is most often transmitted by the parenteral route: blood transfusions; infusions of plasma, fibrinogen, or other blood fractions; contaminated hypodermic needles (a particular problem among IV drug addicts); dental and surgical instruments; and razors. Therefore, there is a high risk of transmission with hemodialysis and transplantation. Transmission may also occur accidentally to health care personnel. In recent years the nearly universal screening of blood donors for HBsAg has significantly reduced the incidence of HBV-induced post-transfusion hepatitis to approximately 10% of all cases; most of the remainder are caused by HCV, as discussed later.

The infection may also be contracted through other routes. The virus may be present in oropharyngeal secretions, in seminal fluid, in menstrual blood, in urine, and in the stool. Infected persons shed virus through literally every orifice, and it is no surprise that intimate personal contact is an important mode of spread. High attack rates occur in spouses and sexual contacts of affected patients, in family members of chronic carriers, among homosexual males, and among institutionalized patients (particularly children with Down's syndrome). Spread by close personal contact may also account for the so-called vertical transmission from mothers who have HBV infection to their infants during the perinatal period. This method of spread is believed to account for the high carrier rate of HBV in some African and Asian populations.

Hepatitis D Virus

Hepatitis D virus (HDV), also referred to as "delta agent," is a unique RNA virus that is replication defective. The virus core contains delta antigen that is surrounded by HBsAg, the coat protein of HBV. Thus, *although taxonomically distinct from HBV, HDV is absolutely dependent upon the genetic information provided by HBV for multiplication and causes hepatitis only in the presence of HBV.* Hepatitis D may occur in two circumstances: (1) when HBV and HDV are acquired concomitantly and (2) when HDV superinfects a chronic HBV carrier. When *acquired together* both viruses are usually cleared although fulminant hepatitis may occur. To what extent coinfection with HDV increases the risk of this complication in HBV-infected persons is not entirely clear. When HDV and HBV infections occur concurrently, in addition to typical markers for HBV infection, antibodies to HDV develop, first IgM followed by IgG. In about 25% of cases, HDAg can be detected prior to the development of antibody. *HDV superinfection in a chronic HBV carrier* may manifest as an acute exacerbation of chronic hepatitis B. More frequently it leads to a chronic delta infection with progressive deterioration of the clinical course. Superinfection of a chronic HBV carrier leads to a transient decrease in HBV replication and circulating HBV. The majority of these persons continue to demonstrate circulating HDAg and develop both IgM and IgG anti-HD.

As might be predicted from the life cycle of HDV, the epidemiology of delta hepatitis parallels that of hepatitis B; like HBV, the delta virus is acquired from blood and secretions. The virus is endemic in the Mediterranean area, the Middle East, the Soviet Union, and parts of Africa, and occurs sporadically around the world. In the United States evidence of infection (as measured by prevalence of antibodies) is uncommon except in certain subgroups of chronic HBsAg carriers, including hemophiliacs and drug abusers (prevalence between 40 and 50%), and dialysis patients, homosexual men, and prisoners (prevalence about 20%).

Hepatitis C Virus

The development of markers of HBV and HAV infections led to the awareness that almost 90% of cases of transfusion-associated hepatitis and many cases of sporadic hepatitis were not caused by either of these viruses. The term "non-A, non-B hepatitis" was coined for such cases. In 1989, using molecular biologic techniques, a small antigen was cloned that led to the characterization of hepatitis C virus (HCV) and the subsequent discovery that this virus is responsible for the vast majority (at least 80%) of cases of non-A, non-B posttransfusion hepatitis and over 50% of sporadic cases of non-A, non-B hepatitis. HCV is a single-stranded RNA virus distantly related to the flaviviruses, which include the agents of both yellow fever and dengue fever.

Similar in many respects to HBV, HCV causes acute and chronic hepatitis and chronic carrier states and is also linked to the causation of hepatocellular carcinoma. As compared with HBV, however, the acute hepatitis caused by HCV is mild, and fulminant hepatitis is much less frequent. In contrast, HCV has a higher propensity for transition to chronicity (in some studies over 50% of patients developed chronic hepatitis). Other similarities to HBV include the epidemiology: exposure to blood products is an important mode of transmission. Thus, high-risk groups include those who receive blood transfusions, patients who receive hemodialysis or renal transplants, IV drug abusers, and medical personnel exposed to blood and blood products. The mode of spread in sporadic cases is unclear; as with HBV, exposure to body secretions brought about by close personal contact is likely to be involved. However, it seems that, as compared with HBV, this form of transmission occurs less readily.

With methods available at the time of writing, anti-HCV antibodies cannot be detected for several months after an acute infection. Furthermore, these antibodies do not neutralize infectious virus, because antibody-containing blood can transmit the virus. Hence, blood banks routinely screen blood for the presence of antibody and exclude anti-HCV antibody-containing blood. This measure has reduced the incidence of posttransfusion HCV hepatitis. However, because of the delayed development of detectable antibodies, the risk of HCV transmission via transfusion has not been eliminated. Therefore, at present it remains unclear how many cases of non-A, non-B posttransfusion hepatitis that develop after transfusion of anti-HCV negative blood are due to HCV or to yet another virus. It must be pointed out that research in this area is proceeding at an extremely rapid pace, and soon improved methods of antibody detection by which infection can be recognized at an earlier stage will be available, making blood transfusions safer and diagnosis more prompt.

The diagnosis of HCV hepatitis may be suspected in cases when other hepatotropic viruses can be excluded and there is a history of blood product transfusion or of intimate association with someone who is a chronic carrier of HCV. A definitive diagnosis requires the detection of specific antibodies in the serum and/or detection of viral RNA by polymerase chain reaction–based assays.

Hepatitis E Virus

Hepatitis E virus (HEV) is an unenveloped single-stranded RNA virus. On the basis of its morphologic and physicochemical properties, it is best characterized as a calicivirus. It causes sporadic and epidemic forms of acute hepatitis that share many features of HAV infection, including transmission by the fecal-oral route and no risk of subsequent chronic liver disease. Its distinguishing clinical feature is the high mortality rate in pregnant women (average 20%) due to the development of fulminant hepatitis.

The epidemic form of hepatitis E occurs primarily in developing countries such as India, other southeast Asian countries, parts of Africa, Mexico, and the Soviet Union. HEV has not been involved in any form of non-A, non-B hepatitis in the United States unless the individual has recently been to an endemic area.

Because there are cases of viral-like hepatitis in the United States that are not associated with any known virus, it is possible that there are other yet unidentified hepatotropic viruses. It should be remembered, however, that drugs, toxins, and other infectious agents can also closely mimic viral hepatitis. Table 16–3 summarizes the important distinguishing features of the hepatitis viruses, including their modes of transmission and clinical outcomes.

PATHOGENESIS

There are two mechanisms of liver injury in viral hepatitis: *(1) a direct cytopathic effect and (2) the induction of immune responses against viral antigens or virus-modified hepatocyte antigens that damage virus-infected hepatocytes.* There is some evidence to suggest that HDV and HCV may be directly cytopathic, while HBV and possibly HAV injuries are immune mediated. The pathogenesis of hepatitis E-induced injury is less clear. As with the related caliciviruses, it likely involves direct liver cell injury.

The mechanism of liver injury has been best studied for HBV. There are several reasons to believe that HBV does not cause direct liver cell injury and that immune mechanisms are important in causing disease. One of the strongest arguments against direct cell injury is that many chronic carriers of the virus have virions in their hepatocytes with no evidence of cell injury. The immune hypothesis is supported by at least two observations. First, during active hepatitis, T cells reactive with HBsAg and HBcAg can be isolated from infected livers. Second, CD8+ T cells are present at sites of liver cell necrosis. Thus, cytotoxic T cells reactive against virus-specific antigens or virus-modified cell membrane antigens could lyse liver cells. It is also conceivable that antibody-coated hepatocytes might be destroyed by antibody-dependent cellular cytotoxicity.

A corollary to the immune-mediated mechanisms of HBV-liver disease is that the variable clinical expressions of infection (i.e., hepatitis, fulminant hepatitis, chronic hepatitis, and the chronic carrier state) with HBV (and possibly with the other viruses) are determined by the strength of the immune response. Thus, a prompt host immune reaction in *acute viral hepatitis* would cause cellular injury but at the same time eliminate the virus. Furthermore, an accelerated and excessive immune response (perhaps related to a large inoculum of the infecting agent) might induce *fulmi-*

nant liver necrosis, but the virus would be totally eliminated. It is relevant that patients who survive massive liver damage caused by HBV seldom become chronic carriers. In contrast, those who mount only a marginal immune response would fail to eliminate the virus, and hepatocytes expressing viral antigens such as HBcAg or virus-modified self antigens would persist, leading to continued low-level destruction expressed as *chronic hepatitis.* Finally, the *carrier state* could be explained as a total failure of the immune response, with perpetuation of the viremia but little or no liver damage. Overall, this view of the pathogenesis of liver injury is supported by the observation that chronic carriers may spontaneously clear their infections and that this event is preceded by a rapid rise in liver enzymes signaling liver cell necrosis with a corresponding loss of viral DNA in the serum. Seductive as the preceding schema may be, it has not been possible to document suppression of specific immune responsiveness in patients who exhibit either chronic hepatitis or the carrier state.

Although cell-mediated immune responses have been invoked as the major mechanism of liver cell injury in HBV hepatitis, antiviral antibodies are undoubtedly involved in the pathogenesis of several extrahepatic manifestations. Circulating immune complexes containing viral antigens and antibodies are responsible for such manifestations as vasculitis, polyarthritis, and immune complex–mediated glomerulonephritis, seen in some patients with acute hepatitis B.

Immune mechanisms also seem to be involved in the pathogenesis of HAV, though the evidence is less strong. This virus does not demonstrate cytopathic effects in vitro. In contrast, both cytotoxic T cells and natural killer (NK) cells can lyse HAV-infected target cells. Immune complex–mediated hypersensitivity reactions have been reported in patients with HAV but much less frequently than with HBV. The mechanism of liver cell injury caused by the recently described HDV, HCV, and HEV is even less clear.

CLINICAL SYNDROMES _____

As indicated, the array of manifestations following exposure to hepatitis virus is great. They can be summarized as follows:

1. Asymptomatic infection (serologic evidence only)
2. Acute hepatitis
   a. Anicteric
   b. Icteric
3. Fulminant hepatitis (submassive to massive hepatic necrosis)
4. Carrier state
5. Chronic hepatitis
   a. Chronic persistent hepatitis
   b. Chronic active hepatitis

As emphasized, not all of the hepatotropic viruses provoke each of these clinical syndromes. Furthermore, for all of these clinical syndromes other infectious, as well as noninfectious, causes can lead to nearly identical syndromes. Drugs and toxins, particularly notable in this regard, will be discussed later (p. 541).

Acute Viral Hepatitis _____

Sporadic attacks of acute hepatitis caused by all of the hepatotropic viruses are clinically indistinguishable but in the United States are most often caused by HAV. When caused by HBV or HCV sporadic cases can be related to these agents only by virologic or serologic criteria. When the infection occurs during an *epidemic outbreak* in the United States, it is highly likely that it is due to HAV. In other countries, where HEV is endemic, it may also be the cause of epidemics. Acute hepatitis can be divided into four stages: (1) an incubation period, (2) a preicteric stage, (3) an icteric stage, and (4) convalescence. As indicated in Table 16–3, hepatitis A and E have relatively short incubation periods (a few weeks), hepatitis B and C, longer ones (many weeks to months). During the incubation period, the person is asymptomatic, but a few weeks before symptoms appear evidence of liver injury can be detected as elevated serum levels of aspartate aminotransferase (AST) and alanine aminotransferase (ALT). In some instances, particularly with hepatitis A, no symptoms, or an extremely mild illness similar to that of many other viral infections, may follow. Probably no more than 5% of cases of hepatitis A become more pronounced than this. In more severe cases, there is a preicteric phase for a few days with malaise, nausea, and loss of appetite, accompanied by a distaste for cigarettes and coffee. Low-grade fever, headaches, muscle aches and pains, vomiting, or diarrhea are less constant findings. In about 10% of patients with HBV, a serum sickness–like syndrome of fever, rash, and arthralgias develops owing to deposition of circulating viral antigen-antibody complexes. Indeed, if these circulating immune complexes persist, glomerulonephritis, arthritis, and systemic vasculitis may develop. Physical examination in the preicteric stage may reveal a mildly enlarged and tender liver. The onset of symptoms tends to be more abrupt in patients with hepatitis A and E than in those with hepatitis B and C. From this point, one of two clinical patterns may emerge. In one, no elevation of the serum bilirubin levels ever appears, and after a period of weeks the patient recovers; this variant is referred to as *anicteric hepatitis.* In the other, the nonspecific symptoms are more marked, with higher fever, shaking chills, and headache, sometimes accompanied by right upper quadrant pain and tender liver enlargement. With this pattern, jaundice develops (*icteric hepatitis*) and, surprisingly, with the appearance of the jaundice the other symptoms begin to abate. The jaundice is usually due to elevated levels of (predominantly conjugated) bilirubin and is accompanied by dark-colored urine related to the presence of conjugated bilirubin. The stools may become light colored because of the onset of cholestasis (cholestatic hepatitis, p. 526), and in some patients the retention of bile salts may cause distressing skin itching (pruritus).

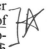

The clinical course of acute icteric hepatitis is variable and is significantly affected by the specific causative viral agent. Typically, with hepatitis A the jaundice and elevated serum enzyme levels begin to subside within two weeks and recovery is complete in four to six weeks. With hepatitis B, the illness is somewhat more protracted, but clinical and biochemical recovery is usually complete within 12 to 16 weeks. Most cases of hepatitis C are mild, with minimal biochemical changes and clinical findings. In some cases of acute hepatitis, as will be further discussed, submassive to massive necrosis or chronic hepatitis supervenes, whereas in others the carrier state develops.

MORPHOLOGY. The anatomic lesions of all the hepatotropic viruses are the same although subtle differences have been described. Indeed, lesions due to certain other viral agents, toxins, and therapeutic agents may appear quite similar to those of hepatitis.

The liver is slightly enlarged and a deeper red than normal, or, if cholestasis is prominent, it demonstrates a greenish discoloration. Histologic features include (1) generalized evidence of injury, as demonstrated by disarray of the usual orderly lobular pattern, (2) focal degeneration and necrosis of single cells or small clusters of cells, (3) Kupffer cell hypertrophy, (4) intralobular and portal mononuclear inflammation, (5) variable degrees of cholestasis, and (6) evidence of hepatocyte regeneration.

The liver cell injury takes the form of diffuse swelling of hepatocytes, referred to as "ballooning degeneration," so that the cytoplasm looks empty and contains only scattered wisps of cytoplasmic remnants. This change is most prominent in the centrilobular areas and is due to marked swelling of the endoplasmic reticulum. Mitochondrial swelling may also be present. Ballooning degeneration may be followed by death of isolated hepatocytes or small nests of cells. Two patterns of cell necrosis are seen. In the first, there appears to be rupture of cell membranes followed by cytolysis. The necrotic cells appear to have "dropped out," with collapse of the reticulin framework where the cells have disappeared. The second pattern of cell death (apoptosis) is more conspicuous and takes the form of condensation and fragmentation of the cell, yielding acidophilic (Councilman) bodies, which are eventually phagocytosed by macrophages. Less frequently, two other patterns, called "piecemeal necrosis" and "bridging necrosis," are seen. Since they are more common in chronic hepatitis, they are described later (p. 540). In the context of acute hepatitis, these uncommon lesions are not considered to be definite indicators of progressive liver disease.

At the height of the disease reactive and inflammatory changes appear. Particularly prominent is marked hypertrophy (and probably hyperplasia) of Kupffer cells and portal macrophages, whose cytoplasm is often filled with lipofuscin pigment. A portal inflammatory infiltrate also appears, composed principally of lymphocytes admixed with macrophages and sometimes plasma cells

and eosinophils (Fig. 16-8). Similar inflammatory cells appear in foci of cell necrosis within the hepatic lobule. Bile stasis may not be present in anicteric hepatitis but may be prominent in icteric patients, in which case droplets of bile pigment are found in ballooned hepatocytes and Kupffer cells and in the form of bile plugs in canaliculi, compressed between swollen liver cells. During the recovery phase, cell regeneration becomes evident, with enlargement of nuclei in surviving liver cells, appearance of mitotic figures, occasional binucleate cells, and liver plates two cells thick.

Complete recovery is the most common outcome, particularly for HAV and HEV (except in pregnancy), and the liver architecture is completely restored over the span of weeks to a few months; the inflammatory infiltrate disappears and the only evidence of a prior infection is the presence of the relevant antibody in the serum. Less happy outcomes are discussed next.

Fulminant Viral Hepatitis

Fulminant hepatitis with submassive to massive necrosis of the liver is, fortunately, one of the infrequent expressions of viral hepatitis. As previously noted, it occurs in fewer than 1% of patients with HAV, 1 to 4% of patients with HBV infection (it is uncertain

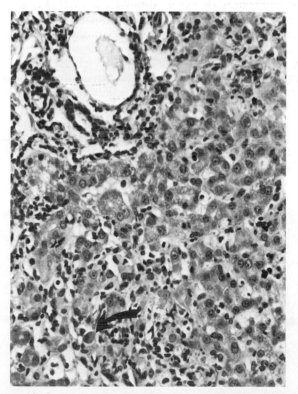

Figure 16-8. Acute viral hepatitis. The portal tract (above) is rimmed with a mononuclear infiltrate. The hepatocytes show focal necrosis and an inflammatory infiltrate. The arrow points to an acidophilic body. (Courtesy of Dr. Edwin Eigenbrodt, Southwestern Medical School, Dallas, Texas.)

whether this complication is more common with a concurrent HDV infection), and in 2 to 5% of patients it is of non-A, non-B origin. Fulminant hepatitis occurs in 0.5 to 3.0% of cases of hepatitis E, but it is far more common in pregnant women (as many as 50%, average 20%). In contrast, although hepatitis A or B acquired in pregnancy is also associated with an increased incidence of fulminant hepatitis, the risk is much less than with HEV. Fulminant viral infection is the most common cause of extensive liver necrosis. Other less common but important agents include toxins and therapeutic agents (p. 541), hepatic venoocclusive syndromes (p. 530), Reye's syndrome (p. 529), and other causes too infrequent to list here.

In the usual case of fulminant viral hepatitis, the onset is marked by rapid deterioration of hepatic function, including coagulopathy, and the onset of hepatic encephalopathy in the setting of an otherwise typical case of acute hepatitis. If this occurs within two weeks of the first symptoms of hepatitis, the term fulminant hepatitis is always used; if the onset is delayed from two weeks to three months after initial hepatic symptoms, the term subfulminant hepatitis may be applied.

MORPHOLOGY. The anatomic changes in the liver depend on the severity of the necrotizing process and duration of survival of the patient. The extent of destruction is extremely variable, as the term "submassive to massive" implies. The process may be limited to patchy foci dispersed throughout the liver, or may involve large (2 to 5 cm) nonconfluent areas, an entire lobe, or even the whole liver.

Early in the course of massive necrosis, the liver is normal in size, but later, as the necrotic areas are resorbed, it is transformed into a shrunken, red-green limp organ with a wrinkled capsule that may weigh as little as 500 gm (Fig. 16–9). With submassive necrosis and survival, regeneration of hepatocytes may produce irregular, firm nodules that bulge above the surrounding surface and may be stained yellow-brown to green, depending on the degree of cholestasis.

Microscopically, in submassive necrosis the coagulative-liquefactive necrosis of cells may be confined to the centers of the lobules, with interconnecting zones of necrosis; sometimes entire lobules are destroyed, with preservation of bile ducts and collapse of the reticulin framework. Surprisingly little inflammatory infiltrate accompanies this extensive destruction. If the patient survives, irregular nodules of regeneration appear. Later there may be surprisingly little residual scarring, although if necrosis has been extensive, pseudolobules of functional hepatocytes separated by bands of fibrous tissue may be formed. Obviously, massive necrosis and early death preclude scarring.

Fulminant hepatitis carries a poor prognosis. Overall, mortality rates are high (70 to 90%); otherwise healthy young adults fare better than children and older persons. The prognosis is best for those with HAV, better in HBV/HDV than in HBV, and poorest with HCV. Fortunately, with the increasing availability of liver transplantation some of these unhappy victims may be rescued. Another hopeful note that can be recorded for these seriously ill patients is that *survivors demonstrate lifelong immunity to the particular infecting virus and tend not to become chronic carriers.*

The Carrier State

As it is applied to most other infectious agents, the carrier state implies that an otherwise healthy person is chronically infected and may transmit the disease. *For the hepatotropic viruses there are two types of carrier states: one in which the carrier is healthy and there is no underlying liver disease and one in which there is evidence of chronic hepatic inflammation* (chronic hepatitis). In this latter group the carrier may not demonstrate any symptoms or signs from liver inflammation and may therefore be labelled "healthy." The carrier state of HBV-infected patients is the best-studied (recall that there is no carrier state for HAV). Epidemiologic evidence indicates a carrier state exists for HDV and HCV (see Table 16–3) but is unknown for HEV.

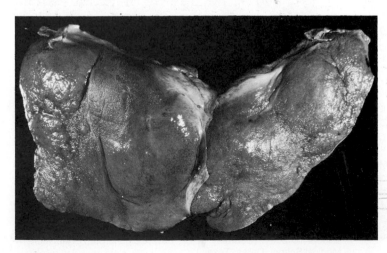

Figure 16–9. Massive hepatic necrosis. The destruction of liver substance has caused irregular collapse and irregular wrinkling of the capsule. The gross lobularity is due to the random areas of preserved hepatic substance.

Carriers of HBV who have no liver disease are usually detected in the course of routine screening of blood donations for the presence of HBsAg. Asymptomatic chronic carriers with underlying liver inflammation are also often identified in the course of screening programs for blood donations. They are also detected when blood is analyzed for liver enzymes in the course of a routine physical examination or for an unrelated illness.

Before the development of HCV antibody tests, HCV carriers were tentatively identified by blood centers that used "surrogate" laboratory testing of donated units of blood. Such tests are based on the assumption that if the blood has elevated levels of hepatic enzymes such as ALT, it is potentially contaminated with a hepatotropic virus, even if there is no serologic evidence of infection. Surrogate testing of donated blood continues to be performed to help exclude *recent* HCV hepatitis because antibodies are not detected until late in the course of infection (p. 535). Such testing also helps prevent transmission of viruses not yet identified.

Perinatal transmission from an HBsAg carrier mother seems to be an important mode of maintenance of the high carrier rate in developing countries. Infected infants tend to carry virus well into adulthood, suggesting that transplacental or neonatal infection produces tolerance to the organism. Transmission from mother to offspring is correlated with the serum titer of HBeAg and inversely related to the serum level of anti-HBeAg. In general, as previously discussed, persons at particular risk of developing the carrier state are those with impaired immune responses, whether constitutional or related to immunosuppressive therapy; patients who have received multiple transfusions or hemodialysis; drug addicts; and mentally retarded persons in institutions. In such high-risk populations the carrier rate may be as high as 15%, even in Western countries.

MORPHOLOGY. In the "healthy" carrier who demonstrates no laboratory evidence of liver cell necrosis, the liver morphology is basically normal; however, striking changes can be seen within hepatocytes containing HBV. The cytoplasm of these hepatocytes has a ground-glass appearance. Ultrastructurally, this can be resolved as proliferation of the endoplasmic reticulum, which is filled with tubular and spherical particles of HBsAg, yielding a strong reaction with specific immunostains. Immunofluorescence techniques may also disclose HBcAg within nuclei. Carriers with chronic liver disease have histologic evidence of liver cell injury (described later) in addition to demonstrating the ground-glass appearance. It is interesting that healthy carriers have more antigen-bearing cells than do those with chronic hepatitis. This observation supports the hypothesis discussed earlier that the healthy carrier state has an inefficient immune response against virus-infected cells.

Although healthy carriers have little or no evidence of liver damage, they have an increased risk of developing hepatocellular carcinoma (p. 558), as do carriers with chronic hepatitis.

Chronic Hepatitis

Chronic hepatitis is defined as the continuation of hepatic inflammation and necrosis for longer than six months. In many cases it presents with evidence of persistent biochemical and symptomatic abnormalities following an episode of acute hepatitis. In others, the onset is insidious and the milder forms are detected only during routine laboratory testing. Traditionally two histologic forms of chronic hepatitis have been distinguished: *chronic persistent hepatitis* (CPH), in which there is minimal necrosis and the course is usually benign, and *chronic active hepatitis* (CAH), which is characterized by progressive liver destruction often leading to cirrhosis, chronic liver failure, and death. For many years CPH and CAH were considered to be two distinctive forms of liver disease; however, recent studies suggest that they represent two ends of the spectrum of chronic hepatitis. With some etiologic agents, CPH represents the initial response to chronic liver injury that gradually evolves into CAH. Conversely, some forms of CAH, with therapy, may revert to CPH.

Most cases of chronic hepatitis are caused by HBV (particularly when HDV infection coexists) and HCV (see Table 16–3), but chronic hepatitis may also be caused by drugs (e.g., oxyphenisatin, α-methyldopa), Wilson's disease, α_1-antitrypsin deficiency, and autoimmunity.

There are no reliable criteria during the stage of acute viral hepatitis to identify persons at risk of developing chronic hepatitis. The severity of the acute attack bears no correlation with the persistence of viral infection. When chronic hepatitis is associated with HBV, findings in the serum suggestive of chronicity include the continued presence of HBsAg, HBeAg, serum HBV-DNA, DNA polymerase, and high titers of anti-HBc. In some patients, after a variable period of 1 to 20 years, the spontaneous appearance of anti-HBe antibodies heralds the control of viremia and cessation of further liver damage. The risk for developing chronic hepatitis following HBV infection is greater for males, very young persons and elders, immunodeficient and immunosuppressed persons, patients on renal dialysis, and those with Down's syndrome.

CHRONIC PERSISTENT HEPATITIS. CPH is characterized clinically by persistence of elevated levels of liver aminotransferase enzymes (AST and ALT) and alkaline phosphatase. Usually there are no symptoms, but some patients may experience relapsing and remitting episodes of malaise, loss of appetite, nausea, and sometimes mild jaundice. In the past, it was thought that CPH almost always followed a benign, self-limited course. Recent studies, however, have begun to cast doubts on this time-honored concept. For example, with certain etiologic agents, e.g., HCV, typical CPH may progress to cirrhosis in a substantial proportion of patients.

Two morphologic patterns exist. In one, lobular architecture is nearly normal but there is a dense portal infiltrate consisting of lymphocytes admixed with plasma cells and macrophages, with no necrosis of hepatocytes. This pattern is most typical of CPH ("usual" CPH). In contrast, in chronic "lobular" hepatitis, the portal tracts are only mildly inflamed and random hepatocytes within the lobules demonstrate the same degenerative and necrotic changes that occur in acute hepatitis. In those cases caused by HBV, ground-glass hepatocytes, seen best in aldehyde fuchsin or orcein stain, are sometimes present (p. 539). Important features of both the usual form of CPH and chronic lobular hepatitis are that the limiting plate (the delimitation between portal connective tissue and periportal hepatocytes) is preserved; unlike full-blown CAH, piecemeal necrosis and fibrosis are minimal or nonexistent.

CHRONIC ACTIVE HEPATITIS. In contrast to the previous condition, CAH is characterized by progressive destruction of hepatocytes over the span of years, continued erosion of the hepatic functional reserve, and in most cases eventual development of cirrhosis.

The major histologic hallmarks of CAH, whether viral or nonviral, are:

● A portal and periportal infiltrate of lymphocytes, plasma cells, and macrophages. The inflammatory cells may appear to spill out into the lobule from the adjacent portal triad (Fig. 16–10). As the disease becomes more chronic, plasma cells become more prominent and lymphoid follicles may appear.

● Active destruction of hepatocytes at the interface between the periportal inflammatory infiltrate and adjacent hepatocytes, leading to a **moth-eaten appearance of the limiting plate** (hence the term piecemeal necrosis; see Fig. 16–10). The liver cell death appears to result from attachment of accumulated lymphocytes to the liver cells, followed by apoptosis and fragmentation of the hepatocytes.

● Destruction of contiguous hepatocytes accompanied by dropout and resulting collapse of the reticulum-supporting framework. In severe forms of CAH this necrosis may connect two central veins, two portal tracts, or a central vein with a portal tract; this is referred to as **bridging necrosis** (Fig. 16–11).

● In the severe forms of CAH, progressive replacement of these bridges and periportal necrotic cells by fibrosis, often developing into cirrhosis.

In summary, the feature that points toward CAH rather than CPH is piecemeal necrosis. Bridging necrosis and fibrosis are present in more severe forms of CAH, which are most likely to progress to cirrho-

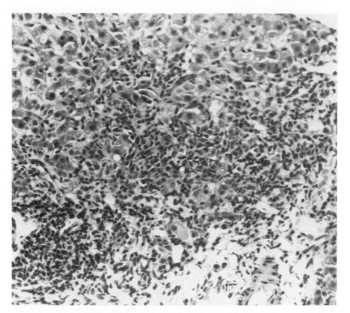

Figure 16–10. Chronic active hepatitis demonstrating piecemeal necrosis. The portal inflammatory infiltrate *(lower left)* is spilling out into the parenchyma, and there is patchy dropout of periportal hepatocytes destroying the usual sharp distinct boundaries between the portal tract and adjacent hepatic parenchyma.

sis. The greater the necrosis, the more likely is the progression to cirrhosis. In addition to all these changes, there may be bile stasis in hepatocytes and canaliculi, variable degrees of intralobular hepatocyte degeneration, necrosis and regeneration, and Kupffer cell hypertrophy and hyperplasia. Kupffer cells may be laden with lipofuscin and bile pigment.

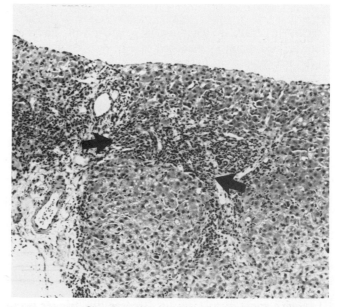

Figure 16–11. Chronic active hepatitis demonstrating bridging necrosis between a portal tract and central vein *(between arrows).*

CAH is associated with highly variable clinical features. About 30% of persons who develop chronic active viral hepatitis previously had an obvious acute attack of icteric hepatitis. In these patients, the signs and symptoms of liver disease persist—fatigue, anorexia, low-grade fever, and sometimes persistent or recurrent jaundice. Some of these patients might initially reveal a picture of CPH on liver biopsy; in others the chronic disease becomes evident with the chance finding of abnormal results of liver function tests without an identifiable prior episode of acute hepatitis. In still others CAH becomes apparent only after cirrhosis is evident; the patient may present with ascites, bleeding esophageal varices, or hepatic failure. Once the diagnosis is made the clinical course also varies. Some patients progress to cirrhosis in a few years. Patients who are positive for both HBsAg and delta agent are particularly prone to develop severe liver injury with diffuse scarring, resulting in a high mortality rate. Some cases, especially those caused by HBV, may revert to CPH following therapy and others spontaneously remit. Overall, with cases of HBV origin, there is a 25 to 50% mortality risk within five years if bridging necrosis is present. An additional hazard for both HBV- and HCV-related CAH is the possible development of hepatocellular carcinoma (p. 558).

AUTOIMMUNE CHRONIC HEPATITIS

Chronic hepatitis unrelated to known viral agents or toxins is frequently ascribed to autoimmunity. Several clinical, genetic, and serologic features serve to distinguish autoimmune chronic hepatitis from that caused by viruses:

- A female predominance, occurring particularly in young and perimenopausal women.
- The absence of serologic markers of infection with hepatotropic viruses.
- Elevated serum IgG levels with the frequent presence of antinuclear antibodies (ANA) and anti–smooth muscle antibodies (ASMA), as well as antibodies against various liver-specific antigens.
- An increased association with other forms of autoimmune disease such as thyroiditis, arthritis, vasculitis, and Sjögren's syndrome.
- A genetic predisposition marked by human leukocyte antigen (HLA)-B8 or -DRw3.
- In many patients, a beneficial response to the administration of steroids. Viral CAH, in contrast, responds less well to steroids.

> Morphologically, autoimmune chronic hepatitis may be indistinguishable from CAH associated with virus infections. As expected, the ground-glass cytoplasm seen in HBV hepatitis does not develop. Less commonly the picture is more like that of CPH.

As with most autoimmune diseases, the trigger event and pathogenesis of the reaction against self are ob-

scure. Cytotoxic T cells and antibody-dependent cellular cytotoxicity have both been implicated, most of the evidence favoring the latter. Some recent reports have incriminated HCV as the trigger for autoimmunity, but others dispute this claim.

DRUG- AND TOXIN-INDUCED LIVER DISEASE

Xenobiotics (i.e., therapeutic agents and environmental toxins) can produce a diverse group of hepatic lesions that mimic virtually any form of hepatic disease, from viral hepatitis and cirrhosis to vascular occlusion and portal hypertension. In contrast to the other diseases, however, the treatment is straightforward: the hepatic injury is often reversed when the agent is removed. Thus, there are few other diseases for which a detailed exposure history is so critical. It is estimated that 5% of cases of jaundice are due to drugs and 25% of cases of fulminant hepatitis are caused by therapeutic agents.

Principles of drug and toxic injury were discussed previously (p. 226). Here it suffices to summarize that drug reactions may be classified as *predictable (intrinsic)* reactions or *unpredictable (idiosyncratic)* ones. Expected drug reactions may occur in anyone who accumulates a sufficient dose; the lag in onset of injury depends on the time required to accumulate a critical concentration of either the drug or its toxic metabolite. Idiosyncratic reactions, on the other hand, are, as implied, unanticipated and mysterious although two influences contribute: (1) the host's propensity to mount an immune response to the offending agent (hypersensitivity reaction) and (2) the rate at which the host metabolizes the agent as compared to the normal population. Immune-mediated injury is suspected if the reaction occurs only after a previous exposure. Although very few drugs have been proven to elicit liver injury as a result of hypersensitivity, this mechanism is likely at work if liver disease is accompanied by symptoms such as fever, rash, eosinophilia, or atypical lymphocytosis and liver biopsy demonstrates eosinophilic infiltrates or granulomas. The second form of idiosyncratic reaction is related to the metabolic handling of the drug by the host. If the drug itself is toxic, slower-than-normal detoxification will cause liver cell injury; conversely if the toxic moiety is a metabolite of the drug, then those who are rapid metabolizers will be prone to sustain hepatic damage.

As mentioned, there is a wide variety of histopathologic responses to drug and toxin injury (Table 16–4). Among the agents listed, *predictable reactions are ascribed to acetaminophen, tetracycline, antineoplastic agents, ethanol, carbon tetrachloride, bromobenzene, and the mushroom* Amanita phalloides *toxin. The drugs that likely cause hypersensitivity reactions are the ones that cause granulomas.* Many of the remaining drugs listed in the table most frequently cause idiosyncratic reactions.

Two agents commonly responsible for adverse reactions, chlorpromazine and halothane, deserve special

TABLE 16–4. DRUG- AND TOXIN-INDUCED HEPATIC INJURY AND COMMONLY INVOLVED XENOBIOTICS

Tissue Reaction	Examples
Hepatocellular Damage	
Microvesicular fatty change	Tetracycline, salicylates, and yellow phosphorus
Macrovesicular fatty change	Ethanol, methotrexate
Centrilobular necrosis	Bromobenzene, CCl₄, acetaminophen, halothane, rifampin
Diffuse or massive necrosis	Halothane, isoniazid, acetaminophen, α-methyldopa, trinitrotoluene, *Amanita phalloides* toxin
Hepatitis, acute and chronic	Oxyphenisatin, α-methyldopa, nitrofurantoin, phenytoin
Fibrosis-cirrhosis	Methotrexate, amiodarone, most drugs that cause chronic hepatitis
Granuloma formation	Sulfonamides, α-methyldopa, quinidine, phenylbutazone, hydralazine, allopurinol
Cholestasis (with or without hepatocellular injury)	Chlorpromazine, erythromycin estolate, anabolic steroids, OC,* and organic arsenicals
Vascular Occlusive Disorder	
Venoocclusive disease	Cytotoxic drugs
Hepatic or portal vein thrombosis	Estrogens, including OC,* and cytotoxic agents
Hyperplasia and Neoplasia	
Adenoma	OC*
Hepatocellular carcinoma	Vinyl chloride, aflatoxin
Angiosarcoma	Vinyl chloride, inorganic arsenic

Handwritten margin notes: "Underlined = predictable rxn", "(others idiosyncratic)"

* Oral contraceptives.

comment because of the frequency with which they cause idiosyncratic reactions. *Chlorpromazine,* an agent widely used in psychiatric medicine, typically produces predominantly intrahepatic cholestasis, with variable amounts of spotty hepatocyte necrosis and portal inflammation. The prognosis of chlorpromazine-induced liver disease is excellent when the drug is withdrawn.

The anesthetic gas *halothane,* on the other hand, is responsible for more serious disease. After viral hepatitis, halothane injury is the most frequent cause of fulminant hepatitis. Two distinct forms of halothane-induced liver injury have been identified. Mild focal hepatocellular necrosis accompanied by an elevation in serum aminotransferase value occurs in as many as 20% of patients following a single exposure to halothane. This reaction, which presumably reflects direct toxicity, is mediated by a metabolite of halothane and is usually noted in the second postoperative week. It is usually mild and completely reversible. Why some persons develop these alterations and others do not is not known. The other more serious and potentially fatal reaction is characterized by massive liver cell necrosis. Virtually all patients who experience the severe reaction have been exposed to halothane on one or more occasions without apparent untoward consequences. This suggests development of hypersensitivity, but conclusive evidence is lacking.

In summary, it should be evident that in the differential diagnosis of any form of liver disease, exposure to a toxin or therapeutic agent should always be on the list of suspected causes.

CIRRHOSIS

The term cirrhosis is applied to a diffuse, fibrosing and nodular condition of the liver associated with a spectrum of clinical findings that include portal vein hypertension and hepatic failure. It is among the top ten causes of death in the Western world, principally owing to the high incidence of alcohol abuse, a major cause of cirrhosis. The many other causes of cirrhosis will be detailed later. Although the histopathology and pathophysiology vary somewhat with the etiologic agent, certain features are common to all (Fig. 16–12):

● Cirrhosis is associated with *diffuse fibrosis* that involves the entire liver and disrupts its normal architecture; focal areas of fibrosis do not constitute the condition. The fibrosis may consist of delicate interlacing bands or dense broad bands. In general, the scarring is *irreversible* although it is known that collagen turns over continuously and in some forms of cirrhosis (e.g., that associated with hemochromatosis) the process may be reversible (p. 554).

● *Nodularity* is a sine qua non of cirrhosis. The fibrous bands may enclose a single lobule by bridging

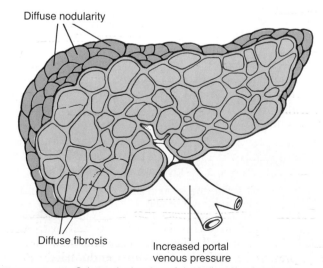

Figure 16–12. Schematic drawing of the hallmarks of cirrhosis.

Labels in figure: Diffuse nodularity; Diffuse fibrosis; Increased portal venous pressure.

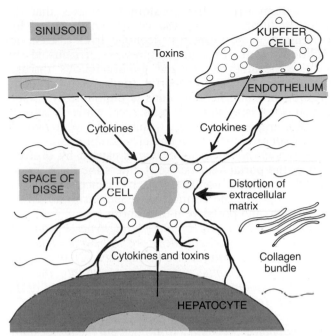

Figure 16-13. Proposed mechanisms for stimulation of collagen production by Ito cells in cirrhosis. Distortion of the extracellular matrix; secretion of cytokines from endothelial cells, Kupffer cells, or hepatocytes; or the direct action of toxins (or their metabolites from adjacent hepatocytes) have all been proposed as possible stimuli for transforming Ito cells (lipocytes) into collagen-secreting myofibroblasts. Not shown are cytokines derived from inflammatory cells, which could also activate Ito cells.

portal tract to portal tract; may traverse the lobule, joining central vein to portal tract to create very small nodules; or may encircle many contiguous lobules to create large nodules. Regeneration of hepatocytes surrounded by fibrous scars may contribute to the nodularity, but often the morphologic evidence of this process may have disappeared by the time the patient comes to study.

● In most instances (largely because its causation cannot be controlled), cirrhosis is a *progressive* disorder that has the potential of leading to portal hypertension and liver failure.

Because progressive fibrosis is the central feature of cirrhosis, it is important to ask what initiates and drives the process and what liver cell is the source of the excess collagen. But first the distribution of collagen in the normal and cirrhotic liver will be reviewed. In normal liver, typical interstitial collagens (types I and III) are concentrated in the portal tracts. Only occasional bundles are seen in the perisinusoidal space of Disse and around central veins. In cirrhosis, however, collagen is deposited not only in the portal tract but also within the lobules: in the spaces of Disse and around central veins. Deposition at these strategic locations is responsible for the hemodynamic derangements characteristic of cirrhosis.

Current evidence suggests that the major source of excess collagen in cirrhosis is the Ito cell (variously called fat-storing cell, lipocyte, perisinusoidal stellate cell), present beneath the sinusoidal endothelial cell in the space of Disse (Fig. 16-13). Ito cells are the

vitamin A storing cells of the liver. During the development of cirrhosis they become activated, lose their retinyl ester stores, and transform into myofibroblasts, the principal collagen-forming cells of the diseased liver. The stimulus for this transformation varies with the type of cirrhosis and includes cytokines and growth factors but in many instances is unknown. In cirrhosis that follows chronic hepatitis, transforming growth factor-β (TGF-β) derived from inflammatory cells is believed to activate Ito cells. Other cytokines such as platelet-derived growth factor, acting in concert with a Kupffer cell–derived factor, are also important stimuli for Ito cells. In addition there is evidence that disturbances in the extracellular matrix of the liver, as might occur in chronic inflammatory liver disease, may also signal the Ito cells to transform into myofibroblasts. A summary of the possible signals that activate collagen production by Ito cells is shown in Figure 16-13.

The *classification* of cirrhosis is unsatisfactory because the cause in many cases is uncertain and there is overlap in the morphology among cases of known cause. Thus, neither an etiologic nor a morphologic classification is entirely satisfactory. Some have attempted to utilize two large categories, *micronodular* and *macronodular*, based on measurement of nodules. The dividing line is usually set at 3 mm for the majority of nodules. It is often difficult to place some cirrhotic livers into either category because the nodules' size varies and it is often extremely difficult to determine their precise dimensions. Furthermore, it is well-recognized that as the disease progresses micronodular cirrhosis may develop into macronodular cirrhosis. Thus, a classification based on cause (when it can be determined) is most often used. In the following list several forms of cirrhosis with an approximate percentage of each type occurring in Western countries is provided. (In South America, Asia, and Africa alcoholism is a much less frequent cause.)

Type	Percent
Cirrhosis associated with alcohol abuse	60–70
Post necrotic cirrhosis	10
Biliary cirrhosis (primary and secondary)	5–10
Pigment cirrhosis (in hemochromatosis)	5
Cirrhosis associated with Wilson's disease	Rare
Cirrhosis associated with α_1-antitrypsin deficiency	Rare
Cryptogenic cirrhosis	10–15

All forms of cirrhosis may be clinically silent. When advanced, systemic symptoms may develop, including anorexia, weight loss, weakness with muscle atrophy, and generalized debilitation. In addition, signs of liver failure, including those outlined previously, develop (p. 526). Portal vein hypertension develops early and often dominates the clinical picture. Because cirrhosis is by far the most common cause of clinically significant portal hypertension it is appropriate to discuss this pathophysiologic syndrome next.

PORTAL HYPERTENSION

Elevation of the pressure in the portal circulation is a serious complication of a variety of disorders that affect the liver and its blood flow. These conditions have been variously classified but can be most simply divided into (1) posthepatic, (2) intrahepatic, and (3) prehepatic ones (Fig. 16–14).

The major *posthepatic* disorders leading to portal hypertension are severe right-sided heart failure, the Budd-Chiari syndrome, constrictive pericarditis, and veno-occlusive disease, all discussed elsewhere.

The dominant *intrahepatic causes of portal hypertension* are the various types of cirrhosis to be considered later. They account for more than 90% of cases of portal hypertension. Less common causes of intrahepatic portal hypertension include (1) chronic active hepatitis, (2) granulomatous disease (tuberculosis and sarcoidosis) involving the portal triads, and (3) schistosomiasis. The pathophysiology of the elevation in portal blood pressure in cirrhosis is complex and not entirely understood, but the major factor is increased resistance in portal blood flow at the level of sinusoids. This increased resistance correlates best with the amount of collagen deposited in the perisinusoidal spaces of Disse and with fibrosis around central veins. Compression of central veins and sinusoids by nodules, and shunting of hepatic arterial blood into the portal

vein system within the anastomotic vessels that develop in fibrous septae, also contribute to portal hypertension in cirrhosis. In alcoholic liver disease, an additional factor may be compression of sinusoids by swollen hepatocytes. In the granulomatous diseases that principally involve portal triads, extrinsic compression of small hepatic veins is undoubtedly important in increasing vascular resistance, while in schistosomiasis impaction of eggs within portal vein radicals creates venous obstruction and elevated pressures.

Prehepatic portal hypertension is caused by obstruction of the portal vein before it enters the liver; causes include extrinsic compression by cancers, enlarged lymph nodes in the connective tissue surrounding the portal vein, and portal vein thrombosis.

Whatever the cause of the portal hypertension, the pathophysiologic consequences are the same. The four most important features are (1) ascites, (2) the formation of bypass channels from the portal into the systemic circulations, particularly in the submucosa of the esophagus (esophageal varices), which may rupture, (3) splenomegaly, and (4) occasionally, hepatic (metabolic) encephalopathy secondary to diffuse parenchymal damage and portosystemic shunting.

ASCITES. Ascites is an intraperitoneal collection of fluid containing protein in the range of 1 to 2 gm/dl. The accumulation of many liters may cause abdominal distention. A scant number of mesothelial cells and

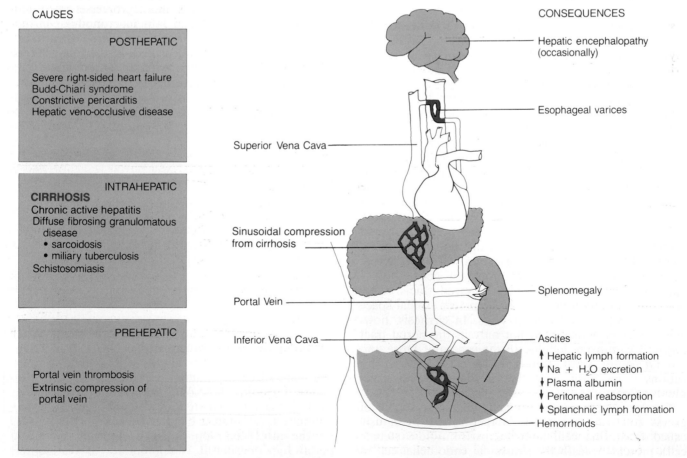

Figure 16–14. The causes of portal hypertension and the major pathophysiologic consequences.

lymphocytes is present, but in uncomplicated cases polymorphonuclear leukocytes or red cells are absent. Glucose, sodium, and potassium concentrations are equal to serum levels. A considerable amount of sodium and albumin may be lost therefore when removal of large volumes of ascites fluid becomes necessary to relieve the abdominal distention.

The mechanisms for the accumulation of ascites are complex (see Fig. 16–14), but three pathways probably play major roles. (1) One is *increased hepatic lymph formation*. The discontinuous endothelial lining of hepatic sinusoids does not restrain plasma proteins, so portal hypertension leads to formation of a protein-rich fluid that weeps through the liver capsule, accounting for the protein content of the fluid. (2) Another is *renal retention of sodium and water*. During the development of ascites there is sodium retention despite a greater than normal total body sodium level. Controversy continues as to whether the sodium and water retention is a renal response to reduced effective circulating volume due to sequestration of fluid in the peritoneal cavity ("underfilling theory") or instead is a primary response (for obscure reasons) marked by salt and water retention with expansion of the blood volume (overfilling theory). (3) Finally, there is *hypoalbuminemia and reduced plasma osmotic pressure*. Diffuse liver diseases impair synthesis of albumin. In the face of portal hypertension this favors extravasation of fluid into the peritoneal cavity. Less important are decreased resorption from the peritoneal surface, and increased lymph formation and seepage from the splanchnic bed (summarized in Fig. 16–14). In about 20% of patients, the ascites fluid passes through transdiaphragmatic lymphatics into the pleural cavities, particularly on the right, to cause *hydrothorax*.

PORTOSYSTEMIC SHUNTS. Capillary beds are shared by the portal vein and systemic venous circulation in the esophagus, the lower rectum, the retroperitoneum, and the falciform ligament of the liver. When portal vein pressure rises, collateral vessels enlarge and blood that ordinarily passes into the portal vein is shunted into the systemic circulation, further enlarging and causing tortuosity of these collateral channels. Where the portal and azygous systems mix in the lower esophagus, this engorged plexus of veins becomes visible beneath the esophageal mucosa as esophageal varices (p. 480). Esophageal varices are prone to rupture; when they do, the bleeding is extremely difficult to control. *Esophageal varices occur in about 67% of patients with advanced cirrhosis* and the massive bleeding causes death in approximately half of these cases. Varices may also develop in the anorectal region, where the superior mesenteric vein of the portal system communicates via the inferior mesenteric system with the hemorrhoidal plexus of the caval system. A third to half of all patients with cirrhosis develop hemorrhoids. Perhaps because the hemorrhoidal communications are remote from the liver, the pressures in these anorectal varices are not as great as those in the esophagus. Serious hemorrhage does not often arise from rupture of hemorrhoids. If the fetal umbilical vein fails to become obliterated, it may communicate with veins about the umbilicus to produce an externally visible vascular pattern called a *caput medusae*.

SPLENOMEGALY. The enlarged spleen in portal hypertension is readily attributed to the prolonged congestion of the spleen, which may attain weights of 1000 gm (normal 150 gm). A variety of hematologic abnormalities may appear secondary to the splenic enlargement, including anemia, leukopenia, and thrombocytopenia. All these hematologic alterations are attributed to *hypersplenism* and may be encountered in any form of spleen enlargement (p. 383). It is important to remember, however, that liver failure itself may lead to anemia and a bleeding diathesis, quite apart from any associated hypersplenism.

With this background, we can turn our attention to the major causes of portal hypertension: the various forms of cirrhosis.

ALCOHOLIC LIVER DISEASE AND CIRRHOSIS

Long-term excessive consumption of alcohol is the single most important cause of liver disease in the United States and much of the Western world. Chronic abuse of alcohol can produce three patterns of change in the liver—fatty liver, alcoholic hepatitis, and cirrhosis. Each one of these may be the sole manifestation of alcoholic liver disease or may coexist with one or both of the others. *Fatty liver*, the most common and innocuous of the three, is often completely asymptomatic and is fully reversible. *Alcoholic hepatitis, on the other hand, is associated with liver cell necrosis and inflammation* and produces clinical manifestations that may mimic viral or toxin-induced hepatitis. Alcoholic hepatitis may be reversible, especially if the initial injury is mild and further exposure to alcohol is avoided; however, repeated bouts of liver cell necrosis with subsequent fibrosis may eventually lead to the final and irreversible stage of alcohol-induced liver disease, *alcoholic cirrhosis*. As will be discussed in greater detail later, alcoholic cirrhosis may also develop without antecedent alcoholic hepatitis.

Alcoholic cirrhosis is the most common form of cirrhosis in North America and Europe and is increasing in frequency. Although at one time this was almost exclusively a male disorder, changing conventions have made it clear that women are also susceptible. The mortality rate among both male and female nonwhites in urban areas in the United States is double that of whites.

The morphology of the three forms of alcoholic liver disease is presented first because this facilitates the consideration of the pathogenesis.

MORPHOLOGY. Because the three patterns of hepatocellular changes associated with alcoholic liver disease may exist independently of each other and do not necessarily represent a continuum of changes, each is described separately.

The fatty liver of chronic alcoholism does not differ from that related to other causes, as described on page 17, but the alcoholic's liver is often much larger, up to 4 to 6 kg, a soft, yellow, greasy, readily fractured organ. The fatty change is initially centrilobular, but in severe cases it may diffusely involve the entire lobule. The majority of hepatocytes demonstrate **macrovesicular steatosis**, seen as the accumulation of large cytoplasmic vacuoles of lipid that displace the nuclei. Occasionally some cells demonstrate microvesicular fatty change, as is seen in Reye's syndrome (p. 529). With excessive fat accumulation the plasma membranes of adjacent hepatocytes may rupture to create **lipogranulomas.** There is little or no obvious increase in fibrous tissue at the outset, but subtle fibrosis, surrounding central veins and in the adjacent perisinusoidal spaces of Disse, develops with continued alcohol abuse. Some argue that these early fibrotic changes predict the development of cirrhosis with continued drinking, although this issue is unsettled. However, certainly **up to the time of appearance of these fibrosing reactions, the fatty change is completely reversible if there is abstention from further alcohol intake.**

Alcoholic hepatitis is the clinical and morphologic constellation of findings that occur in the liver following bouts of heavy alcohol ingestion. It is characterized histologically by (1) **swelling and necrosis of scattered hepatocytes, (2) neutrophilic reaction in and around the foci of necrosis, and, (3) in many patients, the presence of intracytoplasmic hyaline material (Mallory bodies) within the affected liver cells** (Fig. 16–15). The centrilobular areas are the most severely affected but changes occur throughout the lobule. The swelling or ballooning of the liver cells results from the accumulation of fat and water (hydropic change) as well as proteins that are usually exported. A characteristic but not diagnostic feature of alcoholic hepatitis is the presence of **Mallory bodies** appearing as irregular skeins of deeply eosinophilic material often located around the nucleus of swollen or dead hepatocytes. These structures are derived from aggregates of intermediate filaments of prekeratin (cytokeratin) but also contain other proteins of uncertain origin. (The term Mallory bodies is preferable to the term alcoholic hyaline used sometimes, because similar material can occasionally be seen within hepatocytes in such diverse conditions as primary biliary cirrhosis, Wilson's disease, Indian childhood cirrhosis, and hepatocellular carcinoma.) Necrosis of liver cells induces an inflammatory reaction in which neutrophils predominate, with some admixture of lymphocytes as well as macrophages. Deviations from this typical picture occur; the most important is the presence of fibrosis in the centrilobular areas. Perivenular central sclerosis may obliterate the central veins and give rise to portal hypertension without evidence of cirrhosis. In other cases continued alcohol abuse may lead to persistent or recurrent alcoholic hepatitis associated with widespread necrosis, inflammation, and fibrosis, which evolves into alcoholic cirrhosis. In some cases marked intrahepatic cholestasis, manifested by

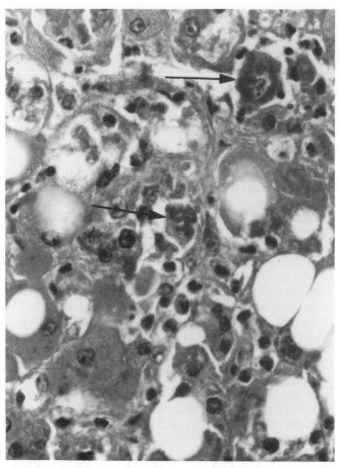

Figure 16–15. Alcoholic hepatitis. There is focal liver cell necrosis and a neutrophilic inflammatory reaction. The irregular, dark masses within the injured liver cells represent Mallory bodies (alcoholic hyaline, *arrows*). At the top of the figure, several liver cells are swollen and vacuolated due to accumulation of fat and water. Other hepatocytes demonstrate confluent globules of fat (macrovesicular steatosis).

bile plugs in distended canaliculi and droplets of bile in swollen hepatocytes and Kupffer cells, may appear.

Alcoholic cirrhosis, the final and irreversible form of alcoholic liver disease, evolves slowly and usually insidiously. At first the liver is fatty and enlarged, with a smooth, yellow-tan, greasy surface that on transection reveals a micronodular pattern of cirrhosis (nodules 1 to 3 mm in diameter, Fig. 16–16). As the fibrosis increases with time, the fat content decreases and the liver becomes browner. In later stages, scattered larger nodules develop, presumably as a consequence of regeneration of liver cells, and nodules may range in size up to 1 cm in diameter. Ultimately, the scars become even larger and may eventually produce a macronodular cirrhosis resembling the postnecrotic pattern (p. 550). Such a liver is shrunken and weighs less than a normal liver. Histologically, the early micronodular stage is character-

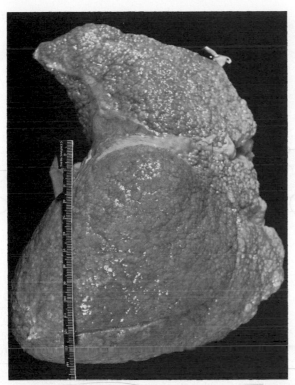

Figure 16–16. Cirrhosis of alcohol abuse, showing the characteristic diffuse micronodularity induced by the underlying fibrous scarring.

On clinical and epidemiologic grounds, there is an unmistakable association between the level and duration of alcohol consumption and the development of cirrhosis of the liver. National surveys document a close correlation between per capita alcohol consumption and mortality from cirrhosis. Because susceptibility to alcohol-induced liver injury varies among individuals, it is difficult to define a "safe" upper limit of alcohol consumption. However, it is clear that with equivalent alcohol consumption (per kilogram of body weight), women are at greater risk of developing cirrhosis than are men. This relationship might be explained on the basis of recent studies that demonstrate that women have a decreased capacity to metabolize alcohol in their gastric mucosa. Thus, as compared with men much more alcohol is delivered to their bloodstream per gram imbibed. It should be pointed out, however, that only 10 to 15% of all alcoholics develop cirrhosis. Individual, possibly genetic, susceptibility must exist, but as yet no genetic markers of susceptibility have been defined.

The *metabolic effects of alcohol* on the liver cell are complex and still incompletely understood. It is possible that alcohol itself can induce toxic effects directly. However, the most likely mechanism for the toxicity of alcohol relates to the intermediate metabolite, acetaldehyde, and the disordered hepatocyte metabolism that results from alcohol detoxification. The liver has two major pathways for alcohol metabolism, the alcohol dehydrogenase (ADH) pathway and the micro-

ized by slender, fibrous septa interconnecting portal areas and bridging portal areas to central veins. Thus, individual lobules may be encased or subdivided. The scarring and regeneration distort the normal lobular architecture. With progression, the fibrosis becomes more marked at the expense of the hepatic parenchyma (Fig. 16–17). Residual hepatocytes still contain some fat, and occasionally changes of alcoholic hepatitis may be present. Portal tracts and central veins become buried within such scars and often aggregate as the intervening parenchyma disappears. A delicate lymphocytic infiltrate and reactive bile duct proliferation are sometimes present within the scarring. In this manner, the histology of advanced alcoholic cirrhosis approaches that of postnecrotic cirrhosis. The spectrum of morphologic changes associated with alcoholic liver disease is schematized in Figure 16–18.

PATHOGENESIS. There is now abundant evidence that alcohol or its metabolites are hepatotoxic—and, indeed, toxic to other cells of the body as well. In addition, secondary malnutrition, which is inevitably associated with chronic alcoholism, contributes to the organ damage initiated by the toxic effects of alcohol, but malnutrition alone cannot be considered a cause of alcohol-related liver injury. The pathogenesis of alcohol-induced liver injury can be conveniently considered within three contexts: (1) clinical and epidemiologic evidence, (2) hepatic metabolism of ethanol, and (3) the mechanism of fibrogenesis.

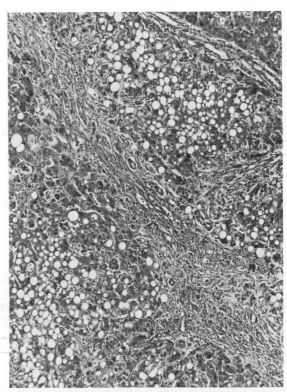

Figure 16–17. A low power view of the cirrhosis associated with alcohol abuse. The fibrous scarring separates islands of hepatocytes, many of which contain fatty vacuoles of varying size.

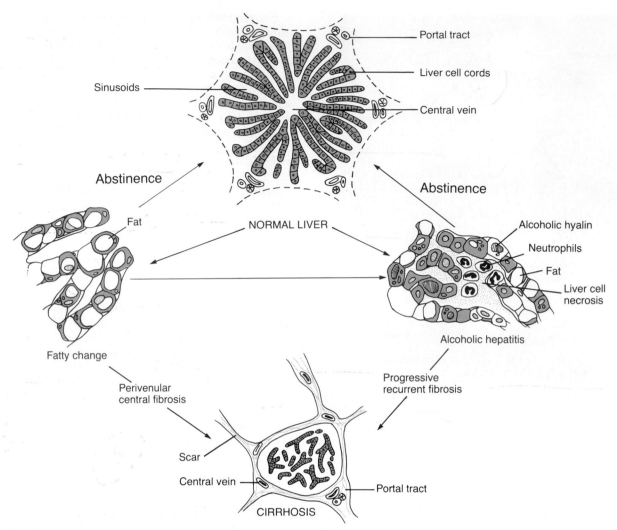

Figure 16–18. Schematic illustration of the changes associated with alcoholic liver disease, their possible interrelationship and their consequences. With abstinence fatty liver and alcoholic hepatitis are reversible, but cirrhosis is not.

somal ethanol-oxidizing system (MEOS). Of these, the ADH-mediated conversion of ethanol to acetaldehyde seems to be the major pathway (Fig. 16–19).

Alcohol is oxidized to acetaldehyde in the cytoplasm and then acetaldehyde is converted to acetate by acetaldehyde dehydrogenase (ALDH), predominantly in the mitochondria. Acetaldehyde causes hepatocyte damage by multiple mechanisms. (1) It can alter the structure and function of mitochondria, thus affecting normal cellular respiration. (2) It may interfere with normal intracellular transport mechanisms by blocking the formation of microtubules from tubulin. (3) Acetaldehyde can also form adducts with proteins, which may alter their function or induce neoantigens that can subsequently initiate an immune response against liver cells. In addition to the possible toxic effects of acetaldehyde, the metabolic process of alcohol oxidation itself has adverse effects on the liver. The conversion of alcohol to acetaldehyde and the subsequent oxidation of acetaldehyde require nicotinamide adenine dinucleotide (NAD), which in turn is reduced to NADH. These reactions alter the NADH-NAD ratio,

leading to an increase in the reducing potential within the cell. This has ripple effects on the metabolism of pyruvates, urates, and fatty acids. In particular, fatty acid oxidation is impaired, which favors the accumulation of free fatty acids and their esterification to triglyceride. Other factors that favor fat accumulation in the liver include increased flux of free fatty acids into the liver and reduced secretion of lipoproteins.

More recently the importance of the MEOS has been recognized in the oxidation of alcohol to acetaldehyde. This pathway seems to assume greater importance with continued (chronic) intake of alcohol. While the ADH pathway produces acetaldehyde and excess hydrogen ions, the MEOS produces acetaldehyde and oxygen radicals. The reactive oxygen produces injury by causing lipid peroxidation, which damages cell membranes. Furthermore, the chronic overuse of the MEOS "up-regulates" the activity of this system, which may secondarily affect other important metabolic activities of the liver because the most important enzyme in the MEOS, a P-450 cytochrome, also oxidizes a number of other compounds. These

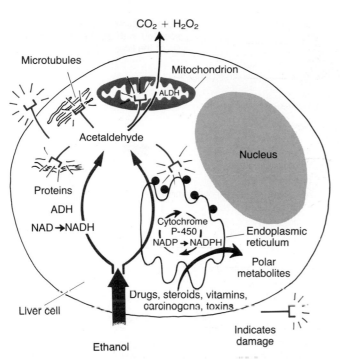

Figure 16-19. The two pathways of ethanol metabolism to acetaldehyde in liver cells. Ethanol is metabolized in the cytoplasm by alcohol dehydrogenase (ADH) and in the endoplasmic reticulum by the microsomal ethanol oxidizing system utilizing cytochrome P-450. The cytochrome P-450 system also metabolizes a number of nonpolar compounds into polar metabolites. Acetaldehyde is further metabolized by acetaldehyde dehydrogenase (ALDH), predominantly in mitochondria. Acetaldehyde damages multiple targets within liver cells.

include (1) various drugs (isoniazid, acetaminophen, many others), (2) toxins (carbon tetrachloride, halothane), (3) vitamins A and D, and (4) carcinogens (aflatoxin, nitrosamines). The products of several of these reactions are often quite toxic. Thus with alcohol-induced increase in the activity of MEOS, the toxicity of several drugs and chemicals is greater. In addition, if therapeutic agents that are metabolized by the MEOS are administered when alcohol levels are high, alcohol may interfere with drug metabolism by competing for the enzymes of the MEOS. As a result of impaired metabolism, the drugs may exceed their therapeutic levels and become dangerously toxic. Thus there are many potentially injurious consequences of ethanol metabolism.

We come finally to the mechanism of fibrosis in alcoholic cirrhosis. The nature of the cells that lay down collagen and the proposed stimuli that trigger fibrogenesis in the liver have been discussed (p. 543). As mentioned earlier, the centrilobular areas are the first to be involved by fibrosis in alcoholic cirrhosis; collagen is secreted by transformed Ito cells (myofibroblasts) in the subendothelium of the central veins and in the perisinusoidal spaces of Disse. The precise signals that activate these mesenchymal cells to produce collagen remain elusive. According to one possibility, acetaldehyde produced by metabolism of alcohol may diffuse out of the hepatocytes and directly stimulate

the collagen-secreting Ito cells (see Figure 16-13). Alternatively, cytokines (such as TGF-β) released by inflammatory cells recruited during alcoholic hepatitis might provide a stimulus for collagen production. The recruitment of these inflammatory cells might be enhanced by the development of autoimmune reactions against the acetaldehyde-altered self-proteins, thus perpetuating both inflammation and fibrosis; however, it should be remembered that cirrhosis may occur insidiously in the absence of liver cell inflammation (alcoholic hepatitis) and simply develop on a background of continuing or recurrent fatty change. How fibrosis is triggered in the absence of inflammation is not clear. Fatty change by itself is not the cause of fibrosis; accumulation of fat in other diseases such as kwashiorkor and marked obesity is not commonly associated with cirrhosis. Clearly factors other than accumulation of fat must come into play in the pathogenesis of alcoholic cirrhosis.

CLINICAL COURSE. There is a broad range of clinical presentations of alcohol-induced liver disease. At one end of the spectrum is the patient with the asymptomatic hepatomegaly of the fatty liver. Infrequently, there is accompanying jaundice. At the other end is the wasted, jaundiced, cirrhotic patient with hepatic failure. And perhaps somewhere in the middle is the patient acutely ill with the toxicity of alcoholic hepatitis.

Alcoholic hepatitis may be mild and virtually asymptomatic. More often, however, it presents in the same manner as viral hepatitis, with nausea, vomiting, anorexia, jaundice, tender hepatomegaly, and fever. Ascites, edema, and, in severe cases, fulminant hepatic necrosis with hepatic encephalopathy may ensue. Alcoholic hepatitis may be superimposed on cirrhosis. Such acute exacerbations may occur at any stage in the development of cirrhosis and may be recurrent. Therefore, it must not be assumed that hepatic insufficiency or failure implies the advanced fibrotic stage of the disease. Each bout of alcoholic hepatitis carries with it a high mortality rate (10 to 20%).

Usually the first signs of cirrhosis relate to portal hypertension, resulting in the classic picture of a grossly distended abdomen filled with ascites fluid along with wasted extremities and a pathetically drawn face. Less frequently, the first manifestation is jaundice; conjugated or unconjugated hyperbilirubinemia occurs concomitantly. Lastly, despite the presence of cirrhosis, a patient may be completely asymptomatic until some stress such as trauma or intercurrent infection upsets the balance and the patient develops symptomatic hepatic insufficiency or even hepatic failure with hepatic encephalopathy. Alternatively, the asymptomatic patient may first present with massive bleeding from esophageal varices and die either as a result of exsanguination or of hepatic encephalopathy precipitated by the metabolism of excess blood in the gastrointestinal tract. Figure 16-20 depicts the various clinical features characteristic of symptomatic alcoholic cirrhosis.

The long-term outlook for patients with cirrhosis is unpredictable. Numerous reports indicate that the dis-

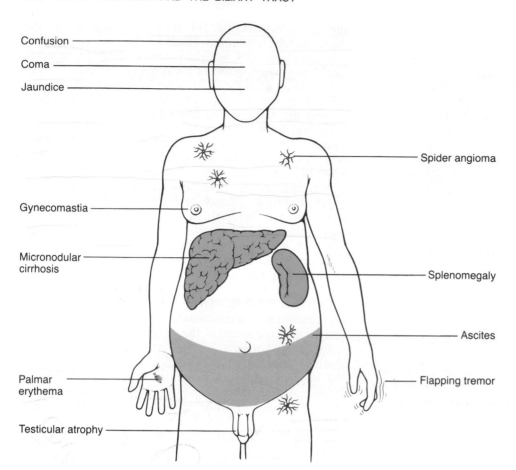

Confusion

Coma

Jaundice

Gynecomastia

Micronodular cirrhosis

Palmar erythema

Testicular atrophy

Spider angioma

Splenomegaly

Ascites

Flapping tremor

Figure 16–20. Clinical features associated with alcohol-induced cirrhosis of the liver.

ease can be arrested if the patient abstains from alcohol. The five-year survival rate approaches 90% in abstainers without jaundice, ascites, or hematemesis but drops to 50 to 60% in those who continue to imbibe. The causes of death are predominantly (1) hepatic failure, (2) intercurrent infection (to which alcoholics are prone), (3) gastrointestinal hemorrhage (often from esophageal varices but also from hemorrhagic gastritis, peptic ulceration, or esophageal laceration, (4) the hepatorenal syndrome, or (5) in 3 to 6% of cases, the development of a hepatocellular carcinoma.

POSTNECROTIC CIRRHOSIS

Postnecrotic cirrhosis is a term applied to cirrhosis of multiple and often unknown causes *characterized grossly by large nodules separated by coarse, irregular scars (macronodular cirrhosis).* Other less frequently used names are "posthepatitic" and "multilobular" cirrhosis. The pathogenesis of postnecrotic cirrhosis usually involves an extensive, sometimes confluent but often irregular loss of liver cells, followed by stromal collapse and fibrosis (Fig. 16–21). About a fourth of cases are caused by chronic active hepatitis B (sometimes accompanied by delta virus infection). The overall incidence of HCV-associated postnecrotic cirrhosis

is not known, but in some regions of the world many cases are caused by HCV. Recall that in chronic active hepatitis piecemeal necrosis and bridging necrosis progressively erode the liver parenchyma, leading to ever-enlarging scars and irregular regenerative nodules. A small number of cases follow chronic active hepatitis caused by the chronic ingestion of certain therapeutic agents (e.g., oxyphenisatin, α-methyldopa, nitrofurantoin, and others). Only infrequently is postnecrotic cirrhosis the result of submassive or fulminant liver necrosis. Either such patients succumb to massive liver destruction, or, if damage is sufficiently limited to permit survival, regeneration of the destroyed hepatocytes ensues, leaving surprisingly little scarring. Nonetheless, massive necrosis, whether it be due to a fulminant viral infection or a hepatotoxic agent (p. 537), may destroy portions of the liver, sparing large tracts. Such instances may be followed by massive scarring. Some would refer to this sequence of events as postnecrotic *scarring* rather than postnecrotic *cirrhosis,* but this is an issue for the purists. Some livers involved by alcoholic micronodular cirrhosis later develop coarse scars and large, irregular nodules so as to merit the morphologic designation postnecrotic cirrhosis. It must be admitted, however, that in the *vast majority of cases no antecedent cause for postnecrotic cirrhosis can be identified.* Such cases, highlighting our ignorance, are dignified by the term "cryptogenic cirrhosis."

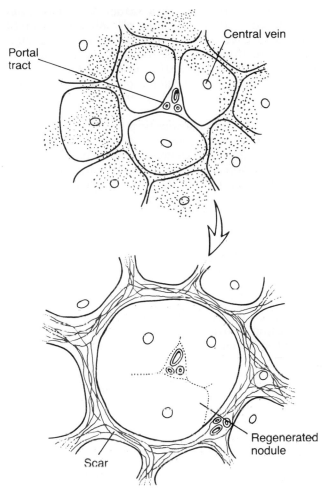

Portal tract

Central vein

Scar

Regenerated nodule

Figure 16–21. Schematic illustration of the pathogenesis of postnecrotic cirrhosis. Note that irregular and large areas of liver cell necrosis *(shaded areas in upper figure)* may leave a surviving island of liver cells, composed of several intact and partially necrotic liver lobules. (Spaces between intact liver lobules in the upper figure are exaggerated for illustrative purpose.) During regeneration, the remnants of the liver lobules merge to form a large nodule surrounded by a dense irregular scar, which replaces the necrotic liver cells.

MORPHOLOGY. The gross appearance of postnecrotic cirrhosis depends on the distribution of the parenchymal destruction and the duration of survival following the necrotizing process. At the outset, the liver may be almost normal in size but more often is slightly shrunken. In time, the scarred areas become progressively larger and eventually contract, leading to liver shrinkage accompanied by accentuation of the nodules. The nodules are of all sizes, but typically some are very large (5 to 8 cm in diameter). Usually, they are the color of normal liver substance, save when retention of bile leads to greenish discoloration. **The diagnostic features of postnecrotic scarring are the large size of the scars and the large nodules enclosed within the scars (macronodular cirrhosis, Fig. 16–22).** With extensive involvement, the liver may be dramatically reduced in size and weight.

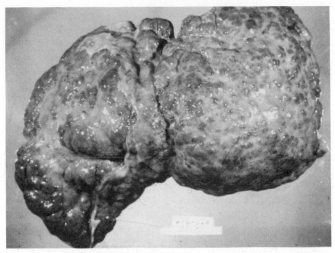

Figure 16–22. Postnecrotic cirrhosis, characterized by irregular, random areas of massive fibrosis alternating with other areas of more delicate scarring, producing nodules of variable size.

Histologically, the classic features are the very broad scars interposed between islands of disorderly regenerating hepatocytes or areas of relatively normal hepatic substance. Within these fibrous bands is an infiltrate of lymphocytes admixed with macrophages and accompanied by proliferating bile ducts and ductules (Fig. 16–23). Where extensive necrosis has occurred, two or

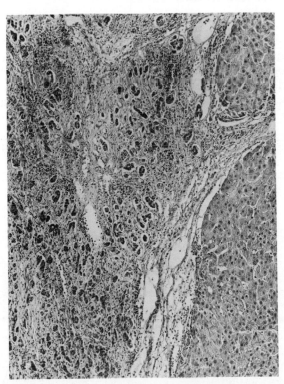

Figure 16–23. A view under low power of postnecrotic cirrhosis of the liver. The massive fibrous scar contains numerous bile ducts, crowded together due to proliferation of the ducts and to destruction of several whole liver lobules. The islands of preserved liver cells on the right are free of fat.

more portal triads may be closely approximated within the scars. At the interface between the scars and hepatocytes, piecemeal necrosis is sometimes present in cases related to chronic active hepatitis of viral origin, indicating the continued activity of the viral infection (p. 540). Surviving hepatocytes may manifest fatty change in cases related to hepatotoxic drugs or chemicals, but more often it is absent.

Clinically, a history of chronic active hepatitis or a well-defined episode of massive liver destruction may be obtained, but *in many cases postnecrotic cirrhosis appears mysteriously.* The signs and symptoms are those expected with other types of cirrhosis. Signs of portal hypertension, such as ascites and splenomegaly, may be the first indication of underlying liver disease. Life-threatening complications such as massive bleeding from ruptured esophageal varices may occur. Liver failure manifested by jaundice, and in severe cases hepatic encephalopathy, are commonly seen, especially in patients with chronic active hepatitis. Most of these patients die within the first year; in others, the disease follows a more indolent course, with slow erosion of hepatic function over the span of three to five years eventuating in hepatic failure. There is an increased risk of developing hepatocellular carcinoma, especially in cases associated with HBV or HCV infection.

BILIARY CIRRHOSIS

This form of cirrhosis develops in association with inflammation or destruction of bile ducts. Thus, fibrosis first involves portal tracts and extends to produce portal tract–to–portal tract fibrotic bridges. Biliary cirrhosis can evolve from at least three different disorders, all of which manifest signs and symptoms of biliary tract obstruction. These patients, therefore, have an elevated serum alkaline phosphatase, jaundice (often associated with pruritus), light-colored stools from failure to secrete bile, dark urine as a result of bilirubinuria, and hepatosplenomegaly. The three disorders are *extrahepatic biliary obstruction* (producing *secondary biliary cirrhosis*), *primary biliary cirrhosis,* and *primary sclerosing cholangitis.* The principal pathogenetic mechanisms accounting for bile duct obstruction in the disorders leading to biliary cirrhosis are depicted in Figure 16–24 and discussed next.

Secondary biliary cirrhosis is considered first because its genesis is clear cut. It is encountered in patients who have had extrahepatic biliary obstruction due to (1) bile stones, (2) strictures, (3) cancers of the bile ducts and head of the pancreas, or (4) extrinsic encroachment caused by enlarged lymph nodes or abdominal masses. Obstruction causes increased pressure within extrahepatic bile ducts and within the intrahepatic biliary tree. The interlobular bile ducts and cholangioles are damaged by the impacted, inspissated bile, and the injury leads to an inflammatory reaction and scarring. Obviously, such patients are jaundiced, sometimes intensely. Subtotal obstruction often leads to an ascending cholangitis (p. 561) as bacteria ascend within or about the ramifications of the biliary tract. Inflammation of the portal triads and periportal scarring ensue in these infected livers without striking evidence of inspissation of bile, and indeed jaundice may be absent. Cirrhosis develops only if the obstruction is not relieved, thus the importance of early recognition.

Primary biliary cirrhosis (PBC) is less clearly understood, but accumulating evidence strongly suggests that it is an immune-mediated disorder. Women are the victims in 90% of cases and onset is usually between age 30 and 65 years. The initial signs and symptoms are typical of bile duct obstruction. Eventually skin xanthomas secondary to hypercholesterolemia and skin

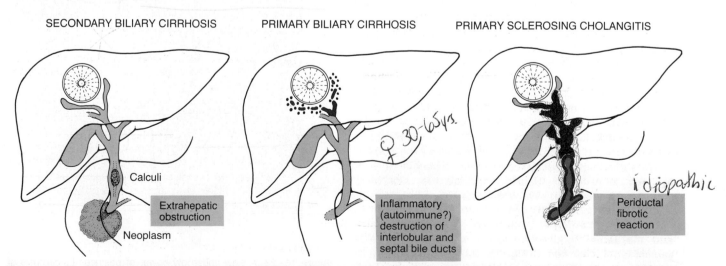

Figure 16-24. Principal pathogenetic mechanisms for bile duct obstruction in the three disorders leading to biliary cirrhosis. In secondary biliary cirrhosis, extrahepatic obstruction is causative. In primary biliary cirrhosis, autoimmune destruction of small intrahepatic ducts occurs. In primary sclerosing cholangitis, idiopathic periductular fibrosis constricts bile ducts, principally the extrahepatic and larger intrahepatic ducts.

pigmentation (as a result of stimulated melanin production) develop. The essential feature of primary biliary cirrhosis is inflammation of small intrahepatic bile ducts, followed by their destruction and eventual disappearance. Full-blown cirrhosis may not be present at the outset but develops as the disease progresses. A variety of abnormalities of both cell-mediated and humoral immunity suggests an autoimmune cause. To begin with, there is an association between primary biliary cirrhosis and other autoimmune diseases, such as scleroderma, Hashimoto's thyroiditis, and Sjögren's syndrome. Derangements of both humoral and cellular immunity are present in almost every patient. Serum immunoglobulins, particularly IgM levels, are elevated, and in addition, over 90% of patients have high concentrations (titers) of IgG antimitochondrial antibody, although this is of obscure significance. Smooth muscle antibody, antinuclear antibodies, and rheumatoid factor are also sometimes present. A variety of abnormalities affecting cellular immunity has been described. These include T- and B-cell lymphopenia, alterations in the ratios of helper and suppressor T cells, and evidence of T-cell sensitization to hepatobiliary antigens. As with other autoimmune disorders, reduced suppressor T-cell function, leading to unbridled activation of autoreactive T and B cells, has been proposed. Despite all this evidence, the possibility cannot be excluded that the immunologic findings are secondary phenomena triggered by some primary cause of damage to interlobular bile ducts. In this connection, it is of interest that patients with primary biliary cirrhosis have high copper concentrations in the liver. As will be seen, the accumulation of copper in the liver is thought to underlie the cirrhosis of Wilson's disease (p. 557) and by analogy could play a role in the causation of PBC; however, once again the question arises, is the elevated copper level primary or secondary, since this metal is largely excreted through the biliary tract. Indeed, impaired bile excretion from any cause increases copper concentrations in the liver.

Primary sclerosing cholangitis is a rare fibroinflammatory condition affecting random segments of both extrahepatic and intrahepatic bile ducts. It is associated with progressive and generalized thickening of the walls of the bile ducts, with segmental narrowing and even focal occlusion. As with primary biliary cirrhosis and extrahepatic bile duct obstruction, cirrhosis is absent early in the course of primary sclerosing cholangitis. The cause and pathogenesis of primary sclerosing cholangitis are obscure. An association with the histocompatibility antigens HLA-B8 and -DR3 suggests an immune origin. Indeed, patients with this disease have elevated levels of immunoglobulins, especially IgM, and possess autoantibodies against both colonic and ductular epithelium. In 50 to 70% of patients there is an associated inflammatory bowel disease, especially ulcerative colitis (p. 501). An interesting possibility is that the periductal capillary network is damaged by absorption of toxins or bacteria from an inflamed gastrointestinal tract. Periductular sclerosis then develops as a reparative reaction.

MORPHOLOGY. All of these disorders are associated with a micronodular cirrhosis. Common to all patterns is a diffuse monotonous, regular, and delicate scarring about each lobule, giving a fine, sandpaper texture to the surface of the liver. The liver is usually dark green owing to cholestasis. Early in the evolution of biliary cirrhosis the liver may be normal in size or even slightly enlarged, but late in the course the progressive scarring may cause a slight reduction in size.

Histologically, the principal characteristics of all forms of biliary cirrhosis are (1) regularity of fibrosis, extending to interconnect portal triads and enclosing regenerative nodules of hepatocytes (micronodular cirrhosis); (2) bile duct and ductule injury, accompanied by proliferation and regeneration within the scars; (3) a mononuclear infiltration, principally of lymphocytes admixed with macrophages, in the scars; and (4) evidence of chronic cholestasis (i.e., pseudoxanthomatous change [foamy, bubbly appearance of liver cells], increased copper, varying amounts of bile pigment, and, sometimes, Mallory bodies). Secondary features relate to the particular pathogenetic mechanism.

In cirrhosis induced by **extrahepatic obstruction**, bile stasis in interlobular ducts, rupture of bile ducts with extravasation of bile, and hepatocyte necrosis ("bile infarct") may be present. Bile infarcts with liquefied bile-stained centers may then develop ("bile lakes"). When obstruction is associated with ascending cholangitis, inflammatory cells, principally polymorphonuclear leukocytes, are scattered within the finer ramifications of the biliary tract.

In **primary biliary cirrhosis,** the characteristic feature is a destructive inflammatory process of the septal and interlobular bile ducts accompanied by a dense infiltrate of lymphocytes, macrophages, occasional plasma cells, and eosinophils. In some cases, poorly formed granulomas are seen in proximity to the damaged ducts and ductules. The destruction of the small ducts is accompanied by portal scarring and irregular duct regeneration, producing abortive ductules and solid cords of cells. Later in the course of primary biliary cirrhosis, when true cirrhosis has developed, well-defined fibrous septa extend from the portal tracts to isolate individual lobules. It should be noted that in these patients there is no evidence of involvement of the larger intra- and extrahepatic biliary ducts.

Histologic changes in **primary sclerosing cholangitis** are distinguished by a milder degree of bile stasis than occurs in secondary obstruction, and by an absence of the duct epithelial injury as seen in primary biliary cirrhosis. The distinctive lesion is periductal fibrosis, particularly of larger bile ducts, extrahepatic ducts, and interlobular ducts, which appears to constrict the lumen. There is very mild accompanying periductal inflammation.

CLINICAL COURSE. The clinical findings are quite variable and depend on the genesis of the liver disease. Some features, such as prominent jaundice and pruritus, are common to all forms of biliary cirrhosis. In addition, deficient flow of bile into the duodenum gives rise to a malabsorption syndrome. Osteomalacia due to malabsorption of vitamin D and calcium is often clinically significant. In most cases of biliary cirrhosis, hepatic failure ultimately ensues. In contrast to the other cirrhoses, *portal hypertension is an uncommon feature,* and the incidence of hepatocellular carcinoma is not increased. The distinguishing features of the three forms of biliary cirrhosis are summarized in Table 16–5 and in the following paragraphs.

When biliary cirrhosis results from *extrahepatic obstruction,* ascending cholangitis is likely to occur and is characterized by right upper quadrant pain and marked leukocytosis. In any patient who presents with evidence of cholestasis, extrahepatic biliary obstruction must be ruled out because prompt surgical intervention often relieves the obstruction and prevents further disease progression. It can be demonstrated by endoscopic retrograde cholangiopancreatography (ERCP), ultrasonography, or computed tomography.

Primary biliary cirrhosis is preceded by a preclinical phase in which there are only biochemical abnormalities such as an elevated alkaline phosphatase value. It usually comes to light with the insidious onset of pruritus; jaundice develops only later. Hypercholesterolemia may be encountered, and in addition to the skin xanthomas previously mentioned severe atherosclerosis may develop. The diagnosis of primary biliary cirrhosis is supported by the demonstration of elevated serum levels of antimitochondrial antibody. Unfortunately, there is no adequate treatment for this condition except liver transplantation.

Patients with *primary sclerosing cholangitis* may initially experience neither clinical nor laboratory abnormalities. With progression, there is laboratory evidence of obstruction, followed by clinical symptoms, and, finally, cirrhosis and liver failure. Diagnosis depends almost entirely on demonstration of the distorted extrahepatic biliary tract with irregular strictures and dilatations, best detected by either percutaneous trans-

hepatic or endoscopic cholangiography. As for primary biliary cirrhosis there is no treatment. Furthermore, 10% of patients develop bile duct carcinoma.

HEMOCHROMATOSIS— PIGMENT CIRRHOSIS

Hemochromatosis is an iron overload disorder that in past years could not be diagnosed until the progressive accumulation of iron caused liver injury. The disease was diagnosed on the basis of a classic triad: (1) a heavily pigmented micronodular cirrhosis (all cases), (2) diabetes mellitus (in 75 to 80% of cases), and (3) skin pigmentation (75 to 85% of cases). The last two features accounted for the older designation *bronze diabetes.* Now the disease can be diagnosed by laboratory studies before cirrhosis and other organ injury occurs, so preventive therapy can be instituted.

The total body iron pool ranges from 2 to 6 gm in normal adults. In hemochromatosis, the iron pool, mainly in the form of ferritin and hemosiderin, may reach 50 to 60 gm. The most common form of iron overload occurs in the genetic disorder called *idiopathic (primary, genetic) hemochromatosis.* The other forms, in which the source of excess iron can be defined, are called *secondary hemochromatosis.* They often are associated with less marked iron overload and, therefore, less evidence of functional or morphologic damage to sites of deposition (Table 16–6).

About 70% of persons who have idiopathic hemochromatosis have HLA-A3, in contrast to 28% of the general population. HLA-B7, -B1, and -Bw35 are closely linked to HLA-A3 and, therefore, are also present in many patients with the idiopathic form of the disease. A hemochromatosis gene is believed to be located on chromosome 6, in close linkage with the HLA locus, and family studies suggest autosomal recessive inheritance of the susceptibility gene. Persons who are homozygous for this mutant gene absorb a

TABLE 16–5. DISTINGUISHING FEATURES OF DISORDERS ASSOCIATED WITH BILIARY CIRRHOSIS

	Secondary Biliary Cirrhosis	Primary Biliary Cirrhosis	Primary Sclerosing Cholangitis
Etiology	Extrahepatic bile duct obstruction (e.g., congenital biliary atresia, gallstones, carcinoma of pancreatic head)	Possibly autoimmune; associated with other autoimmune diseases	Unknown, possibly autoimmune; 50–70% of cases associated with inflammatory bowel disease
Sex Predilection	None	Female-male 9:1	Female-male 1:2
Symptoms and Signs	Pruritus, jaundice, malaise, dark urine, light stools, hepatosplenomegaly	Same as secondary biliary cirrhosis	Same as secondary biliary cirrhosis
Distinctive Pathologic Findings	Prominent bile stasis in interlobular ducts; sometimes PMNs in bile ducts	Lymphocytic infiltrate around and in walls of ducts with evidence of bile duct injury	Periductal fibrosis and segmental stenosis of extrahepatic, (and, often, intrahepatic) ducts
Laboratory Findings	Conjugated hyperbilirubinemia; increased serum alkaline phosphatase, bile acids, cholesterol	Same as secondary biliary cirrhosis plus elevated serum IgM and presence of antimitochondrial antibody	Same as secondary biliary cirrhosis, plus hypergammaglobulinemia, elevated IgM, and auto-antibodies to colonic and ductular epithelium

TABLE 16-6. TYPES OF HEMOCHROMATOSIS

1. Idiopathic (Primary, Genetic) Hemochromatosis

2. Secondary Hemochromatosis
Secondary to anemia with ineffective erythropoiesis
  a. Thalassemia major
  b. Sideroblastic anemia
Secondary to excessive blood transfusions
  a. Aplastic anemia
  b. Chronic anemia of renal failure in hemodialysis patients
Secondary to liver disease
  a. Alcoholic cirrhosis
  b. Postportacaval shunt
Secondary to high oral iron intake
  a. Prolonged ingestion of medicinal iron
  b. Increased intake of iron with alcohol (South African blacks)

large excess of iron from the gastrointestinal tract and develop hemochromatosis; heterozygotes do not manifest evidence of parenchymal organ injury but often have biochemical evidence of mild iron overload in the form of elevated plasma levels of iron, transferrin saturation, and serum ferritin. There is a strong male predominance (5:1 to 7:1), which may be due partly to protection against iron overload afforded by menstrual losses and the drains of pregnancy. It also appears that women with equivalent concentrations of iron in their livers demonstrate lesser degrees of hepatocellular injury, suggesting that additional protective mechanisms are operating.

PATHOGENESIS. It may be recalled that the total body content of iron is normally a closely guarded constant maintained by balancing gastrointestinal absorption with daily limited and fixed losses. The precise mechanisms that control gastrointestinal uptake are not fully understood and were reviewed earlier (p. 345). Most of the available evidence suggests that in primary hemochromatosis the defect lies at the level of the mucosal cells in the duodenum and jejunum, where iron is absorbed from food. It may involve specific membrane receptors, iron-ligand complexes, or intracellular transport proteins (transferrin), all of which are involved in the movement of iron across enterocytes into the plasma.

Alternatively it has been proposed that the basic defect consists of an inability of mononuclear phagocytes to take up or to store iron. Despite overloading of parenchymal cells, macrophages throughout the body, including those in the intestinal mucosa, take up relatively little iron. Conceivably the mononuclear phagocytes cannot deliver a signal to the gut lining cells to turn off iron absorption despite the excess of absorbed iron.

The most common causes of *secondary hemochromatosis* are the hemolytic anemias associated with ineffective erythropoiesis (e.g., thalassemia major, p. 341). In these disorders, the excess iron results not only from transfusions but also from increased absorption of iron, which accompanies ineffective erythropoiesis. Transfusions alone—for example, in aplastic anemias—usually lead to systemic hemosiderosis in

which there is little parenchymal cell injury; however, when more than 60 to 100 units of blood have been received, evidence of iron-induced parenchymal organ toxicity may develop. Persons likely to be so affected include those with chronic renal failure (severe enough to require hemodialysis) and aplastic anemia.

Alcoholic cirrhosis is often associated with an increase in stainable iron within the liver cells. Whether this is due to alcohol-induced increase in iron absorption or to cell necrosis followed by uptake of released iron by surviving liver cells is not clear. In any event, most alcoholics with cirrhosis and increased liver iron stores do not have a significant increase in total body iron and so do not have true hemochromatosis. The small number of alcoholics who do develop gross systemic iron overload and clinical features of hemochromatosis are suspected to be heterozygous for the hemochromatosis gene. Conceivably, in these patients the cumulative effects of alcohol and the hemochromatosis gene on iron absorption lead to significant iron overload and hemochromatosis. A similar speculation applies to the rare cases of hemochromatosis that seem to follow many years of oral (medicinal) iron ingestion. A rather unusual form of iron overload resembling idiopathic hemochromatosis develops in South African blacks who ingest large quantities of alcoholic beverage fermented in iron utensils ("Bantu siderosis"). The increased absorption of iron is possibly due to the combined effect of excessive consumption of alcohol and iron (derived from the iron utensils).

Although iron deposition in the parenchymal cells is fundamental to the pathogenesis of both idiopathic and secondary forms of hemochromatosis, the mechanism of iron toxicity is not fully understood. Currently favored is the view that with progressive iron loading, the capacity of cells to convert iron into ferritin is exceeded, leading thereby to an overload of free iron. This in turn catalyzes the formation of oxygen-derived free radicals that damage the membranes of cell organelles by lipid peroxidation (p. 9). It has also been proposed that iron overload directly stimulates fibrosis.

MORPHOLOGY. The morphologic changes in idiopathic hemochromatosis are characterized principally by (1) the deposition of hemosiderin in the following organs, in decreasing order of severity: liver, pancreas, myocardium, pituitary, adrenal, thyroid and parathyroid glands, joints, and the skin; (2) cirrhosis of the liver; and (3) fibrosis of the pancreas. Fibrosis is relatively rare in the myocardium and other organs.

The evolution of cirrhosis occurs slowly. First, increased amounts of ferritin and hemosiderin accumulate in parenchymal cells. In time, iron deposition extends to Kupffer cells and bile duct epithelium and fibrous septa appear, extending out from portal triads to interconnect portal areas, and sometimes also from central veins to portal areas. Over a span of years, a diffuse, micronodular pigment cirrhosis develops. The liver is usually enlarged, perhaps up to 3 kg, and is dense, radiopaque, and chocolate brown. Iron stains such as the Prussian blue reaction are strikingly positive on transected surfaces of the liver as well as in tissue sections (Fig. 16–25). In 8 to 22% of patients with advanced cirrhosis hepatocellular carcinoma develops.

The **pancreas** is extensively pigmented and often exhibits diffuse interstitial fibrosis. Hemosiderin is found in the acinar cells of the exocrine glands, in islet cells, and in the interstitial stroma. There is some correlation between the levels of siderosis of the pancreas and the occurrence and severity of diabetes mellitus.

The **heart** often demonstrates hemosiderin granules in the myocardial fibers, and in some cases the accumulation is of sufficient magnitude to cause a striking brown color. Any or all of the **endocrine glands** may reveal brownish discoloration because of the accumulation of hemosiderin in parenchymal cells. **Skin pigmentation** is one of the major presenting clinical features of hemochromatosis, and indeed there is hemosiderin deposition in macrophages and fibroblasts about adnexal structures in the dermis. For obscure reasons most of the skin pigmentation results from increased production of melanin within the basal layer of the epidermis rather than from the hemosiderin deposits.

The **joints** may be the site of hemosiderin pigmentation of the synovium in 25 to 50% of cases. The hemosiderin deposition is frequently accompanied by excessive deposition of calcium pyrophosphate, leading to severe articular cartilage damage and sometimes disabling arthritis (pseudogout).

The **testes** usually show little evidence of hemosiderin deposition despite the fact that hypogonadism is sometimes a prominent clinical feature.

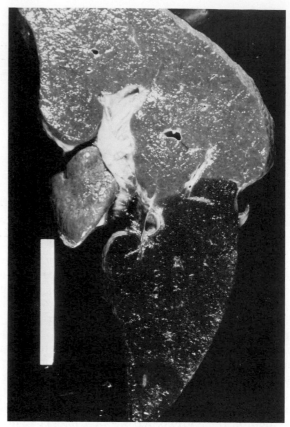

Figure 16–25. Transected surface of a finely nodular liver with pigment cirrhosis. A Prussian blue iron stain has been applied to the lower half, and the contained hemosiderin has produced the discoloration.

CLINICAL COURSE. The clinical manifestations of *idiopathic* hemochromatosis are described here. The findings in the *secondary* variants are similar, depending on the severity of the iron overload and the resultant parenchymal and organ injury. Idiopathic hemochromatosis is primarily a disease of males. It rarely becomes manifest before age 40, apparently requiring this amount of time for the accumulation of the excess iron to result in sufficient organ damage to produce clinical symptoms.

The most common signs and symptoms include skin pigmentation, hepatomegaly, mild diabetes mellitus, and gonadal insufficiency. Splenomegaly and ascites may or may not be present. Cardiac involvement may present as heart failure or as life-threatening arrhythmias. Arthropathy, found in up to 50% of cases, sometimes dominates the clinical course. The major causes of death in untreated patients are cardiac failure, hepatocellular failure, portal hypertension, and liver cancer. The risk of developing hepatocellular carcinoma is particularly high with this form of cirrhosis.

Although the diagnosis can generally be established by the triad of skin pigmentation, diabetes, and hepatomegaly, these are late manifestations. The combination of HLA typing and blood studies can predict the likelihood of idiopathic hemochromatosis with a high certainty, particularly in relatives of known patients. The risk of idiopathic hemochromatosis is 95% in family members who are HLA identical with the index case. Evidence of iron overload can be detected by blood studies: the plasma iron level is elevated, sometimes up to 300 μg/dl (normal 50 to 150 μg/dl), and the transferrin saturation increases from a normal range of 25 to 50%, to 50 to 100% in patients with iron overload. The serum ferritin level is also markedly increased (up to 6000 ng/ml; normal, 10 to 200 ng/ml). Ultimately, in suspected cases a liver biopsy is indicated to determine the level of excess iron in the hepatocytes. With levels of iron above 4 mg per gram of liver, there is a definite risk of cirrhosis.

Once iron overload is established the progression of the disease can be significantly altered by treatment, principally repeated phlebotomy until transferrin saturation and ferritin values fall into the normal range. The use of iron chelators to drain off excess iron is also of value, particularly in patients with secondary or transfusion-associated hemochromatosis. The five-year mortality rate is 11% for those who receive intensive iron-draining therapy but 67% for the untreated group.

WILSON'S DISEASE

Wilson's disease is an autosomal recessive disorder of copper metabolism in which liver disease is a major component. It results in the deposition of toxic levels of copper in many organs, principally the liver, the eye, and the brain—hence the alternate designation, "*hepatolenticular*" *degeneration.*

The molecular basis of the disease, although incompletely understood, hinges on the inability of the liver cells to properly regulate copper metabolism. Ingested copper is absorbed in the stomach and duodenum and rapidly transported to the liver attached to albumin. Free copper is taken up by hepatocytes, where it is complexed to apoceruloplasmin for excretion into the blood. Ceruloplasmin accounts for 90 to 95% of serum copper, and normally it is recycled through the liver, where the ceruloplasmin-copper complex is dissociated and the free copper is released and excreted in the bile. *In Wilson's disease hepatocytes accumulate copper, neither secreting the copper-ceruloplasmin complex into plasma nor secreting free copper into bile.* Eventually, at around five years of age, free copper spills over into blood and is deposited in other sites: brain, cornea, kidneys, bones, joints, and parathyroid glands. Although it was initially postulated that deficient ceruloplasmin synthesis was at the root of the disorder (because serum ceruloplasmin levels are characteristically low), it is now believed that the defect is in the lysosomal degradation of the ceruloplasmin-copper complexes in liver cells. The low ceruloplasmin levels most likely result from hepatocyte damage caused by intracellular accumulation of copper. A second unsettled issue is how copper accumulation causes toxicity. It may result from the ability of excess copper to (1) initiate the formation of free radicals, (2) bind to sulfhydryl groups of cellular proteins, disrupting their function, or (3) displace other metals in hepatic enzymes, interfering with their enzymatic activity. Only when the Wilson's disease gene, mapped to chromosome 13, is cloned and the protein product identified will the molecular basis of this disorder be understood.

MORPHOLOGY. The **liver** often bears the brunt of injury in Wilson's disease. The form of the liver disease varies, depending on whether the patient is seen early or late in the course of the disease. The changes, roughly in the sequence of their evolution are (1) fatty change, (2) acute hepatitis, (3) chronic active hepatitis, (4) cirrhosis, and, rarely, (5) fulminant hepatic necrosis. The histologic changes are similar to those encountered with liver injury of other causes, particularly alcoholic liver disease, except that excess copper deposition can often be demonstrated by special stains (e.g., rhodamine) as reddish cytoplasmic granules representing copper-laden lysosomes. In liver biopsy specimens fatty change and a large number of Mallory bodies may cause confusion with alcoholic liver disease.

In the **brain,** toxic injury primarily affects the basal ganglia, particularly the putamen, which demonstrate atrophy and even cavitation. Nearly all patients with neurologic involvement develop **eye lesions** called **Kayser-Fleischer** rings—green to golden-brown deposits of copper in Descemet's membrane in the limbus of the cornea.

CLINICAL COURSE. The age at onset and the clinical presentation of Wilson's disease are variable, but it rarely manifests before age six years. The most common presentation is liver disease (60%); neuropsychiatric manifestations, often simulating Parkinson's disease, are the initial feature in most of the remaining cases. The diagnosis is readily made in patients with classic Kayser-Fleischer rings and a low serum ceruloplasmin level. In the absence of the rings, a liver biopsy demonstrating excess hepatic copper, together with low ceruloplasmin, establishes the diagnosis. Chelation therapy with D-penicillamine has dramatically altered the usual progressive downhill course.

α_1-ANTITRYPSIN DEFICIENCY

α_1-Antitrypsin (A1AT) deficiency, briefly discussed in an earlier chapter (p. 394), is a genetic disorder that may lead to pulmonary emphysema and hepatic injury. There are many alleles at the A1AT locus. The Z allele is the most common clinically significant variant. Persons who are homozygous for this form (PiZZ) synthesize a protein that differs from the normal A1AT protein by a single amino acid. Although the synthesis of the mutant protein proceeds normally in the liver (the primary source of A1AT), its secretion is impaired. Only 15% of the protein can be secreted by PiZZ homozygotes; the rest accumulates in the endoplasmic reticulum, where it can be seen in the form of round to oval cytoplasmic globular inclusions in hepatocytes. In routine hematoxylin and eosin stains they appear acidophilic and indistinctly demarcated from the surrounding cytoplasm. They are strongly PAS positive (Fig. 16-26). The mechanism by which an A1AT deficiency causes liver disease is not known, but it is likely to be related to the excess intracellular protein. Significantly, only a minority of persons with even the most marked deficiency state develop liver disease.

A variety of hepatic syndromes associated with A1AT deficiency have been recognized. The most common form, occurring in 5 to 17% of those with the PiZZ genotype, is *neonatal hepatitis,* which presents one to eight weeks after birth. Because only a small percentage of patients who have the PiZZ genotype develop neonatal hepatitis, it is likely that a second locus or perhaps environmental factors determine whether liver disease will develop. Family studies suggest that genetic factors are important, and an associa-

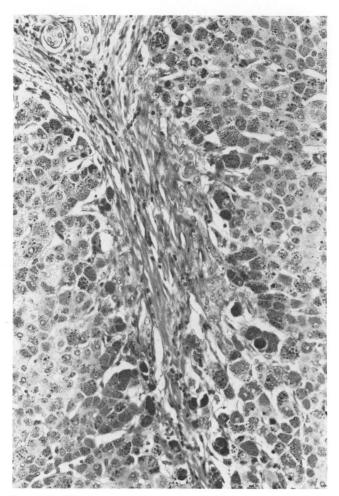

Figure 16–26. Cirrhosis in α_1-antitrypsin deficiency. PAS stain of liver demonstrates the characteristic stained inclusions of the abnormal A1AT protein, producing a granular stippling within the cytoplasm of the hepatocytes. Note the collagen bundles that traverse the hepatic parenchyma.

tion with HLA-DR3 has been reported. The liver changes are characterized by marked cholestasis, liver cell necrosis, mononuclear inflammatory reaction, and cytoplasmic globular PAS-positive inclusions that represent A1AT. The hepatitis subsides in over 80% of cases but in many of the remainder it progresses within 2 to 10 years to cirrhosis and chronic liver failure. Sometimes the initial presentation is cirrhosis in childhood without antecedent hepatitis. Although A1AT deficiency is uncommon, it is a frequent cause of cirrhosis in children.

Liver disease may also develop in adolescents or adults with A1AT deficiency, presenting as either *chronic hepatitis* or *full-blown cirrhosis*. These cases likely reflect smoldering disease with onset in early life. There is some suggestive evidence that the heterozygous state may also increase the risk of chronic liver disease, although this issue is far from settled. Patients who are homozygous for the PiZZ genotype clearly have an increased incidence of *hepatocellular carcinoma.*

TUMORS

The most common hepatic neoplasms are metastatic carcinomas; the colon, lung, and breasts are the most frequent sites of the primary tumor. Metastatic lesions often produce striking hepatomegaly with surprisingly little abnormality of liver functions. As will be discussed, the incidence of primary hepatic malignancies varies with the endemicity of known risk factors. This form of cancer is relatively uncommon in most Western countries. Before discussing primary hepatic carcinomas, brief comments are in order about three benign tumor or tumor-like lesions because of their debated relationship to the use of oral contraceptives, as well as hepatic angiosarcoma, a rare tumor associated with exposure to certain carcinogens.

Cavernous hemangiomas are the most common benign tumors of the liver. These well-circumscribed lesions consisting of endothelial cell–lined vascular channels tend to enlarge during pregnancy or oral contraceptive use, raising the as-yet unanswered question whether they are perhaps induced by female sex hormones. A much less common lesion, *focal nodular hyperplasia,* has also been linked to oral contraceptives, but the evidence is far from convincing. These lesions are in all likelihood hamartomas; they appear as well demarcated but poorly encapsulated nodules with a central stellate scar radiating outward. They contain all the elements of normal liver, including hepatocytes, sinusoids, and proliferating bile ducts. Even less common is *hepatocellular adenoma,* a benign neoplasm that is the most strongly linked to long-term oral contraceptive use. These tumors vary in size from a few centimeters to as large as 30 cm, are usually poorly demarcated from adjacent normal parenchyma, and consist of typical-looking hepatocytes with dilated sinusoids. In contrast to lesions of focal nodular hyperplasia, bile ducts are usually absent. Despite their innocent morphologic appearance, liver cell adenomas may rupture and cause life-threatening hemorrhage.

Hepatic *angiosarcomas* are extremely rare, highly aggressive neoplasms that resemble histologically those that occur in other tissues. They are notable because of their clear association with occupational exposure to vinyl chloride and arsenic and to diagnostic use of the radiographic contrast material Thorotrast (once used in cholangiography).

PRIMARY CARCINOMA

There are three types of primary carcinomas of the liver: (1) hepatocellular carcinoma (HCC, 90%), (2) intrahepatic bile duct carcinoma or cholangiocarcinoma (10%), and (3) mixed hepatocholangiocarcinoma (uncommon). In 60 to 80% of cases, HCC arises in cirrhotic livers; the cholangiocarcinoma, by contrast, is very seldom associated with cirrhosis. The majority of the following discussion will focus on the more common HCC. Cholangiocarcinoma arising from extrahepatic bile ducts is described more fully in a later section (p. 566).

There are striking differences in the frequency of HCC in different nations of the world. In the United States, Canada, and Great Britain, the rates are low, about 1 to 1.5 per 100,000 population for males and about 0.5 for females. The rates are strikingly higher in some African countries such as in Mozambique (104 per 100,000 population for males, 31 for females) and in South African natives (20 to 28 per 100,000 for males, 7 to 10 for females). There is a pronounced male preponderance throughout the world, of the order of about 3:1; this is at least partly related to the greater prevalence of alcoholism, chronic liver disease, and, in particular, hepatitis B infection among males. In high-incidence areas HCC generally arises in early adult life (third to fifth decade), whereas in the low-incidence areas such as the United States it is most often encountered in the sixth and seventh decades.

PATHOGENESIS. The pathogenesis of HCC is not understood but there are three major contributors to the causation: (1) chronic hepatitis B virus infection, (2) hepatocarcinogens in food, and (3) cirrhosis. The recently recognized chronic hepatitis C is also a risk factor for this neoplasm although the strength of this association is still not established.

The voluminous evidence linking HBV and liver cancer is derived from epidemiologic and molecular studies. Epidemiologic evidence shows a direct correlation between the incidence of hepatocellular carcinoma and the frequency of chronic hepatitis B infection. Thus in parts of Africa and in Southeast Asia where the incidence of HBV carriers is very high, liver cancer is extremely common. Prospective studies in Taiwan have demonstrated that HBsAg carriers have a 200 times greater risk of developing HCC than those with no serologic evidence of HBV infection. Conversely, patients who develop HCC are much more likely to have evidence of HBV infection than are controls. In HBsAg-positive patients with HCC, HBV-DNA has been found integrated into the genome of the cancer cells.

Despite all the evidence linking HBV with HCC, it is not proved whether HBV itself causes transformation. This dilemma arises because the HBV genome does not contain any oncogenic sequences. Furthermore, there is no selective site of integration of the viral genome into host DNA, so activation or mutation of a particular protooncogene is precluded. One possibility is that HBV is not directly carcinogenic but renders liver cells susceptible to malignant change by other agents such as aflatoxin. It is interesting to note that in certain regions of the world, such as China and South Africa where HBV is endemic, there is also high exposure to aflatoxins in food. Aflatoxins, derived from *Aspergillus flavus,* are highly carcinogenic in experimental animals and are found in significant quantities in "moldy" grains and peanuts. Recent molecular studies from these geographic locales are particularly revealing. They point to the importance of a specific mutation in the p53 tumor suppressor gene as a factor in the development of HCC. It was previously known that point mutations of the p53 gene were common in HCC, as they are in a number of other forms of cancer. However, in other tumors the p53 mutations are not targeted to a specific site on the gene. In contrast, HCCs from patients in these regions revealed a specific mutation affecting the same codon in the p53 gene. It is worthy of note that the particular point mutation (replacement of G by T or C) is known to occur in experimental animals exposed to aflatoxin. This strongly indicates a pathogenic role for this mutation. Together these observations suggest that in certain settings hepatocyte regeneration that follows HBV-induced liver injury provides a fertile soil for aflatoxin-induced mutations.

Other recent studies implicate HBV more directly in hepatocarcinogenesis (p. 202). The HBV genome encodes a regulatory element called x-protein that acts as a transacting transcriptional activator of many genes. It is conceivable that in liver cells infected with HBV the x-protein disrupts normal growth control by activation of host cell protooncogenes.

As stated earlier, *60 to 80% of hepatocellular carcinomas arise in cirrhotic livers.* The risk of developing cancers is particularly high with postnecrotic cirrhosis associated with HBV infection; somewhat lower with cirrhosis associated with HCV, hemochromatosis, and A1AT deficiency; and lowest with alcoholic cirrhosis. The development of HCC in cirrhosis may be related to long-standing regenerative hyperplastic reactions, with the stimulus for the repair acting as a tumor promoter. There are, however, other possible mechanisms by which the agents that produce cirrhosis may act. For example, chronic alcoholism induces the microsomal P-450 system, which metabolizes several xenobiotic compounds (including aflatoxins) to active carcinogens. Cirrhosis obviously is not a necessary precursor for HCC, since it is not present in 20 to 40% of cases.

It should be noted that none of the influences discussed earlier are pertinent to the causation of cholangiocarcinomas. The only well-documented association is with invasion of the biliary tract by the liver fluke *Opisthorchis sinensis* and related forms.

MORPHOLOGY. HCC and intrahepatic cholangiocarcinoma as well as rare mixed patterns may occur as (1) a solitary massive tumor, which sometimes produces marked hepatomegaly; (2) multiple nodules scattered throughout the liver, inducing less striking hepatomegaly; or (3) a diffuse infiltration of the entire hepatic substance, difficult to discern against the background of an underlying cirrhosis. In all three patterns the tumors are usually yellow-white, but well-differentiated HCC may elaborate sufficient bile to produce a green color (Fig. 16-27). Foci of hemorrhage and necrosis are frequently present in larger masses. Sometimes the margins of cholangiocarcinomas are also bile stained, presumably due to obstruction of bile ducts. In all variants, it may be difficult to differentiate large regenerative nodules of hepatic parenchyma in the cirrhotic liver from small nodules of neoplasm. These cancers (particularly the HCC) have a propensity for invading blood

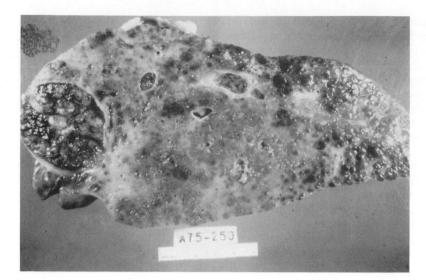

Figure 16–27. A cirrhotic liver involved with hepatocellular carcinoma contains a large number of dark, bilirubin-stained, rounded tumor masses of various sizes, the largest of which is at the left of the photograph.

vessels and may obstruct the hepatic vein, producing the Budd-Chiari syndrome (p. 530), or they may block the portal vein, producing portal hypertension.

Histologically, HCCs range from well-differentiated lesions that virtually reproduce hepatocytes, arranged in cords or small nests (Fig. 16–28), to poorly differentiated lesions, often made up of large multinucleate anaplastic tumor giant cells. **In the better-differentiated variants, globules of bile may be found within the cytoplasm of cells as well as in the pseudocanaliculi between cells.** In addition, acidophilic hyaline inclusions within the cytoplasm may be present, resembling Mallory bodies. There is surprisingly scant stroma in most HCCs, and it is the poor vascularization that leads to the necrosis of central regions of the tumor.

Fibrolamellar carcinoma is a distinctive clinicopathologic variant of HCC. Arising most commonly in non-cirrhotic livers, it usually presents as a single, somewhat circumscribed mass. It is composed of eosinophilic polygonal cells that grow in nests or cords separated by a fibrous stroma. This type of HCC has a better prognosis.

Intrahepatic **cholangiocarcinoma** appears as a more or less well-differentiated adenocarcinoma, typically with an abundant fibrous stroma (desmoplasia). **Bile pigment and hyaline inclusions are not found within cells.** The histologic differentiation of multicentric cholangiocarcinoma from metastatic adenocarcinoma may be treacherous.

Primary carcinomas of the liver tend to remain localized to the organ; at the time of death, only about half have spread to such extrahepatic sites as regional lymph nodes, lungs, bones, adrenal glands, and other sites.

CLINICAL COURSE. Although primary carcinomas in the liver may present as silent hepatomegaly, they are often encountered in patients with cirrhosis of the liver who already have symptoms of the underlying disorder. In these circumstances, rapid increase in liver size, sudden worsening of ascites, or the appearance of

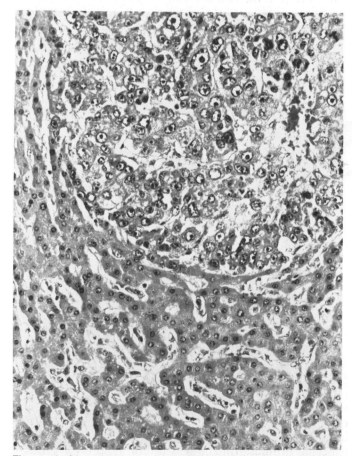

Figure 16–28. Hepatocellular carcinoma occupies most of the upper portion of the photograph. The residual normal hepatic parenchyma is seen below. Tumor cells and their nuclei vary moderately in size and shape but retain their resemblance to normal liver cells.

bloody ascites, fever, and pain calls attention to the development of a tumor. The fever is attributed to resorption of necrotic tumor products. Jaundice may be absent; if present, it is typically mild.

The natural history of primary liver cancer is grim; death, usually within six months of diagnosis, results from profound cachexia, often accompanied by increasing jaundice and other signs of liver failure.

Laboratory studies are helpful but not diagnostic. Thus, 90% of patients with HCC have elevated serum levels of α-fetoprotein; those with cholangiocarcinoma do not. Unfortunately, this tumor marker lacks specificity, because elevated levels are also encountered in a variety of other conditions—cirrhosis, chronic hepatitis, pregnancy, and gonadal germ cell tumors (p. 595) among them. Very high levels, however (above 1000 ng/ml), are relatively specific, so in endemic areas this test is quite useful. An additional serum marker, not yet widely used, is a prothrombin precursor, which is present in high levels in about 90% of patients with HCC. Techniques useful in detecting smaller tumors that might allow curative surgery include ultrasonography, hepatic angiography, CT, and MRI.

The fibrolamellar variant, arising mainly in children and young adults, has a much better prognosis with approximately 60% five-year survival.

The Biliary Tract

Diseases of the biliary tract are extremely common. The overwhelming majority of patients with complaints referable to the biliary tract have *gallstones* (cholelithiasis) or the closely related condition *cholecystitis.* Much less common are *tumors* of the biliary tract. These three entities account for more than 95% of diseases of the biliary tract and together with *cholangitis* (inflammation of the bile ducts) and liver abscesses will be the focus of our discussion.

CHOLANGITIS AND LIVER ABSCESS

Cholangitis should be distinguished from cholangiolitis, which implies inflammation of small bile *ductules,* and may occur in any form of hepatitis, particularly viral hepatitis. Clinically, cholangitis can be readily recognized by Charcot's triad of findings: jaundice, abdominal pain, and fever with chills. The cause is nearly always bacterial infection resulting from bile duct stasis or obstruction, most commonly due to stones, strictures, tumors, and parasitic infections of the biliary tree. Of these, biliary tract stones and strictures account for most cases in the United States. How the bacteria invade the normally sterile biliary tree is not clear. While once it was assumed the infection was almost always ascending, it is now held that spread from adjacent lymphatics, portal venous blood, or even infected gallbladder contents is more likely. The most common infective agents are part of the gut flora, especially *E. coli* and other gram-negative rods, enterococci, and occasionally salmonellae. Rising intraluminal pressure with obstruction facilitates the entry of the bacteria or their products (e.g., endotoxin) into the systemic circulation, which results in the systemic manifestations of the disease (i.e., fever, chills, and leukocytosis). The morphologic changes are typical of acute suppurative inflammation, which may extend upward and produce liver abscess.

Liver abscesses arise most often as complications of acute ascending cholangitis, and as such they are frequently associated with some obstructive disease of the biliary tract such as gallstones or malignancy. The next most common cause is blood-borne infection in a patient with bacteremia, as in association with bacterial endocarditis. Since the advent of antibiotics, extension of infection along the portal vein secondary to intraabdominal sepsis is a much less frequent cause. As might be expected from their frequent association with ascending cholangitis, gram-negative rods such as *E. coli* and *Klebsiella* are commonly isolated from liver abscesses. With improvements in culture techniques it is becoming obvious that liver abscesses are often polymicrobial. Pathogens other than gram-negative rods include anaerobes such as *Bacteroides fragilis* and *Fusobacterium* species as well as microaerophilic streptococci. Staphylococci are also encountered, although less frequently than the other pathogens listed. Liver abscess caused by *Entamoeba histolytica* was described on p. 507.

The lesions vary from microscopic foci to massive areas of suppurative necrosis. In general, they are from 1 to 3 cm in diameter and are usually multiple. Rupture through the capsule may lead to subhepatic or subdiaphragmatic abscesses and peritonitis. On rare occasions, the infection may trek from the subdiaphragmatic location into the thoracic cavity. Liver abscesses may be totally silent if they are small and few in number. When they elicit symptoms, the clinical disease is usually indistinguishable from acute cholangitis, which, of course, is a frequent accompaniment.

CHOLELITHIASIS

Cholelithiasis (gallstones in the gallbladder or biliary tree) is very common, occurring in 8% of men and 20% of women. Gallstones are clinically silent in perhaps 70% of cases, but when they do cause symptoms they usually do so by causing cholecystitis or by passing into one of the excretory ducts, producing excruciating biliary colic. Gallstones only rarely occur in the first two decades of life and have their peak incidence in women in the fourth decade, hence the unflattering mnemonic for the most important risk factors, the "four F's": fat, female, fertile (multiparous), and forty.

Gallstones may arise anywhere in the biliary tract, but the great majority are in the gallbladder. Stones are characterized by their chief chemical component. This distinction is important because the pathogenesis and risk factors vary with the type of stone. Cholesterol is the major component in the vast majority of stones (70 to 85%). Usually they also contain smaller amounts of calcium salts (carbonate, phosphate, and bilirubinate). Whether these should be called *cholesterol stones* or *mixed stones* is a matter of semantics. Most of the remainder (up to 30%) are *pigment stones* composed of calcium bilirubinate and, unlike cholesterol stones, are often fairly "pure." Calcium carbonate occurs in some 10 to 20% of all stones in sufficient concentrations to impart radiopacity, but pure *calcium carbonate stones* are rare.

> The morphology of cholesterol and pigment stones differs. Cholesterol stones are classically 1 to 3 cm in diameter and pale tan or yellow; they may be single but most often are multiple and either round or faceted, owing to apposition to one another. In contrast, pigment stones are smaller (under 1.5 cm), almost never occur singly but rather in large numbers, and are jet black and generally ovoid. The vast majority of gallstones are radiolucent.

PATHOGENESIS AND RISK FACTORS. In considering the causation of cholesterol stones it is necessary to review the components of bile. Bile salts make up approximately two thirds of the solutes in bile (Fig. 16–29). Hepatocytes synthesize two bile salts, cholate and chenodeoxycholate, which are modified in the gut to form deoxycholates, lithocholates, and ursodeoxycholates. The enterohepatic circulation (p. 524) provides the bulk of secreted bile salts and relatively little synthesis of bile salt de novo occurs on a daily basis. Phospholipid, predominantly in the form of lecithin, is another major constituent of bile, whereas cholesterol, proteins, and bilirubin are minor components. Because most bile stones contain cholesterol, this component of the bile deserves special attention. Cholesterol is insoluble in an aqueous medium and its concentration in bile is high enough to create an unstable supersaturated fluid in which crystallization and stone formation might routinely occur. This is normally prevented by the transport of cholesterol in two special physicochemical forms. In one form, cholesterol is contained within the core of micelles whose outer hydrophilic shell is made up of lecithin and bile salts (Fig. 16–30). In the other form it is carried within the lipid bilayers of *vesicles* that are composed largely of lecithin. Stones form when the bile can no longer maintain cholesterol in either of the two soluble forms. This may occur with excess cholesterol secretion in bile or decreased bile salt or lecithin secretion. Indeed, known risk factors (described later) associated with either cholesterol oversecretion or bile salt undersecretion are also associated with cholesterol stone formation; to date lecithin undersecretion has not been demonstrated.

Although cholesterol supersaturation is necessary for gallstone formation it is not sufficient to initiate crystallization. Stone formation requires a nidus (nucleus) to initiate precipitation of cholesterol crystals. This step, called *nucleation,* is followed by the *aggregation* of the crystals into macroscopically visible stones (accretion). Factors that drive these steps are not fully understood but they include an increase in "nucleation" factors such as mucoproteins, or a decrease in "antinucleation" factors (e.g., apolipoprotein AI and

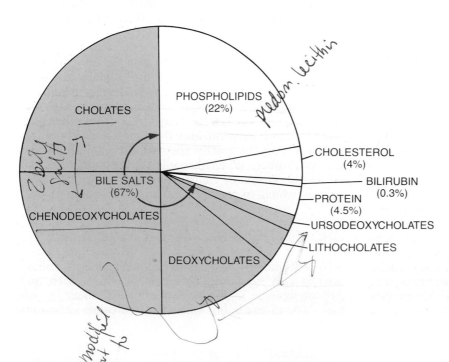

Figure 16–29. Average solute composition of gallbladder and hepatic bile in health. (From Carey, M. C.: Biliary lipids and gallstone formation. In Csomos, G., Thaler, H. (eds.): Clinical Hepatology. Berlin, Springer Verlag, 1983, pp. 52–69. Used by permission.)

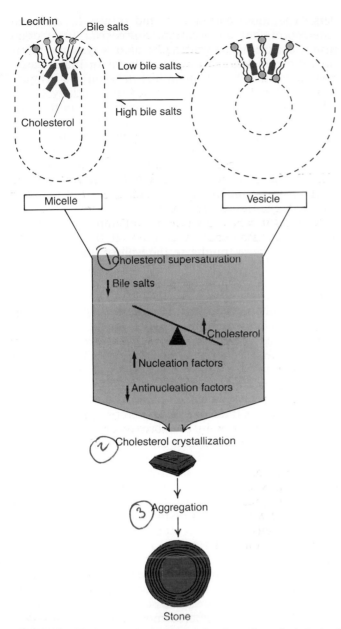

Figure 16-30. Proposed model for the formation of cholesterol stones from cholesterol-containing micelles and vesicles. Three stages are critical: (1) supersaturation, (2) crystallization, and (3) aggregation.

AII) that normally prevent build-up of crystals. A model for cholesterol stone formation is presented in Figure 16-30.

The formation of calcium bilirubinate (pigment stones) is also incompletely understood, although as with cholesterol stones the excess crystallization of an insoluble compound (unconjugated bilirubin) is at the heart of the problem. As a group, patients with pigment stones tend to have higher levels of unconjugated bilirubin in their bile than persons who do not have pigment stones. These observations suggest that in pigment stone disease liver cells secrete excess *unconjugated* bilirubin or that bile contains a deconjugating mechanism, perhaps bacteria with glucuronidases. Neither mechanism has been proved. Infection in the

biliary tree is associated with an increased incidence of pigment stones. In the absence of bacterial infection, some patients with pigment stones have more endogenous glucuronidase activity than controls. It is likely that supersaturation of bile with calcium salts also plays an important role in the formation of pigment stones, because when calcium combines with unconjugated bilirubin the bilirubin is even less soluble. What facilitates calcium salt supersaturation is not known. Once calcium bilirubinate exists in a supersaturated state, nucleation and accretion proceed as with cholesterol stones.

Risk factors, as might be expected, are dependent on the form of stone (Table 16-7). For cholesterol stones, in addition to the four F's already mentioned, several other risk factors have been identified, including an *ethnic* (possibly genetic) predisposition to gallstones. A striking example is the extremely high incidence of cholelithiasis in the Pima Indians of the American Southwest. These people exhibit both decreased bile salt secretion and increased cholesterol secretion. *Malabsorption of bile acids* from the ileum with concurrent decreased bile acid secretion seems to be the basis of an increased risk associated with ileal resection, Crohn's disease, and cystic fibrosis with pancreatic insufficiency. The use of *estrogens,* including those contained in *oral contraceptives,* roughly doubles the risk of gallstone formation. Indeed, the female preponderance of this condition may well be related to an effect of endogenous estrogen. Estrogens are thought to cause excessive cholesterol secretion coupled with defective bile acid synthesis. *Clofibrate,* used in an attempt to lower serum lipids and to inhibit atherogenesis, significantly increases the incidence of gallstones by increasing biliary cholesterol secretion. *Obesity,* as mentioned, also increases the cholesterol content of bile. Perhaps related to obesity is the increased risk of gallstones encountered with *excessive intake of calories and simple sugar. Impaired gallbladder emptying,* as may occur with pregnancy or diabetes mellitus, may

TABLE 16-7. BILIARY COMPOSITION AND RISK FACTORS FOR GALLSTONES

Cholesterol gallstones (70-85%)
Decreased bile acid secretion in bile
Acquired inhibition of synthesis: induced by estrogens in oral contraceptives
Excessive loss: ileal resection, ileal diseases (e.g., Crohn's disease), malabsorption (e.g., cystic fibrosis)
Hereditary defect in synthesis: cerebrotendinous xanthomatosis
Increased cholesterol secretion in bile
Estrogen and oral contraceptive use
Female gender, especially multiparity
Obesity
High-calorie diet
Clofibrate therapy
Pigment (calcium bilirubinate) gallstones (<30%)
Hemolytic anemia
Alcoholic cirrhosis
Ileal resection
Chronic parenteral nutrition
Biliary tract infection

favor lithogenesis, presumably by allowing gallstone growth. In view of the plethora of risk factors, the "social set" will be happy to know that moderate intake of alcohol appears to be protective.

As might be expected, *pigment stones* are more likely to develop in patients with excess hemoglobin breakdown and bilirubin secretion, as occurs in hemolytic anemia. The mechanisms for pigment stones in alcoholic cirrhosis, ileal resection, and chronic parenteral nutrition are largely speculative.

Whatever the type, gallstones may have little or much clinical significance. Approximately 70% of cases of cholelithiasis have no symptoms when the stones are discovered ("silent stones"). The majority of persons who have silent gallstones remain asymptomatic for years or a lifetime, and current medical practice is to simply observe them. In other persons gallstones are not so innocuous. They may:

- Play a role in the induction of cholecystitis and its complications (discussed next)
- Give rise to calculous obstruction of the cystic or common bile duct, manifested by excruciating pain (biliary colic)
- Predispose to acute cholangitis
- Predispose to acute pancreatitis (p. 581)
- Lead to slower-developing obstructive jaundice and the attendant risk of biliary cirrhosis (p. 552)
- Possibly, favor the development of carcinoma of the gallbladder, although this association is somewhat controversial.

The therapy for gallstones has changed in the last five to ten years, reflecting a greater understanding of the pathophysiology of gallstones and technical innovations. For symptomatic patients who are good surgical candidates surgery is usually the best treatment. Alternatives to surgery include (1) oral administration of bile salts; originally thought to increase bile salt secretion, these in fact decrease cholesterol concentration in bile, (2) application of shock waves to dissolve stones (extracorporeal shock wave lithotripsy), and (3) instillation of a gallstone solvent (methyl tert-butyl ether) into the gallbladder via percutaneous transhepatic catheter.

CHOLECYSTITIS ———————————

Inflammation of the gallbladder may be *acute, chronic,* or *acute superimposed on chronic.* In the United States, cholecystitis is one of the most common indications for abdominal surgery. Its distribution in the population closely parallels that of gallstones, and stones are present in 80 to 90% of *all* cases of cholecystitis, but in up to 95% of acute cholecystitis.

ACUTE CHOLECYSTITIS
Even though stones are associated with most cases of acute cholecystitis (*acute calculous cholecystitis*), the exact mechanism of inflammation is not well understood; it is likely to be multifactorial, with contributions from *infection, chemical and mechanical irritation,* and *obstruction of the cystic duct.* Bacteria can be cultured from about 80% of acutely inflamed gallblad-

ders. The most common offenders are *E. coli* and enterococci, but on occasion, *Salmonella typhi* organisms localize in the gallbladder after a systemic infection. Nevertheless, bacteria are absent in many cases, making it unlikely that microbial invasion is a primary causal factor. It has been proposed that initially supersaturation or imbalances in the constituents of the bile, such as high levels of bile salts or acids, results in *chemical inflammation,* which in many cases facilitates secondary invasion by bacteria. Only when cholecystitis develops in the course of a systemic bacterial infection is it likely that bacterial invasion by the microorganism initiates the disease; indeed, in many of these cases gallstones are absent.

Gallstones may contribute to inflammation, chemical and bacterial, in several ways. If they arise first, they might cause trauma to the wall of the gallbladder and predispose to bacterial invasion. More important, they may cause bile duct obstruction. In the majority of cases of acute cholecystitis the cystic duct is obstructed. Bile duct obstruction leads to distention of the gallbladder with an impaired blood supply and compromised lymphatic drainage, which results in ischemia, enhanced chemical damage to the mucosa, and frequently secondary invasion by bacteria. Local prostaglandin synthesis and toxic effects of lysolecithin have been posited as important mediators of acute inflammation in these processes.

Acute cholecystitis in the absence of stones (*acalculous acute cholecystitis*) is more difficult to explain. Its incidence (5 to 10% of all acute cases) is greatest in critically ill adults who are under the stress of recent surgery, trauma, or burns. Investigators speculate that these conditions predispose to transient or prolonged bacteremia, with seeding of the gallbladder and injury to the mucosa.

CHRONIC CHOLECYSTITIS
This may be a sequel to repeated bouts of acute cholecystitis, but in most instances it develops without any history of acute inflammation. Like acute cholecystitis it is almost always associated with gallstones and is therefore encountered most commonly in older, obese women. Despite the strong association with gallstones it is doubtful that stones play a direct role in the initiation of chronic inflammation. More likely, supersaturation of bile predisposes to stone formation as well as to chemical injury of the gallbladder wall. In any event, cholelithiasis and cholecystitis are virtual Siamese twins. Microbial infection, typically caused by *E. coli* and enterococci, is present in only 30% of cases.

> **MORPHOLOGY.** In **acute cholecystitis,** the gallbladder is usually enlarged (two- to threefold), tense, edematous, fiery red, and often covered with a fibrinopurulent exudate. Areas of black, gangrenous necrosis may be evident, sometimes with perforation. The wall is characteristically thickened and edematous, and there is generally extensive inflammatory ulceration of the mucosa (Fig. 16-31). As was mentioned, stones are almost always present, and not infrequently one is impacted in

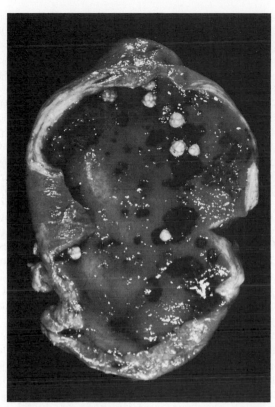

Figure 16–31. Acute cholecystitis. The gallbladder has been opened to show the edematous, thickened wall and the glazed, congested mucosa on which rest some small multifaceted gallstones. The dark, irregular patches are areas of mucosal ulceration.

the neck of the gallbladder, strongly suggesting that it triggered the flare-up. The histologic changes are characteristic of any acute inflammatory response. Sometimes the lumen is filled with pus, creating **empyema of the gallbladder.**

In **chronic cholecystitis,** the gallbladder may be large, but more often it is contracted. The serosa may be smooth and glistening or dulled by subserosal fibrosis. The wall is variably thickened, gray-white, and tough. Stones are usually present; mucosal ulcerations are infrequent. The inflammatory infiltrate is mononuclear, and the submucosa and subserosa are often fibrosed. The changes of chronic cholecystitis are often found accompanying an acute inflammatory reaction in gallbladders removed because of acute cholecystitis.

On occasion, when a stone has been impacted in the neck of the gallbladder or cystic duct for long periods of time, resorption of many bile constituents (excluding the stone) occurs, leaving a clear, mucinous secretion. This pattern is called **hydrops** or **mucocele of the gallbladder.** A second special form of reaction that sometimes follows on the heels of inflammation of the gallbladder is dystrophic calcification in the wall, giving rise to the so-called **porcelain gallbladder.**

CLINICAL COURSE. Cholecystitis has many potential consequences. The acute form announces itself loudly,

with severe, steady upper abdominal pain, often radiating to the right shoulder. Sometimes, when stones are present in the neck of the gallbladder or in ducts, the pain is colicky. Fever, nausea, leukocytosis, and prostration are classic. The right subcostal region is markedly tender and may feel rigid owing to spasm of the abdominal muscles. In approximately a third of cases, a tender, distended gallbladder can be palpated, confirming the diagnosis. Slow penetration of bacteria may yield pericholecystic abscesses, or the gangrenous gallbladder may suddenly perforate, leading to subhepatic abscesses or generalized peritonitis. The bacterial infection may ascend the bile ducts, resulting in intrahepatic ascending cholangitis (p. 561); liver abscesses may follow. The treatment of acute cholecystitis is usually surgical but requires careful assessment of operative risk. The decision whether to operate immediately or wait until the inflammation is quiescent is a difficult one.

The chronic form of the disease does not have the striking manifestations of the acute form but is characterized instead by recurrent attacks of either steady or colicky epigastric or right upper quadrant pain. Nausea, vomiting, and intolerance for fatty foods are frequent accompaniments. Whether these manifestations are intrinsic to the chronic cholecystitis or are secondary to the associated stones is unclear.

The diagnosis of both the acute and chronic cholecystitis often rests on the detection of gallstones, dilatation of the bile ducts, or both, by cholecystography, ultrasonography, CT, or radionuclide imaging.

CARCINOMA OF THE GALLBLADDER

Carcinoma of the gallbladder is the most common cancer of the biliary tract. In 60 to 90% of cases, gallstones are also present, and, indeed, the incidence of this form of neoplasia follows the pattern of cholelithiasis, affecting females about three times as often as males, most often in the 70- to 75-year age group. Many surgeons believe that gallstones play a causal role in the genesis of cancer by producing chronic irritation of the gallbladder mucosa, but this relationship is controversial. It is perhaps significant that certain derivatives of bile acids are powerful experimental carcinogens.

MORPHOLOGY. Most cancers of the gallbladder are adenocarcinomas, some mucin secreting. These grow either in an infiltrative pattern, thickening the gallbladder wall, or as exophytic lesions fungating into the lumen. About 5 to 10% are squamous cell carcinomas or adenoacanthomas. Presumably they arise from metaplastic squamous epithelium. All generally spread by local extension. Direct permeation of the liver is characteristic of those that arise in the liver bed of the gallbladder. Many situated near the neck of the gallbladder produce symptoms highly reminiscent of gallstones or cholecystitis. Some grow along the cystic duct, eventually obstructing the common bile duct. Those arising in the fundus of the gallbladder remain silent until their advance impinges on some structure or function that evokes clinical manifestations. The gallbladder is palpable in about two thirds of patients. Although jaundice eventually develops in most patients, it is relatively mild. Spread to the porta hepatis nodes and liver is frequent. Although widespread metastatic dissemination may occur, it is uncommon.

CLINICAL COURSE. About half the patients come to clinical attention because of complaints referable to the biliary tract. Indeed, the symptoms may be indistinguishable from those of cholecystitis or cholelithiasis —symptoms that may be all too familiar to these patients and, so, not particularly alarming. In the remaining cases, the disease is entirely occult until anorexia and weight loss make their ominous appearance. In most cases, diagnosis is too late for curative surgery and the five-year survival rate is dismal—3%. Survival is most likely in those whose cancers are detected incidentally at surgery for cholelithiasis or in whom early invasion of the cystic duct produces symptoms of biliary obstruction.

CARCINOMA OF EXTRAHEPATIC BILE DUCTS, INCLUDING AMPULLA OF VATER

Carcinomas of the intrahepatic ducts (cholangiocarcinomas) present very much like hepatocellular carcinoma and were discussed with these tumors previously (p. 558). In contrast, cancers arising in the extrahepatic ducts and ampulla of Vater (also called extrahepatic cholangiocarcinomas) are extremely insidious and generally produce painless, progressively deepening jaundice. As mentioned, they are less common than cancer of the gallbladder. In contrast to the situation with gallbladder cancers, men are more frequently affected. The locations of these tumors are as follows:

- The distal common bile duct, including the periampullary region (50%)
- The distal common hepatic duct or proximal common bile duct (30%)
- At or near the bifurcation of the hepatic ducts (20%).

Attempts to relate gallstones to the genesis of these tumors have been unconvincing, and, moreover, gallstones are present in only about a third of cases. As with intrahepatic cholangiocarcinomas, there is an association with coinfections with liver flukes (in the Orient). In addition the presence of inflammatory bowel disease or primary sclerosing cholangitis also increases the risk.

MORPHOLOGY. Almost all are extremely small, presumably because in their strategic locations they produce

extrahepatic obstructive jaundice and hepatic decompensation very early. Accordingly, they rarely metastasize widely but infiltrate locally and sometimes spread to the lymph nodes of the porta hepatis or to the liver. Some infiltrate the wall of the duct, causing thickening and narrowing of the lumen, whereas others fungate directly into the lumen. Almost all are adenocarcinomas, more or less well-differentiated, and some have papillary patterns. Mucin secretion is sometimes present. Rarely they appear as adenoacanthomas. For the most part, fibrous proliferation is a prominent component.

CLINICAL COURSE. In virtually all cases symptoms are related to ductal obstruction and include nausea, vomiting, and weight loss accompanied by progressive jaundice and pale stools. Hepatomegaly is present in about 50%, and a palpable gallbladder in about 25%. As expected, laboratory findings include those of obstructive jaundice, i.e., elevated levels of serum alkaline phosphatase, serum aminotransferases, and urine bilirubin, and prolonged prothrombin time.

The differentiation of obstructive jaundice due to neoplasia from the far more common calculous disease is a major clinical problem. However, the presence of gallstones obviously does not preclude the existence of intercurrent neoplasia, and drainage of ductal secretions by ERCP permitting cytologic study of shed cells or surgical exploration may be necessary to arrive at a diagnosis. Most ductal cancers are not surgically resectable at the time of clinical diagnosis, and the average postoperative survival time is six months to a year. Cancer of the periampullary region, however, has a better prognosis. Depending on the extent of invasion, the five-year survival rate following surgical resection (using a so-called Whipple procedure) is 85% for localized lesions but only 10 to 25% for more infiltrative neoplasms. Overall, the five-year survival rate for extrahepatic cholangiocarcinomas is only 15%.

Bibliography

Bradley, D. W.: Enterically transmitted non-A, non-B hepatitis. Br. Med. Bull. 46:442, 1990. (An overview of the discovery of hepatitis E, including primate studies and the cloning of the virus.)

Choo, Q-L, Weiner, A. J., Overby, L. R., Kuo, G., Houghton, M., Bradley, D. W.: Hepatitis C virus: The major causative agent of viral non-A, non-B hepatitis. Br. Med. Bull. 46:423, 1990. (An overview of the cloning of the viral antigen used in the serologic test and how this test has helped clarify the relationship of hepatitis C to various forms of liver disease.)

Crystal, R. G.: α₁-Antitrypsin deficiency: Pathogenesis and treatment. Hosp Pract.: 26:81, 1991. (A very readable discussion of the genetics of the disease with implications of this knowledge in treating the resulting emphysema and liver disease.)

Edwards, M. S.: Hepatitis B serology—help in interpretation. Pediatr. Clin. North Am. 35:503, 1988. (A clear overview of a complex subject.)

Forbes, A., Williams, R.: Changing epidemiology and clinical aspects of hepatitis A. Br. Med. Bull. 46:303, 1990. (An overview of the changing epidemiology of this virus infection with emphasis on the more developed countries.)

Friedman, S. L., Bissell, D. M.: Hepatic fibrosis: New insights into pathogenesis. Hosp. Pract. 25:43, 1990. (A nicely illustrated and concise overview.)

Hoofnagle, J. H.: Type D (delta) hepatitis. JAMA 261:1321, 1989. (A detailed discussion of the clinical course, methods of diagnosis, epidemiology, and prevention.)

Jones, R. S.: Carcinoma of the gallbladder. Surg. Clin. North Am. 70:1419, 1990. (Brief overview of pathogenesis, histology, diagnosis, and treatment and prognosis.)

Lieber, C. S.: Biochemical and molecular basis of alcohol-induced injury to liver and other tissues. N. Engl. J. Med. 319:1639, 1988. (An excellent review with particular emphasis on the toxic effects associated with the microsomal ethanol-oxidizing system.)

Mondelli, M. U., Manns, M., Ferrari, C.: Does the immune response play a role in the pathogenesis of chronic liver disease? Arch. Pathol. Lab. Med. 112:489, 1988. (A discussion of the role of the immune response in the various forms of hepatitis B–induced liver disease and the autoimmune liver diseases.)

Mullen, K. D.: Benzodiazapine compounds and hepatic encephalopathy. N. Engl. J. Med. 325:509, 1991. (A succinct editorial that summarizes the mechanisms of hepatic encephalopathy.)

Rustgi, V. K. (ed.): Hepatic diseases. Med. Clin. North Am. 73(4), 1989. (A collection of reviews by experts in the field; particularly relevant to topics covered in this chapter are "Hepatic Encephalopathy" by S. H. Gammal and E. A. Jones, "Hemochromatosis" by H. K. Golland and J. U. C. Spivah, "Portal Hypertension" by J. Bosch, M. Navasa, J. C. Garcie-Pagar, A. M. DeLacy, and J. Rodes, and "Conditions Associated with Hepatocellular Carcinoma" by M. Lisker-Mehnan, P. Martin, and J. Hoofnagle.)

Scheuer, P. J.: Classification of chronic hepatitis: A need for reassessment. J. Hepatol 13:372, 1991. (A brief review that provides compelling arguments for reassessing the traditional classification of chronic hepatitis.)

Ueo, C. J., Pitt, H. A., Cameron, J. L.: Cholangiocarcinoma. Surg. Clin. North Am. 70:1429, 1990. (A brief and cogent description of the etiology, pathology, clinical presentation, treatment, and prognosis.)

Wands, J. R., Blum, H. E.: Primary hepatocellular carcinoma. N. Engl. J. Med. 325:729, 1991. (An excellent summary of the epidemiology and molecular pathogenesis of liver cell cancer.)

Zakim, D., Boyer, T. D.: A Textbook of Liver Disease. 2nd ed. Philadelphia, W. B. Saunders, 1990. (A compendium of scholarly, extensively documented chapters on structure, function, and major diseases of the liver. Of special interest are the chapters on "Physiology and Pathophysiology of Bilirubin Metabolism" by N. Blanchart and J. Fevery; "Pathologic Diagnosis of Liver Disease" by J. J. Lefkowitz; and "Pathogenesis and Dissolution of Gallstones" by D. M. Heuman, E. G. Moore, and Z. R. Vlahcevic.)

Zimmerman, H. J., Maddrey, W. C.: Toxic and drug-induced hepatitis. In Schiff, L., Schiff, E. R. (eds): Diseases of the Liver. 6th ed. Philadelphia, J. B. Lippincott, 1987. (A lucid discussion of the basic concepts with comprehensive lists of agents that cause the various types of hepatic injury, e.g., acute hepatitis, granulomas, cirrhosis.)

SEVENTEEN

The Pancreas

ENDOCRINE PANCREAS
DIABETES MELLITUS
ISLET CELL TUMORS
    Beta-Cell Lesions (Hyperinsulinism)
    Zollinger-Ellison Syndrome (Gastrinoma)
EXOCRINE PANCREAS
ACUTE PANCREATITIS
CHRONIC PANCREATITIS
CARCINOMA OF THE PANCREAS

As is well known, the pancreas is in reality two organs in one. Approximately 80 to 85% of the pancreas is an exocrine gland that secretes enzymes necessary for digestion of food. The remaining 10 to 15% of the pancreatic substance consists of the islets of Langerhans, which secrete insulin, glucagon, and a variety of other hormones. These two parts of the pancreas are affected by quite distinctive lesions and so will be considered separately.

Endocrine Pancreas

The endocrine pancreas consists of about 1 million microscopic units, the islets of Langerhans. There are several cell types in the islets of Langerhans that can be differentiated by their staining properties, by the ultrastructural morphology of their granules, and by their hormone content. Of these, the four most important cell types are: B (beta), A (alpha), D (delta), and PP (pancreatic polypeptide) cells. The *B cells* contain insulin and constitute 70% of the islet cell population. *A cells* elaborate glucagon, and account for 20% of the islet. *D cells* contain somatostatin, which suppresses the release of glucagon and insulin. D cells make up 5 to 10% of the islet cell population. *PP cells* are found not only in the islets but also scattered within the exocrine part of the pancreas. Within the islets they constitute 1 to 2% of all cells, and they contain a unique pancreatic polypeptide of unknown physiologic function.

With this background we can turn to the two main disorders of the islet cells, diabetes mellitus and islet cell tumors.

DIABETES MELLITUS

Diabetes mellitus is a chronic disorder of carbohydrate, fat, and protein metabolism. *A defective or deficient insulin secretory response, which translates into impaired carbohydrate (glucose) use, is a charac-*teristic feature of diabetes mellitus, as is the resulting hyperglycemia.

CLASSIFICATION AND INCIDENCE. *Primary, or idiopathic, diabetes mellitus,* by far the most common and important form, will be the focus of our discussion. It must be distinguished from *secondary diabetes,* which includes forms of hyperglycemia associated with identifiable causes in which destruction of pancreatic islets is induced by inflammatory pancreatic disease, surgery, tumors, certain drugs, iron overload (hemochromatosis), and certain acquired or genetic endocrinopathies (Table 17–1).

Primary diabetes mellitus probably represents a heterogeneous group of disorders that have hyperglycemia as a common feature. These can be basically divided into two variants that differ in their pattern of inheritance, insulin responses, and origins (Table 17–2).

● The first is *insulin-dependent diabetes mellitus (IDDM)*, also called *type I diabetes* and previously known as juvenile-onset or ketosis-prone diabetes. This variant accounts for 10 to 20% of all cases of idiopathic diabetes.
● The remaining 80 to 90% of patients have the second variant, *non–insulin dependent diabetes mellitus (NIDDM)*, also called *type II* diabetes and previously referred to as adult-onset diabetes. Type II diabetes is further divided into obese (80% of all cases) and nonobese types.

It should be stressed that while the two major types of

TABLE 17-1. TYPES OF DIABETES

Primary (Idiopathic) Diabetes
Type I (insulin-dependent diabetes mellitus, IDDM)
Type II (non-insulin dependent diabetes mellitus, NIDDM)
   Nonobese NIDDM
   Obese NIDDM
   Maturity-onset diabetes of the young (MODY)
Secondary Diabetes
Chronic pancreatitis
Postpancreatectomy
Hormonal tumors (e.g., pheochromocytoma, pituitary tumors)
Drugs (corticosteroids)
Hemochromatosis
Genetic disorders (e.g., lipodystrophy)

diabetes have different pathogenic mechanisms and metabolic characteristics, the *long-term complications in blood vessels, kidneys, eyes, and nerves occur in both types and are the major causes of morbidity and death from diabetes.*

With an annual mortality rate of about 35,000, diabetes mellitus is the seventh leading cause of death in the United States. It is estimated that 1 to 2% of the adult population have diabetes mellitus. The prevalence of type I diabetes varies widely around the world, probably as a reflection of some as yet obscure environmental factors in the pathogenesis of the disease.

PATHOGENESIS. The pathogenesis of the two types is discussed separately, but first we briefly review normal insulin metabolism, since some aspects of insulin release and action are important in the consideration of pathogenesis.

Normal Insulin Metabolism. The chemical structure, molecular biology, biosynthesis, and secretory pathways of insulin are now understood in elegant detail. The insulin gene is expressed in the beta cells of the pancreatic islets, where insulin is synthesized and stored in granules prior to secretion. Release from beta

TABLE 17-2. TYPE I VS. TYPE II DIABETES

	Type I (IDDM)	Type II (NIDDM)
Clinical	Onset <20 years	Onset >30 years
	Normal weight	Obese
	Decreased blood insulin	Normal or increased blood insulin
	Islet cell antibodies	No islet cell antibodies
	Ketoacidosis common	Ketoacidosis rare
Genetics	50% concordance in twins	90-100% concordance in twins
	HLA-D linked	No HLA association
Pathogenesis	Autoimmunity	Insulin resistance
	Immunopathologic mechanisms	Relative insulin deficiency
	Severe insulin deficiency	
Islet Cells	Insulitis early	No insulitis
	Marked atrophy and fibrosis	Focal atrophy and amyloid deposits
	Beta-cell depletion	Mild beta-cell depletion

cells occurs as a biphasic process involving two pools of insulin. A rise in the blood glucose levels, for example, calls forth an immediate release of insulin, presumably that stored in the beta-cell granules. If the secretory stimulus persists, a delayed and protracted response follows, which involves active synthesis of insulin. *The most important stimulus that triggers insulin release is glucose, which also initiates insulin synthesis.* Other agents, including intestinal hormones and certain amino acids (leucine and arginine), as well as the sulfonylureas, stimulate insulin release but not synthesis.

Insulin is a major anabolic hormone. It is necessary for (1) transmembrane transport of glucose and amino acids, (2) glycogen formation in the liver and skeletal muscles, (3) glucose conversion to triglycerides, (4) nucleic acid synthesis, and (5) protein synthesis. *Its principal metabolic function is to increase the rate of glucose transport into certain cells in the body.* These are the striated muscle cells, including myocardial cells, fibroblasts, and fat cells, representing collectively about two thirds of the entire body weight.

Insulin interacts with its target cells by first binding to the insulin receptor. Since the amount of insulin bound to the cells is affected by the availability of receptors, their number and function are important in regulating the action of insulin. Receptor-bound insulin triggers a number of intracellular responses, including activation or inhibition of insulin-sensitive enzymes in mitochondria, protein synthesis, and DNA synthesis. One of the important early effects of insulin involves translocation of *glucose transport units* (GLUTs) from the Golgi apparatus to the plasma membrane, thus facilitating cellular uptake of glucose. There are several different forms of GLUTs, which differ in their tissue distribution and affinity for glucose. There is increasing evidence that some forms of diabetes may be related to reduced expression and activity of these carrier proteins (p. 573).

Pathogenesis of Type I Diabetes. *This form of diabetes results from a severe, absolute lack of insulin caused by a reduction in the beta-cell mass.* Type I diabetes (IDDM) usually develops in childhood, becoming manifest and severe at puberty. Patients *depend on insulin for survival;* hence the term insulin-dependent diabetes mellitus. Without insulin, they develop serious metabolic complications such as acute ketoacidosis and coma.

Three interlocking mechanisms are responsible for the islet cell destruction: *genetic susceptibility, autoimmunity, and an environmental insult.* A postulated sequence of events involving these three mechanisms is shown in Figure 17-1. It is thought that *genetic susceptibility* linked to specific alleles of the class II major histocompatibility complex predisposes certain persons to the development of *autoimmunity against beta cells* of the islets. The autoimmune reaction either develops spontaneously or, more likely, is triggered by an environmental agent (e.g., a virus or chemical) that causes an initial mild injury to the beta cells. The immune reaction directed against the altered beta cells then causes further beta-cell injury, and eventually,

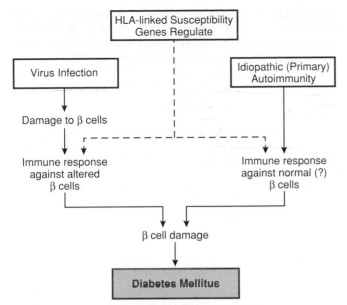

Figure 17–1. A simplified schema to show pathways of beta-cell destruction leading to insulin-dependent (type I) diabetes mellitus.

when most of the cells are destroyed, overt diabetes mellitus appears (Fig. 17–2). With this overview we can discuss each of the pathogenetic influences separately.

Genetic Susceptibility. It has long been known that diabetes mellitus can aggregate in families; however, the precise mode of inheritance of the susceptibility genes for type I diabetes remains unknown. Among identical twins, the concordance rate (i.e., both twins affected) is only approximately 50%. Only 5 to 10% of children of first-order relatives with type I diabetes develop the disease. Environmental factors must therefore play an important role in this type of diabetes, as we shall see.

At least one of the susceptibility genes for type I diabetes resides in the region that encodes the class II antigens of the major histocompatibility complex on chromosome 6 (HLA-D). You will recall (p. 121) that the HLA-D region contains three subregions—DP, DQ, and DR; that the class II molecules are highly polymorphic; and that each has numerous alleles. About 95% of Caucasian patients with type I diabetes have either HLA-DR3 or HLA-DR4 alleles or both, whereas in the general population the prevalence of these antigens is only 40%. Persons who are HLA-DR3 positive have a five times greater risk of developing diabetes, and those with HLA-DR4, a seven times greater risk, compared with those who are HLA-DR3 or -DR4 negative. DR3/4 heterozygotes have an approximately 14.3 greater risk. There is growing evidence that certain HLA-DQ alleles that are in linkage disequilibrium (i.e., inherited together) with previously incriminated HLA-DR alleles are more intimately associated with this increased susceptibility. Precise identification of the diabetogenic DQ alleles has not yet been accomplished with certainty, but an intensive search is in progress at the molecular level. Some investigators have suggested that a single amino acid

difference in the DQ beta chain at position 57, which faces the antigen-binding cleft of the class II molecule, confers increased susceptibility to type I diabetes. This finding, however, has not been confirmed by others. Nevertheless, the notion that a genetic variation in the antigen-binding cleft of a class II molecule may predispose to the development of autoimmunity is attractive. Recall that T cells can recognize an antigen only when the peptide fragment of the antigen binds to the class II molecule and is presented to the T cell on the surface of antigen-presenting cells (p. 122). Conceivably certain class II molecules preferentially bind to beta-cell peptides. Such class II alleles would favor presentation of beta-cell autoantigen to T cells and thus facilitate the induction of pancreatic autoimmunity. Those who inherit these alleles would therefore be prone to develop type I diabetes.

In addition to the established influence of HLA-linked genes in the predisposition of type I diabetes, it is very likely that additional non–HLA-linked genes also play a role in the pathogenesis of this disease.

Autoimmunity. A role for autoimmunity in the pathogenesis of diabetes is supported by several morphologic, clinical, and experimental observations:

- Lymphocytic infiltrate, often intense ("insulitis"), is frequently observed in the islets in cases of recent onset. Both CD4+ and CD8+ T cells are found within such infiltrates. Similar cells are found in animal models of type I diabetes. Furthermore, CD4+ T cells from diseased animals can transfer diabetes to normal animals, thus establishing the primacy of T-cell autoimmunity in type I diabetes.
- As many as 90% of patients with type I diabetes have islet cell antibodies when tested within a year of diagnosis. Asymptomatic relatives of patients with type I diabetes who have a higher than normal risk

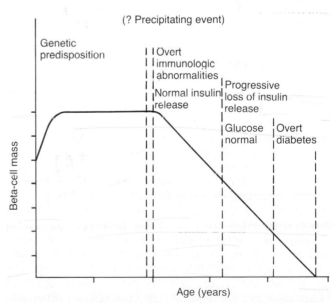

Figure 17–2. Stages in the development of type I diabetes mellitus. The stages of diabetes are listed from left to right, and hypothetical beta-cell mass is plotted against age. (From Eisenbarth, G. E.: Type I diabetes—a chronic autoimmune disease. N. Engl. J. Med. *314*:1360, 1986.)

of developing the disease develop islet cell antibodies months to years before the clinical onset of diabetes. Whether these antibodies participate in causing damage to the beta cells or are formed against sequestered antigens released by T cell–mediated injury is not entirely settled.

- In experimental animals and humans the insulitis is associated with expression of class II major histocompatibility complex (MHC) molecules on the beta cells. Normal beta cells do not possess cell surface class II molecules. This aberrant expression of MHC molecules is most likely induced by locally produced cytokines (e.g., interferon-gamma [IFN-γ]) derived from activated T cells.

- Approximately 10% of persons who have type I diabetes also have other organ-specific autoimmune disorders such as Graves' disease, Addison's disease, thyroiditis, or pernicious anemia. In these patients there appears to be a broad derangement of immunoregulation.

To summarize, overwhelming evidence implicates autoimmunity and immune-mediated injury as causes of beta-cell loss in type I diabetes mellitus. Indeed, immunosuppressive therapy with cyclosporin has recently been shown to prevent the development of or to ameliorate type I diabetes in experimental animals and in children with the disease.

Environmental Factors. Assuming that a genetic susceptibility predisposes to autoimmune destruction of islet cells, what triggers the autoimmune reaction? As mentioned earlier, in a minority of cases the pancreatic autoimmunity is idiopathic (i.e., an immune response occurs against unaltered beta cells as well as several other endocrine cell types). In the majority, however, an environmental insult is believed to trigger autoimmunity by damaging the beta cells. Although no definite environmental agent has been identified, viruses are suspected as initiators of this disease. Several investigators have noted seasonal trends in the diagnosis of new cases; these seasonal trends often correspond to the prevalence of common viral infections in the community. The viral infections implicated include mumps, measles, rubella, coxsackie B virus, and infectious mononucleosis. Although many viruses are beta-cell tropic, direct virus-induced injury is rarely severe enough to cause diabetes mellitus. The most likely scenario is that viruses cause mild beta-cell injury, which is followed by an autoimmune reaction against altered beta cells in persons with HLA-linked susceptibility. One good example is the occurrence of type I diabetes in patients with congenital rubella. About 20% of those infected in utero, almost always those with HLA-DR3 or -DR4 genotype, go on to develop the disease in childhood or puberty. *To summarize, it appears that type I diabetes is a rare outcome of some relatively common viral infection, delayed by the long latency period necessary for progressive autoimmune loss of beta cells to occur and dependent on the modifying effects of MHC class II molecules.*

Pathogenesis of Type II Diabetes. Much less is known, unfortunately, about the pathogenesis of non–insulin dependent diabetes, which, it should be reemphasized, is by far the most common type. Genetic factors are even more important than in type I diabetes, because among identical twins, the concordance rate is more than 90%. *Unlike type I, the disease is not linked to any HLA genes, and there is no evidence that autoimmune mechanisms are involved.*

Two metabolic defects that characterize type II diabetes (NIDDM) are (1) *a derangement in insulin secretion* that is delayed or that is insufficient relative to the glucose load, and (2) an inability of peripheral tissues to respond to insulin *(insulin resistance).* The primacy of secretory defect versus insulin resistance is a matter of continuing debate. In the following discussion each of these two factors is considered separately, beginning with the secretory defect in type II disease.

Early in the course of type II diabetes, *insulin secretion* appears to be normal and plasma insulin levels are not reduced. However, subtle defects in the function of beta cells can be demonstrated. Perhaps the earliest detectable change is in the pattern of insulin secretion. In normal persons, insulin secretion occurs in a pulsatile or oscillatory pattern, whereas in patients with type II diabetes, the normal oscillations of insulin secretion are lost. At about the same time the rapid first phase of insulin secretion triggered by glucose is obtunded, whereas the second phase of insulin release is intact. Despite the loss of early response to glucose, the acute response to other secretagogues such as arginine remains normal. This suggests a *specific abnormality of glucose receptors on beta cells rather than an inadequacy of insulin.* In due course, however, most patients develop mild to moderate deficiency of insulin. Assessment of insulin deficiency in type II diabetes is complicated by the frequent occurrence of obesity in these patients. Obesity, even in the absence of diabetes, is characterized by insulin resistance and hyperinsulinemia; however, when obese type II diabetics are compared with weight-matched nondiabetics, it appears that the insulin levels of obese diabetics are below those observed in obese nondiabetics, suggesting a relative insulin deficiency. Furthermore, in patients with moderately severe type II diabetes (fasting plasma glucose level of 200 to 300 gm/ml), it is possible to demonstrate an absolute deficiency of insulin. We can conclude, therefore, that *most patients with type II diabetes have a relative or absolute deficiency of insulin. However, this insulin deficiency is milder than that of type I diabetes and is not an early feature of this variant of diabetes.*

The pathogenesis of the insulin deficiency in type II diabetes is not entirely clear. Unlike type I, there is no evidence for viral or immune-mediated injury to the islet cells. According to one view, all the somatic cells of diabetics, including pancreatic beta cells, are genetically vulnerable to injury, leading to accelerated cell turnover and premature aging, and ultimately to a modest reduction in beta-cell mass.

Since in most patients with type II diabetes insulin deficiency is not of sufficient magnitude to explain the metabolic disturbances, it is logical to suspect impairment in insulin action. Indeed *there is abundant evi-*

dence that insulin resistance is a major factor in the pathogenesis of type II diabetes. Insulin resistance is a complex phenomenon, not restricted to the diabetes syndrome. In both obesity and pregnancy insulin sensitivity of tissues decreases (even in the absence of diabetes). Hence either obesity or pregnancy may unmask subclinical type II diabetes by increasing the insulin resistance. *Obesity is an extremely important diabetogenic influence, and, not surprisingly, approximately 80% of type II diabetes patients are obese.* In many obese diabetics, especially early in the course of the disease, impaired glucose tolerance can be reversed by weight loss. Although obesity is emphasized as a factor in insulin resistance, such resistance is also encountered in nonobese patients with type II diabetes.

What is the cellular basis for insulin resistance? There is a decrease in the number of *insulin receptors,* and more important, the *postreceptor signaling* by insulin is impaired. You may recall from our earlier discussion (p. 570) that binding of insulin to its receptors leads to translocation of GLUTs to the cell membrane, which in turn facilitates transmembrane diffusion of glucose. It is widely suspected that reduced synthesis and translocation of GLUTs in muscle and fat cells underlies insulin resistance noted in obesity as well as in type II diabetes. Current interest is also focused on the role of *amylin* in the pathogenesis of type II diabetes. This protein is normally produced by the beta cells, copackaged with insulin and cosecreted in the sinusoidal space. For reasons not entirely clear, in patients with type II diabetes amylin tends to accumulate outside the beta cells, in close contact with their cell membranes. It eventually acquires the tinctorial characteristics of amyloid. It is suspected that extracellular deposits of amylin contribute to the disturbance in insulin sensing by the beta cells noted early in the course of type II diabetes. With progressive accumulation, amyloid deposits encroach upon the beta cells.

To summarize, type II diabetes is a complex, multifactorial disorder involving both impaired insulin release and end-organ insensitivity. Insulin resistance, frequently associated with obesity, produces excessive stress on beta cells, which may fail in the face of sustained need for a state of hyperinsulinism. A genetic factor is definitely involved, but how it fits into this puzzle remains mysterious (Fig. 17–3).

PATHOGENESIS OF THE COMPLICATIONS OF DIABETES. The morbidity associated with long-standing diabetes of either type results from complications such as *microangiopathy, retinopathy, nephropathy, and neuropathy.* Hence the basis of these chronic long-term complications is the subject of a great deal of research. Although there are some who think that these complications are a genetic concomitant unrelated to the metabolic abnormalities, *most of the available evidence suggests that the complications of diabetes mellitus are a consequence of the metabolic derangements.* The most telling evidence comes from the finding that kidneys, when transplanted into diabetics from nondiabetic donors, develop the lesions of diabetic nephropathy within three to five years after transplan-

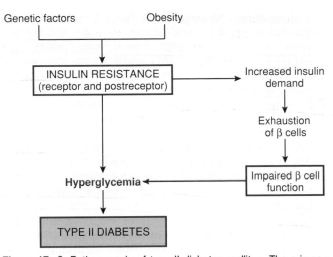

Figure 17–3. Pathogenesis of type II diabetes mellitus. The primacy of insulin resistance versus impaired beta-cell functions is not established. In patients with clinical disease both defects can be demonstrated.

tation. However, if renal transplantation is followed by transplantation of normal pancreas, progression of the lesions in the transplanted normal kidney is halted.

Since hyperglycemia is the most obvious and consistent metabolic abnormality in diabetes mellitus, many mechanisms that link hyperglycemia to the complications of long-standing diabetes have been explored. Currently, two such mechanisms are considered important.

1. Nonenzymatic Glycosylation. This is the process by which glucose chemically attaches to the amino group of proteins without the aid of enzymes. For example, nonenzymatic glycosylation of hemoglobin A (HbA) leads to the formation of HbA_{1c}, which normally constitutes about 4% of hemoglobin in red cells. The degree of nonenzymatic glycosylation is directly related to the level of blood glucose, and therefore the red cell HbA_{1c} levels increase greatly in patients with diabetes mellitus. Since nonenzymatic glycosylation of HbA occurs continuously over the 120-day life span of the red cell, a single measurement of HbA_{1c} level provides an index of the average blood glucose levels over the preceding two to four months. Indeed, measurement of HbA_{1c} levels is a useful adjunct in the management of diabetes mellitus. Although HbA_{1c} is the most investigated glycosylated protein, it is apparent that a variety of other structural and regulatory proteins undergo excessive glycosylation to form advanced glycosylation end-products (AGEs). Examples include serum albumin, collagen, basic myelin protein, and low-density lipoproteins (LDLs). AGEs, it is postulated, alter the function of many proteins, thus contributing to various late complications of diabetes. For example, AGEs attached to collagen in blood vessel walls irreversibly cross-link to plasma proteins, e.g., LDL. In large vessels, such cross-linking retards the normal efflux of LDLs that have entered the vessel wall and thus enhances deposition of cholesterol in the intima. This in turn, accelerates the development of atherosclerosis.

2. Intracellular Hyperglycemia with Disturbances in Polyol Pathways. In some tissues that do not require insulin for glucose transport (nerves, lens, kidney, and blood vessels), hyperglycemia leads to an increase in intracellular glucose. The excess glucose is metabolized to *sorbitol,* a polyol, by the enzyme aldose reductase, and eventually to fructose. These changes have two untoward effects. First, the accumulated sorbitol and fructose lead to increased intracellular osmolarity and influx of water, and, eventually, to osmotic cell injury. In the lens, osmotically imbibed water causes swelling and opacity. Second, sorbitol accumulation is associated with a decrease in myoinositol content and impairment of Na^+/K^+ adenosine triphosphatase (ATPase). This mechanism may be responsible for damage to Schwann cells and to pericytes of retinal capillaries, with resultant peripheral neuropathy and retinal microaneurysms. The possibility that these pathways may contribute to the ocular and neurologic complications of diabetes is supported by experimental studies in which pharmacologic inhibition of aldose reductase prevented the development of cataracts and neuropathy.

METABOLIC DERANGEMENTS. Insulin is a major anabolic hormone in the body and therefore *derangement of insulin function affects not only glucose metabolism but also fat and protein metabolism.* Indeed, all pathways of intermediary metabolism are disrupted to a lesser or greater degree in patients with diabetes mellitus.

The most profound deficiency of insulin and therefore the most severe metabolic derangements are usually encountered in type I diabetes. The utilization of glucose in muscle and adipose tissue is sharply diminished or abolished. Concurrently there is stimulation of glycogenolysis, which is normally inhibited by insulin and favored by glucagon. Fasting blood glucose may reach levels many times greater than normal, and when the level of circulating glucose exceeds the renal threshold, glycosuria ensues. The excessive glycosuria induces an osmotic diuresis and thus polyuria, causing a profound loss of water and electrolytes (Na, K, Mg, P; Fig. 17–4). This obligatory water loss combined with the hyperosmolarity resulting from the increased levels of glucose in the blood tends to deplete intracellular water, as, for example, in the osmoreceptors of the thirst centers of the brain. In this manner, intense thirst (polydipsia) appears. Through poorly defined pathways, increased appetite (polyphagia) develops, thus completing the classic triad of diabetic findings— *polyuria, polydipsia, and polyphagia.* With a deficiency of insulin, the scales swing from insulin-promoted anabolism to catabolism of proteins and fats. Proteolysis follows, and the glucogenic amino acids are removed by the liver and used as building blocks in gluconeogenesis, worsening the deranged carbohydrate metabolism.

Two important acute metabolic complications of diabetes mellitus follow, *diabetic ketoacidosis* and *nonketotic hyperosmolar coma.*

Diabetic ketoacidosis occurs almost exclusively in type I diabetes and is the result of *severe insulin*

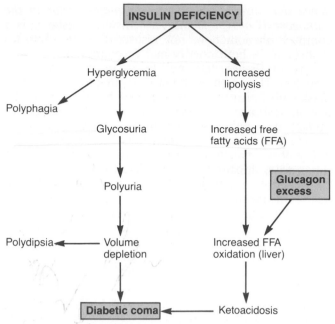

Figure 17–4. Sequence of metabolic derangements in diabetes mellitus.

deficiency coupled with absolute or relative increases of glucagon (see Fig. 17–4). The insulin deficiency causes excessive breakdown of adipose stores, resulting in increased levels of free fatty acids. Oxidation of such free fatty acids within the liver through acetyl CoA produces ketone bodies. *Glucagon* is the hormone that accelerates such fatty acid oxidation. The rate at which ketone bodies are formed may exceed the rate at which acetoacetic acid and β-hydroxybutyric acid can be utilized by muscles and other tissues, thus leading to ketonemia and ketonuria. If the urinary excretion of ketones is compromised by dehydration, the plasma hydrogen ion concentration increases and *systemic metabolic ketoacidosis* results.

In type II diabetes, polyuria, polydipsia, and polyphagia may accompany the fasting hyperglycemia, but ketoacidosis is rare. Adults, particularly elderly diabetics, develop *nonketotic hyperosmolar coma,* a syndrome engendered by the severe dehydration resulting from sustained hyperglycemic diuresis, which is coupled with the inability of these patients to drink water. The absence of ketoacidosis and its symptoms (nausea, vomiting, respiratory difficulties) delays the seeking of medical attention in these patients until severe dehydration and coma occur.

MORPHOLOGY. At death a diabetic may have many morphologic changes suggestive of the diagnosis and a few virtually diagnostic findings, or there may be no lesions that might not also be found in age-matched nondiabetics. This variability is poorly understood, but three factors are probably significant: (1) the duration of the disease, (2) the adequacy of metabolic control, and (3) genetic factors. The duration of diabetes strongly influences the development of anatomic changes. Generally, regardless of the type of diabetes, with disease of 10 to 15 years' duration patients develop dermal, renal, and retinal microangiopathy, as well as atherosclerosis more severe than that found in age-matched controls. Those with poor control of hyperglycemia are at greater risk, for reasons already discussed. Genes other than those responsible for the diabetic state also condition the likelihood of complications. The occurrence of both diabetic nephropathy and retinopathy seems to be related to the genetic background, because some persons seem to be protected despite the long duration of their disease.

Basement Membrane Thickening (BMT) and Microangiopathy. Thickening of basement membrane is characteristic of diabetes mellitus. When it affects capillaries it is referred to as microangiopathy. This microvascular alteration is most evident in the capillaries of the skin, skeletal muscle, retina, renal glomeruli, and renal medulla. However, BMT is also seen in such nonvascular structures as renal tubules, Bowman's capsule, peripheral nerves, placenta, and possibly other sites. The normal basal lamina consists of a relatively uniform layer of extracellular material separating parenchymal or endothelial cells from the surrounding connective tissue stroma. In diabetes this single layer is widened and sometimes replaced by concentric layers of hyaline material composed predominantly of type IV collagen. It should be noted that despite the increase in the thickness of basement membranes, **diabetic capillaries are more leaky than normal** to plasma proteins. This change may be responsible for the glomerular lesions, and possibly neuropathy. It should be noted that indistinguishable microangiopathy can be found in aged nondiabetic patients, but rarely to the extent seen in patients with long-standing diabetes.

Pancreas. Changes in the pancreas are inconstant and only rarely of diagnostic value. Distinctive changes are more commonly associated with type I diabetes than with type II diabetes. Indeed, the pancreas may appear virtually normal in persons with type II diabetes unless precise quantitation of the islet cell mass is attempted. One or more of the following changes may be present: (1) **Reduction in the size and number of islets** is seen most commonly in type I diabetes, particularly with rapidly progressive disease. Most of the islets are so small as to escape detection in routinely stained sections. Subtle reduction in the islet cell mass can be demonstrated in type II disease as well, but doing so requires special morphometric studies. (2) **Increase in the number and size of islets** is especially characteristic of nondiabetic newborns of diabetic mothers. Presumably, fetal islets undergo hyperplasia in response to the maternal hyperglycemia. (3) **Beta-cell degranulation** implies depletion of stored insulin and is most commonly seen in type I disease. (4) **Amyloid replacement** of islets appears as deposits of pink, amorphous material beginning in and around capillaries and between cells. At advanced stages the islets may be virtually obliterated

(Fig. 17–5). This change is often seen in long-standing cases of type II diabetes. As mentioned earlier, the amyloid in this instance is composed of amylin fibrils derived from the beta cells. Similar lesions may be found in elderly nondiabetics. (5) **Two types of leukocytic infiltration are found in the islets,** principally in type I diabetes. The most common pattern is a heavy T-lymphocyte infiltration within and about the islets (insulitis). This is seen early in the course of the disease and results from an immune reaction. Eosinophilic infiltrates may also be found, particularly in diabetic infants who fail to survive the immediate postnatal period.

Vascular System. Diabetes exacts a heavy toll on the vascular system. Whatever the age at onset, **in the course of 10 to 15 years of the disease most diabetics develop significant vascular abnormalities.** Vessels of all sizes are affected, from the aorta down to the smallest arterioles and capillaries.

The aorta and large- and medium-sized arteries suffer from accelerated severe **atherosclerosis. Except for its greater severity and earlier age of onset, atherosclerosis in diabetics is indistinguishable from that in nondiabetics** (p. 279).

Myocardial infarction, caused by atherosclerosis of the coronary arteries, is the most common cause of death in diabetics. Significantly, it is almost as common in diabetic females as in diabetic males. In contrast, myocardial infarction is uncommon in nondiabetic females of reproductive age (p. 308). **Gangrene of the**

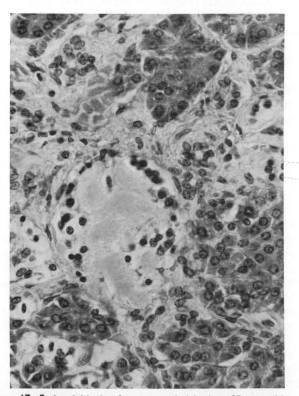

Figure 17–5. Amyloidosis of a pancreatic islet in a 65-year-old male with diabetes of 25 years' duration.

lower extremities, as a result of advanced vascular disease, is about 100 times more common in diabetics than in the general population. The larger renal arteries are also subject to severe atherosclerosis, but the most damaging effect of diabetes on the kidneys is exerted at the level of the glomeruli and the microcirculation. This is the subject of a later discussion.

The bases of accelerated atherosclerosis are not well understood, and in all likelihood multiple factors are involved. About a third to a half of the patients have elevated blood lipid levels, known to predispose to atherosclerosis, but the remainder also have an increased predisposition to atherosclerosis. Qualitative changes in the lipoproteins brought about by excessive nonenzymatic glycosylation may affect their turnover and tissue deposition. Low levels of high-density lipoproteins (HDL) have been demonstrated in type II diabetes. Since HDL is a "protective molecule" against atherosclerosis (p. 279), this could contribute to increased susceptibility to atherosclerosis. Diabetics have increased platelet adhesiveness to the vessel wall, possibly owing to increased thromboxane A_2 synthesis and reduced prostacyclin. In addition to all these factors, diabetics tend to have an increased incidence of hypertension, which is a well-known risk factor for atherosclerosis (p. 280).

Hyaline arteriolosclerosis, the vascular lesion associated with hypertension (p. 462), is both more prevalent and more severe in diabetics than in nondiabetics, but it is not specific for diabetes and may be seen in elderly nondiabetics without hypertension. It takes the form of an amorphous, hyaline thickening of the wall of the arterioles, which causes narrowing of the lumen (Fig. 17–6). Not surprisingly, in the diabetic it is related not only to the duration of the disease but also to the level of the blood pressure. The cause and nature of this vascular change are still uncertain. Although at one time it was attributed to hypertension, so common among diabetics, it can also be seen in diabetics who do not have hypertension. The hyaline material consists of plasma proteins and basement membrane material. It is presumed that the plasma proteins penetrate into the abnormally permeable walls of the arterioles.

Kidneys. The kidneys are prime targets of diabetes. In fact, renal failure is second only to myocardial infarction as a cause of death from this disease. **Four types of lesions, collectively termed "diabetic nephropathy," are encountered:** (1) **glomerular lesions;** (2) **renal vascular lesions, principally arteriolosclerosis;** (3) **pyelonephritis, including necrotizing papillitis;** and (4) **glycogen and fatty changes in the tubular epithelium.**

A variety of forms of glomerular involvement may be present: capillary basement membrane thickening, diffuse glomerulosclerosis, nodular glomerulosclerosis (Kimmelstiel-Wilson lesion), "fibrin caps," and "capsular drops." The last two are sometimes called exudative lesions. The sclerotic lesions of the glomeruli destroy renal function and constitute potentially fatal forms of diabetic nephropathy, but the exudative lesions are largely of diagnostic interest.

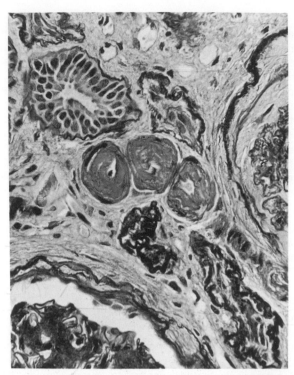

Figure 17–6. Hyaline arteriolosclerosis. Note a markedly thickened, tortuous afferent arteriole (cut in three planes). The amorphous nature of the thickened vascular wall is evident.

Changes in the **capillary basement membrane** take the form of thickening of the basement membranes of the glomerular capillaries throughout their entire length and are part and parcel of diabetic microangiopathy. Under the electron microscope, thickening of the glomerular basement membrane can be detected within a few years of the onset of diabetes, sometimes without any associated change in renal function.

Diffuse glomerulosclerosis is found in most patients with disease of more than 10 years' duration. It consists of a diffuse increase in mesangial matrix along with mesangial cell proliferation and is always associated with basement membrane thickening. These lesions almost always begin in the vascular stalk and sometimes appear to be continuous with the hyaline arteriolosclerosis in the afferent and efferent arterioles (Fig. 17–7). **When the diffuse glomerulosclerosis becomes marked, these patients manifest the nephrotic syndrome (p. 444), characterized by proteinuria, hypoalbuminemia, and edema.**

Nodular glomerulosclerosis describes a glomerular lesion made distinctive by ball-like deposits of a laminated matrix within the mesangial core of the lobule (Fig. 17–8). These nodules tend to develop in the periphery of the glomerulus, and since they arise within the mesangium they push the peripheral capillary loops ahead of them. Often these patent loops create halos about the nodule. This lesion has also been called intercapillary glomerulosclerosis and **Kimmelstiel-Wilson lesion,** after the pioneers who described it. Nodular

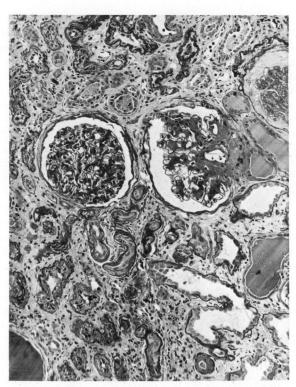

Figure 17-7. Diffuse glomerulosclerosis in a patient who had had diabetes for 16 years. The glomerulus at the right has marked axial thickening, fanning out from the vascular pole. The one on the left, caught in a less advantageous plane, has more delicate, diffuse glomerulosclerosis.

ficient ischemia to cause overall fine scarring of the kidneys, marked by a finely granular cortical surface.

Exudative lesions take two forms. Glassy, homogeneous, strongly eosinophilic deposits in the parietal layer of Bowman's capsule, called capsular drops, may hang into the uriniferous space. Similar-looking deposits, fibrin caps, may develop over the outer surface of glomerular capillary loops. Both the capsular drop and the fibrin cap are attributed to excessive leakage of plasma proteins from glomeruli that were severely injured by either diffuse or nodular glomerulosclerosis. Neither of these two lesions causes any impairment in renal function.

Renal atherosclerosis and arteriolosclerosis constitute only one part of the systemic involvement of vessels in diabetics. The kidney is one of the most frequently and severely affected organs; however, the changes in the arteries and arterioles are similar to those found throughout the body. Hyaline arteriolosclerosis affects not only the afferent but also the efferent arteriole. Such efferent arteriolosclerosis is rarely if ever encountered in persons who do not have diabetes.

Pyelonephritis is an acute or chronic inflammation of the kidneys that usually begins in the interstitial tissue and then spreads to affect the tubules—and, possibly, ultimately the glomeruli. Both the acute and chronic

glomerulosclerosis occurs irregularly throughout the kidney and affects random glomeruli, as well as random lobules within a glomerulus. In advanced disease many nodules are present within a single glomerulus, and most glomeruli become involved. Uninvolved glomeruli and lobules all show striking diffuse glomerulosclerosis. The deposits are PAS-positive and contain mucopolysaccharides, lipids, and fibrils, as well as collagen fibers, as do the matrix deposits of diffuse glomerulosclerosis. Often they contain trapped mesangial cells.

Nodular glomerulosclerosis is encountered in perhaps 10 to 35% of diabetics and is a major cause of morbidity and mortality. Like diffuse glomerulosclerosis, the appearance is related to the duration of the disease but conditioned by the genetic background. Unlike the diffuse form, which may also be seen in association with old age and hypertension, **the nodular form of glomerulosclerosis is, for all practical purposes, highly suggestive of diabetes.**

Progression of diabetic glomerulosclerosis and its constant companion, advanced arteriolosclerosis, usually leads to obliteration of the vascular channels in the glomerulus and to serious, sometimes fatal, impairment of renal function. As a consequence of glomerular sclerosis, the tubules suffer ischemia and are replaced by interstitial fibrous tissue. Both the diffuse and the nodular forms of glomerulosclerosis induce suf-

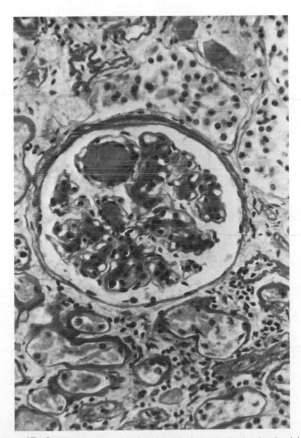

Figure 17-8. Nodular glomerulosclerosis in a patient who had had diabetes mellitus for 17 years. The nodule at the upper left of the glomerulus is surrounded by a patent capillary channel. Note the thickening of the basement membranes of the tubules.

forms of this disease occur in nondiabetics as well as in diabetics; they are described more fully on page 453. These inflammatory disorders are more common in diabetics than in the general population, and once affected, diabetics tend to have more severe involvement.

One special pattern of acute pyelonephritis, **necrotizing papillitis,** is much more prevalent in diabetics than in nondiabetics. It is, however, **not limited to diabetics** but is also seen with obstructions of the urinary tract as well as with analgesic abuse. As the term implies, necrotizing papillitis is an acute necrosis of the renal papillae (Fig. 17–9). Diabetics are particularly prone to develop this lesion, owing to the combination of ischemia resulting from microangiopathy and increased susceptibility to bacterial infection. One or more papillae may be involved, bilaterally or unilaterally. The infarcted papilla may slough off and be excreted in the urine, permitting a clinical diagnosis by examination of the urinary sediment. In diabetics, bilateral necrosis of all papillae is not uncommon. When many papillae are involved, papillary necrosis causes acute irreversible renal failure. This lesion is described more fully on page 454.

Tubular lesions are also encountered in diabetes mellitus. Perhaps the most striking is the deposition of glycogen within the epithelial cells of the distal portions of the proximal convoluted tubules (and sometimes in the descending loop of Henle). This lesion is variously termed glycogen infiltration, glycogen nephrosis, or Armanni-Ebstein cells. The glycogen creates clearing of the cytoplasm of the affected cells. This condition is believed to be a reflection of severe hyperglycemia and glycosuria for a period of days or weeks prior to death. No tubular malfunction has been connected with this tubular change.

Eyes. Visual impairment, sometimes even total blindness, is one of the more feared consequences of long-standing diabetes. This disease is presently the fourth

leading cause of acquired blindness in the United States. **The ocular involvement may take the form of retinopathy, cataract formation, or glaucoma.** Retinopathy, the most common pattern, consists of a constellation of changes that together are considered by many ophthalmologists to be virtually diagnostic of the disease. The lesion in the retina takes two forms— **nonproliferative** or background retinopathy and **proliferative retinopathy.** The former includes intraretinal or preretinal hemorrhages, retinal exudates, edema, venous dilatations, and, most important, thickening of the retinal capillaries (microangiopathy) and the development of microaneurysms. The retinal exudates can be either "soft" (microinfarcts) or "hard" (deposits of plasma proteins and lipids). The **microaneurysms** are discrete saccular dilatations of retinal choroidal capillaries that appear through the ophthalmoscope as small red dots. The pathogenesis of retinal microaneurysms is multifactorial. Selective loss of retinal capillary pericytes occurs early and is believed to be a consequence of changes in the basement membrane. Dilatations tend to occur at focal points of weakening, resulting from loss of pericytes. In addition, retinal edema resulting from excessive capillary permeability might cause focal collapse, making the vessels vulnerable to aneurysmal dilatation.

The so-called **proliferative retinopathy** is associated with neovascularization and fibrosis. This lesion can lead to serious consequences, including blindness, especially when it involves the macula. Vitreous hemorrhages can result from rupture of the newly formed capillaries. It is of interest that about half the patients with retinal microaneurysms also have nodular glomerulosclerosis. Conversely, **patients who have nodular glomerulosclerosis are almost certain to have retinal microaneurysms.**

Nervous System. The central and peripheral nervous systems are not spared by diabetes. The most frequent pattern of involvement is a **peripheral, symmetric neu-**

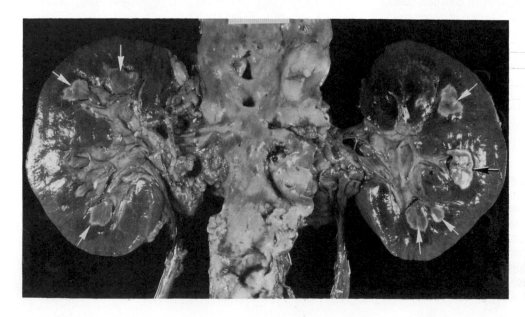

Figure 17–9. Bilateral necrotizing papillitis evidenced by the sharply demarcated areas of pale suppurative necrosis *(arrows)* in many pyramids of both kidneys.

ropathy of the lower extremities that affects both motor and sensory function but particularly the latter. Other forms include: (i) autonomic neuropathy, producing disturbances in bowel and bladder function, and sometimes sexual impotence, and (ii) diabetic mononeuropathy that may manifest as sudden foot drop, wrist drop, or isolated cranial nerve palsies. The neurologic changes may be due to microangiopathy and increased permeability of the capillaries that supply the nerves as well as direct axonal damage caused by alterations in metabolism discussed earlier.

The brain, along with the rest of the body, develops widespread microangiopathy. Such microcirculatory lesions may lead to generalized neuronal degeneration. There is in addition some predisposition to cerebral vascular infarcts and brain hemorrhages, perhaps related to the hypertension and atherosclerosis often seen in diabetics. Degenerative changes have also been observed in the spinal cord. None of the neurologic disorders, including the peripheral neuropathy, is specific for this disease.

Other Organs. Hepatic fatty change (discussed previously on p. 17) is seen in many long-term diabetics. In addition, glycogen vacuolation may be found in the nuclei of hepatic cells in about 10 to 20% of cases. Degenerative changes are encountered in striated muscle, perhaps related to the microangiopathy or to motor nerve degeneration. In addition to the changes already described in the dermal microcirculation, a variety of lesions may be encountered in the skin. **Skin infections,** manifestations of the vascular insufficiency and predisposition to infection of the diabetic, are perhaps the most common. Xanthoma diabeticorum refers to a localized collection in the dermis and subcutis of macrophages filled with lipid (foam cells or xanthoma cells), creating a firm, nontender, usually slightly yellow nodule. They are not specific for diabetes but are associated with all forms of hyperlipidemia.

It is evident that diabetes is associated with widespread anatomic changes, only a few of which are virtually pathognomonic. **Insulitis, nodular glomerulosclerosis, retinopathy, and arteriolosclerosis in the efferent arterioles of the kidney are virtually diagnostic. Marked atrophy, hyperplasia, or amyloid replacement of the islets is strongly suggestive.** Although individually some of these lesions may be found in nondiabetics, when present in combination the anatomic diagnosis of diabetes can be made with a high degree of certainty.

CLINICAL CORRELATION. The clinical manifestations of diabetes derive from the two major aspects of this disease: (1) the metabolic derangement and (2) the vascular and organ involvements. *Type I diabetes,* which begins by age 20 in most patients, is dominated largely by signs and symptoms emanating from the disordered metabolism discussed earlier—polyuria, polydipsia, polyphagia, ketoacidosis. Weight loss and muscle weakness result from widespread catabolic ef-

fects. The combination of polyphagia and weight loss is paradoxical and should always raise the suspicion of diabetes. Plasma insulin is low or absent, and the glucagon level is increased. Glucose intolerance is of the unstable or brittle type, so the blood glucose level is quite sensitive to administered exogenous insulin, deviations from normal dietary intake, unusual physical activity, infection, or other forms of stress. Inadequate fluid intake or vomiting may rapidly lead to significant disturbances in fluid and electrolyte balance. Thus, these patients are vulnerable on the one hand to *hypoglycemic episodes* and on the other to *ketoacidosis. Infection* may precipitate these conditions, and indeed may precede the first manifestations of diabetes in some patients.

Type II diabetes mellitus may also present with polyuria and polydipsia, but unlike type I diabetes, patients are often older (over 40 years) and frequently obese. In some cases medical attention is sought because of unexplained weakness or weight loss. Frequently, however, the diagnosis is made by routine blood or urine testing in asymptomatic persons. Although patients with type II diabetes also have metabolic derangements, these are usually controllable and less severe. In the decompensated state they develop hyperosmolar nonketotic coma, already discussed. *In both forms of long-standing diabetes, atherosclerotic events such as myocardial infarction, cerebrovascular accidents, gangrene of the leg, and renal insufficiency are the most threatening and most frequent concomitants.*

Diabetics are also plagued by *enhanced susceptibility to infections* of the skin and to tuberculosis, pneumonia, and pyelonephritis. Collectively, such infections cause the deaths of about 5% of diabetic patients. The basis for this susceptibility is probably multifactorial; impaired leukocyte function (p. 33) as well as poor blood supply secondary to vascular disease are involved. A trivial infection in a toe may be the first event in a long succession of complications (gangrene, bacteremia, and pneumonia) that ultimately lead to death. Patients with type I diabetes are more likely to die from their disease than those with type II diabetes. The causes of death, in order of importance, are myocardial infarction, renal failure, cerebrovascular disease, atherosclerotic heart disease, and infections, followed by a large number of other complications more common in the diabetic than in the nondiabetic (e.g., gangrene of an extremity or mesenteric thrombosis). Fortunately, hypoglycemia and ketoacidosis are rare causes of death today. It is sad to close with the note that diabetic patients' life expectancy has not improved significantly over the past three decades and, as mentioned at the outset, this disease continues to be one of the top ten killers in the United States. It is hoped that transplantation of pancreas or isolated islets, both still in the experimental stage, will lead to the cure of diabetes mellitus. Even then, the full benefit of islet cell replacement can be derived only early in the course of diabetes, before irreversible vascular complications have set in. Perhaps with good metabolic control it will be possible in the future to postpone the complications of long-standing diabetes until transplantation becomes a practical treatment.

ISLET CELL TUMORS

Tumors of the pancreatic islets are rare in comparison with tumors of the exocrine pancreas (p. 585). They may be hormonally functional or totally nonfunctional. Among the many distinctive clinical syndromes associated with tumors of the islet cells only three are sufficiently common to merit description: (1) hyperinsulinism, (2) hypergastrinemia and the Zollinger-Ellison syndrome, and (3) multiple endocrine neoplasia. The latter is characterized by the occurrence of tumors (generally adenomas) in several endocrine glands and so is described in the chapter on endocrine disease (p. 679).

BETA-CELL LESIONS (HYPERINSULINISM)

Hyperinsulinism, as you know, causes hypoglycemia, and frequently neuropsychiatric disturbances. The hypoglycemic attacks are precipitated by fasting or exercise and promptly relieved by glucose administration or by eating. The critical laboratory findings are hypoglycemia and high circulating levels of insulin, and often increased proportions of circulating proinsulin-like products.

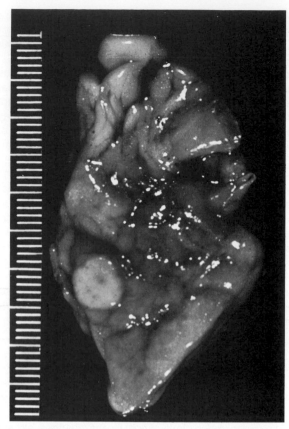

Figure 17-10. A pale beta-cell adenoma of the pancreas *(lower left)*. Despite its small size, the tumor produced hyperinsulinism.

MORPHOLOGY. The morphologic lesions of the beta cells encountered with hyperinsulinism are as follows: solitary adenomas, 70%; multiple adenomas, 10%; diffuse hyperplasia of the islets, usually in newborns or children of diabetic mothers, or adenomas in ectopic pancreatic tissue, 10%; carcinomas, 10%. Multiple adenomas are usually a component of multiple endocrine neoplasia type I syndrome. The solitary adenomas are usually small (rarely more than 5 cm in diameter), encapsulated, pale to red-brown nodules located anywhere in the pancreas (Fig. 17-10). Histologically, these benign tumors look remarkably like giant islets, and there is preservation of the regular cords of cells and their orientation to the vasculature. Not even the malignant lesions present much evidence of anaplasia, and they may also appear deceptively encapsulated. Thus, the diagnosis of cancer rests largely on unmistakable evidence of destructive invasion beyond the pancreas, or, more securely, on metastatic spread to such sites as the regional lymph nodes or the liver. Under the electron microscope neoplastic beta cells, like their normal counterparts, display distinctive granules. They are round and contain polygonal or rectangular dense crystals that are separated from the enclosing membrane by a clear halo. By immunocytochemistry insulin can be localized in tumor cells. Without the identification of the typical granules and their content it is impossible to differentiate beta-cell tumors from other forms of islet cell neoplasia, or indeed to establish the fact that the neoplasms are hormonally active. However, it should be cautioned that granules may be present in the absence of clinically significant hormone activity.

Diffuse hyperplasia of the islets causing hyperinsulinism, as mentioned, is encountered mostly in newborn infants and young children of diabetic mothers. Prolonged exposure to maternal hyperglycemia seems to underlie the development of this lesion.

In closing, it is important to note that there are many other causes of hypoglycemia besides beta-cell lesions. The differential diagnosis of this frequently obscure metabolic abnormality is beyond our scope, but it might include such conditions as insulin sensitivity, diffuse liver disease, the glycogenoses, and ectopic formation of insulin by retroperitoneal or mediastinal fibromas and fibrosarcomas. Indeed, most patients with hypoglycemia have no overt morphologic cause for their disease.

ZOLLINGER-ELLISON SYNDROME (GASTRINOMA)

Marked hypersecretion of gastrin usually has its origin in gastrin-producing tumors (gastrinomas), most often arising in the pancreas but sometimes in the gastrin-producing cells in the duodenum and stomach. Zollinger and Ellison first called attention to the association of pancreatic islet cell lesions with hypersecretion of gastric acid and severe peptic ulceration. At that time, attention was focused on the aberrant location of the peptic ulcers, as, for example, in the jejunum; but since then it has become evident that more often the ulcers occur in the usual sites in the stomach and duodenum. Ulcers are present in 90 to 95% of these persons; the ratio of duodenal to gastric is 6:1 (p. 487).

The cell of origin of the gastrinomas of the pancreas is uncertain. Gastrin cannot be found in any cell of the normal adult islets. By electron microscopy, the tumor cells resemble normal gastrin-producing (G) cells found in the stomach and intestines.

MORPHOLOGY. In a review of a large series of cases of the Zollinger-Ellison syndrome, 60% of the gastrin-producing lesions were malignant, two thirds had metastasized by the time of discovery, 30% were adenomas, and 10% revealed only hyperplasia of the islets. In some instances, multiple adenomas are encountered in patients who have other endocrine tumors, thus conforming to multiple endocrine neoplasia I (p. 679). As with the insulin-secreting lesions of the pancreas, there is rarely marked anaplasia, and the establishment of malignancy requires unmistakable evidence of invasion or spread to lymph nodes and extrapancreatic sites. The peptic ulcers, sometimes multiple, are identical to those found in the general population. They differ only in their intractability to usual modalities of therapy. When they are present in the jejunum, suspicion of the Zollinger-Ellison syndrome should be raised.

In the classic case of the Zollinger-Ellison syndrome, the gastric hyperacidity is associated with peptic ulcers, which in only 25% of the cases occur within the jejunum. Multiple ulcers are found in about 10% of patients. More than 50% of the patients have diarrhea; in 30% it may be the presenting symptom. Treatment of the Zollinger-Ellison syndrome involves control of gastric acid secretion by use of histamine (H_2) receptor blockers and excision of the neoplasm. Surgical resection of malignant invasive neoplasms is difficult. Further surgical difficulty may be occasioned when the lesions, even though benign, are multiple. Total resection of the neoplasm, when possible, eliminates the syndrome.

Exocrine Pancreas

The disorders of exocrine pancreas are relatively uncommon in clinical practice. The three most frequent, to be discussed in the following sections, are acute pancreatitis, chronic pancreatitis, and carcinoma of the pancreas. All of these have clinical importance out of proportion to their prevalence. Acute pancreatitis produces a calamitous acute abdomen, which may lead to death within a few days. Chronic pancreatitis is a cause of less severe abdominal pain, which is nonetheless disabling and at the same time difficult to diagnose. Carcinoma of the pancreas is a silent disease that comes to attention only when far advanced and almost always beyond cure. Thus, pancreatic diseases represent diagnostic clinical challenges that require a constant awareness of their possible occurrence.

ACUTE PANCREATITIS _____

Acute pancreatitis is characterized by the acute onset of abdominal pain due to enzymatic necrosis and inflammation of the pancreas. Typically there is an elevation of pancreatic enzymes in blood and urine. It varies in severity from a mild, self-limited condition called *acute edematous pancreatitis* to a severe life-threatening disorder referred to as *acute hemorrhagic pancreatitis.* In both forms, the release of pancreatic lipases causes *fat necrosis* in and about the pancreas; in the severe form there is damage to the vasculature with resulting hemorrhage into the parenchyma of this organ. Although by no means common, acute pancreatitis can be a life-threatening illness that demands quick diagnosis and prompt treatment.

It is advantageous to consider the morphology of *acute pancreatic necrosis,* also called acute pancreatitis, before exploring its pathogenesis.

MORPHOLOGY. The morphology of acute pancreatic necrosis stems directly from the action of activated pancreatic enzymes that are released into the pancreatic substance. The basic alterations are four: 1 proteolytic destruction of pancreatic substance, 2 necrosis of blood vessels with subsequent hemorrhage, 3 necrosis of fat by lipolytic enzymes, and an associated 4 inflammatory reaction. The extent and predominance of each of these alterations depend on the duration and severity of the process. In the very early stages, only interstitial edema is present. Soon after, focal and confluent areas of frank necrosis of endocrine and exocrine cells are found. Neutrophilic infiltration and interstitial hemorrhage eventually ensue.

The most characteristic histologic lesions of acute

pancreatitis are the focal areas of **fat necrosis** (p. 14) that occur in the stromal, peripancreatic fat, and fat deposits throughout the abdominal cavity (Fig. 17–11). These lesions consist of enzymatic destruction of fat cells, in which **the vacuolated fat cells are transformed to shadowy outlines of cell membranes filled with pink, granular opaque precipitate.** This granular material is derived from the hydrolysis of fat. The liberated glycerol is reabsorbed, and the released fatty acids combine with calcium to form insoluble salts that precipitate in situ and stain basophilic. If the patient survives, milder lesions may resolve completely. Occasionally, liquefied areas are walled off by fibrous tissue to form cystic spaces known as **pancreatic pseudocysts.**

Grossly, acute hemorrhagic pancreatitis is easily recognized. It is characterized by areas of blue-black hemorrhage interspersed with other areas of gray-white necrotic softening, sprinkled with foci of yellow-white, chalky fat necrosis (Fig. 17–12). In individual cases, any of these three components may dominate. Typically there are accompanying changes in the remainder of the abdominal cavity. In the majority of instances, the peritoneal cavity contains a serous, slightly turbid, brown-tinged fluid in which globules of fat can be identified (so-called chicken broth fluid). The liquid fat globules

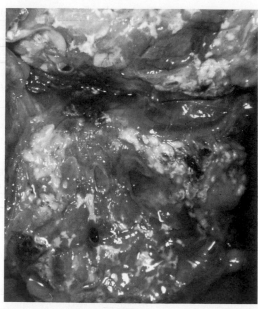

Figure 17–12. Acute pancreatitis. The pancreas has been sectioned across to reveal focal areas of pale fat necrosis and darker areas of hemorrhage.

result from the lipolytic actions of enzymes on adult fat cells. In late cases, this fluid may become secondarily infected to produce suppurative peritonitis. Additionally, foci of fat necrosis may be found in any of the fat depots, such as the omentum, mesentery of the bowel, and periperitoneal deposits. Occasionally, fat necrosis has been described in fat depots outside the abdominal cavity.

ETIOLOGY AND PATHOGENESIS. The pathogenesis of acute pancreatitis is still a mystery. A variety of predisposing conditions have been identified, which can be grouped in four major categories (Table 17–3). Most commonly associated with acute pancreatitis are *gallstones and alcoholism, together responsible for approximately 80% of the cases.* Hypercalcemia and hyperlipoproteinemia (especially types I and IV) are less frequent but important predisposing conditions. Even when all associated and possible contributing influences are taken into account, a significant fraction of cases (10 to 20%) arise without apparent predisposing influences.

The anatomic changes, as pointed out, strongly suggest autodigestion of the pancreatic substance by inappropriately activated pancreatic enzymes. The tissue lesions appear to be the consequence of proteolysis, lipolysis, and weakening of vessels. Thus two questions arise: which of the many pancreatic enzymes initiate the process, and how are they activated? As is well known, pancreatic enzymes are present in the acini in the proenzyme form and have to be activated to fulfill their enzymatic potential. Among many possible activators, a major role is attributed to trypsin, which itself occurs as trypsinogen. Once trypsin is formed, it can

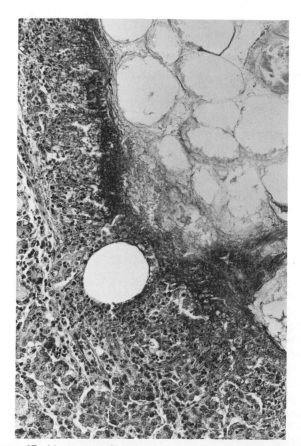

Figure 17–11. Acute pancreatitis. The microscopic field shows a focus of necrosis of the fat cells at upper right, rimmed by an inflammatory hemorrhagic reaction. Preserved pancreatic parenchyma is seen at the bottom left.

TABLE 17–3. ETIOLOGIC FACTORS IN ACUTE PANCREATITIS*

Metabolic
  Alcohol
  Hyperlipoproteinemia
  Hypercalcemia
  Drugs
  Genetic
Mechanical
  Gallstones
  Postoperative (gastric, biliary)
  Posttraumatic
Vascular
  Polyarteritis nodosa
  Atheroembolism
Infectious
  Mumps
  Coxsackievirus

* Modified from Ranson, J. H. C.: Acute pancreatitis: Pathogenesis, outcome and treatment. Clin. Gastroenterol. *13*:843, 1984.

in turn activate other proenzymes such as prophospholipase and proelastase, taking part in the process of autodigestion. The activated enzymes so generated cause disintegration of fat cells and damage to the elastic fibers of blood vessels, respectively. In this manner, fat necrosis and rupture of blood vessels and the ensuing hemorrhage can be explained. Trypsin also converts prekallikrein to its activated form, thus bringing into play the kinin system—and by activation of Hageman factor the clotting and complement systems as well. In this way, the inflammation and small-vessel thromboses (which may lead to congestion and rupture of already weakened vessels) are amplified. *Thus, activation of trypsinogen is an important triggering event in acute pancreatitis.*

As mentioned earlier, even if activated pancreatic enzymes cause the tissue damage, how are they activated and liberated into the pancreatic substance? Endless theories have been proposed, but all are speculative and can be grouped into three categories: (1) duct obstruction, (2) acinar cell injury, and (3) activation of proenzymes within the acinar cells due to defective intracellular transport (Fig. 17–13).

1. Obstruction to the outflow of bile or pancreatic juices or both, along with possible reflux into the pancreas, is considered important in the pathogenesis of acute pancreatitis associated with gallstones. It may be recalled that the common bile duct is joined by the main pancreatic duct in 70% of normal persons. It is proposed that obstruction of the common outflow channel, say by a stone impacted in the ampulla of Vater, raises the intrapancreatic pressure, and, more important, causes *reflux of bile into the pancreas.* The mixture of bile with pancreatic juice may well lead to activation of proenzymes as well as the formation of highly toxic lysolecithin. It is further postulated that increased intraductal pressure consequent to obstruction leads to leakage of activated enzymes into the interstitium. This view is supported by the fact that in 75 to 80% of patients with cholelithiasis and pancreatitis, gallstones can be found in the ampulla or in the stools. When obstructive stones are not found, it is proposed that impaction of gallstones in the ampulla with subsequent passage into the duodenum damages the sphincter of Oddi and allows reflux of the duodenal juices into the pancreas. The enterokinase present within the duodenal juice may then activate the pancreatic enzymes within the substance of the pancreas.

2. Direct injury to the acini may lead to intrapancreatic release and activation of enzymes. This mechanism is most clearly involved in the pathogenesis of acute pancreatitis caused by certain viruses and drugs and following trauma.

3. Derangements of intracellular transport of enzymes

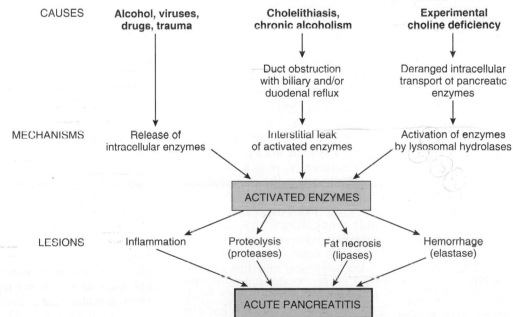

Figure 17–13. Three pathways in the pathogenesis of acute pancreatitis.

may lead to their activation by lysosomal hydrolases. In normal acinar cells digestive enzymes and the lysosomal hydrolases are transported in separate pathways after being synthesized in the endoplasmic reticulum and packaged in the Golgi apparatus. The digestive enzymes make their way through zymogen granules to the cell surface, while lysosomal hydrolases are transported into the lysosomes. In experimental pancreatitis induced by a choline-deficient diet supplemented by ethionine or by infusion of a secretagogue, the *pancreatic enzymes are activated intracellularly as a result of a derangement in their intracellular transport such that they localize within the lysosomes and are then activated by the lysosomal hydrolases* (see Fig. 17–13). A blockage in exocytosis seems to contribute to this deranged transport. It has been suggested that obstruction to the flow of pancreatic juices brought about by gallstones induces a similar derangement in the transport of enzymes. According to this hypothesis, intracellular activation of enzymes plays a dominant role in most forms of acute pancreatitis.

As mentioned earlier, *alcoholism is a strong predisposing factor for acute pancreatitis;* however, the manner by which alcohol precipitates pancreatitis is not known. Increased, transient pancreatic exocrine secretion, contraction of the sphincter of Oddi, and direct toxic effects on acinar cells have all been postulated from experimental studies. Many authorities now think that *most cases of alcoholic pancreatitis are acute exacerbations of chronic asymptomatic pancreatitis rather than acute pancreatitis.* According to this view chronic alcohol ingestion causes secretion of protein-rich pancreatic fluid leading to deposition of inspissated protein plugs and *obstruction of small pancreatic ducts,* followed by degeneration of acini and fibrosis.

CLINICAL COURSE. Abdominal pain is the cardinal manifestation of acute pancreatitis. Its severity varies with the extent of pancreatic injury. It may be mild and tolerable or severe and incapacitating. Localization in the epigastrium with radiation to the back is quite characteristic. Patients with extensive pancreatic necrosis and hemorrhage present with a medical emergency that must be distinguished from other causes of "acute abdomen" such as perforated peptic ulcer, acute cholecystitis, and infarction of the bowel. Shock, a common feature of acute pancreatitis, is caused not only by pancreatic hemorrhage but also by release of vasodilatory agents such as bradykinin and prostaglandins. Elevated serum level of amylase is a very important diagnostic finding. The amylase level rises within the first 12 hours and then often falls to normal within 48 to 72 hours. It should be cautioned that a variety of other diseases may secondarily affect the pancreas and produce elevation of this serum enzyme: perforated peptic ulcer, carcinoma of the pancreas, intestinal obstruction, peritonitis, indeed any disease that secondarily impinges on the pancreas; however, most of these conditions are associated with lesser degrees of elevations. Serum lipase is also increased, and this is more specific for pancreatitis. Direct visualization of the enlarged inflamed pancreas by high-resolution computed tomography (CT) is useful in the diagnosis of

pancreatitis and its complications (such as pseudocysts and suppuration). Hypocalcemia often develops, presumably because calcium is depleted as it binds with fatty acids in the abdomen. Jaundice, hyperglycemia, and glycosuria appear in fewer than half the patients. The mortality rate with severe acute pancreatitis is high, about 10 to 15%. Death is usually caused by shock, secondary abdominal sepsis, or the adult respiratory distress syndrome. Patients who recover must be investigated for the presence of gallstones; if present, cholecystectomy is indicated to prevent future acute attacks.

CHRONIC PANCREATITIS _____

This entity might better be referred to as *chronic relapsing pancreatitis,* since it is characterized by repeated mild bouts of inflammation eventuating in months to years by replacement of much of the pancreatic acinar tissue by fibrous tissue. The disease is protean in its manifestations, as will be discussed later. Middle-aged males, particularly alcoholics, are most frequently affected. Biliary tract disease plays a less important role in chronic pancreatitis than in the acute form of the disease. Hypercalcemia and hyperlipoproteinemia also predispose to chronic pancreatitis. Almost half of the patients have no apparent predisposing influences.

The pathogenesis of chronic relapsing pancreatitis is even more obscure than that of acute pancreatic necrosis. One proposal suggests that chronic ethanol ingestion stimulates protein secretion by the pancreas and that inspissation of the protein-rich secretions causes ductal obstructions. A concurrent decrease in the secretion of a protein that inhibits precipitation of calcium favors calcification of the protein plugs, exacerbates small duct obstruction, and hastens atrophy of the draining pancreatic lobules. Even more obscure is the pathogenesis of special forms of chronic pancreatitis, such as nonalcoholic tropical pancreatitis that is prevalent in parts of India and Africa, and vaguely ascribed to malnutrition.

MORPHOLOGY. Basically, the changes constitute a fibrosing atrophy of the exocrine glands, sometimes with remarkable sparing of the islets. The distribution of these changes permits differentiation of two morphologic variants. In one pattern, the involvement tends to have a lobular distribution and is associated with proteinaceous and calcifying plugs in the ducts within the affected lobules, hence the sometimes-used designation **calcifying pancreatitis.** Sometimes the ducts are extremely dilated and contain grossly visible calcified concretions. The lining epithelium may be atrophic or hyperplastic or may have undergone squamous metaplasia. Pseudocysts similar to those described in acute pancreatic necrosis may appear in this variant of chronic pancreatitis. **This is the pattern most often associated with alcoholism.**

The other variant of chronic pancreatitis shows more widespread atrophic changes, such as would follow obstruction to the main excretory ducts. Although there may be ductal dilatation, it is not usually marked, and calculi and calcifications are infrequent. This pattern of so-called **chronic obstructive pancreatitis** may indeed be associated with a gallstone impacted in the sphincter of Oddi or with stenosis of the sphincter secondary to cholelithiasis.

CLINICAL COURSE. A presentation of the many clinical faces of chronic pancreatitis would far exceed the spatial limitations of this book. It may present as repeated attacks of moderately severe abdominal pain, recurrent attacks of mild pain, or persistent abdominal and back pain. Yet again, the local disease may be entirely silent until pancreatic insufficiency and diabetes develop. In still other instances, the condition may present as recurrent episodes of mild jaundice or vague attacks of indigestion. The diagnosis of chronic pancreatitis requires a high index of suspicion. During an attack of pain, there may be mild elevations of serum amylase and serum lipase levels, but when the disease has been present for a long time, the destruction of acinar cells precludes such diagnostic clues. A very helpful finding is the visualization of calcifications within the pancreas by CT and ultrasonography. These techniques also help to localize pseudocysts and rule out carcinoma of the pancreas, which may also present with vague abdominal complaints. Other, more sophisticated techniques attempt to demonstrate inadequate pancreatic enzyme responses to such stimulants as secretin and cholecystokinin. The condition is more disabling than life threatening but can, as mentioned, lead to severe pancreatic exocrine insufficiency, diabetes mellitus, and the wasting of chronic malabsorption.

CARCINOMA OF THE PANCREAS _____

The term "carcinoma of the pancreas" is meant to imply carcinoma arising in the *exocrine* portion of the gland. (The much less frequent islet tumors were discussed earlier.) Carcinoma of the pancreas is now the fifth most frequent cause of death from cancer in the United States, preceded only by lung, colorectal, prostate, and breast cancers. Moreover, its incidence has been steadily and rather rapidly increasing over the years. Currently 25,000 new patients are identified every year, of whom more than 24,000 are expected to die within five years. These figures are even more distressing when one considers that there are virtually no clues to the cause of pancreatic cancer. Only one significant association has been noted: this form of cancer appears to be two or three times more common in smokers than in nonsmokers. Despite earlier indica-

tions, coffee consumption and diabetes mellitus have not proven to be significant risk factors. The peak incidence occurs between 60 and 80 years of age.

MORPHOLOGY. Approximately 60% of the cancers of this organ arise in the head of the pancreas, 15% in the body, and 5% in the tail; in 20% the tumor diffusely involves the entire gland. Virtually all of these lesions are adenocarcinomas arising in the ductal epithelium. Some may secrete mucin, and many have an abundant fibrous stroma. These desmoplastic lesions therefore present as gritty, gray-white, hard masses. The tumor, in its early stages, infiltrates locally and eventually extends into adjacent structures (Fig. 17–14).

With carcinoma of the **head of the pancreas,** the ampullary region is invaded, obstructing the outflow of bile. In this infiltrative growth, it frequently surrounds and compresses, and less commonly directly invades, the common bile duct or ampulla of Vater. Ulceration of the tumor into the duodenal mucosa may occur. As a consequence of the involvement of the common bile duct, there is marked distention of the gallbladder in about half of the patients with carcinoma of the head of

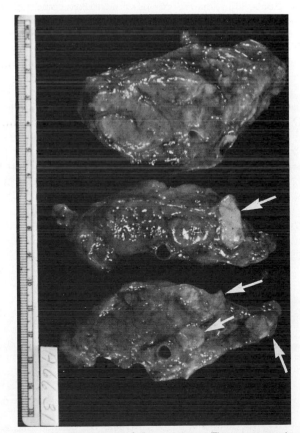

Figure 17–14. Carcinoma of the pancreas. The cross sections of the gland show the nodules of pale tumor that virtually replace the entire gland in the top slice and are evident as nodules *(arrows)* in the lower slices.

the pancreas. Because of the strategic location of these tumors, patients usually die of obstructive jaundice and hepatobiliary dysfunction while the tumor is still relatively small and not widely disseminated.

In marked contrast, **carcinomas of the body and tail of the pancreas** remain silent for some time and may be quite large and widely disseminated by the time they are discovered. They impinge on the adjacent vertebral column, extend through the retroperitoneal spaces, and occasionally invade the adjacent spleen and adrenals. They may extend into the transverse colon or stomach. Peripancreatic, gastric, mesenteric, omental, and porta-hepatic nodes are frequently involved, and the liver is often strikingly seeded with tumor nodules, producing hepatic enlargement two to three times the normal size. Such massive hepatic metastases are quite characteristic of carcinoma of the tail and body of the pancreas and are attributed to invasion of the splenic vein that courses directly along the margins of the pancreas. Distant metastases occur, principally to the lungs and bones.

Microscopically, there is no difference between carcinomas of the head of the pancreas and those of the body and tail of the pancreas. Most grow in more or less well-differentiated glandular patterns (Fig. 17–15). As mentioned, they may be either mucinous or non-mucin–secreting. In some cases, the gland patterns are atypical, irregular, and small, and the glands lined by anaplastic cuboidal to columnar epithelial cells. Other variants grow in a totally undifferentiated pattern.

CLINICAL COURSE. From the preceding discussion, it should be evident that carcinomas in the pancreas remain silent until their extension impinges on some other structure. It is when they erode to the posterior wall of the abdomen and affect nerve fibers that pain appears. There has long been a prevalent misconception that carcinoma of the pancreas is a painless disease. Many large series have clearly documented that pain is usually the first symptom, although unfortunately, by the time pain appears, these cancers have already encroached on adjacent structures. *Those arising in the head of the pancreas eventually cause jaundice, whereas those of the body and tail remain difficult to diagnose until weight loss and pressure on adjacent organs make evident the cause of the pain.* Unfortunately, there are no early signs and symptoms specific enough to offer a clue to the diagnosis. Obstructive jaundice, which is usually severe and progressive, is associated with most cases of carcinoma of the head of the pancreas. Spontaneously appearing *phlebothrombosis,* also called *migratory thrombophlebitis,* is sometimes seen with carcinoma of the pancreas, particularly those of the body and tail (*Trousseau's sign*). But, as was mentioned, this syndrome is not pathognomonic for cancer in this organ (p. 72).

Because of the insidiousness of these lesions, there has long been a search for biochemical tests indicative of their presence. Levels of many enzymes and antigens (e.g., carcinoembryonic antigen, and CA19-9 antigen) have been found to be elevated, but no single marker has proved to be specific for pancreatic cancer. Several imaging techniques such as ultrasonography and CT have proved of great value in diagnosis. With these modalities it is possible to perform percutaneous needle biopsy, obviating the need for exploratory laparotomy. The five-year survival rate is only 2%, and most patients survive less than a year after diagnosis.

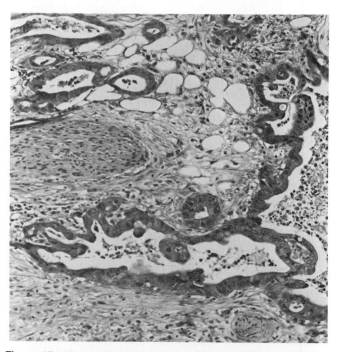

Figure 17–15. Carcinoma of the pancreas. The desmoplastic adenocarcinoma has almost totally replaced the native architecture. Only one normal duct *(below center)* remains. The cancer grows in small nests and strands of cells scattered in an abundant stroma. Occasionally it reproduces gland-like patterns.

Bibliography

Castano, L., Eisenbarth, G. S.: Type I diabetes: A chronic autoimmune disease of human, mouse, and rat. Ann. Rev. Immunol. *8:*647, 1990. (An excellent review of the pathogenesis of type I diabetes.)

Leahy, J. L.: The natural history of β cell dysfunction in NIDDM. Diab. Care. *13:*992, 1990. (A scholarly review of the early and late defects in β-cell function in type II diabetes.)

Merimee, T. J.: Diabetic retinopathy. A synthesis of perspectives. N. Engl. J. Med. *322:*978, 1990. (A succinct discussion of the biochemical mechanisms that underlie complications of diabetes, with emphasis on retinopathy.)

Moller, D. E., Flier, J. S.: Insulin resistance—mechanisms, syndromes, and implications. N. Engl. J. Med. *325:*938, 1991. (An excellent review of insulin action and insulin resistance, with a section on the mechanism of insulin resistance in type II diabetes.)

Saad, M. F., et al.: A two-step model for development of non–insulin-dependent diabetes. Am. J. Med. *90:*229, 1991. (A summary of insights gained into the pathogenesis of type II diabetes by studying Pima Indians. The primacy of insulin resistance is stressed.)

Sarles, H., Bernard, J. P., Gullo, L.: Pathogenesis of chronic pancreatitis. Gut *31:*629, 1990. (A summary of the evidence supporting a role for secretory abnormalities in the causation of chronic pancreatitis.)

Sing, S. M., Reber, H. A.: The pathology of chronic pancreatitis. World J. Surg. *14:*2, 1990. (A clear description of the histologic patterns in chronic pancreatitis.)

Steer, M. L.: Classification and pathogenesis of pancreatitis. Surg. Clin. North Am. *69:*467, 1989. (An excellent overview of the etiology and pathogenesis of acute and chronic pancreatitis; the role of defective intracellular transport of enzymes is emphasized.)

Steffes, M. W., Mauer, S. M.: Toward a basic understanding of diabetic complications. N. Engl. J. Med. *325:*883, 1991. (A brief review of the role of glycosylation in the causation of diabetic complications.)

Unger, R. H.: Role of impaired glucose transport by β cells in the pathogenesis of diabetes. J. NIH Res. *3:*77, 1991. (An excellent review of the role of glucose-transport units [GLUTs] in the pathogenesis of type II diabetes.)

EIGHTEEN

The Male Genital System

PENIS
  Hypospadias and Epispadias
  Phimosis
  Bowen's Disease
  Carcinoma of the Penis
SCROTUM, TESTIS, AND EPIDIDYMIS
  Cryptorchidism
  Klinefelter's Syndrome
  Testicular Tumors
  Inflammations
      Epididymitis and Orchitis
PROSTATE
  Prostatitis
  Nodular Hyperplasia of the Prostate (Benign
    Prostatic Hypertrophy)
  Carcinoma of the Prostate
VENEREAL DISEASE
  Gonorrhea
  Nongonococcal Urethritis and Cervicitis
  Syphilis (Lues)
  Papilloma (Condyloma Acuminatum)
  Chancroid, Granuloma Inguinale, and
    Lymphogranuloma Venereum
  Herpes Genitalis

In this chapter the major anatomic subdivisions of the male genital system—the penis, the scrotum and its contents, and the prostate—will be considered individually. Although there is some overlap, diseases tend initially or predominantly to affect only one of these structures. An exception to this anatomic consideration is the grouping of the venereal diseases together at the end of the chapter. Because the pathologic processes are quite similar in both sexes, and to facilitate comparison, the effects of venereal disease in females are also discussed in this section.

PENIS

The principal lesions of the penis are infectious, congenital, or neoplastic. In most cases they affect the surface of the penis and so are readily visible to the patient. The more important infectious processes are venereally transmitted and are discussed at the end of

the chapter. Remaining to be described here are the congenital anomalies *hypospadias, epispadias,* and *phimosis,* and two neoplastic lesions, *Bowen's disease* (representing carcinoma in situ) and invasive *carcinoma of the penis.*

HYPOSPADIAS AND EPISPADIAS

Among the more frequent congenital anomalies of the penis is termination of the urethra at the ventral surface of the penis (*hypospadias*) or at its dorsal surface (*epispadias*). Because the abnormal opening is often constricted, partial outflow obstruction, with its attendant risk of urinary infection and hydronephrosis, may result. In addition, these anomalies may be causes of sterility when the abnormal orifice is situated near the base of the penis. Frequently, hypospadias and epispadias are associated with failure of normal descent of the testes and with malformations of the bladder; sometimes they are associated with more serious congenital deformities.

PHIMOSIS

When the orifice of the prepuce is too small to permit its retraction over the glans penis, the condition is designated *phimosis.* This may be a congenital anomaly or it may be acquired by inflammatory scarring. In either case, phimosis permits the accumulation of secretions and smegma under the prepuce, favoring the development of secondary infection and further scarring. The nonspecific infection of the glans penis and prepuce that often accompanies phimosis is termed *balanoposthitis.* Forcible retraction of the prepuce may cause constriction, with pain and swelling of the glans penis, a condition known as *paraphimosis.* Urinary retention may develop in severe cases.

BOWEN'S DISEASE

Bowen's disease refers to carcinoma in situ. It is not specific to the penis but may occur on the skin or on mucosal surfaces, including the vulva and the oral cavity. Its importance lies in the potential for its transformation into invasive squamous cell carcinoma.

The frequency of conversion from the premalignant (in situ) stage to frank malignancy is not well established but is considered to be no more than 11%. According to some authors, Bowen's disease is associated with a high incidence of visceral cancer, but others have failed to find such an association.

CARCINOMA OF THE PENIS

In the United States, squamous cell carcinoma of the penis accounts for about 0.25% of cancers in males. Other forms of cancer of the penis are even more rare. This lesion is extremely rare among men who were circumcised early in life. The protection conferred by circumcision has been traditionally ascribed to its effectiveness in preventing accumulation of unidentified carcinogens contained in smegma. However, recent evidence suggests that, as with certain cancers of the female genital tract (p. 613), human papillomavirus (subtypes 16 and 18) may be involved in the causation of penile cancer. It is conceivable, therefore, that the prophylactic effect of circumcision may relate to the associated improvement of general hygiene, thereby lessening exposure to potentially oncogenic viruses. The incidence of this cancer is highest after age 40 years. As mentioned, this form of cancer may be preceded by Bowen's disease.

> Morphologically, squamous cell carcinoma of the penis usually initially appears as a small, grayish, crusted papule on the glans or prepuce, near the coronal sulcus. When the plaque reaches about 1 cm in diameter, the center usually ulcerates and develops a necrotic, secondarily infected base with ragged, heaped-up margins. Less frequently, the tumor takes a papillary form, resembling the benign papilloma that enlarges to produce a cauliflower-like fungating mass. Both patterns are locally destructive and may cause large necrotizing erosions. Histologically, the appearance is that of squamous cell carcinomas occurring anywhere on the skin or mucosa (see p. 210).

Carcinoma of the penis tends to follow a slow, indolent course. Metastases to the inguinal nodes are present in only 25% of patients at the time of diagnosis, although many more have reactive lymphadenopathy. Widespread dissemination is uncommon until late in the course. For all stages, the five-year survival rate is about 70%.

SCROTUM, TESTIS, AND EPIDIDYMIS

The more important disorders of the scrotum and its contents involve the testes. *Some of these disorders produce testes that are smaller than normal, and others cause enlargement.* In the first category are congenital abnormalities that result in failure of the testes to develop normally at puberty. These include *cryptorchidism,* to be described later, and *Klinefelter's syndrome.* In addition, a variety of disorders result in atrophy of previously normal-sized testes.

A number of diseases cause enlargement of the testes. By far the most important are *testicular tumors,* usually associated with insidious painless enlargement. Second in importance are *infections (orchitis).* These usually produce more rapid, painful swelling. A third, relatively infrequent, cause of testicular enlargement is *torsion of the testis.* In this case, violent movement or physical trauma causes twisting of the spermatic cord, with consequent impairment of blood flow to and from the testis. Usually there is some underlying structural abnormality—such as incomplete descent of the testis, absence of the gubernaculum testis, or testicular atrophy—that permits excessive mobility of the testis within the tunica vaginalis. Because the thick-walled arteries are less vulnerable to compression than are the veins, there is intense vascular engorgement and, in severe cases, extravasation of blood into the interstitial tissue of the testis and epididymis, with consequent hemorrhagic infarction. There is usually little doubt about the diagnosis because of the intense pain and rapid swelling, often with bloody discoloration of the scrotum.

It is important to remember that the clinical distinction between enlargement of testicular origin and that due to disorders within the epididymis or scrotum itself is not always easily made. Indeed, swelling due to infection more often originates in the epididymis than in the testis. In addition, abnormal collections of fluid or herniated intestinal loops in the scrotal sac may initially be confused with a testicular mass. Although they are of relatively trivial consequence compared with, say, carcinoma of the testis, these disorders of the scrotum are extremely common. They will be described briefly before discussing testicular tumors and infections in more detail.

A clear serous accumulation within the tunica vaginalis—the serosa-lined sac enclosing the testis and epididymis—is termed a *hydrocele.* It may be a response to neighboring infections or tumors, or it may be a manifestation of generalized edema from any cause. Often, however, it develops slowly and painlessly, without apparent cause. *Hydroceles are frequent and are the most common cause of scrotal enlargement.*

Much less frequent are *hematoceles,* that is, blood in the tunica vaginalis as a result of tissue trauma or bleeding diatheses, and *chyloceles,* an accumulation of lymphatic fluid resulting from lymphatic obstruction.

With an *inguinal hernia,* loops of intestine may descend into the tunica vaginalis, causing marked scrotal enlargement. This is easily differentiated from testicular disease by the presence of bowel sounds in the scrotum and by the reduction of the hernia through the widened inguinal ring. This is also a common cause of scrotal enlargement in children, and is seen in 1% of the pediatric population.

CRYPTORCHIDISM

Normally the testes descend from their initial embryonic position in the coelomic cavity to the pelvic brim in the third month of fetal life, a process termed *internal descent*. During the last two months of intrauterine life, *external descent*, or passage of the testes through the inguinal canals to the scrotal sac, takes place. When either process is incomplete, resulting in the *malpositioning of the testis anywhere along this pathway, the condition is termed cryptorchidism*. It is a common condition, seen in about 0.7% of the adult male population.

Cryptorchidism is best considered a syndrome with various causes. Primary anatomic abnormalities (hereditary or developmental) such as a short spermatic cord or a narrow inguinal canal are observed in some, but in the vast majority of the cases no obvious mechanical factor can be recognized. Because a normally functioning hypothalamic-pituitary-testicular axis is considered essential for testicular development and descent, it is suspected that hormonal factors are primary in most cases.

Cryptorchidism is unilateral in the vast majority of the cases, affecting the right testis somewhat more frequently than the left. Progressive atrophy of the malpositioned testis begins early. Developmental arrest of the germ cells begins as early as two years of age and is evident in most by five to six years. Grossly visible atrophy, characterized by diminution in size and an increase in consistency as a result of progressive fibrosis, is obvious by 13 years of age. Microscopically, the tubules become atrophic, outlined by prominent, thickened basement membranes, and eventually they are virtually totally replaced by fibrous tissue. There may be an accompanying hyperplasia of the interstitial cells of Leydig as well as of the stroma. Surprisingly, histologic evidence of atrophy has also been noted in the contralateral (descended) testis. **Such testicular atrophy is nonspecific and may be seen in many other conditions, including progressive arteriosclerotic encroachment on testicular blood supply, end-stage orchitis, hypopituitarism, prolonged administration of female sex hormones, cirrhosis of the liver, some forms of malnutrition, and obstruction to the outflow of semen, as well as following irradiation.**

It should be apparent that bilateral cryptorchidism, present in 25% of the cases, results in sterility. However, infertility is also noted in a significant number of cases with unilateral cryptorchidism because, as mentioned earlier, the scrotal testis may also be abnormal. In addition, the undescended testis is at much greater risk of developing cancer, so it must be surgically placed in the scrotum (orchiopexy), preferably before two years of age, to prevent progressive atrophy. However, orchiopexy does not preclude the possibility of a cancer developing at a later date, nor can fertility be taken for granted. These results (taken along with abnormalities in the normally placed contralateral testis) suggest that in some cases there is an intrinsic defect in the testis that is unrelated to its position and that cannot be corrected by anatomic repositioning.

KLINEFELTER'S SYNDROME

This syndrome is characterized by primary failure of the testes to develop at puberty, with resultant eunuchoidism (Fig. 18–1). It is responsible for about 3% of cases of infertility in males. This sex-chromosomal disorder is described on page 109.

TESTICULAR TUMORS

Testicular tumors are the most important cause of firm, painless enlargement of the testis. About 95% of testicular tumors arise from germ cells. Almost all of these are malignant. Most of the remaining 5% originate from the interstitial cells of Leydig or the Sertoli cells, and these are usually benign, although they may elaborate steroids and thus cause endocrinopathies. Here we consider only the germ cell tumors.

The average incidence of testicular germ cell tumors in the United States is approximately two per 100,000 males. Their peak incidence is in the 15- to 34-year age group. Moreover, for unknown reasons, in this age group there has been a steady increase in the frequency of these tumors over the past several years.

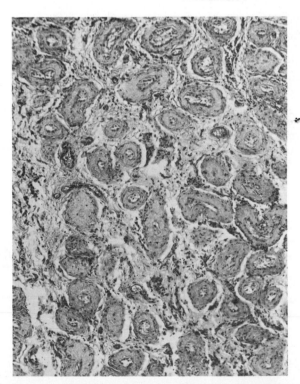

Figure 18–1. Klinefelter's syndrome. The spermatic tubules are totally atrophic and hyalinized and appear as doughnut-shaped masses of collagenous tissue.

The cause of testicular cancer is unknown, but some predisposing factors have been identified. Reference has already been made to the increased incidence of tumors (10- to 40-fold) in undescended testes. Epidemiologic studies suggest that genetic influences also play a role. Blacks in Africa as well as in the United States have an extremely low incidence of germ cell tumors. Among whites in the United States, Jews are affected twice as frequently as non-Jews.

CLASSIFICATION AND HISTOGENESIS. The classification of testicular germ cell tumors has been somewhat controversial. This stems in part from differing views on their histogenesis. Here we present the World Health Organization classification (Table 18–1), most widely used in the United States, followed by the proposed histogenesis of these neoplasms.

Testicular germ cell tumors may be divided into two categories, based on whether they are composed of a single histologic pattern or more than one. Tumors with a *single* histologic pattern constitute about 40% of all testicular neoplasms and are listed in Table 18–1. In approximately 60% of the tumors, there is a *mixture of two or more of the histologic patterns*. The most common mixture is that of teratoma and embryonal carcinoma (*teratocarcinoma*), constituting 14% of all testicular neoplasms. This classification is based on the view that all testicular germ cell tumors arise in totipotential germ cells (Fig. 18–2). *These cells may give rise to a seminoma, reflecting gonadal differentiation, or they may transform into totipotential tumor cells, represented by embryonal carcinoma.* According to this concept, embryonal carcinomas contain the stem cell for all nonseminomatous germ cell tumors. Depending on the degree and the line of differentiation of embryonal carcinoma cells, tumors with different histologic patterns result. The most undifferentiated state is represented by pure embryonal cell carcinoma, whereas choriocarcinoma and yolk sac tumor represent commitment of the tumor stem cells to differentiate into specific extraembryonic cell types. Teratoma, on the other hand, results from differentiation of the embryonic carcinoma cells along all three of the germ cell layers, and therefore teratomas contain the greatest variety of neoplastic cells and tissues. The observation

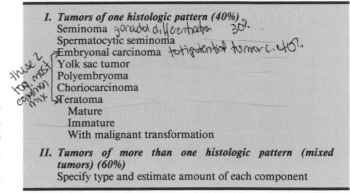

TABLE 18–1. CLASSIFICATION OF TESTICULAR GERM CELL TUMORS

I. Tumors of one histologic pattern (40%)
  Seminoma
  Spermatocytic seminoma
  Embryonal carcinoma
  Yolk sac tumor
  Polyembryoma
  Choriocarcinoma
  Teratoma
    Mature
    Immature
    With malignant transformation

II. Tumors of more than one histologic pattern (mixed tumors) (60%)
  Specify type and estimate amount of each component

that the vast majority of nonseminomatous testicular tumors show a mixed histologic pattern is consistent with this schema of histogenesis. With this background, we present the morphology of the more common individual tumors, to be followed by comments on their clinical course.

SEMINOMA. This common germ cell tumor accounts for approximately 30% of testicular neoplasms. In the great majority of cases it is characterized by sheets or cords of fairly well-differentiated uniform polygonal cells, with distinct cell membranes, central round nuclei, and cleared cytoplasm. Approximately 10% of the cases show syncytial giant cells, which contain human chorionic gonadotropin (HCG). As will be described later, the significance of such admixture is unclear. Typically, there is a variable fibrous stroma with a prominent lymphocytic infiltrate and occasional granulomatous formations. These tumors tend to grow rapidly as large, gray-white, fleshy masses (Fig. 18–3) but remain confined within the tunica albuginea until late in their course.

EMBRYONAL CARCINOMA. In contrast to seminomas, embryonal carcinomas are poorly differentiated. They are generally smaller than seminomas, appearing grossly

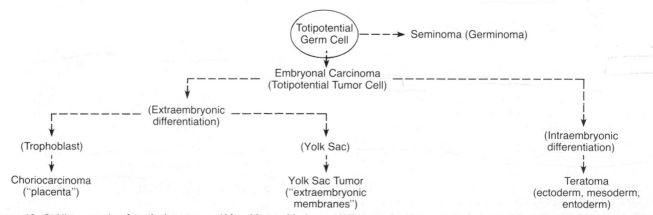

Figure 18–2. Histogenesis of testicular tumors. (After Morse, M. J., and Willet, W. F.: Neoplasms of the testis. *In* Walsh, P. C., et al. [eds.]: Campbell's Urology. 5th ed. Philadelphia, W. B. Saunders Co., 1986, p. 1537.)

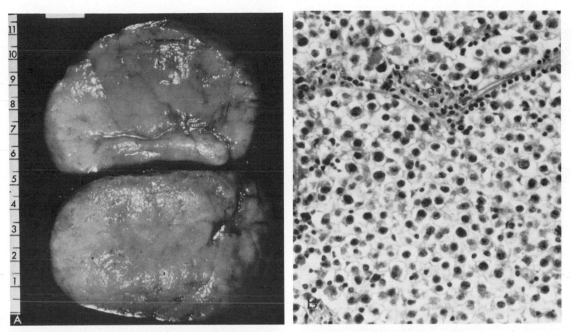

Figure 18-3. *A,* A hemisected seminoma of the testis. The gray-white, fleshy mass totally replaces the testis. Note that its size is approximately 5 × 7 cm and it has therefore caused testicular enlargement. *B,* A high-power detail of a seminoma of the testis, showing sheets of neoplastic cells with clear cytoplasm and regular nuclei. The delicate stroma contains a relatively scant lymphoid infiltrate. (B Courtesy of Dr. Dennis Burns, Department of Pathology, Southwestern Medical School, Dallas TX.)

as gray-white nodules, often with areas of hemorrhage and necrosis. Microscopically, the cells may be completely undifferentiated and arranged in sheets or, alternatively, they may assume an acinar, tubular, or papillary pattern (Fig. 18-4). The neoplastic cells are large and pleomorphic and, unlike seminoma cells, have indistinct cell borders. The stroma is scanty and devoid of lymphocytes. Embryonal carcinomas are said to constitute approximately 40% of testicular germ cell tumors. It should be noted, however, that with histochemical techniques the great majority of apparently "pure" embryonal carcinomas reveal yolk sac cells containing α-fetoprotein (AFP) or syncytial cells containing HCG, or both, and are therefore mixed tumors.

YOLK SAC TUMOR. This tumor is variously known as infantile embryonal carcinoma, endodermal sinus tumor, and orchioblastoma. Although in its pure form the yolk sac tumor constitutes less than 1% of all testicular tumors, it is the commonest tumor affecting the testes of children younger than three years. **Yolk sac elements are frequently found admixed with embryonal carcinoma in adults.** The tumor cells are undifferentiated and vary from endothelium-like to cuboidal or columnar cells. These cells occur in glandular, papillary, or solid formation. With immunoperoxidase techniques it is possible to demonstrate AFP within the tumor cells, a finding highly characteristic of yolk sac tumor but, as you recall, also found in hepatocellular carcinoma (p. 561).

CHORIOCARCINOMA. Choriocarcinoma, a highly malignant neoplasm, accounts for only 1% of testicular cancers in its pure form. The lesion may cause testicular

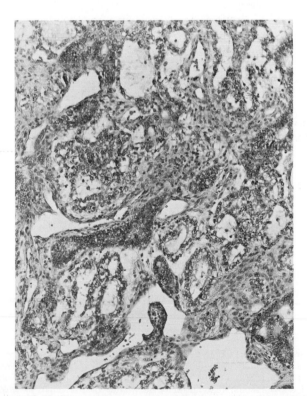

Figure 18-4. Embryonal carcinoma of the testis. An acinar, tubular, and papillary pattern is seen in this neoplasm.

enlargement, but more often the primary tumor is very small and cannot be palpated. Nonetheless, it is highly malignant, metastasizing via the bloodstream early and widely. Histologically, these tumors reproduce the two components of placental tissue—cytotrophoblast, composed of masses of cuboidal cells with central round nuclei, and syncytiotrophoblast, appearing as sheets of syncytial epithelium with an abundant pink, vacuolated cytoplasm and large, pleomorphic nuclei. HCG can be identified within the syncytiotrophoblast. These two cellular elements are not arranged as in placental villi but instead grow in disarray.

TERATOMA. Teratoma of the testis is characterized by a histologic pattern in which tissues from more than one, often from all three, germ cell layer are present. Three variants, based on the degree of differentiation, are recognized. The fully differentiated variant, called the **mature teratoma,** is found most often in children. Microscopically, these tumors are composed of well-differentiated elements such as neural tissue, muscle, cartilage, fat, squamous epithelium, bronchial epithelium, and bits of intestinal wall (Fig. 18–5). These elements lie helter-skelter with no definite pattern or orientation. The **immature teratoma** contains similar elements, which are incompletely differentiated but can be easily identified as embryonic tissues. Although this variant displays malig-

nant behavior, the tissues may not show cytologic features of malignancy. On the other hand, in **teratoma with malignant transformation,** derivatives of one or more of the germ cell layers are frankly malignant. Thus there may be a focus of squamous cell carcinoma, mucin-secreting adenocarcinoma, or sarcoma. Immature and frankly malignant teratomas occur more commonly in adults. Since benign mature teratomas are rare in adults, every teratoma in an adult must be regarded as malignant. Owing to the great variety of tissues present in teratomas, the gross appearance of these tumors is understandably variable. In general, the cut surface reveals cystic areas and a variegated appearance with foci of cartilage, bone, or soft myxomatous tissue. As with embryonal carcinomas, teratomas in adults usually occur in combination with other histologic types.

MIXED TUMORS. Mixed tumors constitute 60% of all testicular tumors and contain combinations of the various histologic patterns already described. Most common is the combination of teratoma and embryonal carcinoma (teratocarcinoma), but all conceivable mixtures have been described. It is important to note that in general the prognosis of a mixed tumor is determined by the more malignant element.

It should be apparent from the foregoing discussion that seminoma is the only tumor that occurs with any appreciable frequency in pure form.

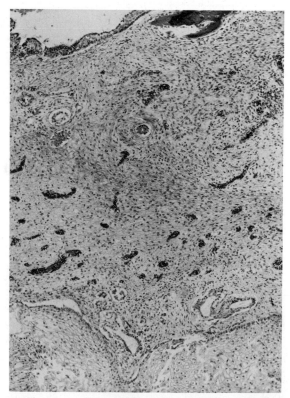

Figure 18–5. Histologic detail of a testicular teratoma. A spicule of bone *(top center)* is immediately to the right of a cystic space lined by columnar ''respiratory-appearing'' epithelium. The center of the field shows areas, resembling white matter of the brain, in which small glands are scattered. At the bottom is a large nest of stratified squamous epithelium.

CLINICAL COURSE. Testicular tumors appear most often as a painless enlargement of the testis. Indeed, the overwhelming majority of intratesticular masses are malignant germ cell tumors. As already pointed out, in some instances the more aggressive variants, such as choriocarcinoma, may present initially with disseminated metastases and a small intratesticular primary lesion. Tumors of the testis have a characteristic mode of spread, the knowledge of which is essential in clinical staging as well as in treatment. In general, testicular tumors spread first to the common iliac and paraaortic lymph nodes and later to the mediastinal and supraclavicular nodes. Clinically, it is important to make the distinction between seminomas and the nonseminomatous tumors. Seminomas typically spread by lymphatics after having remained localized for a long time. Hematogenous spread to the lungs, brain, bones, and other organs is usually a late event. Seminomas are extremely radiosensitive. Even those that have spread can often be cured by radiotherapy. Nonseminomatous germ cell tumors, in contrast, metastasize earlier and also utilize the hematogenous route more frequently. They are much less radiosensitive than seminomas. Choriocarcinomas are the most aggressive, and in most cases lungs and liver are already involved at the time of diagnosis.

Staging of testicular tumors involves several diagnostic techniques, including computed tomography, inferior venacavography, lymphangiography, and studies of tumor markers. Three stages are defined:

● Tumor confined to the testis (stage I).

- Distant spread limited to the retroperitoneal nodes below the diaphragm (stage II).
- Metastases outside the retroperitoneal nodes or above the diaphragm (stage III).

Major advances in the diagnosis and management of testicular cancer have been made possible by the development of sensitive and specific radioimmunoassays for the detection of tumor-associated polypeptides. Two such markers, α-fetoprotein (AFP) and the β subunit of human chorionic gonadotropin (HCG), have proved to be of considerable value. AFP is normally synthesized by fetal tissues (liver, yolk sac, and intestines), whereas HCG is a product of the placental syncytiotrophoblast. As might be expected from the histogenesis and morphology, elevations in the levels of these markers are seen most often in patients with nonseminomatous tumors. All patients with choriocarcinoma have increased levels of HCG, whereas almost 90% of those with embryonal carcinoma or teratocarcinoma have elevated levels of HCG or AFP, or both. In approximately half the patients with teratoma, one or both of these markers are elevated. Seminoma is associated with increased HCG in fewer than 10% of cases. The significance of elevated HCG levels in this group of patients is not clear. In addition to their value in diagnosis, tumor markers are also helpful in studies of staging and follow-up. For example, an elevated serum level following orchiectomy is a clear indication of stage II disease; similarly, an increase in marker levels following therapy can predict recurrences, often well in advance of clinical expression of relapse.

The prognosis of testicular cancer has improved dramatically in the last decade. With the appropriate combination of orchiectomy, radiotherapy, and chemotherapy cure rates between 80 and 100% can be achieved; seminomas have the best prognosis. Table 18–2 summarizes the salient features of testicular tumors.

INFLAMMATIONS

Epididymitis and Orchitis

In general, infections are more common in the epididymis than in the testis but they may ultimately reach the testis by direct or lymphatic spread. Most cases of epididymitis are secondary to urinary tract infection or to prostatitis. In sexually active men younger than 35 years, two sexually transmitted pathogens, *Neisseria gonorrhoeae* and *Chlamydia trachomatis,* are the most frequent causes of epididymitis. On the other hand, after age 35, *Escherichia coli* and *Pseudomonas* are responsible for most of the infections. In addition to these organisms, which cause nonspecific epididymitis, genitourinary tuberculosis may also involve the epididymis and produce typical lesions of tuberculosis. The testis may be infected by an extension of the infection from the epididymis. Thus orchitis may develop in association with gonococcal or tubercular epididymitis. On the other hand, organisms such as *Treponema pallidum* and the mumps virus tend to infect the testis without prior epididymitis. Gonorrhea and syphilis, which are sexually transmitted, are discussed later in this chapter.

With nonspecific infections, the early changes are limited to the epididymis and consist of edema and a nonspecific leukocytic infiltration of the interstitial tissue. Later, the tubules are filled with exudate and there may be abscess formation or a generalized suppurative necrosis. Retrograde spread involves the testis. Any such nonspecific inflammation may become chronic. Pressure within the edematous testis or fibrous scarring of the tubules often leads to sterility. The hardier cells of Leydig are usually spared, so that endocrine function and libido remain intact.

TABLE 18–2. SUMMARY OF TESTICULAR TUMORS

Tumor	Peak Age (yr)	Morphology	Tumor Markers
Seminoma	40–50	Sheets of uniform polygonal cells with cleared cytoplasm; lymphocytes in the stroma	~10% have elevated HCG
Embryonal carcinoma	20–30	Poorly differentiated, pleomorphic cells in cords, sheets, or papillary formation; majority contain some yolk sac and choriocarcinoma cells	90% have elevated HCG or AFP or both
Yolk sac tumor	3	Poorly differentiated endothelium-like, cuboidal, or columnar cells	100% have elevated AFP
Choriocarcinoma (pure)	20–30	Cytotrophoblast and syncytiotrophoblast without villus formation	100% have elevated HCG
Teratoma	All ages	Tissues from all three germ cell layers with varying degrees of differentiation	50% have elevated HCG or AFP or both
Mixed tumor	15–30	Variable, depending on mixture; commonly teratoma and embryonal carcinoma	90% have elevated HCG and AFP

In about 25 to 33% of cases of mumps in postpubertal or adult males an acute interstitial orchitis, usually unilateral but occasionally bilateral, develops about one week after the swelling of the salivary glands. Rarely, cases of mumps orchitis have been described without significant involvement of the salivary glands.

PROSTATE

There are three important lesions of the prostate: *inflammation,* usually as a result of nonspecific infection; *nodular hyperplasia,* commonly known as benign prostatic hypertrophy (BPH); and *carcinoma.* All three cause some degree of enlargement of the prostate. Because the prostate encircles the urethra, any lesion that causes significant prostatic enlargement may easily encroach on the lumen of the urethra. Thus, diseases of the prostate commonly manifest themselves by urinary symptoms. These symptoms are variable but usually include such indications of partial obstruction as frequency of urination, nocturia, and difficulty in initiating or maintaining the stream of urine.

PROSTATITIS

Inflammations of the prostate may be acute or chronic and are further classified on the basis of bacteriologic findings and examination of prostatic secretions obtained by transrectal prostatic massage. *Bacterial prostatitis,* both acute and chronic, is caused by the same microorganisms that are commonly associated with urinary tract infections (UTIs). As might be expected, bacterial infections of the prostate are associated with the presence of inflammatory cells in the prostatic secretions; however, in many patients with symptoms of chronic prostatitis, bacteriologic findings are negative but the presence of prostatic inflammation can be documented by the presence of increased numbers of leukocytes in prostatic secretions. Such *chronic abacterial prostatitis is perhaps the most common form of prostatitis seen today.*

Bacterial prostatitis is caused most commonly by *E. coli,* but other gram-negative pathogens of the urinary tract may also be involved. In acute prostatitis the organisms usually reach the prostate by direct extension from the posterior urethra or the bladder. Chronic bacterial prostatitis may be a sequel to acute prostatitis, but more often it appears insidiously. It is often associated with recurrent UTI. The cause of *chronic abacterial prostatitis* is unclear. Because affected patients are usually 30- to 45-year-old sexually active males, several sexually transmitted pathogens have been implicated. The prime suspects in this group include *C. trachomatis* and *Ureaplasma urealyticum,* which have also been implicated in the causation of nongonococcal urethritis (NGU, p. 602).

Acute prostatitis is characterized by suppuration, either in the form of minute, discrete abscesses or as large, coalescent areas of involvement. Diffuse involvement often leads to soft, boggy enlargement of the entire prostate. Histologically, the gland lumens may become virtually packed with a neutrophilic exudate, and the stroma characteristically contains a nonspecific leukocytic infiltrate.

Because some degree of lymphocytic infiltration of the prostate is a normal accompaniment of aging, the diagnosis of chronic prostatitis should not be made unless other mononuclear leukocytes and neutrophils are also present, along with some evidence of tissue destruction and fibroblastic proliferation.

Granulomas without caseous centers may develop as a nonspecific inflammatory response to inspissated prostatic secretions.

Clinically, both acute and chronic prostatitis may be associated with low back pain, dysuria, frequency, and urgency. Sometimes the prostate is enlarged and tender. With acute disease, systemic signs of acute inflammation, including fever and malaise, may be present. In contrast, many cases of chronic bacterial prostatitis are asymptomatic even when the expressed prostatic secretions contain large numbers of leukocytes. Because most antibiotics penetrate the prostate poorly, bacteria find safe haven in the parenchyma and constantly seed the urinary tract. Thus *in men chronic bacterial prostatitis is the most common cause of recurrent UTI caused by the same pathogen.*

NODULAR HYPERPLASIA OF THE PROSTATE (BENIGN PROSTATIC HYPERTROPHY)

This is an extremely common disorder characterized by the development of large, fairly discrete nodules within the prostate. By long-standing tradition, this entity is known as "benign prostatic hypertrophy" or BPH, although this is a misnomer, since the basic process is hyperplasia rather than hypertrophy and, in either case, the qualification "benign" is redundant.

Beginning in the fifth decade of life, there is a progressive increase in incidence of nodular hyperplasia with age, until about 95% of men beyond age 75 years are affected. Fortunately, most of those affected are not seriously inconvenienced.

The cause of this lesion is unknown, but current opinion favors an endocrine basis. Both androgens and estrogens are involved. Dihydrotestosterone, which is the biologically active metabolite of testosterone, is believed to be the ultimate mediator of hyperplasia. It has been suggested that estrogens "sensitize" the prostatic tissues to the growth-promoting effects of dihydrotestosterone by enhancing the expression of its receptors. This would explain the synergism between estrogens and androgens observed in experimentally induced prostatic hyperplasia in the canine model. In humans, it is postulated that the increase in the level of estrogens that occurs with aging may facilitate the action of androgens within the prostate, even in the face of declining testicular output of testosterone.

MORPHOLOGY. In the typical case, the prostatic nodules weigh between 60 and 100 gm; aggregate weights of up to 200 gm are seen. The nodules characteristically originate around the urethra, arising from glands that drain proximal to the verumontanum. **This distribution is in striking contrast to that of prostatic carcinoma, which usually involves the peripheral zone.** Although the nodules do not have a true capsule, they are well-demarcated on cross section because of the compression of the surrounding parenchyma. The urethra may be compressed to a slit-like orifice by nodules on its lateral aspects. The hyperplastic tissue may project up into the floor of the urethra in a hemispheric mass, sometimes having the effect of a ball valve (Fig. 18–6).

In most cases, the hyperplasia is seen microscopically to result primarily from glandular proliferation, although smooth muscles and fibroblasts are also frequently involved. The new glands are variable in size, often lined by hypertrophic tall columnar epithelium that is characteristically thrown into numerous papillary buds and infoldings. The gland formations are well-developed and are separated from each other by stroma, however scant. Numerous small foci of hyaline concretions, termed corpora amylacea, are nested within these glands. Aggregates of lymphocytes are commonly found within the stroma. Sometimes the hyperplasia is predominantly fibromuscular, and in these cases the nodules may appear microscopically as almost solid masses of spindle cells. Whether glandular or fibromuscular, small areas of ischemic necrosis surrounded by squamous metaplasia involving the glands may be seen within the nodules or in the surrounding prostatic tissue. In addition, squamous metaplasia of the periurethral glands, which may be mistaken for carcinoma, is a common accompaniment of nodular hyperplasia.

CLINICAL COURSE. The clinical significance of nodular hyperplasia lies entirely in its tendency to produce urinary tract obstruction by impinging on the urethra. Despite the prevalence of this disorder, however, not more than 10% of men with this condition require surgical relief of the obstruction. Early symptoms include difficulty in starting, maintaining, and stopping the stream of urine. There may also be frequency and nocturia, presumably because the raised level of the urethral floor leads to retention in the bladder of a large volume of residual urine after micturition. Hydronephrosis may ensue (see p. 466), as may infection, the all too frequent companion of obstruction. It had been suggested that patients with nodular hyperplasia of the prostate have a higher risk of developing cancer; however, current opinion does not favor this view.

CARCINOMA OF THE PROSTATE _____

Carcinoma of the prostate is an extremely common cancer. In 1991 approximately 122,000 new patients were diagnosed in the United States, of whom 32,000 are likely to succumb to their disease. It is the second leading cause of cancer death in males; only lung cancer kills more men. Prostate cancer is a disease of men over the age of 50, reaching a peak incidence around 75 years. In addition to these clinically evident tumors, many more latent, small foci of cancer are found incidentally at autopsy or on histologic examination of glands removed for nodular hyperplasia. As will be discussed later, most of these localized lesions progress so slowly that men who harbor them die of unrelated causes.

ETIOLOGY AND PATHOGENESIS. The etiologic influences responsible for carcinoma of the prostate are not definitely known. As with nodular hyperplasia, its incidence increases with age, and it is speculated that the endocrine changes of old age are related to its origin. Support for this general thesis lies in the inhibition of these tumors that can be achieved with orchiectomy. Neoplastic epithelial cells, like their normal counterparts, possess androgen receptors, which would suggest

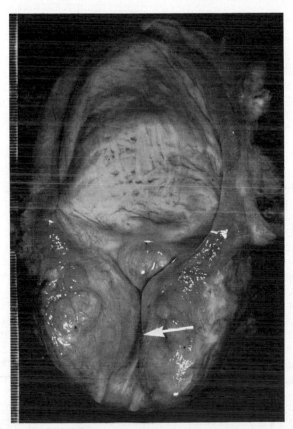

Figure 18–6. Nodular hyperplasia of the prostate. The urinary bladder and prostatic urethra have been opened. The enlargement of the prostate is seen as the two masses flanking the urethra *(arrow)*. A nodule projects under the floor of the bladder as a hemispheric mass.

that they are responsive to these hormones. However, no significant or consistent alterations in the levels or metabolism of the testosterone have been disclosed in any studies. It seems more likely, therefore, that the role of hormones in this malignancy is essentially permissive. Androgens are required for the maintenance of the prostatic epithelium, which is then transformed by agents not yet characterized.

Epidemiologic studies are of interest in seeking the cause of carcinoma of the prostate. The Scandinavian countries show a very high death rate from this form of cancer, whereas at the other extreme, Japanese are relatively free of the disease. The United States occupies an intermediate position. Immigrants from geographic areas of low-risk to areas of high-risk acquire an intermediate risk of developing this tumor, suggesting a role for environmental factors.

Genetic influences also seem to be involved, since there is a tendency toward familial aggregation and in the United States blacks are affected much more frequently than whites.

MORPHOLOGY. Prostate carcinoma usually begins in the peripheral zones of the prostate but can arise anywhere in the gland, usually in multiple foci, which fuse to form a single mass. Grossly, the tumor often blends imperceptibly into the background of the gland, although it may be apparent by its firm, gritty texture or by a somewhat yellower color than the surrounding tissue. Histologically, most of these lesions are adenocarcinomas of varying degrees of differentiation (Fig. 18–7). Stroma in between the glands is sometimes abundant and fibrous. This may be responsible for the hard (scirrhous) consistency. In well-differentiated tumors the acini are smaller than normal, closely spaced (back to back), and lined by a single layer of cuboidal epithelium. The neoplastic epithelium may be thrown into folds, which may fuse and give rise to a cribriform pattern. When gland formation is orderly, it may be difficult histologically to distinguish carcinoma of the prostate from nodular hyperplasia. In these cases, the distinction may rest on the presence of invasion of blood vessels, perineurial and perivascular spaces, or the prostatic capsule. In the undifferentiated tumors the malignant epithelial cells may diffusely infiltrate the stroma without any gland formation. Concomitantly, the cells display obvious cytologic features of malignancy. Several grading systems based on the degree of differentiation, glandular architecture, and extent of cellular atypia have been described. In general there is an excellent correlation between the degree of differentiation, anatomic extent (stage), and prognosis. Hence grading is of considerable value in the treatment of prostate cancer.

Prostate cancer spreads by direct extension and through lymphatics and veins. Local spread frequently involves the seminal vesicles and base of the urinary bladder. Extension into the rectal wall is rare. Metastases to the regional lymph nodes occur early and may often precede vascular spread. Osseous metastases

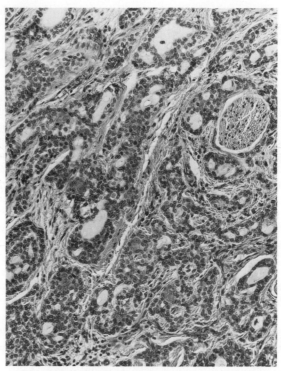

Figure 18–7. Carcinoma of the prostate. The neoplastic glands are small and disorderly and, at the upper right, have encircled and permeated a perineurial space.

constitute the most common form of hematogenous spread. Metastatic lesions in the bones, involving mainly the axial skeleton (pelvis, ribs, spine), may be osteoclastic (destructive) or, more commonly, osteoblastic (bone forming).

CLINICAL COURSE. The symptoms as well as prognosis depend on the anatomic extent and spread of the tumor. Four clinical stages (Table 18–3) are defined. As might be expected, stage A tumors are asymptomatic and discovered on histologic examination of prostatectomy specimens. The incidence of stage A cancers increases with age and approaches 60% or more in men past age 80. Owing to their slow rate of progression, stage A1 lesions are lethal in only a small percentage of patients. Stage A2 lesions, however, are more ominous, leading to death with distant metastases in 20% of untreated cases. Stage B prostate cancers are palpable by rectal digital examination. However, because of their peripheral location and small size, they do not encroach on the urethra, and hence urinary tract symptoms are absent. Approximately 80% of patients present with stage C or D. They usually have urinary symptoms such as dysuria, slow urinary stream, or urinary retention. Local pain in the perineum and rectum are late symptoms. Some patients in stage D may present initially with bone pain produced by osseous metastases.

Careful digital rectal examination is a simple, useful and direct method for detecting early prostatic carci

TABLE 18–3. STAGING OF PROSTATE CANCER*

Stage		Per Cent with Positive Lymph Nodes
A	*Incidental or clinically unsuspected cancer, detected in tissue removed for apparently benign disorders*	
	A1 Well-differentiated lesions occupying less than 5% of resected specimen	2
	A2 More than 5% of cancer in resected specimen or poorly differentiated lesion	23
B	*Tumors palpable by rectal digital examination but confined to prostate*	
	B1 Tumor confined to one lobe	18
	B2 Tumor extending to both lobes	35
C	*Tumors that have extended locally beyond the prostate but not produced clinically evident distant metastases*	
	C1 Tumor not involving seminal vesicles	50
	C2 Extensive periprostatic spread with involvement of seminal vesicles	80
D	*Tumors with distant metastases*	
	D1 Patients who are presumed to have stage A, B, or C disease clinically but are found to have pelvic lymph node metastases at surgery or by cytologic examination of aspirate	100
	D2 Clinical evidence of osseous or distant visceral spread	100

* Modified from Catalona, W. J.: Diagnosis, staging, and surgical treatment of prostatic carcinoma. Arch. Intern. Med. *147*:361, 1987. Other authors use slightly different criteria for staging.

noma, since the posterior location of most tumors renders them easily palpable. Transrectal ultrasonography is an important adjunct for early detection as well as assessment of local spread. A transperineal or transrectal needle biopsy can confirm the diagnosis. Osseous metastases may be detected by x-ray examination or the much more sensitive radionuclide bone scanning. *In males the finding of osteoblastic metastases in bone is virtually diagnostic of prostate cancer.*

Two biochemical markers, prostatic acid phosphatase and prostate-specific antigen, are of value in the diagnosis and management of prostate cancer. Both are produced by normal as well as neoplastic prostatic epithelium. Serum levels of prostatic acid phosphatase are elevated in patients whose tumor has extended beyond the capsule or metastasized, but it is not useful in the diagnosis of localized disease. Elevated blood levels of prostate-specific antigen occur in association with localized as well as advanced prostate cancer. Serum levels are also raised in benign prostatic hyperplasia, although to a lesser extent. However, when used along with rectal examination and/or ultrasonography, measurement of prostate-specific antigen levels is very useful in detection of early cancer. Furthermore, both tumor markers are of great value in following the progress of disease and response to treatment. Immunochemical localization of these markers is also very helpful in deciding whether a metastatic tumor originated in the prostate.

Cancer of the prostate is treated by surgery, radiotherapy, and hormonal manipulations. As might be expected, surgery and radiotherapy are most suited for treatment of patients with localized (stage A or B) disease. Eighty to 90% of patients in this group can expect to live for 10 years. Endocrine therapy is the mainstay for treatment of advanced metastatic carcinoma. Since prostatic cancer cells are dependent on androgens for their sustenance, the aim of endocrine manipulations is to deprive the tumor cells of testosterone. This is readily achieved by orchiectomy or administration of estrogens or synthetic agonists of luteinizing hormone–releasing hormone (LHRH). Estrogens suppress the secretion of pituitary luteinizing hormone (LH), which in turn leads to reduced testicular output of testosterone. Synthetic analogs of LHRH act similarly. Long-term administration of LHRH agonists (after an initial transient increase in LH secretion) suppresses LH release, achieving in effect a pharmacologic orchiectomy. Despite all the treatments, patients with disseminated cancers have a 10 to 40% ten-year survival rate.

VENEREAL DISEASE

The term "venereal disease" refers to disorders that are sexually transmitted. Historically, five classic venereal diseases have been recognized—syphilis, gonorrhea, chancroid, granuloma inguinale, and lymphogranuloma venereum. In the past decade, however, the spectrum of sexually transmitted disease (STD) has widened considerably (Table 18–4). A new group of syndromes primarily affecting homosexual men has emerged. These include infections by enteric pathogens such as *Entamoeba histolytica, Giardia lamblia,* and *Shigella* species, acquired probably by oral-anal contact. In addition, venereal transmission of viral infections such as hepatitis B is also becoming increasingly recognized. Acquired immunodeficiency syndrome (AIDS) has emerged as a major sexually transmitted disease. Epidemiologic studies have revealed a complex interrelationship between human immunodeficiency virus (HIV) infection and other STDs. On the one hand, a number of STDs, especially those associated with genital ulceration (e.g., chancroid, syphilis, genital herpes) facilitate sexual transmission of HIV. On the other hand, by suppressing host immunity HIV infection affects the clinical course of several STDs. For example progression from early syphilis to central ner-

TABLE 18–4. CLASSIFICATION OF IMPORTANT SEXUALLY TRANSMITTED DISEASES*

Pathogens	Disease or Syndrome and Population Principally Affected		
	Males	Both	Females
Viruses			
Herpes simplex virus		Primary and recurrent herpes, neonatal herpes	
Hepatitis B virus	Hepatitis		
Human papillomavirus (genital wart virus)	Cancer of penis (?)	Condyloma acuminatum	Cervical dysplasia and cancer, vulvar cancer
HIV		AIDS	
Chlamydiae			
Chlamydia trachomatis	Urethritis, epididymitis, proctitis	Lymphogranuloma venereum	Urethral syndrome, cervicitis, bartholinitis, salpingitis and sequelae
Mycoplasmas			
Ureaplasma urealyticum	Urethritis		
Bacteria			
Neisseria gonorrhoeae	Epididymitis, prostatitis, urethral stricture	Urethritis, proctitis, pharyngitis, disseminated gonococcal infection	Cervicitis, endometritis, bartholinitis, salpingitis and sequelae (infertility, ectopic pregnancy, recurrent salpingitis)
Treponema pallidum		Syphilis	
Haemophilus ducreyi		Chancroid	
Calymmatobacterium granulomatis		Granuloma inguinale (donovanosis)	
Shigella	†Enterocolitis		
Campylobacter	†Enterocolitis		
Protozoa			
Trichomonas vaginalis	Urethritis, balanitis		Vaginitis
Entamoeba histolytica	†Amebiasis		
Giardia lamblia	†Giardiasis		

* Modified and updated from Krieger, J. N.: Biology of sexual transmitted diseases. Urol. Clin. North Am. *11*:15, 1984.
† Most important in homosexual populations.

vous system involvement, which usually takes years, has been documented after an interval of months. In addition, diagnostic problems arise because HIV-infected persons with syphilis may have negative results of syphilis serologic tests, owing to suppressed humoral immunity (p. 161). Discussion of the entire range of venereal disease listed in Table 18–4 is beyond our scope. Some, such as hepatitis B, are discussed elsewhere (p. 532); others, such as Trichomonas vaginitis, do not cause serious morbidity and are not discussed.

GONORRHEA

With the possible exception of nongonococcal urethritis, gonorrhea is the most frequent of the venereal diseases. It affects approximately 2,000,000 Americans per year, with about 60% of reported cases occurring in males. Most infections occur in the 15- to 30-year age group; the peak is between 20 and 24 years of age.

The organism that causes gonorrhea is *N. gonorrhoeae,* a gram-negative diplococcus identical in appearance to the meningococcus. Much has been learned about the pathogenicity of the gonococcus. Successful invasion of the urogenital mucosa is aided by several cell wall components and occurs in two steps:

- *Attachment:* The ability to attach to epithelial cells is crucial to the pathogenicity and virulence of gono-

cocci. Such anchoring allows the bacteria to multiply in the genital tract despite the flow of mucus. Two components of the bacterial cell wall are believed to mediate adhesion: *pili,* which are seen as filamentous protrusions under the electron microscope, and one of the outer membrane proteins (p. 270). Because of the importance of pili in the pathogenicity of gonococci, pilus-associated proteins are considered to be promising candidates for vaccine development.

- *Mucosal invasion:* Following attachment, gonococci are internalized by a process resembling endocytosis. This is facilitated by an outer membrane protein that is distinct from that required for attachment. Once inside the cell, viable organisms sequestered in vacuoles are transported across the epithelium and discharged into the subepithelial space.

Several additional factors contribute to virulence and help the bacteria to evade host defenses. Gonococci release immunoglobulin A (IgA) proteases that serve to inactivate antibacterial IgA antibodies present in urethral and vaginal secretions. Like all other gram-negative bacteria, gonococci possess endotoxin, which decreases ciliary activity and damages the ciliated epithelial cells. Some membrane proteins inhibit the action of neutrophils; others render them resistant to the action of complement. Strains that can escape antibody- and complement-mediated lysis are particularly prone to systemic dissemination. Like the other pyogenic cocci, gonococci evoke a nonspecific, neutrophilic inflammatory reaction manifested by the production of copious amounts of yellow pus.

MORPHOLOGY. Two to seven days after exposure, the anterior urethra and meatus of the male become hyperemic and edematous and exude a mucopurulent material. At this stage the major symptoms are dysuria and increased frequency. Symptomatic men who seek treatment are easily cured and the disease does not progress any further. **Males with mild symptoms who fail to obtain treatment become the major reservoir of infection.**

Unless there is prompt and adequate therapy, gonorrhea tends to spread upward in the genital tract. In males, the prostate, seminal vesicles, and epididymides may become involved, producing marked perineal or scrotal pain and fever. The testes, however, are relatively resistant to gonococcal infection. Untreated gonococcal urethritis may lead to urethral strictures, sometimes leading to hydronephrosis and serious secondary pyelonephritis. Most of these complications are very uncommon in countries that have adequate health care delivery systems.

In the female, the initial involvement is in the urethra and the endocervical canal. Reddening and edema of the urethral meatus, however, is less conspicuous than in males. Bartholin's and Skene's glands are also involved early in the course of infection. The mature squamous epithelium of the vagina is resistant to infections, so vaginitis does not occur in adults, but newborns and infants may be susceptible. The symptoms of gonorrhea in the female reflect the involvement of the lower urogenital tract and include dysuria, vaginal discharge, and intermenstrual bleeding. As in the male, untreated gonorrhea tends to spread upward and in the female involves one or both fallopian tubes. Approximately 30% of women with gonorrhea develop salpingitis. The lumens of the affected oviducts become filled with purulent exudate, creating a **pyosalpinx** (pus tube). At first, the exudate may leak out of the tubal fimbriae, but often the fimbriae become sealed, sometimes against the ovary, producing a **salpingo-oophoritis.** As pus collects in these sealed tubes, they become distended, occasionally attaining a diameter of 10 cm or more. A localized pelvic peritonitis commonly is present, with a tendency toward formation of extensive adhesions. This pattern of inflammatory involvement in the female is known as **pelvic inflammatory disease (PID).** Since gonococcal salpingitis is just one of a number of causes of PID, this entity is also described in Chapter 19. Permanent sterility almost always results when gonorrhea is neglected in either sex.

In homosexual males, and less frequently in heterosexual males or females, anorectal and pharyngeal infections may be the initial site of infection.

Disseminated gonococcal infection (DGI), representing hematogenous spread, occurs in 1 to 3% of recently infected patients and can occur in two settings. Most often it occurs in women and is caused by strains of gonococci that are uniquely resistant to complement-mediated lysis by antibodies present in normal serum. The other affected group is persons who are genetically deficient in late-acting complement components C6, C7, and C8. Hematogenous seeding usually occurs during the menstrual period. The most common manifestation of disseminated disease is the **arthritis-dermatitis syndrome,** in which joint involvement takes the form of suppurative arthritis or tenosynovitis and skin lesions take the form of petechiae, pustules, or hemorrhages. Other manifestations of DGI include endocarditis and meningitis. A tragic complication of gonorrhea that has become rare, thanks to the use of prophylactic antibiotics, is gonococcal **ophthalmia neonatorum,** caused by contamination of an infant's eyes as it passes through the birth canal of its infected mother.

In summary, gonorrhea may be an asymptomatic infection or may produce local symptoms in the lower urogenital tract, which can be readily treated without any long-term sequelae. Approximately 80 to 90% of the cases remain uncomplicated in the United States. Local complication in the urogenital tract is uncommon but leads to serious morbidity. The spectrum of gonococcal infections is depicted in Figure 18–8. The diagnosis of gonorrhea rests on identification of typical gram-negative diplococci within the leukocytes in Gram-stained smears obtained from discharge or by culture. By these techniques almost 100% of the cases can be diagnosed.

Penicillin has been the mainstay of treatment for several decades, but owing to the increasing prevalence of penicillinase-producing gonococci other antibiotics are employed much more commonly.

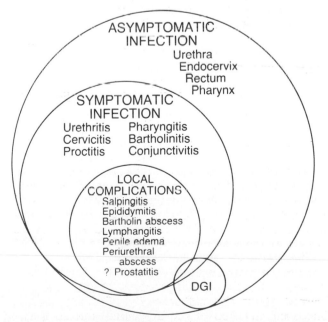

Figure 18–8. Clinical spectrum of gonococcal infection. DGI = disseminated gonococcal infection. (From Holmes, K. K., et al. [eds.]: Sexually Transmitted Diseases. 2nd ed. New York, McGraw-Hill Information Services Co., 1990, p. 152.)

NONGONOCOCCAL URETHRITIS (NGU) AND CERVICITIS

Among STDs, NGU, in males, and nongonococcal cervicitis, in females, are perhaps the most common of all. They mimic gonorrhea and must be distinguished from it because the treatment differs.

Various organisms have been implicated in the causation of these conditions. C. trachomatis, by far the most common culprit, can be identified in approximately 50% of cases. In males, U. urealyticum (a mycoplasma) is suspected to be the agent in some 30% of cases, but firm evidence is lacking.

It should be recalled that the chlamydiae are obligate intracellular bacteria (p. 263), but their life cycle distinguishes them from most other bacteria. They exist in two forms: the elementary body, which is the infectious extracellular particle, and the reticulate body, which represents the replicating intracellular phase of the organism. Chlamydiae require tissue culture techniques for isolation. The diseases caused by chlamydiae are listed in Table 18–5. Only the urogenital diseases caused by C. trachomatis are briefly described in this section. Lymphogranuloma inguinale is described later in this chapter (p. 605).

The clinical features of chlamydial NGU resemble those of gonococcal urethritis, already discussed; however, the symptoms are usually milder and serious complications are much less common. NGU, unlike gonorrhea, responds to tetracyclines but not to penicillin; this makes it important to distinguish between the two conditions.

Postgonococcal urethritis (PGU) refers to residual chlamydial infection in patients who have simultaneous gonococcal and C. trachomatis infection. It presents as persistent urethritis following successful treatment for gonorrhea or as recrudescence of symptoms after a brief asymptomatic period.

TABLE 18–5. HUMAN DISEASES CAUSED BY CHLAMYDIA

Chlamydia Species	Serotype	Disease
C. psittaci	Many unidentified serotypes	Psittacosis
C. trachomatis	L-1, L-2, L-3	Lymphogranuloma venereum
C. trachomatis	A, B, Ba, C	Endemic trachoma
C. trachomatis	D, E, F, G, H, I, J, K	Inclusion conjunctivitis (adult and newborn), NGU, cervicitis, salpingitis, proctitis, epididymitis, and pneumonia of newborns
C. pneumoniae	—	Community-acquired pneumonia in adults

From an epidemiologic point of view mucopurulent cervicitis is considered to be the equivalent of NGU in men. Most commonly it is asymptomatic but may be associated with a copious yellow mucopurulent discharge containing many neutrophils. As with gonococcal infections there may be associated urethritis. Much more ominous is ascending infection causing endometritis, salpingitis, pelvic inflammatory disease (PID), and their sequelae such as infertility and ectopic pregnancy.

Because of the significant overlap between the symptoms and signs of chlamydial and gonococcal infections it is essential to distinguish them by laboratory techniques. Gonococcal infection is readily established by demonstration of gram-negative diplococci within leukocytes and by culture. Positive identification of C. trachomatis is more involved. Chlamydiae can be cultured in mammalian cell lines, but this is a cumbersome and expensive technique that may not be available in all laboratories. Chlamydial antigens in secretions can be detected with monoclonal antibodies. Under appropriate clinical circumstances, antigen detection assays are quite sensitive and specific.

SYPHILIS (LUES)

Syphilis is far less common than gonorrhea, and efforts to control it have been more successful. Its incidence in the United States increased dramatically during World War II; then, with the advent of penicillin and the return to peacetime conditions, it declined to a low point in 1977. A resurgence involving mainly homosexual and bisexual males began in 1978 and reached a peak in 1982. The recognition that AIDS was predominantly an STD led to adoption of safer sex practices by homosexual men and resulted in a decline of new cases between 1982 and 1986. Unfortunately a precipitous increase began in 1987 among heterosexual men and women. This new epidemic is confined largely to urban areas and involves primarily the Hispanic and black populations. Epidemiologically it seems to be linked to illicit drug use (both parenteral and nonparenteral) and the associated increase in promiscuous sexual activity.

The causative organism of syphilis is the spirochete T. pallidum, which is transmitted primarily by venereal contact and, less commonly, by an infected mother to the fetus in utero. The extreme vulnerability of Treponema to drying probably precludes any other mode of transmission. These organisms can rapidly traverse intact mucous membranes and abraded skin, but little is known about their precise mechanism of toxicity. No toxins have been isolated and characterization of treponemal antigens has been seriously hampered by the inability to culture these bacteria in vitro. The immune responses and immune-mediated protection against syphilis have remained enigmatic. Those who develop an initial infection (primary syphilis) usually heal spontaneously and develop resistance to reinfections. Yet most of these apparently "resistant" individuals go on to develop disseminated (secondary) syphilis. The presence of a humoral immune response can be inferred from the appearance of two distinct antibodies in the serum: (1) a *nontreponemal antibody*, which by long tradition is called reagin, although it is not an IgE, and which reacts with a lipid antigen derived from beef heart (cardiolipin), and (2) *specific antibodies to treponemal antigens*. These antibodies are not protective, but their detection is an important step in the diagnosis of syphilis. The reaginic antibody is commonly detected by a flocculation test, called the VDRL (Venereal Disease Research Laboratory) test, and the rapid plasma reagin test. These tests are not specific, and there are a number of biologic false-positive (BFP) results with other disorders such as infectious mononucleosis, mycoplasma pneumonia, autoimmune diseases (e.g., systemic lupus erythematosus), and nearly any acute febrile illness. One method commonly used for detecting specific treponemal antibody is the fluorescent treponemal antibody (FTA) test. The FTA is based on indirect immunofluorescence. False-positive test results are relatively infrequent.

> **MORPHOLOGY.** Syphilis may affect nearly any organ or tissue in the body. **In all sites, it evokes one of two morphologic patterns of tissue injury.** One of these is a type of vasculitis, termed obliterative endarteritis, which is characterized by concentric endothelial and fibroblastic proliferative thickening of the small vessels in an involved area and a surrounding mononuclear (principally plasma cell) inflammatory infiltrate, known as perivascular cuffing.
>
> The second pattern of tissue injury, seen years after the initial infection, is a lesion known as a **gumma,** which, on occasion, may be difficult to distinguish from the lesions of tuberculosis. Gummas consist of a center of coagulative necrosis in which the native cells are barely discernible as shadowy outlines. This focus is surrounded by macrophages (some resembling epithelioid cells) admixed with mononuclear leukocytes (principally plasma cells) and enclosed by a fibroblastic wall. The small vessels in the enclosing inflammatory wall may show obliterative endarteritis and perivascular cuffing. With difficulty, treponemes may be demonstrated in the reactive inflammatory zone. Gummas are infrequent late lesions and may occur in any site of the body, most often in the liver, bones, and testes. They vary in size from microscopic defects to grossly visible tumorous masses of necrotic material. Erosion of a cutaneous or mucosal gumma may yield a persistent, shaggy ulcer that shows a surprising resistance to local therapeutic measures.

CLINICAL COURSE. *Clinically, acquired (untreated) syphilis is characterized by three fairly distinct stages,* which are discussed separately. The disease is infectious only in the first two stages. Congenital syphilis may be regarded as a fourth distinct entity.

Primary Syphilis. This stage is marked by the development of a *chancre* at the site of inoculation, usually on the penis or on the vulva or cervix, within a week to three months after exposure. Usually there is an accompanying painless, nonspecific regional lymphadenopathy. The primary chancre begins as a single indurated, button-like papule, up to several centimeters in diameter, which erodes to create a clean-based, shallow ulcer on an elevated base. The most distinctive histologic feature, deep within the base, is the obliterative endarteritis with perivascular plasma cell cuffing so characteristic of lues. The more superficial reaction consists of a nonspecific diffuse mononuclear leukocytic infiltrate. Although a systemic spirochetemia occurs within a day of infection and persists for several weeks, the patient feels well at this stage. The results of nontreponemal antibody tests are positive in approximately 25, 50, and 75% of the patients within the first, second, and third weeks, respectively. *Because the serologic test results may be negative in early cases, direct demonstration of the treponemes by dark-field examination of the exudate is extremely important in the diagnosis of primary syphilis.* The chancre slowly heals spontaneously. Approximately 50% of female patients and 30% of males do not notice the primary lesion.

Secondary Syphilis. One to three months after the development of the primary chancre, a *widespread patchy or diffuse mucocutaneous rash* ensues, accompanied by a generalized, nonspecific lymphadenopathy. Secondary syphilis results from hematogenous dissemination of the treponemes and the host response to their presence, primarily in the skin. The lesions that constitute the rash are extremely variable. Most commonly, they are bilaterally symmetric and maculopapular; each red-brown lesion is 5 to 10 mm in diameter. In other cases, however, follicular, pustular, annular, or scaling lesions may be seen. Histologically, the lesions show typical vasculitis, perhaps with a less marked mononuclear infiltrate, and spirochetes are present. In the external genital and anogenital regions the lesions may take the form of large, elevated plaques, designated *condylomata lata.* Constitutional symptoms such as fever, malaise, and weight loss may also be experienced. Hepatitis, arthritis, and meningeal involvement are seen in only a small minority of cases. By this stage serologic test results are positive in almost all patients.

Latent Syphilis. Virtually all untreated cases of secondary syphilis remit spontaneously within four to 12 weeks and enter a phase called *latent syphilis.* During this period patients are asymptomatic, but serologic markers of previous syphilitic infection remain positive. The outcome of latent syphilis is extremely variable. Some patients develop relapses of secondary syphilis; others remain asymptomatic for several years before they develop lesions characteristic of tertiary or late syphilis. Relapses of secondary syphilis usually occur within one year, a period referred to as *early latent syphilis.* During this phase patients are potentially infectious to sex partners. During early or late phase of latent syphilis, pregnant females may transmit the infection to their offspring, who are born with congenital syphilis. The vast majority, however, remain asymptomatic and never develop progressive disease.

Tertiary Syphilis. In only about a third of patients with untreated syphilis does the disease ever progress to this stage, and, of these, about half remain asymptomatic. Typically tertiary syphilis develops after a period of latency lasting from one to 30 years but in patients with AIDS the latent period may be much shorter. It may affect any part of the body, but it shows a predilection for the cardiovascular system (80 to 85%) and the central nervous system (5 to 10%). Cardiovascular syphilis and its complications are discussed on page 295. Other organs may be involved, singly or concurrently, giving rise to truly protean and often confusing clinical findings. In the liver, gummas may produce the coarsely nodular pattern of cirrhosis, termed *hepar lobatum* because of the simulation of multiple irregular lobes by the deep scars. Bone and joint gummas lead to areas of cortical and articular destruction. Pathologic fractures and joint immobilization may result. Testicular gummas often cause painless enlargement of the affected testis, thus simulating a tumor. In general, tertiary syphilis is becoming increasingly rare.

Congenital Syphilis. Syphilis may be transmitted to the fetus by an infected mother for a variable period of months to years after she contracts the disease, presumably until the spirochetemia has abated. Transmission may occur at any time during gestation, but the stigmata of congenital syphilis develop only in fetuses affected after the fourth month, when immune competence begins to develop. This suggests that the lesions of congenital syphilis result from the host response to the spirochetes. Depending on the magnitude of the infection, the fetus may die in utero or soon after birth or it may survive. Surviving infants usually show a widespread, rather fulminant infection with spirochetemia that differs from any of the classic stages of acquired syphilis. The most striking lesions affect the mucocutaneous surfaces and the bones. A diffuse maculopapular rash develops, which differs from that of acquired syphilis by its tendency to cause extensive desquamation of the skin. Generalized osteochondritis and perichondritis are present. Destruction of the vomer of the nose produces the characteristic *saddle deformity,* inflammatory proliferation of the anterior surface of the tibiae causes the typical anterior bowing of *saber shins,* and dental malformations create wedge-shaped notched incisors (hutchinsonian incisors) and "mulberry molars." A diffuse interstitial inflammatory reaction with prominent fibrosis may affect any organ of the body. In particular, the liver and lungs are frequently involved and can exhibit severe functional impairment. The eyes commonly show an interstitial keratitis or a choroiditis, and sometimes there are areas of abnormal pigmentation of the retina.

Occasionally, congenital syphilis remains latent until early adulthood and then simulates tertiary syphilis in its manifestations, with the formation of gummas and the frequent development of neurosyphilis.

PAPILLOMA (CONDYLOMA ACUMINATUM) _____

This STD takes the form of a benign tumor and is caused by human papillomavirus (subtypes 6 and 11). It is related to the common wart (verruca vulgaris) and may occur on any moist mucocutaneous surface of the external genitals of males or females. It should not be confused with the condyloma latum of secondary syphilis.

In males, most often the tumors are seen about the coronal sulcus and inner surface of the prepuce, and they range from minute sessile or pedunculated excrescences of 1 mm in diameter to large, raspberry-like masses several centimeters in diameter. Histologically, there is a villous connective tissue stroma covered by hyperplastic epithelium that shows perinuclear vacuolization (**koilocytosis**, p. 609). Such cells are characteristic of human papillomavirus infection. The basement membrane is intact, and there is no evidence of invasion of the underlying stroma. Malignant transformation to carcinoma of the penis, although reported in some cases, is uncommon.

CHANCROID, GRANULOMA INGUINALE, AND LYMPHOGRANULOMA VENEREUM _____

These are three distinct venereal diseases caused by three different infectious organisms. The diseases, however, are often confused because of their *common tendency to produce ulcerative lesions of the external genitalia and sometimes tender inflammatory swelling* (buboes) *of the inguinal lymph nodes.*

CHANCROID (SOFT CHANCRE). This is an acute process caused by the gram-negative coccobacillus *Haemophilus ducreyi.* It is characterized by the development of a necrotic ulcer at the site of inoculation on the genitals and by suppurative inflammation in the regional lymph nodes. Its incidence has been increasing steadily in the last few years. This disease is more common in males.

Within three to seven days after exposure, a small maculopapular lesion appears on the penis or vulva, followed over the next few days by rapid pustule formation and sloughing of the overlying skin, producing an ulcer between 1 and 3 cm in diameter. This bears a superficial resemblance to the chancre of syphilis, but unlike the syphilitic "hard chancre" it is painful and lacks induration. Histologically, the superficial necrotic debris covers a zone of granulation tissue and vasculitis, and this in turn overlies a zone of chronic inflammatory changes, with fibroblastic proliferation and mononuclear leukocytic infiltration. Often, autoinoculation produces multiple lesions. In about 50% of cases, within two weeks after the appearance of the ulcer the inguinal lymph nodes become enlarged and exquisitely tender. The histologic changes in the lymph nodes are essentially similar to those of the skin ulcer. There may be central abscess formation. Sometimes these abscesses drain to the surface.

Diagnosis is by tissue biopsy and identification of the organisms by culture. The course is usually self-limited, leaving only fibrous induration of the affected nodes and a scar at the site of the skin lesion.

GRANULOMA INGUINALE. In contrast to chancroid, this is a chronic rather than an acute process, caused by the gram-negative coccobacillus *Calymmatobacterium granulomatis*. It is distinctive in its tendency to produce large, irregular ulcers that form keloid-like scars upon healing. Lymph nodes are generally spared; however, the extensive scarring may eventually produce lymphatic obstruction, which results in elephantiasis of the external genitalia. Although the sexual partners of patients are not always affected, it is thought to be a venereal disease, possibly of relatively low infectivity.

The initial lesion is a papule at the site of inoculation, usually on the external genitalia, which develops into a spreading, necrotic ulcer with a raised inflammatory border. Microabscesses form in the advancing margin of the lesion, and satellite papules and ulcers may appear along the course of lymphatic drainage. The lesion is characterized histologically by nonspecific acute and chronic inflammation accompanied by an exuberant granulation tissue. The most distinctive finding is of large, vacuolated macrophages containing many faintly blue, "safety pin" like phagocytized organisms, termed Donovan bodies.

Diagnosis is by the demonstration of Donovan bodies, either in smears or in tissue biopsy specimens.

LYMPHOGRANULOMA VENEREUM (LYMPHOGRANULOMA INGUINALE). This disorder is caused by *C. trachomatis*. As seen in Table 18–5 (p. 602), lymphogranuloma venereum and NGU are caused by distinct serotypes of the same organism.

The disease is characterized by ulceration of the external genitalia, but in contrast to donovanosis there is prominent involvement of the lymph nodes. In most cases the genital ulcers are small and inconspicuous and the patients present initially with lymphadenopathy. Histologically, the lesions show a granulomatous reaction with central suppuration. In late stages the lymph nodes become matted and lymphatic obstruction leads to elephantiasis of the genitalia. The late sequelae tend to be much more serious in females. Whereas in males the nodal involvement remains limited to the inguinal region, in females vaginal or posterior perineal lesions lead to involvement of the perirectal and deep pelvic nodes. Such involvement produces chronic fibrosis about the rectum, with resultant rectal strictures.

Lymphogranuloma venereum, then, should be considered when rectal obstruction in the female is evaluated. The laboratory diagnosis depends on a complement fixation test. The Frei skin test is less sensitive and no longer widely used.

HERPES GENITALIS _____

Herpes genitalis is caused by the herpes simplex virus (HSV). Although most (75 to 80%) patients are infected by HSV type 2, some cases are caused by the closely related HSV-1, which is commonly associated with oral infections (p. 474). As such, genital herpes is the venereal counterpart of oral "fever blisters" or gingivostomatitis. Along with NGU, herpes genitalis is now an extremely common STD. Its prevalence correlates fairly closely with the sexual activity of the population under study. Three clinical forms are recognized. *First-episode primary herpes* refers to initial infection in persons who were not previously exposed to HSV, as indicated by lack of antibodies; *first-episode nonprimary herpes* occurs in seropositive patients with previous asymptomatic exposure; and *recurrent herpes* refers to reactivation of infection in patients with a history of symptomatic infection. All are associated with vesicular and ulcerative lesions; however, owing to the absence of any immunity, the lesions in the first-episode primary herpes are numerous, bilateral, and more painful; they are associated with tender inguinal lymphadenopathy and systemic signs such as fever, headache, and malaise. In contrast, nonprimary and recurrent lesions are less extensive and milder and systemic illness usually is not noted.

In both sexes herpetic lesions are found on the external genitalia. In women, the cervix is involved in more than 90% of the primary infections. Involvement of the urethra may also occur. Extragenital lesions, resulting from autoinoculation of the virus, may be found on the thighs, buttocks, or fingers. Proctitis may be the presenting feature in homosexual males. Grossly, the lesions appear as small vesicles, 1 mm or more in diameter, surrounded by marked erythema and edema. These rapidly rupture to form shallow ulcerations. *Histologically, the hallmark of the herpetic infection is the presence of multinuclear giant cells of epithelial origin that contain intranuclear inclusions.* Such cells are found in Papanicolaou smears, indicating herpetic cervicitis. The clinical manifestations of primary herpes genitalis last three to four weeks. *Recurrent* herpes genitalis is characterized by the periodic development of vesiculoulcerative lesions on an erythematous base. There is less edema and inflammatory response than with the primary disease, and the lesions disappear within a week to 10 days. More than 80% of the patients with HSV-2 genital herpes have one or more recurrences yearly for several years.

A grave complication of herpes genitalis in pregnant women is transmission to neonates. About 50% of pregnant women infected near the time of delivery transmit the infection (*neonatal herpes*) to newborns delivered vaginally. This is a severe, generalized disease that is often fatal.

Bibliography

Coffey, D. S., Walsh, P. C.: Clinical and experimental studies of benign prostatic hyperplasia. Urol. Clin. North Am. *17:*461, 1990. (An excellent discussion of the hormonal basis of benign prostatic hyperplasia.)

Gittes, R. F.: Carcinoma of the prostate. N. Engl. J. Med. *324:*236, 1991. (An up-to-date and concise presentation of the important aspects of prostate cancer.)

Hutchinson, C. M., Hook, E. W. III: Syphilis in adults. Med. Clin. North Am. *74:*1389, 1990. (A modern summary of this well-described disease.)

Jacobsen, G. K.: Pathology and cytochemistry of germ cell tumors. *In* Oliver, R. T. D., Blandy, J. P., Hope-Stone, H. F. (eds.): Urologic and Genital Cancer. Oxford, Blackwell Scientific Publications, 1989, p. 322. (A modern review of the histopathology of testicular germ cell tumors.)

Landy, H. J., Grossman, J. H.: Herpes simplex virus. Obstet. Gynecol. Clin. North Am. *16:*495, 1989. (A review of genital herpes in females.)

Martin, D. H.: Chlamydial infections. Med. Clin. North Am. *74:*1367, 1990. (A concise review of genitourinary chlamydial diseases: nongonococcal urethritis, cervicitis, and lymphogranuloma venereum.)

Osterling, J. E.: Prostate specific antigen: A critical assessment of the most useful tumor marker for adenocarcinoma of the prostate. J. Urol. *145:*907, 1991. (An extensive review of the chemistry and clinical utility of prostate-specific antigen.)

Stephens, D. S.: Gonococcal and meningococcal pathogenesis as defined by human cell, cell culture, and organ culture assays. Clin. Microbiol. Rev. *2:*S104, 1989. (A discussion of microbial factors that are responsible for the pathogenesis of gonorrhea.)

NINETEEN

Female Genital System and Breast

VULVA
VULVITIS
NON-NEOPLASTIC EPITHELIAL DISORDERS
CYSTS OF THE VULVA
TUMORS
    Condylomas
    Paget's Disease of the Vulva
    Carcinoma and Vulvar Intraepithelial Neoplasia

VAGINA

CERVIX
CERVICITIS
TUMORS OF THE CERVIX
    Polyps
    Carcinoma of the Cervix

BODY OF UTERUS
ENDOMETRITIS
ADENOMYOSIS
ENDOMETRIOSIS
DYSFUNCTIONAL UTERINE BLEEDING AND
ENDOMETRIAL HYPERPLASIA
    Dysfunctional Uterine Bleeding
    Endometrial Hyperplasia
TUMORS OF ENDOMETRIUM AND
MYOMETRIUM
    Endometrial Polyps
    Leiomyoma and Leiomyosarcoma
    Carcinoma of the Endometrium

FALLOPIAN TUBES

OVARIES
FOLLICLE AND LUTEAL CYSTS
POLYCYSTIC OVARIES
TUMORS OF THE OVARY
    Surface Epithelial – Stromal Tumors
        Serous Tumors
        Mucinous Tumors
        Endometrioid Tumors

        Cystadenofibroma
        Brenner Tumor
    Germ Cell Tumors
        Teratoma
        Dysgerminoma
        Choriocarcinoma
    Sex Cord – Stromal Tumors
        Granulosa-Theca Cell Tumors
        Fibroma
        Sertoli-Leydig Cell Tumors
        (Androblastomas)
    Clinical Correlations for All Ovarian Tumors
    Tumors Metastatic to the Ovary

DISEASES OF PREGNANCY
PLACENTAL INFLAMMATIONS AND INFECTIONS
ECTOPIC PREGNANCY
GESTATIONAL TROPHOBLASTIC DISEASE
    Hydatidiform Mole
    Invasive Mole
    Choriocarcinoma

BREAST
FIBROCYSTIC CHANGES
    Simple Fibrocystic Change: Cysts and Fibrosis
    Proliferative Fibrocystic Change
    Sclerosing Adenosis
    Relationship of Fibrocystic Changes to Breast
    Carcinoma
INFLAMMATIONS
TUMORS OF THE BREAST
    Fibroadenoma
    Phyllodes Tumor
    Intraductal Papilloma
    Carcinoma
MALE BREAST
    Gynecomastia
    Carcinoma

Vulva

The vulva is less frequently a site of disease than is the cervix, uterus, or ovary. The major pathologic changes of the vulva can be conveniently divided into the following categories: inflammatory disorders (vulvitis), epidermal hyperplasias or atrophy (dystrophy), cysts, and tumors (benign and malignant). The first three categories can be distressing to the patient because frequently they are associated with either intense itching or painful intercourse, but fortunately they are not life threatening. Malignant neoplasms, on the other hand, are uncommon but too often lethal. The only congenital anomaly worthy of mention is imperforate hymen; it may be unnoted until menstrual flow is impounded and collected within the vagina *(hematocolpos)* and the uterus *(hematometria).*

VULVITIS

The moist hair-bearing skin and delicate membrane of the vulva are vulnerable to many nonspecific microbe-induced inflammations and dermatologic disorders. Intense itching (pruritus) and subsequent scratching often exacerbates the primary condition. There are also many specific forms of microbial vulvitis related to the sexually transmitted diseases. These often evoke distinctive findings such as the suppurative infections of the vulvovaginal glands, caused by gonococci and other agents; the chancre of syphilis; the ulcerative infections of donovanosis, lymphogranuloma venereum (with its prominent lymphadenopathy), and chancroid; the characteristic gray-white curdy exudate of monilial infection; and the vesicular eruption of herpesvirus. Details on most of these venereal diseases are given on page 599.

NON-NEOPLASTIC EPITHELIAL DISORDERS (VULVAR DYSTROPHIES)

The epithelium of the vulvar mucosa may undergo atrophic thinning or hyperplastic thickening. For want of a better term, these alterations were collectively referred to as *dystrophies* but are now simply referred to as *non-neoplastic epithelial disorders* (NNED) to differentiate them from the premalignant dysplasias discussed later. All variants may appear macroscopically as depigmented white lesions, referred to in the past as *leukoplakia.* However, similar white patches or plaques are seen with (1) vitiligo (loss of pigment) of the skin, (2) a variety of benign dermatoses such as psoriasis and lichen planus, (3) carcinoma in situ, (4) Paget's disease (described later), and (5) invasive carcinoma. Thus *leukoplakia is merely a descriptive term that gives no indication of its underlying nature.* Only biopsy and microscopic examination can differentiate among these similar-looking lesions.

Other than the inflammatory dermatoses and infections, two varieties of NNED need to be considered: *lichen sclerosus,* a characteristic disorder manifested by epithelial thinning and subepithelial fibrosis, and *squamous hyperplasia,* characterized by epithelial hyperplasia and hyperkeratosis. The two forms may coexist in different areas of the vulva.

LICHEN SCLEROSUS. Lichen sclerosus occurs in all age groups but is most common in postmenopausal women. These epithelial alterations may also be encountered elsewhere on the skin. The pathogenesis is unknown. The changes are thinning of the epidermis and disappearance of rete pegs accompanied by dermal fibrosis with a scant perivascular, mononuclear inflammatory cell infiltrate (Fig. 19–1). Macroscopically, the lesions appear as smooth, white plaques or papules that in time may extend and coalesce. The surface of the lesions appears smoothed out and sometimes parchment-like. When the entire vulva is affected, the labia become somewhat atrophic and stiffened and the vaginal orifice constricted.

SQUAMOUS HYPERPLASIA. Previously called "hyperplastic dystrophy," this lesion constitutes hyperplasia of the squamous epithelial lining, frequently with hyperkeratosis. The epithelium is thickened and may show increased mitotic activity in both the basal and prickle cell layer. Leukocytic infiltration of the dermis is sometimes pronounced. The hyperplastic epithelial changes show no atypia, but if they do, the current trend is to consider the lesions as *dysplasia* (p. 610).

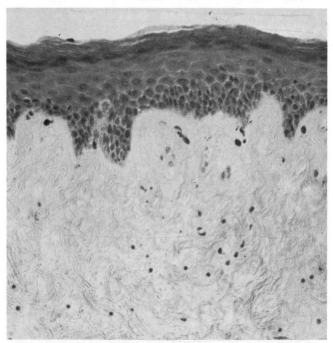

Figure 19–1. Lichen sclerosus illustrating atrophy of epidermis and dense sclerosis of dermis with total atrophy of dermal adnexal structures. (Courtesy of Dr. Arthur Hertig.)

CYSTS OF THE VULVA _____

Cysts, sometimes multiple, may arise in the subclitoral or periurethral areas or in the regions of Bartholin's glands of the vulva in women of any age. More often they occur as single lesions, usually in relation to Bartholin's glands. Those that arise in the Bartholin's glands or their excretory ducts may reach a diameter of 5 cm and are most often the result of obstruction of one of the major excretory ducts and subsequent progressive accumulation of mucinous secretion. Such cysts are lined by either the transitional or cuboidal epithelium of the ducts, which may become markedly flattened or almost disappear, owing to the intracystic pressure. Besides causing local pain and discomfort, these cysts are vulnerable to secondary infection, producing a *Bartholin's abscess.* Cysts in other locations are thought to arise from embryonic rests; they are generally small (1 to 2 cm diameter) and are lined by columnar to cuboidal mucinous or ciliated epithelium that occasionally undergoes metaplastic change into squamous epithelium. Not having connections with the vulvar vestibule, these cysts rarely become infected.

TUMORS _____

CONDYLOMAS _____

Condylomas are essentially anogenital warts, but in the moist environment of the vulva they tend to be large. Most fall into two distinctive biologic forms, but rarer types also exist. *Condylomata lata,* rarely seen today, are flat, moist, minimally elevated lesions that occur in secondary syphilis. The more common *condylomata acuminata* may be papillary and distinctly elevated or somewhat flat and rugose. They occur anywhere on the anogenital surface, sometimes singly but more often in multiple sites. On the vulva they range from a few millimeters to many centimeters in diameter and are red-pink to pink-brown. The histologic appearance of these lesions was described earlier (p. 604), but *particularly significant is the characteristic cellular morphology, namely perinuclear cytoplasmic vacuolization with nuclear angular pleomorphism— koilocytosis (Fig. 19–2). Such cells are considered to be hallmarks of human papillomavirus (HPV) infection.* Indeed, there is a strong association with at least two genotypes (6 and 11) of the HPV, closely related to the virus causing common warts. The HPV can be transmitted venereally; identical lesions occur in men on the penis and around the anus. Vulvar condylomas are not precancerous but may coexist with foci of intraepithelial neoplasia in the vulva and cervix. As discussed later (p. 610), the genotypes of HPV isolated from the cancers differ from those most often found in condylomas.

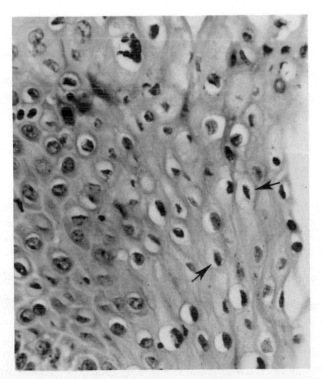

Figure 19–2. A high-power detail of koilocytes with cytoplasmic clearing and striking angulated nuclear pleomorphism *(arrows).*

PAGET'S DISEASE OF THE VULVA _____

Vulvar Paget's disease is a rare form of intraepithelial carcinoma that is analogous to the more common Paget's disease of the breast (p. 639) and so is often referred to as "extramammary Paget's disease." It sometimes extends into the perianal region. Clinically, it presents as an indurated or nodular, fairly well-defined area of varying shades of red, usually on the labia majora. Sometimes the lesions have a scaling or even eroded surface. This appearance invites the misdiagnosis of dermatitis. Only infrequently can a small underlying tumor be palpated. *The histologic hallmarks of Paget's disease in all locations are large anaplastic cancer cells lying singly or in small clusters within the epidermis (Paget's cells). These anaplastic cells have perinuclear cleared cytoplasm (produced by vacuoles of periodic acid–Schiff [PAS]-positive polysaccharides), creating the appearance of a halo around the nucleus* (Fig. 19–3). Sometimes these cells extend down into the intraepithelial segments of the secretory ducts of the adnexal appendages, but in most cases the tumor cells are restricted to the epidermis, and indeed may persist in this location for decades without invading the dermis. Such lesions are amenable to curative resection, but because of lateral intraepithelial spread, recurrence may follow incomplete removal. Infrequently they become invasive. In a few cases there is a well-defined small cancer of apparently apocrine- or sweat gland origin that underlies the epidermis. *When there is well-defined invasion or a subepithelial tumor, the prognosis is poor.*

The origin of Paget's cells in the vulva remains unclear, but they are thought to arise from primitive intraepithelial precursors capable of differentiation along multiple cell lines.

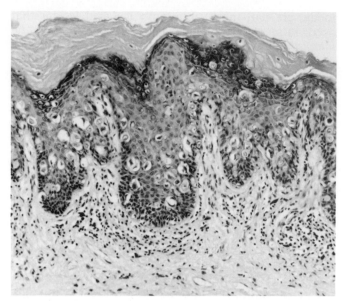

Figure 19-3. Paget's disease of the vulva, showing the intraepithelial cancer cells accentuated by their cleared "halos."

CARCINOMA AND VULVAR INTRAEPITHELIAL NEOPLASIA (DYSPLASIA)

Carcinoma of the vulva, an uncommon malignancy, represents about 3% of all genital cancers of females. Eighty-five per cent are squamous cell carcinomas and the remainder basal cell carcinomas, melanomas, or adenocarcinomas.

Frequently, the squamous cell carcinomas are preceded by atypical epithelial proliferations called vulvar dysplasia or vulvar intraepithelial neoplasia (VIN). These are characterized by nuclear and epithelial atypia, increased mitoses, and lack of surface differentiation. The spectrum of dysplastic changes ranges from mild dysplasia (VIN I), to moderate dysplasia

(VIN II), to severe dysplasia and *carcinoma in situ* (VIN III). Carcinoma in situ, called Bowen's disease by dermatologists, is an intraepithelial squamous cell carcinoma that presents as either white (leukoplakia) or dark lesions. Identical lesions are encountered in the male (p. 589).

The lesions of VIN are maculopapular, white, and in 70% of patients multicentric. The incidence of VIN is increasing particularly in younger women. About 30% coexist with foci of in situ or invasive *cervical* or *vaginal carcinoma,* suggesting a common carcinogen. HPV (types 16, 18, and others) is present in about 90% of cases of VIN, whether in situ or invasive. VIN uncommonly progresses to invasive carcinoma and then principally in those who are elderly or immunosuppressed.

> Any region of the vulva may be affected by VIN or carcinoma. Carcinomas begin as small areas of epithelial thickening, but in the course of time progress to firm, indurated, **exophytic** tumors or ulcerated and endophytic lesions. Histologically, most cancers are well-differentiated squamous cell carcinomas, with the formation of keratohyaline pearls and prickle cells. The tumors infiltrate locally and tend to metastasize at a relatively early stage to the regional nodes. Such nodal metastasis is correlated more with the size and age of the lesion than with the degree of differentiation of the squamous cell growth. Ultimately, lymphohematogenous dissemination involves the lungs, liver, and other internal organs.

The clinical manifestations evoked are chiefly pain, local discomfort, itching, and exudation, because superficial secondary infection is common. Lesions less than 2 cm in diameter are associated with a 60 to 80% five-year survival rate after treatment; larger lesions with lymph node involvement with less than a 10% five-year survival rate.

Vagina

The vagina of the adult is seldom the site of primary disease. More often, it is secondarily involved in the spread of cancer or infections arising in close proximity (e.g., cervix, vulva, bladder, rectum). The only primary disorders that merit brief comment are a few congenital anomalies, vaginitis, and primary tumors.

Congenital anomalies of the vagina are fortunately uncommon—entities such as total absence of the vagina, a septate or double vagina (usually associated with a septate cervix and, sometimes, uterus), and congenital small lateral *Gartner's duct cysts* arising from persistent embryonic remnants.

Vaginitis—inflammation of the vaginal mucous membrane that often involves the cervix and vulva—

is by far the most common primary disorder of the vagina. It occurs mainly in infants or in young women during active reproductive life. These infections account for about 5 to 10% of patient visits to gynecologists. The most common causes are cited in Table 19-1. Any of these agents, most notably herpes simplex virus (HSV), HPV, and chlamydia (a frequent cause of urethritis in males), can be sexually transmitted. But many of the agents, such as the candidal species and *Trichomonas gardnerella,* are normal inhabitants of the vagina; *Candida* organisms, for example, can be found in about a third of apparently healthy women. Thus it is uncertain whether an attack of monilial vaginitis implies sexual transmission of

TABLE 19–1. CAUSES OF VAGINITIS*

Causes	Comments
In Newborns	
Neisseria gonorrhoeae	Now uncommon because of postdelivery prophylaxis
In Infants and Young Children	
N. gonorrhoeae	May be epidemic in nurseries, schools—indirect spread by contaminated articles
In Young Adults	
Common agents:	
Gardnerella vaginalis	Normal commensal—may require mixed flora
Trichomonas vaginalis	Normal commensal—may require predisposing influence
Candida spp.	Normal commensal—may require predisposing influence
Less common agents:	
Chlamydia trachomatis	
Mycoplasma hominis	
Herpesvirus type II	Associated vesicular genital herpes
Human papillomavirus	Associated condylomata
Staphylococci (exotoxic strains)	Toxic shock syndrome (rash, fever, hypotension, multisystem involvement)

* From Cotran, R. S., Kumar, V., Robbins, S. L.: Robbins Pathologic Basis of Disease. 4th ed. Philadelphia, W. B. Saunders, 1989.

new strains to which prior immunity is lacking or instead reflects accentuation of some predisposing influence (e.g., diabetes mellitus, marked sexual activity, pregnancy, exposure to broad-spectrum antibiotics or oral contraceptives).

Although most attacks of vaginitis are more uncomfortable than serious, some have particular importance. Herpetic infections of the genital tract may lead to serious infections in the newborn. The toxic shock syndrome (rash, fever, hypotension, multisystem involvement) has been traced (most often) to the growth of exotoxin-producing strains of staphylococci that flourish in certain types of vaginal tampons saturated with menstrual flow. It should be noted that *Neisseria gonorrhoeae* is not responsible for primary vaginitis in adults because the mature vaginal mucosa is resistant

to this pathogen. Nonetheless (as has been detailed on p. 599), it often induces suppurative inflammation involving vulvar and endocervical glands and so may produce a vaginal discharge that must be differentiated from primary vaginitis. In newborns and infants it can cause suppurative vulvovaginitis.

Whatever the causative agent, the local changes consist of erythema and sometimes superficial erosions of the vaginal mucosa. The clinical symptoms are nonspecific and include excessive vaginal discharge (sometimes purulent—leukorrhea), itching, and localized discomfort. Although certain features of the infection may be clinically distinctive, such as the vesicular eruption of herpes in the vagina and on the vulva, the curdy white exudate of candidiasis, and the sometimes frothy yellow-green exudation of trichomoniasis, the differential diagnosis ultimately depends on identification of the causative agent.

Specific infections may also occur in postmenopausal women, but nonspecific vaginitis is more common because atrophy of the vaginal mucosa, secondary to diminished estrogen function, induces increased vulnerability.

Neoplasms are fortunately rare. Among these rarities, *squamous cell carcinoma* is most common. Of particular interest is the vaginal *clear cell adenocarcinoma*, encountered usually in girls in their late teens whose mothers had taken diethylstilbestrol during pregnancy. Sometimes these cancers do not appear until the third or fourth decade of life. The overall risk is one per thousand or less of those exposed in utero. In about a third of the instances these cancers arise in the cervix. Much more frequently, perhaps in one third of the population at risk, small glandular or microcystic inclusions appear in the vaginal mucosa—*vaginal adenosis*. These benign lesions appear as red granular foci and are lined by mucus-secreting or ciliated columnar cells. It is from such inclusions that the rarer clear cell adenocarcinoma arises.

Sarcoma botryoides, producing soft polypoid masses, is another fortunately rare form of primary vaginal cancer that is encountered usually in infants and children before age five. It is basically a subtype of rhabdomyosarcoma, which may occur in other sites, such as the urinary bladder and bile ducts.

Cervix

The cervix lives a troubled life: it must serve as a barrier to the ingress of air and the microflora of the vagina yet must permit the escape of menstrual flow and sustain the mild buffeting of intercourse and the trauma of childbirth. No small wonder it is often the seat of disease. Fortunately, most of its lesions are relatively banal inflammations—cervicitis—but it also is the site of one of the most common cancers in

women—squamous cell carcinoma, which is responsible for 2 to 5% of all cancer deaths.

CERVICITIS

Inflammations of the cervix are extremely common. Traditionally, they have been divided into specific infections (those caused by the agents responsible for the sexually transmitted diseases, discussed on p. 599) and nonspecific infections (those caused by all other organisms, many of which are normal inhabitants of the vagina). Among the specific pathogens *Chlamydia trachomatis* has replaced the gonococcus as the leading cause of specific cervicovaginal infections. Infectious cervicitis is pivotal to the spread of sexually transmitted diseases by ascending infection to the uterus and ovaries and by vertical transmission through the placenta to the fetus.

Much more common is the relatively banal *nonspecific cervicitis,* which is present to some degree in almost every multiparous woman. Although this baffling infection is known to be associated with a variety of organisms and factors (trauma of childbirth, hormonal imbalances), its pathogenesis is poorly understood.

Nonspecific cervicitis may be either **acute** or **chronic.** Excluding gonococcal infection, which causes a specific form of acute disease, the relatively uncommon **acute nonspecific** form is limited to postpartum women and is usually caused by staphylococci or streptococci. The **chronic** form is the nearly ubiquitous entity usually referred to by the unqualified term "nonspecific cervicitis."

Grossly, chronic cervicitis appears as a reddening, swelling, and granularity around the margins of the external cervical os. Histologically, the infiltration is largely mononuclear. Inflammatory stenosis of the cervical glands may yield cystic dilatations designated as **nabothian cysts.**

The cervical epithelium may show hyperplasia and **reactive atypia,** characterized by epithelial disorganization and nuclear alterations not to be confused with the changes of dysplasia. In the course of these changes, the epithelial cells are depleted of their normal content of glycogen.

In certain cases, in the region of the external os, tongues of stratified squamous epithelium may extend down from the surface mucosa into the endocervical glands. These changes are designated **squamous metaplasia of endocervical glands.**

Nonspecific chronic cervicitis commonly comes to attention on routine examination or because of marked leukorrhea. When the lesion is severe, differentiation from carcinoma may be difficult even with colposcopy and may require a biopsy. Cervicitis per se is not a precancerous lesion, but the secondary epithelial dysplastic changes may constitute a favorable subsoil for carcinogenic influences such as viruses (p. 613). Severe cervicitis may lead also to sterility through deformation and exudative blocking of the cervical os while simultaneously producing an unfavorable environment for sperm.

TUMORS OF THE CERVIX

Although a wide variety of tumors may develop in the cervix uteri, all are rare except the relatively unimportant polyp and squamous cell neoplasia and its sometimes accompanying condylomas.

POLYPS

Although *polyps* occur in 2 to 5% of adult females they are innocuous, occasionally being important as a cause of abnormal bleeding that must be differentiated from that due to more ominous causes.

These lesions typically arise within the endocervical canal. They may be sessile, hemispheric masses or pedunculated, spherical lesions up to 3 cm in diameter. Those with long stalks may be seen on clinical examination, hanging down through the exocervical os and causing dilatation of the cervix. Characteristically, cervical polyps are soft, almost mucoid. Their histologic nature is that of a loose fibromyxomatous stroma containing cystically dilated endocervical glands. Although the covering epithelium is usually columnar and secretes mucus, superimposed chronic inflammation may lead to squamous metaplasia and ulcerations.

CARCINOMA OF THE CERVIX

The decline in the number of deaths caused by cancer of the cervix in the United States and in other developed nations is a dramatic and gratifying testament to the benefits of early diagnosis. Once one of the leading causes of cancer death, cervical cancer now ranks seventh or eighth among the killer cancers of females in the United States, causing about 4000 deaths yearly, according to a 1991 estimate. In sharp contrast, there are still more than 13,000 new cases of invasive cancer and 50,000 of carcinoma in situ every year. It is evident that *well over half of invasive cancers are cured by effective therapy and, even more important, most lesions are discovered while still in situ and amenable to eradication by timely and appropriate treatment.* These dramatic gains in discovery and treatment are owed largely to the effectiveness of the Papanicolaou cytologic test in detecting cervical carcinoma during its incipiency and by the fortuitous accessibility of the cervix to colposcopy and biopsy. The widespread application of the "Pap smear" in mass screening programs and in routine physical examinations, followed by biopsy to evaluate and confirm abnormal cytologic findings, has documented that carcinoma of the cervix arises in a series of incremental epithelial changes ranging from progressively more severe dysplasia (also called *cervical intraepithelial neoplasia* [CIN]) to invasive carcinoma.

INCIDENCE AND EPIDEMIOLOGY. Both in situ and invasive carcinomas are diagnosed now at younger ages than in past decades. Indeed, CIN is now being discovered in teenagers and young adults! The peak incidence is at about 30 years of age. Similarly, invasive carcinoma is now appearing as early as the third decade of life with a peak incidence at about age 40 (i.e., about 10 to 15 years later). Deaths begin in the fourth decade, and the mortality rate rises throughout life. Only a few decades ago, all of these unfortunate events were delayed at least 10 years, strongly suggesting that oncogenic influences (as will be noted later) are now at work earlier in life.

Many risk factors for cervical carcinoma have been identified. Among them, the following are most important:

● Early age at first intercourse
● Multiple sexual partners
● High-risk male sexual partners—i.e., those who are promiscuous, who have a former wife with cervical cancer, or who have a history of penile condylomas.

All other risk factors can be related to these three influences, such as the higher incidence of cervical carcinoma in lower socioeconomic groups, the higher incidence among married women (increasing with the number of marriages and children), the rarity of cervical carcinoma in virgins, and the high incidence in prostitutes. No longer considered significant risk factors are cigarette smoking, birth control pills, vague agents in semen, and lack of circumcision in the male sexual partner (implicating some putative carcinogen in smegma).

ETIOLOGY AND PATHOGENESIS. The epidemiology of cervical cancer strongly suggests sexual transmission of an oncogen, and particularly incriminated is HPV (Fig. 19–4). This virus is known to cause the venereally transmitted vulvar condyloma acuminatum and is suspected to be an oncogenic agent in squamous cell tumors of skin and mucous membranes. DNA sequences of HPV are detected in 75 to 100% of patients with cervical condylomas, precancerous cervical dysplasia, and invasive carcinoma.

The cervical condylomas can be verrucous, like those of the vulva, but much more often they are flat lesions (flat condylomas). Although there is overlap in the HPV types present in various lesion, *HPVs 6 and 11 (low-risk HPVs)* are found most frequently in condylomas associated with the typical viral changes of *koilocytosis* (p. 609). In contrast, lesions exhibiting epithelial atypia (carcinoma and high-grade dysplasia) contain *HPVs 16, 18, and 31 (high-risk HPVs)*.

The precise reasons for the difference in oncogenicity between low- and high-risk HPVs are still unclear. Currently it is thought that the low-risk HPVs lead to productive infection associated with unintegrated episomal viral DNA, characterized by cell proliferation, cell maturation, koilocytosis, and other features distinctive of condylomas. High-risk HPVs are associated with a greater proportion of viral DNA becoming integrated into the host genome, but it is not clear that this property correlates with malignant transformation. Current interest is in the interaction of the proteins encoded by the E6 and E7 open reading frames of these high-risk HPV types with p53 and the retinoblastoma gene product, respectively. The p53 gene and the retinoblastoma gene, as you recall (p. 190), are tumor suppressor genes involved in oncogenesis.

Although the evidence is persuasive, it is, of course, incomplete, and all the associations cited might be independent consequences of promiscuity or may indeed follow the earliest precancerous lesion. In this manner these viruses may act in concert with other carcinogens (co-carcinogens) to give rise to cervical carcinoma. Co-carcinogens could be other viruses, such as HSV type II (which is known to occur with high frequency in patients with cervical cancer), and other environmental agents.

Although the cause of cervical carcinoma is still uncertain, there is agreement that this form of cancer is derived from dysplastic epithelial changes or CIN. These changes begin with *mild dysplasia (grade I CIN)* either in the usual cervical epithelium or in a *flat condyloma* marked by koilocytotic changes. The dysplasia becomes more disorderly and may be associated with some variation in cell and nuclear size and with normal-looking mitoses above the basal layer of either the usual cervical mucosa or flat condyloma; this stage is designated *moderate dysplasia (grade II CIN)*. The superficial layer of cells is still well-differentiated but in some cases shows koilocytotic changes. The next step in the sequence is *severe dysplasia (grade III CIN)*, marked by greater variation in cell and nuclear size, disorderly orientation, hyperchromasia, and mitoses, normal or abnormal, sometimes near the surface layer (Fig. 19–5). Differentiation of surface cells and koilocytotic changes have usually disappeared or are found very uncommonly. In grade III CIN the atypical epithelium has not invaded the underlying stroma but may extend into endocervical glands; this stage represents *carcinoma in situ*. The next stage is invasive

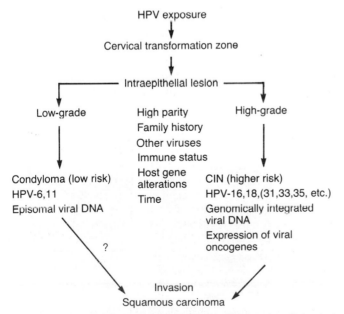

Figure 19–4. Postulated steps in the pathogenesis of cervical neoplasia. The conditions listed *(center)* are possible risk factors for cancer. (Courtesy of Christopher Crum, M. D., Brigham and Women's Hospital, Boston.)

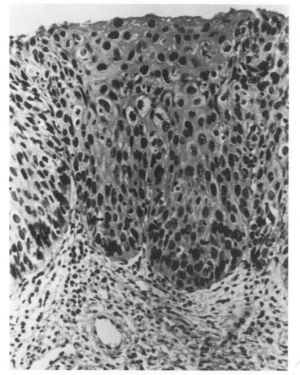

Figure 19-5. Focus of carcinoma in situ of the cervix (CIN grade III) shows markedly atypical cells that occupy the full thickness of the epithelium. (Courtesy of Dr. D. Antonioli, Beth Israel Hospital, Boston.)

cancer (Fig. 19-6). Sequential biopsies and the epidemiologic data cited earlier document that the progression from mild dysplasia to carcinoma in situ to invasive cancer evolves slowly over the span of many years (10 to 15). *The rates of progression, however, are by no means uniform, and in general, it is difficult, if not impossible, for a clinician using any technique to predict the outcome in an individual patient.* Careful follow-up is the only recourse. Regression does occur, but only in very mild lesions and flat condylomas.

Epithelial atypicalities and carcinoma of the cervix almost always begin at or close to the squamocolumnar junction of the external os. **In the CIN stages no changes are visible to the naked eye,** but atypical cells can be detected by cytologic examination in most cases. In addition, colposcopy provides a magnified look at the cervix and often reveals abnormal areas not visible to the naked eye. Foci of epithelial changes can also be rendered more apparent by either painting the cervix with iodine solution—the Schiller test (the normal mucosa stains red-brown owing to the glycogen content of the cells but the atypical cells are glycogen depleted and appear pale)—or with dilute acetic acid, which for unknown reasons renders abnormal foci pale white. Ultimately, biopsy is required and histologic examination reveals changes that range from mild dysplasia to carcinoma in situ, as has been amply detailed.

Invasive carcinoma takes one of three distinct macroscopic forms. The most frequent is a **fungating** tumor, which begins as a nodular thickening of the epithelium and eventually appears as a cauliflower-like mass projecting above the surrounding mucosa, sometimes completely encircling the external os (Fig. 19-7). The second is an **ulcerative** form, characterized by sloughing of the central surface of the tumor. The least frequent variety is **infiltrative,** which tends to grow downward into the underlying stroma rather than outward. With time these forms tend to merge as they infiltrate the underlying tissue, obliterate the external os, grow upward into the endocervical canal and lower uterine segment, and eventually extend into and through the wall of the fundus into the broad ligaments. Advanced lesions may extend into the rectum or base of the urinary bladder, sometimes to obstruct one or both ureters. Only relatively late is there involvement of lymph nodes or distant metastases. Distant metastases, when present, usually affect the lungs, bones, and liver.

The histologic character of 95% of carcinomas of the cervix is that of a typical **squamous cell carcinoma** of varying differentiation. The remaining 5% are **adenocarcinomas,** presumably arising in the endocervical glands or mixed squamous and adeno- forms, termed **adenosquamous carcinomas.**

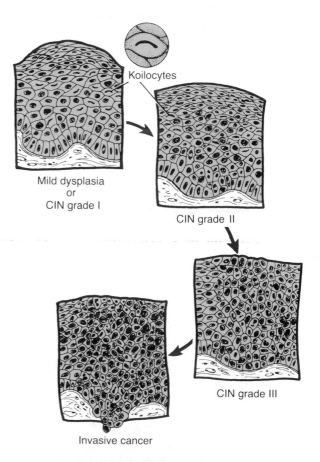

Koilocytes

Mild dysplasia
or
CIN grade I

CIN grade II

CIN grade III

Invasive cancer

CIN = Cervical intraepithelial neoplasia

Figure 19-6. Representation of the progressive evolution of dysplasia (CIN) to invasive carcinoma of the cervix.

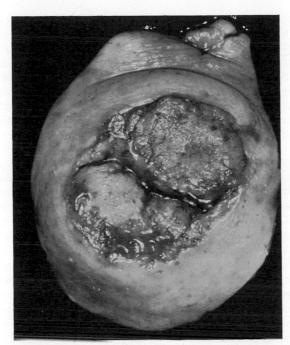

Figure 19–7. Carcinoma of the cervix, well advanced.

Both a grading system, based on the degree of cellular differentiation, and a staging system, based on tumor spread, have been devised. Grades I through III refer to progressively less differentiated lesions. The details of the currently used staging system are beyond our needs. In brief, it recognizes stage 0—carcinoma in situ—and then stages 1 to 4, based on whether the carcinoma is strictly confined to the cervix (stage 1) or has extended beyond the cervix ultimately to reach

stage 4, marked by extension beyond the uterus into the pelvis and by involvement of adjacent organs or metastatic dissemination.

CLINICAL COURSE. Results of a Pap smear may first become abnormal with mild dysplasia in asymptomatic teenagers or young adults. Even frank carcinoma in situ is usually asymptomatic except possibly for the presence of some leukorrhea, which is more often related to concurrent cervicitis or vaginitis. The cervix may still appear normal to the naked eye, but colposcopy and the Schiller or acetic acid test may disclose an abnormal area. When invasive carcinoma appears, usually in the fourth or fifth decade of life or sometimes later, it is often associated with irregular vaginal bleeding, leukorrhea, painful coitus, and dysuria. Biopsy is always necessary to confirm the cytologic findings and to evaluate the depth of penetration of the lesion.

The mortality from this form of cancer is more often related to its local effects (i.e., obstruction of the ureters or penetration into the bladder or rectum) than to distant metastases. Death from this disease is a particularly lamentable tragedy because at least a decade elapses between the in situ and invasive stages providing ample opportunity for early diagnosis. Neither is there any need for hasty ill-considered treatment. If the interpretation of a biopsy is in doubt, there is time to permit the lesion to declare itself.

Survival with this disease, assuming appropriate management (usually surgery, radiotherapy, or both), depends largely on the stage when first discovered, as the following data on five-year survival indicate: stage 0, 100%; stage 1, 85–95%; stage 2, 70–75%; stage 3, 35%; stage 4, 10%.

Body of Uterus

The corpus with its endometrium is the principal seat of female reproductive tract disease. Many disorders of this organ are common, often chronic and recurrent, and sometimes disastrous. Only the more frequent and significant ones are considered.

ENDOMETRITIS

The endometrium is relatively resistant to infections. Acute reactions are virtually limited to bacterial infections that arise following parturition or miscarriage. Retained products of conception are the usual predisposing influence. The inflammatory response is chiefly limited to the interstitium and is entirely nonspecific. Removal of the retained gestational fragments by curettage is followed by prompt remission of the infection. *Chronic endometritis* occurs in the following settings: (1) in association with chronic gonorrheal

pelvic disease; (2) in tuberculosis, either from miliary spread or more commonly from drainage of tuberculous salpingitis; (3) in postpartal or postabortal endometrial cavities, usually due to retained gestational tissue; (4) in patients with intrauterine contraceptive devices (IUDs); and (5) spontaneously, without apparent cause in 15% of patients. Histologically, chronic endometritis is manifested by the irregular proliferation of endometrial glands and the presence of chronic inflammatory cells: plasma cells, macrophages, and lymphocytes in the endometrial stroma.

ADENOMYOSIS

Adenomyosis refers to the growth of the basal layer of the endometrium down into the myometrium. Nests of endometrial stroma or glands, or both, are found well down in the myometrium between the muscle bundles. In the fortuitous microscopic section, continuity between these nests and the overlying endometrium can be established. As a consequence, the uterine wall often becomes thickened. Cyclic bleeding into the penetrating nests, producing hemosiderin pigmentation, is extremely unusual because the stratum basalis of the endometrium, from which the penetrations arise, is nonfunctional. Marked involvement may produce menorrhagia, dysmenorrhea, and pelvic pain prior to the onset of menstruation.

ENDOMETRIOSIS

Endometriosis is a far more important clinical condition than adenomyosis; it often causes infertility, dysmenorrhea, pelvic pain, and other problems. _The condition is marked by the appearance of foci of more or less recognizable endometrial tissue in the pelvis (ovaries, pouch of Douglas, uterine ligaments, tubes, and rectovaginal septum), less frequently in more remote sites of the peritoneal cavity, and about the umbilicus._ Uncommonly, the lymph nodes, lungs, and even heart or bone are involved. Three possibilities (not mutually exclusive) have been invoked to explain the origin of these dispersed lesions (Fig. 19–8). (1) The _regurgitation theory_ proposes menstrual backflow through the fallopian tubes and subsequent implantation. Indeed, menstrual endometrium is viable and survives when injected into the anterior abdominal wall; however, this theory cannot explain lesions in the

lymph nodes or lungs, for example. (2) The _metaplastic theory_ proposes endometrial differentiation of coelomic epithelium, which in the last analysis is the origin of the endometrium itself. This theory, too, cannot explain endometriotic lesions in the lungs or lymph nodes. (3) The _vascular or lymphatic dissemination theory_ has been invoked to explain extrapelvic or intranodal implants. Conceivably, all pathways are valid in individual instances.

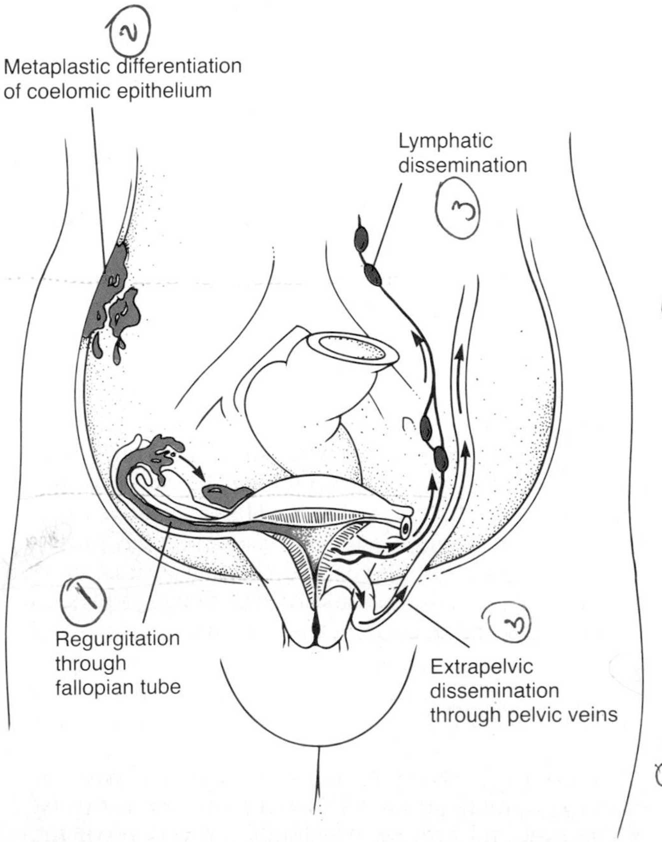

> In contrast to adenomyosis, **endometriosis almost always contains functioning endometrium, which undergoes cyclic bleeding.** Because blood collects in these aberrant foci, they usually appear grossly as red-blue to yellow-brown nodules or implants. They vary in size from microscopic to 1 to 2 cm in diameter and lie on or just under the affected serosal surface. Often, individual lesions coalesce to form larger masses. When the ovaries are involved, the lesions may form large blood-filled cysts that are transformed into so-called **chocolate cysts** as the blood ages (Fig. 19–9). Seepage and organization of the blood leads to widespread fibrosis, adherence of pelvic structures, sealing of the tubal fimbriated ends, and distortion of the oviducts and ovaries. The histologic diagnosis at all sites depends on finding within the lesions two of the following three features: endometrial glands, stroma, or hemosiderin pigment.

The clinical manifestations of endometriosis depend on the distribution of the lesions. Extensive scarring of the oviducts and ovaries often produces discomfort in the lower quadrant and eventually causes sterility. Pain on defecation reflects rectal wall involvement, and dyspareunia (painful intercourse) and dysuria reflect involvement of the uterine and bladder serosa, respectively. _In almost all cases, there is severe dysmenorrhea and pelvic pain as a result of intrapelvic bleeding and periuterine adhesions._

DYSFUNCTIONAL UTERINE BLEEDING AND ENDOMETRIAL HYPERPLASIA

By far the most common problem for which women seek medical attention is some disturbance in menstrual function—_menorrhagia_ (profuse or prolonged bleeding at the time of the period), _metrorrhagia_ (irregular bleeding between the periods), or _ovulatory (intermenstrual) bleeding._ Common causes include polyps, leiomyomas, endometrial carcinoma, endometritis, endometriosis, and, of interest here, dysfunctional uterine bleeding, and endometrial hyperplasias.

DYSFUNCTIONAL UTERINE BLEEDING

Abnormal bleeding in the absence of a well-defined organic lesion in the endometrium or uterus is called

Metaplastic differentiation of coelomic epithelium

Lymphatic dissemination

Regurgitation through fallopian tube

Extrapelvic dissemination through pelvic veins

Figure 19–8. The potential origins of endometrial implants.

Figure 19–9. Endometriosis. The ovaries are converted into enlarged, irregular masses by large "chocolate cysts." (Courtesy of Dr. Arthur Hertig.)

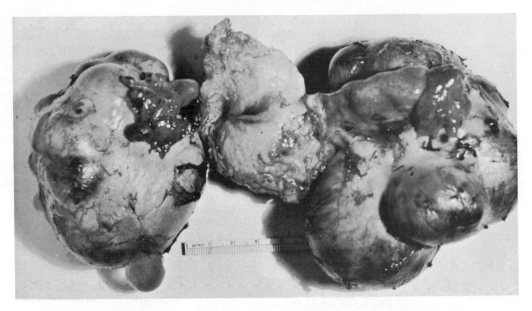

dysfunctional uterine bleeding. In many cases it arises from normal secretory endometrium and then is attributed to excessive fibrinolytic activity or changes in prostaglandin production within the uterus. The most common cause, however, is failure of ovulation and anovulatory bleeding. As a consequence there is no luteal or secretory phase of the endometrium, and under the influence of prolonged estrogen activity, the proliferative endometrium develops mild hyperplasia characterized by persistent mitotic activity and an increase in gland size. The diagnostic feature is a proliferative endometrium in the last half of the menstrual cycle when secretory changes would be expected.

Anovulatory cycles are most common at menarche and premenopausally, but they can occur throughout life. Oral contraceptives also block ovulation, but the combination of contained estrogens and progestogens is intended to prevent the development of the endometrial changes seen in dysfunctional uterine bleeding. In most instances, in the absence of oral contraceptives, anovulatory cycles are of obscure origin, but a number of endocrine-metabolic derangements alter ovulation: pituitary, adrenal, and thyroid disease; functioning ovarian tumors (p. 626); marked obesity; chronic inanition; and emotional stress or excessive physical activity like that of marathon runners and ballet dancers. Whatever the cause, longstanding anovulatory endometrial changes are associated with an increased incidence of endometrial carcinoma, presumably because of the unbalanced estrogen stimulation.

ENDOMETRIAL HYPERPLASIA _____

Endometrial hyperplasia is not only a cause of abnormal bleeding but also, in its more severe expression, a forerunner of endometrial carcinoma. Hyperplasia represents a spectrum of proliferative alterations which are divided into subtypes. The mildest form is called *simple hyperplasia*. More advanced changes are termed *complex hyperplasia*, and the most severe form is called *atypical hyperplasia*. Because these patterns represent a continuum, considerable importance attaches to the severity of the hyperplastic changes, since the "bad" end of the spectrum progresses to carcinoma. Despite some confusion in terminology, most authors agree that *increased cancer risk correlates best with the degree of cytologic (cellular) atypia* associated with hyperplasia. Thus, 2% of untreated hyperplasias *without* cellular atypia develop carcinoma, whereas 23% with atypical hyperplasia do. Cellular atypia is usually but not always associated with a *complex glandular architecture.*

Encountered most often in perimenopausal women, hyperplasias are caused by relative or absolute hyperestrinism, such as is seen with polycystic ovaries, chronic failure of ovulation, functioning estrogenic ovarian tumors, adrenocortical hyperfunction, and prolonged use of exogenous estrogens. Oral contraceptives are not implicated, presumably because of their progestogen content.

Simple hyperplasia without atypia (also known as cystic or mild hyperplasia) is characterized by the presence of glands of various sizes, including many that are cystic (Fig. 19–10A). The epithelial lining may be cuboidal or tall columnar, and occasionally multilayered. Mitoses are scant, but typical proliferative endometrium may be admixed with the dilated glands. **These lesions rarely progress to adenocarcinoma.** A new World Health Organization (WHO) classification recognizes a subtype of **simple hyperplasia with atypia,** but its precancerous potential is unknown.

Complex hyperplasia (also known as moderate or adenomatous hyperplasia without atypia) exhibits an increase in the number and size of endometrial glands, which vary in size and irregularity of shape. The glands

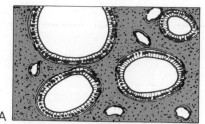

Simple (cystic) hyperplasia

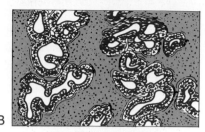

Complex hyperplasia

Figure 19–10. Glandular patterns in simple and complex hyperplasia. Atypical hyperplasia is much more frequent in the complex type.

are crowded. Papillary buddings into the glands are formed, as are finger-like outpouchings into the adjacent endometrial stroma. The lining epithelium is hyperplastic, and frequently there is stratification of the epithelium surrounding the lumens (Fig. 19–10B). **In the absence of cytologic atypia,** fewer than 5% of these lesions develop into carcinoma.

Atypical hyperplasia is also known as **complex hyperplasia with atypia.** In addition to glandular crowding and complexity, the distinguishing feature is **cellular atypia** of the hyperplastic epithelium, consisting of cytomegaly, loss of polarity, hyperchromatism, prominence of nucleoli, and altered nuclear-cytoplasmic ratio. This atypia could be mild, moderate, or severe, and the **risk of cancer correlates with the degree of atypia.**

Not only is curettage necessary to control the abnormal bleeding caused by endometrial hyperplasia, it is also required to establish the nature and severity of the glandular changes, which in some cases must be monitored over time by repeated endometrial biopsy or curettage to ascertain possible recurrence or progression.

TUMORS OF THE ENDOMETRIUM AND MYOMETRIUM

The most common neoplasms are *endometrial polyps, leiomyomas,* and *endometrial carcinomas.* In addition, exotic mesodermal tumors are encountered, such as the stromal sarcoma botryoides (also encountered in the vagina), described on page 611. *All tend to produce bleeding from the uterus as the earliest manifestation.*

ENDOMETRIAL POLYPS

These are sessile, usually hemispheric (rarely pedunculated) lesions, 0.5 to 3 cm in diameter. Larger polyps may project from the endometrial mucosa into the uterine cavity. On histologic examination, they are covered with columnar cells; some have an edematous stroma with essentially normal endometrial architecture, but more often they have cystically dilated glands similar to those seen with cystic hyperplasia.

Although endometrial polyps may occur at any age, they develop more commonly at the time of menopause. Probably their only clinical significance lies in the production of abnormal uterine bleeding.

LEIOMYOMA AND LEIOMYOSARCOMA

Benign tumors that arise in the myometrium are properly termed "leiomyomas," although often they are referred to as "fibroids." *These are the most common benign tumors in females, developing in about one in four women during active reproductive life.* Although the cause and pathogenesis are unknown, leiomyomas, once developed, seem to be estrogen dependent, as evidenced by their rapid growth during pregnancy and their tendency to regress following menopause.

Leiomyomas usually occur as multiple, sharply circumscribed but unencapsulated, firm, gray-white masses, with a characteristically **whorled cut surface.** They vary in size from barely visible seedings to massive tumors that may simulate a pregnant uterus. They may be embedded within the myometrium **(intramural)** or be **subserosal** or lie directly beneath the endometrium **(submucosal);** (Fig. 19–11). Subserosal lesions may become pedunculated and, rarely, become attached to a loop of bowel, develop a blood supply from it, and then, by attenuation of the original stalk, free themselves from the uterus to become "parasitic leiomyomas." The submucosal tumors may project as polyps into the uterine cavity. Larger leiomyomas can undergo necrosis and cystic degeneration. After menopause they tend to shrink, become firmer and more collagenous, and sometimes undergo partial or even complete calcification. Histologically, the tumors are characterized by whorling bundles of smooth muscle cells, duplicating the normal muscle bundles of the myometrium. Foci of fibrosis, calcification, ischemic necrosis with hemorrhage, and more or less complete proteolytic digestion of dead cells may be present. After menopause, the smooth muscle cells tend to atrophy, eventually being replaced by fibrous tissue.

Leiomyomas of the uterus are often entirely asymptomatic and are discovered on routine pelvic examination as a mass or asymmetry of the uterine fundus. The most frequent manifestation is menorrhagia, with or without metrorrhagia. Large masses may produce a dragging sensation in the pelvic region.

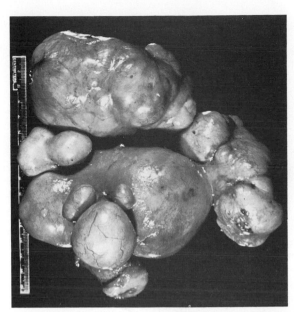

Figure 19–11. Leiomyomas of the uterus. The multiple subserosal, pedunculated, irregular tumors are viewed in the removed uterus. The uterine corpus is distorted beyond recognition. Only the cervix is identifiable as the lowermost projection.

Leiomyosarcomas arise from the myometrium directly. Whether or not uterine leiomyomas ever undergo malignant transformation to become leiomyosarcomas is a controversial point. If they do, such transformation is indeed rare, because the benign tumors are commonplace but their malignant counterparts are rare.

Grossly, **leiomyosarcomas** develop in several distinct patterns: as bulky masses infiltrating the uterine wall; as polypoid lesions projecting into the uterine cavity; or as structures with deceptively discrete margins that masquerade as large benign leiomyomas. Histologically, they show a wide range of differentiation, from well-differentiated growths approaching the leiomyomas to wildly anaplastic lesions approximating undifferentiated sarcomas. The well-differentiated tumors may be difficult to differentiate from cellular leiomyomas. Histologic features indicative of leiomyosarcoma include (1) more than ten mitoses per ten high-power fields (hpf), with or without cellular atypia; and (2) five to ten mitoses per ten hpf with cellular atypia.

The five-year survival rate with overt malignancy is about 20 to 40%. After surgical removal, leiomyosarcomas show a striking tendency toward local recurrence, and some metastasize widely.

CARCINOMA OF THE ENDOMETRIUM _____

The incidence of this disease has remained at about the same level for many years. Although invasive carcinoma of the cervix was once much more common than cancer of the endometrium, the dramatic control that has been seen with the former (p. 612) has not been achieved with endometrial carcinoma, so it is now almost as common as invasive cervical carcinoma. Cytologic diagnosis with endometrial carcinoma is less effective than with cervical cancers; however, endometrial lesions tend to arise postmenopausally and cause irregular bleeding, permitting them to be diagnosed while they are still confined to the uterus and therefore curable by surgery or radiotherapy.

Carcinoma of the endometrium is uncommon in women before age 40. The peak incidence is in the 55- to 65-year age range. *An increased frequency of this form of neoplasia is seen with: (1) obesity; (2) diabetes or, merely, glucose intolerance; (3) infertility; and (4) hypertension.* Infrequently, both endometrial and breast carcinomas arise in one patient.

PATHOGENESIS. The evidence is quite convincing that endometrial carcinoma arises as a progression from ever more florid endometrial hyperplasia under the influence of prolonged estrogen stimulation. The supporting observations can be summarized as follows:

* Complex hyperplasia progressing to atypical hyperplasia (clearly related to hyperestrinism) frequently antedates the appearance of endometrial carcinoma.
* Exogenous estrogens, particularly when used to control menopausal symptoms, are associated with a modestly increased risk.
* Estrogen-secreting ovarian neoplasms (e.g., granulosa cell tumors) increase the risk of endometrial carcinoma.
* Obesity predisposes because of increased synthesis of estrogens in fat depots from adrenal and ovarian precursors.
* The cancer is more common in infertile women, related to ovulatory failure and prolonged estrogen stimulation unopposed by postovulatory progestins.

MORPHOLOGY. Endometrial carcinomas assume one of two macroscopic appearances: either they infiltrate, causing diffuse thickening of the affected uterine wall, or they assume an exophytic form (Fig. 19–12). In both cases, they eventually fill the endometrial cavity with firm to soft, partially necrotic tumor tissue, and in time they extend through the myometrial wall to the serosa and thence by direct extension to periuterine structures. Late in the course metastasis to regional lymph nodes, and later to distant organs, occurs.

In about 85% of these tumors, the histologic form is that of an **adenocarcinoma,** with well-defined gland patterns lined with anaplastic cuboidal to columnar epithelial cells. Ten to twenty percent of endometrial carcinomas contain foci of squamous differentiation. Squamous elements most commonly are histologically benign in appearance (called **adenocarcinoma with squamous metaplasia or adenoacanthoma,)** but they are sometimes frankly malignant (sometimes termed **adenosquamous carcinoma** if more than 10% of the tumor is squamous) (Fig. 19–13). Since the behavior of these tumors is largely dependent on the grade of **glandular** differentiation, WHO classifies all simply as **adenocarcinoma with squamous differentiation.**

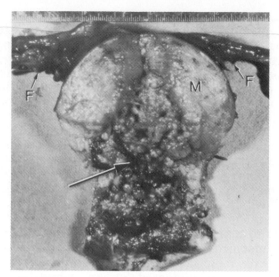

Figure 19-12. Endometrial carcinoma, presenting as a fungating mass in the fundus of the uterus *(arrow)*. (M, myometrium; F, fallopian tubes.)

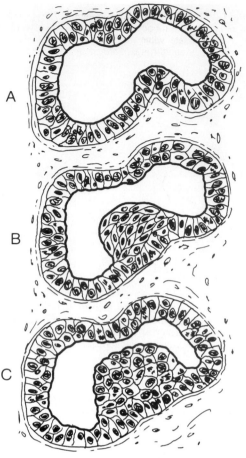

Figure 19-13. *A*, adenocarcinoma, *B* and *C*, adenoacarcinoma with squamous differentiation.

Like most cancers, endometrial carcinoma is graded according to cellular differentiation and staged according to the extent of the disease at diagnosis. The grades are I to III, from well-differentiated to undifferentiated. The following staging system is most widely used: stage I, confined to uterine corpus; stage II, involvement of corpus and cervix; stage III, extension outside of uterus but not outside true pelvis; stage IV, extension beyond stage III.

CLINICAL COURSE. The first clinical indications of endometrial carcinoma are usually marked leukorrhea and irregular bleeding. This reflects erosion and ulceration of the endometrial surface. With progression, the uterus may be palpably enlarged, and in time it becomes fixed to surrounding structures by extension of the cancer beyond the uterus. Fortunately, these are usually late-metastasizing neoplasms, but dissemina-

tion eventually occurs with involvement of regional nodes and more distant sites. With therapy, stage I carcinoma is associated with a 90% five-year survival rate. This rate drops to 30 to 50% in stage II and to less than 20% in stages III and IV.

Fallopian Tubes

These should be treasured organs to the pathology student because they are so seldom the site of primary disease. Their most common afflictions are inflammations, almost always as part of pelvic inflammatory disease. Much less often they are affected by ectopic (tubal) pregnancy (p. 628), followed in order of frequency by endometriosis (p. 616) and the rare primary tumors. Only a few comments on salpingitis and tumors are necessary.

Inflammations of the tube are almost always bacterial in origin. With the declining incidence of gonorrhea, nongonococcal organisms such as chlamydia, *Mycoplasma hominis,* coliforms, and, in the postpar-

tum setting, streptococci and staphylococci are now the major offenders. The morphologic changes produced by gonococci conform to those already described (p. 600). Nongonococcal infections differ somewhat, inasmuch as they are more invasive, penetrating the wall of the tubes and thus tending more often to give rise to blood-borne infections and seeding of the meninges, joint spaces, and sometimes the heart valves. Rarely, tuberculous salpingitis is encountered, almost always in combination with involvement of the endometrium. All forms of salpingitis may produce fever, lower abdominal or pelvic pain, and pelvic masses when the tubes become distended with either

Figure 19-14. Tubo-ovarian inflammation. The uterus is flanked by large bilateral tuboovarian masses resulting from the accumulation of exudate within the sealed-off tubes and ovaries. Note the shaggy hemorrhagic surface responsible for pelvic adhesions.

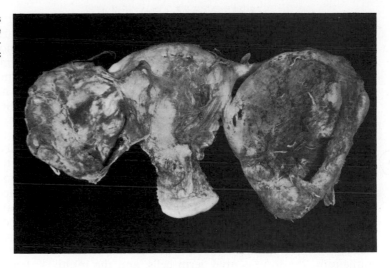

exudate or later burned-out inflammatory debris and secretions (*hydrosalpinx;* Fig. 19-14). Even more serious is the potential for obstruction of the tubal lumens, which sometimes produces permanent sterility.

Primary adenocarcinomas may arise in the tubes. They are curiosities that usually are not discovered until they spread. In time they may cause death.

Ovaries

The ovaries are infrequently the primary site of any disease except, notably, neoplasms. Indeed, carcinomas of the ovaries account for more deaths (about 12,000 per year) than cancers of the cervix and uterine corpus together. It is less their frequency than their lethality that makes them so evil. Nonneoplastic cysts are commonplace but generally are not serious problems. Primary inflammations of the ovary are rarities, but salpingitis of the tubes frequently causes a periovarian reaction called salpingo-oophoritis. As discussed earlier, the ovary is frequently secondarily affected in endometriosis. Only the nonneoplastic cysts and neoplasms merit further consideration.

FOLLICLE AND LUTEAL CYSTS _____

Follicle and luteal cysts in the ovaries are so commonplace as almost to constitute physiologic variants.

These innocuous lesions originate in unruptured graafian follicles or in follicles that have ruptured and have immediately sealed. Such cysts are often multiple and develop immediately subjacent to the serosal covering of the ovary. Usually they are small—1 to 1.5 cm in diameter—and are filled with clear serous fluid, but occasionally they accumulate enough fluid to achieve diameters of 4 to 5 cm and may thus become palpable masses and indeed produce pelvic pain. They are lined by granulosa lining cells or luteal cells when small, but as the fluid accumulates under pressure it

may cause atrophy of these cells. Thus, the larger cysts often have only a compressed stromal enclosing wall. On occasion, these cysts rupture, producing intraperitoneal bleeding and acute abdominal symptoms.

POLYCYSTIC OVARIES _____

Oligoamenorrhea, hirsutism, infertility, and sometimes obesity may appear in young women, usually in postmenarchal girls, secondary to excessive production of estrogens and androgens (mostly the latter) by multiple cystic follicles in the ovaries. This condition is also called *polycystic ovaries,* or *Stein-Leventhal syndrome.*

The ovaries are usually twice normal in size, are gray-white with a smooth outer cortex, and are studded with subcortical cysts 0.5 to 1.5 cm in diameter. Histologically, there is a thickened fibrosed outer tunica, sometimes referred to as "cortical stromal fibrosis," beneath which are innumerable cysts lined by granulosa cells with a hypertrophic and hyperplastic luteinized theca interna. There is a conspicuous absence of corpora lutea.

The principal biochemical abnormalities that can be identified in most patients are excessive production of androgens, high levels of luteinizing hormone (LH), and low levels of follicle-stimulating hormone (FSH). It is now believed that the ovarian and hormonal changes are probably the result of unbalanced or asynchronous release of FSH and LH by the pituitary, which is in turn related to some disruption of hypothalamic control of pituitary secretion. Reduction in size of the ovarian mass by wedge resections corrects the condition because it reduces the volume of ovarian tissue that can respond to pituitary hormones.

TUMORS OF THE OVARY _____

Ovarian neoplasms come in an amazing variety of histogenic types and shapes. This diversity is attributable to the three cell types that make up the normal ovary—the multipotential surface (coelomic) covering epithelium, the totipotential germ cells, and the multipotential sex cord—stromal cells (Fig. 19–15). You recall that coelomic epithelium lines the embryonic furrows that form the müllerian ducts and covers the ovaries. Thus tumors of the coelomic epithelium may be composed of epithelium recapitulating the lining of the fallopian tubes (ciliated and serous columnar cells), the endometrial lining (nonciliated columnar cells), or the endocervical glands (columnar mucus-secreting nonciliated cells). These neoplasms of *surface epithelial*

origin account for about 65 to 70% of all primary ovarian tumors and, in their malignant forms, for almost 90% of all ovarian cancers. The totipotential germ cells give rise to a variety of neoplasms, ranging from teratomas (mature and immature) to other forms of neoplasia, which represent unidirectional differentiation of the germ cells and account collectively for about 15 to 20% of all ovarian tumors but only 2 to 4% of ovarian cancers. The sex cord–stromal cells may differentiate along granulosal, thecal, fibromatous, and Sertoli-Leydig cell lines, as well as others representing 5 to 10% of all ovarian tumors and 2% of ovarian cancers. Only the more common among this large array of neoplasms will be considered. Nulliparity and a positive family history increase the risk for ovarian cancer.

All ovarian neoplasms pose formidable clinical challenges because they produce no symptoms or signs until they are well advanced. Indeed, many are discovered on routine gynecologic examination. Thus the cancers often are not discovered until they have extended beyond the ovaries. Unlike the case with cancers of the cervix, deaths from malignant neoplasms of the ovary have not declined in frequency over the years and now rank fourth among the killer cancers of women (behind those of the lung, breast, and large intestine).

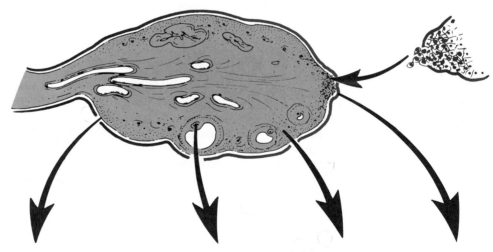

Origin	Surface epithelial cells (Surface epithelial–stromal cell tumors)	Germ cell	Sex cord–stroma	Metastasis to ovaries
Frequency	65–70%	15–20%	5–10%	5%
Age group affected	20 + years	0–25 + years	All ages	Variable
Types	• Serous tumor • Mucinous tumor • Endometrioid tumor • Clear cell tumor • Brenner tumor • Cystadenofibroma	• Teratoma • Dysgerminoma • Endodermal sinus tumor • Choriocarcinoma	• Fibroma • Granulosa–theca cell tumor • Sertoli-Leydig cell tumor	

Figure 19–15. Derivation of various ovarian neoplasms and some data on their frequency and age distribution.

TABLE 19–2. FREQUENCIES OF MALIGNANT TUMORS

Type of Tumor	Approximate Proportion of Ovarian Cancers (%)
Serous tumors	40
Endometrioid tumors	20
Mucinous tumors	10
Undifferentiated carcinoma	10
Granulosa cell tumors	5
Metastatic	6
Clear cell carcinoma	5
Teratoma	1
Dysgerminoma	1
Others	2

SURFACE EPITHELIAL–STROMAL TUMORS

Previously called common epithelial tumors, these neoplasms are derived from the coelomic epithelium. They can be strictly epithelial (e.g., serous, mucinous tumors) or can have a distinct stromal component (cystadenofibroma, Brenner tumor). Although it is traditional to divide neoplasms into benign and malignant categories, the surface epithelial tumors establish an intermediate—borderline—category. The latter appear to be low-grade cancers with limited invasive potential. Thus they have a better prognosis than their uglier cousins, as will be evident.

Serous Tumors

These most frequent of the ovarian tumors are usually encountered between ages 30 and 40 years. Although they may be solid, they are usually cystic, so they are commonly known as *cystadenomas* or *cystadenocarcinomas. About 60% are benign, 15% borderline, and 25% malignant.* Combined borderline and malignant lesions account for about 40% of all ovarian cancers.

Grossly, serous tumors may be small (5 to 10 cm in diameter) but most are large, spherical to ovoid, cystic structures, up to approximately 30 to 40 cm in diameter. **About 25% of the benign forms are bilateral, whereas 66% of the more aggressive lesions are bilateral.** In the benign form, the serosal covering is smooth and glistening. In contrast, the covering of the cystadenocarcinoma shows nodular irregularities, which represent penetration of the tumor to or through the serosa. On transection, the small cystic tumor may reveal a single cavity, but larger ones are usually divided by multiple septa into a multiloculated mass (Fig. 19–16). The cystic spaces are usually filled with a clear serous fluid, although a considerable amount of mucus may also be present. Jutting into the cystic cavities are polypoid or papillary projections, which become more marked in malignant tumors (Fig. 19–17).

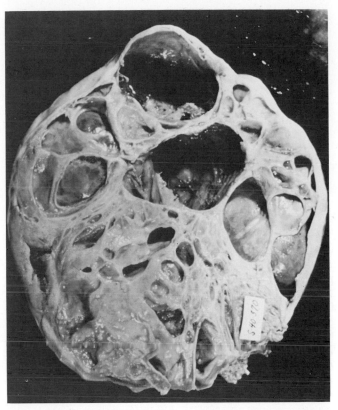

Figure 19–16. Multilocular serous cystadenoma of the ovary, on cross section.

Histologically, the benign tumors are characterized by a single layer of tall columnar epithelium which lines the cyst or cysts. The cells are in part ciliated and in part dome-shaped secretory cells. Psammoma bodies (concentrically laminated concretions) are common in the tips of papillae. When frank carcinoma develops, microscopic examination discloses most importantly anaplasia of the lining cells. Invasion of the stroma is usually readily evident, and papillary formations are complex and multilayered with invasion of the axial fibrous tissue by nests or totally undifferentiated sheets of malignant cells. Between these clearly benign and obviously malignant forms are the so-called **tumors of borderline malignancy** with obvious epithelial anaplasia and little stromal invasion. The overt carcinomas tend to spread contiguously within the pelvis and, by seeding the frequently associated ascites fluid, implant throughout the peritoneal cavity. Spread to regional lymph nodes is frequent, but distant lymphatic and hematogenous metastases are infrequent.

The prognosis for the patient with clearly invasive serous cystadenocarcinoma after surgery, which is sometimes followed by radiation and chemotherapy, is poor and depends heavily on the stage of the disease at the time of diagnosis; an overall 10-year survival rate is only 13%. In contrast, the borderline cancers are associated with an overall 10-year survival rate of about

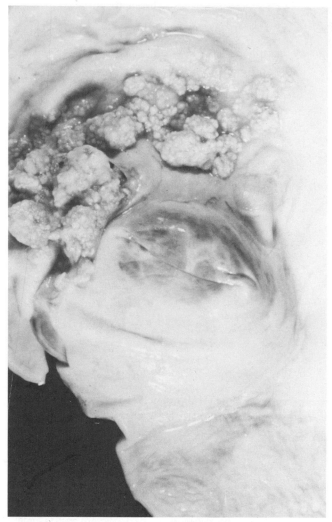

Figure 19–17. Multilocular serous cystadenocarcinoma of the ovary —close-up of the papillary excrescences that have penetrated the covering serosa.

Only about 5% of benign and 20% of malignant tumors are bilateral, a much lower incidence than for their serous counterparts. On gross examination, they may be indistinguishable from serous tumors except by the mucinous nature of the cystic contents. However, **they are more likely to be larger and multilocular, and papillary formations are less common. Prominent papillation, serosal penetration, and solidified areas point to malignancy.**

Histologically, these mucinous tumors are identified by the apical vacuolation of the tall columnar epithelial cells and by the absence of cilia. Two histologic types have recently been differentiated: **endocervical-like** (müllerian) and **intestinal-type,** depending on the resemblance to endocervical or colonic epithelium, respectively. Malignant lesions are identified by the presence of stromal invasion, which is sometimes difficult to assess in the mucinous lesions. Metastasis or rupture of mucinous cystadenocarcinomas may give rise to the clinical condition designated **pseudomyxoma peritonei.** The peritoneal cavity becomes filled with a glairy mucinous material resembling the cystic contents of the tumor. Multiple tumor implants are found on all the serosal surfaces, and the abdominal viscera become matted together. This form of pseudomyxoma peritonei is analogous to that encountered with rupture of a carcinomatous mucocele of the appendix (p. 521). Pseudomyxoma peritonei can also occur with histologically borderline tumors, and in the case of intestinal-type borderline tumors is associated with a poor prognosis.

The prognosis of mucinous cystadenocarcinoma is better than that for the serous counterpart. The overall 10-year survival rate is about 35%. Borderline mucinous tumors are associated with an 85% 10-year survival rate.

Endometrioid Tumors

These tumors are characterized by the formation of tubular glands, similar to those of the endometrium, within the linings of cystic spaces. Although benign and borderline forms exist, endometrioid tumors are usually malignant. They are bilateral in about 30% of cases, and _15 to 30% of patients with these ovarian tumors have a concomitant endometrial carcinoma._

Grossly, the ovarian lesion may be solid or cystic. The cystic forms are usually indistinguishable on gross inspection from the serous and mucinous lesions just described. Sometimes these tumors develop as a mass projecting from the wall of an endometriotic cyst filled with chocolate-colored fluid. Microscopically, the cells lining the glandular formations are usually columnar, producing an _adenocarcinoma._ Sometimes, foci of metaplastic squamous cells or mucin-secreting epithelium may be seen. Varying degrees of anaplasia are present.

80%. Forty per cent of patients with borderline serous lesions, however, have extraovarian foci of _peritoneal implants_ of serous neoplasia, and almost 40% of such women eventually die of their tumors. Presence of invasion in these implants is a particularly ominous prognostic finding.

Mucinous Tumors

They are in most respects entirely analogous to the serous tumors, differing essentially in that the epithelium consists of mucin-secreting cells similar to those of the endocervical mucosa. These tumors occur in patients in the same age range as those with serous tumors, but mucinous lesions _are considerably less likely to be malignant, accounting for about 10% of all ovarian cancers._ Benign lesions (_cystadenomas_) account for 80%; borderline represent 10%; and malignant (_cystadenocarcinomas_), 10%.

When these tumors are relatively well-differentiated, there is a 62% five-year survival rate; with the more aggressive carcinomas it is 23%.

Cystadenofibroma

The cystadenofibroma is essentially a variant of the serous cystadenoma in which there is more pronounced proliferation of the fibrous stroma that underlies the columnar lining epithelium. These benign tumors are usually small and multilocular and have rather simple papillary processes that do not become so complicated and branching as those in ordinary cystadenomas. The epithelial lining is usually quite regular. Carcinomatous transformation is rare. Borderline lesions with cellular atypia also occur, but their malignant potential is much less than that of borderline serous tumors.

Brenner Tumor

The *Brenner tumor* is an uncommon ovarian, solid, usually benign tumor consisting of an abundant stroma *containing nests of transitional epithelium resembling that of the urinary tract*. It thus belongs to the *transitional cell tumor* subgroup of surface epithelial–stromal cell tumors. Occasionally the nests are cystic and are lined by columnar mucus-secreting cells. Brenner tumors generally are smoothly encapsulated and gray-white on transection and range from a few centimeters to 20 cm in diameter. These tumors may arise from the surface epithelium, but it is also hypothesized that they spring from urogenital epithelium trapped within the germinal ridge.

GERM CELL TUMORS

Tumors of germ cell origin constitute about 15 to 20% of ovarian neoplasms. More than half arise in the first two decades of life and, unfortunately, the younger the patient, the greater the likelihood of malignancy. About 90 to 95% are benign cystic mature teratomas that are readily identified morphologically. Most of the residual represent immature (and often malignant) teratomas, dysgerminomas, choriocarcinomas, or other lines of development of germ cells. Only the better-defined lesions are discussed here.

Teratoma

Teratomas, you recall, contain elements representative of more than one germ layer. Similar tumors may also arise in the testis—and, rarely, in extragonadal sites (p. 173). In the ovary 99% differentiate mainly along ectodermal lines and, fortunately, are benign cystic teratomas. The small remainder of immature teratomas are much more likely to be malignant.

BENIGN (MATURE) CYSTIC TERATOMA. These interesting neoplasms are marked by ectodermal differentiation with the formation of cysts, which are, to all appearances, lined by normal-appearing skin that is often replete with adnexal appendages; hence the common designation "dermoid cysts." About 80% occur between 20 and 30 years of age.

Most are unilateral, most often on the right, but in 10% of cases they are bilateral. Typically, they are smaller than 10 cm in diameter and are covered by a glistening serosa. On sectioning there is a thin cystic wall lined by well-differentiated skin having adnexal glands, including hair. The cystic space is filled with a thick, sebaceous secretion containing matted hair (Fig. 19–18). Sometimes teeth protrude from a nodular projection and (children take note) they are unbrushed and may be carious! Occasionally, foci of bone, cartilage, nests of bronchial or gastrointestinal epithelium, and other recognizable structures are present in the nodular projection.

Excision of these tumors is almost always curative. In about 1% of dermoid cysts there is malignant transformation of one of the tissue elements, usually taking the form of a squamous cell carcinoma. Of interest, *torsion of the tumor occurs in about 10 to 15% of cases, producing an acute surgical emergency.*

IMMATURE TERATOMA. As the name indicates, this often malignant neoplasm is composed of random mixtures of immature tissue derived from any or all of the three germ layers. Sometimes immature teratomas also have components representing other types of germ cell neoplasia, such as foci of choriocarcinoma or dysgerminoma. Immature teratomas occur in patients younger than 40 years, and a significant number occur before puberty.

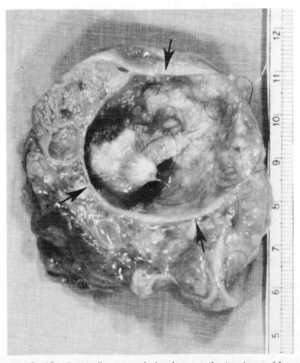

Figure 19–18. A small, opened, benign cystic teratoma (dermoid cyst) of the ovary. Note the hair and sebaceous material in the lumen.

They are generally unilateral, often cystic, masses up to 25 cm in diameter. The external surface is smooth and the cut surface is of varying consistency (reflecting the contained tissue elements) and red to pink with areas of hemorrhage and necrosis. Microscopically, there is a wide range of cellular differentiation, with varying degrees of tissue maturation. Most have immature but recognizable cartilage, bone, and, particularly, neuroepithelial and glial elements. But many other tissues, such as gastrointestinal, bronchial, and squamous epithelium, may be identified. Tumors having more or less well-differentiated components may remain confined to the ovary, but with progressive immaturity (most often within the neuroepithelial elements) penetration through the capsule and metastases may appear.

The prognosis is dependent on the most immature component having the greatest degree of anaplasia, the presence of metastases, and the level of anaplasia in the metastases. Unfortunately, most of these neoplasms grow rapidly and extend beyond the ovary, yielding about a 25 to 30% five-year survival rate. The better-differentiated lesions confined to the ovary can be cured by excision.

MONODERMAL (SPECIALIZED) TERATOMAS. These merit brief comment only because they are medical curiosities. Very rarely teratogenous, unidirectional differentiation produces an ovarian mass composed of red-brown thyroid tissue *(struma ovarii).* These lesions are of interest because the ectopic tissue has in some cases participated along with the thyroid gland in causing hyperthyroidism. Equally exotic is the *carcinoid,* which occasionally induces the carcinoid syndrome.

Dysgerminoma

This uncommon, usually malignant ovarian tumor is composed of primordial germ cells and so is the counterpart of the seminoma of the testis (p. 592). It occurs in children and young adults, generally as a solid unilateral (90%) mass ranging up to 25 cm in diameter. Most are quite distinctive histologically, having nests and aggregates of large vesicular cells with clear cytoplasm and centrally placed nuclei separated by trabeculae that have a lymphocytic infiltrate and, occasionally, syncytial-type giant cells and granuloma formations.

Although the tumors are invasive and have a propensity for early spread to regional and then para-aortic nodes before metastasizing elsewhere, they respond to radiotherapy (and some to chemotherapy), yielding a 65 to 95% five-year survival. A well-defined association with congenital malformations of the genitals and with Turner's syndrome (p. 110) has been noted.

Choriocarcinoma

This rare tumor is analogous anatomically to its counterparts in the testis (p. 593) and in the placenta

(p. 630). When primary in the ovary, it is usually part of a mixed germ cell tumor; "pure" choriocarcinoma is most often a metastasis from a tumor arising in the placenta.

SEX CORD–STROMAL TUMORS

These neoplasms are composed of varying combinations of sex cord and stromal derivatives capable of differentiating in an "ovarian direction" (granulosa cells, theca cells), in a "testicular direction" (Sertoli cells, Leydig cells), or in the "stromal direction," to remain fibromatous. Neoplasms in this category account for about 5 to 10% of all ovarian tumors but only about 2% of cancers. Nonetheless, they are clinically important because many elaborate steroid hormones, which are usually estrogenic but sometimes androgenic.

Granulosa-Theca Cell Tumors

This designation embraces ovarian neoplasms composed of varying proportions of granulosa cells and theca cells, which may be luteinized. At one end of the spectrum are tumors composed almost entirely of granulosa cells, *granulosa cell tumors,* and at the other are pure *thecomas.* Collectively, these neoplasms account for about 3% of all ovarian tumors. Although they may be discovered at any age, approximately two thirds occur in postmenopausal women.

Granulosa cell tumors are usually unilateral and vary from microscopic foci to large, solid, and cystic encapsulated masses. Tumors that are endocrinologically active have a yellow coloration to their cut surfaces, produced by contained lipids. The pure thecomas are firm to solid tumors.

The granulosa cell component of these tumors has one of many histologic patterns. The small, cuboidal to polygonal cells may grow in anastomosing cords, sheets, or strands. In occasional cases, small, distinctive, gland-like structures filled with an acidophilic material recall immature follicles (Call-Exner bodies; Fig. 19–19). In the thecoma component, the cells may be disposed in large sheets of cuboidal to polygonal cells that gradually change into plump spindle cells resembling the theca lutein cells.

Pure thecomas are composed of large sheets or poorly defined areas of plump spindle cells that closely resemble those of the fibroma. Characteristically, theca cells contain lipid droplets, but only clinical or biochemical evidence of hormone production by the tumor distinguishes functional theca cells from fibroblasts.

These tumors are clinically important for two reasons: (1) their potential elaboration of large amounts of estrogen and (2) the definite hazard of malignancy in the granulosa cell forms. Functionally active tumors in prepubertal girls have certain characteristic histologic

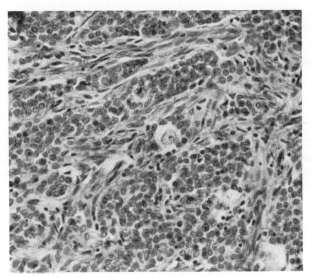

Figure 19–19. Granulosa cell tumor.

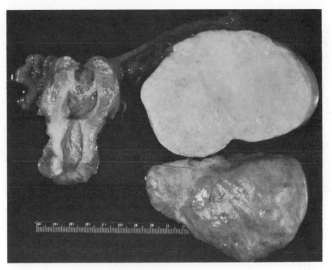

Figure 19–20. Large bisected fibroma of ovary apparent as a white, firm mass *(right)*. The uterus is to the left.

features (juvenile granulosa cell tumor) and may produce precocious sexual development. In adult women, they may be associated with endometrial hyperplasia, cystic changes of the breast, and endometrial carcinoma. All these tumors are potentially malignant. The estimates of clinical malignancy (recurrence, extension) range from 5 to 25%. The 10-year survival rate is approximately 85%.

Fibroma

Fibromas arising in the ovarian stroma are a relatively common form of ovarian neoplasm and account for about 4% of all types. Some are pure fibromas, but others contain theca elements and are termed fibrothecomas. Pure fibromas are nonfunctioning.

> The fibromas of the ovary are unilateral in about 90% of cases and usually are solid, spherical, or slightly lobulated, encapsulated, hard, gray-white masses covered by glistening, intact ovarian serosa (Fig. 19–20). Histologically, they are composed of well-differentiated fibroblasts with a more or less scant collagenous connective tissue interspersed between the cells.

In addition to the relatively nonspecific findings of pain and pelvic mass, the tumors may be accompanied by *ascites.* Uncommonly, there is also hydrothorax, usually only on the right side. This combination of findings — *ovarian tumor, hydrothorax,* and *ascites* — is designated *Meigs' syndrome.* Its cause is unknown.

Sertoli-Leydig Cell Tumors (Androblastomas)

These tumors recapitulate, to a certain extent, the cells of the testis at various stages of development.

They commonly produce masculinization, or at least defeminization.

> The tumors are unilateral, gray-white, and solid. Histologically, the well-differentiated tumors exhibit tubules composed of Sertoli cells or Leydig cells interspersed with stroma. The intermediate forms show only outlines of immature tubules and large, eosinophilic Leydig cells. The poorly differentiated tumors have a sarcomatous pattern with a disorderly disposition of epithelial cell cords. Leydig cells may be absent. The tumors recur or metastasize in fewer than 5% of cases.

CLINICAL CORRELATIONS FOR ALL OVARIAN TUMORS

The clinical presentation of all ovarian tumors is remarkably similar despite their great morphologic diversity, except for the functioning neoplasms that have hormonal effects. Ovarian tumors are usually asymptomatic until they become large enough to cause local pressure symptoms, (e.g., pain, gastrointestinal complaints, urinary frequency). Indeed, about 30% of all ovarian neoplasms are discovered incidentally on routine gynecologic examination. Larger masses, notably the "common epithelial tumors," may cause an increase in abdominal girth. Smaller masses, particularly dermoid cysts, may become twisted on their pedicles (torsion), producing severe abdominal pain and an acute abdomen. Fibromas and malignant serous tumors often cause ascites, the latter owing to metastatic seeding of the peritoneal cavity, so that tumor cells can be identified in the ascitic fluid. Mucinous cancers may literally fill the abdominal cavity with a gelatinous neoplastic mass (pseudomyxoma peritonei). Functioning ovarian tumors often come to attention because of the endocrinopathies they induce.

The major challenge is the early detection of ovarian cancers. To this end an intense search has been made for circulating tumor antigens. Regrettably, only a few (such as CA-125) have proved to have limited value because of difficulties with sensitivity and specificity. Their principal utility is in monitoring possible recurrences in patients who had elevated levels prior to therapy.

Despite all efforts to achieve early diagnosis and effective methods of treatment, the overall five-year survival rate for the surface epithelial–stromal cancers is a disappointing 30 to 35%. These poor results are attributable in large part to the fact that (as in years past) more than half of these cancers are advanced at the time of discovery.

TUMORS METASTATIC TO THE OVARY _____

Metastases to the ovary most often arise from the gastrointestinal tract or nearby pelvic organs. The term _Krukenberg tumor_ refers to bilateral ovarian metastases characterized by mucin-secreting "signet ring" cells. Commonly, such lesions are primary in the stomach, but they may also be metastatic from the colon, breast, or, indeed, any other organ that has mucin-producing cells.

Diseases of Pregnancy

Diseases of pregnancy and pathologic conditions of the placenta are important causes of intrauterine or perinatal death, congenital malformations, intrauterine growth retardation, maternal death, and a great deal of morbidity for both mother and child. Here we shall discuss only a limited number of disorders in which knowledge of the morphologic lesions contributes to an understanding of the clinical problem.

PLACENTAL INFLAMMATIONS AND INFECTIONS _____

Infections reach the placenta by two pathways: (1) ascending infection through the birth canal and (2) hematogenous (transplacental) infection. _Ascending infections_ are by far the most common; in most instances, they are bacterial and are associated with premature rupture of the membranes. The chorioamnion shows leukocytic polymorphonuclear infiltration associated with edema and congestion of the vessels. When the infection extends beyond the membranes, it may involve the umbilical cord and placental villi and cause acute vasculitis of the cord.

Uncommonly, bacterial infections may arise by the _hematogenous spread_ of bacteria; histologically, the villi are most often affected (villitis). _Syphilis, tuberculosis, listeriosis, toxoplasmosis, candidiasis, and various viral (rubella, cytomegalovirus, herpes simplex) and mycoplasma infections_ can also affect the placenta.

ECTOPIC PREGNANCY _____

Ectopic pregnancy is implantation of the fertilized ovum in any site other than the normal uterine location. The condition occurs in as many as 1% of pregnancies. _In more than 90% of these cases, implantation is in the oviducts (tubal pregnancy); other sites include the ovaries, the abdominal cavity, and the intrauterine portion of the oviducts (interstitial pregnancy)._ Any hindrance that retards passage of the ovum along its course through the oviducts to the uterus predisposes to an ectopic pregnancy. In about half of the cases such hindrance is based on chronic inflammatory changes in the oviduct, although intrauterine tumors and endometriosis may also hamper passage of the ovum. In approximately 50% of tubal pregnancies, no anatomic cause can be demonstrated. Ovarian pregnancies probably result from those rare instances of fertilization with trapping of the ovum within its follicle just at the time of rupture. Gestation within the abdominal cavity occurs when the fertilized egg drops out of the fimbriated end of the oviduct and implants on the peritoneum.

In all sites, ectopic pregnancies are characterized by fairly normal early development of the embryo, with the formation of placental tissue, amniotic sac, and decidual changes. An abdominal pregnancy is occasionally carried to term. With tubal pregnancies, however, the invading placenta eventually burrows through the wall of the oviduct, causing **intratubal hematoma, intraperitoneal hemorrhage,** or both (Fig. 19–21). The tube is usually locally distended up to 3 to 4 cm by a contained mass of freshly clotted blood in which may be seen bits of gray placental tissue and fetal parts. The histologic diagnosis depends on the visualization of placental villi or, rarely, of the embryo. Less commonly, poor attachment of the placenta results in death of the embryo, with spontaneous proteolysis and absorption of the products of conception.

Until rupture occurs, an ectopic pregnancy may be indistinguishable from a normal one, with cessation of menstruation and elevation of serum and urinary placental hormones. Under the influence of these hormones, the endometrium (in about 50% of cases) undergoes the characteristic hypersecretory and deci-

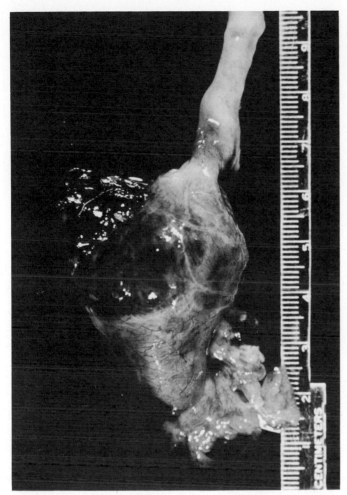

Figure 19–21. Tubal pregnancy with marked dilatation and rupture of distal end of tube by the contained pregnancy and subsequent hemorrhage.

dual changes. *However, the absence of elevated gonadotropin levels does not exclude this diagnosis, because poor attachment with necrosis of the placenta is common.* Rupture of an ectopic pregnancy may be catastrophic, with the sudden onset of intense abdominal pain and signs of an acute abdomen, often followed by shock. Prompt surgical intervention is necessary.

GESTATIONAL TROPHOBLASTIC DISEASE

Traditionally, *the gestational trophoblastic tumors have been divided mainly into three overlapping morphologic categories—hydatidiform mole, invasive mole, and choriocarcinoma.* They range in level of aggressiveness from the hydatidiform moles, most of which are benign, to the highly malignant choriocarcinomas. All elaborate human chorionic gonadotropin (HCG), which can be detected in the circulating blood and urine at titers considerably higher than those found during normal pregnancy, the titers progressively rising from hydatidiform mole, to invasive mole, to chorio-

carcinoma. In addition to aiding diagnosis, the fall or, alternatively, rise in the level of the hormone in the blood or urine can be used to monitor the effectiveness of treatment. Clinicians therefore prefer the term "gestational trophoblastic diseases" because the response to therapy as judged by the hormone titers is significantly more important than any arbitrary anatomic segregation of one lesion from another. Nonetheless, it is necessary to understand their individual characteristics to appreciate the spectrum of lesions.

HYDATIDIFORM MOLE

The typical hydatidiform mole is a voluminous mass of swollen, sometimes cystically dilated, chorionic villi covered by varying amounts of banal to highly atypical chorionic epithelium and appearing grossly as grape-like structures. Two distinctive subtypes of moles have been segregated, *complete* and *partial* moles. *The complete hydatidiform mole never contains fetal parts. All the chorionic villi are abnormal, and the chorionic epithelial cells are diploid (46XX or uncommonly, 46XY). The partial hydatidiform mole contains fetal parts, has some normal chorionic villi, and is almost always triploid (e.g., 69XXY;* Table 19–3, see Fig. 19–18).

The incidence of complete hydatidiform moles is about 1 to 1.5 per 2000 pregnancies in the United States and other Western countries. For unknown reasons, there is a much higher incidence in Asian countries. They are much more common before age 20 and after age 40. They usually present clinically with painless vaginal bleeding, on average 16 to 17 weeks after conception. The uterus is "too large for dates," and no fetal parts or heart sounds are present. Elevated levels of HCG are present in maternal blood and urine, and ultrasonography provides a positive diagnosis.

When discovered, usually in the fourth or fifth month of gestation, the uterus is larger than anticipated for the duration of the pregnancy. The uterine cavity is filled with a delicate, friable mass of thin-walled, translucent,

TABLE 19–3. FEATURES OF COMPLETE VERSUS PARTIAL HYDATIDIFORM MOLE

Feature	Complete Mole	Partial Mole
Karyotype	46,XX (46,XY)	Triploid
Villous edema	All villi	Some villi
Trophoblast proliferation	Diffuse; circumferential	Focal; slight
Atypia	Often present	Absent
Serum HCG	Elevated	Less elevated
HCG in tissue	++++	+
Behavior	2% choriocarcinoma	Rare choriocarcinoma

cystic, grape-like structures (Fig. 19–22). Fetal parts are rarely seen in complete moles but are common in partial moles.

Microscopically, the **complete mole** shows hydropic swelling of chorionic villi and virtual absence of vascularization of villi. The central substance of the villi is a loose, myxomatous, edematous stroma. The chorionic epithelium almost always shows some degree of proliferation of both cytotrophoblast and syncytial trophoblast. The proliferation may be mild but in many cases there is striking circumferential hyperplasia. Histologic grading to predict clinical outcome of moles has been supplanted by careful following of the HCG levels. In **partial moles,** the villous edema involves only some of the villi, and the trophoblastic proliferation is focal and slight.

Overall, 80 to 90% of moles remain benign after thorough curettage. Ten per cent become invasive moles, and not more than 2 to 3% give rise to choriocarcinoma. Monitoring the postcurettage blood and urine levels of HCG, particularly the more definitive beta subunit of the hormone, permits detection of incomplete removal or a more ominous complication and the institution of appropriate therapy, including in some cases chemotherapy, which is almost always curative.

INVASIVE MOLE

Biologically, *an invasive mole is intermediate between a benign mole and choriocarcinoma.* It is more invasive locally, but it does not have the aggressive metastatic potential of a choriocarcinoma.

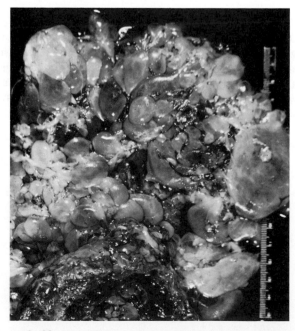

Figure 19–22. Hydatidiform mole evacuated from the uterus. The "bunch-of-grapes" appearance of the lesion is readily apparent.

An *invasive mole retains hydropic villi,* which penetrate the uterine wall deeply, possibly causing rupture and sometimes life-threatening hemorrhage. Local spread to the broad ligament and vagina may also occur. Microscopically, the epithelium of the villi is markedly hyperplastic and atypical, with proliferation of both cuboidal and syncytial components.

Although the marked invasiveness of this lesion makes removal technically difficult, metastases do not occur. Hydropic villi may embolize to distant organs, such as the lungs or the brain, but these emboli do not constitute true metastases and may actually regress spontaneously. Owing to the greater depth of invasion of the myometrium, an invasive mole usually is not removed completely by curettage, and therefore HCG levels remain elevated. This alerts the clinician to the need for further treatment. Fortunately, in most cases cure is possible by chemotherapy.

CHORIOCARCINOMA

This very aggressive malignant tumor arises either from gestational chorionic epithelium or, less frequently, from totipotential cells within the gonads or elsewhere. Choriocarcinomas are rare in most Western cultures and in the United States occur in about one in 30,000 pregnancies. They are much more common in Asian and African countries, reaching a frequency of one in 2000 pregnancies. The risk is somewhat greater before age 20 and is significantly elevated after age 40. *In about 50% of cases, it follows a complete hydatidiform mole but only rarely a partial mole. About 25% arise after an abortion, and most of the remainder occur in a previously normal pregnancy.* Stated in another way, the more abnormal the conception, the greater the hazard of developing gestational choriocarcinoma. Most cases are discovered by the appearance of a bloody brownish discharge accompanied by a rising titer of HCG, particularly the beta subunit, in blood and urine and by the absence of marked uterine enlargement such as would be anticipated with a mole. In general, the titers are much higher than those associated with a mole. In those instances that follow abortion or pregnancy, the fact that maternal age influences the frequency of this neoplasm suggests origin from an abnormal ovum rather than retained chorionic epithelium.

Choriocarcinomas appear usually as very hemorrhagic, necrotic masses within the uterus. Sometimes the necrosis is so complete as to make anatomic diagnosis difficult because there is deceptively little recognizable viable neoplasm. Indeed, the primary lesion may self-destruct and only the metastases tell the story. Very early, the tumor insinuates itself into the myometrium and into vessels. **In contrast to the case with hydatidiform moles and invasive moles, chorionic villi are not formed; instead, the tumor is purely epithelial, composed of anaplastic cuboidal cytotrophoblast and** syncytiotrophoblast (Fig. 19-23). However, identification of such atypicality can be difficult because normal chorionic epithelium is so variable in cytomorphology.

By the time most neoplasms are discovered, widespread dissemination via the blood is usually present, most often to the lungs (50%), vagina (30 to 40%), brain, liver, and kidneys. Lymphatic invasion is uncommon.

Despite the extreme aggressiveness of these neoplasms, which made them nearly uniformly fatal in the past, present-day chemotherapy has achieved remarkable results. Nearly 100% cures have been obtained with neoplasms that have not spread beyond the pelvis, vagina, and lungs. Almost a 75% remission rate has been achieved with even widely disseminated neoplasms. Equally remarkable are the many reports of healthy infants borne by these survivors. By contrast, there is relatively poor response to chemotherapy in choriocarcinomas that arise in the gonads (ovary or testis).

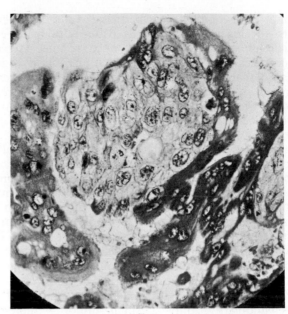

Figure 19-23. High-power detail of choriocarcinoma illustrates the two types of epithelial cells—cytotrophoblast and syncytiotrophoblast. (Courtesy of Dr. Arthur Hertig.)

Breast

Lesions of the female breast are much more common than lesions of the male breast, which is remarkably seldom affected. These lesions usually take the form of palpable, sometimes painful, nodules or masses. Fortunately, most are innocent, but as is well known, breast cancer was the foremost cause of cancer deaths in women in the United States until 1986, when it was supplanted by carcinoma of the lung. The following discussion deals largely with lesions of the female breast. The conditions to be described should all be considered in terms of their possible confusion clinically with a malignancy. This problem is most acute with fibrocystic change because it is the most common cause of breast "lumps" and because of the continuing controversy about the association of particular variants with breast carcinoma.

An overall perspective of the frequency of various breast problems can be gained from an analysis of a large series of patients with breast complaints who were seen in a surgical outpatient department. About 30% of the women were considered, after careful evaluation, to have no breast disease. Almost 40% were diagnosed as having fibrocystic changes. Slightly more than 10% had biopsy-proven cancer, and about 7% had a benign tumor (fibroadenoma). The remainder were suffering from a miscellany of benign lesions (Fig. 19-24). Three features of this study deserve particular note: (1) *a significant proportion of women who have no recognizable breast disease have sufficient irregularity of the "normal" breast tissue to cause concern and*

to necessitate clinical evaluation; (2) fibrocystic changes are the dominant breast problem; and (3) cancer unfortunately is all too frequent.

FIBROCYSTIC CHANGES _____

This designation is something of a catch-all term, since it is applied to a miscellany of changes in the female breast that range from those that are entirely innocuous to the patterns associated with an increased risk of breast carcinoma. The only unifying feature is that all these alterations—stromal fibrosis, concurrent

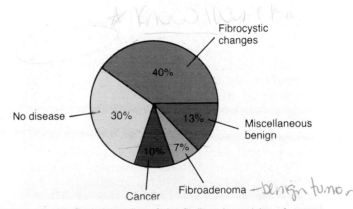

Figure 19-24. Representation of the findings in a series of women seeking evaluation of apparent breast "lumps."

stromal and epithelial hyperplasia (often inducing micro- or macrocysts), various patterns of banal epithelial hyperplasia, and the more serious atypical hyperplasias—produce palpable "lumps." It is widely accepted that *this range of changes is the consequence of an exaggeration and distortion of the cyclic breast changes that occur normally in the menstrual cycle.* Estrogenic therapy and oral contraceptives do not appear to increase the incidence of these alterations.

In years past, these breast alterations were called fibrocystic disease; however, physicians have expressed much dissatisfaction with this term on two levels. First, it is extremely difficult to draw a line between "physiologic nodularity," most prominent during the menstrual cycle, and changes that merit the appellation "disease." Various reports in the past have cited histologic evidence of "fibrocystic disease" in 60 to 90% of autopsies on women. Second, most of the changes encompassed within the diagnosis of "fibrocystic disease" have little clinical significance except that they cause nodularity; only a small minority represent forms of epithelial hyperplasia that are clinically important. Thus the term "fibrocystic changes" is preferred, since it does not stigmatize the subject with "a disease." Despite this semantic controversy, it should not be overlooked that there are valid lesions that are properly encompassed under the rubric of fibrocystic changes; they sometimes produce masses that must be distinguished from cancer, and the distinction between the trivial variants and the not so trivial ones can be made only by biopsy and histologic evaluation. In a somewhat arbitrary manner, these alterations are here subdivided into three dominant patterns: (1) cysts and/or fibrosis *without* epithelial cell hyperplasia, known as *simple fibrocystic change;* (2) cysts and/or fibrosis with epithelial cell hyperplasia, known as *proliferative fibrocystic change;* and (3) *sclerosing adenosis.* All tend to arise during reproductive life but may persist after the menopause.

SIMPLE FIBROCYSTIC CHANGE: CYSTS AND FIBROSIS _____

This is the most common type of alteration, characterized by an increase in fibrous stroma associated with dilatation of ducts and formation of cysts of various sizes.

Grossly, a single large cyst may form within one breast, but the disorder is usually multifocal and often bilateral. The involved areas show ill-defined, diffuse increased density and discrete nodularities. The cysts vary from smaller than 1 cm to 5 cm in diameter. Unopened, they are brown to blue (blue dome cysts) and are filled with serous, turbid fluid. Histologically, in smaller cysts, the epithelium is more cuboidal to columnar and is sometimes multilayered in focal areas. In larger cysts, it may be flattened or even totally atrophic (Fig. 19–25). Occa-

sionally, epithelial proliferation leads to piled-up masses or small papillary excrescences. Frequently, cysts are lined by large polygonal cells that have an abundant granular, eosinophilic cytoplasm, with small, round, deeply chromatic nuclei, so-called **apocrine metaplasia;** this is virtually always benign.

The stroma surrounding all forms of cysts is usually compressed fibrous tissue, having lost its normal, delicate, myxomatous appearance. Stromal lymphocytic infiltrate is common in this and all other variants of fibrocystic change.

PROLIFERATIVE FIBROCYSTIC CHANGE _____

The terms "epithelial hyperplasia" and "proliferative fibrocystic change" encompass a range of proliferative lesions within the ductules, terminal ducts, and sometimes the lobules of the breast. Some of the epithelial hyperplasias are mild and orderly and carry little risk of carcinoma, but at the other end of the spectrum are the more florid atypical hyperplasias that carry a significantly greater risk, commensurate with the severity and atypicality of the changes. The epithelial hyperplasias often are accompanied by other histologic variants of fibrocystic change, but nonetheless they may be the dominant pattern morphologically.

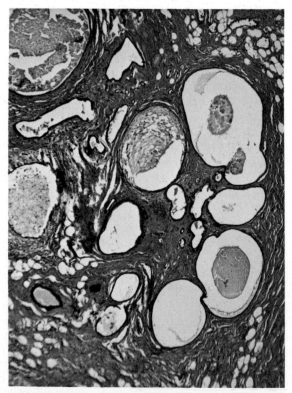

Figure 19–25. Cystic change of the breast. The microscopic view shows numerous small cysts, some containing inspissated secretions. The epithelium is flattened and inactive.

The gross appearance of epithelial hyperplasia is not distinctive and is often dominated by coexisting fibrous or cystic changes. Histologically, there is an almost infinite spectrum of proliferative alterations. The ducts, ductules, or lobules may be filled with orderly cuboidal cells, within which small gland patterns can be discerned (**cribriform pattern**). Sometimes the proliferating epithelium projects in multiple small papillary excrescences into the ductal lumen (**ductal papillomatosis**). The degree of hyperplasia, manifested in part by the number of layers of intraductal epithelial proliferation can be mild, moderate, or severe (Fig. 19–26).

In some instances the hyperplastic cells are more multilayered and disorderly and vary in nuclear and cell size and exhibit slight hyperchromasia; in short, they have changes approaching those of carcinoma in situ (p. 637). Such irregular hyperplasia is called **atypical**. The line separating the epithelial hyperplasias without atypia from atypical hyperplasia is poorly defined, just like the line demarcating atypical hyperplasia from carcinoma in situ, but these distinctions are important, as will soon become clear.

Atypical lobular hyperplasia is the term used to describe hyperplasias of the terminal duct and ductules (acini) that have some but not all the features of lobular carcinoma in situ, described on page 637. Cytologically, the atypical cells resemble those of lobular carcinoma in situ but do not fill or distend more than 50% of the terminal duct units. Atypical lobular hyperplasia is associated with an increased risk of invasive carcinoma.

Epithelial hyperplasia per se does not often produce a clinically discrete breast mass. Occasionally it produces microcalcifications on mammography, raising doubts about cancer. Such nodularity as may be present usually relates to other concurrent variants of fibrocystic disease; however, florid papillomatosis may be associated with a serous or serosanguineous nipple discharge.

SCLEROSING ADENOSIS _____

This variant is less common than cysts and hyperplasia but is significant because its clinical and morphologic features may be deceptively similar to those of carcinoma. There is in this lesion marked intralobular fibrosis and proliferation of small ductules and acini.

Grossly, the lesion has a hard, rubbery consistency, similar to that of breast cancer. Histologically, sclerosing adenosis is characterized by proliferation of small ducts and ductules yielding masses of small gland patterns within a fibrous stroma (Fig. 19–27). Aggregated glands or proliferating ductules may be virtually back to back, with single or multiple layers of epithelial cells in contact with one another (**adenosis**). Always associated with the adenosis is marked stromal fibrosis, which may compress and distort the proliferating epithelium, hence the designation "sclerosing adenosis." **This overgrowth of fibrous tissue may completely compress the lumens of the acini and ducts, so that they appear as solid cords of cells.** This pattern then may be difficult to distinguish histologically from an invasive scirrhous carcinoma. Helpful in suggesting a benign diagnosis is the presence of double layers of epithelium and the identification of myoepithelial elements.

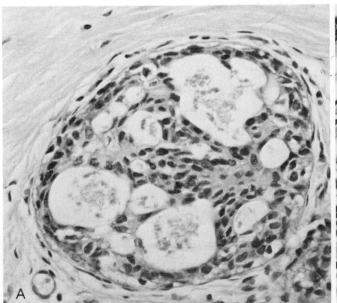
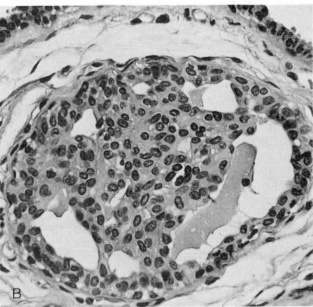

Figure 19–26. *A,* Moderate duct epithelial hyperplasia. Note cells fill part of the duct lumen. *B,* More florid duct epithelial hyperplasia, with irregular lumina at the periphery, so called fenestrations. (Courtesy of Dr. Noel Weidner.)

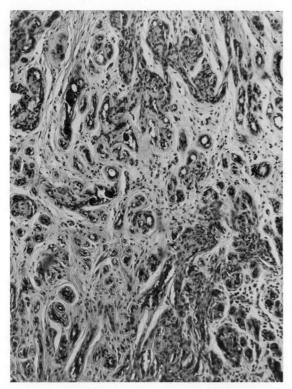

Figure 19–27. Sclerosing adenosis of the breast. The epithelial hyperplasia has produced the nests of cells, which appear quite disorderly. The overgrowth of fibrous tissue enmeshes and partially obliterates many of the epithelial nests, creating a pattern very similar to the infiltrative growth of a cancer.

Although sclerosing adenosis is sometimes difficult to differentiate clinically and histologically from carcinoma, it is associated with only a minimally increased risk of progression to carcinoma.

RELATIONSHIP OF FIBROCYSTIC CHANGES TO BREAST CARCINOMA

Here we enter a stormy arena filled with claims and counterclaims. Only some reasonably supportable summary statements are possible. Clinically, although certain features of fibrocystic change tend to distinguish it from cancer, the only certain way of making this distinction is biopsy and histologic examination. With respect to the relationship of the various patterns of fibrocystic change to cancer, the following statements currently represent the best-informed opinion:

- *Minimal or no increased risk of breast carcinoma:* Fibrosis, cystic changes (micro- or macroscopic), apocrine metaplasia, sclerosing adenosis, mild hyperplasia
- *Slightly increased risk (1.5 to 2 times):* Moderate to florid hyperplasia, ductal papillomatosis
- *Significantly increased risk (5 times):* Atypical hyperplasia, ductular or lobular with duct involvement
- *A family history of breast cancer increases the risk in all categories* (e.g., to about 10-fold with atypical hyperplasia).

Only about 5% of biopsy specimens exhibit atypical epithelial hyperplasia. Thus the great majority of women who have lumps related to fibrocystic change can be reassured that there is little or no increased predisposition to cancer. The need to differentiate among the many variants and the grounds for dissatisfaction with the unqualified terms "fibrocystic changes" or, even worse, "fibrocystic disease" are apparent. The risks inherent in the various patterns are shown in Figure 19–28.

INFLAMMATIONS

Inflammations of the breast are uncommon and during the acute stages usually cause pain and tenderness in the involved areas. However, in the later healing or healed stage they become painless and sometimes leave residual scarring that is palpable as a breast lump. Included in this category are several forms of mastitis and traumatic fat necrosis, none of which is associated with increased risk of cancer.

Acute mastitis develops when bacteria gain access to the breast tissue either through the ducts when there is inspissation of secretions, or through fissures in the nipples, which usually develop during the early weeks of nursing, or from various forms of dermatitis involving the nipple.

Staphylococcal infections induce single or multiple abscesses accompanied by the typical clinical acute inflammatory changes when they are near the surface. They are usually small, but when sufficiently large they may leave in the course of healing residual foci of scarring that are palpable and as localized areas of induration. **Streptococcal infections generally spread throughout the entire breast, causing pain, marked swelling with enlargement, and breast tenderness.** Resolution of these infections rarely leaves residual areas of induration.

Mammary duct ectasia (periductal or plasma cell mastitis) is a nonbacterial inflammation of the breast associated with inspissation of breast secretions in the main excretory ducts. Ductal dilatation with ductal rupture leads to reactive changes in the surrounding breast substance. It is an uncommon condition usually encountered in women who have borne children in their 40s and 50s.

Usually the inflammatory changes are confined to an area drained by one or several major excretory ducts opening into the nipple. There is increased firmness of the tissue and, on cross section, dilated ropy ducts are apparent from which thick, cheesy secretions can be extruded. Histologically, the ducts are filled by granular debris, sometimes containing leukocytes, principally lipid-laden macrophages. The lining epithelium is gener-

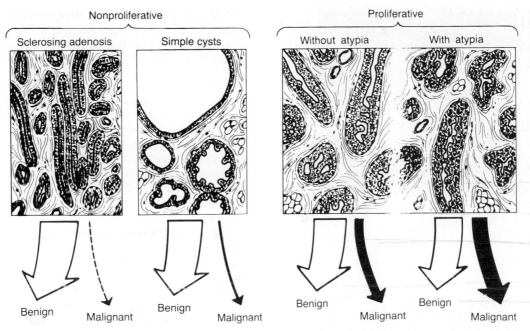

Figure 19-28. An attempt to depict, by the sizes of the arrows, the risk of malignant transformation of the various patterns of fibrocystic change.

ally destroyed. **Most distinguishing is the prominence of the lymphocytic and plasma cell infiltration and occasional granulomas in the periductal stroma.**

Mammary duct ectasia is of principal importance because it leads to induration of the breast substance and, more significantly, to retraction of the skin or nipple, mimicking the changes caused by some carcinomas.
Traumatic fat necrosis is an uncommon and innocuous lesion that is significant only because it produces a mass. Most but not all patients report some antecedent trauma to the breast.

During the early stage, the lesion is small, often tender, rarely more than 2 cm in diameter, and sharply localized. It consists of a central focus of necrotic fat cells surrounded by neutrophils and lipid-filled macrophages, and, later, by an enclosing wall of fibrous tissue and mononuclear leukocytes. Eventually, the necrosis is replaced by scar tissue or the debris becomes encysted within the scar. Calcifications may develop in either scar or cyst wall.

TUMORS OF THE BREAST

Tumors are the most important lesions of the female breast. Although they may arise from any of its component tissues (i.e., connective tissue and epithelial structures), it is the latter that give rise to the common breast neoplasms. Here we will describe fibroadenoma,

phyllodes tumor, papilloma and papillary carcinoma, and carcinomas of the breast.

FIBROADENOMA

The encapsulated fibroadenoma is by far the most common benign tumor of the female breast. An absolute or relative increase in estrogen activity is thought to play a role in its development, and indeed, similar lesions, perhaps less discretely encapsulated, may appear with fibrocystic changes *(fibroadenosis)*. Fibroadenomas usually appear in prepubertal girls and in young women; the peak incidence is in the third decade of life.

The fibroadenoma occurs as a discrete, encapsulated, usually solitary, freely movable nodule, 1 to 10 cm in diameter. Rarely, multiple tumors are encountered. Grossly, they are firm, with a uniform gray-white color on cut section, punctuated by softer yellow-pink specks representing the glandular areas. Histologically, there is a loose fibroblastic stroma containing duct-like, epithelium-lined spaces of various forms and sizes. These duct-like or glandular spaces are lined with single or multiple layers of cells that are regular and have a well-defined, intact basement membrane. Although in some lesions the ductal spaces are open, round to oval, and fairly regular (the **pericanalicular fibroadenoma**), others are compressed by extensive proliferation of the stroma so that on cross section they appear as slits or irregular, star-shaped structures (**the intracanalicular fibroadenoma**) (Fig. 19-29).

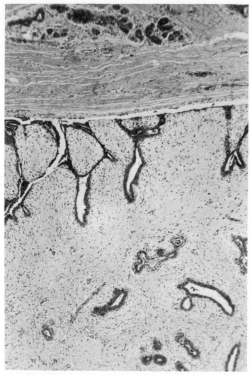

Figure 19–29. Fibroadenoma of the breast. The margin of the nodule shows clear demarcation from the compressed breast substance above. The tumor is in part intracanalicular, particularly near the capsule. Toward the bottom of this view, the pattern is pericanalicular.

Clinically, fibroadenomas usually present as solitary, discrete, movable masses. They may enlarge late in the menstrual cycle and during pregnancy. Postmenopausally they may regress and calcify.

PHYLLODES TUMOR

Rarely, fibroadenomas grow to massive proportions, reaching diameters of 10 to 15 cm (*giant fibroadenomas*). Some of these become lobulated and cystic and on gross section exhibit leaflike clefts and slits (phyllodes), in which case they are designated phyllodes tumors. In the past they had the tongue-tangling name cystosarcoma phyllodes," an unfortunate term, because these tumors are usually benign though some become malignant. The most ominous change is the appearance of increased stromal cellularity with anaplasia, and high mitotic activity, accompanied by rapid increase in size, usually with invasion of adjacent breast tissue by malignant stroma. Malignant lesions may recur, but they tend to remain localized. In time, metastasis to distant sites occurs in about 15% of cases.

INTRADUCTAL PAPILLOMA

This is a neoplastic papillary growth within a duct. Most lesions are solitary and are found within the principal lactiferous ducts or sinuses. They present clinically as a result of (1) the appearance of serous or bloody nipple discharge; (2) the presence of a small subareolar tumor a few millimeters in diameter; and (3) rarely, nipple retraction.

> The tumors are usually less than 1 cm in diameter and consist of delicate, branching growths within a dilated duct or cyst. Histologically, the tumor is composed of multiple papillae, each having a connective tissue axis covered by cuboidal or cylindrical epithelial cells that are frequently double layered, the outer epithelial layer overlying a myoepithelial layer.

These lesions should be differentiated from papillary carcinoma, which lacks a myoepithelial component and shows severe cytologic atypia and abnormal mitotic figures. Complete excision of the duct system should be performed in order to avoid local recurrences. *Multiple intraductal papillomas* should be distinguished from intraductal papillomas, since the former are more likely to recur and are associated with an increased risk of development of carcinoma.

CARCINOMA

As noted earlier, carcinoma of the breast has lately been supplanted as the number one cause of cancer deaths in females in the United States; this is also likely to occur in other Western countries. Unhappily, this fall from predominance reflects an alarming increase in the frequency of lung cancer in women rather than a decline in the death rate from carcinoma of the breast, which has held steady for many years. Carcinoma of the breast continues to account for about 20% of cancer deaths in women in the United States. The only happy note is that many women who develop an invasive carcinoma are being cured of their disease. In contrast, breast carcinoma is extremely rare in men.

EPIDEMIOLOGY. The following risk factors for carcinoma of the breast have been identified:

- *Geographic influences:* Five times more common in the United States than in Japan and Taiwan.
- *Genetic predisposition:* Well-defined: the risk is proportional to the number of close relatives with breast cancer and inversely proportional to the age at which their cancers developed. Bilateral cancers are also associated with greater genetic predisposition. There are uncommon high-risk families in which there is apparent autosomal dominant transmission and familial association of breast and ovarian carcinomas.
- *Increasing age:* Breast carcinoma is uncommon before age 20, but then a steady rise to the time of menopause is followed by a slower rise throughout later life.
- *Length of reproductive life:* Risk increases with early menarche and late menopause.
- *Parity:* More frequent in nulliparous than in multiparous women.

- *Age at first child:* Increased risk when over 30 at time of first child.
- *Obesity:* Increased risk attributed to synthesis of estrogens in fat depots.
- *Exogenous estrogens:* Still controversial, but some data show moderately increased risk with high-dose therapy for menopausal symptoms (p. 228).
- *Oral contraceptives:* No clearly increased risk with present use; this is attributed to balanced content of estrogens and progestins in currently used formulations (p. 228).
- *Fibrocystic changes with atypical epithelial hyperplasia:* Increased risk, as noted in earlier discussion of this condition.
- *Carcinoma of the contralateral breast or the endometrium:* Increased risk.

ETIOLOGY AND PATHOGENESIS. Extensive studies have failed to discover the ultimate origin or origins of breast carcinoma. The only clues point to genetic influences, hormone imbalances, and possibly environmental factors. The former enthusiasm for oncogenic viruses, which clearly cause mammary tumors in animals, has waned.

Genetic predisposition undoubtedly exists, as the afore-mentioned data indicate. Of great interest is the recent demonstration of an inherited mutation of the tumor suppressor gene p53 in a rare form of familial breast cancer associated with the Li-Fraumeni syndrome. Mutations affecting a different gene (also mapped on chromosome 17) seem to be involved in the pathogenesis of the more common forms of familial breast cancer.

Endogenous hyperestrinism is thought to play a significant role. Many of the risk factors mentioned— long reproductive life, nulliparity, and late age at first child—all imply increased exposure to the estrogen peaks during the menstrual cycle. There are the additional findings of the association with fibrocystic epithelial hyperplasia (presumed to reflect estrogen influences), the modestly increased (albeit disputed) risk imposed by exogenous estrogens, and the rarity of breast carcinoma in girls castrated before puberty. There are hints of how the estrogens might act. It is well known that normal breast epithelium possesses estrogen and progesterone receptors. These have been identified in some but not all breast cancers. A variety of growth factors (TGF-α, PDGF) are secreted by human breast cancer cells. Production of these growth factors is estrogen dependent, and it is possible that interactions between circulating hormones, hormone receptors on cancer cells, and autocrine growth factors induced by tumors cells play a role in breast cancer progression. Receptor assays of tissue biopsies are now being used in an attempt to predict the responsiveness of particular neoplasms to hormone therapy, as we will discuss later. Of the *environmental influences,* the effect of diet is controversial, but there are ardent advocates of the thesis that a large proportion of dietary fat is associated with a significant predisposition. Moderate alcohol consumption is associated with a 1.5-fold increased risk of breast cancer.

The role of viruses in human breast cancer has been pursued since Bittner's brilliant discovery in 1936 that a filterable agent, transmitted through the mother's milk, causes breast cancer in suckling mice. The virus, mouse mammary tumor virus (MMTV), was later identified as a retrovirus. Subsequently there were many hints of the existence of an analogous virus in breast cancer of humans, but the findings have not been conclusive.

MORPHOLOGY. Cancer of the breast affects the left breast slightly more often than the right. In 4 to 10% of patients there are bilateral primary tumors or a second primary tumor develops subsequently. The locations of the tumors within the breast are as follows:

	Per Cent
Upper outer quadrant	50
Central portion	20
Lower outer quadrant	10
Upper inner quadrant	10
Lower inner quadrant	10

Tumors may arise in the ductal epithelium (90%) or within the lobular epithelium (10%). Unless otherwise specified, the term "breast carcinoma" implies ductal origin. Both ductal and lobular cancers are further divided into those that have not penetrated the limiting basement membranes **(noninfiltrating)** and those that have done so **(infiltrating)**. Thus, the chief forms of carcinoma of the breast can be classified as follows:

A. Noninfiltrating
   1. Intraductal carcinoma (comedocarcinoma)
   2. Intraductal papillary carcinoma
   3. Lobular carcinoma in situ
B. Infiltrating (invasive) ductal carcinoma
   1. Not otherwise specified (NOS)–scirrhous *most common
   2. Invasive lobular carcinoma
   3. Medullary carcinoma
   4. Colloid (mucinous) carcinoma
   5. Paget's disease
   6. Tubular carcinoma

Of these, the infiltrating ductal (scirrhous) carcinoma is by far the most common. The morphology of each type will be discussed separately.

Intraductal Carcinoma (Comedocarcinoma). This type represents about 5% of carcinomas of the breast. The tumor may present as a clinically palpable mass (up to 5 cm in diameter) or as ropy cords within the breast created by proliferation of the ductal epithelium, which tends to grow within the ducts without invading the ductal basement membrane and underlying breast tissue. Eventually, the ducts become filled with cheesy necrotic tumor tissue, which can be extruded with slight pressure when the ducts are transected (hence the name **comedocarcinoma**). Histologically, the neoplastic cells may initially assume a glandular pattern or pile up within the ducts to create irregular excrescences. Often the proliferating cells form bridges that traverse the duct or, alternatively, create large arches about the circumference. Continued replication fills the ducts with compressed tumor cells until all architectural detail is lost. At this point they appear as solid cords of anaplastic cells. Whether all intraductal cancers are fated in time to become invasive is at present not clear. Twenty-eight per cent of women treated with biopsy alone develop invasive cancer within 15 years. Whether the remainder would in time become invasive is moot.

Infiltrating Ductal Carcinoma (NOS). This most common form of breast cancer accounts for roughly 75% of carcinomas of the breast. Clinically, it is a deceptively delimited mass, rarely over 3 to 4 cm in diameter, of stony hard consistency, hence the commonly used designation **scirrhous carcinoma** (Fig. 19–30). On cut section, the tumor is obviously infiltrative and retracted below the surrounding fibrofatty tissue, and it has a gritty texture that produces a grating sound when the tumor is scraped with a knife. Foci of chalky white necrosis and sometimes calcification are often evident on the cut surface. Extension of the growth may cause dimpling of the skin, retraction of the nipple, or fixation to the chest wall. Histologically, the lesion is composed principally of dense fibrous stroma in which are found widely scattered nests or cords of tumor cells (Fig. 19–31). These are round to polygonal, or compressed, and contain fairly uniform, small, dark nuclei with remarkably few mitotic figures. At the margins of the tumor, the neoplastic cells can be seen infiltrating the

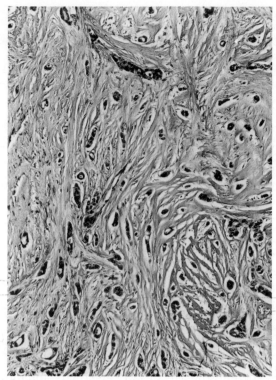

Figure 19–31. A high-power detail of a scirrhous adenocarcinoma of the breast. The scattered islands of cancer cells are trapped in the striking desmoplastic stromal overgrowth.

surrounding tissue and frequently invading perivascular and perineurial spaces as well as blood vessels.

Medullary Carcinoma. Medullary carcinoma represents about 1% of breast carcinoma. The morphology of these tumors is in sharp contrast to that of the usual breast carcinoma. They tend to be soft and fleshy rather than stony hard and often become large (up to 10 cm in diameter). On cut section, the tumor bulges above the surrounding tissue, rather than retracting below it. The reason for these differences is apparent on histologic examination. Unlike the scirrhous carcinoma, the medullary carcinoma has a scant stroma. The tumor cells grow in large, irregular sheets of undifferentiated polygonal to spindled cells, although occasionally well-differentiated gland formations are present, meriting the designation medullary adenocarcinoma. There is usually moderate to marked lymphocytic infiltration between the tumor cells and particularly in the margins of the tumor mass. This feature is presumed to represent a host response to the tumor, and, correspondingly, these tumors have a distinctly better prognosis than the usual infiltrating breast carcinoma.

Colloid (Mucinous) Carcinoma. This form is even more uncommon than the medullary carcinoma. It is charac-

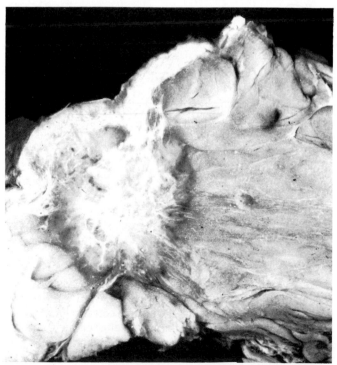

Figure 19–30. Carcinoma of the breast, infiltrating. The cut surface illustrates the lack of demarcation, the fixation to the skin, and the chalky foci of necrosis within the mass.

terized by the production of mucin, intracellularly and extracellularly. Grossly, these lesions are extremely soft, bulky, gray-blue masses with the consistency of gelatin. Histologically, there are two patterns of growth. In the first pattern, the tumor cells are seen as small islands, or even isolated cells, floating in a large lake of basophilic mucin that flows into contiguous tissue spaces and planes of cleavage. In the second pattern, the neoplastic cells grow in well-defined glandular arrangements, the lumens of which contain mucinous secretions. In both patterns, the neoplastic cells may be vacuolated, containing mucin. The prognosis of these variants is better than that of the usual infiltrative neoplasm.

Paget's Disease of the Breast. This is an unusual form of ductal breast cancer that affects women in a slightly older age group than the other forms. It begins as a typical intraductal carcinoma but involves the main excretory ducts, from which it extends to infiltrate the skin of the nipple and areola. As a consequence, eczematoid changes in the nipple and areola antedate the formation of any palpable mass in the breast. The involved areolar and periareolar skin is frequently fissured, ulcerated, and oozing. There are surrounding inflammatory hyperemia and edema, and superimposed bacterial infections are common. The histologic hallmark of this tumor is the invasion of the epidermis by pathogenomonic neoplastic cells termed **Paget cells**—large, hyperchromatic cells surrounded by a clear halo, which represents intracellular accumulation of mucopolysaccharides. In other respects the morphology of Paget's disease is similar to that of an intraductal carcinoma, and despite extension to the skin, has a favorable prognosis.

Lobular Carcinoma. Lobular carcinoma arises from the acini or terminal ductules of the lobule. Not only does it differ from the ductal carcinomas in its origin, but it is characterized by a peculiar tendency to multicentricity within the same breast and by a high incidence (20%) of bilaterality. Two forms are described, **lobular carcinoma in situ and infiltrating lobular carcinoma. Lobular carcinoma in situ** is impalpable and can be defined only histologically. With the microscope, an entire lobule reveals acini (terminal ductules), which are distended with neoplastic cells (Fig. 19–32). The cells are somewhat larger than normal and loosely cohesive, and they have oval or round nuclei and small nucleoli. In general, mitotic figures and pleomorphism are lacking. The distention of the acini (terminal ductules) is a particularly characteristic feature. The significance of lobular carcinoma in situ lies in the possibility of transition to infiltrating carcinoma. About 30% of patients develop carcinoma in the same or the **contralateral** breast. Curiously, the invasive carcinomas that develop can be either lobular or ductal.

Infiltrating lobular carcinoma is poorly circumscribed and usually rubbery in consistency. Sometimes the lesion may be hard and scirrhous. Histologically, in the classic form strands of tumor cells often one cell in width (Indian file pattern) are loosely dispersed in a

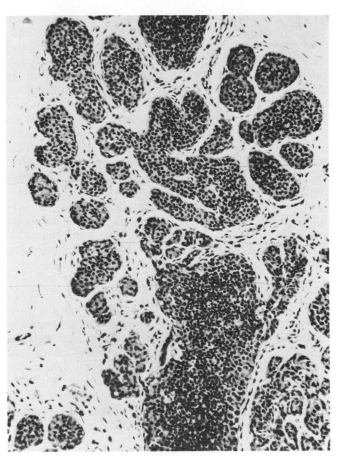

Figure 19–32. Lobular carcinoma in situ. Note proliferation of tumor cells in terminal ducts and acini.

fibrous stroma. In most cases, the tumor cells are small and uniform, with little pleomorphism. Occasionally, they surround normal-appearing acini or ducts, the so-called bull's eye pattern, which is considered characteristic. Not uncommonly, the tumors have histologic features of both ductal and lobular patterns. It is therefore difficult to determine the precise incidence of infiltrating lobular carcinoma. Most studies report that they account for 5 to 10% of breast carcinomas. Despite their infrequent occurrence, these tumors are considered important owing to the high incidence of bilaterality, which mandates a careful clinical and histologic evaluation (by biopsy) of the contralateral breast.

FEATURES COMMON TO ALL INVASIVE CANCERS. In all of the forms of breast cancer discussed previously, progression of the disease leads to certain local morphologic features. These include a tendency to become adherent to the pectoral muscles or deep fascia of the chest wall, with consequent *fixation* of the lesion, as well as adherence to the overlying skin, with *retraction* or *dimpling* of the skin or nipple. The latter is an important sign, because it may be the first indication of a lesion, observed by the patient herself during self-examination. Involvement of the lymphatic pathways may cause localized *lymphedema*. In these cases the skin becomes thickened around exaggerated hair follicles, a change known as *peau d'orange* (orange peel). Sometimes, particularly in pregnancy, the tumor spreads so rapidly that it excites an acute inflammatory reaction with swelling, redness, and tenderness. This picture has been referred to as "*inflammatory carcinoma.*" The advent of mammography as a diagnostic tool has called attention to the frequency of microcalcifications in breast carcinoma. Although certain variants (e.g., intraductal carcinoma) only infrequently have such calcifications, they are common in the usual infiltrative scirrhous lesion, so that overall, they are found in 60 to 80% of breast cancers. They may also be present in the epithelial proliferation of fibrocystic changes.

Spread eventually occurs through lymphatic and hematogenous channels. Nodal metastases are present in about two thirds of cases at the time of diagnosis. Outer quadrant and centrally located lesions typically spread first to the axillary nodes. Those in the inner quadrants often involve the lymph nodes along the internal mammary arteries. The supraclavicular nodes are sometimes the primary site of spread but may become involved only after the axillary and internal mammary nodes are affected. More distant dissemination eventually ensues, with metastatic involvement of almost any organ or tissue in the body. Favored locations are the lungs, skeleton, liver, and adrenals and, less commonly, the brain, spleen, and pituitary. But no site is exempt. *Metastases may appear many years after apparent therapeutic control of the primary lesion, sometimes 15 years later.* However, with each passing year the scene brightens. Breast cancer is an ugly lesion for many reasons, not the least being its potential to reappear so many years later.

GRADING AND STAGING. These neoplasms have been graded on the basis of their level of anaplasia (grades I to III) and have been divided into three categories based on their biologic aggressiveness:

Nonmetastasizing: Intraductal carcinoma without stromal invasion; in situ lobular carcinoma

Uncommonly metastasizing: Colloid carcinoma; medullary carcinoma with lymphocytic infiltration; infiltrating papillary carcinoma

Moderately to aggressively metastasizing: All other types

In addition, there are staging systems; regrettably, too many are currently in use. All attempt to create stages based on the size of the primary lesion, the possible presence of nodal metastases, and the possible presence of distant dissemination. One of those widely used is shown in Table 19–4.

CLINICAL COURSE. Breast cancer is often discovered by the patient or her physician as a deceptively discrete, solitary, painless, and movable mass. At this time the lesion is typically less than 4 cm in diameter, although, as mentioned, involvement of the regional lymph nodes (most often axillary) is already present in about two thirds of patients. With increasing fre-

TABLE 19–4. AMERICAN JOINT COMMITTEE ON CANCER STAGING OF BREAST CARCINOMA*

Stage Tis	In situ cancer (in situ lobular, pure intraductal, and Paget's disease of the nipple without palpable tumor)
Stage I	Tumor 2 cm or less in greatest diameter and without evidence of regional or distant spread
Stage II	Tumor more than 2 cm but not more than 5 cm in greatest dimension, with regional lymph note involvement but without distant spread
Stage III (A)	Tumor of up to and more than 5 cm in diameter with or without homolateral regional (local) spread that may or may not be fixed, but without distant spread
Stage III (B)	Tumor of up to and more than 5 cm in diameter with homolateral metastatic supraclavicular and intraclavicular nodes
Stage IV	Tumor of any size with or without regional spread but with evidence of distant metastases

* From Beahrs, O. H.: Staging of cancer of the breast as a guide to therapy. Cancer *53*:592, 1984.

quency, an occult lesion is detected by a routine mammogram. Admittedly, "mammos" incur increased costs and worry produced by questionable findings (calcifications are also seen with fibrocystic changes). Nonetheless, currently there is an apparent consensus for mammography every one or two years beginning at about age 40 unless there is a family history of cancer or a history of atypical hyperplastic fibrocystic change, in which case screening should begin earlier and be performed more frequently. This technique is well-established as a valuable diagnostic modality in the differentiation of cancerous from benign breast masses.

The prognosis of breast cancer is influenced by many factors. Obvious poor prognostic signs include extensive edema or multiple nodules in the skin of the breast, fixation to the chest wall, spread to internal mammary or supraclavicular lymph nodes, inflammatory carcinoma and, of course, distant metastases. In early breast cancer, when these signs are not apparent, prognosis is affected by the following variables:

1. *The size of the primary tumor.* Tumors smaller than 2 cm are associated with favorable prognosis.
2. *Lymph node involvement and the number of lymph nodes involved by metastases.* With no axillary lymph node involvement the five-year survival rate is close to 80%. The disease-free survival rate falls off to 21% in the presence of four or more involved nodes.
3. *The histologic type and grade of tumor.* The 30-year survival rate for various types is as follows: intraductal carcinoma, 74%; papillary carcinoma, 65%; medullary carcinoma, 58%; colloid, 58%; infiltrating lobular, 34%; and infiltrating ductal, 29%.
4. *The presence or absence of estrogen and progesterone receptors.* The number of estrogen receptors in breast cancer cells can be large or moderate, or there may be none; it is proportional to the degree

of cell differentiation and of the potential responsiveness of the tumor to antiestrogen ablation by oophorectomy or chemotherapy. The highest response rates to endocrine ablation are in patients with tumors that contain both estrogen and progesterone receptors.

5. *The proliferative rate, and the presence of aneuploidy* (increased and scattered DNA values) as measured by flow cytometry. The tumor's nuclear DNA content—specifically, larger fractions of cells scattered outside the modal peaks of DNA histograms—is a strong indicator of poor outcome.
6. *The presence of amplified or activated oncogenes.* Breast cancer shows consistent associations with activation of *myc* and *neu* oncogenes and loss of Rb and putative cancer suppressor genes. Amplification of the c-*neu* gene has in fact been correlated with aggressive behavior.
7. The presence of *substantial angiogenesis* or *high cathepsin D levels* in the tumor (p. 198).

Current therapeutic approaches include combinations of simple mastectomy or segmental resection of the mass (lumpectomy) with or without lymph node dissection, postoperative irradiation, and chemotherapy.

The overall five-year survival rate for stage I cancer is 80%; for stage II, 65%; for stage III, 40%; and for stage IV, 10%. It should be noted that recurrence may appear late, even after 10 years, but with each passing year free of disease, the prognosis improves. Overall, the 10-year survival rate for breast cancers is still no more than 50%.

MALE BREAST

The rudimentary male breast is relatively free from pathologic involvement. Only two disorders occur with sufficient frequency to merit consideration—*gynecomastia* and *carcinoma.*

GYNECOMASTIA

Like females, male breasts are subject to hormonal influences, but they are considerably less sensitive than female breasts. Nonetheless, enlargement of the male breast, or *gynecomastia,* may occur in response to absolute or relative estrogen excesses. *Gynecomastia, then, is the male analog of fibrocystic change in the female.* The most important cause of such hyperestrinism in the male is cirrhosis of the liver, with consequent inability of the liver to metabolize estrogens. Other causes include Klinefelter's syndrome, estrogen-secreting tumors, estrogen therapy, and occasionally,

digitalis therapy. Physiologic gynecomastia often occurs in puberty and in extreme old age.

The morphologic features of gynecomastia are similar to those of intraductal hyperplasia. Grossly, a button-like, subareolar swelling develops, usually in both breasts but occasionally in only one.

CARCINOMA

This is a rare occurrence, with a frequency ratio to breast cancer in the female of 1:125. It occurs in advanced age. Because of the scant amount of breast substance in the male, the tumor rapidly infiltrates the overlying skin and underlying thoracic wall. Both morphologically and biologically, these tumors resemble invasive carcinomas in the female. Surprisingly, considering the size of the male breast, almost half spread to regional nodes and more distant sites by the time they are discovered.

References

Berkowitz, R. S., Goldstein, D. P.: Gestational trophoblastic disease. *In* Moosa, A. R., et al. (eds.): Comprehensive Textbook of Oncology. Baltimore, Williams & Wilkins, 1989.

Breast Cancer. vol. 1. New England Journal of Medicine Reprint Collection, 1991.

Carter, D.: Interpretation of Breast Biopsies. 2nd ed. New York, Raven Press, 1991. (Thorough description of the microscopic interpretation of mammary lesions.)

Crum, C., Nuovo, G. J.: Genital Papillomaviruses and Related Neoplasms. New York, Raven Press, 1991. (A monograph devoted to the role of HPV in gynecologic tumors.)

Harris, J. R., et al. (ed.): Breast Diseases. 2nd ed. Philadelphia, J. B. Lippincott Co., 1991. (A multiauthor comprehensive book of clinical, pathologic, and therapeutic aspects of breast diseases, including breast cancer.)

Hertig, A. T., Sommers, S. C.: Genesis of endometrial carcinoma. I. Study of prior biopsies. Cancer 2:964, 1949. (A classic early study of the relationship between endometrial hyperplasia and carcinoma.)

Kurman, R. (ed.): Blaustein's Pathology of the Female Genital Tract. 3rd ed. New York, Springer-Verlag, 1987. (A comprehensive book of gynecologic and obstetric pathology.)

Lage, J. M.: Flow cytometric analysis of nuclear DNA content in gestational trophoblastic disease J. Reprod. Med. 36:31, 1991.

Page, D. L., Anderson, T. J.: Diagnostic Histopathology of the Breast. New York, Churchill-Livingstone, 1988.

Recent Advances in Gynecologic Pathology. Human Pathology 22:737 and 22:847, 1991. (Includes brief up to date reviews of recent work on the pathology of gynecologic tumors and tumor-like conditions.)

Sternberg, S. S., Mills, S. E.: Surgical Pathology of the Female Reproductive System and Peritoneum. New York, Raven Press, 1991. (An illustrated handbook.)

Visscher, D. W., Sarkar, F. H., Crissman, J. D.: Clinical significance of non-traditional parameters in carcinoma of the breast. *In* Advances in Pathology 5, 1992. (A recent summary of the prognostic significance of DNA ploidy, proteinases, and oncogenes in breast cancer.)

TWENTY

Diseases of the Endocrine System

PITUITARY GLAND
HYPERPITUITARISM—ADENOMAS
   General Features
   Types
HYPOPITUITARISM
POSTERIOR PITUITARY SYNDROMES

THYROID GLAND
HYPOTHYROIDISM
   Cretinism
   Myxedema
THYROTOXICOSIS (HYPERTHYROIDISM)
GRAVES' DISEASE
DIFFUSE (SIMPLE) AND MULTINODULAR GOITER
   Diffuse (Simple) Goiter
   Multinodular (Toxic or Nontoxic) Goiter
THYROIDITIS
   Hashimoto's Thyroiditis
   Subacute (DeQuervain's, Granulomatous) Thyroiditis
   Chronic (Silent) Thyroiditis
TUMORS
   Adenoma
   Carcinoma
      Papillary Carcinoma
      Follicular Carcinoma
      Anaplastic Carcinoma
      Medullary Thyroid Carcinoma
   Metastases to the Thyroid

PARATHYROID GLANDS
HYPERPARATHYROIDISM
   Primary Hyperparathyroidism
      Adenoma
      Primary Hyperplasia
      Carcinoma of the Parathyroids
   Secondary Hyperparathyroidism
HYPOPARATHYROIDISM

ADRENAL CORTEX
ADRENAL CORTICAL HYPERFUNCTION (HYPERADRENALISM)
   Cushing's Syndrome
   Hyperaldosteronism
   Adrenogenital Syndromes—Congenital Adrenal Hyperplasia
ADRENAL CORTICAL HYPOFUNCTION
   Chronic Adrenocortical Insufficiency— Addison's Disease
   Acute Adrenocortical Insufficiency
ADRENOCORTICAL NEOPLASMS

ADRENAL MEDULLA
PHEOCHROMOCYTOMA
NEUROBLASTOMA

THYMUS
HYPERPLASIA
THYMOMA

MULTIPLE ENDOCRINE NEOPLASIA

Pituitary Gland

A few details of normal cytology may be helpful in clarifying the nomenclature of anterior lobe tumors. Electron microscopy and immunocytochemistry have made it clear that the simple subdivision of the adenohypophysis into acidophils, basophils, and chromophobes is inadequate and oversimplified. The various functional secretory cells bear cytoplasmic granules of the particular tropic hormone produced by the cell. It is possible, then, to unmistakably identify the cells of origin of the various pituitary hormones in immunostains using specific antisera to the various pituitary hormones (Table 20–1).

Although most functional cells produce a single hormone, it is evident that gonadotrophs produce both

TABLE 20–1. CELL TYPES OF THE ADENOHYPOPHYSIS AND THEIR FUNCTION

Cell Type	Frequency (%)	Secretory Product
Somatotroph	~50	Growth hormone (GH)
Mammotroph (lactotroph)	10–20	Prolactin (PRL)
Corticotroph	15–20	Corticotropin (ACTH)
Gonadotroph	~10	Luteinizing hormone (LH) and follicle-stimulating hormone (FSH)
Thyrotroph	~5	Thyrotropin (TSH)

luteinizing hormone (LH) and follicle-stimulating hormone (FSH), and some stem cells may elaborate both growth hormone (GH) and prolactin (PRL) or other combinations. This virtuosity is not surprising, since all the secretory cells of the adenohypophysis derive from a common stem cell. The cells vary from densely to sparsely granulated. Sometimes there are very few granules or even none in functionless cells; such cells conform to the "chromophobes" of the past and are now sometimes called "null cells." Although the secretory granules associated with particular hormones differ in size (50 to 1000 nm), there is considerable overlap and indeed variability in granule size within a cell, so that size is not a reliable indicator of the nature of the hormone. With this brief survey of the normal cells, we can turn to the major disorders of the anterior lobe, which can be conveniently considered under the headings of hyper- and hypopituitarism.

HYPERPITUITARISM—ADENOMAS

Excess hormone production by the anterior pituitary, unless proven otherwise, is caused by a pituitary adenoma. Carcinomas of the gland and hyperfunction owing to nontumorous hyperplasia of particular cell types are both rare. Equally rare are hypothalamic lesions (hamartomas, gliomas, gangliocytomas) and visceral cancers (e.g., small cell bronchogenic, thyroid medullary carcinoma) that produce releasing factors that secondarily initiate pituitary hyperfunction. So hyperpituitarism almost always implies an adenoma. Most are monoclonal and produce only a single hormone (i.e., monohormonal), but not so infrequently an adenoma is associated with excess GH and PRL. Sometimes both cell types are apparently present in the tumor (biclonal), but occasionally the adenoma is monoclonal despite bihormonal function. Other unexpected combinations are also encountered. Table 20–2 presents the approximate frequency of the various types of adenoma as encountered in unselected surgical biopsy specimens of a large series of patients.

GENERAL FEATURES

Some morphologic and clinical features are common to all adenomas; these will be presented before particular secretory types are characterized.

TABLE 20–2. PREVALENCE OF ADENOMAS IN UNSELECTED SURGICAL BIOPSY SPECIMENS*

Cell Type	Approximate Prevalence (%)
Somatotroph (GH cell) adenoma	
Densely granulated	7
Sparsely granulated	7
Mammotroph (PRL cell) adenoma	
Densely granulated	<1
Sparsely granulated	27
Mixed GH cell–PRL cell adenoma	5
Monomorphic bihormonal adenoma	3
Corticotroph cell adenoma	8
"Silent cortocotrophin" adenoma	6
Gonadotroph adenoma	7
Nonsecretory adenoma (including null cell adenoma)	25
Plurihormonal (usually pluricellular) adenoma	4

* Modified from Horvath, E., Kovacs, K.: Pituitary gland. Pathol. Res. Pract. *183*:129, 1988.

Functional adenomas vary in size from large tumors approaching 10 cm in diameter to microadenomas less than 10 mm in diameter (Fig. 20–1). Most large neoplasms are discretely encapsulated and tend to expand the sella turcica, erode the anterior clinoid processes, and produce pressure defects in the optic chiasm or optic nerves. Some rupture through their capsules and diaphragma sellae to expand along broad fronts into the contiguous brain or cavernous and nasal sinuses, thus

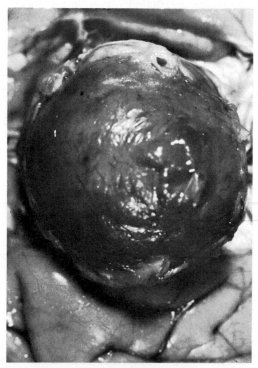

Figure 20–1. Close-up detail of a pituitary adenoma still attached to the brain. Compressed vessels and nerves are apparent about the periphery.

giving the false impression of cancerous invasion. On transection they are usually soft red-brown but frequently have areas of ischemic necrosis, cystic softening, and sometimes hemorrhages (**pituitary apoplexy**). Occasional large adenomas undergo virtually total infarction as the expansile pressure compresses their blood supply. The nonneoplastic anterior lobe may be markedly attenuated, to the point where it may virtually disappear. Microadenomas, on the other hand, may be so small as to not be visible to the naked eye, may have a poorly developed capsule or none, and may therefore be difficult to differentiate from a focus of hyperplasia.

The polygonal cells in most adenomas are more or less uniform in size with basically central round nuclei surrounded by an abundant cytoplasm. They are dispersed in sheets, trabeculae, or nests separated by a delicate vascularized stroma. Only immunochemical reactions using monoclonal antibodies to specific tropic hormones permit segregation of one type of secretory adenoma from another.

Clinically, adenomas may cause manifestations because of (1) the mass effect of the neoplasm when large, (2) the secretory function, or (3) both. The mass effects include: visual field defects, headaches, nausea and vomiting (all reminiscent of a brain tumor), and suppression of the hormonal function of the nontumorous pituitary. In addition, the findings of enlargement of the sella turcica, erosions of the bony enclosure of the sella, and expansion through the diaphragma sellae by radiography, computed tomography (CT) or magnetic resonance imaging (MRI) are major markers of a pituitary lesion (Fig. 20–2). Among these effects, most typical is bilateral homonymous hemianopsia or some other field defect re-

sulting from pressure encroachment on the optic chiasm or optic nerves. However, approximately half of all hyperfunctioning tumors are microadenomas marked by excess hormone production in the absence of any localizing manifestations.

TYPES

Somatotroph tumors tend to be the largest of the adenomas because they are discovered late. They are about evenly divided into densely and sparsely granulated types. Electron microscopy reveals within the densely granulated tumors: spherical secretory granules ranging widely in size but averaging 500 nm in diameter. Such cells appear acidophilic with routine dyes, and the granules yield a strong positive reaction to growth hormone with immunoperoxidase methods. By contrast, the sparsely granulated lesions: might be faintly acidophilic or chromophobic and be weakly reactive or nonreactive on immunoperoxidase stains.

GH-producing adenomas are usually large because the clinical manifestations are at first very subtle and come to attention only after many years to decades. Hence mass effects are frequently present. Eventually, functioning granulated tumors produce gigantism in the prepubertal child, or much more often acromegaly in adults, or sometimes both when the lesion has been present since childhood. Sparsely granulated lesions may yield no manifestations of excess GH but instead features of hypopituitarism as the nontumorous pituitary becomes attenuated by pressure (p. 647). Avoiding much detail, gigantism is exemplified by the tragic circus giants of the past, whose height sometimes

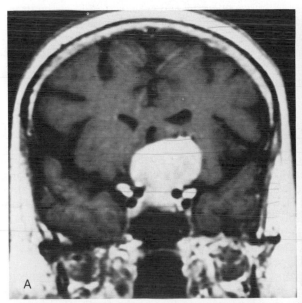
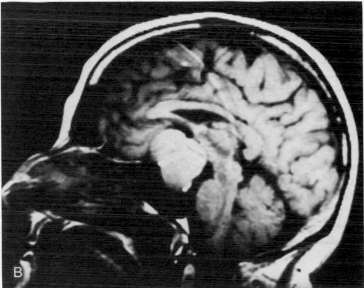

Figure 20–2. *A*, Coronal and *B*, sagittal magnetic resonance images of a large somatotroph adenoma in a 56-year-old woman. The mass has expanded the sella turcica and pushed up through the diaphragma sellae. (Courtesy of Dr. David Bloom, Department of Radiology, Brigham and Women's Hospital.)

exceeded 8 feet and who exhibited proportionate enlargement of viscera, facial features, tongue, hands, and feet. These unfortunate victims prematurely become tottering, arthritic hulks. Acromegaly, on the other hand, is a more insidious syndrome characterized by enlargement and coarsening of the facial features, hands, and feet ("megaly" of the acral parts). Frequently glucose intolerance or diabetes mellitus, osteoporosis, and hypertension are also present. To be remembered, hypothalamic tumors (mainly gangliocytomas) and various visceral neoplasms, such as pancreatic islet cell tumors, carcinoids, and medullary carcinomas of the thyroid, may produce GH-releasing factor and in turn hyperplasia and hyperfunction of GH cells yielding syndromes identical to those associated with primary pituitary neoplasms.

About a third of tumors that produce excess GH are bihormonal, also producing PRL. Most often both distinctive cell types can be identified by immunoelectron microscopy, but rarely both types of secretory granules are found in the same stem cells. The resultant clinical syndrome is a complex of the two hormones, but usually the features related to GH dominate.

Prolactinomas are the most common hyperfunctioning tumors of the pituitary. The overwhelming majority are sparsely granulated. They range from microadenomas to large, expansile masses that produce mass effects. The cytologic characteristics are somewhat different from those of GH-cell adenomas. The cells tend to have more abundant rough endoplasmic reticulum (RER) and somewhat smaller secretory granules under the electron microscope (Fig. 20–3). Stained with usual aniline dyes most of these tumors are chromophobic or slightly acidophilic. Only appropriate immunoperoxidase methods identify with certainty the nature of the granules. Microcalcifications are present in about 10 to 15% of the lesions.

Adenomas that produce excess PRL induce the characteristic *amenorrhea-galactorrhea syndrome in women.* Because these manifestations come to attention very early, prolactinomas of women tend to be very small or microadenomas. In contrast, in males and older females, they are usually discovered only when large enough to cause local effects. To be noted, the many other causes of the amenorrhea-galactorrhea syndrome (e.g., lesions in the hypothalamus, estrogen therapy, and drugs such as methyldopa and reserpine) must be ruled out in these cases.

Corticotroph adenomas, when autonomous within the pituitary, are usually small microadenomas, but patients who have had bilateral adrenalectomy also develop secondary corticotroph adenomas, and in this circumstance the tumors are often large and invade adjacent tissue. In all adenomas, the cells tend to be large, ovoid, and

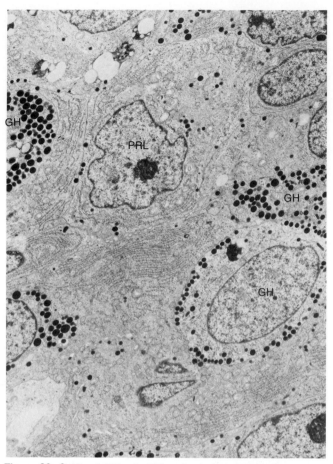

Figure 20–3. Mixed GH cell–PRL cell adenoma associated clinically with acromegaly and hyperprolactinemia. The GH cells are densely granulated as compared with the sparsely granulated PRL cells, which contain abundant RER. (Kindly provided by Dr. Eva Horvath, Department of Pathology, St. Michael's Hospital, Toronto.)

angular, arranged singly and in clumps. With aniline dyes they are basophilic and PAS positive. Electron microscopy reveals secretory granules of varying size and density (averaging about 300 nm in diameter) that are reactive to monoclonal antibodies to adrenocorticotropic hormone (ACTH).

Primary autonomous corticotroph adenomas, with excess elaboration of ACTH, produce *Cushing's disease* (discussed on p. 666) owing to excess secretion of adrenal cortical steroids. However, for obscure reasons, some well-granulated corticotroph adenomas revealing ACTH with immunostains are clinically "silent." Conceivably, the cells might elaborate the antigenically reactive precursor molecule of proopiomelanocortin and are unable to process it into its fragments of ACTH, endorphins, and β-lipotropin.

Secondary corticotroph adenomas in adrenalectomized patients produce *Nelson's syndrome.* The neoplasms develop owing to loss of the feedback-inhibiting effect of adrenal steroids on corticotroph function. In the absence of the adrenal glands, the pituitary tumor cannot cause Cushing's disease but instead comes to attention because of hyperpigmentation or enlargement with local mass effects.

FSH, LT

Gonadotroph adenomas represent about 10 to 20% of macroadenomas in middle-aged men and women. Generally there are no disturbances in gonadal function or other manifestations, so these tumors are generally large by the time they are discovered and come to clinical attention only because of their mass effect. The cells are usually arranged in cords, but follicle formation is fairly common. Often there is great variability in cell size and shape. In some adenomas, the cells are small, polyhedral, basophilic, and have scanty, undistinctive secretory granules. At the other end of the scale, the cells are polyhedral, elongated, and have well-defined secretory granules up to 250 nm in diameter.

Diagnosis depends on the detection of gonadotropic hormone, mainly FSH or LH, in the serum or excised tissue or their α or β subunits. These neoplasms produce no distinctive clinical syndromes and generally grow large enough, as noted, to cause local mass effects. Occasionally they are identified by elevated serum concentrations of FSH, one of its subunits, or, more rarely, LH.

Other types of tumors that elaborate thyroid-stimulating hormone (TSH) are too uncommon for characterization, and nonsecretory neoplasms are described under hypopituitarism.

Primary carcinomas of the anterior lobe are, as mentioned, exceedingly uncommon. Moreover, they are usually sufficiently undifferentiated so that they only rarely elaborate hormones and so no particular cell type of origin can be identified. Cytologically they may have some features of anaplasia, but many cannot be reliably differentiated from benign neoplasms, so the only criterion for malignancy is metastasis, mainly to regional lymph nodes in the head and neck, to the liver, and to bones.

HYPOPITUITARISM

Hypofunction of the anterior pituitary results most often from destruction of at least 80 to 90% of the adenohypophysis. Rarely it is related to a developmental defect. In some instances it is secondary to a hypothalamic lesion (e.g., gangliocytoma, glioma, craniopharyngioma, or germ cell tumor) that destroys the source or blocks the delivery of the pituitary hormone–releasing factors. The lesions that damage the pituitary or hypothalamus may also directly injure the posterior lobe to interfere with the synthesis or release of vasopressin (antidiuretic hormone) and oxytocin. Here our attention is focused on the hypopituitarism that derives from direct destruction of the adenohypophysis related in more than 90% of instances to (1) nonsecretory adenomas, (2) pituitary necrosis, or (3) the empty sella syndrome. Infrequent

causes of pituitary destruction are sarcoidosis or infections that sometimes arise in the meninges; surgical or radiation ablation of the pituitary; metastases to the pituitary; and disruption of the blood supply by cavernous sinus thrombosis or some form of arteritis. Deficiencies of the tropic hormones usually develop in the following temporal sequence: GH, FSH/LH, TSH, ACTH, and lastly PRL. Rarely hypopituitarism manifests as a monohormonal deficiency. A deficiency of GH is associated with no distinctive clinical syndrome in adults, but in prepubertal children it produces pituitary dwarfism. In males depressed levels of the gonadotropins induce testicular atrophy, sterility, and loss of axillary and pubic hair. In females they produce amenorrhea, atrophy of the ovaries sometimes with sterility, atrophy of the external genitalia, and loss of axillary and pubic hair. A deficiency of TSH or ACTH would lead to anticipated hypofunction of the relevant target endocrine glands. With this brief introduction we can turn to the major causes of anterior pituitary hypofunction.

Nonsecretory (null cell, chromophobe) adenomas are the commonest cause of hypopituitarism. About 25 to 30% of clinically demonstrable adenomas are nonfunctional. They come to attention either because the expanding mass produces compressive atrophy of the nontumorous pituitary and hypopituitarism or because of the local mass effects described earlier (p. 645). Histologically they are composed of small, sometimes clear cells bearing scant, small cytoplasmic granules. With usual staining techniques such cells conform to the chromophobes of the past. Immunoelectron microscopy, however, reveals that frequently the granules yield positive reactions for LH, FSH or its α or β subunit. Occasionally the secretory granules apparently contain GH or ACTH. Why such apparent secretory function does not become clinically manifest is not understood, but it may be a quantitative phenomenon or some qualitative defect in the processing and release of the synthesized hormone. In about a third of these tumors the granules in the cells fail to react with antisera to any of the known tropic hormones. A minority of nonsecretory adenomas are composed of large acidophilic cells having granular cytoplasm imparted by closely packed, large mitochondria (oncocytic adenomas). Occasionally the oncocytes have sparse secretory granules, which usually fail to react with any of the known pituitary tropic hormones.

Sheehan's syndrome (postpartum pituitary necrosis) is the second most common cause of hypopituitarism. This syndrome is the consequence of sudden infarction of most of the anterior lobe, triggered most often by obstetric hemorrhage or shock. The anterior lobe normally enlarges during pregnancy, thereby compressing its already tenuous vascular supply and rendering it extremely vulnerable to any significant drop in perfusion pressure. Indeed, incidental microinfarcts are common even in the absence of pregnancy. However, pituitary necrosis may also be seen in males, since there are many potential nonobstetric causes such as disseminated intravascular coagulation (DIC), sickle cell anemia, cavernous sinus thrombosis, some form of arteritis, profound hypotension from any cause, and traumatic injury to the vascular supply. As noted earlier, the infarction must cause destruction of most of the anterior lobe to produce manifestations of hypopituitarism. How soon the hormone deficiency becomes apparent is extremely variable. Sometimes it occurs so rapidly as to cause failure of lactation after delivery. At other times, perhaps with less destruction of the anterior lobe, the condition may be asymptomatic or become apparent after a long delay as the resultant fibrous scarring encroaches on residual functional cells. With replacement therapy or incomplete destruction of the anterior lobe, long survival is possible, as, indeed, is childbearing. In some instances, postmortem examination of the pituitary fossa years later reveals only a small nubbin of fibrous tissue attached to the posterior lobe.

Empty sella syndrome is a curious, poorly understood condition. Special radiographic techniques demonstrate the apparent absence of the pituitary. At autopsy, any stage of pituitary atrophy or compression may be found up to virtual total absence of the anterior lobe (Fig. 20–4). The pathogenesis may be related to herniation of the arachnoid through a defect in the diaphragma sellae permitting cerebrospinal fluid (CSF) pressure to cause slowly progressive atrophy of the pituitary, and sometimes enlargement of the sella (highly reminiscent on x-ray or scans of a pituitary tumor). Other possible bases for Sheehan's syndrome are total infarction of an adenoma followed by fibrous scarring, irradiation, and surgical ablation of the pituitary. In most instances, sufficient functioning parenchyma is preserved to prevent hypopituitarism, but occasionally a deficiency of one or more of the tropic hormones is manifested or at other times, paradoxically, hyperprolactinemia.

POSTERIOR PITUITARY SYNDROMES

These disorders are exceedingly rare and most often are produced by suprasellar hypothalamic tumors such as gangliocytoma, craniopharyngioma, glioma, and germ cell neoplasms, and even less frequently by posterior lobe destruction by metastatic tumor or infection. A significant minority of cases are idiopathic. One of two conditions may result: (1) a deficiency of antidiuretic hormone (ADH) causing diabetes insipidus (polyuria and polydypsia) or (2) inappropriate release of ADH (abnormal reabsorption of glomerular filtrate and consequent retention of water). The more common cause of inappropriate ADH secretion is ectopic production by nonendocrine tumors. Oxytocin, the other posterior lobe secretion, is involved only in the potentiation of uterine contractions during labor and contraction of the ducts in the lactating breast.

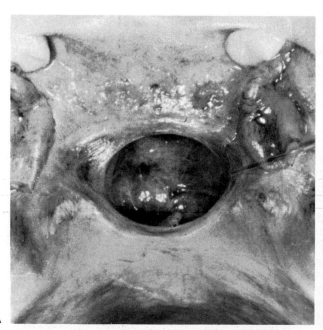
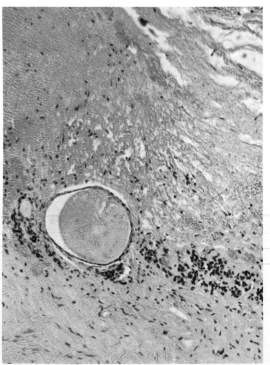

A   B

Figure 20–4. View of sella turcica *A*, in situ in a patient dying of far-advanced pituitary insufficiency. Residual gland substance remains in situ and can be seen as a minute nubbin of tissue protruding from midline of posterior wall of sella *(below)*. *B*, Microscopic view of anterior lobe of pituitary illustrated in *A*. Complete fibrous atrophy of anterior lobe is evident above pars intermedia, indicated in photograph by cystic space. Posterior lobe, below, appears normal.

Thyroid Gland

Disorders of the thyroid come to clinical attention because of (1) enlargement of the gland (goiter), which may be diffuse and symmetric, asymmetric, multinodular, or focal; (2) oversupply of thyroid hormone to the tissues of the body (thyrotoxicosis); or (3) inadequate hormone production (hypothyroidism). Often two or all of these derangements are present, either concurrently or in the course of the disease. Thus patients who have a goiter may also be thyrotoxic, and quite often a period of hyperfunction is followed by hypofunction. Because hypofunction and hyperfunction are common threads that run through most thyroid disorders, these clinicopathologic states are presented first.

HYPOTHYROIDISM

This syndrome is caused by any structural or functional derangement that interferes with the synthesis of sufficient amounts of thyroid hormone to maintain normal homeostasis. The major implicated clinical disorders are cited in Table 20–3.

About 95% of cases of hypothyroidism are caused by one of three conditions: (1) surgical or radiation ablation of the gland incident to therapy of Graves' disease or thyroid cancer, (2) Hashimoto's thyroiditis, and (3) primary idiopathic hypothyroidism, very likely of autoimmune origin with thyroid-stimulating hormone (TSH) receptor–blocking antibodies. When the thyroid insufficiency is present during infancy and childhood *cretinism* results. Hypothyroidism at a later age causes *myxedema.*

CRETINISM

At one time cretinism was endemic in iodine-deficient regions of the world such as areas of Nepal, China, inland Africa, and surprisingly in mountainous

areas even in well-developed countries, but the widespread iodination of salt and other foodstuffs has reduced the prevalence of this condition. Sometimes cretinism is sporadic and related to hereditary metabolic derangements in synthesis of thyroid hormone, such as the lack of a critical enzyme in the biosynthetic pathway, or it is related to hypoplasia or agenesis of the thyroid gland.

Depending on the age when the hormone deficiency appears, two patterns of cretinism may result: (1) neurologic cretinism or (2) myxedematous cretinism. The former is seen in iodine-deficient areas because of depressed maternal thyroxine and triiodothyronine (T_4, T_3) levels in early pregnancy, before the fetal thyroid has developed. Normally maternal hormones pass the placenta and are critical to fetal brain development, which organ is known to have specific receptors for thyroid hormones. In contrast, a reduction in maternal T_4 and T_3 levels later in pregnancy, after fetal thyroid development has occurred, permits relatively normal brain development but stunts somatic development.

The clinical manifestations may be evident at birth but usually do not become apparent for several months; they may take the form of marked retardation of mental development (e.g., delay in the appearance of the normal milestones of infant behavior) or less severe mental impairment accompanied by short stature, coarse facial features with protruding tongue, delayed dentition, dry skin, and protuberant abdomen. Unfortunately in such cases, the physical abnormalities may not become overt until the intellectual impairment has become irreversible. Only a high index of suspicion and the finding of low serum T_4 and T_3 or elevated TSH levels (unless the basic defect is suprathyroidal) permit early enough diagnosis for appropriate therapy to be maximally useful.

MYXEDEMA

In older children and adults the manifestations of thyroid hormone deficiency appear insidiously and are often subtle. They usually begin with lethargy, cold intolerance, and, in females, profuse menstrual flow. Over the span of months, slowing of mentation, speech, and movement become evident and are often accompanied by distinctive myxedema, particularly noticeable about the eyes. The skin becomes cool, rough, and doughy. Other systems share in the hypodynamic state, and constipation sometimes progresses to adynamic ileus. The cardiac output is reduced, and typically the heart becomes enlarged. The enlargement is caused mostly by chamber dilatation as the myocardium becomes flabby owing to an increase of interstitial mucopolysaccharide-rich edema (*myxedema heart*). Pericardial and pleural effusions may appear. Respiratory depression can become serious. Unless the condi-

TABLE 20–3. CAUSES OF HYPOTHYROIDISM

Insufficient Thyroid Parenchyma
  Developmental
  Radiation injury (radioiodine, external radiation)
  Surgical ablation
  Hashimoto's thyroiditis
Interference with Thyroid Hormone Synthesis
  "Primary" hypothyroidism (?immune blockade of TSH receptors)
  Heritable biosynthetic defects
  Iodine deficiency
  Drugs (lithium, iodides, *p*-aminosalicylic acid, others)
  Hashimoto's thyroiditis
Suprathyroidal
  Pituitary lesions reducing TSH secretion
  Hypothalamic lesions that reduce thyrotropin-releasing hormone delivery

tion is corrected, the patient with advanced hypothyroidism ultimately becomes stuporous and may even go into fatal coma. The diagnosis can be established at any point in the course by low levels of serum total and free T$_4$ and T$_3$. The TSH level is compensatorily elevated unless the condition is due primarily to some hypophyseothalamic dysfunction.

With this overview of the systemic consequences of thyroid dysfunction, we can turn to the various lesions of the thyroid itself.

THYROTOXICOSIS (HYPERTHYROIDISM)

Thyrotoxicosis is the term applied to the hypermetabolic state induced by an oversupply of active thyroid hormone to the tissues of the body. *When the oversupply arises because of hyperfunction of the thyroid, it is referred to as hyperthyroidism;* however, in certain conditions (for example, some types of thyroiditis), the oversupply is related to excessive release of preformed thyroid hormone and not hyperfunction of the gland. Thus, hyperthyroidism is only one category of thyrotoxicosis. *The principal causes of excess circulating thyroid hormone (i.e., thyrotoxicosis), accounting for more than 90% of all cases, are primary diffuse toxic hyperplasia (Graves' disease), toxic multinodular goiter, and toxic adenoma.* Most of the remaining cases of thyrotoxicosis are referable to certain forms of thyroiditis and are typically self-limited. Rarely, thyroid hyperfunction is secondary to a TSH-producing pituitary adenoma or increased production of thyrotropin-releasing hormone (TRH) by the hypothalamus.

Whatever its origin, the major manifestations of thyrotoxicosis are nervousness, menstrual changes, emotional instability, fine tremors of the hands, warm skin with excessive sweating, heat intolerance, weight loss despite an increased appetite, and loss of strength. Most patients have characteristic widened palpebral fissures (responsible for the prominent stare) and frequently lid lag. Other more serious eye changes (exophthalmos) are sometimes also present in patients with Graves' disease. Cardiopulmonary symptoms may also be prominent: dyspnea, rapid pulse, palpitations, and more importantly atrial fibrillation. Despite the distinctive signs and symptoms of thyrotoxicosis, the diagnosis must always be confirmed by laboratory tests. Most characteristic are elevated serum levels of free T$_4$ and T$_3$ and depressed TSH levels. To ascertain whether the increased level of hormone relates to thyroid hyperfunction rather than to abnormal release, a radioactive iodine uptake (RAIU) test can be performed. Assays for circulating antibodies may be used in certain situations, for reasons that will soon become clear. In instances of suspected hyperfunctioning tumors or foci, a radionuclide scan may be helpful to evaluate the locus or distribution of the hyperfunction, but sometimes fine-needle aspiration or open biopsy is required.

The morphologic changes induced by excess thyroid hormone are surprisingly scanty and for the most part vague. They are more often seen with Graves' disease than in the other forms of thyrotoxicosis, because this disease tends to produce the most severe and protracted elevations of thyroid hormone. Most prominent is cardiomegaly. Sometimes there are myocardial foci of lymphocytic and eosinophilic infiltration, mild interstitial fibrosis, and, occasionally fatty change (collectively designated **thyrotoxic cardiomyopathy**). The pathogenesis of these cardiac changes remains uncertain. Extracardiac alterations that are sometimes seen include variable atrophy and fatty infiltration of skeletal muscles, sometimes with focal interstitial lymphocytic infiltrates; generalized lymphoid hyperplasia with lymphadenopathy; occasionally, a mild nonspecific lymphocytic periportal infiltration and fatty change in the liver; and, even more rarely, osteoporosis.

GRAVES' DISEASE

Graves' disease is the most common cause of thyrotoxicosis. *Although the cause of the hyperfunction is not known, there is compelling evidence that the pathogenesis involves a variety of thyroid cell autoantibodies interacting with various epitopes on the TSH receptor or closely related membrane domains.* An infiltrative ophthalmopathy causing exophthalmos and infiltrative dermopathy sometimes accompany the hyperthyroidism. Although these two features, when coupled with the hyperthyroidism, are referred to as the classic triad of Graves' disease, overt ophthalmopathy is encountered in only about a third of patients, and more subtle ocular changes in another third. Moreover, the ophthalmopathy may precede or follow the onset of the hyperthyroidism, raising the possibility that it may be a distinct entity rather than being integral to the hyperthyroidism, and the dermopathy is encountered even less frequently and has an equally uncertain relationship to the thyroid changes. Ultimately the diagnosis of Graves' disease therefore hinges on the documentation of thyrotoxicosis related to a diffusely hyperplastic, hyperfunctioning thyroid gland.

Graves' disease may occur at any age but is most common in the third and fourth decade; females are affected ten times more frequently than males. A strong association with human leukocyte antigen (HLA) DR3 suggests a genetic predisposition. Indeed, a well-defined familial predisposition has been noted (about 50% concordance in identical twins). Interestingly, Hashimoto's thyroiditis is also an autoimmune disorder, but it is associated with HLA-DR5. In some patients features of both disorders are present ("hashitoxicosis"). Not surprisingly, Graves' disease and Hashimoto's thyroiditis commonly occur along with the same autoimmune disorders, such as pernicious anemia, systemic lupus erythematosus, rheumatoid arthritis, insulin-dependent diabetes mellitus, and Addison's disease.

PATHOGENESIS. The evidence that Graves' disease is of autoimmune origin is quite convincing. Nearly all patients have a variety of autoantibodies, some of which are directed against the TSH receptor or closely related membrane domains. Other antibodies are directed against microsomes (peroxidase), thyroglobulin, T_4, T_3, as well as other thyroid targets. Of particular importance are those that interact with the TSH receptor. These are of two types: one mimics the action of TSH by activating the adenylcyclase and phosphoinositol pathways, thereby inducing hypersecretion of thyroid hormone. These are called *thyroid-stimulating immunoglobulins (TSI)*. The other receptor antibodies initiate growth of thyrocytes; these are called *thyroid growth–stimulating immunoglobulins (TGI)*. Thus comes about the hyperplastic, hyperfunctioning thyroid of Graves' disease (Fig. 20–5). But the story is even more complex, other autoantibodies have been identified that appear to block TSI and TGI and still others that may block the TSH receptor itself by binding to it.

What initiates these autoimmune reactions? Although the answer is still speculative, genetic, immune, and possibly environmental influences are proposed. The strong association between Graves' disease and HLA-DR3 suggests that the DR-region genes that code for class II molecules regulating helper T-cell responses in these persons in some way permit the unregulated formation of thyroid autoantibodies. It is speculated that "DR3 persons" have a genetic defect in antigen-specific suppressor T-cell function, which permits uncontrolled helper T-cell participation in antibody formation. But thyrocytes do not normally express class II antigens. Several scenarios are proposed. Conceivably there is ectopic expression of class II molecules, permitting helper T-cell recognition; chance mutation might produce autoreactive B cells that cannot be held in check because of the suppressor cell dysfunction. A viral infection or some other stimulus might lead to the intrathyroidal production of interferon-γ which is known to induce class II molecule expression on epithelial cells. Certain microbes (e.g., *Yersinia*) have a high affinity for TSH and could evoke antibodies that cross-react with the TSH receptor. Much is uncertain, but the autoantibody participation in the disease seems well-established.

The pathogenesis of the exophthalmos (proptosis) ascribed to an infiltrative ophthalmopathy is even more obscure. As noted previously, it appears in only some, not all, patients and could represent a related condition or be a parallel but unrelated association. Many hints point toward an immune-mediated attack on retroorbital tissues such as a marked lymphocytic infiltration and swelling of the extraocular muscles and fibrofatty tissue, thus producing the proptosis. A unique class of TSI has been described that simultaneously stimulates fibroblasts in vitro. The elaboration of hydrophilic glycosaminoglycans by the proliferating fibroblasts could contribute to the swelling of the retrobulbar tissues. Other autoimmune hints include a putative circulating autoantibody against soluble eye muscle antigens, but it must suffice that much is speculative and even more so for the dermopathy.

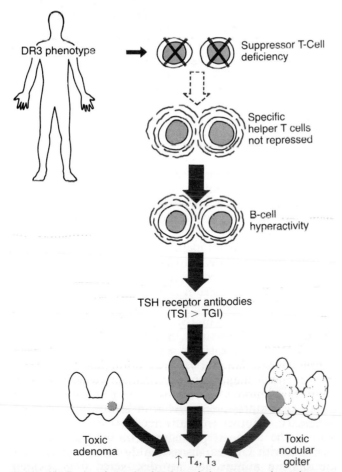

Figure 20–5. A schematic drawing of the presumed autoimmune origin of Graves' disease. The two other major causes of thyrotoxicosis are also shown. (TSI, thyroid-stimulating immunoglobulins; TGI, thyroid growth immunoglobulins.)

DR3 phenotype → Suppressor T-Cell deficiency → Specific helper T cells not repressed → B-cell hyperactivity → TSH receptor antibodies (TSI > TGI) → Toxic adenoma, ↑ T_4, T_3, Toxic nodular goiter

MORPHOLOGY. The thyroid gland is usually diffusely and symmetrically enlarged, but rarely more than three times normal size. It has a red-brown, muscle-like appearance on transection. **The cardinal histologic features in the untreated case are "too many follicular cells and too little colloid"** (Fig. 20–6). The epithelial cells become columnar, crowded, and often buckle into the thyroid follicles to form small papillae. While there is some slight variation in size and shape of the cells, there is no significant atypia. The colloid is more or less resorbed and has a thin, almost watery appearance when present, but many follicles are devoid of it. There is a marked diffuse lymphocytic infiltrate in the interfollicular stroma along with lymphoid hypertrophy throughout the body, which causes enlargement of lymph nodes, thymus, and spleen. Increased vascularity of the gland is also present.

The classic histologic changes are significantly altered by preoperative medication. Iodides block lysis of the thyroglobulin-containing colloid and promote colloid storage, and the increased size of the follicles compresses

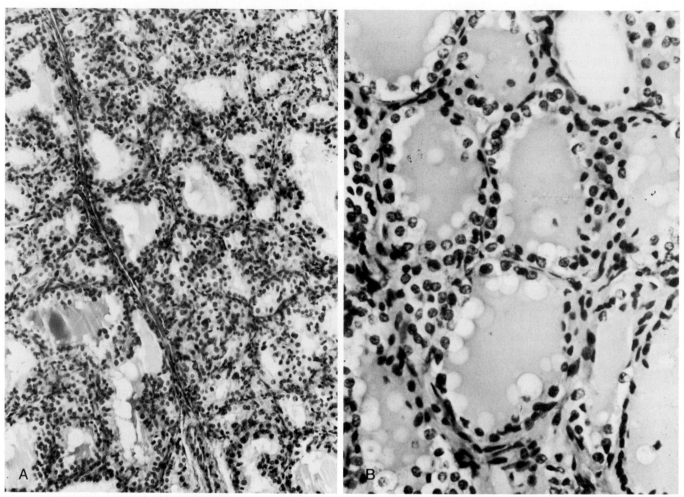

Figure 20–6. Diffuse hyperplasia of the thyroid *(left)*. Despite the marked hypercellularity of the glands and resorption of colloid, there is no anaplasia. Compare with normal thyroid *(right)*.

the vascularization. Thioureas, on the other hand, suppress thyroid hormone synthesis, leading to a compensatory increase in TSH, which augments the hypercellularity.

When present, the exophthalmos is related to the swelling and lymphocytic infiltration of the extraocular muscles and retroorbital tissues described. The dermopathy, taking the form of localized swelling, usually involves the dorsum of the legs or feet and so is incongruously termed "pretibial myxedema." These changes are attributed to the dermal and subcutaneous accumulation of glycosaminoglycans accompanied by a lymphocytic infiltration.

The heart may be enlarged and exhibit the changes previously described as **thyrotoxic cardiomyopathy** (p. 650).

CLINICAL COURSE. When the thyrotoxicosis is associated with ophthalmopathy and dermopathy the diagnosis of Graves' disease is almost certain, but as already noted the eye and skin changes frequently are not present. As you know, thyrotoxicosis may also be produced by other conditions, such as toxic multinodular goiter, a hyperfunctioning thyroid adenoma, TSH-producing pituitary adenoma, or as will be pointed out, several forms of thyroiditis, principally Hashimoto's disease. However, none of these conditions causes the ophthalmopathy and dermopathy seen in patients with Graves' disease. In most instances the diagnosis is confirmed by one or more of the following findings: increased serum levels of total or free T_4 and T_3, increased levels of RAIU, and when needed increased serum levels of TSI.

The thyrotoxicosis can be successfully controlled by various forms of medical and surgical treatment, but unfortunately the proptosis does not respond to such therapy and may even progress to corneal injuries, ulcerations, and infections leading possibly to blindness. Decompressive surgical measures may become necessary. Another (recently recognized) serious problem is the 5 to 10% incidence of thyroid cancer in patients with Graves' disease. Although many of these tumors are minute and are discovered only incidentally in thyroid tissue surgically resected for the treatment of Graves' disease, some turn out to be clinically significant.

DIFFUSE (SIMPLE) AND MULTINODULAR GOITER

These two patterns of thyroid enlargement (goiter) have common origins; the multinodular variant arises over time as an extension of the diffuse goiter. Underlying these conditions is some basis for deficient thyroid hormone output. As the thyroid's size increases in diffuse goiter, the hormone output increases, culminating, in most cases, in a euthyroid state, but following this early period of thyroid hyperplasia, colloid involution sets in. Hence the diffuse form is sometimes referred to as *colloid goiter.*

DIFFUSE (SIMPLE) GOITER

In this disorder, the thyroid gland is usually diffusely and more or less symmetrically enlarged, and although it may be associated with hypofunction early in the course, in most instances normal thyroid hormone output ultimately is achieved. *It is seen in both endemic and sporadic distributions.*

The designation *endemic goiter* implies that more than 10% of the regional population have similar lesions. The principal cause of this condition is deficient iodine intake, which is estimated to affect 800 million persons worldwide, particularly in the goitrous regions mentioned on page 649. With severe iodine deficiency in the mother the developing fetus may be affected, leading to cretinism (p. 649). The iodine deficit leads to decreased synthesis of thyroid hormone and a compensatory rise in the serum TSH level, which in turn causes follicular cell hypertrophy and hyperplasia. Iodination of salt and other foodstuffs has largely corrected the condition in many previously deficient locales around the world, but the problem has not been eradicated.

Other influences that may play roles in the development of this form of goiter are dietary substances referred to collectively as *goitrogens.* Calcium and fluorides in the water supply, lithium and thiocyanates in foods, and drugs have all been identified as being goitrogenic in animals and so could be associated with diffuse goiter in humans. Particularly implicated in the human diet are cabbage, cauliflower, cassava, Brussels sprouts, turnips, and other vegetables belonging to the Brassica and Cruciferae families.

Sporadic diffuse goiter is one tenth as common as the endemic variety. There is a striking female preponderance, with a peak incidence in puberty or young adult life, ages when there is increased demand for thyroid hormone. The cause of the inadequate thyroid function is evident only seldom, but in some cases it results from a well-defined hereditary biosynthetic defect inherited as an autosomal recessive familial trait blocking or impairing some critical step in T_4 and T_3 synthesis. Depending on the completeness of the biosynthetic block, cretinism (p. 649) or mild to moderate hypothyroidism in a child or adult may result, goiter being present in most instances. Hereditary defects account for only a fraction of the sporadic cases and

recently autoimmune mechanisms have been proposed as the basis for the "primary" hypothyroidism and goiter formation. Postulated are the appearance (for mysterious reasons) of TGIs but not the TSI mentioned previously in the discussion of Graves' disease. However, the relationship of autoimmunity to the genesis of simple goiter is still somewhat controversial.

MORPHOLOGY. With **diffuse colloid goiter,** the thyroid is firm and symmetrically enlarged, up to 200 to 300 gm, which is 10 times its normal size. The capsule is usually not involved. The transected surface is pale, brown-gray, glistening, brittle, and gelatinous. On histologic examination, large colloid-filled follicles are seen, lined by flattened epithelial cells and separated by a scant stroma. Sometimes there is evidence of preexisting hyperplasia in the form of occasional small acini lined by cuboidal to tall columnar cells or small papillary epithelial buds projecting into the colloid.

CLINICAL COURSE. Simple goiter may come to attention because of manifestations of hypothyroidism in the infant, child, or adult with only mild thyroid enlargement or because of overt thyromegaly usually in a euthyroid or at most mildly hypothyroid individual. In most cases euthyroidism is achieved as the goiter increases in size. The thyroid enlargement may be subtle or simply represent a cosmetic defect, but uncommonly, when sufficiently large, it can compress the trachea, esophagus, or vessels in the neck. Early in the course the goiter sometimes responds to iodine therapy, but if not corrected it may in time become multinodular.

MULTINODULAR (TOXIC OR NONTOXIC) GOITER

In time most diffuse goiters become transformed into nodular goiters. Only a single nodule may develop, but more often the gland becomes multinodular; the nodules may be nontoxic (i.e., associated with euthyroidism) or be toxic (toxic multinodular goiter) and induce thyrotoxicosis. Strangely, scintiscans often reveal that the hyperfunction is restricted to one or only a few of the discrete nodules. Whatever their functional state, multinodular goiters account for the most extreme thyroid enlargements.

Because of their relationship to diffuse goiters, the nodular variants appear in both endemic and sporadic settings, but the basis for the transformation is mysterious. There is evidence that normal thyrocytes vary in their metabolic activity, replicative capacity, and abilities to respond to TSH. Conceivably this variation in cell growth potential could result in nodule formation with long-term exposure to increased levels of TSH. Studies indicate that unlike monoclonal adenomas, the nodules are polyclonal. Varying levels of TSH over time with repeated cycles of hyperplasia and involution, the physical stresses and encroachment on the

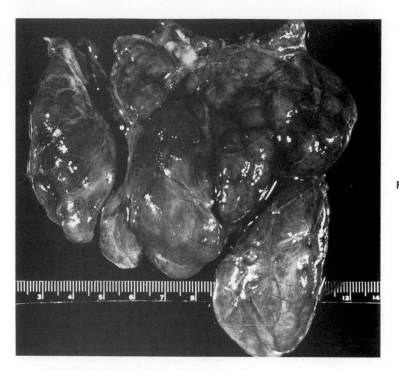

Figure 20-7. A completely distorted multinodular goiter.

vascularization induced by variations in growth of one locus relative to another, and the possibility of areas of cell death with subsequent fibrosis and compensatory generation of new follicles may all contribute to the multinodularity. Whatever the basis, the nodules once they appear may slowly increase in size in some areas while other areas may undergo involution or scarring and contraction. Not surprisingly, then, the thyroid gland shows much histologic variability.

A multinodular goiter can weigh as much as 1000 gm. Some are huge masses producing asymmetric thyromegaly that may fill the thoracic inlet and compress the structures that pass through it (Fig. 20-7). Some extend or expand downward behind the sternum (so-called **plunging goiter**). The variation in the size of the nodules may make one so dominant that it gives the clinical impression of a solitary thyroid mass. Although the capsule is usually not involved, subcapsular hemorrhage sometimes causes adhesion to surrounding structures. Perhaps the most important histologic feature is the extreme variability of the tissue in these glands. Nodules of hyperplasia exist side by side with nodules composed of dilated, colloid-filled follicles. Grossly, this appears as meaty, red-brown parenchyma alternating with pale, gelatinous areas punctuated by small cysts, foci of red-brown hemorrhage, and pale fibrotic scars (Fig. 20-8). Calcification is common in the scarred areas. **Although the nodules may give the false impression of encapsulation on gross examination, they are actually merely surrounded by compressed stromal tissue.** It is frequently difficult, then, to differentiate a single nodule from a poorly encapsulated adenoma (as is discussed later), and impossible to judge the degree of function of a nodule histologically. Thus, morphologic examination does not permit the differentiation of nontoxic goiter from the toxic multinodular type.

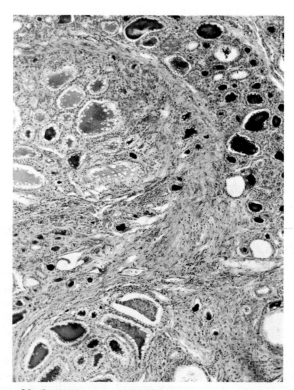

Figure 20-8. Multinodular goiter illustrates scarring and variation in size of follicles.

CLINICAL COURSE. Nodular goiters are most often encountered in elders because they evolve slowly from diffuse goiters. They are clinically important because of (1) their size and location, (2) the possible development of hyperfunction, and (3) the need to differentiate them from neoplasms.

As potentially massive lesions, multinodular goiters may cause dysphagia or respiratory difficulty or compress the large vessels passing through the thoracic inlet and so induce a superior vena caval syndrome (p. 299).

Approximately half of patients become thyrotoxic (*toxic nodular or multinodular goiter*). The thyrotoxicosis tends to be less marked than with Graves' disease and moreover is not accompanied by the infiltrative ophthalmopathy and dermopathy sometimes encountered with it. Nonetheless, the other features of hypermetabolism and cardiac disease previously described (p. 650) may be present. Scintiscans of the gland reveal either multiple patchy foci of radioiodine accumulation, indicative of hot areas; alternatively the hyperfunction may be restricted to one or several "hot" nodules.

The clinical differentiation of nodular goiter from a thyroid tumor is a challenging problem both anatomically and clinically. More will be said later about histologic criteria for separating discrete thyroid nodules from adenomas, but sometimes the line is a fine one. Moreover, the recognition that some nodules develop a degree of autonomy blurs the line even more. Analogously, the clinical differentiation of the nodular goiter from neoplasia may be extremely difficult, particularly when there is asymmetric enlargement and a single dominant nodule. It is beyond our needs to venture onto this slippery slope; it suffices to point out that ultrasonography, CT or MRI scans, response of the nodule to suppression of TSH by the administration of thyroid hormone, and fine-needle aspiration (FNA) or excisional biopsy may be required.

THYROIDITIS

This generic term is applied to thyroid disorders marked by prominent infiltration of the gland by leukocytes, fibrosis, or both changes. There are three distinctive forms of thyroiditis that merit description: Hashimoto's, subacute granulomatous, and chronic painless thyroiditis. Before these are described, several uncommon variants should be mentioned. Involvement of the thyroid by sarcoidosis or microbes, most often bacteria, is uncommon. The resultant inflammatory changes are those encountered in any other localization of the particular offender, and in most instances the involvement is self-limited. Equally rare is *Riedel's fibrous thyroiditis,* in which the gland is virtually replaced by dense fibrosis, of unknown cause. Some systemic dysfunction may underlie this lesion, because on occasion it is accompanied by mediastinal and retroperitoneal fibrosis.

HASHIMOTO'S THYROIDITIS

Hashimoto's thyroiditis (HT) is characterized by widespread replacement of much of the thyroid gland by an intense lymphoplasmacytic infiltration. There is abundant evidence that this most common form of thyroiditis is autoimmune in origin. It can arise at any age, but there is a strong female preponderance (10:1 to 20:1). Typically, the condition occurs in middle age, but it may arise earlier or later. It usually presents with variable goitrous enlargement, and in its fully developed stage with hypothyroidism. However, the patient may have been euthyroid earlier, or sometimes thyrotoxic, possibly representing concurrent Graves' disease (giving rise to the term "hashitoxicosis").

There is considerable clinical overlap between Graves' disease and HT. Both conditions are thought to be autoimmune in origin, share many types of autoantibodies, and frequently are associated with the same constellation of autoimmune diseases cited earlier (p. 650). However, it should be noted that persons who have HT have an increased frequency of HLA-DR5, whereas Graves' disease is associated with HLA-DR3. HT is also more common in patients with chromosomal abnormalities such as Down's and Turner's syndrome, which is not true of Graves' disease.

PATHOGENESIS. HT is the archetype of organ-specific autoimmune diseases, marked by lymphocytes sensitized to thyroid antigens and a panoply of autoantibodies to various thyroid antigens, most of which were mentioned in the consideration of Graves' disease. Among the autoantibodies most consistently present (about 95% of cases) are antimicrosomal (antiperoxidase) antibodies. Less frequent are antithyroglobulin antibodies and others directed against T_4 and T_3 themselves. In addition, most patients have autoantibodies targeted on the TSH receptors or on closely related membrane domains. Some of these receptor autoantibodies stimulate thyroid function, the TSI mentioned in the discussion of Graves' disease, whereas others stimulate thyroid growth (TGI, Fig. 20–9). *In Graves' disease the TSIs dominate; in HT the TGIs predominate.* To increase the complexity, blocking antibodies to each of these subsets may be present as well as receptor-binding antibodies that may also block the actions of TSI and TGI. How all these autoantibodies play out is uncertain, and indeed the titers may vary during the course of the disease, but the bottom line appears to be that HT is characterized mainly by TGIs inducing goitrous enlargement of the gland whereas TSIs either are not produced in significant amount or are suppressed by blocking antibodies, possibly accounting for the progressive development of hypothyroidism in this condition.

What initiates these autoimmune reactions in HT is as mysterious as it is with Graves' disease. It is proposed that persons bearing HLA-DR5 have a predisposition to the formation of thyroid autoantibodies, presumably as a consequence of some genetic antigen-specific suppressor T-cell defect associated with unregulated helper T-cell participation in the B-cell synthesis of autoantibodies.

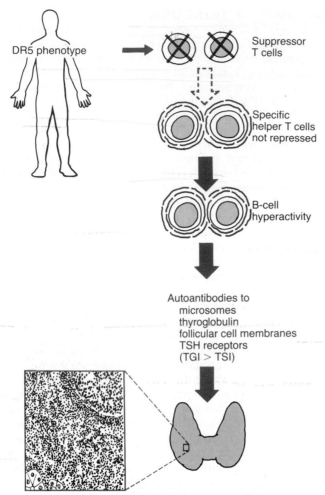

Figure 20–9. A schematic representation of the autoimmune origin of Hashimoto's thyroiditis. (TSI, thyroid-stimulating immunoglobulins; TGI, thyroid growth immunoglobulins.)

The trigger event that initiates the autoimmune attack on the thyroid gland remains unknown. Conceivably, a viral infection results in the local production of interferon-γ in the thyroid, initiating the appearance of class II molecules on the thyrocytes converting them into T-cell antigenic targets, but it is not clear whether cytotoxic T cells, antibody-dependent cellular cytotoxicity, activated complement, or more than one of these mechanisms are involved in the follicular cell destruction.

MORPHOLOGY. Typically, the gland is modestly enlarged, symmetric, firm, rubbery, and discrete. It may, however, be normal in size and even be contracted when there is significant fibrosis. Sometimes the enlargement is asymmetric and seemingly lobular. On transection, the normal red-brown, meaty, thyroidal substance is replaced by a pale, gray-white tissue that can even arouse concern at surgery about the possibility of a neoplasm, but the thyroid capsule remains intact. The classic features become evident microscopically. **There is extensive replacement of the thyroid architecture**

by lymphocytes (sometimes forming germinal centers), plasma cells, immunoblasts, and macrophages. Indeed, entire microscopic fields may resemble a lymph node. However, here and there are isolated follicles or clusters of distorted follicles (Fig. 20–10). Frequently, the residual follicular epithelium is transformed into brightly acidophilic Hürthle cells (oncocytes) that have abundant granular cytoplasm. A delicate or fairly significant fibrosis is present, but the fibrosing reaction does not extend beyond the capsule.

CLINICAL COURSE. Classically, this condition presents as a nontender goiter in association with mild to significant hypothyroidism. In this circumstance the serum T_4 and T_3 levels are low and the TSH level elevated; however, early in the disease the patient may be euthyroid, since the hypofunction develops slowly over the course of years. As noted earlier, occasionally a patient manifests thyrotoxicosis at the outset, but it is transient and self-limited and is either the result of an episode of concurrent Graves' disease or incident to excessive release of thyroid hormones from injured follicular epithelium. Infrequently, the clinical findings are not distinctive, particularly when there is asymmetric involvement of the gland and needle biopsy is required. The hypothyroidism progresses only very slowly or may plateau for years, so HT is most often a benign condition, although patients are at significantly increased risk of developing a B-cell lymphoma.

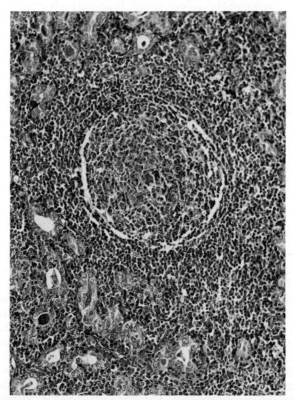

Figure 20–10. Hashimoto's thyroiditis. The microscopic field shows a prominent lymphoid follicle and a diffuse lymphocytic and plasma cell infiltrate interspersed between the atrophic thyroid follicles.

SUBACUTE (DEQUERVAIN'S, GRANULOMATOUS) THYROIDITIS

This acute to subacute inflammatory disorder is marked clinically by thyroid pain, swelling, and tenderness and histologically by granulomatous inflammation with multinucleate giant cells. Although the disease may occur at any age, the peak incidence is in the middle years, females being affected twice as often as males. There is suggestive evidence that it is of viral origin since it is frequently preceded by an upper respiratory infection and is associated with prodromal symptoms typically associated with a systemic viral infection—malaise, fever, and muscle aching. A number of viruses have been implicated, particularly those causing mumps, measles, and influenza. There is no convincing evidence for an autoimmune origin.

The thyroid is usually somewhat enlarged (two to three times normal), often asymmetrically, with patchy foci of gray-white necrosis or fibrosis. Histologically there are random foci of disruption and necrosis of the follicles, surrounded at first by a nonspecific acute to subacute inflammatory infiltrate, which later changes to a granulomatous pattern. The centers of the granulomas often contain irregular fragments of colloid surrounded by a foreign body giant cell reaction, suggesting disruption of a follicle. The giant cells are of monocyte-histiocyte origin. Still later, the reactive foci undergo fibrosis with a residual lymphocytic infiltrate.

This condition is self-limited. At the outset, the thyroid is somewhat enlarged, perhaps irregularly tender and painful, and there may be signs and symptoms of thyrotoxicosis resulting from release of stored hormone. At this stage the serum concentrations of T_4 and T_3 are elevated. Within weeks, these manifestations abate as the patient becomes euthyroid; a few have a transient phase of hypothyroidism marked by elevated serum levels of TSH. The great majority of cases resolve completely with no residual sequelae.

CHRONIC (SILENT) THYROIDITIS

A better designation for this entity would be the cumbersome term "lymphocytic, painless thyroiditis with transient thyrotoxicosis" since it specifies the cardinal morphologic and clinical features. It accounts for 10 to 20% of cases of thyrotoxicosis. Occurring at any age, it is somewhat more common in young females (ratio 2:1). Many patients bear the HLA-DR5 antigen. The cause of this condition is thought to be some variation of the Graves/Hashimoto story because silent thyroiditis may be difficult to differentiate from its close cousins, but the details are still unclear. However, relevant autoantibodies have not been identified.

The gland is normal in size or sometimes modestly enlarged, usually symmetrically. The transection may reveal no changes or subtle foci of pallor. Histologically, the dominant findings are a diffuse or focal lymphocytic infiltration with injury to follicles in the areas of involvement but little fibrosis and no formation of germinal centers. The lymphoid infiltrate is less dense than that of Hashimoto's disease and lacks plasma cells. Granulomas such as those seen in subacute thyroiditis are not present. Ultimately, the changes resolve. Many of the residual follicle cells are converted into oncocytes.

Clinically, the disease appears silently with manifestations of thyrotoxicosis; indeed this condition is said to account for 20% of all cases of thyrotoxicosis. Ophthalmopathy does not appear. The gland is neither tender nor painful and at most only slightly enlarged. The serum levels of T_3 and T_4 are elevated, and the major condition in the differential diagnosis is the hyperthyroidism of Graves' disease. Critical in distinguishing these two conditions is measurement of RAIU, which is uniformly suppressed in painless thyroiditis but elevated in Graves' disease. Thus, the thyrotoxicosis arises from inappropriate release rather than production of hormones. In the usual case, the thyrotoxic phase passes in 4 to 8 weeks and is followed by euthyroidism. However, a minority of cases have a subsequent transient phase of thyrotoxicosis, or less commonly hypothyroidism. Ultimately, the condition resolves with no sequelae.

TUMORS

Nodules of the thyroid have always commanded a great deal of attention because of the fear that they might be cancerous. However, the fraction of nodules that proves to be cancerous is extremely small. Indeed thyroid cancer is uncommon in the United States; it accounted for only about 1000 deaths in 1990 (lung cancer causes almost 130,000 deaths and breast cancer 50,000). Thus thyroid nodules and their relationship to cancer must be viewed within the following framework:

- Many benign conditions may present as a thyroid nodule—adenomas, multinodular goiters, thyroiditis, cysts, malformations of the thyroid, focal granulomatous disease.
- More than 50% of clinically apparent single nodules prove to be multinodular goiters or thyroiditis.
- Among the clinically documented solitary nodules only about 1 or 2 in a thousand prove to be malignant.
- The likelihood of a nodule harboring cancer is markedly increased by previous exposure of the neck region to ionizing radiation.

Despite all these data, neither the nodule nor the patient is a statistic.

ADENOMA

Clinically apparent solitary nodules are present in 4 to 7% of the adult population of the United States. Most, as noted above, prove not to be adenomas. The true incidence of adenomas is nearer 1 to 3%, but accurate unselected data are scant. The frequency increases with age, and they are distinctly more common in women than in men. Prior radiation exposure, as mentioned earlier, increases the prevalence of thyroid adenomas, and indeed of thyroid cancer. Most true adenomas are solitary lesions, but rarely more than one is present. Apparent multiple adenomas prove most often to be discrete nodules of a multinodular goiter. Differentiation of one from the other is not only difficult clinically but also anatomically, as will become apparent. Very uncommonly a solitary nodule proves to be a thyroid cyst, perhaps arising from cystic degeneration of a preexisting adenoma.

Thyroid adenomas are usually spherical, completely encapsulated, and rarely exceed 4 cm in diameter (Fig. 20–11). On transection, they vary from gray to brown, but a central focus of fibrosis, and sometimes calcification, may be present. Some lesions undergo cystic degeneration. True adenomas are derived from the epithelium of the follicle, and in the overwhelming majority there are readily recognized follicles on microscopy,

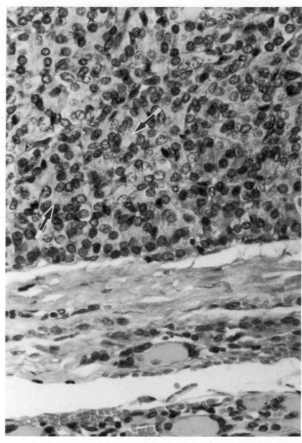

Figure 20–12. The capsular margin of a follicular adenoma reveals the so-called embryonal pattern of closely packed cells, sometimes forming abortive follicles (arrows). Note the normal follicles outside the capsule (bottom). (Courtesy of Dr. Merle Legg, New England Deaconess Hospital, Boston, Massachusetts.)

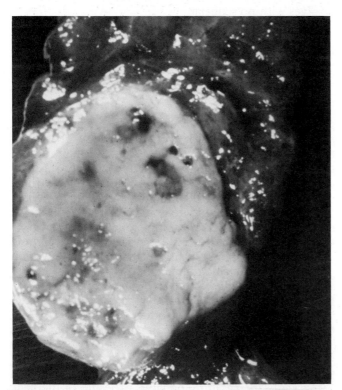

Figure 20–11. A transection of the thyroid reveals a pale, solitary, discrete adenoma clearly demarcated from the surrounding darker normal gland. (Courtesy of Dr. Merle Legg, New England Deaconess Hospital, Boston, Massachusetts.)

so almost all could be designated **follicular adenomas.** Sometimes, however, they are divided into macrofollicular and microfollicular categories. They have been more elaborately subdivided according to the relative amounts of colloid and cellularity. **A colloid adenoma** is composed of large follicles with abundant colloid and scant interfollicular stroma. The **simple adenoma** has colloid-bearing follicles of normal size with scant stroma. **Fetal adenomas** have microfollicles separated by an abundant interfollicular loose connective tissue. In **embryonal or trabecular adenomas,** the cells are disposed in cords or sheets with scattered abortive follicles (Fig. 20–12). In addition, there are encapsulated nodules that have well-developed papillary formations; experience teaches that such lesions behave as papillary carcinomas. One additional variant is the Hürthle cell adenoma composed of acidophilic granular cells (oncocytes), usually disposed in trabeculae.

Helpful in the differentiation of an adenoma from a nodule of a multinodular goiter are the following criteria. **(1) Adenomas are generally well encapsulated, whereas the apparent encapsulation of a nodule is imperfect. (2) The architecture within the adenoma is homogeneous, is distinctly different from that of the** surrounding thyroid substance, and does not have the variability typical of a nodule within a multinodular goiter. (3) The adenoma produces compression of the more or less normal surrounding follicles.

Adenomas with well-developed follicles uncommonly show microinvasion of their capsules and seemingly vascular invasion. It is frequently very difficult to differentiate these "angioinvasive adenomas" from one variant of follicular carcinoma, as will be apparent later. Microinvasion is more often encountered with the more cellular, embryonal, or trabecular patterns of adenoma. While some experts contend that such aggressiveness portends transformation into carcinoma, the clinical course rarely bears this out. The weight of opinion favors the view that adenomas do **not** give rise to thyroid carcinomas.

Most adenomas are "silent," and are discovered by chance, either by the patient or on routine physical examination. Rarely, they become large enough to cause local pressure symptoms or be disturbing cosmetically. Equally rarely, intralesional hemorrhage may produce painful enlargement. The paramount— and not simple—clinical problem is to differentiate them from carcinomas. Basically four approaches are used: (1) ultrasonography, (2) TSH suppression, (3) radionuclide scans, and (4) fine-needle aspiration (FNA) biopsy. Sometimes, however, surgical excision is necessary to provide the final diagnosis. High-resolution ultrasonography can visualize nodules as small as 1 mm in diameter. Thus, it sometimes reveals other nodules in the gland, favoring the likelihood of a multinodular goiter rather than tumor. Ultrasonography can also disclose the contour of the lesion and its internal architecture. While the findings may point in one or another direction, ultimately ultrasound cannot reliably distinguish benign from malignant lesions. TSH suppression is predicated on the concept that benign lesions are more dependent on TSH stimulation than malignant lesions, and hence if the TSH levels in the patient were suppressed by the administration of thyroid hormone, shrinkage of a nodule over time would favor "benignancy" over malignancy. Unfortunately, adenomas later proven benign fail to "suppress," and contrariwise some cancers appear to decrease in size at least for some period of time. Scintigraphy for uptake of radioiodine or pertechnetate tends to determine how avidly the nodule is able to trap iodine or an analogous isotope, on the theory that such function is more characteristic of benign adenomas than cancers. However, "hot" nodules that avidly bind the isotope sometimes prove later to be cancers, and only about 10% of "cold" nodules prove to be malignant. FNA biopsy has emerged as a valuable diagnostic tool. The reported diagnostic accuracy ranges from 50% to over 95% and depends largely on the adequacy of the aspiration and the expertise of the histocytopathologist. Even in the best of hands, however, about 35% of FNA results are indeterminate. Ultimately, excision may be necessary.

CARCINOMA

Thyroid carcinoma is an uncommon form of cancer in the United States, representing in 1989 only about 1% of all forms of cancer and responsible for only about 0.2% of all cancer deaths, or numerically about 1000 per year. In contrast, it is estimated that about 12,000 new cases will be diagnosed; it is evident many must be cured. Occult carcinomas (by definition smaller than 1 cm in diameter) can, however, be discovered in 3 to 30% of thyroids, depending on diagnostic criteria and the rigor of the search. With this frequency, it is evident that most are incidental findings rather than biologically significant lesions.

There are several anatomic categories of thyroid carcinoma, each with its own clinical behavior and significance (Table 20–4). The two most prevalent variants, papillary and follicular carcinoma (collectively referred to as well-differentiated cancers), account for 80 to 85% of all thyroid cancers; they have a much more favorable prognosis than the "poorly differentiated" carcinomas.

PATHOGENESIS. Ionizing radiation has been clearly established as a major carcinogenic influence for the thyroid. Between 1920 and 1960, children and young adults often received radiotherapy to the head, neck, and upper thorax for a variety of benign conditions— acne, cervical lymphadenopathy, tinea capitis, and putative thymic enlargement. As many as 7% of them developed thyroid carcinoma, sometimes 50 years later (mean about 22 to 25 years). Similarly, the Japanese survivors of the atomic bombs have experienced a thirtyfold excess rate of thyroid cancer. The risk is dose related, but even the very small exposures involved in diagnostic fluoroscopy have increased the risk. Fortunately, the use of radioiodine for diagnostic or therapeutic purposes has not been implicated to date. The peak of this postradiation complication appears to have passed and with it a lowering of the prevalence of thyroid cancer.

Not surprisingly, overexpressed or mutated oncogenes have been identified in some thyroid cancers. The three *ras* genes have been involved. Of interest, activation of *ras* genes has also been reported in so-called follicular adenomas, although the possibility that these lesions were well-differentiated follicular car-

TABLE 20–4. CLASSIFICATION OF THYROID MALIGNANCIES

Type	Frequency (%)
Papillary carcinoma (including mixed papillary and follicular types)	60–70
Follicular carcinoma (including clear cell, Hürthle cell, and insular types)	20–25
Medullary (C-cell) carcinoma	5–10
Undifferentiated carcinoma (including small cell, giant cell, and spindle cell types)	10
Epidermoid carcinoma	<1
Other tumors (lymphoma, sarcoma, metastatic carcinoma)	<1

cinomas cannot be excluded. Alternatively, despite earlier contrary statements (admonitions that adenomas do not give rise to cancers), some follicular adenomas rarely may become carcinomatous. Overexpression of c-*myc* and c-*fos* has also been observed. In addition, c-*erb* B and c-*erb* B2/*neu* oncogenes have also been found to be overexpressed in thyroid carcinomas. Of interest, the c-*erb* B oncogene encodes the receptor for epidermal growth factor and transforming growth factor-α, raising the possibility that this oncogene may be a link that involves growth factors in the development of carcinomas of the thyroid. Finally, mention should be made of the increased incidence of carcinoma in the diffuse thyroid hyperplasia of Graves' disease and of lymphoma in Hashimoto's thyroiditis.

Papillary Carcinoma

The designation "papillary carcinoma" is applied to any thyroid malignancy that has "pure" papillary or mixed papillary and follicular architecture or to all cancers composed of cells having "ground-glass," optically clear nuclei, whether papillary formations are present or not. So defined, papillary carcinomas constitute about 60 to 70% of all thyroid cancers. Most radiation-induced cancers and most occult lesions are of this type. In the past, extremely well-differentiated papillary lesions have been called "papillary adenoma," but time has proven that these lesions are best considered cancerous, so the entity "papillary adenoma" has largely been discarded. The following comments relate to clinically overt tumors, but you recall that occult foci of papillary cancer are quite common but of doubtful clinical significance.

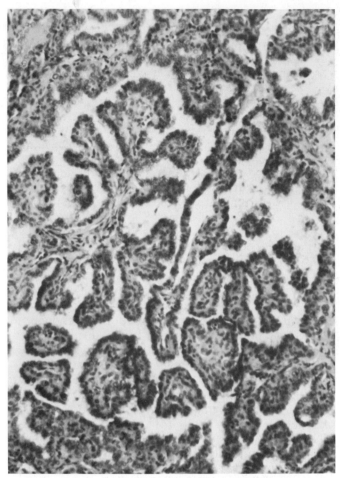

Figure 20-13. A moderately well-differentiated papillary carcinoma shows the complex branching papillae. (Courtesy of Dr. Merle Legg, New England Deaconess Hospital, Boston, Massachusetts.)

Most significant papillary carcinomas are poorly delineated unencapsulated focal masses located anywhere within the thyroid, but sometimes there are multiple foci. Rare variants are encapsulated, and equally rare are sclerotic infiltrative tumors that diffusely involve a whole lobe. Sometimes the tumors appear multifocal but are actually interconnected. Advanced tumors may penetrate the thyroid capsule into surrounding structures. The neoplastic foci are gray to brown and firm and sometimes have a furry appearance on transection. Some are almost entirely papillary. **True papillae, when present, have a central fibrovascular stalk covered by a single or multiple layers of cuboidal to low columnar epithelial cells** (Fig. 20-13). Most are well-differentiated; uncommonly, the cells are somewhat anaplastic, but mitoses are rare. **Usually the cells have ground-glass nuclei**—the nuclear membranes are distinct, the nucleoli are small and marginated, and the nucleoplasm contains finely divided chromatin, imparting a clear appearance to create so-called orphan Annie eye nuclei. Invaginations of the cytoplasm may in cross section give the appearance of nuclear inclusions. Tumors having true papillae are regarded as papillary carcinomas even if they do not have ground-glass nuclei. At the other extreme are the tumors that are almost purely follicular but are categorized as papillary carcinoma because of the ground-glass nuclei. Other microscopic features that may be present include psammoma bodies within the tips of papillae, cystic changes rarely found in other types of thyroid cancer, foci of squamous metaplasia, and lymphoid infiltration of the stroma. Uncommonly, there is vascular invasion, which makes the outlook bleaker.

In more than 50% of cases, by the time they are discovered these neoplasms have already spread through lymphatics to lymph nodes, usually within the neck, and sometimes even when the primary lesion is undetectable. Hematogenous spread is less common, but nonetheless 5 to 10% have metastasized to the lungs by the time of diagnosis. Spread to more distant sites (e.g., bones) is unusual unless the primary tumor has invaded beyond the thyroid.

This form of carcinoma may arise at any age and is the commonest form before age 40 years, particularly when there has been prior radiation. Females are affected twice as often as males. Not infrequently, such a tumor comes to attention when a metastasis is discovered in an enlarged lymph node in the neck. Indeed, in about 20% of cases, pulmonary or other metastases are present at the time of diagnosis. These may change little, if at all, over a period of years. These cancers are, on the whole, indolent lesions, yielding an overall 70 to 85% 10-year survival rate. Surprisingly, the initial presence or subsequent development of cervical lymph node metastases does not significantly influence the prognosis, because the nodal lesions too are indolent and readily excised. *Favorable prognostic features are young age, small tumor size, well-differentiated tumor cells, and encapsulation.* Conversely, unfavorable indicators are multicentricity, extrathyroid extension, and, obviously, distant metastases.

Follicular Carcinoma

The term "follicular carcinoma" is applied to cancers composed of cells that form follicles or are disposed in cords or islands with microfollicles that have no papillae, no ground-glass nuclei, nor psammoma bodies. As noted above, when any of these features is present the lesion is considered a papillary carcinoma, both anatomically and biologically. Follicular carcinomas, the second most common form of thyroid cancer, more often affect women and usually at a later age (45 to 60 years) than papillary lesions.

Macroscopically, **they may take the form of either an encapsulated gray-white nodule up to several centimeters in diameter or a massive, obviously invasive neoplasm that shows extension into perithyroid structures** (Fig. 20–14). The encapsulated pattern obviously mimics an adenoma. There is much histologic variation among these cancers. The cells range from well-differentiated to markedly anaplastic. Rare neoplasms are composed largely or entirely of Hürthle cells. The better levels of differentiation tend to be seen in lesions that produce follicles. Vascular and capsular invasion may be present in both the encapsulated and infiltrative variants, but it is more characteristic of the infiltrative lesion.

The differentiation of the small, encapsulated, well-differentiated follicular cancers from adenomas or even nodules in multinodular goiter may be difficult. Although much stress has been placed on capsular and vascular invasion as a marker of malignancy, rarely adenomas may have foci of apparent capsular invasion and occasional vessels seemingly penetrated by tumor cells, so caution is required to avoid overdiagnosis of angioinvasive lesions. **Almost always when the capsular and vascular invasion have biologic significance, the capsule has been completely penetrated, the tumor cells fill the vascular lumen, and there is accompanying cytologic atypia, providing support for the diagnosis of malignancy.** When follicular carcinomas disseminate, it is usually hematogenously, most often to the lungs, bone, liver, or brain (strangely, sparing regional lymph nodes).

Large, invasive lesions with extrathyroidal extension usually can readily be recognized clinically as cancers, but the small encapsulated pattern may defy clinical differentiation from an adenoma until biopsy. Better-differentiated lesions may elaborate thyroid hormone and induce hyperthyroidism. The outlook depends on the size and extent of the tumor (i.e., capsular and vascular invasion). But even the small encapsulated lesions slowly enlarge and extend, though of course not as rapidly as the infiltrative kind. Overall there is a 70% mortality rate at five years. More hopeful is the fact that follicular carcinomas often avidly take up iodine and so sometimes respond to the radiation provided by radioiodine.

Anaplastic Carcinoma

In contrast to the two types of well-differentiated thyroid cancer described previously, this is a poorly differentiated, highly malignant tumor that almost always causes death within two years. It affects older persons, usually between ages 60 and 80 years. About 10% of thyroid carcinomas fall into this category.

By the time it is brought to medical attention, anaplastic carcinoma is usually a bulky mass that has obviously extended beyond the thyroid capsule. The histologic pattern is extremely variable, but three variants can be identified (1) giant cell, (2) spindle cell, and (3) squamoid. So-called small cell undifferentiated tumors are likely to be lymphomas or medullary carcinomas. In about a third of the tumors, areas reminiscent of better-differentiated carcinomas can be found, suggesting origin of the anaplastic cancer in a papillary or follicular carcinoma. Cytokeratin or CEA can often be identified within the tumor cells, confirming the epithelial origin of even the most anaplastic lesions.

Rapid increase in size, extension beyond the thyroid, and widespread metastases, all occurring within one year, are characteristic of these aggressive neoplasms.

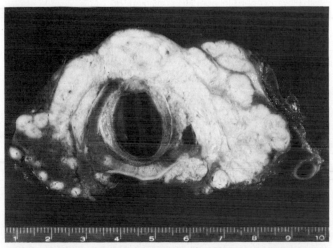

Figure 20–14. A diffusely infiltrative follicular thyroid carcinoma viewed at autopsy on transection of the gland and trachea.

Medullary Thyroid Carcinoma _____

The origin of this uncommon form of thyroid cancer has been ascribed classically to the neuroendocrine calcitonin-secreting parafollicular C cells of the thyroid. However, most of these tumors elaborate thyroglobulin, raising the possibility that they may also arise in follicular cells. Whatever their histogenesis, they are capable of elaborating a large panoply of bioactive products, including calcitonin, CEA, serotonin, neuron-specific enolase, prostaglandins, somatostatin, and many others. Calcitonin is the major product secreted by 80 to 90% of medullary thyroid carcinomas (MTCs); it can often be identified in the serum, providing a biochemical screening test for this form of cancer. Modification and precipitation of the calcitonin within some tumors yields a form of amyloid laid down in the stroma about and between cells, accounting for the designation *"medullary amyloidotic carcinoma."*

About 80 to 85% of MTC are sporadic. The remainder occur in association with multiple endocrine neoplasia (MEN) syndromes IIa and IIb, discussed on page 679, in which the MTC occurs along with pheochromocytoma, parathyroid hyperplasia or adenoma, and extraendocrine changes. Both these MEN syndromes are transmitted by autosomal dominant inheritance; the gene responsible for MEN IIa has been mapped to chromosome 10. So it is expected that soon molecular probes will permit the identification of this condition even before the endocrine tumors have appeared.

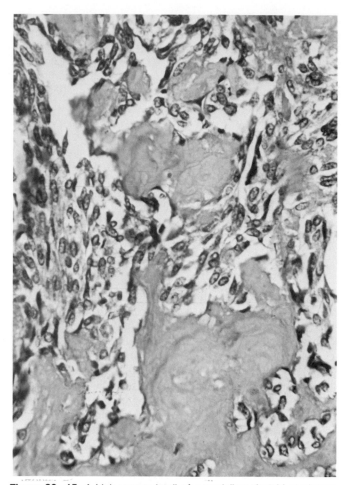

Figure 20–15. A high-power detail of a medullary thyroid carcinoma reveals the spindled tumor cells interspersed between masses of amyloid.

The anatomic changes in the thyroid depend on whether the tumor occurs as a sporadic neoplasm or in a familial setting. **Sporadic tumors** are solitary, gray-white to yellow-brown, sometimes seemingly encapsulated masses, ranging up to many centimeters in diameter, arising in one lobe. Occasionally a second isolated mass is also present, probably representing intrathyroid spread or metastasis. As they enlarge, these tumors tend to develop foci of necrosis or hemorrhage, and some invade beyond the capsule of the gland. By contrast, **familial tumors** tend to be multicentric, presenting many small neoplasms scattered throughout the thyroid gland; necrosis, hemorrhage, and penetration of the capsule are much less frequent. Both variants are alike microscopically, presenting basically polygonal or spindle cells with central round to ovoid nuclei and small nucleoli disposed in nests, cords, or trabeculae separated by a fibrovascular stroma. By electron microscopy there are abundant cytoplasmic neurosecretory granules. Amyloid may be found within the stroma of about 90% of these tumors (Fig. 20–15). Uncommonly, MTC has areas of tubular or follicular differentiation, raising questions about the histogenesis of these neoplasms. Occasionally, the tumor cells are extremely anaplastic.

In sporadic MTC, venous invasion may be prominent and may also be present to a lesser degree in the familial tumors. In the latter, outside of the neoplasm(s) there are often foci of C cell hyperplasia. Indeed, in occasional instances, only hyperplasia but no well-defined tumors can be found. Immunohistochemical procedures disclose one or more of the bioactive products in the cytoplasm, cited earlier, but particularly useful is the demonstration of calcitonin or CEA, at least one of which is present in over 90% of tumors.

Most sporadic tumors present as a painless thyroid mass, sometimes associated with lymphadenopathy, usually in the fifth or sixth decade of life. Occasionally one of the products produces a paraneoplastic syndrome such as diarrhea related to calcitonin or prostaglandins, or the carcinoid syndrome attributable to serotonin. Familial lesions are identified much earlier in the second or third decade because they are often called to attention by symptoms induced by the pheochromocytomas. In such cases, as pointed out, the lesions are usually multifocal and bilateral. Strongly supporting the diagnosis of MTC is an elevated level of serum calcitonin and CEA, but other nonthyroid neoplasms (e.g., carcinomas of the lung, breast, and pancreas) may also induce elevated CEA levels. The overall survival rate for patients with sporadic disease is

40% at 10 years. Favorable indicators are young age, small tumor, few mitoses, and somatostatin production. The prognosis for familial medullary carcinoma is significantly better: an 85% 10-year survival rate. In large part this improved outlook can be attributed to earlier diagnosis, owing to periodic screening of family members for elevated serum levels of calcitonin.

METASTASES TO THE THYROID _____

Metastatic implants into the thyroid gland occur in the dissemination of many forms of cancer, notably those arising in the lung and breast, and particularly malignant melanoma.

Parathyroid Glands

All the disorders of these glands can be considered under the headings of hyper- and hypoparathyroidism.

HYPERPARATHYROIDISM _____

HPT is categorized as primary when some intrinsic disorder of the parathyroids is responsible for hypersecretion of parathormone (PTH), producing in turn hypercalcemia and hypophosphatemia. Secondary HPT, by contrast, is marked by hypersecretion of PTH as the result of some disorder outside the parathyroids that causes hypocalcemia. It is evident that in both primary and secondary HPT there are increased serum levels of PTH, but the former is associated with hypercalcemia whereas there is hypocalcemia with the latter, which indeed is the major stimulus to the secondary HPT.

PRIMARY HYPERPARATHYROIDISM _____

The most consistent feature of primary HPT is hypercalcemia, secondary to excess secretion of PTH by either a parathyroid adenoma or primary hyperplasia of the glands. Although in the past adenomas were thought to account for at least 80% of the cases and primary hyperplasia for almost all of the remainder, an increasing number of reports suggest that hyperplasia is more common than adenomas. There is, however, agreement that parathyroid carcinoma accounts for fewer than 1% of cases. Rarely, primary HPT is a part of one of the MEN syndromes, type I or type IIA described on page 679.

The hypercalcemia in primary HPT is largely attributable to the following effects of the raised serum levels of PTH:

- Increased osteoclast-mediated mobilization of calcium from bones
- Increased renal tubular reabsorption of calcium filtered through the renal glomerulus
- Increased gastrointestinal absorption of calcium in collaboration with $1,25(OH)_2D$
- Increased excretion of phosphate in the urine, lowering the serum phosphorus level.

Although hypercalcemia is characteristic of HPT, in about 40% of instances it is not related to parathyroid disease. The long list of possible causes is offered in Table 20–5.

Among the nonparathyroid causes, cancers with or without osseous metastases are in the forefront. Indeed, although hypercalcemia in ambulatory settings is more often related to HPT in hospitalized patients it is most often related to malignant tumors. The basis for the malignancy-associated hypercalcemia was discussed on page 207, so it suffices here that it is either attributable to direct destruction of bone by osseous metastases or to the ectopic elaboration by the cancers of a variety of osteoclast-activating factors, including PTH-related peptides, transforming growth factor-α, interleukin 1 (IL-1), tumor necrosis factors, and other cytokines.

Primary HPT is one of the most common endocrinopathies (prevalence 5 to 50 per 10,000 population) in the United States. The disorder is much more common after age 40 years and has a 3:1 female predominance. The clinical manifestations have undergone considerable change over the years. At one time it was

TABLE 20–5. CAUSES OF HYPERCALCEMIA*

Primary hyperparathyroidism
Malignancy, with or without bone metastases
Other endocrine disorders
  Hyperthyroidism
  Pheochromocytoma
  Vipoma
Vitamin D toxicity
Granulomatous diseases
  Sarcoidosis
  Tuberculosis
  Histoplasmosis
  Coccidioidomycosis
  Leprosy
Lymphomas, with ectopic production of 1,25-dihydroxy-vitamin D
Drugs
  Thiazide diuretics
  Lithium
  Estrogens/antiestrogens
  Milk alkali syndrome
  Vitamin A, Vitamin D toxicity
Immobilization
Acute and chronic renal disease

* Modified from Petti, G. H.: Hyperparathyroidism. Otolaryngol. Clin. North Am. *23*:339, 1990.

characterized as "painful bones, renal stones, abdominal groans, and psychic moans." The painful bones, formerly found in most cases, reflect the mobilization of skeletal calcium with the development of osteomalacia or osteoporosis (p. 682), and in more marked cases osteitis fibrosis cystica (p. 684) leading to microfractures. Prolonged calciuria led to nephrocalcinosis and nephrolithiasis in more than 75% of cases. The abdominal and mental changes are less clearly understood. However, today most cases are discovered at a very early stage by the chance finding of hypercalcemia on routine laboratory testing, so bone disease has become uncommon and renal stones are found in only 15 to 20% of cases. Today the presentation of HPT is usually quite subtle, with nonspecific fatigue, weakness, musculoskeletal complaints, constipation, depression, and in some cases symptoms arising from one of the following commonly associated conditions: (1) peptic ulcer, (2) hypertension, (3) cholelithiasis, (4) pancreatitis, and (5) gout and pseudogout. Some of these related conditions are attributable to the hypercalcemia, but the origin of others is less certain. In addition, the prolonged hypercalcemia may lead to metastatic calcifications in blood vessels, soft tissues, and joints (chondrocalcinosis), as discussed on page 23. Ultimately the diagnosis rests on the demonstration of elevated serum calcium and PTH levels.

Adenoma

Adenomas, as noted earlier, are, at the least, one of the two most common causes of primary HPT. Almost always a single tumor arises in one of the parathyroid glands. Rarely, there are two or more, but in such cases asymmetric primary hyperplasia (discussed later) must be ruled out as well as a familial MEN syndrome (p. 679). Earlier concepts notwithstanding, recent studies clearly establish that adenomas are monoclonal, as are most neoplasms. There has long been a question, however, about the possible origin of adenomas from antecedent parathyroid hyperplasia as a fertile soil for the chance development of a somatic mutation. This sequence of an adenoma arising on a background of hyperplasia is sometimes referred to as "tertiary hyperparathyroidism" and while of interest, it remains a somewhat "speculative" entity.

For unknown reasons, the majority of adenomas occur in the lower glands. They are discrete, encapsulated, yellow-brown masses that can weigh less than 100 mg or more than 5 gm (mean about 1 gm, Fig. 20–16). Sometimes they are found in such odd locations as the thyroid, thymus, or adjacent neck tissues, much to the distress of the surgeon. Most are composed predominantly of solid sheets of uniform polygonal, chief cells (the major source of PTH and progenitor of the other cell types) that have regular central nuclei, but foci of larger acidophilic oxyphil and clear cells (containing more glycogen) are commonly present. Typically there is no stromal fat or it is markedly decreased when compared

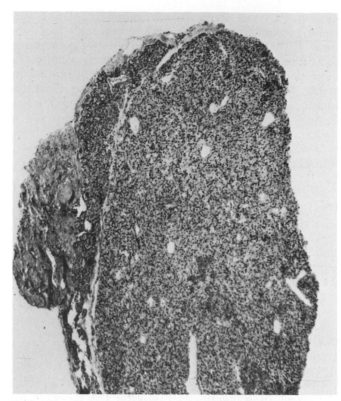

Figure 20–16. An encapsulated parathyroid chief cell adenoma is clearly demarcated from the residual gland at left.

with the surrounding normal parathyroid outside the capsule. **A clear-cut histologic difference between the tissue within and outside of the capsule comprises one of the major features differentiating adenomas from primary hyperplasia.** Moreover, typically with an adenoma, the activity of the other parathyroid glands is suppressed and they may be shrunken and have normal or increased amounts of fat. Occasionally there is follicle formation, producing a striking resemblance to thyroid tissue, and even more rarely the adenoma is composed predominantly of oxyphils. Whatever the cell type, they are uniform in size and shape and mitoses are rare.

Surgical removal of the adenoma is followed promptly by return to normal of the serum calcium level. The nephrolithiasis becomes inactive but the stones persist. The skeletal changes of osteitis fibrosa cystica, if not far advanced, are reversible within a year or two. With removal of a solitary adenoma, recurrence of HPT is rare.

Primary Hyperplasia

This designation implies diffuse hyperplastic enlargement, usually of all four parathyroid glands, in the absence of known provocation, such as a hypocalcemic condition. The glandular enlargements may be uneven and sometimes only two or three of the glands are affected, and rarely only one. It is obvious that when only one or two of the parathyroids are enlarged it is extremely difficult clinically to rule out the possibility that the enlargements represent adenomas. The differentiation is more than academic, since excision of one or two adenomas usually cures the HPT, but in the case of asymmetric primary hyperplasia, removal of one or two enlarged glands is often followed at some later date by recurrence of the hyperfunction in the remaining glands.

The stimulus for primary hyperplasia is not known. Infrequently it is a part of familial MEN syndrome I or IIa (p. 679). Recently a circulating growth factor was identified in MEN I, but no similar observation has been made in any of the other settings. Other speculations have included elevation of the set point at which serum calcium suppresses parathyroid function, calling therefore for hyperplastic enlargement of the glands to produce more hormone. Yet another speculation postulates end-organ resistance to PTH. Whatever its origins, primary hyperplasia vies with adenoma as the most common cause of primary HPT.

The individual hyperplastic glands vary in weight between 50 mg and 4 gm (mean about 500 mg). There may be much asymmetry among the four glands — as much as a tenfold difference. Histologically, the most common pattern is chief cell hyperplasia, which may involve the gland diffusely or take the form of scattered hyperplastic nodules (Fig. 20–17). Often there is an admixture of oxyphils and clear cells. Stromal fat is decreased in proportion to the magnitude of the hyperplasia, and so may be completely or largely absent. Infrequently the enlarged glands show principally clear cell hyperplasia, usually without the nodularity seen in the chief cell hyperplasias. The cells in this variant may be disposed in cords, trabeculae, or sheets. The clear cell hyperplasia may be associated with more striking glandular enlargement than is seen in the chief cell patterns. An important feature that differentiates primary hyperplasia from adenomas is the lack of a well-defined capsule in the former that separates the changes from a rim of normal parathyroid tissue.

Surgically, the differentiation of asymmetric hyperplasia from one or several adenomas is both important and difficult. Here, the condition of the seemingly uninvolved glands becomes important. With an adenoma, the other glands are suppressed and should therefore be atrophic and possibly contain larger amounts of stromal fat. With hyperplasia, despite the lack of glandular enlargement there is no atrophy and often focally increased cellularity and diminished fat; but ultimately the ice is thin. Recurrence is much more common with primary hyperplasia than with one, or even two, adenomas.

Carcinoma of the Parathyroids _____

Carcinoma of the parathyroids is an extremely rare cause of HPT, accounting for fewer than 1% of cases.

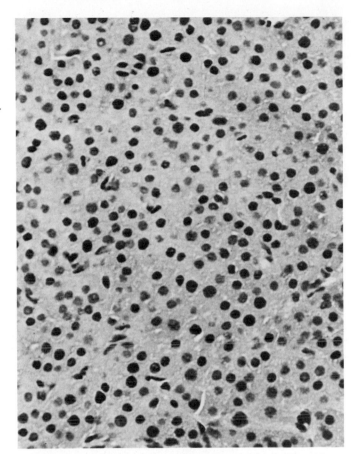

Figure 20–17. Marked chief cell hyperplasia of the parathyroids.

Brevity is, therefore, indicated. The malignant neoplasms grow and spread slowly and present as hard, gray-white masses, rarely weighing more than 10 gm. Like all malignancies, they invade the surrounding tissues, metastasize first to regional nodes, and rarely spread to distant sites. *The differentiation of a small, localized carcinoma from an adenoma is difficult, and so three required criteria have been established: (1) evidence of local invasion; (2) metastasis to cervical lymph nodes or distant sites, such as lung, liver, and bone; and (3) well-defined cellular atypia accompanied by capsular or vascular invasion.* The last-mentioned criterion is a slender thread and so is discounted by many experts on the grounds that some cellular atypia is present in occasional adenomas and the interpretation of capsular and vascular invasion is difficult, so only metastasis is left. Some carcinomas are nonsecretory but, when functioning, tend to induce more marked hypercalcemia with more prominent "bone and stone" disease.

SECONDARY HYPERPARATHYROIDISM _____

Compensatory hyperfunction and hyperplasia of the parathyroids occurs with hypocalcemia or peripheral resistance to PTH. The most common setting for secondary HPT is chronic renal insufficiency, with its attendant hyperphosphatemia and hypocalcemia. Less common associations are calcium malabsorption, osteomalacia, and deficient or deranged vitamin D metabolism.

With chronic renal disease the pathophysiology of the secondary hyperparathyroidism (HPT) is not simply hyperphosphatemia with its attendant hypocalcemia. The loss of functional renal tissue produces a quantitative decrease in the synthesis of 1,25-$(OH)_2$D. With the decline in this active metabolite there is decreased absorption of calcium from the intestine. The hyperphosphatemia also depresses the activity of the renal 1-α-hydroxylase, further impairing synthesis of 1,25-$(OH)_2$D, as does the acidosis of renal failure. Although the major stimulus to hyperplasia of the parathyroid is reduced serum calcium, there is some evidence that hyperphosphatemia and a deficiency of 1,25-$(OH)_2$D may directly stimulate PTH secretion and hyperplasia. Surprisingly, the hyperfunction and hyperplasia sometimes continue to progress despite normalization of the serum calcium level, raising the possibilities of end-organ resistance to PTH or elevation of the set point at which the parathyroid glands are "turned off" by the serum calcium level.

The glandular enlargement may be somewhat asymmetric, but usually all four glands are involved. Aggregate weights in excess of 15 gm have been recorded. Usually there is diffuse chief cell hyperplasia, but it may be nodular and accompanied by scattered foci of oxyphils, clear cells, or both. Because the serum calcium levels usually return to nearly normal levels, metastatic calcifications are rare, but skeletal changes sometimes appear in long-standing secondary HPT caused by chronic renal

disease. The bony changes in this setting, referred to as **renal osteodystrophy,** are described on page 684.

Unlike primary hyperplasia the secondary parathyroid changes are usually reversible if the underlying disorder can be corrected, e.g., renal transplantation in patients who have chronic renal insufficiency. However, with long-standing secondary hyperplasia, complete reversion may not occur, raising the possibility of transformation into tertiary hyperplasia.

HYPOPARATHYROIDISM

Hypoparathyroidism is basically a metabolic disorder characterized by hypocalcemia and consequent neuromuscular and mental changes, related either to inadequate secretion of PTH or secretion of biologically ineffective PTH. Anatomic consequences are exceedingly scant; they are intracranial calcifications, cataract formation, and disturbed dentition when the disorder affects very young children. The major causes of parathyroid insufficiency are unintentional removal of glands during thyroid or parathyroid surgery, radiation injury, developmental failure as in DiGeorge's syndrome (p. 155), and "idiopathic" hypoparathyroidism. The last mentioned, in some instances, is familial and accompanied by other endocrine deficiencies and autoimmune disorders. Often there is an associated predisposition to mucocutaneous candidiasis, strongly suggesting some defect in T-cell function. Thus, "idiopathic" hypoparathyroidism is attributed to deranged cell-mediated immunity and autoimmunity.

Adrenal Cortex

Disorders of the adrenal cortex will be considered under the headings of adrenal cortical hyperfunction, adrenal cortical hypofunction, and neoplasms (since these may be functional or nonfunctional).

ADRENAL CORTICAL HYPERFUNCTION (HYPERADRENALISM)

As you well know, the cortical steroids can be divided into glucocorticoids, mineralocorticoids, and adrenal androgens. Disorders related to hyperfunction of the cortex fall into three more or less distinctive syndromes, depending on which category of steroids is produced in excess. *Thus, overproduction of cortisol, the principal glucocorticoid, results in Cushing's syndrome; an excess of aldosterone, the principal mineralocorticoid, induces, not surprisingly, hyperaldosteronism; and excess adrenal androgens, usually arising in*

congenital adrenal hyperplasia, induce adrenal virilism. Just as there are overlaps in the function of the three categories of steroids (e.g., glucocorticoids have weak effects on electrolyte metabolism), so are there sometimes overlaps in the three clinical syndromes they produce.

CUSHING'S SYNDROME

This syndrome is caused by a chronic excess of glucocorticoids, mostly cortisol. It is seen most often as an exogenous iatrogenic condition because of the widespread therapeutic use of glucocorticoids. In addition there are three categories of endogenous Cushing's syndrome. These are uncommon and are associated with a variety of conditions (Fig. 20–18).

Somewhat more than half of the cases of spontaneous endogenous Cushing's syndrome are of pituitary

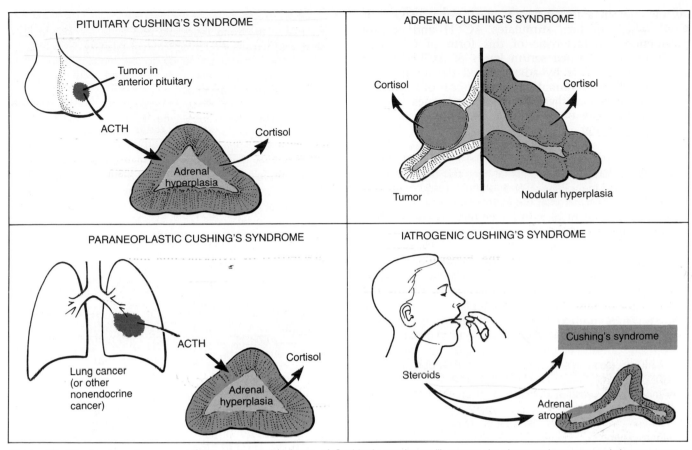

Figure 20-18. A schematic representation of the varied forms of Cushing's syndrome illustrates the three endogenous and the exogenous (iatrogenic) categories.

origin and related hypersecretion of ACTH (and so, might be referred to as pituitary Cushing's syndrome). Because this pattern was first described by the neurosurgeon Harvey Cushing it is sometimes called, confusingly, "Cushing's *disease*" meaning one variant of Cushing's *syndrome.* In the great majority of cases, there is a corticotropin-releasing pituitary basophil adenoma, usually a microadenoma smaller than 10 mm diameter. In the remaining small minority of cases there are multiple foci or diffuse hyperplasia of basophils, or rarely no obvious anatomic abnormality. Occasionally, these pituitary lesions are related to hypothalamic stimulation of corticotropin release. Whatever the fundamental defect or lesion, all cases of Cushing's disease are marked by bilateral adrenal cortical hyperplasia (sometimes quite modest); excess glucocorticoid secretion (mainly cortisol), and in most cases demonstrable elevation of the plasma level of ACTH. Women are affected much more often than men (5:1) usually in the third or fourth decade of life. The hypercortisolism of Cushing's disease can be alleviated by large doses of corticosteroids (e.g., dexamethasone) which, in classic feedback fashion, suppress the anterior lobe release of ACTH, thus providing a clinical diagnostic test of the pituitary origin of the syndrome.

Primary adrenal tumors, or less commonly bilateral nodular hyperplasia, accounts for about 30% of cases of spontaneous Cushing's syndrome. This pattern is best termed *"adrenal Cushing's syndrome."* Because the tumors and the nodular hyperplasia autonomously hypersecrete cortisol, this variant is sometimes also called *"ACTH-independent Cushing's syndrome."* The neoplasms may be benign or malignant in adults, but in young children they are more often malignant. The uncommon cases of diffuse nodular hyperplasia are poorly understood. It is suspected that the adrenal changes may have been initiated by excess ACTH or CRF (corticotropin-releasing factor) secretion; but in time the hyperplasia becomes autonomous. It may take either a macronodular or (less often) micronodular form. The micronodular disease occurs as an autosomal dominant, familial condition (primary pigmented nodular adrenal hyperplasia) seen mostly in children and young adults. Characteristic of adrenal Cushing's syndrome, whatever the underlying glandular lesion, is a low serum ACTH level and failure of administered dexamethasone to suppress the hypercortisolism. When there is a hyperfunctioning neoplasm, the low level of ACTH leads to atrophy of the uninvolved ipsilateral cortex and the contralateral gland.

About 15% of cases of endogenous Cushing's syndrome relate to ectopic ACTH or CRF secretion by a non-endocrine-producing tumor, most often a small cell bronchogenic carcinoma, but also implicated are malignant thymoma, medullary thyroid carcinoma, bronchial carcinoids, islet cell tumors, and prostate carcinoma. In most cases, these neoplasms elaborate

ACTH, but in a few instances the ectopic product is CRF, which in turn stimulates ACTH and cortisol production. Characteristic of this form of Cushing's syndrome are elevated serum levels of ACTH, which are not suppressible by administered dexamethasone. Because of the dominating importance of bronchogenic carcinoma in these "ectopic syndromes," males are affected more often than females (3:1) usually in middle life or later.

MORPHOLOGY. The fundamental anatomic changes are restricted to the pituitary and adrenal glands. In all variants of the syndrome, the increased serum levels of cortisol, whether of exogenous or endogenous origin, produce apparent feedback effects on the nontumorous corticotrophs (and sometimes those within adenomas), a phenomenon referred to as **Crooke's hyaline degeneration of the basophils.** The usual cytoplasmic granularity imparted by the ACTH-containing granules is patchily or completely obscured by a basophilic hyalinization, which can be resolved under the electron microscope as densely aggregated intermediate filaments of cytokeratin (normally present in small numbers). In the pituitary variant of Cushing's syndrome, a corticotroph (basophilic) adenoma, more usually a microadenoma (p. 646), is most often present, but, as noted earlier, sometimes there is only diffuse or nodular hyperplasia of the basophils, or rarely no anatomic change except the hyaline degeneration.

The changes in the adrenals take one of the following forms: (1) diffuse hyperplasia, (2) nodular hyperplasia, (3) a benign or malignant adrenal cortical tumor, or (4) bilateral adrenal cortical atrophy as a result of exogenous glucocorticoid administration or in the uninvolved and contralateral gland when there is a functioning cortical neoplasm. A modest **diffuse hyperplasia** involving mainly the zona reticularis and zona fasciculata is seen with excess ACTH whether of pituitary or ectopic origin. The hyperplasia tends to be modest with the pituitary syndrome and more marked with ectopic ACTH, sometimes exceeding a combined weight of 20 g (normal 8 to 10 g). **Nodular hyperplasia** is much less common than the diffuse type. Most often there is a substrate of diffuse hyperplasia of the zona reticularis and zona fasciculata and in addition diffuse macronodularity. The nodules, composed of fasciculata clear cells, may achieve diameters of 1 to 3 cm, producing a combined weight in excess of 50 gm (Fig. 20–19). The rare familial form of hyperplasia is marked by micronodules of fasciculata cells laden with lipofuscin, accounting for the brown-black pigmentation of the nodules. **The adrenal adenomas and carcinomas** associated with Cushing's syndrome are not distinctive macroscopically or microscopically from nonfunctioning neoplasms. On the whole, the adenomas tend to be quite large (up to 50 gm). The carcinomas also tend to be large, although only the clinical manifestations and biochemical proof of steroid synthesis distinguish them from their nonfunctioning counterparts.

CLINICAL COURSE. The patient with Cushing's syndrome may be recognizable from a distance, or the manifestations may be extremely subtle. The major features are (1) obesity with a distinctive distribution of fat: round, moon facies, truncal obesity, and deposition of fat at the back of the neck (buffalo hump), (2) hypertension, (3) polyuria and polydipsia related to the development of diabetes, (4) hirsutism, (5) thin skin often marked by purple or red abdominal striae and a tendency to bruise easily, (6) menstrual dysfunction, (7) proximal muscle weakness, (8) osteoporosis, and (9) depression and sometimes frank psychosis. When the

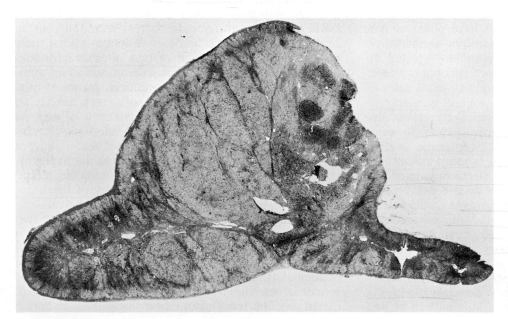

Figure 20–19. Irregular, nodular, adenomatous hyperplasia of an adrenal from a patient with Cushing's syndrome.

Cushing's syndrome relates to ectopic ACTH secretion by a rapidly growing malignant tumor, the clinical course is truncated and is frequently dominated by muscle wasting and the cachexia of advanced cancer. Although the diagnosis of endogenous Cushing's syndrome can be suspected from the clinical presentation, many of the changes are nonspecific and additional evidence is necessary, first to confirm the diagnosis of Cushing's syndrome and second to identify its cause. The diagnosis rests mainly on the 24-hour free cortisol level, and the loss of the normal diurnal pattern of cortisol secretion. Identifying the cause of the syndrome is much more difficult and beyond our scope, but for the most part it depends on suppression tests and imaging techniques.

HYPERALDOSTERONISM

As you recall, aldosterone promotes potassium excretion and sodium retention and so expands blood and extracellular fluid volume. Thus *increased production of aldosterone is marked by hypokalemia, hypernatremia, and hypertension.* When the aldosterone excess appears without an apparent physiologic need it is called "*primary hyperaldosteronism.*" In contrast, in *secondary hyperaldosteronism* it occurs as an appropriate compensatory reaction in conditions marked by stimulation of the renin-angiotensin system with elevated circulating levels of renin (e.g., normal pregnancy, unilateral renal ischemia [renal artery stenosis], congestive heart failure, and marked hypoalbuminemia). Further comments about the *secondary pattern* are not required, except to point out that the hyperaldosteronism is the consequence of *elevated plasma levels of renin activity.* In contrast, in *primary hyperaldosteronism, the plasma renin activity is depressed* because sodium retention expands the blood volume, serving to down-regulate renin release. Thus *primary hyperaldosteronism is sometimes called low renin hypoaldosteronism.* The sodium retention and expansion of the extracellular fluid volume contribute to the development of hypertension, and headaches, usually mild, but sometimes severe, are a frequent complaint. In addition, the low level of potassium may induce proximal muscle weakness, paralysis, and disturbances in cardiac function.

In about 80% of cases of primary hyperaldosteronism the excess steroid production derives from a functioning adrenal adenoma. Most of the remaining cases are attributable to primary bilateral adrenal hyperplasia (**idiopathic hyperaldosteronism**). Rarely, an adrenal carcinoma or some uncommon variant such as unilateral hyperplasia, glucocorticoid suppressible hyperplasia, or idiopathic hyperaldosteronism underlies the excess aldosterone production. When an adenoma is present the condition is referred to as **Conn's syndrome.** The adenoma is more often located on the left, is usually smaller than 2 cm in diameter, is well encapsulated, and is composed of cells resembling those of the zona glomerulosa or zona fasciculata, or sometimes hybrid forms. In idiopathic hyperaldosteronism, with its bilateral, diffuse, sometimes nodular hyperplasia, the adrenals are often several times normal size owing to diffuse or focal hyperplasia of zona glomerulosa cells, which are sometimes admixed with fascicular cells. In the **glucocorticoid-suppressible variant** the glomerulosa and fasciculata zones are replaced by a transitional zone of hybrid cells that has features of the cells in both zones. These hybrids are in part under the control of ACTH and, so, are suppressible by administration of dexamethasone to the patient.

Primary hyperaldosteronism is a rare condition responsible for about 0.5 to 1% of cases of hypertension, but it is a major basis for "curable hypertension" by the simple expedient of removing a benign adrenal tumor. The adenomas appear mainly in women (2:1) in midlife. The cases of hyperplasia are more common in children and young adults and are amenable only to drug therapy. The diagnosis of primary hyperaldosteronism depends heavily on the laboratory evidence of high serum aldosterone levels that fail to fall after the administration of salt, but differentiating an adenoma from primary hyperplasia is difficult.

ADRENOGENITAL SYNDROMES—CONGENITAL ADRENAL HYPERPLASIA

The adrenogenital (AG) syndromes are a rare group of autosomal recessive inborn errors of metabolism, all characterized by excess production of adrenal androgens secondary to enzyme defects blocking the synthesis of cortisol. As a consequence of the lowered cortisol level, ACTH release is stimulated, leading to increased production of precursors proximal to the block, which are ultimately channeled into androgens that have virilizing effects. The most frequently encountered enzyme defects involve the 21-hydroxylase (21-HD), the 11-β-hydroxylase, or the 3-β-hydroxysteroid dehydrogenase. The first is by far the most common, and further comments are restricted to it. The consequences of a 21-HD deficiency depend on its severity (partial or complete) and on whether the enzyme deficit is restricted to the zona fasciculata, and so affects only cortisol and androgen synthesis, or also involves the zona glomerulosa with deficient synthesis of mineralocorticoids. Given these variables there are at least three different clinical forms of 21-HD deficiency:

- Classic salt-losing AG syndrome results from a complete lack of the enzyme in the zona glomerulosa and fasciculata (Fig. 20–20).
- Simple virilizing AG syndrome reflects complete enzyme lack that is, however, restricted to the zona fasciculata alone.
- Late onset 21-HD deficiency syndrome results from partially deficient function of the enzyme.

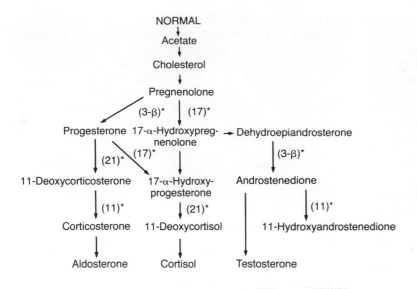

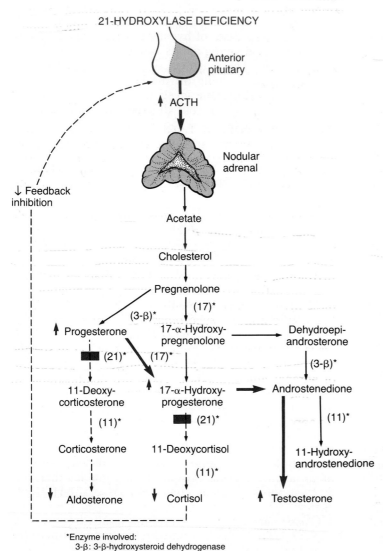

*Enzyme involved:
  3-β: 3-β-hydroxysteroid dehydrogenase
  11: 11-hydroxylase
  17: 17-hydroxylase
  21: 21-hydroxylase

Figure 20–20. A flow chart of normal steroidogenesis *(above)* and of the consequences of a complete 21-hydroxylase deficiency indicated by blocked pathways *(below)* producing deficient synthesis of cortisol and aldosterone and increased production of testosterone. The lowered cortisol levels lead to elevated ACTH and secondary adrenal hyperplasia.

Depending on the severity of the enzyme lack, the clinical manifestations may appear at birth, before or after puberty, or in adult life. Neonatal manifestations, which occur only when enzyme is totally lacking, may take the form of masculinization of female infants (i.e., transformation of the clitoris into a penis and fusion of the labial folds so that the external genitalia resemble those of a male infant); male infants may exhibit no overt manifestations, but occasionally the genitalia appear abnormally large or precocious virilization appears later. When a deficiency of mineralocortocoids, particularly aldosterone, is added, there are excessive salt losses and life-threatening electrolyte crises. With less severe deficiencies of the hydroxylase, the manifestations of excess androgen production may not appear until just before, or sometimes after, puberty, as progressive virilization in girls and precocious puberty in boys. With even milder enzyme defects, the major consequences for women are hirsutism, oligomenorrhea, and infertility and for men, oligospermia.

In all forms of AG syndromes, the componsatory increase in ACTH leads to adrenal hyperplasia and in its most severe expressions can produce glands 10 to 20 times normal weight owing to diffuse or nodular cortical hyperplasia. There are no diagnostic or distinctive histologic features to permit recognition of an enzyme lack, and only biochemical analysis permits differentiation of this form of adrenal hyperplasia from those encountered, for example, in Cushing's syndrome or primary hyperaldosteronism.

Remarkable strides have been made recently in unraveling the molecular genetics underlying the several types of 21-HD deficiency, which are probably allelic. The human genome has duplicated 21-HD genes in tandem with the duplicated genes for the fourth component of complement, all located on the short arm of chromosome 6 between the HLA-DR and B loci. The mutations affect the CYP-21 structural gene for the 21-HD. Homozygous marked modifications of the two 21-HD genes result in severe congenital adrenal hyperplasia (i.e., the simple virilizing or classic salt-losing syndrome). The nonclassic, milder, later-appearing form of the disease may be the result of less extreme alterations of the two alleles or of one mildly and one severely affected allele. The close relationship with the HLA system reveals linkage disequilibrium between the salt-losing and simple virilizing forms of hydroxylase deficiency with Bw47 and the late-onset, nonclassic disease with B14DR1, suggesting heterogeneity in the responsible mutations. HLA typing may therefore point to the possible existence of these metabolic errors. More specifically, the mutant gene from a patient with nonclassic disease has been cloned recently, the specific nucleotide identified, and an oligonucleotide probe for the mutant DNA constructed. Prenatal identification of the fetus at risk is likely soon to be possible for all forms of the AG syndrome by HLA typing and DNA analysis of amniotic cells.

ADRENAL CORTICAL HYPOFUNCTION

Inadequate adrenal cortical function may reflect extensive cortical destruction of both glands (primary adrenocortical insufficiency) or inadequate release of ACTH secondary to some hypophyseothalamic derangement such as a nonsecretory adenoma of the pituitary (secondary adrenocortical insufficiency). Primary hypoadrenalism may further be subdivided into chronic insufficiency, better known as Addison's disease, or acute insufficiency.

CHRONIC ADRENOCORTICAL INSUFFICIENCY— ADDISON'S DISEASE

Clinically overt Addison's disease is an uncommon condition seen only when more than 90% of the adrenal cortical mass is destroyed. Subclinical disease with less extensive cortical destruction is much more common but only surfaces when stress increases the need for corticosteroids. Whatever the severity, most cases are seen in persons between ages 20 and 50 years with no sex predilection.

The major causes of Addison's disease, clinical and subclinical, along with their relative contributions to the pool, are cited in Table 20–6. It is evident that autoimmune disease and tuberculosis account for the great majority of cases of Addison's disease. At one time, the latter was the dominant cause, but today it is much less common than autoimmune adrenal insufficiency.

Autoimmune adrenalitis, sometimes called idiopathic adrenal atrophy, may appear as a sporadic disorder or be familial, often in association with a number of other autoimmune diseases, including Hashimoto's thyroiditis, pernicious anemia, type I diabetes mellitus, and idiopathic hypoparathyroidism. Combinations of these involvements, frequently comprise the "polyglandular autoimmune syndromes" often associated with HLA-DR3. The pathogenesis of autoimmune adrenalitis is attributed to an immunogenetic defect in specific suppressor T cells that permits unregulated production of adrenal autoantibodies. These are demonstrable in the majority of patients with this condition and in some cases have been identified months to years before the appearance of a functional deficit.

TABLE 20–6. CAUSES OF ADDISON'S DISEASE

Condition	Relative Contribution (%)
Major contributors	
Autoimmune adrenalitis	50–65
Tuberculosis	5–30
Metastatic disease	5–10
Minor contributors	
Systemic amyloidosis	Rare
Fungal infections	Rare
Hemochromatosis	Rare
Sarcoidosis	Rare

Tuberculosis and fungal disease (histoplasmosis, coccidioidomycosis, blastomycosis) are the principal infections that may cause chronic adrenal cortical insufficiency. In the United States, tuberculous adrenalitis has become relatively uncommon except among native Americans and impoverished groups, however, it still accounts for a third or more of cases of Addison's disease in developing and Third World countries. Almost always there is concurrent tuberculosis elsewhere, most frequently in the lungs or genitourinary system. Histoplasmosis is the most frequent of the fungal diseases, involving the adrenals when that infection becomes disseminated.

Among the many other potential causes of Addison's disease, metastatic cancer merits first consideration. Indeed, autopsy studies indicate that approximately a quarter of all patients with disseminated malignancy have adrenal involvement. In most instances the metastatic disease does not destroy enough of the functioning cortical tissue to produce clinically overt insufficiency, but occasionally only a marginal reserve persists, producing subclinical Addison's disease. The cancers most frequently implicated are bronchogenic and breast carcinoma, malignant melanoma, Hodgkin's disease, and lymphoma, but any metastatic cancer may be involved. Amyloidosis, usually seen following some chronic destructive disease such as rheumatoid arthritis, bronchiectasis, or tuberculosis, has now become a rare cause of Addison's disease, as is also true of the many other conditions cited at the outset.

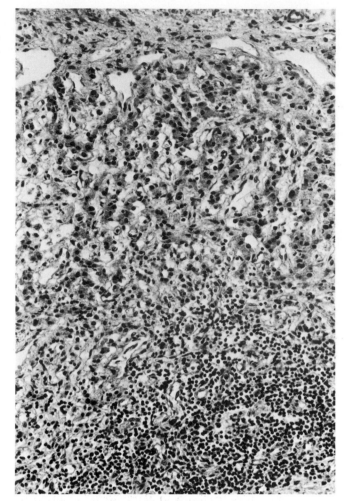

Figure 20–21. Autoimmune adrenalitis. In addition to loss of all but a subcapsular rim of cortical cells there is an extensive mononuclear cell infiltrate.

MORPHOLOGY. Autoimmune adrenalitis, when fully expressed, reveals small, irregularly contracted adrenal glands, with a combined weight as low as 2.5 gm. On sectioning, the cortex may appear to have collapsed around an otherwise normal medulla. The histologic changes are variable and include atrophy and destruction of the cortical cells with replacement by fibrous scarring, accompanied by a lymphocytic infiltrate (Fig. 20–21). The few remaining viable cells may be enlarged, with an eosinophilic, lipid-poor cytoplasm (compact cells). The medulla is not affected.

Tuberculous adrenal glands and those involved by histoplasmosis, on the other hand, are enlarged, firm, and nodular, with a thickened capsule. Histologically, the changes are characteristic of the infections in any site, with confluent areas of necrosis and granuloma formation throughout the cortex extending into the medulla. Focal calcifications of the granulomatous lesions may provide useful radiologic clues to these infections, but special stains and cultures are necessary to differentiate among them. When metastatic cancer causes Addison's disease, the adrenals are converted into cancerous masses with apparently total obliteration of the native architecture. But in general functional insufficiency secondary to adrenal metastases is uncommon because sufficient cortex usually persists between the implants to maintain adequate steroid production. Addison's disease caused by amyloidosis is also associated with enlargement of the adrenal glands, sometimes up to a combined weight of 40 gm. Grossly, the glands are firm and pale gray. On microscopic examination, most of the cortex is replaced by amyloid deposits.

CLINICAL COURSE. Clinically overt Addison's disease typically appears insidiously and often is ill defined. The first indications are usually vague weakness and fatigability. *As the negative feedback on the hypothalamic-pituitary axis is abolished, ACTH (and perhaps β-lipotropin) levels rise, with a consequent increase in pigmentation of the skin, particularly over the extensor surfaces, mucous membranes, areolae, and surgical scars.* The presence of pigmentation is helpful in differentiating primary adrenocortical hypofunction from the secondary pattern, which results from pituitary lesions. The latter is associated with low ACTH levels and no hyperpigmentation. Most patients develop gastrointestinal disturbances, including anorexia with weight loss, nausea, vomiting, and diarrhea. Blood sugar is low, and hypoglycemic symptoms may occasionally occur. Although some degree of hypotension is characteristic, actual syncope is uncommon. The heart becomes smaller, possibly because of its lighter work load as a result of chronic hypovolemia and hypotension.

When Addison's disease is full blown the diagnosis is generally apparent from the distinctive signs and symptoms. But the clinical manifestations may be extremely subtle in earlier phases, when the diagnosis is most important because the adrenal dysfunction is correctable with exogenous steroids even though the underlying disease persists or progresses. Confirming the diagnosis are the lack of a normal steroid response to administered ACTH and hyponatremia with hyperkalemia owing to aldosterone deficiency. CT or MRI may offer valuable diagnostic clues to the specific cause of the adrenal destruction.

Although patients with Addison's disease may continue indefinitely in their subactive precarious existence, any stress such as surgery, infection, or injury may precipitate an acute crisis, characterized by the sudden appearance about 12 hours later of profound weakness, hyperpyrexia progressing to hypothermia, coma, and vascular collapse. Without prompt steroid therapy, death may ensue.

ACUTE ADRENOCORTICAL INSUFFICIENCY _____

Acute adrenocortical steroid insufficiency may be caused by (1) sudden withdrawal of long-term steroid therapy, (2) stress in patients with Addison's disease (see previous discussion), or (3) massive hemorrhagic destruction of the glands. Hemorrhage into the adrenals is seen in the newborn incident to the trauma of childbirth, during anticoagulant therapy either spontaneously or following minor trauma, during the postoperative period, and most importantly, with overwhelming septicemia (*Waterhouse-Friderichsen syndrome*) (Fig. 20–22). Implicated most often are meningococci,

but sometimes pneumococci, staphylococci, or *Haemophilus influenzae* type B. The basis for the adrenal hemorrhage in these infections is unclear, but speculations include bacterial toxemia, direct vascular injury, a Schwartzman reaction, and DIC. It is the overwhelming sepsis rather than the acute steroid insufficiency that threatens life. Small medullary hemorrhages may occur in any of the bleeding diatheses but they must be massive to produce acute steroid insufficiency. Thus even with the Waterhouse-Friderichsen syndrome, in which the hemorrhage appears to have converted the adrenals into bags of blood, sufficient islands of cortical cells often survive to maintain adequate adrenal function.

ADRENOCORTICAL NEOPLASMS _____

As has been pointed out in previous discussions, a functional cortical adenoma—or carcinoma, or hyperplasia—may be the source of one or more excess steroids in all hyperadrenal syndromes. However, all adenomas and carcinomas do not elaborate steroids, and, regrettably, it is not possible by morphologic examination alone to determine whether a tumor is functional or which steroids it is elaborating. Biochemical analysis of the lesion, its venous efflux, or the plasma drawn from the patient is necessary to identify any or all specific products. Thus on morphologic grounds "a tumor is a tumor is a tumor," so adenomas and carcinomas have not been well characterized to this point.

Adenomas are common at autopsy and only rarely are associated with one of the hyperadrenal states. Nonetheless, they are the commonest cause of primary hyperaldosteronism and on rare occasion underlie Cushing's syndrome. They are discrete, encapsulated, yellow-brown nodules within the cortex that often project into the medullary cavity or under the capsule

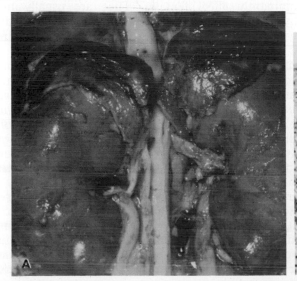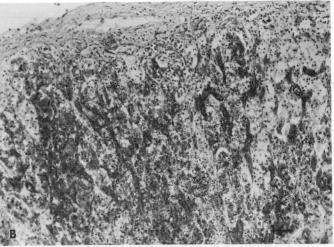

Figure 20–22. *A*, The kidneys and adrenals in situ in a child with the Waterhouse-Friderichsen syndrome. The dark adrenals are markedly hemorrhagic. *B*, On low-power section the cortical cells between the extravasated blood have undergone ischemic necrosis.

and sometimes appear to be extracapsular. They range up to 3 cm in diameter (average 1 to 2 cm). The smaller lesions are usually composed of lipid-laden cells resembling those of the fasciculata, having clear cytoplasm and regular, small nuclei (Fig. 20–23). Occasionally, the cells have less lipid, a granular cytoplasm, and resemble those of the zona reticularis. Larger tumors may have areas of hemorrhage, cystic necrosis, and more variation in cell and nuclear size, with nuclear hyperchromasia and scattered mitoses. The line between such an "atypical" adenoma, particularly when poorly encapsulated, and a carcinoma is vague, but as a rule of thumb—*tumors smaller than 3 cm in diameter are benign unless they have marked cellular atypia and numerous mitoses* or are unmistakably aggressive (invasive or disseminated). Unhappily, flow cytometry has not proved useful in separating adenomas from carcinomas, since both may be aneuploid. Equally difficult is the differentiation of a focus of nodular hyperplasia from an adenoma, particularly when there are multiple small adenomas. Here the rule of thumb is: when well-encapsulated or unilateral the lesions are adenomas. Ultimately, however, the nodule and the adenoma may well be the same lesion, since many larger adenomas may have arisen in a focus of nodular hyperplasia.

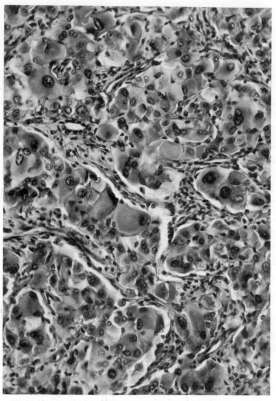

Figure 20–24. Adrenal carcinoma. There is marked anaplasia and pleomorphism of the neoplastic cells.

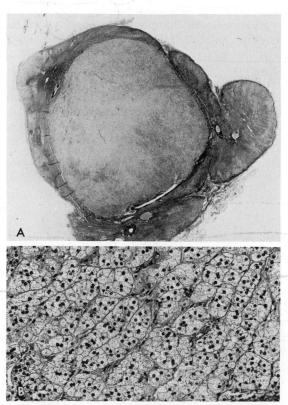

Figure 20–23. *A,* A slightly enlarged whole-organ mount of a section of an adrenal bearing an adenoma. The tumor has expanded into the medulla and is enclosed within a rim of adrenal cortex. *B,* The lipid-laden cortical cells are arranged in nests.

Cortical carcinomas, in contrast to adenomas, are usually functional, particularly in children, and therefore they are associated with one of the hyperadrenal syndromes described previously. Whether functional or not, they are exceedingly uncommon; they may arise at any age in either sex, but in childhood they predominantly affect females. They are usually bulky, obviously invasive masses that have obliterated the involved gland and have extended into the periadrenal fat, and sometimes the adjacent kidney. The rare smaller lesion may appear deceptively encapsulated and be difficult to differentiate from an adenoma. On transection cortical carcinomas present a variegated surface with areas of yellow, viable tumor surrounded by hemorrhage, necroses, and cystic foci. Histologically, they range from well-differentiated carcinomas having mild degrees of atypia, not unlike that seen in some larger adenomas, to wildly anaplastic neoplasms composed of bizarre giant cells with extremely hyperchromatic pleomorphic nuclei that often bear mitoses (Fig. 20–24). Invasion of the veins, sometimes with extension into the vena cava, and permeation of lymphatics leads to widespread metastases to the lungs, liver, periaortic lymph nodes, and bones, accounting for a median survival time of about one or two years.

Adrenal Medulla

Disease primary in the medulla is very uncommon and is almost always a tumor. Nonetheless, these neoplasms have great importance, for reasons that will become clear.

PHEOCHROMOCYTOMA _____

Arising in chromaffin cells, pheochromocytomas elaborate catecholamines (as well as other secretory products) and so characteristically produce hypertension that can be fatal. Although only about 0.1% of all patients with diastolic hypertension have such a tumor, it remains unsuspected in about 20% of cases, depriving these patients of potential cure of their disease. In about 90% of cases there is a sporadic solitary neoplasm in one of the adrenals; rarely there are bilateral tumors. Most of these patients are in the third to fifth decade of life (although the tumor may arise at any age) and there is no sex predilection. In the remaining 10%, multiple or extraadrenal pheochromocytomas arise in one of the familial syndromes cited in Table 20–7. In these well-defined familial syndromes the neoplasms may be located anywhere from the base of the skull to the perineum (including the bladder), arising in paraganglionic cells distributed along the aorta, most frequently within the organ of Zuckerkandl at the bifurcation of the aorta. These extraadrenal pheochromocytomas are frequently called paragangliomas. The tumors, in association with one of the familial syndromes, tend to appear in the first or second decade of life. Although only about 10 to 15% of sporadic adrenal pheochromocytomas are malignant, the incidence of cancer in the extraadrenal lesions rises to about 40%.

Wherever they arise, pheochromocytomas elaborate mostly epinephrine and norepinephrine, and occasionally dopamine; those in the adrenals produce principally epinephrine; the extraadrenal neoplasms, mostly norepinephrine. In addition, pheochromocytomas may also produce chromogranins, ACTH, somatostatin, calcitonin, endorphins, and other secretory products. When any of these products is elaborated in addition to the catechols, the clinical picture obviously becomes much more complicated. Were these complexities not sufficient, it has lately been observed that pheochromocytomas may also elaborate neuropeptide Y (NPY), which is normally produced in small amounts in the adrenal medulla and in the central and peripheral nervous system. NPY is important because it potentiates the vasopressor actions of the catecholamines, thereby contributing to the hypertension.

MORPHOLOGY. Pheochromocytomas range from massive neoplasms that weigh several kilograms to minute lesions that probably represent focal areas of hyperpla-

TABLE 20–7. FAMILIAL SYNDROMES WITH PHEOCHROMOCYTOMA*

Syndrome	Components
Multiple endocrine neoplasia (MEN), type II or IIA	Medullary thyroid carcinomas and C cell hyperplasia
	Pheochromocytomas and adrenal medullary hyperplasia
	Parathyroid hyperplasia
Multiple endocrine neoplasia (MEN), type III or IIB	Medullary thyroid carcinomas and C cell hyperplasia
	Pheochromocytomas and adrenal medullary hyperplasia
	Mucosal neuromas
	Marfanoid features
von Hippel-Lindau	Renal, hepatic, pancreatic, and epididymal cysts
	Renal cell carcinomas
	Pheochromocytomas
	Angiomatosis
	Cerebellar hemangioblastomas
von Recklinghausen	Neurofibromatosis
	Café au lait skin spots
	Schwannomas, meningiomas, gliomas
	Pheochromocytomas
Sturge-Weber	Cavernous hemangiomas of fifth cranial nerve distribution
	Pheochromocytomas

* From Silverman, M. L., Lee, A. K.: Anatomy and pathology of the adrenal glands. Urol. Clin. North Am. *16*:417, 1989.

sia. Sporadic tumors tend to be solitary (about 10% are bilateral), arise in the adrenal glands, and usually weigh 50 to 150 gm. These lesions tend to be discretely encapsulated. In contrast, the lesions of the familial syndromes mentioned previously are frequently multicentric, bilateral, and smaller than the sporadic variety, and often even when there is a well-defined neoplasm there are additional small hyperplastic nodules in the remaining medulla and contralateral gland. Whatever their size, they are gray-pink in cross section; larger masses often have central areas of hemorrhage, necrosis, and cystic softening. Treatment of the cross section with dichromate solution turns it dark brown, hence the term chromaffin tumor.

Histologically, the tumor cells range from large to small, and typically they are irregular in shape or polygonal. They are disposed in nests or cords separated by a vascularized connective tissue stroma creating "zell-ballen" (ball-like aggregates) (Fig. 20–25). Less frequently the cells are spindle shaped or pseudoglandular. In all tumors they vary considerably in size and shape

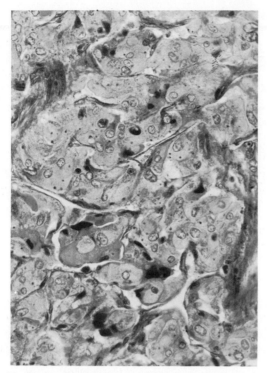

Figure 20–25. Pheochromocytoma. High-power cellular detail shows "zellballen," irregular nuclei and abundant granular cytoplasm. The chromatin pigment is not visible in the photograph.

and have marked nuclear pleomorphism, sometimes with bizarre lobulations creating the appearance of multiple nuclei. In contrast, the cells in the hyperplastic nodules are rarely encapsulated and tend to resemble those of the normal adrenal medulla. Electron microscopy of pheochromocytomas reveals variable numbers of distinct membrane-bound cytoplasmic granules in the neoplastic cells. Those that contain epinephrine have a less electron-dense matrix enclosed within a tight-fitting membrane, whereas those that contain norepinephrine are more electron dense with a loose-fitting membrane. The content of the granules can be confirmed by immunohistochemical staining.

Capsular and vascular invasion are not uncommon in clinically proven benign tumors. **Moreover, the cytologic features of benign and malignant tumors overlap, so the only reliable criteria for malignancy are metastases (usually to related nodes, lungs, liver, and bones) and extensive local invasion. About 10% prove to be malignant.**

CLINICAL COURSE. The clinical signs and symptoms may be so characteristic as to shout *pheochromocytoma* or so mild and atypical that the tumor goes undetected, as noted earlier. The major presenting features are hypertension, headache, palpitations, sweating, pallor, chest pain, anxiety, tremor, and sometimes attacks of weakness or even syncope. It is obvious that many of these manifestations can be confused with a panic reaction. Although classically the hypertension is said to be paroxysmal, this occurs in fewer than half of the patients; in the remainder, the hypertension is sustained, or rarely there is no elevation of the blood pressure when the neoplasm secretes mostly dopamine. Typically there is postural hypotension (orthostatism), manifest as a significant drop in blood pressure on standing. In the most classic presentation, patients have paroxysmal attacks of headache, palpitation, anxiety, and precipitous elevation in the blood pressure, all of which abate between attacks. Many patients, however, present with only sustained hypertension without the accompanying symptoms, or they may present with chest pain simulating a myocardial infarction or with heart failure resulting from catecholamine-induced cardiomyopathy or seemingly diverse manifestations that result from the ectopic production by the neoplasm of other bioactive products. Ultimately, therefore, laboratory tests are required to document elevated blood levels of total catecholamines or elevated levels of metabolites such as vanillylmandelic acid (VMA) or metanephrines in the urine. After the biochemical diagnosis is established there comes the difficult problem of locating the pheochromocytoma and determining whether it is a solitary neoplasm or multiple and bilateral lesions, as is likely in the familial syndromes. Excision of solitary lesions can be curative, but with the familial syndromes it is often necessary to fall back on medical treatment of the hypertension.

NEUROBLASTOMA _____

This neoplasm is the most common extracranial childhood solid tumor; it accounts for about 15% of all childhood cancer deaths. Most (80 to 90%) are found in children younger than five years—sometimes in the first year of life. Some neoplasms diagnosed in infancy are thought to be neuroblastomas in situ, which sometimes undergo spontaneous regression. About 10 to 15% of neuroblastomas arise between ages five and 15 years, but some of these may represent look-alikes or closely related neoplasms such as primitive neuroectodermal tumors.

Of neural crest origin, neuroblastomas may arise anywhere in the sympathetic nervous system from the head to the pelvis. About 75% arise within the abdomen: about half in the adrenal glands and the other half in the abdominal paravertebral autonomic ganglia. Similar neoplasms rarely arise in the brain. Although neuroblastomas have been reported in peripheral locations, many are closely related tumors but not neuroblastomas. The great majority occur sporadically, but a few are familial with autosomal dominant transmission, and in such cases the neoplasms may involve both adrenals or multiple primary autonomic sites.

These tumors range from microscopic nodules (usually in infants) to masses that virtually fill the abdomen. Smaller tumors may appear to be circumscribed or even encapsulated, but larger masses often grow into nearby organs (kidney, liver, pancreas). Advanced disease frequently invades the renal vein, often extending into the inferior vena cava. On cross section they are gray-white, soft, friable, and often have areas of hemorrhage, necrosis, cystic degeneration, and calcification.

Histologically, the cells, growing in solid sheets, are round to ovoid and primitive looking with large, hyperchromatic nuclei surrounded by scant cytoplasm. It is evident that such total lack of differentiation makes it difficult to distinguish these neoplasms from lymphomas, Ewing's sarcoma, peripheral neuroectodermal tumors, and other highly undifferentiated cancers; however, more characteristic features can often be identified in neuroblastomas—e.g., rosettes (Homer-Wright pseudo-rosettes) in which the tumor cells are arranged about the periphery of a central space filled with fibrillar extensions of the cells. Other helpful features are immunochemical reactions for neuron-specific enolase and small, membrane-bound, catecholamine-containing cytoplasmic secretory granules.

Larger tumors, generally found in children aged two to five years, are extremely aggressive lesions that invade not only adjacent organs locally but also metastasize widely through the hematogenous and lymphatic system, particularly to liver, lungs, and bones. Neoplasms with extensive bony metastases, particularly to the skull and orbit, create what is called Hutchinson's syndrome; lesions that involve primarily the liver, and possibly the lungs, Pepper's syndrome.

Staging of neuroblastomas (Table 20–8) assumes great importance in establishing a prognosis. Special note should be taken of stage IV-S, because, as will be seen, the outlook for these patients is excellent despite the spread of the disease.

CLINICAL COURSE. At the time of diagnosis most children are already extremely ill, having disseminated metastases. Thus, they present with weight loss, weakness, protuberant abdomen owing to an abdominal mass, bone pain from bony metastases, and generalized malaise related to resorption of necrotic products. With metastasis to the liver and hepatic enlargement, ascites may develop. A cerebellar encephalopathy is often responsible for progressive ataxia and jerking movements of the eyes. On the other hand, tumors in the chest, neck, and other extraabdominal sites may produce few symptoms other than those related to the local mass. About 90% of neuroblastomas, wherever located, produce catecholamines (similar to those associated with pheochromocytomas), which are an important diagnostic feature, (elevated blood levels of catecholamines and elevated urine levels of metabolites, vanillylmandelic acid [VMA], and homovanillic acid [HVA]). Despite the elaboration of catecholamines, hypertension is much less frequent with these neoplasms than with pheochromocytomas.

Many factors influence the prognosis, but most important are the age of the patient and the stage of disease. Children younger than two years have a much more favorable outlook than older children at comparable stages of the disease. Some of this improved outlook may be related to the fact that tumors discovered in infancy have a tendency to regress spontaneously or differentiate into benign ganglioneuromas. There has been no satisfactory explanation of this curious behavior, but some speculations will be mentioned later. The stage of the neoplasm profoundly influences outlook. With stage IV-S, the two-year survival rate is almost 100%, with stages I and II nearly 90%, but with stages III and IV, despite all forms of treatment, 20 to 30%.

Molecular genetic analyses of neuroblastomas, mostly in stages III and IV, have revealed some very distinctive chromosomal changes—deletions or translocations of the short arm of chromosome 1 at band 32 (1p32), homogenous-staining regions at this specific site or sometimes elsewhere in the cell genome, and double minute chromosomes (Fig. 20–26). Further analysis disclosed that the homogeneous-staining regions represent multiple copies of the protooncogene N-*myc*. There is a correlation between the number of N-*myc* copies and the aggressiveness of the tumor. It is intriguing that neoplasms at stages I, II, and IV-S do not reveal the marker chromosome 1, homogeneous-staining regions, or double minutes but instead are hyperdiploid or nearly triploid. Thus, there is a suggestion that there are two dissimilar subsets of neuroblastomas, the highly malignant one accounting for the tumors in stages III and IV, and the other much less aggressive one, which is nonetheless capable of metastasis, accounting for stages I, II, and IV-S. The latter subset may well express distinctive tumor antigens that evoke an immune response that causes the spontaneous regression or maturation of tumors in stages I and IV-S. Admittedly, the concept of two subsets of neuroblastoma is speculative, but it could explain some of the well-documented behavioral enigmas of these neoplasms.

TABLE 20–8. STAGING OF NEUROBLASTOMAS*

Stage	
I	Tumor confined to organ of origin
II	Tumor extends in continuity beyond organ of origin but does not cross midline. Ipsilateral lymph nodes may or may not be involved
III	Tumor extends in continuity beyond the midline. Ipsilateral lymph nodes may or may not be involved
IV	Metastatic disease to viscera, distant lymph nodes, soft tissue, and skeleton
IV-S	Patients who would be stage I or II but who have distant disease of liver, skin, or bone marrow (without evidence of bone involvement)

* From Silverman, M. L., Lee, A. K.: Anatomy and pathology of the adrenal glands. Urol. Clin. North Am. *16*:417, 1989.

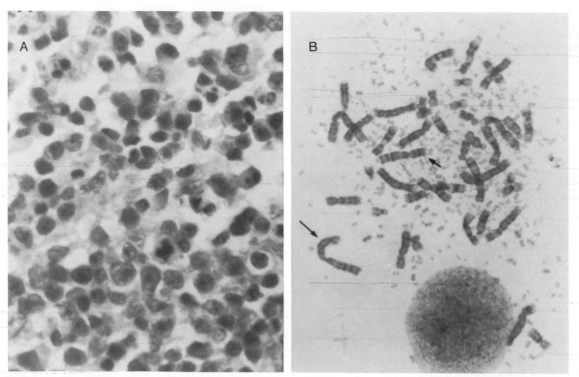

Figure 20–26. The small round cell histology, _A,_ and karyotype, _B,_ of a neuroblastoma in a three-year-old boy. The normal chromosome 1 is indicated by the long arrow. The homologous chromosome 1 with a short arm deletion is indicated by the short arrow. Numerous double minute chromosomes are also present. The changes are characteristic of a poor prognosis neuroblastoma. (From Fletcher, J. A., et al.: Diagnostic relevance of clonal cytogenetic preparations in malignant soft tissue tumors. N. Engl. J. Med. _324:_436, 1991.)

Thymus

Thymic hyperplasia and thymomas, the two most frequent (albeit uncommon) disorders of the thymus, are of particular interest because of their association with a variety of systemic disorders. Thymic lymphomas were discussed on page 363.

HYPERPLASIA

The weight of the thymus is of little use in establishing the diagnosis of hyperplasia. There is wide individual variation in the weight of the normal thymus, and the progressive atrophy during life pursues a variable course. Thus _hyperplasia of the thymus is best characterized by the appearance of lymphoid follicles within the medulla._ The normal thymus is devoid of lymphoid follicles. Immunochemical staining techniques reveal that the follicles are rich in immunoglobulins. Thymic hyperplasia is present in the great majority of patients with myasthenia gravis and also present in various other autoimmune diseases such as systemic lupus erythematosus and rheumatoid arthritis. The relationship between the thymus and myasthenia gravis is discussed in detail on page 698; for now it suffices that T cells generated in the thymus and sensitized to

its myoid cells cooperate with B cells in the lymphoid follicles to produce the autoantibodies that underlie the autoimmune reaction to acetylcholine receptors at the neuromuscular junction, a characteristic of this grave neuromuscular disorder. Significantly, removal of a hyperplastic thymus is beneficial early in the disease.

THYMOMA

Although the normal thymus is a lymphoepithelial organ, _the term thymoma is restricted to tumors in which epithelial cells constitute the neoplastic element._ Scant or abundant thymic lymphocytes may also be present in these tumors, but they are essentially normal thymocytes and not neoplastic. Lymphomas arising in the lymphoid elements of the thymus gland are therefore not classified as thymomas. Numerous subtypes of thymoma have been established, based on cytologic and biologic criteria. For our purposes _it suffices that they be divided into benign (representing about 90% of thymic tumors) and malignant thymomas,_ omitting the other more rare, more aggressive malignancies called thymic carcinomas.

Both benign and malignant thymomas are gray-tan, lobulated neoplasms that have much histologic diversity. As noted, all have neoplastic epithelial cells and a variable lymphocytic infiltrate. In most neoplasms, the epithelial cells resemble their normal counterparts, having poorly defined cytoplasmic outlines and large, pale nuclei. Less commonly, the epithelial cells are oval- to spindle-shaped and sometimes appear squamoid. Hassall's corpuscles are most frequently found in the squamoid neoplasms. Whatever their shape, the cells are disposed in sheets but sometimes arranged in isolated nests separated by sparse or abundant lymphocytes. **Based on the intensity of the lymphoid infiltrate, the tumors are sometimes further subdivided into epithelial predominance; lymphoid predominance; and mixed lymphoepithelial composition.** Benign thymomas range up to 10 to 15 cm in diameter and are enclosed in a well-defined capsule. Their malignant counterparts extend beyond the capsule and are usually larger. They range up to 20 cm in diameter and sometimes metastasize. To be noted, **the diagnosis of malignant thymoma is not based on cytologic atypia but rather on the basis of capsular invasion or metastasis.** Infrequently, a neuroendocrine carcinoid tumor arises in the thymus, resembling its counterparts elsewhere both morphologically and functionally.

All thymomas are rarities, the malignant more so than the benign. They may arise at any age but typically occur in middle adult life. In a large series about 30% were asymptomatic; 30 to 40% produced local manifestations such as a CT-demonstrable mass in the anterior superior mediastinum associated with cough, dyspnea, and superior vena caval syndrome, and the remainder were associated with some systemic disease, principally myasthenia gravis. Some 15 to 20% of patients with this disorder have a thymoma. Removal of the tumor often leads to improvement in the neuromuscular disorder. There is the suggestion, then, that the thymic neoplasm in some way contributes to the production of the autoantibody found in this condition (p. 698). Additional associations with thymomas include hypogammaglobulinemia, systemic lupus erythematosus, various cytopenias, and nonthymic cancers. The survival rate following resection of a localized thymic neoplasm is about 80% at 10 years, but associated disease, when present, may exact its toll. The 10-year survival rate is about 20% for malignant thymomas.

Multiple Endocrine Neoplasia

There are three autosomal dominant MEN syndromes, or as some authors prefer to call them, multiple endocrine adenopathy (MEA) syndromes, all characterized by hyperplastic or neoplastic involvement of at least two endocrine glands, and sometimes associated nonendocrine lesions. The essential features of each are presented in Table 20–9.

The MEN I (Wermer's) syndrome is most prominently marked by the parathyroid involvement producing hypercalcemia, but it is the pancreatic involvement that is most important, responsible for the deaths of well over half of all patients. Islet cell tumors elaborate one or more of the following products, in descending order of frequency: gastrin, insulin, vasoactive intes-

TABLE 20–9. MEN SYNDROMES

	MEN I (Wermer's Syndrome)	MEN II or IIa (Sipple's Syndrome)	MEN IIB or III
Pituitary	Adenomas		
Parathyroid	Hyperplasia+++ Adenomas+	Hyperplasia+	
Pancreatic islets	Hyperplasia+ Adenomas++ Carcinoma+++		
Adrenal	Cortical hyperplasia++	Pheochromocytoma++	Pheochromocytoma+++
Thyroid	C-cell hyperplasia±	Medullary carcinoma+++	Medullary carcinoma++
Extraendocrine changes			Mucocutaneous ganglioneuromas Marfanoid habitus
Mutant gene locus	11q13	10 (near centromere)	Unknown

Relative frequency: +, uncommon; +++, common.

tinal peptide, glucagon, and sometimes others. The hypersecretion of gastrin is often associated with the Zollinger-Ellison syndrome and peptic ulcerations. The pancreatic lesions are almost always multiple and include hyperplasia, adenoma formation, and carcinoma; sometimes all three are present in a single patient. The carcinomas are frequently disseminated by the time of diagnosis because the hypercalcemia often goes undetected for years and the significance of the peptic ulceration is not immediately apparent. This syndrome seldom is diagnosed before age 20 years and may go undetected until late in life.

The MEN II or IIa (Sipple's) syndrome is more easily remembered as the medullary thyroid carcinoma–pheochromocytoma syndrome. Sometimes there is also parathyroid hyperplasia. Thyroid tumors are present in virtually all patients; frequently they are multicentric and bilateral, and sometimes they have spread to regional nodes by the time of diagnosis. The pheochromocytomas are less consistently present, but as noted earlier (p. 675), they are frequently bilateral and have a greater tendency to be extraadrenal. As you would expect, these patients usually present with hypertension or with a thyroid mass, but ectopic production of other products such as ACTH, gastrin, or prolactin by the thyroid tumor may produce confusing clinical complexes. Age at diagnosis ranges from early childhood to the late decades.

MEN IIb or III is very similar to MEN II, and is also characterized by medullary carcinoma and pheochromocytoma, but in addition, there is a marfanoid habitus, and typically multiple mucocutaneous ganglioneuromas in the lips, oral cavity, eye, upper respiratory tract, bladder, skin, and elsewhere. Notable in this syndrome is the absence of parathyroid involvement.

Despite the phenotypic overlaps, the three syndromes are genetically quite distinct, MEN I being characterized by a mutation located on chromosome 11 band 13 of the long arm, MEN II by a mutation near the centromere of chromosome 10, but the mutation that accounts for MEN III is at this point undetected. The relationship of the identified mutations to the pathogenesis of the multiglandular involvement is unknown, but there is speculation that oncogene activation occurs with the production of some growth-promoting, circulating product. There is recent evidence that the inherited germinal mutation is recessive and is unmasked by a second somatic mutation that eliminates the normal counterpart—a scenario like that of retinoblastoma and certain other neoplasms.

BIBLIOGRAPHY

Aasland, R., et al.: Expression of oncogenes in thyroid tumours: Coexpression of c-erbB2/neu and c-erbB. Br. J. Cancer *57:*358, 1988. (A brief insight into some of the molecular genetics underlying thyroid neoplasms.)

Barzilay, J. I., Pazianos, A. G.: Adrenocortical carcinoma. Urol. Clin. North Am. *16:*457, 1989. (A brief review of the essential morphologic and clinical aspects with emphasis on treatment.)

Beall, G. N.: Immunologic aspects of endocrine diseases. JAMA *258:*2952, 1987. (A very brief and helpful analysis of the immunology of various endocrine diseases of the thyroid, adrenals, and pancreatic islets.)

Bilezikian, J. P.: Etiologies and therapy of hypercalcemia. Endocrinol. Metab. Clin. North Am. *18:*389, 1989. (Good for differential diagnosis of hypercalcemia.)

Bravo, E. L.: Primary aldosteronism. Urol. Clin. North Am. *16:*481, 1989. (Emphasis here is on the pathophysiology and diagnostic problems.)

Carcangiu, M. L., et al.: Papillary thyroid carcinoma: A study of its many morphologic expressions and clinical correlates. Pathol. Annu. *20:*1, 1985. (An authoritative coverage of the morphology of these tumors.)

Clark, O. H., Duh, Q.-Y.: Primary hyperparathyroidism. Endocrinol. Metab. Clin. North Am. *18:*701, 1989. (Strong on clinical features with brief morphologic considerations.)

Cutler, G. B., Laue, L.: Congenital adrenal hyperplasia due to 21-hydroxylase deficiency. N. Engl. J. Med. *323:*1806, 1990. (A brief, clinically oriented article with excellent pathophysiology.)

Franssila, K. O., et al.: Follicular carcinoma. Semin. Diagn. Pathol. *2:*101, 1985. (A detailed analysis of the morphologic and relevant differential features of follicular carcinomas of the thyroid.)

Kannan, C. R.: Diseases of the adrenal cortex. Disease-a-Month *34:*601, 1988. (Excellent comprehensive coverage of the major forms of hyper- and hypoadrenalism.)

Kohn, L. D., et al.: Monoclonal antibody studies defining the origin and properties of autoantibodies in Graves' disease. Ann. N.Y. Acad. Sci. *475:*157, 1986. (A good review of the immunology of Graves' disease.)

Kovacs, K., Horvath, E.: Pathology of pituitary tumors. Endocrinol. Metab. Clin. *16:*529, 1987. (An authoritative morphologic review, by acknowledged experts, devoted mainly to pituitary adenomas.)

Lever, E. G., et al.: Inherited disorders of thyroid metabolism. Endocrinol. Rev. *4:*213, 1983. (A superb review of these rare conditions—an excellent reference source.)

McNicol, A. M.: Pituitary adenomas. Histopathology *11:*995, 1987. (An excellent, relatively brief presentation of the functional and specialized features of these tumors.)

Nakano, M.: Adrenal cortical carcinoma. A clinicopathological and immunohistochemical study of 91 autopsy cases. Acta Pathol. Jpn. *38:*163, 1988. (A detailed anatomic consideration with excellent immunohistochemical considerations.)

Nelkin, B. D., et al.: The molecular biology of medullary thyroid carcinoma. A model for cancer development and progression. JAMA. *261:*3130, 1989. (Good brief overview of this form of cancer—includes brief details on morphology and molecular genetics.)

Pittman, C. S., Menefee, J. K.: Pathophysiology of Graves' disease. Hosp. Pract. *22:*99, 1987. (A succinct and basic overview of the clinical and pathophysiologic features.)

Rojeski, M. T., Gharib, H.: Nodular thyroid disease. Evaluation and management. N. Engl. J. Med. *313:*428, 1985. (A good presentation of the clinical problems of sifting out the cause of a nodular thyroid.)

Schteingart, D. E.: Cushing's syndrome. Endocrinol. Metab. Clin. North Am. *18:*311, 1989. (A brief discussion of the pathophysiology, clinical features, and diagnostic approaches.)

Schwartz, M. R.: Pathology of the thyroid and parathyroid glands. Otolaryngol. Clin. North Am. *23:*175, 1990. (Excellent capsule characterizations of the major disorders of both glands.)

Strakosch, C. R.: Thyroiditis. Aust. N.Z. J. Med. *16:*91, 1986. (An excellent overview of the pathophysiology of the major forms of thyroiditis with clinical and diagnostic considerations.)

Van Dop, C.: Pseudohypoparathyroidism: Clinical and molecular aspects. Semin. Nephrol. *9:*168, 1989. (Very complete analysis of this uncommon disorder.)

TWENTY-ONE

The Musculoskeletal System

BONES
HEREDITARY AND CONGENITAL DISORDERS
METABOLIC DISEASES
    Osteoporosis
    Rickets and Osteomalacia
    Osteitis Fibrosa Cystica (Hyperparathyroid
      Skeletal Disease, von Recklinghausen's
      Disease of Bone)
    Renal Osteodystrophy
INFECTIONS
    Pyogenic Osteomyelitis
    Tuberculosis of Bone
PAGET'S DISEASE (OSTEITIS DEFORMANS)
FIBROUS DYSPLASIA
HYPERTROPHIC OSTEOARTHROPATHY
TUMORS
    Osteochondroma
    Chondroma (Enchondroma)
    Osteoid Osteoma
    Giant Cell Tumor
    Osteosarcoma
    Chondrosarcoma
    Ewing's Sarcoma
JOINTS
OSTEOARTHRITIS—DEGENERATIVE JOINT
DISEASE

SUPPURATIVE ARTHRITIS
LYME DISEASE
BURSITIS

SKELETAL MUSCLE
MUSCLE ATROPHY
MYOSITIS
MUSCULAR DYSTROPHY
MYASTHENIA GRAVIS
TRICHINOSIS

SOFT TISSUE TUMORS
COMMENTS ON SELECTED TUMORS

This chapter is divided into disorders of bones, joints, and muscles, followed by a section on soft tissue tumors that arise in the supporting tissues of the skeleton. The many diseases involving these "bits and pieces" range from the exotic to those that vie in frequency with gray hair. Only the more frequent ones are considered, interspersed with a few less common entities that offer elegant insights into recent advances in understanding the origins of some musculoskeletal diseases.

Bones

Bone is a remarkably ingenious and complex tissue that has great structural stability despite being in constant turnover. It is composed of a large and varied cell complement in its cancellous and cortical compartments, all of which are subject to disease. The disorders of the marrow cells are discussed in Chapter 12, among them plasma cell myeloma, the most common of the primary tumors of bone. Most disorders of bone are quite uncommon, and so the following discussions with a few notable exceptions can be brief.

HEREDITARY AND CONGENITAL DISORDERS

A large number of bone disorders are of genetic origin, either hereditary and familial or related to new mutations. They range from the innocuous (e.g., extra digits) to the extreme (e.g., *achondroplasia*, an autosomal dominant condition characterized by impaired epiphyseal cartilaginous growth resulting in abnormally short limbs but head and torso of normal size). Another, fortunately uncommon, genetic disorder provides an example of the remarkable advances mentioned earlier. Not so long ago, *osteogenesis imperfecta* (OI), also known as "brittle bone disease," was thought to be virtually always devastating because affected infants sustained multiple fractures, sometimes in utero or during birth, and as a consequence usually were stillborn or died in infancy. Now we appreciate that there is a wide range of severity, owing to varying abnormalities in the synthesis of type I collagen (which constitutes about 90% of the bone matrix). These are due to a large variety of gene mutations that alter either the rate of synthesis or molecular structure of type I procollagen. It is awesome to realize that a single base substitution in the genetic code may yield a lethal skeletal and connective tissue (e.g., scleral) disorder. Some of the mutations that produce the more lethal forms of OI are indeed hereditary but other patterns compatible with life appear to be related to newly acquired mutations and therefore have no relevance to future siblings.

METABOLIC DISEASES

OSTEOPOROSIS

Osteoporosis is an extremely common disorder characterized by a reduction in the bone mass that may prejudice its structural integrity and predispose to fractures. Asymptomatic at the outset, eventually microfractures and skeletal distortion become painfully disabling. However, the "too little" bone that remains is of normal composition (i.e., has normal proportions of protein matrix and minerals). The condition may be encountered under a variety of clinical circumstances (Table 21–1) but preponderantly is associated with aging, and particularly the menopause. The frequency of postmenopausal osteoporosis accounts for the overall female-to-male ratio of 2:1 to 3:1. About 25% of women sustain a fracture by age 65, and 50% by age 90. This form of osteopenia (too little bone) is said to be responsible annually in the United States for over a million fractures (mainly of the vertebrae, hips, and wrists) with the approximately 300,000 hip fractures exacting a mortality of 15 to 20% among very elderly persons.

PATHOGENESIS. Over 95% of cases of osteoporosis are of the primary type—a euphemism for of unknown cause. As you know, bone remodeling occurs throughout life. Normally there is an exquisite balance between the bone resorption by osteoclasts and subsequent restoration of the bone by osteoblasts. A number of factors produced locally may participate in this process, among them interleukin 1 (IL-1), tumor necrosis factor (TNF), platelet-derived growth factor (PDGF), tumor growth factor-β, and insulin growth factor-I, some of which stimulate osteoclastic activity, others osteoblastic activity, and some with varying circumstances have one or the other action. It appears that in osteoporosis the loss of bone results from an imbalance between bone resorption and bone forma-

TABLE 21–1. CLASSIFICATION OF OSTEOPOROSIS

Primary (of unknown cause)
  Aging (postmenopausal)
  Juvenile idiopathic
Secondary
  Endocrinopathy
    Hypercortisolism, exogenous, and Cushing's disease ↓ bone formation
    Hyperthyroidism
    Hypogonadism
    Diabetes mellitus
    Hyperparathyroidism ↑ bone resorption
    Hyperprolactinemia
  Malignancy
    Multiple myeloma
    Leukemia
    Lymphoma
    Systemic mastocytosis
  Drugs
    Anticonvulsants
    Heparin
  Alcohol
  Cigarette smoking
  Immobilization
  Primary biliary cirrhosis
  Malabsorption
    Protein deficiency
    Calcium deficiency

tion. In health, formation outpaces resorption until about age 25 to 30, when peak bone mass is achieved. Between 35 and 40 years, the resorption and formation are exquisitely balanced with no net gain or loss. After age 40 years, resorption outpaces formation: both women and men lose about 0.3 to 0.5% of bone mass annually, owing largely to increased osteoclastic mobilization of bone and in some part to reduced osteoblastic formation. In the few years prior to and following the menopause, the imbalance worsens measurably, and women may lose 2 to 5% of bone mass annually. Thereafter the rate of loss slows. The aging-related losses are much slower in men of comparable age. Moreover, women are particularly vulnerable because on average their skeletons are more delicate than men's throughout life.

The precise basis for this accelerated bone loss in elders is unclear, but it is likely to be multifactorial. Most important appears to be estrogen deficiency in women and androgen deficiency in men. The evidence is more dramatic with estrogens and takes such forms as the well-defined increased rate of bone loss in young women after surgical oophorectomy, and the ability of estrogen replacement therapy to prevent bone loss in the postmenopausal years. Significantly, once osteoporosis appears, administered estrogens have very little effect (i.e., may not restore the lost bone), although some would still debate this issue. How estrogen acts is still unknown; although bone cells can be shown in vitro to have estrogen receptors, they are not demonstrable in vivo. Conceivably, estrogen acts indirectly by either inhibiting local synthesis by bone cells, lymphocytes, and monocytes of osteoblast-activating factors mentioned earlier or by promoting the release of osteoblast-activating factors.

Many other influences may contribute to bone loss, but they are generally not considered to have major roles, e.g., hereditary predisposition, increased level of parathormone (PTH), decreased level of calcitriol, dietary deficiency of vitamin D, and decreased level of physical activity. Somewhat better established is that inadequate intake of calcium speeds the loss and conversely adequate intake and absorption of calcium slows it.

The many forms of secondary osteoporosis are so uncommon that only the following few comments are indicated. Hyperparathyroidism, as discussed on page 663, is a well-known cause of increased bone resorption, but the anatomic changes are not identical to those of osteoporosis. Increased levels of glucocorticoids, whether administered exogenously or produced by a condition such as Cushing's syndrome, suppress bone formation. The basis for the bone loss with malignancies is less clear and is vaguely attributed to synthesis by tumor cells of osteoclast-activating factors.

MORPHOLOGY. Except when it is secondary to prolonged immobilization of localized parts, osteoporosis is a systemic disorder affecting the entire skeleton. Nevertheless, bone loss is most severe in areas of the skeleton that contain relatively large amounts of trabecular bone and that are subject to most weight-bearing stress. Thus, the vertebrae and wrists are early targets and, as the disease advances, the femoral necks. These are often the sites of fractures. The cancellous bone plates are resorbed, converting them to slender spicules that are sometimes split or transected, and the cortical bone is thinned (Fig. 21–1). Nevertheless, osteoporotic bone, although reduced in mass, has the same composition as normal bone, with no evidence of inadequate mineralization, increased amounts of osteoid (unmineralized matrix), or widened osteoid seams. Although some increased osteoclastic activity may be evident, there is no great disproportion between "blasts" and "clasts."

CLINICAL COURSE. Bone pain, especially backache, is a common complaint of patients with osteoporosis. This results from microfractures and collapse of fractured vertebral bodies, accounting for the expression "vertebral crush fracture syndrome." Other common sites of fracture are the lower end of the radius, and in the later years (after age 70) the femoral neck. Often these follow trivial trauma. Radiographs may show an increase in radiolucency of bone, but this method of diagnosis is insensitive because nearly half of bone mineral must be lost before it can be detected by routine radiography. Newer, more sensitive techniques such as single- or dual-photon absorptiometry more accurately quantitate the mineral content of bone and help differentiate this form of osteopenia from such other forms as osteomalacia and osteitis fibrosa. Serum levels of alkaline phosphatase, calcium, and phosphorus are characteristically within normal limits, and also help differentiate osteoporosis from osteomalacia. Several agents that retard bone resorption or favor

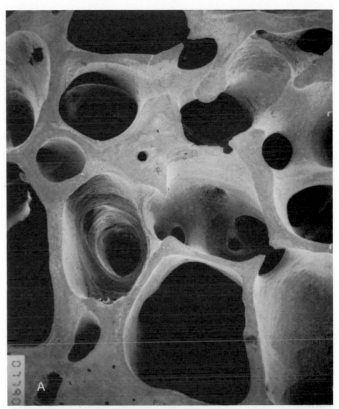

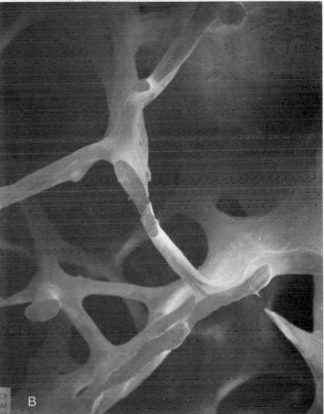

Figure 21–1. Scanning electron micrographs of iliac crest biopsies from, *A,* a normal female and, *B,* a younger female with marked osteoporosis. (From Dempster, D. W., Shane, E., Horbert, W., Lindsay, R.: A simple method for correlative light and scanning electron microscopy of human iliac crest bone biopsies: Qualitative observations in normal and osteoporotic subjects. J. Bone Miner. Res. *1:*15, 1986.)

osteogenesis are used in the prevention of primary osteoporosis: calcium supplementation, estrogens, and etidronate (a biphosphonate). Fluorides are of doubtful value. No agent has yet been proven to unequivocally reverse established changes.

RICKETS AND OSTEOMALACIA

Rickets and osteomalacia (discussed on page 247 in detail) are both characterized by deficits in the mineralization of newly formed bone matrix, resulting in soft, osteopenic bones. Before the epiphyses have closed, the mineralization deficit induces rickets, with skeletal deformities such as bowing of the legs and rib deformities. After growth has ceased in adults, osteomalacia, a much more subtle disorder, develops. It is marked principally by osteopenia, with inadequately mineralized bone susceptible to pseudofractures and fractures, often accompanied by proximal muscle weakness. The major causes of rickets and osteomalacia are cited in Chapter 8, page 250.

The basic morphologic change in rickets and osteomalacia resulting from the defective mineralization is an excess of osteoid. The excess involves both the thickness and proportion of trabecular surface covered, along with widening of osteoid seams. Thus, overall, bone is poorly mineralized (osteopenic) and subject to deformation during skeletal growth and to fracture or pseudofracture (incomplete fracture) in adults.

OSTEITIS FIBROSA CYSTICA (HYPERPARATHYROID SKELETAL DISEASE, VON RECKLINGHAUSEN'S DISEASE OF BONE)

The causes of hyperparathyroidism are discussed in Chapter 20; here the focus is on its skeletal consequences. Because of the wider use of laboratory screening tests that can detect the elevated serum levels of calcium in hyperparathyroidism, the condition is being diagnosed much earlier in its course, before skeletal changes develop. Only late in the course of primary hyperparathyroidism is there generalized resorption of bone, yielding a form of osteopenia. The increased circulating level of PTH mobilizes calcium from the skeleton and recruits increased numbers of osteoclasts and osteoblasts, causing increased bone turnover with a net loss of well-formed bone.

MORPHOLOGY. Histologically, there is increased osteoblast activity, with laying down of increased amounts of osteoid, and increased osteoclast activity with resorption lacunae and tunneling defects in the cortex and thinning, dissection, or complete resorption of trabeculae. The increased osteoid is poorly mineralized, so as a net effect bone formation does not keep pace with the resorption. At the same time the marrow spaces become filled with delicate fibrous tissue containing micro- or macroscopic cysts. These changes result at first in only demineralization, indistinguishable from osteomalacia or osteoporosis. In time, more fully evolved osteitis fibrosa cystica appears with the following features that distinguish it from the other osteopenic conditions: (1) Subperiosteal resorption of bone in the phalanges and distal clavicles is accompanied by loss of the lamina dura about the tooth sockets. (2) Bone resorption may result in multiple, localized, cystic lesions that may expand and sometimes deform the basic architecture but rarely erode through the cortical surface. (3) Sometimes these cystic spaces have a background of a loose fibrous stroma and contain hemorrhage with deposits of hemosiderin. Resorption and repair of the hemorrhage by uninuclear and multinucleate cells produce reparative giant cell granulomas (unfortunately referred to as "brown tumors").

Control of the hyperparathyroidism, as by removal of a parathyroid adenoma, arrests the progression of the skeletal disease and, over the course of years, permits restoration to a considerable extent of the normal skeletal architecture.

RENAL OSTEODYSTROPHY

Chronic renal failure, particularly in patients maintained on dialysis, is often associated with a complex of skeletal changes embracing osteitis fibrosa cystica admixed with osteomalacia, often complicated by the changes resulting from aluminum toxicity. This melange of bone changes, termed *renal osteodystrophy,* is attributed in part to the secondary hyperparathyroidism associated with chronic renal failure, in part to hypocalcemia, and in some part to the direct effect of aluminum toxicity on bone mineralization.

The basis for the secondary hyperparathyroidism was discussed on page 665. The hypocalcemia has complex origins but is attributable mainly to a reduction in the synthesis of 1,25-dihydroxyvitamin D incident to the loss of functioning renal parenchyma. The lower level of the vitamin reduces intestinal calcium absorption and the calcium-mobilizing action of PTH on bones. Phosphate retention in renal failure also contributes to decreased synthesis of $1,25\text{-}(OH)_2D$, as does the accompanying acidosis. The hyperphosphatemia itself induces hypocalcemia, stimulating parathyroid activity to normalize the serum calcium level. The role of aluminum toxicity is less clear. The source of the aluminum is oral ingestion of aluminum-containing phosphate binders and the very small amounts contained in dialysis fluid. Aluminum directly suppresses osteoblast function and new bone formation so that osteoblasts are reduced in number and appear inactive; it also hampers mineralization, thus contributing to a low turnover and an osteomalacia-like condition. In passing, it should be noted that aluminum also has been implicated as the cause of "dialysis encephalopathy" and microcytic anemia in patients with chronic renal failure.

INFECTIONS

The two most important types of infection are pyogenic osteomyelitis and tuberculosis of bone.

PYOGENIC OSTEOMYELITIS

Pyogens may "set up housekeeping" in bones (1) by hematogenous spread, (2) from a contiguous infection, or (3) by direct traumatic introduction (including orthopedic surgical procedures). Hematogenous seeding is most common in the developing world and in drug addicts or in generally young, otherwise vulnerable hosts, whereas the last two pathways account for most cases in developed countries (e.g., osteomyelitis of the jaw initiated by a periapical tooth abscess or a compound fracture with penetration of the skin by bone fragments). Hematogenous osteomyelitis is caused principally by *Staphylococcus aureus* and less frequently by species of *Pseudomonas* or *Klebsiella*, *Escherichia coli*, or other pyogens. Mixed infections are more common in osteomyelitis following compound fractures, and anaerobes frequently participate in instances associated with dental problems. Antibiotic-resistant microbes such as *Pseudomonas* species are growing in importance and are often encountered in drug addicts. For reasons unknown, salmonellae are often implicated in patients with sickle cell disease.

In children, the infection most often begins in the metaphyseal region of the long bones, where capillary flow is least active (Fig. 21-2). In adults, the jaw or the spine is often the site of infection. Wherever located, a characteristic suppurative reaction ensues, which in the course of its build-up compromises the vascular supply to the area, adding an element of ischemic necrosis. The inflammation may then penetrate the endosteum and traverse the haversian system to reach the periosteum (periostitis), creating, possibly, a **subperiosteal abscess.** Further extension may lead to single or multiple sinus tracts into the soft tissue, and sometimes through the skin. In adults, the periosteum is tightly attached to the articular margin, so extension into the joint space is uncommon; however, in infants the periosteum is attached more loosely and the epiphyseal plate is vascularized, so infection may spread either directly into the joint space or track along the periosteum. Detachment of large areas of the periosteum may cause necrosis of a small or large fragment of bone, known as a **sequestrum.** In occasional instances, the infection becomes walled off, creating a localized (Brodie's) abscess that may undergo spontaneous sterilization or become a chronic nidus of infection. Under such circumstances, reactive osteoblastic activity leads to new bone formation, producing an **involucrum** that encloses the inflammatory focus.

Essentially similar changes occur in vertebral osteomyelitis with possible subligamentous spread to adjacent vertebral bodies. Penetration into the sheaths of the psoas muscles may yield infections that track into the inguinal regions. The intervertebral disks are remarkably resistant.

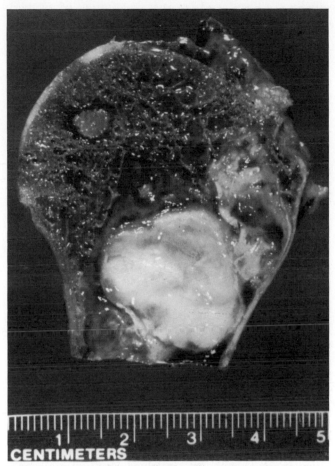

Figure 21-2. The transected head of the humerus of a young adult reveals a large focus of osteomyelitis near the line of resection and a smaller focus close to the articular surface.

CLINICAL COURSE. In children, hematogenous osteomyelitis usually manifests as an acute febrile illness with pain and tenderness referable to the local lesion. In time there may be redness and swelling, but these are usually advanced changes. The presentation may be much more subtle in infants or adults with few localizing findings. The diagnosis is confirmed by radiographic evidence of bone destruction, which in the early days may be so subtle as to require radionuclide scans to document the aggregation of white cells. Blood cultures demonstrate the pathogen in more than half of the cases. Although spontaneous healing may occur, in the absence of adequate therapy, chronicity is likely, and with it the risk of metastatic dissemination of infection. Amyloidosis is a potential complication of neglected chronic infections.

TUBERCULOSIS OF BONE _____

Tuberculous osteomyelitis is no longer a significant clinical problem except in developing countries, where the incidence of tuberculosis is high. Seeding of the bones usually occurs by the hematogenous route, but in many cases a primary focus in the lungs or elsewhere may not be identifiable. Unlike pyogenic osteomyelitis, tuberculous osteomyelitis tends to arise insidiously and to extend into joint spaces. Often it is not noted until destruction is widespread. The long bones of the extremities and the spine *(Pott's disease)* are the favored sites of localization. In the spine, tuberculous osteomyelitis can lead to serious deformities (kyphosis, scoliosis) due to the destruction and malalignment of the vertebrae. The histologic reaction is typical of all tuberculous lesions and will not be repeated here.

PAGET'S DISEASE (OSTEITIS DEFORMANS) _____

Paget's disease is a fairly common disorder of uncertain cause, characterized basically by uncoordinated bone resorption and bone formation, leading ultimately to skeletal deformation. *The condition has three recognizable stages: (1) an initial osteolytic phase, followed in time by (2) a mixed stage of frenzied osteolysis and osteogenesis, culminating in (3) a final inactive, burned-out sclerotic phase* (Fig. 21–3). The changes may be confined to a single bone (monostotic); more often many bones are involved (polyostotic), and, rarely, the entire skeleton. Rare before age 40 years, Paget's assumes a frequency of 1 to 3% in Caucasians after age 50, reaching 10% among very elderly persons, but it is rare in blacks and Asians. There is a modest male preponderance.

PATHOGENESIS. More than a century ago, Sir James Paget considered this condition to be inflammatory, hence the designation "ost*eitis* deformans." This idea was discarded until recently; virus-like particles of measles-type or adenovirus type have been seen by several independent observers in both osteoclasts and osteoblasts of pagetic bone. It has been proposed, therefore, that Paget's disease is a slow virus infection akin to the slow virus disease of the central nervous system—subacute sclerosing panencephalitis—which is related to the same family of viruses. Subsequent studies have disclosed paramyxovirus antigens of both measles and respiratory syncytial viruses in the nuclei and cytoplasm of pagetic osteoclasts but not in similar cells of uninvolved bone. The agent(s) cannot be isolated from these cells, however, and could represent "an uninvited, unimportant guest."

MORPHOLOGY. Monostotic Paget's disease tends to involve, in descending order of frequency, tibia, iliac bone, femur, skull, and vertebra. In contrast, in the polyostotic disease, the spine is most often involved (70%), followed closely by the pelvis (65%), and then in

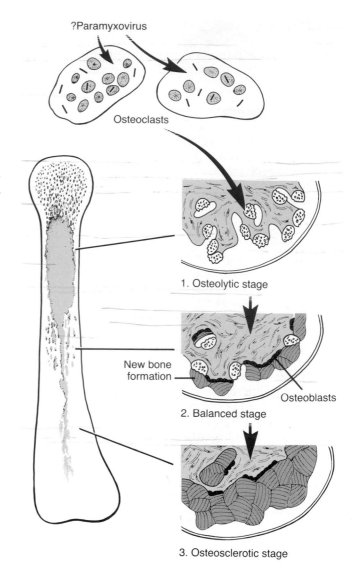

Figure 21–3. A diagrammatic representation of the three stages of Paget's disease, beginning with a putative viral infection of osteoclasts.

descending order, femur, skull, sacrum, tibia. Any bone **may** be affected.

The initial osteolytic phase is marked at first by replacement of the marrow by a richly vascularized fibrous tissue. This is followed by a disordered patchwork of areas of resorption produced by an increased number of overly active, very large osteoclasts, some containing as many as a hundred nuclei. As mentioned, these cells may contain microcylindrical apparent viral inclusions. In the mixed phase, resorption is closely followed by new bone formation, which at first forms irregular islands of woven bone filling the resorption lacunae. In time the woven bone is replaced by lamellar bone. In the course of this erratic resorption and new bone formation, a disordered mosaic resembling the pieces of a jigsaw puzzle is created, rendered visible because of the persistence of cement lines demarcating the individual islands of newly formed bone. **This mosaic pattern is**

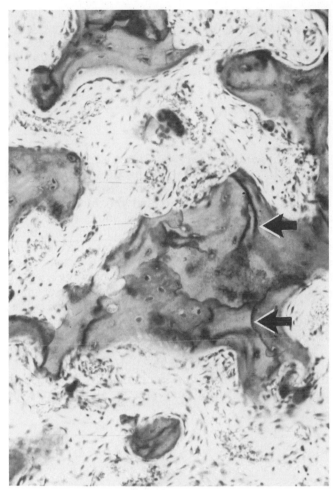

Figure 21–4. Paget's disease of bone shows the classic mosaic pattern *(arrows)* and fibrosis of the intertrabecular spaces.

pathognomonic of Paget's disease (Fig. 21–4). In the course of this frenzy, the cortex is thickened, as are the trabeculae of cancellous bone. In this manner the skull may become abnormally thickened with expansion of its external diameter, as occurs with all affected bones (Fig. 21–5). Despite the fact that there is "too much bone," it is soft and porous and has the consistency of dried bread, leading to anterior bowing of the femur and tibia under weight bearing, coarsening of the facial features, narrowing of the foramens through which the cranial nerves pass, and collapse of the vertebrae to produce marked kyphosis. In time, although the activity burns out, the mosaic persists, and the bones become densely sclerotic, but they lack structural strength and are brittle and vulnerable to "chalk-stick fractures."

CLINICAL FEATURES. Depending on the extent and stage of the disease, it may be entirely asymptomatic (80 to 90% of patients) and be discovered only by chance radiography. The most common symptoms, when there are any, are pain or deformity related to the skeletal changes. Headache, pain in the face, deafness, or visual disturbances may result from impingement on cranial nerves by enlarging skull bones. The long bones of the legs, particularly the tibiae, may become bowed under the stress of weight bearing. Back pain may become disabling because of compression fracture of vertebrae and narrowing of the foramens of spinal roots. Often the patient first becomes aware of the condition by the appearance of unusual warmth over an involved bone or because of a progressive increase in hat size. X-ray examination can be diagnostic, especially during the osteolytic and mixed phases. Although the serum calcium and phosphate levels are often normal, usually the serum levels of alkaline phosphatase and osteocalcin (the major calcium-binding protein of bone matrix) are elevated and

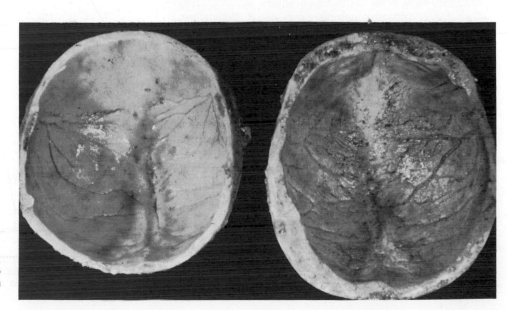

Figure 21–5. Paget's disease of skull. Irregular thickening of the right calvarium is well brought out by comparison with normal control on left.

urinary hydroxyproline excretion increased, all reflections of increased bone turnover.

Two complications may arise. (1) About 1% of patients develop a sarcomatous change in an involved bone, most often an osteogenic sarcoma but sometimes another type. (2) Rarely, high-output cardiac failure develops owing to the increased vascularity of the subcutaneous tissue overlying the involved bones, which in effect speeds venous return and overloads the heart.

FIBROUS DYSPLASIA _____

An uncommon disease of unknown cause, *fibrous dysplasia is marked by focal areas of disordered maturation of bone leaving a loose, whorled fibrous tissue punctuated by haphazard islands and strands of woven bone, and rarely foci of cartilage.* The changes suggest a developmental disorder. It appears in three patterns: (1) monostotic (about 70% of cases), affecting either sex, involving, in descending order of frequency, ribs, femur, tibia, maxilla, mandible, calvarium, humerus, and other bones; (2) a polyostotic form, in either sex (about 25% of cases), in which there is unilateral involvement of more than one of the mentioned bones but rarely all; (3) principally in females, polyostotic disease with associated endocrinopathy, rendered distinctive because the unilateral bone lesions are often accompanied by large, irregular, cafe au lait skin pigmentations confined to the same half of the body as the bone lesions and frequently overlying them. The most common endocrinopathy is precocious sexual development, the *McCune-Albright syndrome,* but less frequent associations are hyperthyroidism, Cushing's syndrome, acromegaly, and other endocrinopathies.

> **MORPHOLOGY.** Whatever the setting, the individual lesions arise in the medullary cavity and erode the adjacent cortex but rarely rupture through it. As the process expands, new bone formation maintains an enclosing shell, but considerable deformity may result. Sometimes large tracts of the bone may be affected, particularly in craniofacial involvement with considerable distortion of the facial features, seen in 10% of cases of monostotic disease and 50% of cases of polyostotic involvement. Lesional tissue is generally gray-pink and soft but may be gritty and is amenable to evacuation by curettage. Histologically, mature connective tissue encloses abundant to scant islands and random trabeculae of woven bone and sometimes islands of partially calcified cartilage.

CLINICAL COURSE. Monostotic lesions may be asymptomatic, but sometimes cause bone deformity or predispose weight-bearing bones to fracture. With disseminated disease there is a greater tendency to facial and other deformities and a greater vulnerability to fracture. There is a general correlation between age of onset and rate of progression of the condition. Radio-

graphs are distinctive, revealing round or ovoid, lucent lesions having a ground-glass appearance. A rare complication is sarcomatous transformation, usually in areas that were previously irradiated, so bone grafting or conservative excision is recommended.

HYPERTROPHIC OSTEOARTHROPATHY _____

This mysterious entity has three separate components: (1) "clubbing" of the fingertips, (2) periostitis with new bone formation at the distal ends of long bones as well as the carpals and proximal phalanges, and (3) swelling and tenderness of joints (Fig. 21–6). These changes may appear in a multitude of clinical settings, most commonly lung cancer, chronic lung sepsis (for example, bronchiectasis), and chronic interstitial pneumonia. Clubbing alone may develop in patients with congenital cyanotic heart disease, infective endocarditis, biliary cirrhosis, ulcerative colitis, Crohn's disease, chronic myelogenous leukemia, or thyroid cancer.

The changes involved in clubbing are edema and fibrovascular overgrowth at the tips of the fingers and in the nail bed, causing rounding or "watchglass" deformity of the nail. When present, clubbing may be

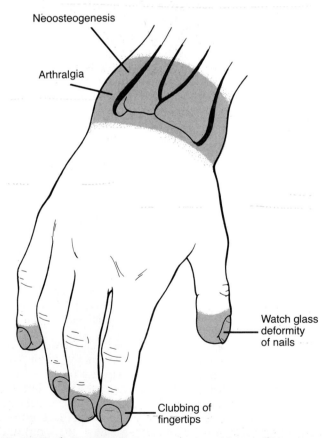

Figure 21–6. The three major components of hypertrophic osteoarthropathy: (1) clubbing of the fingertips, (2) periostitis with new bone formation at the distal ends of bones, and (3) swelling and tenderness of joints.

a valuable diagnostic clue to some underlying serious condition, most often bronchogenic carcinoma. The periosteal bone changes are seen radiographically as barely visible tufting or a completely enclosing layer of new bone.

Although the mechanism or mechanisms that produce these changes are obscure, correction of the underlying condition (e.g., resection of the lung tumor) is soon followed by their regression.

TUMORS

The great majority of tumors in bone are metastatic. Although any extraosseous cancer may be implicated, those most commonly involved (in descending order of frequency) are carcinomas of the prostate, breast, lung, kidney, colon, and thyroid. The vertebral column is by far the most frequent site of implantation, followed by ribs, skull, and pelvis, but no bone is immune. The great majority of these implants are osteolytic, but a few, specifically metastases from the breast or prostate, may stimulate bone formation (are osteoblastic).

Primary tumors of bone are by contrast uncommon, but they have a disproportionate importance for several reasons:
- Excluding multiple myeloma, which is discussed on p. 374, about 40% are malignant, certain types being among the most aggressive of all neoplasms.
- They most often attack young persons, in the early decades of life, sometimes the first.
- Approximately 80% occur about the knee, and while formerly amputation was necessary, current methods of therapy that employ combinations of conservative excision, chemotherapy, and radiotherapy have saved not only limbs but also lives.

Large clinics that treat these neoplasms report the following distribution (excluding multiple myeloma):

Benign		*Malignant*	
Osteochondroma	(30%)	Osteosarcoma	(30%)
Giant cell tumor	(20%)	Chondrosarcoma	(15%)
Chondroma	(10%)	Ewing's tumor	(10%)
Osteoid osteoma	(10%)	Malignant lymphoma	(10%)

Only these most common neoplasms will be described; the lymphomas are presented on page 354.

OSTEOCHONDROMA

These benign lesions, also known as *exostoses,* are probably developmental aberrations rather than true neoplasms. They arise from aberrant lateral growth of epiphyseal cartilage or cartilaginous remnants left behind, producing mushroom-shaped, lateral projections, usually metaphyseal, from the contours of long bones, most often the femur. The stalks (3 to 4 cm long) and heads of these lesions are composed of orderly bone, having thin cortical layers in continuity with the cortex of the attached bone enclosing cancellous bone. The expanded heads are capped by a layer of normal-looking cartilage. While most appear as sporadic solitary lesions, they may occur in profusion in an uncommon autosomal dominant disorder termed *osteochondromatosis*. The solitary lesions are usually asymptomatic and are discovered by chance, or they may be locally tender because of pressure on overlying soft tissue, but rarely they give rise to chondrosarcomas, the risk being substantially greater in the hereditary syndrome.

CHONDROMA (ENCHONDROMA)

This benign neoplasm, almost always located within the interior of a bone (hence enchondroma), is composed of mature hyaline cartilage. Like the osteochondroma, it is believed to arise from remnants of epiphyseal cartilage left behind. They occur at any age, most often singly, but they are also seen in two systemic syndromes marked by great numbers of these lesions. Typically they arise in the small bones of the hands, and less often the feet, but sometimes in other sites. By slow growth they may erode the adjacent cortex and expand the contours of the bone; rarely do they rupture into the soft tissue. The lesional tissue is gray-blue, translucent, and well-demarcated. Histologically the cartilage cells within their lacunae are mature but irregularly dispersed. Foci of calcification or ossification may be present and punctuate the classic osteolytic radiographic appearance.

Solitary tumors arising in the small bones of the hands and feet are almost always innocuous, but in other locations they rarely transform into osteosarcomas. By contrast in the systemic syndromes, with their profusion of tumors, the frequency of sarcoma reaches 30 to 50%.

OSTEOID OSTEOMA

These benign neoplasms are of interest because they rarely exceed 1.5 cm in diameter but are exquisitely painful. Most occur in the first two decades of life, with a male-female ratio of 3:1. They tend to arise within the cortex of the tibia and femur (near the ends), but any other bone including the vertebrae may be involved. The center of such a lesion (the nidus) is characterized early in the course by interlacing trabeculae of osteoid, which later are partially converted into poorly mineralized woven bone enclosed within vascularized connective tissue. In time the bony trabeculae become densely packed. The surrounding bone is stimulated into neoosteogenesis, creating a densely sclerotic enclosing shell. Radiographs reveal the characteristic radiolucent nidus enclosed within a sclerotic shell. Near the periosteum this neoosteogenesis may deform the external contour. Recognition of these lesions is important because virtually all are cured by local excision. On occasion there is recurrence, but rarely malignant transformation.

GIANT CELL TUMOR

The giant cell tumor is usually benign but it is locally aggressive with a tendency to recur following incomplete excision, carrying with it the risk (albeit rarely) of transformation into a sarcoma. About 1 to 3% of the more anaplastic tumors, difficult to segregate morphologically, are malignant de novo and capable of widespread invasion and metastases. To further complicate matters, a rare innocent-looking lesion has produced sparse indolent metastasis to the lungs or elsewhere without affecting longevity. Thus, the clinical behavior of this particular type of lesion is more difficult to predict from histologic evaluation than that of any other type of bone tumor.

Typically, these tumors occur between age 20 and 40, in the epiphyseal region, most commonly in the distal femur, proximal tibia, distal radius, and proximal humerus. Less often other bones are involved (e.g., sacrum or small bones of hands and feet). Persons of other ages and other locations are sometimes affected, but almost never do the lesions arise in skeletally immature patients. There is no well-defined sex preponderance.

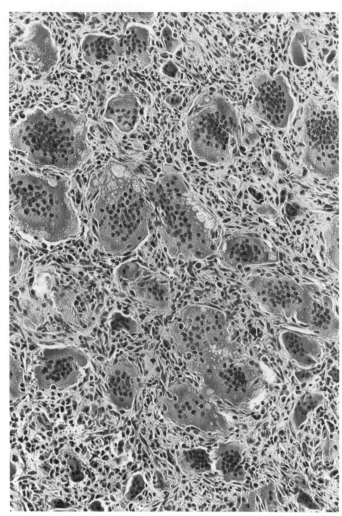

Figure 21-8. Giant cell tumor of bone. The large multinucleate osteoclast-like giant cells are separated by a scant, benign-looking spindle cell stroma.

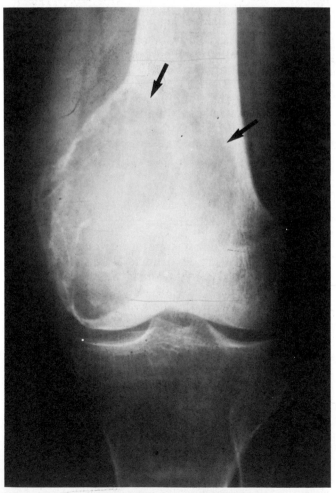

Figure 21-7. A lytic giant cell tumor in the lower epiphysis of the femur. The contour of the bone is expanded and the neoplasm abuts the articular cartilage and extends to the arrows.

MORPHOLOGY. Grossly, the tumor is gray-brown, well-vascularized, and may have areas of hemorrhage, necrosis, and cyst formation. They appear as eccentric lytic lesions in the epiphysis and may extend into the metaphysis but rarely into the adjacent joint (Fig. 21-7). The contour of the bone may be expanded, but a thin shell of subperiosteal new bone persists. Very infrequently these tumors arise in multicentric foci within several bones.

All are characterized by an abundance of multinucleate giant cells resembling osteoclasts dispersed throughout a stroma of round to ovoid, to spindle-shaped mononuclear cells, some of which appear to be fibroblastic in lineage while others have monocyte-macrophage markers (Fig. 21-8). It is the stromal cells that are the neoplastic element of these neoplasms. When anaplasia appears, it involves the stromal cells, but in the great preponderance of lesions the cells are uniform in size and shape and benign looking. In rare tumors the stroma is more anaplastic.

The presenting complaint is usually pain. The radiograph is quite characteristic and has been likened to a lytic cluster of "soap bubbles." Acknowledging the difficulties in characterizing the behavior of these tumors, it suffices to say that the more benign-looking ones are managed conservatively by curettage or local resection, sometimes followed by radiotherapy preserving joint and limb function; unhappily the more anaplastic lesions require more radical procedures.

OSTEOSARCOMA *malig.*

The hallmark of osteosarcomas is the direct formation of osteoid or bone by tumor cells. The amount of osteogenesis among tumors is variable, and some are largely fibroblastic; others may show some chondroid differentiation; still others are highly vascular (telangiectatic), and some densely sclerotic because of abundant bone formation. As noted, excluding multiple myeloma, osteosarcomas are the most common primary cancer of bone. Moreover, they are generally aggressive lesions that are capable of widespread metastasis and require as early diagnosis as possible and expert treatment.

So-called *primary osteosarcomas* arise in the apparent absence of underlying bone disease or predisposing influences, most often in the second decade of life, with a definite male preponderance. Most of these neoplasms are situated in the central metaphyseal region of long tubular bones (i.e., distal femur, proximal tibia, proximal humerus). Much less commonly, so-called *secondary osteosarcomas* occur on a background of some predisposing influence such as Paget's disease of bone or prior irradiation, and in other locations (e.g., jaws), usually later in life.

Convincing evidence implicates genetic factors in the origins of some (possibly all) osteosarcomas. Patients who have a hereditary predisposition for or develop a retinoblastoma (p. 189) have a markedly increased risk of developing an osteosarcoma, much greater than persons with sporadic retinoblastomas and control subjects. These individuals are known to have homozygous deletions on chromosome 13q14, the so-called Rb (retinoblastoma) locus. About a third of patients with osteosarcomas have such a loss of heterozygosity at the Rb locus, whether retinoblastoma is present or not. The Rb gene is a well-known tumor suppressor gene whose role in carcinogenesis was discussed in an earlier chapter (p. 190).

MORPHOLOGY. The tumor arises, usually in the metaphyseal cancellous bone, and progressively extends in all directions, eventually eroding the cortex and often invading the adjacent soft tissues, producing an obvious extraosseous mass (Fig. 21–9). Cartilage appears to be resistant, and therefore invasion of the joint space through the epiphyseal plate is uncommon. When it penetrates the cortex, the tumor sometimes lifts the periosteum, and a characteristic "Codman's triangle"

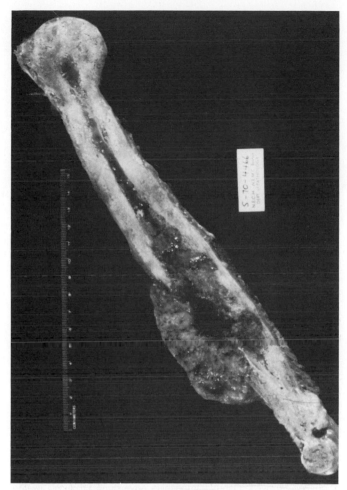

Figure 21–9. Osteosarcoma of the humerus with obvious erosion of the cortex and extension into the surrounding soft tissues.

can be visualized radiographically—the angle between the plane of the outer surface of the cortex and the elevated periosteum. Although characteristic, this triangle is not diagnostic of osteosarcoma. The cut surface is gray-white with areas of hemorrhage and cystic necrosis. The consistency depends on the amount of partially mineralized tumorous osteoid and cartilage. **The histologic hallmark is the formation of osteoid directly by tumor cells.** Thus anaplastic cells are found within lacunae of the osteoid, simulating osteocytes. It is the anaplastic fibroblastic stroma that is the cutting edge of the neoplasm and determines the degree of aggressiveness of the lesion. The most malignant prototypes show marked hyperchromasia, abnormal mitoses, and bizarre-looking giant tumor cells in the fibroblastic component (Fig. 21–10).

The bloodstream is the major route of spread and the lungs the most frequent site of metastases, although other organs may be involved. In the great majority of cases, these neoplasms kill by widespread hematogenous dissemination.

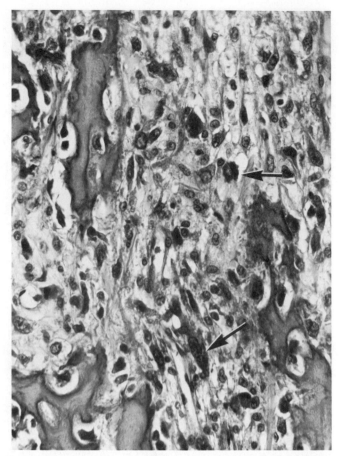

Figure 21–10. Osteogenic sarcoma. The high-power detail illustrates the anaplastic fibrous tissue with mitoses and tumor giant cell formation (arrows). Osteoid trabeculae have been produced by the neoplastic cells, and anaplastic tumor cells are found lying within apparent bone lacunae.

CLINICAL FEATURES. The demonstration by radiography of a lytic or patchily blastic, invasive, often locally painful, metaphyseal tumor that produces a detectable mass with calcifications outside of the bony contour is highly characteristic of osteosarcoma in the individual of appropriate age. As noted, sometimes Codman's triangle can be demonstrated. These tumors tend to grow rapidly and early metastasis is typical. The findings must be confirmed by biopsy and histologic examination.

Advances in treatment have substantially improved the prognosis. Amputation may be necessary, but combined conservative surgery, radiation, and chemotherapy have yielded about a 60% five-year disease-free survival rate, and very few incremental losses over the succeeding years. In general, so-called primary osteosarcomas yield better results than the secondary lesions.

CHONDROSARCOMA _____

This malignant cartilaginous skeletal tumor is next to osteosarcoma in frequency. It differs from osteosarcoma in several respects. Chondrosarcomas rarely arise before age 35, their growth tends to be much slower,

and the prognosis is therefore much better. Males are affected twice as often as females and most tumors arise in the pelvis and long bones, particularly the femur and humerus. Although the great majority arise de novo, some originate from malignant transformation of enchondromas (particularly the multiple lesions in the systemic enchondromatoses) or from osteochondromas.

MORPHOLOGY. These tumors begin within the medullary portion of the bone and progressively extend within the medullary cavity as well as encroaching on the cortex. Frequently new bone formation in advance of the cortical penetration produces a radiographically demonstrable enclosing shell. The cut surface shows gray-white gelatinous tumor punctuated by foci of calcification and areas of hemorrhage or necrosis.

Microscopically there is great variability. Some tumors are very well differentiated and difficult to distinguish from enchondromas. At the other end of the spectrum are tumors with obvious signs of malignancy, such as extremely plump chondroblasts showing atypical large nuclei, multinucleate cells, and occasionally two or more cells lying within a lacuna (Fig. 21–11). Very helpful in differentiating malignant from benign tumors is the tendency for chondrosarcoma to cause erosive endosteal scalloping as well as microscopic extension into the intertrabecular spaces with progressive erosion of the trabeculae.

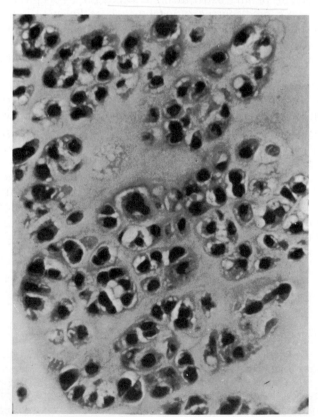

Figure 21–11. Anaplastic chondrocytes within a chondrosarcoma.

Varying with the level of differentiation, these tumors tend to grow slowly, but eventually they metastasize via the hematogenous route, typically to the lungs. Whatever the level of anaplasia, all require complete surgical excision; otherwise they stubbornly recur, sometimes five to ten years later. The five-year survival rate ranges from about 90% for well-differentiated lesions to less than 40% for the most anaplastic.

EWING'S SARCOMA

This relatively uncommon and aggressive malignant tumor most often arises in the long bones of children between ages 10 and 15 years; however, some cases arise in the bones of the head and neck and an even smaller number in extraosseous soft tissues of the trunk, extremities, and elsewhere. Rarely, such unexpected origins as the orbit, genitourinary tract, and meninges are encountered.

Grossly, most of these rapidly growing neoplasms arise within the medullary cavity, often within the metaphysis. However, at the time of presentation they diffusely permeate the cortex without causing large cortical defects and extend into the adjacent soft tissue. As the tumor progressively expands, subperiosteal new bone formation may produce multiple radiographically visible, "onionskin" layers about the shaft of the bone. Microscopically, they are composed of sheets of closely packed, round to ovoid cells of uncertain genealogy, having uniform, monotonous round nuclei and no other distinguishing features. The cells often form broad ribbons disposed about blood vessels with necrosis of

intervening large tracts of cells. More anaplastic variants display greater cell size and variability. Cytoplasmic PAS-positive glycogen granules are usually present in well-preserved cells.

Ewing's sarcoma must be differentiated from the many other round cell tumors—neuroblastoma, lymphoma, rhabdomyosarcoma. Indeed, this problem has challenged pathologists for decades, despite modern immunohistochemical and immunocytologic techniques. Somewhat helpful is the demonstration of glycogen within cells; but some tumors do not contain glycogen (attributed to improper fixation of tissue), and moreover, glycogen is a feature of other forms of neoplasia. Most helpful is the demonstration of a reciprocal translocation between chromosomes 11 and 22. This translocation is a virtually absolute marker of Ewing's sarcoma, since it is not found in the more common round cell tumors. The same chromosomal translocation, however, has been reported in several rare primitive neuroepitheliomas.

The dominant presenting features of Ewing's sarcoma are local pain and tenderness and fever. Sometimes these tumors masquerade as osteomyelitis until their true aggressiveness becomes apparent. With radiographic evidence of a permeating medullary tumor that extends into the soft tissue producing onion-skin layering about the bone, the diagnosis is reasonably certain.

Although there is great variability, in general these are rapidly growing neoplasms that disseminate through the bloodstream to many organs, including lungs and brain. With combinations of chemotherapy, radiotherapy, and surgery, approximately 75% of patients now survive five years or longer.

Joints

The joints are among the most frequently affected parts of the body, but one condition, osteoarthritis (OA), is responsible for the overwhelming majority of these involvements. Rheumatoid arthritis (RA, p. 145) and gouty arthritis (p. 99) are much less common but nonetheless important. The few other conditions included here are not common but crop up in clinical practice frequently enough to merit brief consideration.

OSTEOARTHRITIS—DEGENERATIVE JOINT DISEASE

This extremely common disabling form of arthritis is one of the major challenges in medicine. Nearly everyone who lives long enough is afflicted, its cause and pathogenesis remain unknown, and there is no entirely

satisfactory method for preventing it or reversing it. Uncommon before age 40 years, the prevalence of OA in both men and women increases steeply with age, to reach about 75% at 75 years, climbing to over 90% after 80 years of age. Basically, it is characterized by slow, progressive, focal erosion and later more extensive destruction of articular cartilage, followed by subchondral sclerosis and the formation of large bony spurs or protrusions (osteophytes) at the margins of affected joints. The large weight-bearing joints—spine, knees, hips—and the small joints of the hands and feet are most often involved. The osteophytes may contribute to pain and disability, but they never fuse to cause ankylosis of the joint. When they occur at the distal interphalangeal joints, they are called "Heberden's nodes."

In the great majority of instances, OA, which is

most often monoarticular but may be oligoarticular or generalized, arises without obvious predisposing influences and so is called *primary.* Less often, affected joints have been predisposed by previous trauma, congenital deformity, some other form of bone and joint disease, or a metabolic or endocrine disorder (ochronosis, hemochromatosis, diabetes), and in these circumstances the OA is referred to as *secondary.* The variation in the particular joint or number of joints involved and the diverse clinical settings in which this condition appears have raised the possibility that OA is in fact a common end-point of a variety of disorders.

ETIOLOGY AND PATHOGENESIS. Although both remain unknown, some associations are well founded.

- The pervasiveness of OA in very elderly persons raises a number of questions: Is this condition merely a natural part of aging, as is graying of hair? Does slowing of metabolic or cellular reparative processes contribute? Is it the price humans pay for getting up off our forefeet?
- Gender influences the distribution of joint involvement. After age 55 the knees and hands are affected more commonly in women than in men of comparable age, and conversely the hips in men. There is also a tendency for the disease to appear earlier in men than in women.
- Heredity (probably autosomal dominant transmission) strongly influences the development of Heberden's nodes.
- Trauma to a joint predisposes to OA, whether it be a previous major injury with disturbance of the joint mechanics or congruence of the articular surfaces or repeated abnormal stresses (microtrauma, witness the high frequency of OA in the shoulders and elbows of baseball pitchers, ankles of ballet dancers, and knees of basketball players). Obesity plays a contributing role, perhaps because of the increased impact loading of weight-bearing joints. However, the fact that one hip or one knee may be more affected than the other (the condition is often monoarticular) argues somewhat against an important role for aging alone.

How these influences translate into the development of the anatomic changes characteristic of OA remains "a small black box." There is general agreement that an early change is an increase in the water content of the articular cartilage, suggesting some weakening of the intrinsic collagen network (type II collagen). This alteration is accompanied by a diminution in the proteoglycan concentration within the matrix as well as some shifts in the concentration of particular types of glycosaminoglycans and an increase in the levels of collagenase and proteoglycan-degrading enzymes. Accompanying these regressive changes are focal areas of proliferation of chondrocytes (cloning) with active synthesis of glycosylated macromolecules indicative of reparative efforts. At the outset the reparative activities are able to keep pace with the cartilage deterioration, but eventually the degradation dominates.

Still unknown is the key initial event. Is it repair of aging microfractures or microinjuries to subchondral bone with thickening of trabeculae and decreased resil-

iency that leads in turn to increased stress on chondrocytes and cartilage degradation? Alternatively, does the slowing of chondrocyte reparative and metabolic capabilities with aging reduce the resiliency of cartilage as the key initial event and is bone injury secondary? By either pathway it is postulated that the articular surface is damaged, a mild synovitis develops, and with it secondary mediators of inflammation come into play such as prostaglandins, IL-1, TNF-α, and transforming growth factor-β, which have the net effect of releasing lytic enzymes from chondrocytes and inhibiting matrix synthesis. Much is speculative, and indeed more than one pathway may lead to OA, perhaps explaining its near ubiquitousness (Fig. 21–12).

MORPHOLOGY. The initial changes observable in experimental models of OA are swelling of cartilage with loss of matrix proteoglycans; the first alteration to be seen in patients is fibrillation of the cartilage (i.e., cracks parallel to the articular surface). These changes reflect degradation of the collagen network that maintains the normal integrity of cartilage. At about this stage, there are focal areas of cloning of chondrocytes with increased synthesis of proteoglycans and other areas

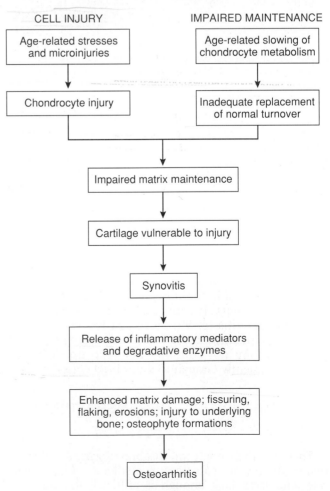

Figure 21–12. Putative pathogenic pathways of osteoarthritis.

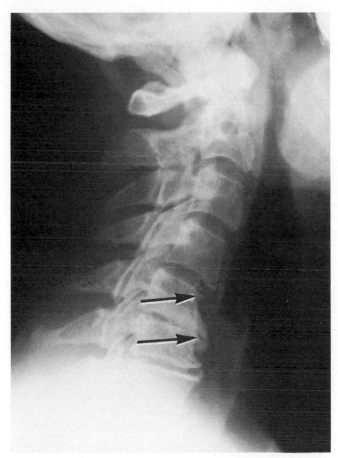

Figure 21-13. Osteoarthritis of the cervical vertebrae. Note the narrowing of the intervertebral space between C5 and C6 and the prominent osteophytes *(arrows)* on these vertebrae.

where chondrocytes are lost. The net regressive changes lead to extension of the cracks into deeper layers of the cartilage, which tend to become more vertically oriented until finally erosion or fragmentation of

cartilage appears, producing pits and surface irregularities. These changes potentiate injury to the synovium, initiating a nonspecific synovitis that is generally mild. Progressive loss of cartilage exposes the underlying bone, which becomes eburnated (thickened and polished by motion over time). The subchondral sclerosis is accompanied by thickening of the subjacent bony trabeculae, rendering the bone less elastic and less capable of absorbing impact loading. Small subchondral bone cysts may form as synovial fluid seeps through cartilage defects. As the disease advances, osteoblasts and chondroblasts at the lateral edges of the joint space form "osteophytes." These account for the so-called "lipping" seen by x-ray in the involved vertebrae overlapping the edges of the intervertebral discs and also account for the formation of Heberden's nodes (Fig. 21-13). Despite the sometimes extensive damage to the joint surfaces and the protruding osteophytes, ankylosis and fixation of joints does not occur.

CLINICAL COURSE. In its developmental stages, OA is asymptomatic. When sufficiently advanced, aching pain (at first mild), stiffness (at first transient), and decreased mobility (most prominent in the morning on arising) become evident, usually referred to a region of the spine, knee(s), or hip(s). In women, Heberden's nodes may be an early manifestation followed later by flexion and lateral deformity of the fingers. With progression, the pain on motion and disability become more marked and may be accompanied by joint crepitation with some limitation of joint mobility. Swelling of affected joints and effusion may or may not be present.

The diagnosis can be confirmed by x-ray, revealing narrowing of the joint spaces and the characteristic osteophytes. Regrettably, the only relief is symptomatic or replacement with an artificial joint. The major anatomic features that differentiate OA from rheumatoid arthritis (p. 145) are shown in Figure 21-14.

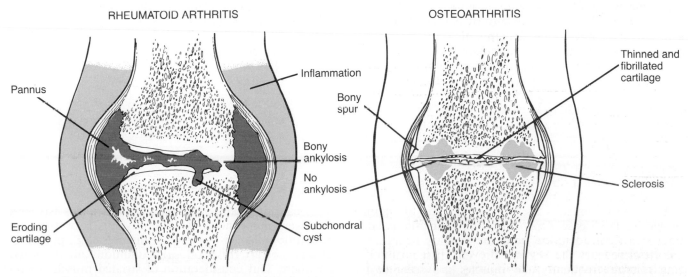

RHEUMATOID ARTHRITIS   OSTEOARTHRITIS

Pannus

Inflammation

Bony spur

Thinned and fibrillated cartilage

Bony ankylosis

No ankylosis

Eroding cartilage

Subchondral cyst

Sclerosis

Figure 21-14. Some of the more important morphologic features that differentiate osteoarthritis from rheumatoid arthritis.

SUPPURATIVE ARTHRITIS _____

This form of arthritis is characterized by pus in the joint space. It may be acute or chronic and may be caused by bacterial seeding through the hematogenous pathway, spread of a neighboring infection, a perforating injury, or intraoperative contamination.

At least 50% of cases are caused by *Staphylococcus aureus*. Another important culprit is blood-borne gonococci, capable of causing two forms of arthritis: (1) a mono- or oligoarticular suppurative arthritis from which organisms can be recovered or (2) an acute polyarticular pattern of arthritis, seemingly related to some form of hypersensitivity reaction and therefore sterile. Ultimately, any organism may cause suppurative arthritis, particularly in a vulnerable, debilitated, or immunosuppressed host.

The joints most frequently affected are the large joints—knee, hip, ankle, shoulder, and for obscure reasons, the sternoclavicular joints. The anatomic changes are, as expected with suppuration, acute inflammation of the synovial membrane and, with chronicity, ulceration of the synovia and possibly the underlying articular cartilage. Thus, chronic suppurative arthritis has the potential for joint destruction, fibrous ankylosis with calcifications, and permanent impairment of joint mobility.

LYME DISEASE _____

This relatively uncommon condition is caused by the spirochete *Borrelia burgdorferi,* which is transmitted to humans by the bite of the tick *Ixodes dammini* (or related ticks). The reservoirs for *I. dammini* are white-footed mice and white-tailed deer. The appropriate vectors are prevalent in the northeastern United States, but Lyme disease now has been reported worldwide.

Typically, the infection begins with an expanding, ringlike rash known as *erythema chronicum migrans* at the site of the bite, sometimes accompanied by fever, chills, malaise, and meningeal symptoms (stage I). This is followed weeks to months later by cardiac or neurologic involvement, often accompanied by migratory joint pain (stage II), and months to years later by oligoarthritis (stage III) and sometimes various neurologic sequelae.

Multiple joints may be involved in stage II by a nonspecific transient arthralgia, but about 50% of patients develop more significant arthritis in stage III, typically involving the knees, though both large and small joints are sometimes affected. The acute arthritis is marked by swelling and redness that reflects histologically an acute nonspecific synovitis. Infrequently, these attacks fail to clear and are followed by a chronic arthritis months to a few years later in the large joints with cartilage erosion and changes closely resembling those of rheumatoid arthritis (p. 145). In a small subset the arthritis may recur repeatedly for years. These individuals tend to have human leukocyte antigen (HLA)-DR4 or -DR2. Only rarely can the pathogen be identified in the inflammatory synovium, so the late-appearing arthritis is thought to be immune complex mediated in immunogenetically predisposed patients.

BURSITIS _____

This more painful than significant condition is well known to every weekend athlete. The bursa is a fibrous, membranous sac that develops over bony prominences (e.g., shoulder and elbow) as a consequence of the sliding motions of the overlying tendons and muscle sheaths. For obscure reasons (generally assumed to be excessive trauma) these sacs may become inflamed.

Early, the bursa is distended by a serous or mucoid fluid. With persistence of the acute inflammation or recurrent attacks, the bursal wall undergoes fibrous thickening and the space becomes filled with granular, brown, inspissated changed blood admixed with gritty, calcific precipitates. Histologically, as might be anticipated, during the acute phase the wall shows only mild edema and scattered, mostly mononuclear inflammatory cells, but in the chronic stages there is marked infiltration by lymphocytes, plasma cells, and macrophages accompanied by increased vascularization of the wall, sometimes producing hemangiomatoid aggregations of vascular channels. Basophilic calcium precipitates may be visualized in chronic calcific bursitis.

The only hazard imposed by these lesions is a tendency to double-fault in tennis and develop a bad slice in golf.

Skeletal Muscle

The skeletal muscles are not often a site of significant primary disease. Only a few nonneoplastic conditions merit consideration here; the primary neoplasms are described in the section on soft tissue tumors. Much more frequently the muscles are secondarily affected (for example, in central nervous system diseases causing death of upper motor neurons [strokes] or lower motor neurons [poliomyelitis]), or they are sometimes affected in systemic diseases (e.g., polymyositis or polyarteritis nodosa), conditions all discussed elsewhere. Our consideration of striated muscle, therefore, can be brief.

MUSCLE ATROPHY

Whenever skeletal muscles are unused, suffer from general malnutrition, are deprived of their blood supply, or are denervated, they undergo atrophy. The individual muscle fibers become smaller and assume an angulated cross-sectional appearance, particularly with denervation atrophy as the denervated fibers are compressed by adjacent innervated fibers. Despite the loss of myofilaments and other organelles, the marginal sarcolemmal nuclei persist and therefore appear to be increased in number as the fiber shrinks. In time, interstitial fibrosis develops along with volume shrinkage of the affected muscle.

The denervation atrophy caused by upper motor neuron disease, wasting, and disuse tends to affect mainly type II "fast twitch" myofibers involved in rapid contractions; these fibers, which stain darkly with ATPase at a pH of 9.4, are scattered among type I slow-twitch fibers involved in maintaining posture that preferentially stain with ATPase at a pH of 4.2. Type I and type II fibers cannot be differentiated in ordinary hematoxylin and eosin sections. In contrast in lower motor neuron disease (e.g., poliomyelitis) both types of fibers are affected.

MYOSITIS

Inflammation of muscles may be encountered in diverse clinical settings. Direct invasion by blood-borne microbes is infrequent. One specific pattern, trichinosis, is described later. Bacterial toxins such as those produced by *Botulinum perfringens* may literally proteolyze large areas of exposed muscle. The most important forms of myositis are seen in the collagen vascular diseases, e.g., polymyositis (Chapter 6) and polyarteritis nodosa described in Chapter 10.

MUSCULAR DYSTROPHY

The muscular dystrophies constitute a family of genetically determined myopathies that range in clinical severity from those that cause mild motor weakness, permitting a relatively normal life (Becker type), to those of great severity that cause progressive incapacity and early death (Duchenne's dystrophy). The latter condition, the most common and devastating of the dystrophies, is now known to be caused by a mutation of a gene located on the short arm of the X chromosome. Most patients are sons of carrier mothers, but some acquire mutations de novo, and rarely females with unfortunate lyonization of the normal X chromosome are affected. The normal gene at this locus synthesizes a protein named "dystrophin" that is present in small quantities in muscle. Dystrophin has considerable homology with a cytoskeletal α-actinin, and like α-actinin is membrane associated. A mutation of this gene in Duchenne's dystrophy lowers the level of dystrophin, leading to some perturbation in cell contraction and progressive muscle weakness.

MORPHOLOGY. The involvement is most marked in the muscles around the shoulder girdles, pelvis, and then progressively those of the extremities. Affected muscles show vacuolation, fragmentation, and coagulation necrosis of individual myofibers, followed by invasion by phagocytic macrophages. Some of the injured muscle fibers undergo a brisk regenerative response rendered distinctive by cytoplasmic basophilia and enlargement and internalization of sarcolemmal nuclei. Other fibers are totally removed and replaced by fibrofatty tissue, while unaffected fibers become hypertrophic, the two changes more than compensating for the muscle loss and accounting for pseudohypertrophy, particularly in calf muscles. In the late stages, as more myofibers degenerate, affected muscles shrink and become pale and flabby as they are virtually replaced by fibrofatty tissue (Fig. 21–15).

CLINICAL COURSE. In Duchenne's dystrophy signs appear in early childhood in the form of difficulty in standing, walking, and getting out of a chair. The muscle weakness is progressive, most evident in the lower extremities, but eventually the upper extremities

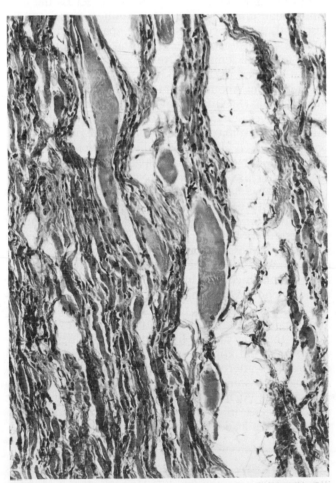

Figure 21–15. Advanced muscular dystrophy with marked atrophy of most of the myofibers. Only a few identifiable muscle cells remain. Note the fatty replacement.

may also be affected. Despite the motor weakness, there is often prominence of the calf muscles owing to pseudohypertrophy. Involvement of trunk muscles leads to progressive spinal curvature sometimes encroaching on respiratory function. By age 12 years most patients are confined to a wheelchair, and death usually occurs by age 20, precipitated most often by pulmonary infections related to weakness of the muscles of respiration and difficulties in swallowing with aspiration of food. In addition, degenerative changes in the myocardial cells may lead to cardiac failure, and the deficiency of dystrophin may also affect the membrane cytoskeleton of neuronal cells, accounting for the intellectual impairment often manifested by these patients.

The diagnosis can be suspected by the distinctive clinical features, markedly elevated serum muscle enzymes, particularly creatine kinase, and by electromyography, and can be confirmed by biopsy.

MYASTHENIA GRAVIS _____

In this autoimmune disease, antibodies are produced to the acetylcholine receptors (AChR) of the muscle endplate of the neuromuscular junction that impair transmission of the acetylcholine signal across the neuromuscular junction. They thus induce muscle weakness and pronounced fatigability, particularly of the muscles in most active use. The peak age of onset is 20 years; affected females outnumber males 3:1, but a second smaller peak, predominantly male, occurs in late adult life. About two thirds of patients with myasthenia gravis (MG) have thymic hyperplasia, about 15 to 20% have a thymoma, and the remainder have no thymic abnormality. In addition, some patients have other associated autoimmune diseases such as systemic lupus erythematosus (SLE), Sjögren's syndrome, rheumatoid arthritis, and hyperthyroidism.

PATHOGENESIS. Although circulating autoantibodies to AChR are demonstrable in nearly 90% of patients with MG, they may be absent in those with milder manifestations of the disorder. These antibodies lead to muscle weakness by one of several mechanisms, including increased degradation of cross-linked receptors, complement-mediated lysis of receptors, and inhibition of acetylcholine binding (Fig. 21–16). What initiates this abnormal humoral response and what role thymic abnormalities play remain unclear; however, it is known that the thymic hyperplasia is frequently associated with the appearance on some thymic epithelial cells and scattered myoid cells of AChR epitopes. Analogously, some neoplastic epithelial cells in thymomas express AChR. It is assumed without proof that these antigens in some way sensitize helper T cells, which in turn lead to the autoantibody production.

MORPHOLOGY. Despite the profound motor disability, there are surprisingly few histologic changes. Only immunocytochemical or immunofluorescent stains disclose

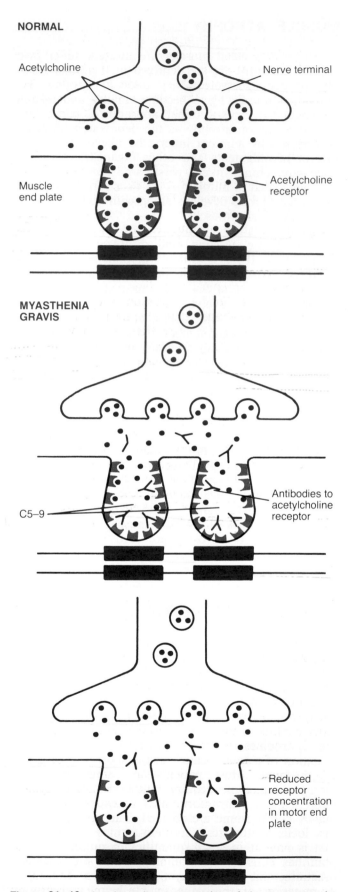

Figure 21–16. A schematic representation of the neuromuscular junction in myasthenia gravis shows cross-linking of acetylcholine receptors by specific antibodies and complement activation.

complement and IgG in the neuromuscular junctions, and electron microscopy reveals simplification along with a dramatic reduction in the number of AChRs in affected muscles. The loss of these receptors impairs reception of the neural acetylcholine signal, leading to the muscle weakness and fatigability.

There is wide variation in the clinical course of patients with early-onset MG. The presence of a thymoma and high titers of circulating AChR antibodies are unfavorable portents. The weakness and fatigability first become manifest in the muscles in most active use (e.g., the extraocular muscles and those in the face, tongue, and extremities). Although the condition pursues a somewhat unpredictable course, in severely affected patients there is progressive involvement of other muscle groups, including those required for speech and swallowing. Eventually trunk and limb muscles become involved, inducing motor incapacity. A major threat to life is respiratory compromise and increased vulnerability to pulmonary infections. However, as indicated, there are milder expressions of the disease, manifested possibly only by mildly increased fatigability of the extraocular muscles and those of the face.

The natural course of this condition, however severe or mild, is improved by thymectomy, in cases of hyperplasia, or by removal of a thymic tumor. In addition, a variety of drugs, such as anticholine esterases or immunosuppressive agents, have been beneficial. Overall there is about a 10% ten-year mortality rate, representing those with severe generalized disease. Children born of affected mothers often have transient myasthenic syndromes.

TRICHINOSIS

Worldwide in distribution, trichinosis is caused by ingestion of inadequately cooked meat containing viable cysts of *Trichinella spiralis*. Smoked meats also constitute a potential hazard. Although several carnivores and omnivores may harbor trichinae, for humans the major vector is pork. The disease has become uncommon in the United States because of stringent regulations on commercially produced pork and pork products (e.g., sterilization of garbage to be fed to pigs and deep freezing of pork).

Animals ingest adult worms with contaminated food. These produce larvae that preferentially localize within striated muscles and encyst within a myofiber. On ingestion of contaminated meat by humans, the cyst wall is digested, and the parasites attach to the small intestinal wall, mature, and copulate, after which the female releases larvae that penetrate into the intestinal lacteals, thus gaining entrance to the circulation. Although the larvae may be trapped in the lungs to produce an interstitial eosinophilic pneumonitis and similarly may be trapped in the central nervous system (CNS) to cause meningitis and gliosis about small

capillaries, the most important localization is within skeletal muscles, where the larvae penetrate a muscle cell, become encysted, and in this manner may survive in a dormant state for years without producing a significant host response (Fig. 21–17). Death of the larva and its "nurse cell" incites a mononuclear inflammatory reaction, followed in time by calcification of the larva. The most intense parasitization is found in the most active muscles of the body, which have the richest blood supply—the diaphragm, extraocular muscles, intercostal muscles, and those of the extremities. The myofibers of the heart may also be parasitized, evoking interstitial myocarditis, but the larvae do not become encysted since they undergo necrosis.

During the period of invasion of the intestinal mucosa, vomiting, diarrhea, and features suggestive of "food intoxication" may appear. Dissemination to the skeletal muscles is marked by widespread muscle aches and pains and fever, often with periorbital and facial edema. Extensive seeding of the lungs by trapped larvae along with involvement of the respiratory muscles may induce respiratory manifestations. Involvement of the brain may cause headaches, disorientation, and, indeed, symptoms suggestive of encephalitis. With myocardial involvement cardiac failure may ensue.

Although the diagnosis can be suspected on the basis

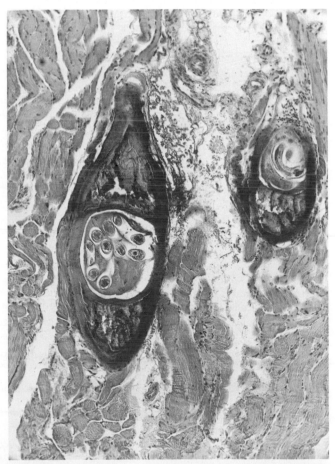

Figure 21–17. Trichinosis with encysted larvae in two of the skeletal muscle fibers.

of the clinical features along with eosinophilia, confirmatory tests are necessary, including serologic evidence of the infection, skin sensitization, and ultimately muscle biopsy and histologic examination. Although the mortality rate is usually low, severe parasitemia can be fatal.

Soft Tissue Tumors

By convention, soft tissue tumors (STTs) are a collection of neoplasms that arise in fat, fibrous tissue, skeletal muscle, smooth muscle, and the neurovascular elements that support these components, excluding those that arise in the supportive structures of parenchymal origin. STTs are grouped together because they often present in similar fashion, tend to appear in the same locations, and are difficult to differentiate from each other on clinical grounds, by imaging techniques, and indeed often on histologic examination. Although they may occur anywhere in the body, about 40% arise in the soft tissues of the lower extremities, 20% in the upper extremities, 10% in the head and neck region, and 30% in the trunk and retroperitoneum. The benign forms far outnumber the malignant, and indeed soft tissue sarcomas are relatively uncommon, accounting for slightly fewer than 2% of all forms of cancer. Although the sarcomas may occur in childhood, about 75% appear in adult life. The present consideration of STTs is restricted largely to general comments about these neoplasms as a group; only selected details about some of the more common ones are offered.

CLASSIFICATION. STTs, like most other tumors, are classified on the basis of their histogenesis (i.e., presumed cell of origin), although admittedly in some instances, such as the fibrous histiocytoma and synovial sarcoma, the histogenesis remains uncertain. The more common types of these neoplasms are presented in Table 21–2, excluding those of neural and vascular origin, which are considered in other chapters. A few tumor-like conditions are also included, because they

TABLE 21–2. COMMON SOFT TISSUE TUMORS AND TUMOR-LIKE LESIONS

Designation	Common Locations	Comments
Benign		
Lipoma	Subcutaneously on back, shoulders, abdomen, or proximal extremities; intestinal tract	Mostly in adults
Fibroma	Ovary, along nerve trunks (neurofibroma)	Fibromatoses more common (see below)
Fibrous histiocytoma	Skin (dermatofibroma, fibroxanthoma, sclerosing hemangioma)	
Rhabdomyoma	Head and neck region; heart; vagina; vulva	Less frequent than rhabdomyosarcomas; ?hamartomatous
Leiomyoma	Uterus, gastrointestinal tract, subcutaneously from blood vessel walls	Uterine are most common tumor in females
Granular cell tumor	Tongue, subcutaneously in trunk and upper extremities	
Malignant		
Liposarcoma	Retroperitoneum, lower extremities; less often inguinal canal, mediastinum, omentum, chest wall	Less common than lipomas
Fibrosarcoma	Thigh, knee, trunk, forearms, wherever fibrous tissue is found	Tend to involve deeper structures rather than subcutaneous fibrous tissue
Malignant fibrous histiocytoma	Skeletal muscle of extremities, retroperitoneum, subcutaneous tissue, elsewhere	Most common soft tissue sarcoma in adults
Rhabdomyosarcoma	Head and neck region, genitourinary tract, retroperitoneum, extremities	Most common soft tissue sarcoma of children and adolescents; rare after age 45
Leiomyosarcoma	Uterus, gastrointestinal tract, abdomen, retroperitoneum, blood vessel walls	Principally in adults; rare in children; even extrauterine more common in women
Synovial sarcoma	About but not within joint cavities, parapharyngeal region, mediastinum, abdominal wall	No benign counterpart
Tumor-like lesions		
Superficial fibromatoses	Palms (Dupuytren's contracture), soles of feet, penis (Peyronie's disease)	Collagenous strictures
Deep fibromatoses (desmoids)	Anterior abdominal wall in women; musculature of shoulder, chest wall, back, and thigh; abdomen in both sexes	Lie in the interface between nonneoplastic proliferation and fibrosarcoma
Nodular (pseudosarcomatous) fasciitis	Subcutaneously in upper extremities of adults, trunk, back, elsewhere; in infants, head and neck	Commonly mistaken clinically for a neoplasm

often present as tumorous masses that must be differentiated both clinically and pathologically.

STAGING AND GRADING. The staging and grading of an STT, along with its location and therefore resectability, are major determinants of its prognosis. Most critical of course is whether it is benign or malignant, but, as was pointed out earlier, sometimes this judgment is difficult. For example, there are cellular leiomyomas that look and behave more aggressively than the usual leiomyoma; thus the desirability of grading even benign tumors. But the major importance of staging and grading relates to sarcomas. Many factors are involved:

- *Histogenesis of the tumor.* Synovial sarcoma, for example, has a bleak outlook. Fewer than 20% of patients survive ten years, despite current modes of therapy. In contrast, childhood rhabdomyosarcoma, even when advanced at time of diagnosis, permits survival in 75% of cases with appropriate therapy.
- *Tumor size.* In general, the smaller the primary neoplasm, the better the outlook, with less likelihood of metastasis or anatomic extension beyond the limits of resectability.
- *Grading.* Elaborate proposals have been made to semiquantitate the apparent aggressiveness of neoplasms based on the level of differentiation of the tumor cells. Built into these various estimates are the number of mitoses per high-power field (hpf), cell and nuclear size, pleomorphism, level of hyperchromasia, amount of necrosis within the tumor (as a reflection of rate of growth), and cellularity relative to connective matrix. Generally considered to be more significant are the number of mitoses per hpf and the level of pleomorphism. Based on these variables, neoplasms have been graded I to IV (least to most aggressive) or more simply as low grade to high grade.
- *Staging.* The assigned stage of an STT expresses an estimate of the size and extent of the neoplasm, based at first on clinical and imaging parameters and later possibly on histologic examination. Most important is the presence or absence of nodal involvement and more distant metastasis. Particularly important with an STT is tumor size, which bears on the issue of whether the lesion has remained confined to its anatomic compartment (defined by natural barriers such as fascia, bone, tendon) or has penetrated these natural barriers. The intracompartmental neoplasm is obviously much more amenable to complete surgical excision.

Several systems for incorporating these variables have been proposed. Perhaps the simplest is the following one:

Stage I
Histologically low-grade, well-differentiated, few mitoses.
A. Intracompartmental
B. Extracompartmental
Stage II
Histologically high-grade, frequent mitoses, nuclear atypia, areas of necrosis, high cell-matrix ratio.

A. Intracompartmental
B. Extracompartmental
Stage III
Metastases to regional nodes or remote sites (lymphatic, pulmonary, visceral, or osseous).

COMMENTS ON SELECTED TUMORS ⸻

Lipomas and *liposarcomas* are dissimilar in more ways than levels of aggressiveness. The lipoma is the most common of the soft tissue tumors; the liposarcoma on the other hand is uncommon. A lipoma is a delicately encapsulated mass of adult fat that grossly and histologically looks like nonneoplastic fat. Occasionally they contain admixtures of fibrous tissue (fibrolipoma) or proliferating blood vessels (angiolipoma) or bone marrow elements (myelolipoma). The last variant is most often encountered in the adrenal glands. Liposarcomas, on the other hand, are usually encapsulated, more often small than large, invasive, pale gray neoplasms that have the "fish-flesh" appearance of most sarcomas. In one variant, the well-differentiated liposarcoma, there may be vestiges of yellowish fatty areas that correspond to well-defined, large, fatty vacuoles within the neoplastic cells. But other variants of liposarcoma have only scant traces of their lipoblastic origins and are composed of immature mesenchymal cells, sometimes dispersed in a myxoid background.

Fibromas are much less common than *fibrosarcomas*. Many lesions heretofore called fibromas have been reclassified as fibromatoses. Fibromas of the ovary, the prime site for these rarities, are described on page 627. Fibrosarcomas also constitute infiltrative "fish-flesh" masses, but rarely they may appear deceptively encapsulated. The latter pattern often discloses well-differentiated fibroblastic cells bordering on a cellular fibroma. However, all fibrosarcomas have some level of anaplasia, with few or many mitoses, but sometimes the lack of differentiation renders identification of the nature of the lesion difficult or impossible. Immunocytochemical features such as the identification of vimentin by monoclonal antibodies are by no means specific to these tumors, but they may help to exclude some look-alikes.

The *benign and malignant fibrous histiocytomas* are both composed of a mixture of cells that resemble fibroblasts and histiocytes, with many hybrid forms. Additional features include scattered, lipid-laden xanthomatous cells and occasional multinucleate giant cells. The benign tumors, predominantly in the skin, may contain sufficient lipid to justify the designation fibroxanthoma or xanthohistiocytoma. The malignant fibrous histiocytoma (MFH) is the most common of the soft tissue sarcomas. These usually appear as unencapsulated but circumscribed, gray-white, fleshy lesions that have been divided into many histologic variants, which are well beyond our scope. It suffices to say that all have the basic cell types described and reveal some level of pleomorphism, anaplasia, and mitotic activity.

In the more typical tumors, the spindled fibroblasts may be arrayed in a radial cartwheel (storiform) pattern, often about slit-like vessels (Fig. 21–18). Characteristic of all MFHs is an abundant vascular background, sometimes disposed in a so-called chicken wire pattern. Immunocytochemical reactions characteristic of histiocytes (e.g., lysozyme, α_1-antichymotrypsin) are often helpful in differentiating MFH from other sarcomas.

Rhabdomyosarcomas are the most common soft tissue sarcoma in children; they are relatively uncommon in adults but surprisingly are still more frequent than *rhabdomyomas*. The benign lesions that occur in the heart are probably not true neoplasms (see p. 331). Extracardiac rhabdomyomas are too rare to merit further consideration. Rhabdomyosarcomas in most locations are nondescript, gray, sometimes myxoid, infiltrative masses indistinguishable from other sarcomas. Sometimes they occur in the vagina or vulva, and then they may appear as protruding, grape-like clusters of lobules directly beneath or penetrating the mucosa of the underlying organ *(sarcoma botryoides)*. There is a wide range in the histologic appearance of these

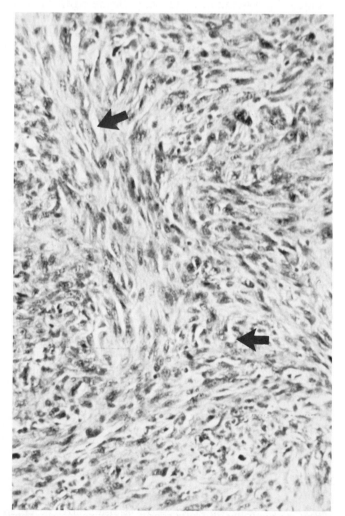

Figure 21–18. Malignant fibrous histiocytoma. The plump spindle cells are arrayed in swirling fascicles. There are numerous, barely visible vascular channels *(arrows)* and occasional giant cells.

tumors. At one end of the spectrum are recognizable, ribbon-like skeletal muscle cells complete with transverse striations; at the other end are the highly pleomorphic lesions that present exceedingly few recognizable rhabdomyoblasts. Indeed, so-called embryonal rhabdomyosarcomas are made up of small, dark, undifferentiated tumor cells that may be exceedingly difficult to distinguish from other so-called round cell neoplasms. The use of monoclonal antibodies for desmin and muscle actins as well as molecular probes are frequently of much help in identifying these neoplasms.

Leiomyomas and *leiomyosarcomas* at the extreme ends of the spectrum may be very different, but in the middle is a gray zone where the line between benign and malignant is ill defined. The classic benign leiomyoma is described on page 618 as being made up of inactive-looking, spindled, smooth muscle elements. There are, however, some circumscribed, seemingly benign tumors made up of plump smooth muscle cells with some variation in cell and nuclear size, sometimes referred to as cellular leiomyomas or leiomyoblastomas. The appearance of these tumors is close to that of a well-differentiated leiomyosarcoma, which may also be deceptively discrete. On the other hand, the more anaplastic variants, difficult to differentiate from fibrosarcomas, are infiltrative, gray-white, and fleshy. As with all sarcomas, with increasing anaplasia there is greater pleomorphism, hyperchromasia, and more frequent mitoses (Fig. 21–19). Immunoreactions for desmin and electron microscopic features (bundles of thin cytofilaments) may help to identify the leiomyosarcoma.

The *synovial sarcoma,* despite its designation, does not arise from synoviocytes; rather it derives from mesenchymal cells about joint cavities, and indeed in sites totally removed from joints. They range from the quite small, deceptively circumscribed, to the characteristic infiltrative sarcomatous masses. Histologically, however, they can be distinctive by virtue of a biphasic pattern that has an epithelial component forming glands, microcystic spaces, or nests of cells interspersed in a spindle-cell pattern replicating fibroblast-like sheets. Less commonly, the synovial sarcoma may be monophasic and composed entirely of epithelioid elements that resemble a carcinoma or, alternatively, spindle cells that are difficult to distinguish from other sarcomas. Immunocytochemical reactions for keratin, epithelial membrane antigen, and vimentin, in combination, may be helpful but more definitive is the (X;18) (p11.2;q11.2) chromosomal translocation.

Nodular (pseudosarcomatous) fasciitis is a reactive lesion that is commonly mistaken for a neoplasm because of its aggressive-looking histologic appearance. These lesions tend to appear as discrete, unencapsulated masses, rarely larger than 2 cm in diameter, usually subcutaneous but sometimes attached to or within skeletal muscle. *They begin as basically myxoid lesions that become progressively cellular and ultimately fibrosed.* During the stage of peak cellularity, they are composed of plump spindled cells of varying size and shape, some having large, seemingly "anaplastic" nuclei arrayed in broad interlacing ribbons creat-

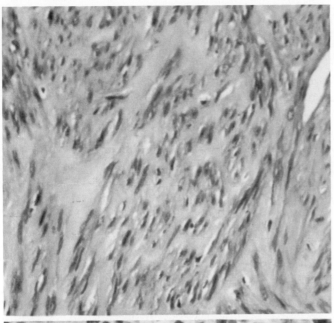

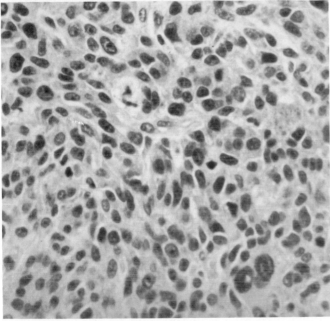

Figure 21–19. A comparison between a leiomyoma *(above)* composed of inactive spindled smooth muscle cells and a cellular pleomorphic leiomyosarcoma *(below).*

ing a vaguely spoke-wheel pattern. Intermixed are mononuclear inflammatory cells, lipid-laden histiocytes, and occasionally benign-looking giant cells. As the lesions mature, the centers become fibrosed. Because of the "florid" histologic pattern and the infiltrative nature of the periphery of the lesion it is understandable that they are readily overdiagnosed as sarcomas, hence the descriptor "pseudosarcomatous." Recurrence following even incomplete excision almost never occurs.

Desmoid tumors are better called aggressive fibro-matoses. These fibroblastic proliferations have been referred to as fibrosarcomas grade one-half. They tend to occur in the second to fourth decades of life in one

of three locations: (1) in the musculature of the abdominal wall, particularly in women during or following pregnancy, (2) in the musculature of the shoulder, chest wall, back, or thigh in men or women, and (3) rarely within the abdomen in patients who have Gardner's syndrome (p. 513). They present as large, infiltrative masses of mature fibroblasts, often embedded within abundant collagen, with only moderate variation in cell and nuclear size and shape. Anaplasia and pleomorphisms are generally absent, but trapped muscle cells may appear as multinucleate giant cells. Because of their tendency to infiltrate surrounding structures, they are readily mistaken for low-grade fibrosarcomas, but they do not metastasize. However, they stubbornly recur after incomplete excision.

Benign STTs and lesions usually can be differentiated on the basis of location and histology. The differential problem is far more difficult with the more anaplastic sarcomas, since recognizable cytologic features may be lost and one type of anarchic cell looks much like another. Sometimes the only diagnosis that can be rendered is undifferentiated anaplastic sarcoma. However, here is where special procedures for the identification of characteristic markers are sometimes very helpful—the use of monoclonal antibodies in immunochemical reactions to identify specific constituents, ultrastructural examination for cytofilaments and other details, and if possible karyotype analysis for distinctive alterations such as the translocation (X;18) (p11.2;q11.2) in synovial sarcoma. But ultimately, the appropriate categorization of an STT is in part art as well as science.

BIBLIOGRAPHY

Agamanolis, D. P., et al.: Tumors of skeletal muscle. Hum. Pathol. 17:778, 1986. (A detailed authoritative review of the morphology of rhabdomyosarcomas, rhabdomyomas, and desmoid fibromatoses arising within skeletal muscle.)

Arnaud, C. D., Sanchez, S. D.: The role of calcium in osteoporosis. Ann. Rev. Nutr. 10:397, 1990. (A lucid discussion of the important role of an adequate calcium intake in preventing the development of osteoporosis.)

Cole, W. G., et al.: New insights into the molecular pathology of osteogenesis imperfecta. Quart. J. Med. 70:1, 1989. (A brief review of the remarkable molecular insights that have been gained into the origins of this condition.)

Conrad, E. U. III, Enneking, W. F.: Common soft tissue tumors. Clin. Symp. 42:2, 1990. (A simplified presentation of the general nature of soft tissue tumors and capsule descriptions of some; not complete.)

Drachman, D. B., et al.: Humoral pathogenesis of myasthenia gravis. Ann. N.Y. Acad. Sci. 505:90, 1987. (A presentation of the new understanding of the origins of myasthenia gravis.)

Eckardt, J. J., Grogan, T. J.: Giant cell tumor of bone. Clin. Orthop. 204:45, 1986. (An excellent clinicopathologic analysis of this unpredictable neoplasm.)

Eisman, J. A.: Osteomalacia. Bailliere's Clin. Endocrinol. Metab. 2:125, 1988. (Good coverage of the various origins of rickets and osteomalacia.)

Enneking, W. F., Conrad, E. U. III: Common bone tumors. Clin. Symp. 41:3, 1989. (A very well-illustrated general overview high lighting the major pathologic and clinical features.)

Fallon, M. D., Schwamm, H. A.: Paget's disease of bone. An update on the pathogenesis, pathophysiology, and treatment of osteitis deformans. Pathol. Annu. 24(part 1):115, 1989. (An extremely thorough, lucid presentation.)

Finn, H. A., Simon, M. A.: Staging systems for musculoskeletal neoplasms. Orthopedics *12:*1365, 1989. (A presentation of the major systems of staging soft tissue tumors.)

Greenspan, A.: Tumors of cartilage origin. Orthop. Clin. North Am. *20:*347, 1989. (Extensive review of both benign and malignant cartilaginous tumors—good for morphologic details.)

Hamerman, D.: The biology of osteoarthritis. N. Engl. J. Med. *320:*1322, 1989. (A detailed analysis of the many mechanisms that may be involved in the pathogenesis of osteoarthritis.)

Klein, M. J., et al.: Osteosarcoma. Clinical and pathological considerations. Orthop. Clin. North Am. *20:*327, 1989. (Good detail on the many anatomic variants of these neoplasms along with the surgical, but not other, treatment options.)

Kunkel, L. M., Hoffman, E. P.: Duchenne/Becker muscular dystrophy: A short overview of the gene, the protein, and current diagnostics. Br. Med. Bull. *45:*630, 1989. (A brief overview of the exciting advances that have been made in the genetics and pathogenesis of this disorder.)

Merkow, R. L., Lane, J. M.: Paget's disease of bone. Orthop. Clin. North Am. *21:*171, 1990. (A good comprehensive overview covering pathogenesis, pathology, and clinical aspects.)

Miettinen, M.: Immunohistochemistry of soft-tissue tumors. Possibilities and limitations in surgical pathology. Pathol. Annu. *25*(part 1):1, 1990. (A comprehensive survey of the usefulness and limitations of cellular markers in the differential diagnosis of these neoplasms.)

Parisien, M., et al.: Bone disease in primary hyperparathyroidism. Endocrinol. Metab. Clin. North Am. *1:*19, 1990. (A brief but complete overview of the complex features of this condition.)

Pritchard, D. J.: Small round cell tumors. Orthop. Clin. North Am. *20:*367, 1989. (A concise overview of Ewing's sarcoma with brief considerations of morphologically similar lesions.)

Raisz, L. G.: Local and systemic factors in the pathogenesis of osteoporosis. N. Engl. J. Med. *318:*818, 1988. (A succinct survey of the many factors possibly involved in the causation of osteoporosis.)

Schajowicz, F., McGuire, M. H.: Diagnostic difficulties in skeletal pathology. Clin. Orthop. *240:*281, 1989. (Broad anatomic coverage of benign and malignant bone-forming, cartilage-forming, and Ewing's tumors of bone.)

Sherrard, D. J.: Renal osteodystrophy. Semin. Nephrol. *6:*56, 1986. (A detailed analysis of the pathogenesis of this condition.)

Witkin, G. B., et al.: A biphasic tumor of the mediastinum with features of synovial sarcoma. A report of four cases. Am. J. Surg. Pathol. *13:*490, 1989. (An excellent overview of the morphologic features of these neoplasms.)

TWENTY-TWO

The Nervous System

JAMES H. MORRIS, D. Phil., M.B.B.C.H.

BASIC REACTIONS OF NEURONS AND
GLIAL CELLS
    Neurons
    Astrocytes
    Oligodendrocytes
    Ependymal Cells
    Microglia
COMMON PATHOPHYSIOLOGIC
COMPLICATIONS
    Increased Intracranial Pressure and Cerebral
      Herniation
    Cerebral Edema
    Hydrocephalus
INFECTIONS
    Meningitis
      Acute (Purulent) Meningitis
      Acute Lymphocytic (Viral) Meningitis
      Chronic Meningitis
    Encephalitis
      Cerebral Abscess
    Viral Encephalitis
      Acute Viral Encephalitis
      Slow Virus Diseases
      Unconventional Agent (Spongiform)
        Encephalopathies
    Other Infections
VASCULAR DISEASE
    Ischemic (Hypoxic) Encephalopathy
    Cerebral Infarction
    Intracranial Hemorrhage
      Intraparenchymal Hemorrhage
      Subarachnoid Hemorrhage
      Mixed Intraparenchymal and Subarachnoid
        Hemorrhage (Vascular Malformations)
TRAUMA
    Epidural Hematoma
    Subdural Hematoma
    Parenchymal Injuries

TUMORS
    Primary Intracranial Tumors
      Astrocytoma
      Oligodendroglioma
      Ependymoma
      Medulloblastoma
      Meningioma
    Metastatic Tumors
DEGENERATIVE DISEASES
    Alzheimer's Disease
    Huntington's Disease
    Parkinsonism
      Idiopathic Parkinson's Disease (Paralysis
        Agitans)
    Motor Neuron Disease (Amyotrophic Lateral
      Sclerosis Complex)
DEMYELINATING DISEASES
    Multiple Sclerosis
NUTRITIONAL, ENVIRONMENTAL, AND
METABOLIC DISORDERS
    Nutritional Diseases
      Thiamine Deficiency
      Cobalamin Deficiency
    Environmental Diseases
    Metabolic Encephalopathy
      Hepatic Encephalopathy
INBORN ERRORS OF METABOLISM
    Leukodystrophies
THE PERIPHERAL NERVOUS SYSTEM
    Peripheral Neuropathy
      Acute Idiopathic Polyneuropathy (Landry-
        Guillain-Barré Syndrome)
      Diabetic Neuropathy
    Peripheral Nerve Tumors
      Schwannomas (Neurilemmomas) and
        Neurofibromas

The brain has a number of unique physiologic and anatomic features that markedly influence the expression of disease in the nervous system. The most important of these are as follows:

1. *Function is localized within the nervous system.* This is the most important difference between the brain and other organs, and it has a number of pathologic consequences.
   a. *The nervous system is inherently vulnerable to small focal lesions* that can produce selective deficits in specific functions, for example, speech. This is quite different from other organs such as the liver or the lung, where a large fraction of the organ can be destroyed without compromising any particular function.
   b. A given type of focal lesion (e.g., a tumor) produces quite different clinical syndromes in different parts of the nervous system.
   c. Pathologically, since the brain has only a limited repertoire of responses, one type of pathologic change (e.g., neurofibrillary tangle formation) may occur in more than one disease. In this circumstance *diagnosis often rests on the localization (distribution) of the pathologic change in the nervous system.*
2. *The brain has a number of unique anatomic features that confer protection against one form of pathologic assault while rendering it more vulnerable to another.* For example, the skull protects against trauma but makes possible the development of increased intracranial pressure. Similarly, the cerebrospinal fluid (CSF) cushions the brain against trauma but is the medium for the development of hydrocephalus and the dissemination of microorganisms and tumors.
3. Although most diseases of the brain have their counterparts in other organs, some disease categories, notably, neuronal degenerations and diseases of myelin, are unique to neuropathology.

BASIC REACTIONS OF NEURONS AND GLIAL CELLS

The brain parenchyma is composed of neurons embedded in a specialized supporting framework of glial cells—astrocytes, oligodendrocytes, and ependyma cells—and the so-called microglia. The feltwork of the cytoplasmic processes of all these cells (neurons and glia) is known as the neuropil.

NEURONS

Pathologically, neurons undergo a variety of more or less specific types of degenerative change, such as neurofibrillary tangle formation and Lewy body formation. These are described with the respective diseases.

ASTROCYTES

In damaged brain, astrocytes produce a dense feltwork of cellular processes that form a glial "scar." An important difference between gliosis and the fibrosis that occurs in other organs is that astrocytes do not produce collagen or an equivalent extracellular protein, and glial scars are composed entirely of cellular processes.

In response to gross tissue damage, *reactive (gemistocytic) astrocytes* develop which have conspicuous eosinophilic cytoplasm with the nucleus often being displaced to one side of the cell. With resolution of the pathologic process, the astrocyte cytoplasm becomes less conspicuous, yielding so-called *fibrillary astrocytes*. *Rosenthal fibers* are elongated, densely eosinophilic structures that form in astrocytic processes. They are found chiefly in slow-growing pilocytic astrocytomas and around chronic irritative lesions such as cavernous angiomas that have bled multiple times.

OLIGODENDROCYTES

Oligodendrocytes are the central nervous system (CNS) equivalents of Schwann cells and produce CNS myelin. Their principal involvement in disease is in the demyelinating diseases and the leukodystrophies.

EPENDYMAL CELLS

Ependymal cells line the cerebral ventricles. Focal destruction of ependymal cells is followed by compensatory proliferation of astrocytes and the production of ependymal granulations. Ependymal cells may be the target of infectious agents, notably cytomegalovirus (CMV).

MICROGLIA

Notwithstanding their name, microglia are not of neural origin but are the CNS representatives of the monocyte-macrophage system. When stimulated by cerebral damage their nuclei enlarge and elongate (*rod cells*), and with more severe damage they may become actively phagocytic and form foamy macrophages (*gitter cells*), although most such cells are derived from the blood.

COMMON PATHOPHYSIOLOGIC COMPLICATIONS

Increased intracranial pressure, cerebral herniation, cerebral edema, and hydrocephalus are pathophysiologic complications that occur in many different diseases. They are also interrelated in that both cerebral edema and hydrocephalus are among the causes of increased intracranial pressure and may also produce cerebral herniation. All these complications occur because the brain is confined within a rigid skull that, while it protects against trauma, by its nature also restricts expansion of the intracranial contents.

INCREASED INTRACRANIAL PRESSURE AND CEREBRAL HERNIATION ___

Although small expansions of the intracranial contents can be accommodated by shifts of CSF and reduction in venous volume, further increases produce raised intracranial CSF pressure. With small increases, cerebral blood flow is maintained by compensatory elevation in arterial blood pressure, but persistent intracranial pressures above 20 mm Hg result in a drop in cerebral perfusion pressure and blood flow and lead to cerebral ischemia.

Focal space-occupying lesions such as tumors, hemorrhages, and abscesses are obvious causes of increased intracranial pressure, as are more diffuse processes such as edema, hydrocephalus, and meningitis.

Cerebral herniation is an ominous complication that occurs when focal tissue expansion displaces brain from its normal intracranial location. There are three major types (Fig. 22–1):

1. *Subfalcine (cingulate) herniation* of the cingulate gyrus underneath the falx cerebri.

2. *Uncinate (uncal, transtentorial) herniation,* in which the uncus of the temporal lobe is displaced mediad and downward through the incisura of the tentorium cerebelli. This displacement also stretches the oculomotor (third cranial) nerve and produces pupillary dilatation on the same side as the lesion.

3. *Tonsillar herniation* is displacement of the cerebellar tonsils through the foramen magnum. This compresses the medulla and its respiratory center, which if not promptly relieved causes respiratory irregularity, and eventually apnea and death.

A further consequence of swelling of the cerebral hemispheres is downward displacement of the brainstem in uncinate herniation that may rupture blood vessels in the mesencephalon and produce Duret hemorrhages.

CEREBRAL EDEMA ___

Because the brain is sensitive to small volume changes, it is severely affected by cerebral edema, which exacerbates both the local effects of lesions and any increase in intracranial pressure. Its effects are enhanced by the absence of cerebral lymphatics to remove accumulated edema fluid. There are two major types of cerebral edema.

Vasogenic edema is the accumulation of extracellular fluid, principally in white matter. It results from bulk fluid leakage across damaged or incompetent cerebral capillaries and may be general or focal. Typically, it is most apparent around mass lesions that are necrotic or that exhibit marked capillary proliferation (metastatic implants and abscesses), since newly formed capillaries do not have a properly functioning blood-brain barrier.

Cytotoxic edema is an intracellular accumulation of excess fluid. It affects gray matter more than white and results from processes such as ischemia or toxic exposure that impair the function of the cell membrane or ion pump and allow uncontrolled ingress of water or other molecules into the cell.

Although they are described separately both types of edema often occur together, for example, in an infarct that damages both cells and capillary function.

HYDROCEPHALUS ___

Hydrocephalus is the term for a marked increase in the volume of CSF with expansion of the cerebral ventricles. It is a result of obstruction of CSF flow and the consequent rise in CSF pressure proximal to the obstruction. The hydrocephalus is called *noncommunicating* when the obstruction is within the ventricular system. If the obstruction is in the subarachnoid space or is caused by damage to the arachnoid villi the result is *communicating hydrocephalus.*

In infants and children, before fusion of the cranial sutures, hydrocephalus produces enlargement of the head; in adults the principal effect is increased intra-

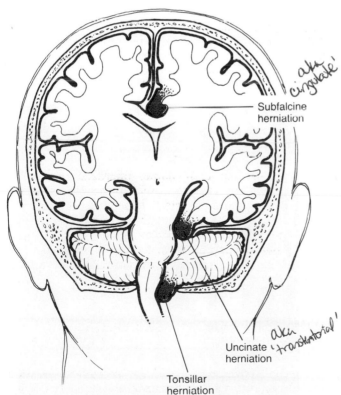

aka 'cingulate'

aka 'transtentorial'

Figure 22–1 Herniations of the brain: subfalcine (cingulate), uncinate (uncal, transtentorial), and tonsillar. (Adapted from Fishman, R. A.: Brain edema. N. Engl. J. Med. *293*:706, 1975. Adapted, with permission, from The New England Journal of Medicine.)

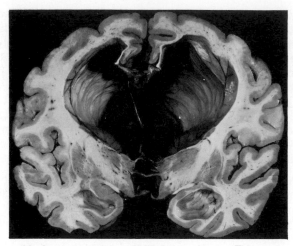

Figure 22-2. Hydrocephalus of moderate degree. This was associated with an Arnold-Chiari malformation. The basal ganglia have been displaced downward and laterally, and the overlying corpus callosum has been thinned.

cranial pressure. There are many causes of hydrocephalus. Examples include congenital malformations such as the Arnold-Chiari malformation (displacement of cerebellar tonsils into the cervical canal), infections that cause aqueductal stenosis or fibrotic adhesions in the subarachnoid space, trauma, and subarachnoid hemorrhage (Fig. 22-2). Space-occupying lesions, adjacent to the fourth ventricle or aqueduct, may also produce hydrocephalus.

Hydrocephalus ex vacuo is really just another term for brain atrophy and refers to the compensatory enlargement of the ventricles and increased CSF volume that accompany reduction in brain volume.

INFECTIONS _____

The nervous system is susceptible to infection by numerous bacteria, fungi, and viruses, as well as to occasional higher organisms such as amebae. Most pathogens reach the brain through the *blood.* Some viruses, notably herpes simplex and rabies, ascend through *peripheral nerves. Penetrating trauma* may be followed by infection. Very infrequently, medical procedures (usually lumbar puncture) may introduce pathogenic microorganisms. *Infections in adjacent structures,* such as sinuses or middle ear, may erode through the bone and involve either the meninges or the brain.

It is clinically and pathologically convenient to divide infections into (1) those of the meninges and CSF (meningitis) and (2) those of the brain parenchyma (encephalitis). However in most encephalitides the inflammatory infiltrate spills over into the CSF, and, conversely, meningitis may invade the brain.

MENINGITIS _____

Meningitis, an inflammation in the leptomeninges and subarachnoid space, is usually caused by an infec-

tion, but chemical meningitis also occurs. Once infection is established it is rapidly disseminated throughout the CSF, this being one of the major negative side effects of the protective function of CSF against trauma.

Infectious meningitis can be broadly classified as acute pyogenic (usually bacterial), acute lymphocytic (viral), and chronic (bacterial or fungal).

Acute (Purulent) Meningitis _____

The most frequent causes of these infections are *Escherichia coli* in the neonate and, particularly, the neonate with a neural tube defect; *Haemophilus influenzae* in infants and children; *Neisseria meningitidis* in adolescents and young adults (which is also the most frequent cause of epidemic meningitis, since it is a mouth commensal and can be transmitted through air); and the *pneumococcus,* particularly in the very young and old and in meningitis following trauma.

> Acutely, the brain and spinal cord are swollen and congested. The subarachnoid space contains exudate (Fig. 22-3), which varies in location. In meningitis caused by *H. influenzae,* for example, the exudate is usually basal, but in pneumococcal meningitis it is more often located over the cerebral convexity, near the longitudinal sinus. From the areas of greatest accumulation, tracts of pus can be followed around the blood vessels. Even in those areas where there is no gross exudate, the leptomeninges are opaque and congested. When the process is fulminant, and especially if it is prolonged, the inflammation may extend to the ependymal surface of the ventricles and produce ventriculitis.

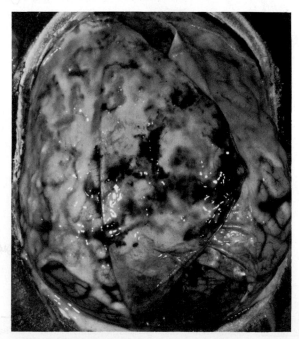

Figure 22-3. Pyogenic meningitis. A heavy layer of suppurative exudate is disclosed by folding back the dural covering.

Microscopically, the subarachnoid space contains a neutrophilic exudate that has varying amounts of fibrin. At its most severe, the entire subarachnoid space is filled with polymorphs, whereas in less severe cases, only the tissue around the leptomeningeal blood vessels contains cells. In fulminant infections, the inflammatory cells infiltrate the walls of the leptomeningeal veins, producing a vasculitis that may result in venous occlusion and hemorrhagic infarction of the cortex and underlying white matter.

Clinically, patients have a fever, the general signs of infection, and, in addition, the symptoms and signs of meningeal irritation (i.e., headache, photophobia, irritability, clouding of consciousness, and a stiff neck). A spinal tap yields cloudy or frankly purulent CSF, under increased pressure, with up to 90,000 polymorphs per microliter, a raised protein level, and a strikingly *reduced sugar content*. In fulminant infections, bacteria may sometimes be visible on smear or be readily cultured for a few hours before polymorphs appear.

Acute Lymphocytic (Viral) Meningitis _____

In viral meningitis the signs and symptoms of meningeal irritation are less pronounced than in bacterial meningitis and the infection is self-limiting, having none of the life-threatening complications of bacterial meningitis. In the CSF there is a lymphocytic pleocytosis (an increased number of cells in the CSF), the protein elevation is only moderate, and the sugar content is normal. A large number of different viruses may be involved: mumps, echoviruses, coxsackieviruses, Epstein-Barr (EBV), and herpes simplex virus (HSV) type II, but the pathogenic virus is often difficult to identify, and at best, a specific agent is identified in only about two thirds of the cases of presumed viral meningitis.

Chronic Meningitis _____

The major causative agents of chronic meningitis are bacteria such as *Mycobacterium tuberculosis, Treponema pallidum* (syphilis), and *Brucella* species, and fungi such as *Coccidioides* and *Candida* organisms. Although the details of the clinical presentation differ with the different organisms, the pathologic reactions have many similarities.

MORPHOLOGY. The subarachnoid space is filled with a gelatinous or fibrinous exudate that is usually most obvious around the base of the brain and extending into the lateral sulci. In late cases there may be a dense fibrous adhesive arachnoiditis. Microscopically, the exudate is composed of varying mixtures of lymphocytes, plasma cells, histiocytes, and fibroblasts. Granulomas, with or without necrosis, and giant cells may be present. Arteries in the subarachnoid space often show obliterative endarteritis with inflammatory infiltrates in their walls and marked intimal thickening.

The CSF findings are variable but there is usually only moderate CSF mononuclear pleocytosis (up to 1000 cells per microliter), a moderately reduced sugar content, and often a strikingly increased protein level.

The most significant complications of chronic meningitis are a result of the continuing inflammatory reaction in the subarachnoid space. The arachnoid fibrosis may cause hydrocephalus. The obliterative endarteritis can result in ischemia or infarction of the brain, with consequences that depend on which artery is occluded. They may be catastrophic, as for example with occlusion of the anterior spinal artery. The cranial and peripheral nerves may also be affected in their passage through the subarachnoid space.

Cryptococcal meningitis merits special mention because of its clinical and pathologic variability. Depending on the immune status of the patient, cryptococci in the CSF may provoke only a trivial inflammatory response in those with depressed immunity, even in the presence of large numbers of organisms in the subarachnoid and perivascular Virchow-Robin spaces, or there may be a marked chronic meningitis. Clinically the course may be fulminant or fatal in as little as two weeks or indolent over months or even years.

ENCEPHALITIS _____

Encephalitis is the general term for parenchymal infections of the brain. Pathologically they range from focal necrotizing processes exemplified by bacterial cerebritis and abscesses to viral infections that cause only individual cell death.

Bacterial parenchymal infections of the nervous system most frequently produce focal acute cerebritis with necrosis that leads to abscess formation. Other bacterial parenchymal infections include syphilis in its manifestations as general paresis and gumma formation and *M. tuberculosis* when it produces a tuberculoma.

Cerebral Abscess _____

Abscesses may arise from *direct implantation* of organisms by trauma, *extension from an adjacent infectious focus* (e.g., mastoiditis), or *hematogenous spread*, usually from a primary source in lung, heart or bone. Notable predisposing causes are chronic pulmonary sepsis (bronchiectasis) and cyanotic congenital heart disease where a right-to-left shunt allows blood to escape pulmonary filtration. The microflora of abscesses is varied and includes many anaerobic organisms (streptococci and *Bacteroides fragilis*) as well as aerobic streptococci and staphylococci.

MORPHOLOGY. Abscess formation in the brain is basically the same as in other organs: a collagen capsule forms around a focus of necrotising cerebritis. Since astrocytes do not produce collagen, the abscess wall is produced by fibroblasts derived from the blood vessels that proliferate around the margin of the necrotic brain. Capsule formation is therefore less vigorous and slower than in other organs. The vascular proliferation is also associated with pronounced local edema. Outside the capsule there is reactive astrocytosis and, often, perivascular inflammatory infiltrates that spill over into the CSF.

Abscesses are so destructive that focal neurologic signs are almost always present together with increased intracranial pressure. A systemic or local source is usually detectable, but a small systemic source may not be detectable by the time the patient presents with brain involvement.

Mass effect and herniation may be fatal, and rupture can lead to ventriculitis, meningitis, or sinus thrombosis. Surgery and antibiotics have reduced the rate of the otherwise inevitable mortality to less than 20%.

VIRAL ENCEPHALITIS _____

The CNS can be infected by many viruses, an event that has usually been preceded by primary infection elsewhere. In varicella-zoster the primary infection is another recognized disease, but it is more often non-specific, as in the gastroenteritis of poliomyelitis, or even unknown, as in progressive multifocal leukoencephalopathy, where there is only serologic evidence of prior exposure to the virus. In rabies and herpes simplex the virus enters the CNS through inoculation into and ascent up peripheral nerves.

Immunosuppression, particularly in acquired immunodeficiency syndrome (AIDS), has emerged as a major factor in the appearance of a number of unusual viral diseases, notably progressive multifocal leukoencephalopathy (PML) and CMV, herpes zoster, and uncommonly measles encephalitis.

The most characteristic histologic change in acute viral diseases is a mononuclear cell infiltrate (lymphocytes, plasma cells, and macrophages), generally located around blood vessels (Fig. 22–4). The presence of **glial nodules** and **neuronophagia** (individual neuron necrosis and phagocytosis) also suggest viral disease. A more direct expression of viral involvement is the presence of intranuclear or intracytoplasmic **inclusion bodies** in some forms of viral infection. A well-known diagnostic inclusion is the intracytoplasmic **Negri body** of rabies.

A particularly striking feature of viral infections of the nervous system is the degree of tropism exhibited by some viruses. Herpes zoster and poliomyelitis virus, for example, affect only specific subpopulations of neurons

—the dorsal root ganglion cells and the anterior horn motor neurons, respectively. Other viruses affect whole classes of cells; the virus of PML infects primarily oligo-dendrocytes, and rabies virus attacks only neurons. HSV, although it infects all types of neural cells, is "geographically" restricted, affecting principally the temporal lobes. The basis for these different specificities is not clear, but they probably reflect surface receptor compatibility between the host cells and the infecting virus.

The capacity of some viruses for *latency* is important in viral diseases of the nervous system. HSV and varicella-zoster virus can remain latent in their host cells in the nervous system, to be reactivated months or years after the initial infection.

Infections, overt or otherwise, do not make up the full gamut of viral effects on the nervous system. Systemic viral infections may occasionally be followed by an immune-mediated *perivenous encephalitis* or *polyneuritis* with no viral penetration of the nervous system. *Reye's syndrome,* a condition of unknown but possibly toxic origin, occurs most frequently after viral infection (usually influenza or chickenpox) and is associated with severe, often fatal brain edema. Some *congenital malformations* can also be attributed to intrauterine viral infection, as occurs with rubella.

Virus infections of the brain can be divided into two general categories: (1) acute viral infections and (2) slow virus diseases.

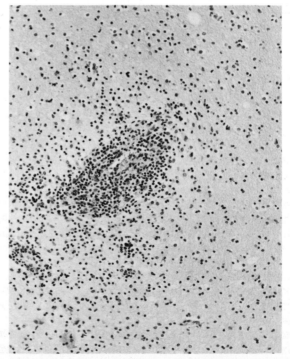

Figure 22–4. Microscopic detail of cerebral white matter in viral encephalitis. There is marked perivascular cuffing with lymphocytes, some of which have invaded the adjacent parenchyma.

Acute Viral Encephalitis

Many acute viral infections are widespread in the brain (panencephalitis). The agents most frequently responsible for this type of encephalitis are the arboviruses (*ar*thropod-*borne*), transmitted by biting insects and typified by eastern and western equine, Venezuelan, St. Louis, and California encephalitis. Also included in this category are the diseases in which encephalitis is an occasional, though sometimes severe, complication of another disease. Examples include EBV, mumps, measles, rubella, and chickenpox, although at least the last three of these are more often examples of allergic perivenous encephalitis rather than true viral infection of the CNS.

Pathologically the true viral infections all exhibit meningoencephalitis characterized by perivascular and parenchymal lymphoplasmacytic inflammatory infiltrates with neuronophagia (phagocytosis of damaged neurons), microglial nodules, and sometimes inclusion bodies. Some, such as eastern equine encephalitis, may also have a polymorph and vasculitis component. Depending on the pathogen there is considerable variation in pathologic and clinical severity of disease and in distribution of the most severe pathologic lesions in the brain.

HERPES SIMPLEX VIRUS. HSV I encephalitis typically involves principally the inferior and medial regions of the temporal lobes and the orbital gyri of the frontal lobes. The infection produces hemorrhagic necrosis with mononuclear perivascular infiltrates. Intranuclear inclusion bodies may be found in neurons and glial cells. It may occur at any age but is most frequent in children and young adults. The diagnosis is made by immunocytochemical or ultrastructural demonstration of the virus or by its isolation in biopsy material. Treatment with acyclovir has reduced the mortality rate from 70 to 30%, although some survivors have a striking memory loss, because of the destruction of the temporal lobes, as well as other neurologic deficits. Outcome in this disease is markedly influenced by the clinical state of the patient at the start of treatment.

HSV II also produces disease in the nervous system; it is responsible for most cases of herpetic viral meningitis. More ominously it causes a generalized and very severe encephalitis in neonates that occurs in as many as 50% of neonates born by vaginal delivery to women with primary genital HSV II infection. The risk to the infant with recurrent genital herpes is reported to be very much lower.

ACQUIRED IMMUNODEFICIENCY SYNDROME. The nervous system is a major target for the human immunodeficiency virus (HIV-1). At least four syndromes have been ascribed to the direct effects of the virus: acute aseptic meningitis or encephalitis, subacute encephalitis, vacuolar myelopathy, and peripheral neuropathies.

The *aseptic meningitis* resembles a viral meningitis and occurs in about 10% of patients with HIV infection, usually around the time of seroconversion.

Subacute encephalitis is characterized histologically by variable degrees of myelin rarefaction associated with microscopic foci of multinucleate giant cells, macrophages, and lymphocytes intermixed with microglial cells and reactive astrocytes (Fig. 22–5). These changes are pathognomonic for HIV-1. Virus particles and viral proteins are present in at least some of the multinucleate giant cells. These lesions are most common in cerebral and cerebellar white matter and deep gray matter and are found in about 30% of patients who die of AIDS. In addition there may be some evidence of neuronal loss; however it is still uncertain whether all these changes are adequate to explain the AIDS dementia complex sometimes observed. Their presence is correlated with the AIDS dementia syndrome, but the lesions themselves do not always produce either the type or degree of damage that would be expected to cause dementia.

Vacuolar myelopathy is found in 20 to 30% of patients at autopsy, about half of whom have clinical evidence of spinal cord dysfunction. Many also have the AIDS dementia syndrome. Pathologically, there is

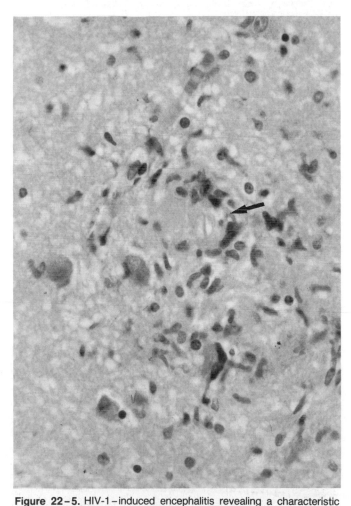

Figure 22–5. HIV-1–induced encephalitis revealing a characteristic cerebral focus of reactive astrocytes, macrophages, and lymphocytes, intermixed with microglial cells. A poorly formed giant cell *(arrow)* is centrally located. (Courtesy of Dr. Matthew Frosch, Department of Pathology, Brigham and Women's Hospital and Harvard Medical School.)

vacuolation of the myelin and accumulation of lipid-laden macrophages very similar in character and distribution to that seen in vitamin B_{12} deficiency (subacute combined degeneration). In mild cases the axons are preserved, but with severe disease there is also disruption of axons. These changes are extremely rare in childhood AIDS.

Peripheral neuropathy in AIDS is very common and highly variable. It may be demyelinating or axonal or both and have a predominantly sensory or motor expression. This variation probably reflects different pathogenic mechanisms, but in at least some cases it is associated with the presence of HIV in the affected nerves.

Infection with HIV-1 is also associated with a significantly higher risk of opportunistic infection of the nervous system, notably CMV, varicella-zoster, herpes simplex encephalitis, PML (see below), cryptococcosis, and toxoplasmosis. There is also a much greater risk of developing a primary CNS lymphoma that is unusually high grade and aggressive, and relatively resistant to treatment.

Slow Virus Diseases

The slow virus diseases are infections with a very long latent period that evolve at a pace so much slower than usual infections that they do not clinically resemble an infectious process.

The two major slow virus diseases are subacute sclerosing panencephalitis (SSPE) and PML. SSPE is a complication of measles that appears when there is accumulation of a defective measles virus. Its incidence has been greatly reduced by widespread immunization against measles, making the condition too rare for further comment.

PROGRESSIVE MULTIFOCAL LEUKOENCEPHALOPATHY. PML is a viral infection of oligodendrocytes that causes demyelination. It occurs in immunosuppressed patients, particularly in association with hematologic malignancies and AIDS. Almost all cases are caused by a papovavirus called JC (the initials of a patient and not connected to Creutzfeldt-Jakob disease). About 65% of normal persons have antibodies to this virus, but it is not known whether the disease is a rekindling of a latent infection or a new infection in a susceptible host.

MORPHOLOGY. The affected white matter is soft and has a gray, translucent appearance. Microscopically, there are numerous areas of demyelination, ranging in size from minute foci to huge confluent regions affecting whole lobes. The infected oligodendrocytes are grossly enlarged and contain intranuclear inclusion bodies which range from violet smudges to discrete homogeneous eosinophilic masses. They are most frequent at the edges of the lesions. There are also characteristic bizarre giant astrocytes with irregular, hyperchromatic, and sometimes multiple nuclei. Numerous foamy macrophages contain myelin debris, but there is little or no inflammatory reaction; in some cases the axons traversing the lesion are strikingly preserved. Electron microscopy shows numerous papovavirus particles in the oligodendrocyte nuclei.

Clinically, patients develop protean but focal and relentlessly progressive neurologic symptoms and signs. Both computed tomography (CT) and magnetic resonance imaging (MRI) show multifocal lesions in white matter with relative sparing of the cortex. No effective treatment is currently known.

Unconventional Agent (Spongiform) Encephalopathies

This is a small group of diseases that includes Creutzfeldt-Jakob disease, Gerstmann-Straussler syndrome, and kuru in humans and scrapie in sheep. In all there is tissue accumulation of a 30-kd protein that is a modification of a normally occurring cell protein. The diseases are transmissible by an extract containing this modified protein, which has been called a "prion" (from proteinaceous infective agent) by one major research group. However, it has not been unequivocally established that there is no nucleic acid associated with the infectious extract, and the exact mechanism of disease transmission and pathogenesis has not yet been established.

SUBACUTE SPONGIFORM ENCEPHALOPATHY (CREUTZFELDT-JAKOB DISEASE). This is a rare but well-characterized form of rapidly progressive dementia. Despite the demonstrated transmissibility of its causative agent, it is sporadic in occurrence, with a worldwide incidence of about one per million and no apparent pattern of exposure in the patients. The natural mode of transmission is unknown, although a few cases of iatrogenic transmission (e.g., corneal transplantation, pituitary-derived human growth hormone) have occurred. Familial clusters of Creutzfeldt-Jakob disease exist with apparent autosomal dominant transmission. In some of these patients, as well as in unrelated victims, molecular genetic studies have found single nucleotide changes in at least one copy of the gene for the prion protein.

Because the progress of the disease is usually rapid, despite the degree of neuronal loss there may be little if any grossly apparent atrophy of the brain. **Microscopically, the pathognomonic feature is vacuolization in the neuropil (spongiform change) in the cortex and sometimes the basal ganglia.** There is no associated inflammatory infiltrate. The later stages of the disease are characterized by severe neuronal loss and marked reactive astrocytosis.

The clinical picture is usually quite typical: initial subtle changes are followed by a rapidly progressive dementia, often accompanied by a pronounced startle myoclonus. The disease is uniformly fatal: average life expectancy is only a few months, although occasional patients survive for several years.

OTHER INFECTIONS _____

Protozoal diseases such as malaria, toxoplasmosis, amebiasis, and trypanosomiasis; rickettsial infections (typhus, Rocky Mountain spotted fever); and metazoal diseases such as echinococcosis and cysticercosis may also involve the CNS. Of these, cerebral toxoplasmosis merits a brief additional mention because in its acquired form in adults it occurs only in immunosuppressed persons, is particularly common in AIDS, and is treatable. Pathologically it is a rapidly progressive, multifocal, necrotizing, and often hemorrhagic encephalitis with a predilection for gray matter. The organisms are present both as characteristic pseudocysts and free tachyzoites in the tissue, and they are usually most easily seen at the margins of the necrotic areas.

In this brief summary of infections there has been a considerable bias toward diseases encountered in western European and North American practice. However, outside these privileged areas, cerebral malaria, cysticercosis, and tuberculosis are probably the most common infections of the nervous system.

VASCULAR DISEASE _____

Vascular disease of the brain, in spite of a recent and gratifying reduction in its incidence, remains a very important cause of neurologic morbidity and mortality, with personal and social consequences extending far beyond the acute medical phase of the illness. It is hoped that the continued treatment of hypertension and progress in understanding the causes of atherosclerosis will further control these all too common disorders.

Cerebrovascular disease is most easily thought of in three general categories: (1) *general reductions in blood flow without vascular occlusion—ischemic encephalopathy and boundary zone infarcts;* (2) *local cessation of blood flow caused by vascular occlusion—thrombotic and embolic infarcts, and venous obstruction;* (3) *hemorrhages—within the brain (intraparenchymal hemorrhages), in the subarachnoid space (subarachnoid hemorrhages), or in both areas.*

ISCHEMIC (HYPOXIC) ENCEPHALOPATHY _____

The brain has a remarkably constant level of metabolic activity, and autoregulation of the cerebral circulation normally ensures the maintenance of cerebral perfusion pressure, and hence blood flow, over a wide range of systemic blood pressure and intracerebral pressure. In normal persons, blood flow to the brain is adequate down to a systolic blood pressure of about 50 mm Hg.

Reductions in pressure below this level induce increasing tissue ischemia and subsequent ischemic encephalopathy. In the brain, the cells most vulnerable to ischemia are the neurons, and they suffer first reversible and then irreversible damage. **For obscure reasons, some types of neurons, notably the pyramidal cells of the hippocampus and the Purkinje cells of the cerebellum, are more susceptible than others,** and consequently they are often the first to be lost.

The changes seen in the brain depend on the duration and intensity of the ischemia and on the length of survival. When the insult has been slight, the nerve cells will recover function and no anatomic change occurs. In patients who survive only a few minutes or hours, no changes are seen regardless of the severity of the insult. The first demonstrable change is seen after survival for 12 to 24 hours. **All forms of ischemia initially result in either swelling or shrinkage of neurons.** Shortly thereafter, affected neurons may develop **ischemic cell change,** characterized by strikingly eosinophilic cytoplasm and a small pyknotic nucleus (red neurons). In the cortex, the process is usually widespread but not completely uniform; clusters of damaged cells may be found next to unaffected cells, even in the same cortical lamina. Subsequently, the nerve cells die and disappear, to be replaced by fibrillary gliosis. Frank cortical necrosis followed by gliosis occurs in areas of greater destruction, so that **laminar necrosis** interrupts the normal continuity of the cerebral cortex. In long-term survivors, the degree of cortical atrophy is proportional to the amount of cortical destruction. In generalized reductions of cerebral perfusion, the most severe ischemia is suffered by tissue supplied by the most distal branches of the arteries. This may be severe enough to result in wedge-shaped areas of tissue necrosis in the junctional zones between the major arterial territories, called **border-zone or watershed infarcts.** In the cerebral hemispheres, the border zone between the territories for the anterior and middle cerebral arteries seems to be most at risk. Damage to this region produces a linear parasagittal infarction, usually with some expansion over the lateral occipital gyri; the precise geometry of the infarct is governed by the degree of ischemia and the extent of narrowing of local vessels in the affected region. Border-zone infarcts are almost invariably seen in the context of a generalized severe ischemic encephalopathy.

The clinical expression of ischemic encephalopathy depends on the severity and duration of the period of ischemia. In mild cases, there may be only a transient postischemic confusional state and subsequent complete recovery, whereas more severely affected patients will be comatose, with loss of most cortical functions. Prolonged ischemia, which for the brain may be as little as four minutes, results in generalized neuronal death.

CEREBRAL INFARCTION

Cerebral infarction occurs as a result of vascular occlusion; *the issue of whether infarction will or will not occur, and its size and shape, are determined by which vessel is occluded and the pattern and degree of anastomotic connections among the cerebral arteries.* In the case of the large internal carotid and vertebral arteries, the circle of Willis may provide a total functional anastomosis. The middle-sized intracranial arteries, such as the middle and anterior cerebral, have a partial anastomosis of their distal branches, so that, although a quite severe stenosis in one artery can be tolerated, complete occlusion always causes an infarct that is smaller than the territory supplied by the obstructed vessel. In the small parenchymal arteries, such as the lenticulostriate and cortical penetrating arteries, there is little or no arterial anastomosis, and occlusion of these vessels always results in an infarct.

Clinically, the symptoms generated by vascular occlusion are called "strokes." *Stroke* is one of those old-fashioned clinical terms that is frequently used but is pathologically imprecise. *It implies the usually sudden onset of a focal neurologic syndrome,* such as a hemiparesis (weakness of the limbs on one side of the body) secondary to some sort of vascular event. This event may be either an occlusion, producing a focal infarct, or a hemorrhage, which also causes local destruction of tissue. Other types of disease processes that cause local destruction (for example, tumors) may also occasionally present with a focal syndrome of rapid onset, mimicking a stroke.

Cerebral vascular occlusions are either thrombotic or embolic. **Thrombotic occlusions are almost invariably atherosclerotic,** and most occur either in the internal carotid artery at the carotid bifurcation or in the vertebrobasilar system. The consequence of a carotid occlusion depends largely on the function of the circle of Willis. If it is functioning normally, carotid occlusion may be asymptomatic, as indeed it is in many patients. If the anastomotic capacity of the circle of Willis is reduced by atherosclerosis or there is an abnormal pattern of circulation an infarction may occur that can range in size from a small distal infarction in the territory of the middle cerebral artery to a catastrophic infarct of a whole hemisphere.

The posterior circulation is not afforded the same level of anastomotic protection, and occlusion of the basilar artery is invariably seriously incapacitating and often fatal. Occlusion of a vertebral artery may be asymptomatic.

Before total occlusion occurs, ephemeral focal neurologic symptoms and signs, called **transient ischemic attacks** (TIAs), often point to significant atherosclerotic cerebrovascular disease. Although atherosclerosis is by far the most frequent basis of thrombotic occlusions, other causes exist, notably arteritis. This usually results

in occlusion of arteries smaller than those obstructed by atherosclerosis.

Cerebral emboli have a wide range of origins and, probably for hemodynamic reasons, a marked tendency to impact in the territory of the middle cerebral artery. They are often small enough to affect only a part of the vascular territory of this artery (Fig. 22–6).

Some types of emboli tend to fragment or lyse, allowing reflow of blood into ischemically damaged vessels, which leak, thereby converting an ischemic infarct into a hemorrhagic one. The hemorrhage is petechial and restricted to the cortex unless the patient is taking anticoagulants, in which case the hemorrhage may be massive and sometimes difficult to distinguish from a lobar hemorrhage.

No matter what their cause, cerebral infarcts have a similar pattern of pathologic evolution. Grossly, ischemic infarcts are first detectable at about 12 hours because of slight discoloration and softening of the gray matter, but within 48 to 72 hours the softening and discoloration become more apparent, and with large infarcts, marked swelling of the infarcted region appears. Reperfusion hemorrhage may accentuate the changes (Fig. 22–7). This tissue expansion may be sufficient to cause herniation. As resolution of the infarct proceeds, there is tissue liquefaction, with cystic degeneration that is most pronounced in large infarcts. Around the infarct there is marked glial reaction and the overlying meninges often become thickened and opaque.

Microscopically, the changes seen in infarcted brain are much like those in other organs, except for the important difference that **no fibrous scar is formed.** There is an initial loss of basophilic staining of neurons and large numbers of red (ischemic) neurons may be seen. By 24 to 48 hours, there is a variable neutrophil infiltration, that by 72 to 96 hours is beginning to be replaced by the macrophages that are the main agent of tissue breakdown. The length of time required for complete resolution of the infarct is variable and largely dependent on the volume of infarcted tissue. Large infarcts require many months, but even years later scattered macrophages may be present in the interstices of old lesions. In the tissue around the infarct there is a marked reactive astrocytosis that is prominent from about the second week. After resolution, the residual cyst is surrounded by a zone of fibrillary gliosis. Hemorrhage within the infarct does not affect the process of infarct resolution.

Lacunae (little lakes) are small cystic lesions (up to 15 mm diameter) that are most commonly found in the basal ganglia, internal capsule, thalamus, basis pontis, and hemispheric white matter. They may be multiple and they are particularly associated with systemic arterial hypertension. They are thought to be the result of occlusion of small deep arterioles, either by emboli or hypertensive hyalinization of the vessels. Most often asymptomatic, they may become clinically

Figure 22-6. An old hemorrhagic infarct involving the superior lip of the sylvian fissure in the territory of the middle cerebral artery. The gyral pattern has been lost, the infarcted area has a yellow-brown discoloration, and there is gliotic scarring.

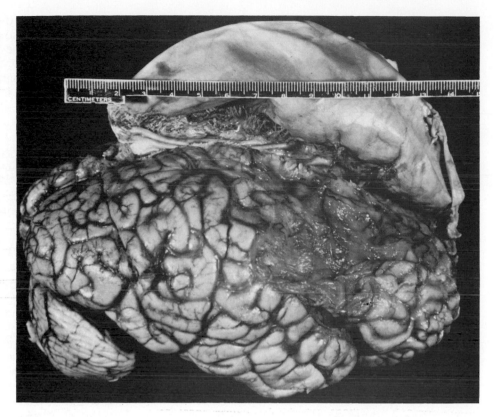

apparent when critically located (e.g., in the internal capsule or basis pontis).

INTRACRANIAL HEMORRHAGE _____

Spontaneous (nontraumatic) intracerebral hemorrhage falls into three basic categories: (1) intraparenchymal hemorrhage, (2) subarachnoid hemorrhage, and (3) mixed hemorrhage.

Intraparenchymal Hemorrhage _____

Most intraparenchymal hemorrhages result from rupture of one of the small intraparenchymal arteries. Their occurence is particularly associated with a history of hypertension and, it is thought, the formation of microaneurysms called *Charcot-Bouchard* aneurysms that burst and cause the bleeding. Rupture destroys the aneurysms and leads to hemorrhage into the immediately adjacent brain tissue. Studies of hypertensive patients without hemorrhage have shown that the occurrence of these microaneurysms in the arteries of the brain increases with age and with length of history of hypertension.

The aneurysms, and therefore the hemorrhages, occur most frequently in the basal ganglia (Fig. 22-8), the pons and cerebellar hemispheres (Fig. 22-9), and less frequently in the hemispheric white matter. Bleeding in this last location is often called a lobar hemorrhage.

CT and MRI have revealed smaller hemorrhages, often in unusual locations. Many of these are the result of bleeding from small cavernous angiomas. These bleeds tend to be symptomatic when located in sensitive regions such as the pons or internal capsule.

Overall with cerebral hemorrhage, there is an initial mortality rate of about 40%; most of these patients suffer extension of the hemorrhage into the cerebral ventricles. Those who survive have a relatively good prognosis for recovery of function, perhaps because

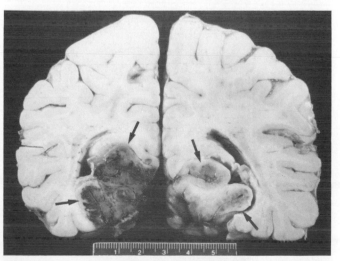

Figure 22-7. Coronal cross-section of the brain reveals infarcts (more hemorrhagic on left) several days old involving both posterior cerebral artery territories.

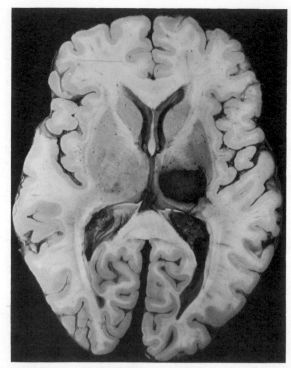

Figure 22–8. An intraparenchymal hemorrhage involving the basal ganglia and the posterior limb of the internal capsule.

hemorrhages tend to separate tissue planes rather than destroy the tissue, so that resolution of the mass of the hematoma may be accompanied by restitution of function. Generally, recurrent hemorrhage is rare, in contrast to the situation in subarachnoid hemorrhage, in which rebleeding is a major risk.

Gross inspection of the brain of a patient with, for example, a hemorrhage in the basal ganglia often shows obvious expansion of the affected hemisphere and flattening of the gyri. Frequently there is uncinate herniation (p. 707) and displacement of the midbrain to the side opposite the hemorrhage. If the hemorrhage has erupted into the ventricles, a blood clot may be present in the subarachnoid space and is often present around the foramina of Luschka and Magendie, where the ventricles communicate with the subarachnoid space.

The cut surface of the brain typically shows the blood clot expanding and separating the tissues of the basal ganglia. The parenchyma immediately adjacent to the clot is usually edematous and often discolored by degradation products of blood pigment, especially if the hemorrhage is some days old. **The mass effect of the blood clot causes distortion of the cerebral ventricles;** the ipsilateral one is usually compressed, but there may also be acute hydrocephalus if the aqueduct of Sylvius or either of the foramina of Monro is occluded by the ventricular distortion. Sometimes the hemorrhage

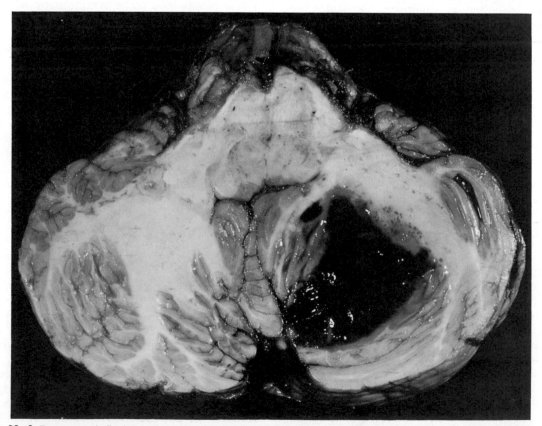

Figure 22–9. Recent cerebellar hemorrhage that has produced distortion of the vermis and compression of the fourth ventricle.

ruptures into a ventricle and fills it. Resolution of a hemorrhage begins with the appearance of macrophages that, over a period of months, remove the clot and leave a slit-like cavity surrounded by a zone of fibrillary gliosis that contains scattered hemosiderin-laden macrophages.

Since in about 80% of cases there is a history of hypertension, vascular changes are also found in other parts of the brain. The most frequent is arteriolar sclerosis, with thickening and hyalinization of the walls of the arterioles, seen most conspicuously in the deep white matter of the hemispheres. In the basal ganglia there is often arterial thickening, focal atherosclerosis, and expansion of the Virchow-Robin spaces with perivascular gliosis. Atherosclerosis of the larger arteries is also often severe but is not a necessary accompaniment to hypertensive hemorrhage.

Supratentorial hemorrhages tend to present as progressive hemiplegias. In the posterior fossa, cerebellar hematomas produce symptoms such as intractable vomiting. Whatever the location of the hemorrhage, if there is substantial bleeding and mass effect, the signs of raised intracranial pressure, coma, and the syndromes of herniation rapidly come to dominate the clinical picture.

Subarachnoid Hemorrhage

Bleeding into the subarachnoid space usually results from rupture of either an aneurysm or, much less frequently, an arteriovenous malformation. *Aneurysms are divided into berry (congenital), arteriosclerotic, and mycotic, berry aneurysms being the most common.*

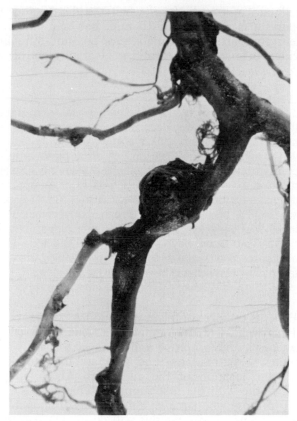

Figure 22–11. A berry aneurysm of the middle cerebral artery. The vessels have been dissected away from the brain.

Berry aneurysms occur at bifurcations of cerebral arteries: the most common sites are (1) the junction of the carotid and posterior communicating arteries, (2) the anterior communicating artery connecting the two anterior cerebral arteries, and (3) the major division of the middle cerebral artery in the sylvian fissure. In 20 to 30% of cases they are multiple. Together these three sites account for at least 90% of ruptured aneurysms (Fig. 22–10); almost all the remainder are in the posterior circulation. Although often called congenital aneurysms, *they are not present at birth and develop at sites of medial weakness at arterial bifurcations.* The arterial wall bulges out through the muscular defect at this point to form a thin-walled sac composed only of fibrous tissue, in which there may be additional local degeneration and calcification (Fig. 22–11). Laminated blood clot and fibrin may be deposited on this attenuated wall. Rupture of aneurysms may be associated with acute rises in intracranial pressure, such as may be caused by straining at stool or lifting heavy weight.

Although acute elevation of blood pressure is often implicated in subarachnoid hemorrhage, there is no established association between chronic hypertension and either the development or the rupture of berry aneurysms. Conditions particularly associated with berry aneurysms include fibromuscular dysplasia, polycystic kidney disease, and cerebral arteriovenous malformations, but most are sporadic. There is clear evidence that aneurysms enlarge with time, and the

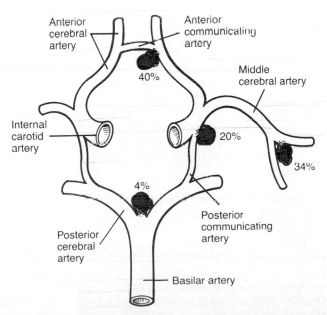

Figure 22–10. Common sites of berry aneurysms in the circle of Willis.

likelihood of rupture rises when the diameter of the aneurysm is greater than 10 mm; however, not every aneurysm bursts, and small ones are not infrequent incidental findings on carotid angiography and at autopsy.

The most common site of rupture in an aneurysm is the thin-walled fundus, with consequences that depend on its orientation. If the fundus is pointing toward or applied to the surface of the brain, the escaping blood at high pressure may tunnel its way into the brain, sometimes reaching a ventricle and producing as much intraparenchymal as subarachnoid bleeding. This occurs in some 15 to 40% of patients and is particularly common in those who die within the first week after rupture. Alternatively, the blood may leak straight into the subarachnoid space and produce the more typical clinical presentation of a subarachnoid hemorrhage.

Patients usually complain of a sudden, severe, occipital headache and may rapidly lose consciousness. In most cases, they improve and are awake again within minutes. Arteriography (and CT) are used to determine the location of the aneurysm. About 50% of patients die with the first rupture. Rebleeding is common in those who survive; although it is impossible to predict in which patient this will occur, when it does, the prognosis is much more grave. Other complications include infarction, hydrocephalus, herniation, and brain stem hemorrhage.

Four to nine days after rupture, some patients develop additional neurologic deficits due to arterial vasospasm. About 40% of patients with ruptured aneurysms have arterial spasm that can be demonstrated arteriographically, but not all become symptomatic. Postmortem examination of patients dying with vasospasm frequently discloses infarcts in the territories supplied by the affected vessels. Experimentally, platelet products and red cell lysates cause constriction in cerebral vessels, but whether these play a role clinically is unknown.

Mixed Intraparenchymal and Subarachnoid Hemorrhage (Vascular Malformations)

Arteriovenous malformations (AVMs) constitute about 1% of intracranial tumors. When they rupture, they bleed into both the brain and subarachnoid space in about two thirds of the cases, into only the subarachnoid space in about 25% of cases, and solely into the CNS in the remainder. They consist of tangles of abnormal vessels of varying sizes, many of which have a structure intermediate between arteries and veins. Ninety per cent of AVMs are in the cerebral hemispheres; about half are predominantly located on the surface of the brain, and the other half are more deeply situated. The abnormal vessels within the brain substance are separated by gliotic tissue in which there is either recent hemorrhage or evidence of old bleeding, in the form of hemosiderin-laden macrophages.

Irregular, often grossly enlarged arteries supply the vascular tangle, and veins that drain the malformation can usually be found.

Bleeding from AVMs is clinically most frequent between the ages of 10 and 30 years; after 60 it is rare. Males are affected twice as often as females. Subarachnoid and intracerebral hemorrhage associated with seizures is the most common clinical presentation. Other forms of vascular malformation that are clinically less significant than AVMs include cavernous angiomas, venous angiomas, and capillary telangiectases.

TRAUMA

Cerebral trauma is most frequent in young males, who may survive with varying degrees of incapacity for many years. It is estimated that in the United States more than 400,000 persons have a major persisting handicap following head injury. Thus, as with cerebrovascular disease, trauma is an area of neuropathology with high costs to society as well as to the individual.

The most important anatomic feature that influences the effects of trauma on the brain is the skull. Although it protects against moderate forces, in more severe trauma it can turn into a weapon against the brain.

Injuries affecting the brain fall into three groups: (1) epidural hematomas, (2) subdural hematomas, and (3) parenchymal injuries.

EPIDURAL HEMATOMA

Epidural hematomas develop after rupture of one of the meningeal arteries, usually the middle meningeal, that run between the dura and the skull. Since the dura is, in part, the periosteum of the skull and is therefore firmly attached to it, a skull fracture is usually present (Fig. 22–12). Because they are a product of _arterial_ bleeding, epidural hematomas accumulate quickly and cause a rapid and progressive rise in intracranial pressure, which usually develops within minutes to a few hours of the trauma. _Typically, patients recover from the initial trauma, the so-called lucid interval, only to slip back into a progressively deepening coma._ Epidural hematomas are surgical emergencies that, if not immediately drained, produce in rapid succession uncinate herniation, tonsillar herniation, medullary compression, respiratory paralysis, and death.

SUBDURAL HEMATOMA

In contrast to epidural hematomas, which are the result of arterial bleeding, most subdural hematomas occur after rupture of some of the bridging veins that connect the venous system of the brain with the large venous sinuses that are enclosed within the dura. Since the brain in its bath of CSF can move, whereas the venous sinuses are fixed, the displacement of the brain

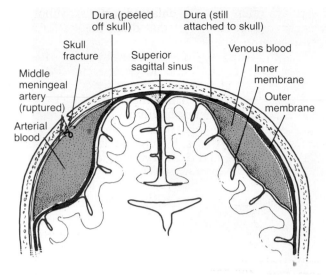

Dura (peeled off skull)
Dura (still attached to skull)
Skull fracture
Superior sagittal sinus
Venous blood
Middle meningeal artery (ruptured)
Inner membrane
Outer membrane
Arterial blood

A. Epidural hematoma   **B. Subdural hematoma**

Figure 22-12. *A,* Epidural hematoma, in which rupture of a meningeal artery, usually associated with a skull fracture, leads to accumulation of arterial blood between the dura and the skull. *B,* In a subdural hematoma, damage to bridging veins between the brain and the superior sagittal sinus leads to the accumulation of blood between the dura and the brain.

that occurs in trauma can tear some of these delicate veins at the point where they penetrate the dura, with subsequent bleeding into the subdural space between the dura and the arachnoid (see Fig. 22-12). Subdural hematomas occur most frequently over the convexities of the hemispheres, where the freedom of movement of the brain is greatest, and are relatively infrequent in locations such as the posterior fossa, where little movement is possible. They may be either acute or chronic.

Acute subdural hematomas are usually associated with obvious trauma, and frequently with a laceration or contusion of the brain. *In contrast to the case with epidural hematomas, the onset of symptoms is generally delayed and is manifested clinically by fluctuating levels of consciousness.* The outcome of an acute subdural hematoma depends not only on the effectiveness of surgical treatment but also on whether the adjacent brain is injured.

Chronic subdural hematomas are much less obviously symptomatic. Older persons and alcoholics are frequent victims. In such patients, there is usually some atrophy of the brain and consequently an increased range of movement of the brain within the skull cavity. This increased freedom of movement translates into an increased risk of rupture of the bridging veins, and in these patients subdural hematomas, often bilateral, may develop slowly after insignificant or even unnoticed trauma. The symptoms such as confusion, inattention, and progressive obtundation are often vague and insidious in onset, although more rarely seizures or progressive hemiparesis may occur. A source of clinical difficulty is that these protean symptoms may either mimic or be masked by concomitant

disease, such as cerebrovascular disease or dementia. CT has greatly simplified this diagnostic problem.

Histologically, these hematomas consist of accumulations of blood encased by an outer membrane underlying the dura and an inner membrane that separates the blood from the adjacent arachnoid. Both subdural membranes are composed of granulation tissue derived from the dura. Electron microscopy shows that the vascular channels within the membranes have incompletely endothelialized walls. This makes them very susceptible to rebleeding with only minimal trauma, resulting in progressive enlargement of the hematoma. The circumscribed mass of blood may cause marked compression and molding of the contiguous cerebral hemispheres (Fig. 22-13). Treatment consists of surgical drainage, but rebleeding from the membranes sometimes necessitates craniotomy for their removal.

PARENCHYMAL INJURIES _____

Trauma to brain itself can be grouped under five headings: (1) concussion, (2) contusions and lacerations, (3) diffuse axonal injury, (4) pure traumatic intracerebral hemorrhage, and (5) complications, which may be early or late.

Concussion is a transient loss of consciousness following head trauma. The duration of unconsciousness is usually short but may last for some hours. There is usually complete recovery. There are no established anatomic changes or explanations for its occurrence, but one hypothesis is that torsion of the midbrain may temporarily disrupt the activating action of the reticular formation and may cause ensuing loss of consciousness.

Contusions and lacerations of the brain are traumatic lesions analogous to those of other soft tissues (p. 236).

Contusions occur when blunt trauma crushes or bruises brain tissue without rupturing the pia. The most common sites of contusions are either directly related to the trauma, in which case they may be at the site of impact (**coup lesions**) or at a point opposite (**contrecoup lesions**), where the brain in motion strikes against the inner surface of the skull, or at irregularities of the skull (e.g., the wing of the sphenoid and the orbital ridges, which produce contusions at the frontal and temporal poles and on the orbitofrontal gyri). The occipital poles are rarely damaged by this mechanism. Contusions usually damage only the crowns of the gyri, leaving the depths of the sulci intact. Histologically, acute contusions show foci of hemorrhagic necrosis. Later, macrophages remove dead tissue, and the area gradually resolves into an irregular, yellow-brown crater with a floor of glial tissue that is often covered by leptomeningeal fibrosis. Because of their color, these old contusions are referred to as "plaques jaunes." **Lacerations** are tears produced by severe blunt trauma, sometimes with an associated fracture followed by hemorrhage and

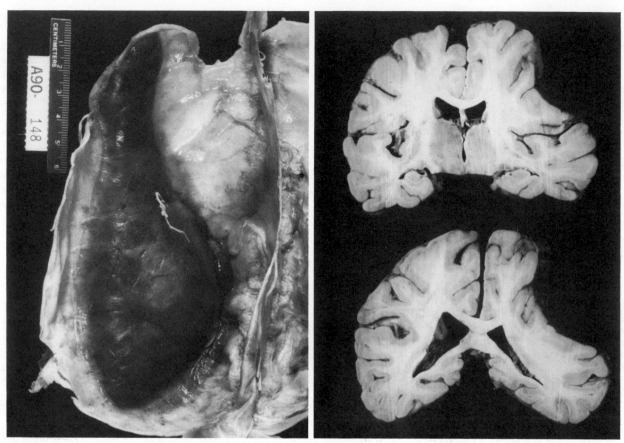

Figure 22–13. On the left, a large organizing subdural hematoma producing marked pressure molding of the cerebral hemispheres seen on cross-section at right. (Courtesy of Dr. Matthew Frosch, Department of Pathology, Brigham and Women's Hospital and Harvard Medical School.)

necrosis. Resolution of lacerations is similar to that of contusions, except that it results in an irregular, yellow-brown, gliotic scar that involves not only cortex but also the underlying structures.

Diffuse axonal injury is present in some patients who have severe neurologic impairment without massive, grossly visible brain damage. Typically these patients are deeply comatose from the moment of injury and recover only to the point of a persistent vegetative state. Microscopically, there is diffuse damage to the white matter with widespread rupture of axons. With long survival there is a microglial reaction, myelin degeneration, and sometimes microcavitation. The most likely explanation is that the shearing forces produced by the distortion of the brain during acceleration and deceleration cause actual physical rupture of axons.

Pure traumatic intracerebral hemorrhages are often multiple and most often involve the frontal and temporal lobes and the deep structures. They may be accompanied by contusions, lacerations, or acute axonal injury. Like the latter, they are probably the result of shearing forces causing direct rupture of intracerebral vessels at the time of trauma.

Complications of trauma may develop in those who survive the initial insult. *Acute complications* include *brain edema,* particularly in children, which may be followed by *herniation, brainstem compression,* and *Duret hemorrhages.* Less frequently, skull fractures provide a path for *infection,* particularly from the ear or nose, and *hydrocephalus* may follow hemorrhage or infection in the ventricular system, aqueduct, or subarachnoid space. There are also a few patients who die shortly after trauma with no apparent brain damage. *Delayed complications* include *posttraumatic epilepsy,* which usually follows a cortical contusion or laceration, and rarely *delayed intracerebral hemorrhage (spät apoplexy).*

TUMORS

A somewhat simplified classification of tumors affecting the nervous system is given in Table 22–1. For operational purposes it is most convenient to divide tumors into three groups: (1) primary intracranial tumors of CNS parenchymal cells. (2) primary intracranial tumors that originate within the skull cavity but are not derived from the brain parenchyma itself, and (3) metastatic tumors.

In the *primary parenchymal tumors* each type of cell in the nervous system gives rise to its own particular type or types of tumor, and there are some additional

TABLE 22-1. TUMORS OF THE NERVOUS SYSTEM*

Primary Parenchymal Tumors
   Tumors of neuroglia
      Astrocytes
         Astrocytoma
         Anaplastic astrocytoma
         Glioblastoma multiforme
         Pilocytic astrocytoma
      Oligodendrocytes
         Oligodendroglioma
      Ependymal cells
         Ependymoma and its homologues
   Tumors of neurons
      Neuroblastoma (p. 676)
      Ganglion cell tumors
         Ganglioneuroma
         Ganglioma
   Tumors of primitive cells
      Medulloblastoma
   Tumors of mesenchymal cells
      Lymphoma, primary and secondary
      Hemangioblastoma
      Vascular malformations
Primary Nonparenchymal Tumors
   Meningeal tumors
      Meningioma
      Hemangiopericytoma
      Hemangioblastoma
      Meningeal sarcoma
   Pineal tumors (nonneuroectodermal)
   Pituitary tumors (adenohypophyseal)
   Malformative tumors
      Craniopharyngioma
      Dermoid cyst
      Epidermoid
Metastatic Tumors

* Tumors in light italics are discussed in the text.

mixed, primitive, and mesenchymal tumors. The *primary nonparenchymal tumors,* as distinct from primary brain tumors, derive mostly either from the meninges or from adjacent structures such as the pituitary and pineal glands.

PRIMARY INTRACRANIAL TUMORS

There are four general features of primary brain tumors that distinguish them from tumors elsewhere in the body.

1. Histologically benign brain tumors can kill the patient if they are located in a position where they cannot be completely resected (e.g. an ependymoma growing from the floor of the fourth ventricle).
2. Parenchymal brain tumors in general, and astrocytomas in particular, have a marked propensity for infiltrative growth into adjacent normal brain tissue and usually do not have grossly or microscopically definable margins. Consequently, curative resection of such tumors is effectively impossible, even if the neurologic damage that would ensue were deemed acceptable.

3. Even the most histologically malignant brain tumors rarely metastasize to the rest of the body. In the rare instances when this occurs it is usually from a glioblastoma or medulloblastoma. Surgical procedures that breach the dura are occasionally followed by systemic metastasis; however, dissemination of tumor within the nervous system via the CSF can be seen. With some tumors, notably medulloblastomas, it is almost the rule rather than the exception.
4. Some types of tumor have a predilection for specific sites. Medulloblastomas, for example, are confined to the cerebellum. There are also age preferences. Medulloblastomas are most frequent in the first decade of life, whereas anaplastic astrocytomas and glioblastomas tend to occur in middle-aged and older patients.

The most frequent and important primary parenchymal tumors are astrocytomas, oligodendrogliomas, ependymomas, and medulloblastomas.

Astrocytoma

Collectively, astrocytomas are the most frequent type of brain tumor, and most examples fall into one of three clinicopathologic groups: (1) astrocytomas, including glioblastoma multiforme, (2) brainstem gliomas, and (3) pilocytic astrocytoma.

Astrocytomas in the cerebral hemispheres are frequently classified into three grades of increasing pathologic anaplasia and rapidity of clinical progression: astrocytoma, anaplastic astrocytoma, and glioblastoma multiforme. Together they account for 80 to 90% of all the glial tumors of adults. They are most frequent in middle age, anaplastic astrocytomas having a peak incidence in the sixth decade and glioblastomas about ten years later.

A clinically important feature of these neoplasms is that astrocytomas have a marked tendency to become more anaplastic with time, so that a tumor initially diagnosed as an astrocytoma may develop into a glioblastoma. A major problem in the interpretation of small biopsy specimens from these tumors is that in a single neoplasm different areas may have quite different histologic appearances and examination of a biopsy specimen may underestimate the grade of the tumor.

Astrocytomas are usually ill-defined, gray-white, infiltrative tumors that expand and distort the underlying brain. They are solid and, depending on their fibrillary content, may be firm or soft and gelatinous (Fig. 22-14). They range from a few centimeters in diameter to enormous lesions that replace the major part of a cerebral hemisphere and extend through the commissures into the opposite hemisphere.

Histologically they are composed of a mixture of astrocytic forms such as protoplasmic, fibrillary, and gemistiocytic astrocytes, as well as many that do not fall into one of the named types. Among the cells is usually

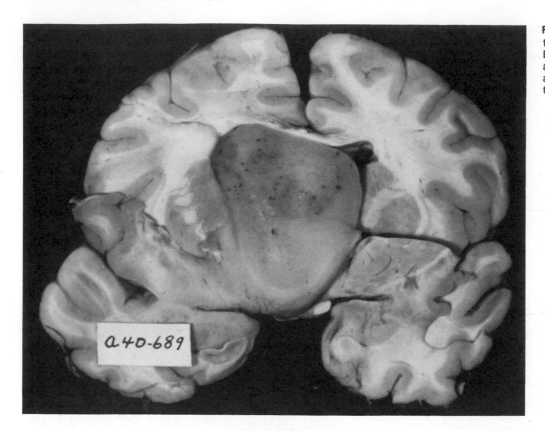

Figure 22–14. A large astrocytoma arising near the midline. Both lateral ventricles have been almost completely obliterated, and there is some distortion of the adjacent basal ganglia.

a highly characteristic fibrillary background of astrocytic processes of varying density and caliber.

Anaplastic astrocytomas are not grossly distinguishable from astrocytomas. Microscopically they have typical anaplastic features, such as hypercellularity, nuclear and cytoplasmic pleomorphism, and nuclear hyperchromatism. The presence in an astrocytoma of either vascular endothelial proliferation or a mitotic rate greater than one per 10 high-power fields suggests this diagnosis.

Grossly, **glioblastoma multiforme** can be usually distinguished from the other astrocytomas by its variegated appearance, hence the designation multiforme. Some regions may be white and firm, others yellow and soft, and foci of necrosis, cysts, and hemorrhages are often seen (Fig. 22–15). **Microscopically, they are distinguished from anaplastic astrocytomas by the presence of necrosis.** As with anaplastic astrocytomas, vascular endothelial proliferation and mitoses are frequently seen (Fig. 22–16). In spite of the presence of these anaplastic features, areas of lower-grade tumor are usually present, intermixed with the more malignant regions, underscoring the hazards of interpreting a small biopsy specimen. Both anaplastic astrocytomas and glioblastomas are occasionally disseminated through the neuraxis via the CSF.

Clinically, astrocytic neoplasms present with general or local signs and symptoms, or both, depending largely on the location of the tumor. The symptoms may remain static or progress only slowly for a num-

ber of years. Eventually, however, patients usually enter a period of more rapid clinical deterioration that is generally correlated with the development of anaplastic features and more rapid growth in the tumor.

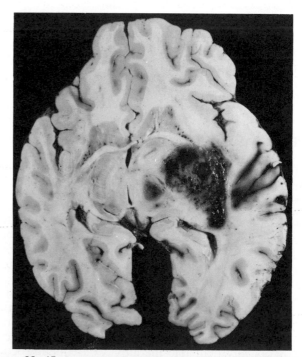

Figure 22–15. A glioblastoma multiforme showing hemorrhage into an area of cystic softening. The tumor and the surrounding edema have produced marked expansion of the affected hemisphere and a shift of the midline.

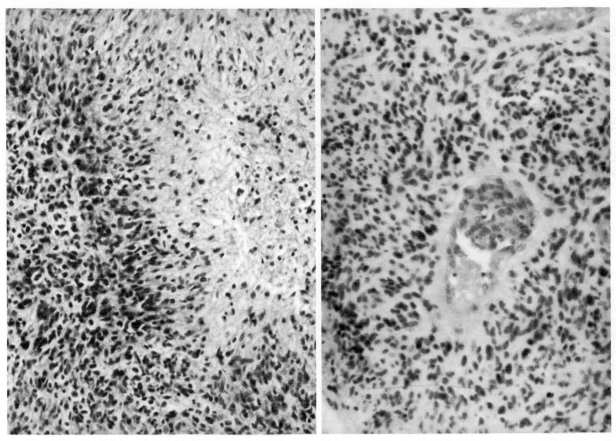

Figure 22–16. Two microscopic views of a glioblastoma multiforme showing on the left an area of ischemic necrosis surrounded by crowded anaplastic astrocytes, and on the right a vessel with striking endothelial proliferation. (Courtesy of Dr. Matthew Frosch, Department of Pathology, Brigham and Women's Hospital and Harvard Medical School.)

Current treatment consists of palliative resection when feasible together with radiotherapy and steroids, and mean survival time is only 8 to 10 months; fewer than 10% of patients are alive after two years, although a fortunate few survive much longer. The more anaplastic the tumor, the more grim the outlook. Survival is substantially shorter with increasing age.

Most *brainstem gliomas* occur in the first two decades of life and account for about 20% of the primary brain tumors in persons of this age group. Histologically they resemble the astrocytomas in the hemispheres, and at autopsy about 50% prove to be glioblastomas. The prognosis is variable, depending on the location and aggressiveness of the tumor, but survival is often less than one year.

Pilocytic astrocytomas are distinguished from other astrocytomas by a distinctive pathologic appearance and *their almost invariably benign biologic behavior.* Typically, they occur in children and young adults and are usually located in the cerebellum, but they are also found in the floor and walls of the third ventricle, the optic chiasm and nerves, and occasionally in the cerebral hemispheres.

Grossly, they often manifest as a mural nodule in the wall of a cyst, but if solid they may be well-circum-

scribed or apparently infiltrative. Microscopically they are only moderately hypercellular and are composed of pilocytic astrocytes, which are bipolar cells with thin, hairlike processes. Rosenthal fibers (p. 706) and microcysts are also characteristic. Vascular endothelial proliferation is often seen, but in this tumor, unlike other astrocytomas, it does not imply an unfavorable prognosis, and other features of anaplasia are almost never seen.

These tumors are extremely slow growing and have the best prognosis of all brain tumors; patients have survived more than 40 years after incomplete resection.

Oligodendroglioma

These tumors account for about 5% of gliomas. They are most frequent in middle life and are found mostly in the cerebral hemispheres.

Grossly, they are well-circumscribed, gelatinous gray masses, often with cysts, focal hemorrhages, and calcifications. **The calcification is often a valuable radiologic diagnostic clue.** As with other gliomas, there is occasionally extension of tumor into the subarachnoid space and dissemination through the CSF. Microscopically, **the tumor is composed of sheets of regular cells with spherical nuclei that contain finely granular chromatin** surrounded by a clear cytoplasmic halo that, although regularly present, is an artifact of fixation. Typically, a delicate vascular network of anastomosing capillaries separates the tumor cells into clusters. The calcifications range from microscopic foci to massive depositions. As many as 50% of these tumors contain foci of astrocytoma that, if anaplastic, determine the prognosis.

Clinically, these tumors have a widely variable prognosis that, according to some experts, depends on the level of anaplasia (grade of the tumor).

Ependymoma

Ependymomas are derived from the single layer of epithelium that lines the ventricles and extends down the center of the spinal cord as the remnant of the central canal. Although they may occur at any age and anywhere in this epithelium, they are particularly likely to occur in the first two decades of life and in the fourth ventricle; they account for some 5 to 10% of primary brain tumors of this age group. In middle life, the spinal cord is their most likely site of occurrence and, in this site, they comprise a large fraction of the intraparenchymal neoplasms.

Grossly, in the fourth ventricle they are typically **solid or papillary masses erupting from the floor of the ventricle and, although often well-demarcated from the adjacent brain, their proximity to the vital medullary and pontine nuclei usually makes complete removal impossible.** With intraspinal tumors this sharp separation makes total removal, and therefore cure, sometimes possible. Microscopically, they are composed of elongated cells with rather regular round to oval nuclei that have abundant granular chromatin. Among the cells there is a fine fibrillary background, which may be very dense. The principal diagnostic features are **ependymal canals** and **rosettes,** in which the tumor cells form epithelial rings and surfaces that closely resemble ependyma, and perivascular **ependymal pseudorosettes,** in which there is a dense array of long, delicate ependymal processes inserted into the wall of the blood vessel, leaving a prominent nucleus-free halo around the vessel. Most tumors are well differentiated, but occasionally they are more anaplastic and may even resemble glioblastomas.

Medulloblastoma

Medulloblastomas occur in the cerebellum and are overwhelmingly tumors of the first two decades of life.

Grossly, they are gray-white expansile lesions that sometimes appear to be quite well-demarcated. In young children they are typically located in the vermis, but in older patients they are more often found laterally in the hemispheres. **Dissemination through the CSF with extensive ependymal and subarachnoid growth often occurs.** Microscopically, medulloblastomas are very cellular tumors with small but moderately pleomorphic nuclei containing variable densities of chromatin and very little, if any, visible cytoplasm. Some do not exhibit any form of differentiation, but in a few, neuronal differentiation occurs, whereas other tumors show glial (spongioblastic) differentiation in the form of spindle cells, with delicate processes containing the specific glial fibrillary acidic protein. Occasionally, both types of differentiation are present in the same tumor. Usually, but not invariably, there are many mitoses in these rapidly growing tumors.

Clinically, patients tend to present with either hydrocephalus or progressive cerebellar signs (such as motor incoordination or unsteadiness of gait), or both. Because of the high frequency of CSF dissemination, treatment generally involves chemotherapy and/or radiation of the entire neuraxis. Currently, about 50% survival at 5 years and 25% at 10 years is achieved, but virtually no long-term survival.

Meningioma

Meningiomas develop from the meningothelial cells of the arachnoid and are thus outside the brain. They comprise about 20% of all primary tumors within the cranial cavity. *Their most common sites of occurrence are in the front half of the cranial cavity—the hemispheric convexity, the falx, the lesser wing of the sphenoid bone, and the olfactory groove.* Other rarer but clinically important locations include inside the cerebral ventricles, the cerebellopontine angle, the foramen magnum, and around the spinal cord. Although they are usually solitary, multiple tumors may occur and are particularly likely in von Recklinghausen's neurofibromatosis type 2. The gene for this disease is located on chromosome 22, and loss of heterozygosity (deletion or reduplication) of a segment of this chromosome is frequent in sporadic menigioma. Intracranial meningiomas are generally tumors of middle and later life and are more common in women (3:2 ratio of women to men). Some tumors grow rapidly during pregnancy.

Grossly, meningiomas are usually irregular, bosselated masses that are firmly attached to the dura and indent the surface of the brain but rarely invade it. Growth occasionally occurs in a plate-like fashion, producing the so-called **meningioma en plaque.** Hyperostosis of the overlying bone is frequently seen, and occasionally superficial invasion of it. The tumors are usually firm and solid, often with a whorl-like pattern on their cut surfaces.

Microscopically, the three major histologic types (**syncytial, fibroblastic,** and **transitional**) form a spectrum. **Syncytial** meningiomas tend to recapitulate the normal appearance of meningothelial cells, with prominent cellular whorls, nodules, and indistinct cell borders. **Fibroblastic** meningiomas have spindle-shaped bipolar cells arranged in interwoven bands and swaths, with more elongated nuclei and denser chromatin. **Transitional** meningiomas express intermediate characteristics and often contain **psammoma bodies** which are roughly spherical, laminated, calcified structures (Fig. 22-17). Psammoma bodies are also often found in small numbers in both syncytial and fibroblastic meningiomas.

Other histologic configurations, such as microcystic variants, are occasionally seen, as are various forms of degenerative change, such as xanthomatous degeneration and bone (or more rarely, cartilage) formation. None of these histologic variants has prognostic significance; all previously described patterns are slow growing and histologically benign. In contrast, meningiomas with papillary architecture have a more aggressive clinical course. Malignant meningiomas do occasionally occur, either as rather ordinary-looking tumors with a high mitotic rate and brain invasion or as more frankly sarcomatous lesions that resemble fibrosarcomas.

METASTATIC TUMORS _____

About 25 to 30% of tumors in the brain are metastatic. They are more frequent in older people, and carcinomas of the lung, breast, skin (melanomas), kidney, and gastrointestinal tract comprise (in descending order of frequency) 80% of the total. Some tumors (e.g., choriocarcinomas) are quite rare but are very likely to metastasize to the brain; others, such as prostate cancers hardly ever do so, even when disseminated to adjacent bone.

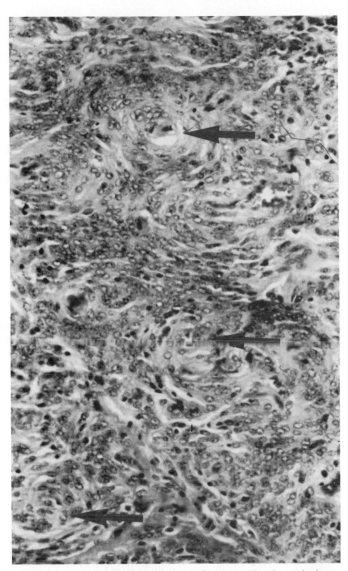

Figure 22-17. A microscopic view of a transitional meningioma disclosing prominent whorls *(arrows)* separated by spindle-shaped, fibroblastic-looking cells. (Courtesy of Dr. Matthew Frosch, Department of Pathology, Brigham and Women's Hospital and Harvard Medical School.)

Typically, metastases are multiple, well-circumscribed, roughly spherical masses, often located at the cortex–white matter junction and surrounded by zones of edematous white matter. Solitary metastases are generally unusual, although with some tumors, notably renal cell carcinomas, single lesions are relatively frequent. **Meningeal carcinomatosis,** with tumor nodules studding the surface of the brain, cord, and intradural nerve roots, is an occasional complication, particularly of small cell and adenocarcinomas of the lung, and carcinoma of the breast. Microscopically, most metastases resemble the primary tumor. In difficult cases, the sharp demarcation between metastatic tumor and the surrounding reactive brain helps to distinguish them from the usually infiltrative primary tumors.

The symptoms and signs are those of any intracranial mass. Occasionally, and particularly with carcinoma of the lung, they may even be the presenting features. In general, treatment is symptomatic and palliative, although the precision attainable with modern neuroimaging and neurosurgical procedures makes resection of some metastases a therapeutic option that gives substantial benefit to some patients.

DEGENERATIVE DISEASES _____

Unlike most other categories of disease such as infections or trauma that may share etiologic origins, the degenerative diseases are unified only by some general clinicopathologic features. Currently, almost all are of obscure origin, and there is no compelling reason to suppose that they have the same, or even a similar type of cause.

There are two major common features of degenerative diseases. (1) They are diseases of neurons and selectively affect one or more functional systems of neurons while they leave others intact. For example, in Parkinson's disease there is selective degeneration of the striatonigral dopaminergic system. (2) They are marked generally by symmetric and progressive involvement of the CNS.

In other ways these diseases differ among themselves quite sharply: some have a clear pattern of heritability, others are sporadic; some exhibit intracellular abnormalities of greater or lesser specificity, whereas in others the pathological process is atrophy and loss of the affected neurons without specific features.

Degenerative diseases that affect similar regions of the brain tend to produce clinical syndromes with many similarities, so that, for example, disease of the cortex may manifest as dementia, and similarly, disorders of the basal ganglia as extrapyramidal movement disorders. A specific diagnosis can often be made only by correlating the clinical and pathologic findings.

For ease of description it is most convenient to group these diseases according to the part or parts of the brain that are *principally* affected, and an abbreviated list is given below. No etiologic connection among the diseases in each group is implied. Only a few of the more important entities (in *italics*) are discussed.

Diseases predominantly affecting the cortex	1. *Alzheimer's disease* (AD) 2. Pick's disease
Diseases of the basal ganglia and brainstem	1. *Huntington's disease* 2. *Idiopathic Parkinson's disease* 3. Postencephalitic Parkinson's disease 4. Striatonigral degeneration 5. Progressive supranuclear palsy 6. Shy-Drager syndrome
Spinocerebellar degenerations	1. Olivopontocerebellar degeneration 2. Friedreich's ataxia 3. Ataxia-telangiectasia
Motor neuron diseases	1. *Motor neuron disease (amyotrophic lateral sclerosis complex)* 2. Werdnig-Hoffman disease 3. Kugelberg-Welander syndrome

The major degenerative diseases with a large cortical component are AD and Pick's disease, and their principal clinical manifestation is *dementia.* There are many other causes of dementia, including cerebrovascular disease, encephalitis, hydrocephalus, Creutzfeldt-Jakob disease, and metabolic diseases.

ALZHEIMER'S DISEASE

Alzheimer's disease (AD) is by far the most common cause of senile dementia; other major causes are cerebrovascular disease and Parkinson's disease. Onset of AD before age 50 is rare. The most frequent initial complaints are impairment of concentration, memory, and other higher intellectual functions. Eventually, usually over the course of five to ten years, progressive memory loss, disorientation, and language dysfunction lead to a mute, immobile state. Death usually results from intercurrent infection. Although at least 10% of cases are clearly familial, most are sporadic.

Grossly, there may be widening of the cerebral sulci, usually most pronounced in the frontal and temporal lobes (Fig. 22–18), with compensatory ventricular enlargement (hydrocephalus ex vacuo). The significant microscopic features are **neurofibrillary tangles** and **senile plaques.**

Neurofibrillary tangles are composed of paired helical filaments (PHF) in the neuronal cytoplasm that encircle and displace the nucleus and are best visualized by silver stains. They are very insoluble and may remain as visible and stainable "ghost" tangles long after the death of the parent neuron. Although characteristic of AD, they are not specific, being found in different regions of the brain in other conditions (e.g., progressive supranuclear palsy).

Senile plaques are found most frequently in the cerebral cortex and limbic structures and range from 20 to 150 μm in diameter. In their classical form, they are composed of focal collections of dilated, tortuous, silver-staining neurites that often contain PHF, arranged around a central amyloid core (Fig. 22–19). This Congo red–positive core is composed primarily of a specific

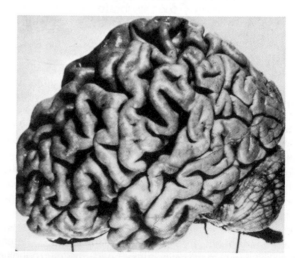

Figure 22–18. Alzheimer's disease. Cerebral atrophy is demonstrated by narrowed gyri and sulcal widening that is particularly marked in the frontal and superior temporal lobes. (Courtesy of Dr. Robert D. Terry.)

The number of plaques and tangles is roughly correlated with the severity of the dementia, but the mechanisms underlying their formation are not yet clear. Biochemically, the most consistent abnormalities are deficiencies of acetylcholine and its associated enzymes (choline acetyl transferase and acetylcholinesterase) in cerebral cortex, hippocampus, and amygdala. The major cholinergic innervation of these structures comes from the nucleus basalis of Meynert, which is severely involved in AD. Deficiencies in other neurotransmitters may be present as well, reflecting the widespread cortical and subcortical damage of the disease.

The basic pathogenic defect in AD remains unclear, although much current work is focused on the βAPP. The gene for this protein is located on chromosome 21, which is also the site of the genetic locus for some cases of familial AD. Recent studies have shown a point mutation in the βAPP gene in some patients with the inherited disease, and mice transgenic for a fragment of βAPP develop features of AD. Interestingly, patients with trisomy 21 reliably develop the pathologic changes of AD and comparable cognitive decline at a relatively young age.

HUNTINGTON'S DISEASE

This disease usually first appears in persons between 20 and 50 years of age and is characterized by extrapyramidal or choreiform movements combined with progressive dementia. It is inherited as an autosomal dominant condition, with the interesting but unexplained feature that those who inherit the disease from their fathers tend to manifest it much earlier in life than those who inherit from their mothers. *This combination of autosomal dominant inheritance with symptomatic onset that is often delayed until middle life turns this disease into a medical sword of Damocles over the heads of the children of affected persons.* For these offspring, an already difficult personal situation is exacerbated by the dilemma as to whether they themselves should have children, and perhaps pass on the disease. Although the defective gene has not yet been isolated, it has been assigned to chromosome 4 on the basis of a closely linked marker that permits presymptomatic diagnosis by analysis of restriction fragment–length polymorphisms. Antenatal diagnosis cannot be far away, putting to rest the dangling sword.

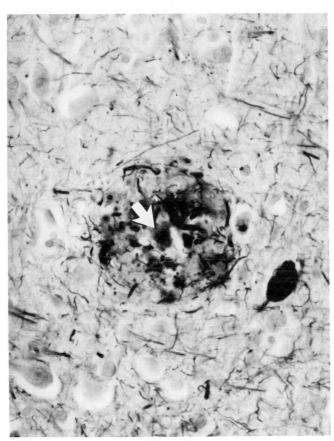

Figure 22-19. Alzheimer's disease. A microscopic detail of a senile plaque composed of tangled, silver-staining neurites about a central amyloid core *(arrow)*. (Courtesy of Dr. Matthew Frosch, Department of Pathology, Brigham and Women's Hospital and Harvard Medical School.)

and unique molecule, the β-amyloid peptide. The β peptide is a fragment of a much larger amyloid precursor protein (βAPP), the normal function and source of which have not yet been elucidated. Formation of β peptide appears to represent the product of one of several possible cleavage patterns of βAPP.

Amyloid angiopathy of the subarachnoid and cortical arteries of the brain is a constant accompaniment to AD, although it varies greatly in its severity. The amyloid, the same as that found in the plaque core, is distinct from proteins associated with the various other systemic amyloidoses (Fig. 22-20).

It is important to appreciate that some plaques and tangles can be found in the brains of older patients who did not show appreciable intellectual impairment. **It is the number and distribution of plaques and tangles that allows the diagnosis of AD to be made, rather than their mere presence.** In AD, plaques and tangles are found throughout the neocortex (with relative sparing of the primary sensory areas) and in the hippocampus and amygdala. Subcortically, there is neuronal depletion from and tangle accumulation in the nucleus basalis of Meynert (cholinergic neurons), the periaqueductal gray matter, and the locus ceruleus.

Grossly, the brain is small (usually less than 1000 gm) with marked caudate and putamen atrophy and conspicuous dilatation of the frontal poles of the lateral ventricles, which, because of the caudate atrophy, have a characteristic concave lateral border. There may be secondary atrophy of the globus pallidus, and there is variable but sometimes conspicuous cortical atrophy. Microscopically, there is severe loss of both large and small neurons from the caudate and putamen that is

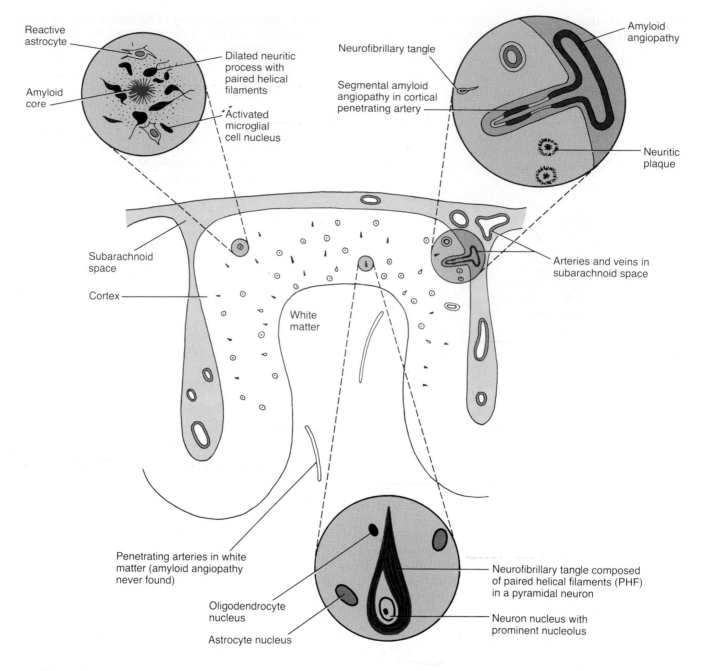

Figure 22-20. Diagrammatic representation of the major microscopic changes in the cortex in Alzheimer's disease. The cortex contains both neuritic plaques and neurofibrillary tangles, and amyloid angiopathy is present in subarachnoid and intracortical arteries and arterioles.

most conspicuous in the dorsal regions of these nuclei (with marked relative preservation of the nucleus accumbens in the inferior striatum). Generally, loss of small neurons seems to precede that of the larger ones. There is also a very marked fibrillary gliosis.

The disease is relentlessly progressive, with an average course of 15 years to death. The precise genetic defect and the pathogenesis of the striatum degeneration are unknown, but recent work on the effects of excitotoxins that can produce selective cell death sug-

gests that these effects may play a role in producing some of the otherwise puzzling morphologic and biochemical changes of this disease.

PARKINSONISM

Parkinsonism is a disturbance of motor function characterized by expressionless faces, stooped posture, slowness of voluntary movements, festinating gait (progressively shortened, accelerated steps), rigidity, and in most cases a characteristic tremor. This type of motor disturbance is seen in a number of different disease states that have in common damage to the nigrostriatal dopaminergic system. It may also be produced by drugs, particularly dopamine antagonists and toxins.

Idiopathic Parkinson's Disease (Paralysis Agitans)

This sporadic, progressive disorder, by far the most common form of Parkinson's disease, has onset between 50 and 80 years of age. The incidence increases with age.

> Grossly, there is only visible depigmentation of the substantia nigra and locus ceruleus. Microscopically, there is loss of melanin-containing neurons from these regions, with extraneuronal pigment deposition and the presence of **Lewy bodies** in some of the remaining neurons. Lewy bodies are intracytoplasmic, eosinophilic, round or elongated inclusions that often have a dense core surrounded by a paler rim.

The loss of the dopamine-containing neurons from the substantia nigra results in dopamine depletion in the striatum because this is the principal site of their axonal projections. The severity of the parkinsonian syndrome is proportional to the severity of the dopamine deficiency. This deficiency, at least in part, can be compensated for by replacement therapy with L-dopa (the precursor of dopamine). Recent studies have also suggested that treatment with monoamine oxidase inhibitors can slow the progression of clinical symptoms in idiopathic Parkinson's disease.

MOTOR NEURON DISEASE (AMYOTROPHIC LATERAL SCLEROSIS COMPLEX)

In this disease complex, neuronal degeneration is concentrated in the upper and lower motor neurons of the pyramidal motor system. The upper motor neurons (UMNs) are in the motor cortex and their axons traverse the internal capsule and corticospinal tract to synapse on the lower motor neurons (LMNs) in the cranial motor nerve nuclei and the motor neurons in the anterior horn of the spinal cord.

> Pathologically, degeneration of UMNs produces axonal loss, atrophy, and pallor on myelin stains of the corticospinal tracts in the lateral columns of the spinal cord. LMNs in the anterior horns and lower cranial nerve nuclei degenerate and the resulting loss of motor axons from the anterior (motor) roots makes them atrophic and gray. In affected muscles there is widespread denervation atrophy of muscle fibers.

The neurologic symptoms exhibited by the patients include UMN (spasticity, hyperreflexia) and LMN (muscle atrophy and weakness) signs. Clinically, the balance and distribution of symptoms and signs reflect the varying distribution and degree of upper and lower motor neuron loss in the different parts of the pyramidal motor system. About two thirds of patients exhibit combined UMN and LMN involvement.

Most cases are sporadic, and there is about a 2:1 male predominance. Onset is typically in late middle age, with a progressive course that invariably has a fatal outcome in 2 to 6 years. The cause and pathogenesis of motor neuron disease are unknown, and there is no known treatment.

DEMYELINATING DISEASES

The major pathologic process in the demyelinating diseases is loss of the myelin sheath that surrounds and insulates the axon. The axons themselves are relatively preserved. *Demyelination results either from damage to the oligodendrocytes that produce the myelin or a direct, usually immunologic or toxic assault on the myelin itself.* The demyelinating diseases, like the degenerative diseases, are a group of conditions bound together by a common pathologic process rather than causal association. However, unlike the degenerative diseases, advances in understanding have allowed the transfer of many disorders previously included in the demyelinating diseases to more explicit etiologic categories. The most important diseases still remaining in this category are *multiple sclerosis* and its variants, and the *acute disseminated encephalomyelitides.* The *leukodystrophies* (inborn errors of metabolism). *PML* (slow virus disease) and *central pontine myelinolysis* (toxic metabolic disorder) are examples of diseases in which the principal pathologic process is demyelination but that are now more appropriately included in other etiologic categories.

MULTIPLE SCLEROSIS

Since multiple sclerosis (MS) was first described by Charcot in 1868, it has been the subject of exhaustive but inconclusive study. The onset is between 20 and 40 years of age in about two thirds of cases, and it is rare before age 15 or after 50 years. The natural history of the disease is as varied as the number and distribution of the "plaques" of demyelination in the brain. *A relapsing and remitting course over many years is by far the most frequent pattern, but some patients have only a few brief episodes of mild disability, whereas others have a relentless downhill course to death in weeks or months.* Common early manifestations are paresthesias, retrobulbar neuritis, mild sensory or motor symptoms in a limb, or cerebellar incoordination. Intellectual deterioration is not usually an early feature. As the disease progresses, remissions become less complete. Although not all patients become totally disabled, the end stage is often marked by unsteadiness of gait, incontinence, and paralysis due to widespread cerebral and spinal cord demyelination.

There is no effective treatment, though ACTH, and sometimes other immunosuppressive agents, are often administered during relapses, with some benefit.

The external appearance of the brain and spinal cord is usually normal. On cut section, multiple, irregularly shaped, sharp-edged areas of demyelination called "plaques" are seen (Fig. 22–21). Their appearance varies with their age; they are initially slightly pink and swollen but later become gray, sunken, and opalescent. Less frequently plaques have a diffuse rather than a sharp border, and they may be only faintly visible (shadow plaques). They occur in gray and white matter, range from barely visible to many centimeters in diameter, and may be sparsely scattered or involve a large fraction of the brain and spinal cord. Although they have a predilection for the angles of the ventricles, they may occur anywhere in the CNS, but often they are bilaterally distributed in a relatively symmetrical fashion.

Microscopically, the earliest loss of myelin is seen around small veins and venules (perivenous demyelination). Mononuclear cells and lymphocytes are present around these vessels (Fig. 22–22). **As the demyelination progresses, the perivenular foci expand to form the macroscopically visible plaques.** In actively enlarging plaques, there is a lymphocytic inflammatory infiltrate at the border between the demyelinated and normal areas. Within the plaque, there is loss of oligodendrocytes but a pronounced reactive astrocytosis and numerous neutral lipid-laden macrophages. The axons traversing the plaque are conspicuously spared. Old inactive plaques have sharply defined edges, profound myelin loss, almost total absence of oligodendrocytes, and scattered fibrillary astrocytes. Although axons are relatively preserved, some loss is often detectable.

Epidemiologically, there is a slight excess of females in the patient population. The disease is also much more prevalent in the temperate latitudes of both the northern and southern hemisphere. It is most frequent in populations of European descent, there being a

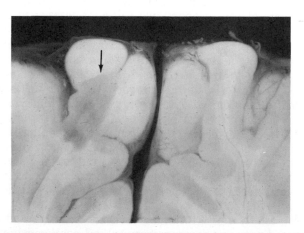

Figure 22–21. A plaque of multiple sclerosis in the subcortical white matter of a cerebral gyrus.

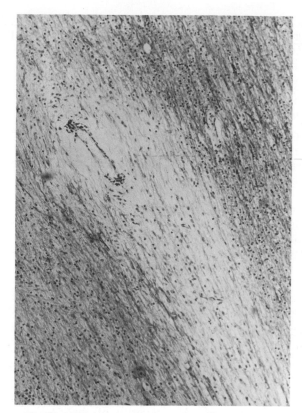

Figure 22–22. Multiple sclerosis. A myelin stain reveals demyelination adjacent to a small vessel in the white matter.

notably low incidence of MS in Oriental, African, and native peoples. Migration studies have indicated that persons who move from regions of high incidence to lower-risk tropical areas (and conversely) tend to retain the risk of their birthplace if they move after about age 15 years but "adopt" the risk of their new home if they move as children.

In isolated communities there is evidence of epidemic outbreaks of MS, notably in the Faroe Islands. This suggests exposure to an environmental agent that can predispose to later development of MS. Much effort has been devoted to the search for a viral association, so far without success.

Genetic studies demonstrate a higher incidence of disease in first-degree relatives, a finding strongly corroborated by the much higher concordance of disease in identical twins than in fraternal twins. There is also an excess of human leukocyte antigens (HLA)-A3, -B7, and -DW2 in northern European and white American patients.

As has been described, the demyelination in MS is marked by a prominent lymphocyte infiltration of both helper (CD4) and suppressor (CD8) cells into the lesions. Current areas of investigation are focused on the repertoire of T-cell receptors used by these lymphocytes, as well as the spectrum of epitopes that they recognize. The precise immunopathogenesis of demyelination in MS is not yet defined, but the evidence suggests that the immunoglobulin oligoclonal bands in the CSF in MS are probably epiphenomena that result from the presence of trapped activated B cells in the

CSF. Although diagnostically helpful, the immunoglobulins are probably not etiologically significant.

The evidence relating to the pathogenesis of MS, although incomplete, suggests a role for genetic, infective, and immune mechanisms, perhaps operating at different times during the patient's life.

NUTRITIONAL, ENVIRONMENTAL, AND METABOLIC DISORDERS

NUTRITIONAL DISEASES

The major vitamin deficiences that affect the adult nervous system involve *thiamine* and *cobalamin.*

Thiamine Deficiency

A deficiency of thiamine has many systemic effects (p. 252) but in addition may result in the Wernicke-Korsakoff syndrome, a peripheral neuropathy, or both conditions. Clinically, these complications are most often but not exclusively encountered in alcoholics but are not solely a toxic effect of the alcohol itself. *Wernicke's encephalopathy* is an acute syndrome with confusion, eye movement abnormalities, and cerebellar signs that rapidly progress to coma but are completely reversible with thiamine if it is administered in time. *Korsakoff's psychosis* is a chronic memory disorder that causes an inability to form new memories or retrieve old ones. Both states are characterized by lesions in the mamillary bodies and the walls of the third ventricle (and sometimes other locations), in which in the early stages there is prominent dilatation of small vessels, sometimes ringed by hemorrhages, and hyperplasia of endothelial cells in the affected regions, replaced later by focal gliosis with hemosiderin deposition. It is probable that the principal effect of the deficiency is on the vessels rather than the nervous system itself.

Cobalamin Deficiency

An inadequacy of vitamin B_{12} (cobalamin), if prolonged, results in pernicious anemia (p. 347) and its *subacute combined degeneration of the cord,* marked by a characteristic vacuolation and degeneration of both axons and myelin in the dorsal columns and lateral white columns of the spinal cord. The gray matter is unaffected.

ENVIRONMENTAL DISEASES

The central and peripheral nervous systems are the target of a very large number of environmental agents, so large indeed that not even a basic outline can be given here. Among the major categories of neurotoxic substances are *metals,* examples of which are lead, mercury, and arsenic; a wide variety of *industrial chemicals,* including aromatic hydrocarbon solvents, organophosphates, methyl alcohol, and carbon disulfide; and a range of *naturally occurring toxins* such as botulinum toxin and the chickpea toxin that causes lathyrism.

Therapeutic agents are an additional important and expanding category of neurotoxins; some of the many types of adverse effects are *peripheral neuropathies* (vinca alkaloids, isoniazid), *tardive dyskinesias* (neuroleptics), and *convulsions* (metronidazole). Many neurotoxic effects have occurred after antitumor treatment. *Ionizing radiation,* as it does in other organs, can cause a vasculopathy leading to tissue ischemia and infarction. *Radiation-chemotherapy leukoencephalopathy* is particularly associated with the combination of radiation and intrathecal or large-dose intravenous methotrexate, and it consists of irregularly shaped, necrotic lesions in the white matter. Even saline solution can have neurotoxic effects. *Central pontine myelinolysis* is associated with overly rapid correction of a low serum sodium level, a therapeutic maneuver made possible by the availability of hypertonic saline solutions. The demyelination can be extensive enough to involve the whole of the basis pontis and may cause complete paralysis.

Ethyl alcohol is a widely used, and abused, neurotoxin. Acutely, it causes CNS depression that can be fatal. With chronic abuse, in addition to the Wernicke-Korsakoff syndrome and a peripheral neuropathy that are associated with thiamine deficiency, there is also a cerebellar vermis degeneration that may be a direct toxic effect of the alcohol (p. 233), or may also be nutritional in origin.

METABOLIC ENCEPHALOPATHY

The blood-brain barrier protects the CNS neurons from all but large or prolonged changes in the levels of electrolytes and metabolites in the blood. When deviations from the norm produce disturbances in cerebral function, it is referred to as a *metabolic encephalopathy.* Frequently encountered causes include diabetes, in which *exogenous insulin-induced hypoglycemia* produces an acute confusional state that can be rapidly reversed by the administration of glucose. *Hyperglycemic coma* is more complicated, with additional changes in pH, electrolytes, and osmotic pressure all contributing to a cerebral dysequilibrium that can persist for several days after the serum levels have been restored to normal. This persistence of dysfunction presumably reflects the time required to reestablish intracellular biochemical normality. Other frequent causes of a more chronic metabolic encephalopathy are uremia, hypercalcemia, and hepatic failure (p. 526). Despite the sometimes profound disturbance in cerebral function, there is often little or no morphologic change, a finding that reflects the predominantly biochemical nature of the cerebral disorder.

Hepatic Encephalopathy

Patients with hepatic failure exhibit a characteristic clinical picture that includes a peculiar flapping tremor of the extremities, called *asterixis,* and a disturbance in consciousness that progresses to coma and even death in severe cases. The course of the encephalopathy parallels that of the hepatic failure. A similar encephalopathy can be produced, and marginally compensated patients precipitated into encephalopathy, by portacaval shunting. Although the severity of the encephalopathy is generally correlated with the raised blood ammonia level seen in hepatic failure, it is probably not a simple toxic effect of the hyperammonemia (p. 528).

Pathologically, *the only consistent abnormality is a proliferation of protoplasmic astrocytes that have enlarged, watery, deformed nuclei, each containing a "glycogen dot" (Alzheimer II astrocytes).* They are found predominantly in gray matter and are especially prominent in the lenticular nucleus, thalamus, red nucleus, substantia nigra, and the deeper layers of the cerebral cortex. Nuclei that are similar but without the glycogen dot can be seen in patients with many of the other metabolic encephalopathies.

Severe and long-standing hepatic encephalopathy can lead to a cerebral degeneration morphologically similar to that seen in Wilson's disease.

INBORN ERRORS OF METABOLISM

The variety and range of effects of the inborn errors of metabolism on the nervous system are legion. Many of these diseases have effects both inside and outside the nervous system; it is the balance of these effects that determines whether they present clinically as diseases of the nervous system or as systemic diseases. For example, in *Wilson's disease* some patients present with hepatic failure with little nervous system involvement, whereas others present with choreoathetosis and dementia, diseases of the brain. In *phenylketonuria* (p. 91), although the inborn error affects all tissues, the clinical manifestations are overwhelmingly in the nervous system. In this section only the neurologic features of the *leukodystrophies* will be considered.

LEUKODYSTROPHIES

These are diseases of white matter in which the inborn error is known, or presumed, to be in the pathways of myelin metabolism. In all the leukodystrophies in which the biochemical defect has been identified, it is a deficiency of a lysosomal degradative enzyme. *Pathologically, the principal process is demyelination, but there may also be some neuronal storage.* From their biochemical origin it might be expected that all leukodystrophies would become manifest in early childhood as symmetric disorders of myelination, affecting the entire neuraxis. In many cases (e.g., the childhood form of metachromatic leukodystrophy) this is so, but in other conditions (e.g., adrenoleukodystrophy) there is marked phenotypic variation in spite of the apparent uniformity of the biochemical defect.

The major leukodystrophies are *metachromatic leukodystrophy,* in which a deficiency of arylsulphatase A leads to the accumulation of galactosyl sulphatides; *globoid cell leukodystrophy* (Krabbe's disease), in which galactocerebroside accumulates because of a lack of galactocerebroside β-galactosidase; and the *adrenoleukodystrophy-adrenomyeloneuropathy* complex, in which the enzyme deficiency is not known but there is defective handling of long-chain fatty acids that leads to a raised C26:C20 fatty acid ratio in many tissues.

THE PERIPHERAL NERVOUS SYSTEM

Unlike the brain, in which there is effectively no regeneration, both *degeneration* and *regeneration* can occur in the peripheral nervous system (PNS). There are three basic degenerative processes: *wallerian degeneration, axonal degeneration,* and *segmental demyelination.*

Wallerian degeneration follows peripheral transection of the axon. Proximal to the site of transection there is degeneration back to the nearest node of Ranvier and, if the transection is sufficiently proximal, there will be chromatolysis in the cell body of the transected axon. Distal to the transection there is degeneration of the axon and its myelin sheath, both of which are digested by the Schwann cells, which proliferate to accomplish this task.

Axonal degeneration occurs when neuronal dysfunction renders the neuron unable to maintain its axon, which therefore starts to degenerate. The degeneration begins at the distal, or peripheral, end of the axon and proceeds back toward the cell body, a process called dying back. There is often chromatolysis of the cell body. Schwann cell proliferation occurs in the region of active axonal degeneration, although it is less pronounced than that seen in wallerian degeneration.

If the neuronal dysfunction can be halted or reversed, regeneration and some recovery of nerve function can occur.

Regeneration occurs by the outgrowth of multiple sprouts from the distal ends of the surviving segments of the axons. If there is no obstruction to their growth, the regenerating axons grow back down the nerve trunk at a rate of about 1 mm per day in association with the Schwann cells, which remain after digesting the degenerated axon. If, as is frequently the case in wallerian degeneration secondary to a traumatic injury, hematoma or fibrous scar prevents the regenerating sprouts from entering the distal stump of the nerve, the obstructed regenerating axons form a tangled, often painful mass of intertwined nerve fibers called an *amputation,* or *traumatic neuroma.*

Segmental demyelination is analogous to demyelination in the brain and is the selective loss of individual myelin internodes with preservation of the underlying axon (Fig. 22–23). After an episode of demyelination, remyelination can be accomplished by the remaining Schwann cells, which proliferate. Repeated episodes of

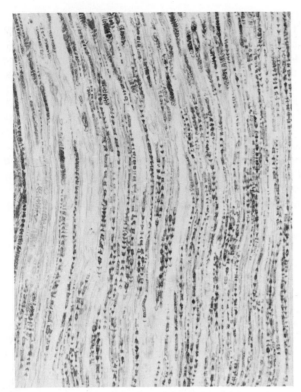

Figure 22–23. Demyelinating neuropathy. A myelin stain reveals focal loss of myelin in a peripheral nerve.

demyelination and remyelination can occur and generate concentric arrangements of alternating Schwann cell processes and collagen, called "onion bulbs," which are found in the hypertrophic neuropathies.

PERIPHERAL NEUROPATHY _____

Both diffuse demyelination and axonal degeneration tend to affect the longest axons first and produce a syndrome called a *polyneuropathy.* Polyneuropathies are typically symmetric and present with distal signs and symptoms in the limbs, such as motor weakness and loss of deep tendon reflexes or a "glove-and-stocking" sensory loss. If the autonomic system is affected, there may be postural hypotension, constipation, and impotence. When there is muscle weakness, axonal degeneration will be accompanied by muscle fasciculation and wasting; in demyelination, where there is conduction failure but no denervation, these are not present. Clinically, different etiologic agents preferentially tend to affect axons of different diameters or to affect sensory, motor, and autonomic axons to different degrees. The balance of symptoms and signs reflects the axons principally involved. Neuropathies may also be mild or severe; they may be acute, subacute, or chronic and may have relapses and remissions.

While many etiologic agents produce generalized damage, there are also pathologic processes that are focal (e.g., vasculitis) and affect only individual nerves, producing a *mononeuropathy* or, if more than one

nerve is affected, a *mononeuropathy multiplex.* When they are widespread, even pathologically focal processes may present, usually asymmetrically, as a *polyneuropathy.*

Most clinical classifications of peripheral neuropathies are based on the type of clinical syndrome that develops. A simplified version of a widely used one is given in Table 22–2, which includes an indication in each clinical category of the predominant pathologic process encountered.

In most clinical series, between 25 and 70% of peripheral neuropathies remain undiagnosed in etiologic terms. Intensive evaluation of a series of such cases has shown that at least 40% were probably hereditary and 20% were inflammatory or demyelinat-

TABLE 22–2. PRINCIPAL NEUROPATHIC SYNDROMES*

Acute ascending motor paralysis with variable sensory disturbance — **Acute demyelinating neuropathies**
  Acute idiopathic polyneuropathy (Landry-Guillain-Barré syndrome)
  Infectious mononucleosis with polyneuropathy
  Hepatitis and polyneuropathy
  Diphtheritic polyneuropathy
  Toxic polyneuropathies (e.g., triorthocresyl phosphate)
Subacute sensorimotor polyneuropathy
  (1) Symmetric — *Mostly axonal neuropathies*
    Alcoholic polyneuropathy and beriberi
    Arsenic polyneuropathy
    Lead polyneuropathy
    Vinca alkaloids and other intoxications
  (2) Asymmetric — *Axonal neuropathies with focal and/or diffuse pathology*
    Polyarteritis nodosa and other arteritides
    Sarcoidosis
Chronic sensorimotor polyneuropathy
  (1) Acquired — *Axonal neuropathies with focal and/or diffuse pathology*
    Carcinomatous
    Paraproteinemias (demyelinating)
    Uremia
    Diabetes
    Connective tissue diseases
    Amyloidosis
    Leprosy
  (2) Inherited — *Mostly chronic demyelination with hypertrophic changes*
    Peroneal muscular atrophy (Charcot-Marie-Tooth disease)
    Hypertrophic polyneuropathy (Déjérine-Sottas disease)
    Refsum's disease
Chronic relapsing polyneuropathy — **Mixed pathology**
  Idiopathic polyneuropathy
  Porphyria
  Beriberi and intoxications
Mono or multiple neuropathy — **Focal axonal or demyelinating pathology**
  Pressure palsies
  Traumatic palsies
  Serum neuritis
  Zoster
  Tumor invasion with neuropathy
  Leprosy

* Adapted from Adams, R. D., Asbury, A. K.: Diseases of the peripheral nervous system. *In* Petersdorf, R. G., et al. (eds.): Harrison's Principles of Internal Medicine. 10th ed. New York, McGraw Hill Book Co., 1983, p. 2158.

ing, but that a significant number remained undiagnosed. In this section only two examples of peripheral neuropathy will be discussed.

Acute Idiopathic Polyneuropathy (Landry-Guillain-Barré Syndrome)

This acute demyelinating neuropathy has been associated with a bewildering variety of antecedent events. About 40% of the cases are associated with a "viral prodrome," with mycoplasma infection in about 5% of the cases, with allergic phenomena in 10%, and with a wide variety of other associations, including surgery, in 25%; the residual 20% of cases have no known antecedent event. It presents as a rapidly progressive motor neuropathy that has variable sensory features. In severe cases, the muscle weakness may be so profound and proceed so far proximally as to produce potentially fatal respiratory paralysis and facial diplegia. The CSF often, but not invariably reveals a strikingly raised protein level and a normal or only slightly raised cell count.

Pathologically, focal inflammatory lesions marked by demyelination and an accumulation of lymphocytes and macrophages are scattered throughout the peripheral nerves, although there is some predilection for the proximal nerve trunks. Ultrastructurally, the earliest visible change is splitting of the myelin lamellae. Later, the myelin is apparently stripped off the axon and digested by macrophages, leaving the Schwann cells intact. This demyelination occurs without, apparently, the direct participation of the lymphocytes.

Diabetic Neuropathy

Peripheral neuropathy frequently develops in diabetes and is often one of its most troublesome complications. One of its outstanding clinical features is its seemingly capricious occurrence—sometimes it is not present even after 40 years of poorly controlled juvenile-onset diabetes, whereas in other cases it may even antedate measurable hyperglycemia. However, most cases occur late in the course of the disease. Clinically, _it is a distal, symmetric, predominantly sensory polyneuropathy, and, pathologically, it is principally an axonopathy_ but with features suggesting the presence of a demyelinating component.

PERIPHERAL NERVE TUMORS

Schwannomas (Neurilemmomas) and Neurofibromas

Despite their usually quite distinct clinical presentations and histologic features, both these tumors derive from Schwann cells. They may occur singly and sporadically or usually multiply in the autosomal dominant neurofibromatosis (p. 88).

Grossly, both types of tumor have a white to gray color and a firm texture, but schwannomas are typically solitary, circumscribed, and encapsulated lesions that are **eccentrically located on proximal nerves or spinal nerve roots.** By contrast, neurofibromas are more often multiple and usually but not invariably unencapsulated; they appear as **fusiform enlargements of distal nerves.** Many are subcutaneous. Microscopically, **schwannomas are distinguished by the presence of areas of high and low cellularity called Antoni A and B tissue, respectively.** In the Antoni A tissue there may be foci of palisaded nuclei called **Verocay bodies.** Blood vessels in schwannomas often have **hyaline thickening,** around which there may be pseudopalisading of the tumor nuclei. **Neurofibromas have none of these features and usually consist of a loose pattern of interlacing bands of delicate spindle cells with elongated, slender, and sometimes wavy nuclei.** In both types of tumor there may be quite marked nuclear pleomorphism and irregularity, and even occasional giant cells, but these are not necessarily ominous findings. Myxoid or xanthomatous degeneration may also be seen. **In schwannomas, no nerve fibers are present in the body of the tumor, although the residual nerve of origin of the tumor may be seen compressed to one side. In neurofibromas, nerve fibers are found scattered throughout the tumor mass, as though it had arisen by expansion of the entire nerve fascicle.** This distinction has practical significance, as the compression of the nerve to one side in a schwannoma may permit its removal without requiring transection of the nerve, a course of action not possible with neurofibromas, in which the entire nerve is involved in the tumor process.

Malignant transformation may occur in both types of tumor, but it is much less frequent in schwannomas. It is characterized by hypercellularity, pleomorphism, mitoses, and blood vessel proliferation, so that the tumor resembles a fibrosarcoma. **Most cases of malignant neurofibroma are encountered in patients with von Recklinghausen's neurofibromatosis** (p. 88).

Except in von Recklinghausen's disease, these are usually tumors of adults, presenting most frequently in the fifth and sixth decades. The most serious symptoms are those produced by schwannomas on the cranial and spinal nerve roots. Patients with acoustic (VIII nerve) schwannomas typically present with complaints of deafness and tinnitus, associated, if the tumor is large enough, with pressure palsies of the adjacent fifth and seventh cranial nerves or evidence of brainstem compression and hydrocephalus. Those with spinal root neurilemmomas may present with signs of slowly progressive cord compression or a cauda equina syndrome. With more distal tumors on nerve trunks there may be local complaints in the territory of the affected nerve, and, finally, there are the ubiquitous subcutaneous "lumps and bumps," which, if of neural origin, usually prove to be neurofibromas.

Bibliography

Agid, Y.: Parkinson's disease: Pathophysiology. Lancet *337:*1321, 1991. (An excellent overview of the pathogenetic theories and morphology of this condition.)

Burns, D. K., Risser, R. C., and White, C. L.: The neuropathology of human immunodeficiency virus infection. The Dallas, Texas, experience. Arch. Pathol. Lab. Med. *115:*1112, 1991. (A large autopsy series from a major metropolitan area of the U.S. that documents the spectrum of opportunistic infections and HIV-related changes in the brain of patients with AIDS.)

Chataway, S. J.: What's new in the pathogenesis of multiple sclerosis? A review. J. Roy. Soc. Med. *82:*159, 1989. (Comprehensive survey of the many factors possibly involved in the causation of this disease.)

Harriman, D. G. F.: Bacterial infections of the central nervous system. *In* Blackwood, W., Corsellis, J. A. N. (eds.): Greenfield's Neuropathology. 4th ed. London, Arnold Ltd., 1984, pp. 236–259. (A comprehensive chapter on CNS infections in a classic text on neuropathology. Includes both bacterial and viral agents.)

Hseuh, C., Reyes, C. V.: Progressive multifocal leukoencephalopathy. Am. Fam. Physician *37:*129, 1988. (A succinct clinical overview with excellent morphologic details.)

Hsiao, K., et al.: Mutation of the prion protein in Libyan Jews with Creutzfeldt-Jakob disease. N. Engl. J. Med. *324:*1091, 1991. (An exciting new report bearing on the strange etiology of Creutzfeldt-Jakob disease and supporting the critical role of prion protein.)

Joachim, C. L., et al.: Clinically diagnosed Alzheimer's disease: Autopsy results in 150 cases. Ann. Neurol. *24:*50, 1988. (An authoritative analysis with careful microscopic evaluation of the characteristic findings in classic cases.)

Kawabata, S., Higgins, G. A., and Gordon, J. W.: Amyloid plaques, neurofibrillary tangles and neuronal loss in brains of transgenic mice overexpressing a C-terminal fragment of human amyloid precursor protein. Nature *354:*476, 1991. (This report and the accompanying editorial [on page 432 of the same journal] provide compelling evidence for the primacy of amyloid deposition in the pathogenesis of AD.)

Klatzo, I.: Pathophysiological aspects of brain edema. Acta Neuropathol. *72:*236, 1987. (A brief consideration of this important condition contrasting the important distinction between vasogenic and cytotoxic edema.)

Meissen, G. J., et al.: Predictive testing for Huntington's disease with use of a linked DNA marker. N. Engl. J. Med. *318:*535, 1988. (One of the milestones in the process of identifying the precise gene responsible for this dread disease.)

Poser, C. M.: Notes on the pathogenesis of subacute sclerosing panencephalitis. J. Neurol. Sci. *95:*219, 1990. (A brief but thoughtful consideration of the possible etiology and pathogenesis of this condition.)

Prusiner, S. B., et al.: Novel mechanisms of degeneration of the central nervous system—prion structure and biology. Ciba Found. Symp. *135:*239, 1988. (A detailed characterization of the putative novel cause of Creutzfeldt-Jakob disease with brief discussions of its possible mechanism of action and effects on the brain.)

Ransohoff, R. M.: Multiple sclerosis: New concepts of pathogenesis, diagnosis, and treatment. Compr. Ther. *15:*39, 1989. (Good state-of-the-art discussion of the most likely pathways leading to the anatomic changes, with excellent clinical correlation.)

Russell, D. S., Ruberstein, L. J.: Pathology of Tumors of the Nervous System. 5th ed. Baltimore, Williams & Wilkins, 1989. (A classic text on brain tumors with detailed morphology and abundant high-quality illustrations.)

Vinken, P. J., Bruyn, G. W., Klawans, H. L., Matthews, W. B.: Handbook of Clinical Neurology. Vol. 51. Neuropathies. Amsterdam, Elsevier Science Publishers, 1987. (A comprehensive review of the major causes of nerve damage and their morphologic consequences. An inclusive reference resource.)

Vinken, P. J., Bruyn, G. W., Klawans, H. L., Toole, J. F. (eds.): Handbook of Clinical Neurology. Vols. 53, 54, 55. Vascular Diseases, Parts I, II, and III. Amsterdam, Elsevier Science Publishers, 1989. (An all-inclusive monumental compendium of all forms of vascular disease of the CNS. Excellent as a reference source for particular problems.)

Vinken, P. J., Bruyn, G. W., Klawans, H. L., Braakman, R. (eds.): Handbook of Clinical Neurology. Vol. 56. Viral Disease. Amsterdam, Elsevier Science Publishers, 1989. (A scholarly collection of all the major viruses that infect the brain with up-to-date material on AIDS and the CNS.)

Vinken, P. J., Bruyn, G. W., Klawans, H. L., Braakman, R. (eds.): Handbook of Clinical Neurology. Vol. 57. Head Injury. Amsterdam, Elsevier Science Publishers, 1990. (A comprehensive epidemiologic, morphologic, clinical, and diagnostic review of all forms of head injury.)

Index

Note: Page numbers in *italics* refer to illustrations; page numbers followed by (t) refer to tables.

A

ABO incompatibility, 343
Abrasion, 236
Abscess, 44
  amebic, 507
  Bartholin's gland, 609
  breast, 634
  Brodie's, 685
  cerebral, 709–710
  hepatic, 561
  pulmonary, 411(t), 424–425
  subperiosteal, 685
Acalculous cholecystitis, 564
Accumulation(s), intracellular, 17–19
Acetaminophen, adverse effects of, 229
Acetylcholine receptors, antibodies to, 698
Acetylsalicylic acid, adverse effects of, 229
Achalasia, of esophagus, 478–479
Acoustic neuroma, 88
Acquired immunodeficiency syndrome (AIDS), 157–165. See also
  Human immunodeficiency virus (HIV) infection.
Acromegaly, 646
Actinomycosis, 416
Activated oxygen species. See *Oxygen-derived free radical(s).*
Adaptation, cellular, 3, *4*, 20–23
Addison's disease, 671(t), 671–673
Adenocarcinoma. See also under specific organs.
  definition of, 173
Adenohypophysis, 643–648. See also *Pituitary gland.*
Adenoma. See also under specific organs.
  definition of, 172
Adenomyosis, of uterus, 615–616
Adenosine deaminase, deficiency of, 156
Adenosis, of vagina, 611
  sclerosing, of breast, 633–634, *634*
ADH (antidiuretic hormone), deficiency of, 648
Adhesins, bacterial, *270*, 270–271
ADP (adenosine diphosphate), release of, by platelets, 67
Adrenal cortex, 666–674
  adenoma of, 673–674, *674*
    Cushing's syndrome and, 668
    hyperaldosteronism associated with, 669
  carcinoma of, 674, *674*
    Cushing's syndrome and, 668
  histoplasmosis of, 672
  hyperfunction of, 666–671
    and adrenogenital syndromes, 669–671
    and Cushing's syndrome, 666–669, *667, 668*
    and hyperaldosteronism, 669
  hyperplasia of, congenital, 669–671
    Cushing's syndrome and, 668, *668*
    diffuse, 668

Adrenal cortex *(Continued)*
    nodular, 668, *668*
  hypofunction of, 671–673
    acute, 671–673
    and Addison's disease, 671–673
    chronic, 673
  in shock, 80
  tuberculosis of, 672
  tumors of, 673–674
Adrenal medulla, 675–677
  neuroblastoma of, 676–677, 677(t)
  pheochromocytoma of, 675(t), 675–676, *676*
  tumors of, 675–677
Adrenalitis, autoimmune, 671, 672, *672*
Adrenocortical insufficiency, acute, 673
  chronic, 671–673
Adrenogenital syndromes, 669–671
Adrenoleukodystrophy, 732
Adult polycystic kidney disease, 464–465, *465*
Adult respiratory distress syndrome (ARDS), 399(t), 399–401, *400*
Adult T-cell leukemia/lymphoma, 360
  HTLV-1 in, 201, *202*
Aflatoxin, as carcinogen, 200, 559
Agammaglobulinemia, Swiss-type, 155–156
  X-linked, 154–155
Aganglionic megacolon, 494–495, *495*
Aging, 10–11
  and amyloidosis, 167, 169
  and atherosclerosis, 278
  and cancer, 182
Agranulocytosis, 351
AIDS (acquired immunodeficiency syndrome), 157–165. See also
  Human immunodeficiency virus (HIV) infection.
AIDS-related complex, 163
Air embolism, 75
Air pollution, 218(t), 218–219, 219(t)
Albinism, 93
Albright's syndrome, 688
Alcohol, metabolism of, 232–233, *233*, 547–549, *549*
  neurotoxicity of, 731
Alcohol-induced injury, 233–234
  to liver, 545–550
Alcoholic cirrhosis, 545–547, *547*, 549, *550*
Alcoholic hyaline, 17, 546, *546*
Alcoholic liver disease, 545–550, *546–548*
Alcoholic pancreatitis, 584
Alcoholism, 233
Aldosteronism, 62, 669
Allergy, 126. See also *Hypersensitivity.*
Alpha$_1$-antitrypsin deficiency, 557–558, *558*
  emphysema associated with, 394
Alpha-fetoprotein, 210, 561, 595

Alpha-thalassemia, 339, 340(t)
Alveolitis, allergic, 405
Alveolus (alveoli), pulmonary, diffuse damage to, 399(t), 399–401, *400*
Alzheimer's disease, 17, 726–727, *726–728*
Amebiasis, 506–507
Amenorrhea-galactorrhea syndrome, 646
Amniotic fluid embolism, 75
Ampulla of Vater, carcinoma of, 566
Amylin, 573
Amyloid, 165–166, *166*. See also *Amyloidosis.*
Amyloidosis, 165–170
    cerebral, 167, 727
    classification of, 167(t)
    clinical aspects of, 170
    diagnosis of, 170
    heredofamilial, 167, 167(t), 168
    immunocyte dyscrasias with, 166–167, 167(t), 376
    localized, 167, 167(t)
    morphologic changes in, 168–169
    pancreatic, in diabetes mellitus, 575, *575*
    pathogenesis of, 167–168, *168*
    primary, 166, 167(t)
    reactive systemic, 167, 167(t)
    secondary, 167, 167(t)
    systemic, 166–167, 167(t)
Amyotrophic lateral sclerosis complex (motor neuron disease), 729
Analgesic(s), adverse effects of, 229
Analgesic nephritis, 456–457
Anaphylactic type hypersensitivity (type I hypersensitivity), 122–126, 123(t), *124*
    clinical manifestations of, 125–126
    mast cells in, 123, *124*, 125, 125(t)
    mediators of, 125(t)
        primary, 123, *124*, 125
        secondary, *124*, 125
Anaphylatoxins, 36
Anaphylaxis, local, 126
    systemic, 125–126
Anaplasia, 175, *175*, 176, *176*, 177
Anasarca, 61, 63
Androblastoma, 626
Anemia, 334(t), 334–350
    aplastic, 349–350
    blood loss and, 334
    chronic disease and, 346
    cobalamin deficiency, 347–349, *349*
    folate deficiency, 347
    hemolytic, 334–345
        drug-induced, 341, 342
        glucose-6-phosphate dehydrogenase deficiency and, 341
        hereditary spherocytosis and, 335–336
        immune, 342(t), 342–343
        malaria and, 344
        microangiopathic, 344
        neonatal (erythroblastosis fetalis), 343–344
        paroxysmal nocturnal hemoglobinuria in, 342
        sickle cell, *336*, 336–337, *337*
        thalassemia and, 338–341
    hemorrhage and, 334
    immunohemolytic, 342(t), 342–343
    iron deficiency, 345–346
    megaloblastic, 346–349
    myelophthisic, 350
    pernicious, 347–349, *349*
        chronic gastritis and, 485
        neurologic changes in, 731
    sickle cell, *336*, 336–337, *337*
    vitamin B_{12} deficiency, 347–349, *349*
Anemic infarct (white infarct), 76
Aneuploidy, 104
Aneurysm(s), 294–298
    aortic, 294–298
        in Marfan's syndrome, 86
        atherosclerotic, *294*, 294–295

Aneurysm(s) *(Continued)*
    berry, 717, *717*
    cerebral, 715, 717, *717*
    Charcot-Bouchard, 715
    dissecting, *296*, 296–298
    syphilitic (luetic), *295*, 295–296
    ventricular, 311
Angina pectoris, 307–308
Angiodyplasia, intestinal, 498
Angiogenesis (neovascularization), 52, *53*
    in tumor growth, 194–195
Angioma, 300
Angiosarcoma, 301
    of liver, 558
Ankylosing spondylitis, 149(t)
    HLA-B27 and, 122, 139
Anorexia nervosa, 244
Anterior pituitary, 643–648. See also *Pituitary gland.*
Anthracosis, pulmonary, 221–222
Antibody-dependent hypersensitivity (type II hypersensitivity), 123(t), 126–127, *127*
Anticoagulant(s), 68–69
Antidiuretic hormone (ADH), deficiency of, 648
Antigen(s), carcinoembryonic, 210, 516–517
    class I, 120–121
    class II, 121, 122
    histocompatibility. See *HLA complex.*
    oncofetal, 204
    tumor-associated, 204
    tumor-specific, 203
Antigen-antibody complexes. See *Immune complex* entries.
Anti–glomerular basement membrane nephritis, *441*, 441–442
Antinuclear antibodies, 139
    in autoimmune diseases, 141(t)
Antiphospholipid antibodies, in systemic lupus erythematosus, 140
    in thrombogenesis, 70
Antithrombin(s), 68
Antral gastritis, 485
Aorta, aneurysm of, 294–298
        Marfan's syndrome and, 86
        atherosclerosis of, *283*, *285*, 294, *294*
        coarctation of, 318
        cystic medionecrosis of, 297, *297*
        dissection of, *296*, 296–298
        rupture of, 64, 86, *237*
        syphilitic lesions of, *295*, 295–296
        thrombi in, *70*
Aortic dissection, *296*, 296–298
Aortic valve, bicuspid, 318
    calcific stenosis of, *23*, 318–319, *319*
    disease of, 319(t)
    infective endocarditis of, *324*
Aortitis, syphilitic, *295*, 295–296
Aphthous ulcers, 474
Aplastic anemia, 349–350
Aplastic crisis, in hereditary spherocytosis, 336
    in sickle cell anemia, 338
Apocrine metaplasia, 632
Apoplexy, pituitary, 645
Apoptosis, 4, *14*, 14–15, *15*
Appendicitis, 520, *520*
Appendix, 519–521
    carcinoid of, 517
    inflammation of, 520, *520*
    tumors of, 521
Arachidonic acid, 36
    metabolism of, cyclooxygenase pathway of, 36, *37*
        in inflammation, 36–37, *37*
        in type I (anaphylactic) hypersensitivity, 125
        lipoxygenase pathway of, 36–37, *37*
ARDS (adult respiratory distress syndrome), 399(t), 399–401, *400*
Argentaffinoma, 325, 517–519, *518*
Arnold-Chiari malformation, 70
Arterial disorders, 277–298
Arteriolosclerosis, 278

Arteriolosclerosis *(Continued)*
    hyaline, 462, *463*
        in diabetes mellitus, 576, *576*
    renal, 462, *463*
        in diabetes mellitus, 577
Arteriosclerosis, 277–285. See also *Atherosclerosis.*
Arteritis, Takayasu's (pulseless disease), 291–292
    temporal (cranial, giant cell), 286(t), 290–291, *291*
Artery (arteries), disorders of, 277–298
    emboli in, 74
    sclerosis of, 277–285. See also *Atherosclerosis.*
    thrombi in, 70, 71
Arthritis, degenerative (osteoarthritis), 693–695, *694, 695*
    gonococcal, 601
    gouty, 99, 101, *101*, 102, 103
    Lyme disease and, 696
    rheumatoid, 145–149, *146, 148*
    suppurative, 696
Arthritis-dermatitis syndrome, 601
Arthropathy, psoriatic, 149(t)
    reactive, 149(t)
Arthus reaction (local immune complex–mediated hypersensitivity), 129–130
Artificial heart valves, complications of, 325, 344
Asbestos bodies, 225, *225*
Asbestosis, 221(t), 223–226, *225*
    and mesothelioma, 432
Aschoff bodies, 320–321, *322*
Ascites, 544–545
Ascorbic acid (vitamin C), 245(t)
    deficiency of, 245(t), 255–256, *256*
Aspergillosis, 424
Aspiration bronchopneumonia, 414
Aspirin, adverse effects of, 229
Asteroid bodies, in sarcoidosis, 403, *404*
Asthma, 389–391, *390*
Astrocytes, 706
Astrocytoma, 721–723, *722, 723*
Atelectasis, 386, *386*
Atherosclerosis, 278–285
    aneurysm due to, *294*, 294–295
    aortic, *283*, 285, 294, *294*
    arterial thrombi in, 73
    diabetes mellitus and, 280, 575, 576, 577
    endothelial injury and, 280–281, *281*
    fatty streak in, *282*, 283, *283*
    foam cells in, 282, *282*
    pathogenesis of, 280
    plaques in, *284*, 284–285, *285*
Atopic asthma (allergic asthma), 389, 390, *390*
Atopy, 126
Atresia, biliary, extrahepatic, 529
    esophageal, 479
    small intestinal, 494
Atrial septal defect, 316–317, *317*
Atrophic gastritis, 486
Atrophic glossitis, in pernicious anemia, 348
    in riboflavin deficiency, 254, *254*
Atrophy, 20–21
    brown, 21
    cerebral, *20*
        in Alzheimer's disease, *726*
        in Huntington's disease, 727
    muscular, 697
    pituitary, 648, *648*
    testicular, in cryptorchidism, 591
        in Klinefelter's syndrome, 109, 591, *591*
Atypical pneumonia, 411(t), 415–416
Autoantibodies, 136
Autoimmune adrenalitis, 671, 672, *672*
Autoimmune chronic hepatitis, 541
Autoimmune diseases, 40, 136(t), 136–154. See also specific disorders.
    antinuclear antibodies in, 141(t)
    genetic factors in, 139

Autoimmune diseases *(Continued)*
    mechanisms of, 138–139
    microbial agents in, 139
Autoimmune sialadenitis, 477
Automobile accidents, 236
Autophagy, *15*, 15–16
Autosomal dominant diseases, 85(t), 85–88. See also specific disorders.
Autosomal recessive diseases, 85(t), 88–98. See also specific disorders.
Autosplenectomy, in sickle cell anemia, 337
Axonal degeneration, 732
Azo dyes, as carcinogens, 200
Azotemia, 438

B
B cell(s), 118
    antigen-induced transformation of, *356*
    differentiation of, *355*
    in AIDS, 161, 162(t)
    in Burkitt's lymphoma, 202
    in chronic lymphocytic leukemia, 369–370
    in Epstein-Barr virus infection, 202
    in HIV infection, 161, 162(t)
    in lupus erythematosus, 141
    in non-Hodgkin's lymphoma, 355
    in rheumatoid arthritis, 147
    in systemic lupus erythematosus, 141
B-cell tolerance, 137
Bacterial adhesins, *270*, 270–271
Bacterial endocarditis, 71, 323–324, *324*
Bacterial endotoxins, 271
Bacterial epiglottitis, 434
Bacterial exotoxins, 271–272
Bacterial infection(s), 262(t), 262–263
    AIDS and, 164(t)
    cell injury in, 270–272
    diarrhea due to, 504(t)
    gastrointestinal, 266
    pyogenic, 44, 272
    shock due to, 78, 78(t), 81
Bacterial pneumonia, 411(t), 411–414, *412, 413*
Bacterial prostatitis, 596
Bacterial sialadenitis, 477
Balanoposthitis, 589
Bantu siderosis, 555
Barbiturates, effects of, on smooth endoplasmic reticulum of liver, 16, *16*
Barlow's disease, 319
Barr body (sex chromatin), 107
Barrett's esophagus, 482
Bartholin's gland, abscess of, 609
    cysts of, 609
Basal cell carcinoma, of skin, 211–212, *212*
Basement membrane, glomerular, 438
    antibodies to fixed antigens in, 441
    in repair, 47
    in spread of cancer, *197*, 197–198
    thickening of, in diabetes mellitus, 575, *576*
Basic fibroblast growth factor, 52
Basophils, Crooke's hyaline degeneration of, 668
bcl-2 oncogene, 187, 189
Benign hypertension, 459
Benign nephrosclerosis, 462, *463*
Benign prostatic hypertrophy, 596–597, *597*
Benign tumor(s), 172, 174–179
    vs. cancer, 174–179, 180(t)
Berger's disease (IgA nephropathy), 451
Beriberi, 253, *253*
Berry aneurysm, 717, *717*
Berylliosis, 221(t), 226
Beta$_2$-amyloid protein, 166
Beta cell lesions, 580, *580*
Beta-globin gene, 338–339, *339*
Beta$_2$-microglobulin, 166

Beta-thalassemia, 338–339, *340*, 340(t), 341
Bile, 562, *562*
Bile infarcts, 553
Biliary atresia, extrahepatic, 529
Biliary cirrhosis, *552*, 552–554, 554(t)
Biliary tract, 561–566
  extrahepatic, atresia of, 529
    obstruction of, and cirrhosis, 552, 553, 554
  intrahepatic, carcinoma of, 559, 560
  obstruction of, 526
    and cirrhosis, 552, 553, 554
Bilirubin, conjugated, 526
  elevated serum levels of, 525(t), 525–526, 527(t)
  metabolism of, 525, *525*
    disorders of, 524–526, 525(t). See also *Jaundice (icterus)*.
      hereditary, 526, 527(t)
  unconjugated, 525
    elevated serum levels of, 525, 525(t), 527(t)
Biotin, 245(t)
  deficiency of, 245(t)
Birbeck granules, 377
Blackwater fever, 345
Bladder, urinary, carcinoma of, 469–470, *470*
    infection/inflammation of (cystitis), 455
    papilloma of, 469
    stones in, 466
    tumors of, *469*, 469–470
Blastomycosis, 424
Bleeding. See *Hemorrhage*.
Blood cell(s), disorders of, 334–377
  red, disorders of, 334–350
  white, disorders of, 350–377. See also *Leukocyte(s)*.
Blood clot. See *Coagulation*.
Blood flow, and thrombogenesis, 69
Blood pressure. See also *Hypertension*.
  regulation of, 460, *460*
    kidney in, 460–461
    renal vasodepressor substances in, 461
    renin-angiotensin system in, 460, *460*
    sodium homeostasis in, 460–461
Blood transfusion, adverse reaction to, 126
Blood vessels, diseases of, 277–304. See also *Vascular diseases*.
  formation of, 52, *53*
    in tumor growth, 194–195
Bone, 681–693
  congenital diseases of, 681–682
  deficit in mineralization of, 684
  fibrous dysplasia of, 688
  hereditary diseases of, 681–682
  in Albright's syndrome, 688
  in Brodie's abscess, 685
  in hypertrophic osteoarthropathy, *688*, 688–689
  in osteomalacia, 248, 684
  in osteoporosis, 682(t), 682–684, *683*
  in rickets, 247, 684
  infections of, 685–686
  metabolic diseases of, 682–684
  multiple myeloma involving, 375, *375*
  Paget's disease of, *686*, 686–688, *687*
  parathyroid disease affecting, 684
  renal disease affecting, 684
  tuberculosis of, 686
  tumors of, 689–693
  von Recklinghausen's disease of, 684
Bone marrow, fibrosis of, 373
  in agranulocytosis, 351
  in aplastic anemia, 349
  in folate deficiency anemia, 347
  in hemolytic anemia, 334
  in iron deficiency anemia, 346
  in leukemia, 370, *370*
  in neutropenia, 351
  in pernicious anemia, 348
  in polycythemia vera, 372
  transplantation of, 135
Borrelia burgdorferi infection, 696

Bowel. See *Intestine*.
Bowen's disease, of penis, 589
  of vulva, 610
Bradykinin, 34
Brain, 706–732
  abscess of, 709–710
  AIDS involving, *161*, 164–165, 711
    pathogenesis of, 162–163
  amyloid deposition in, 167, 727
  aneurysms in, 715, 717, *717*
  arteriovenous malformations in, 718
  astrocytoma of, 721–723, *722*, *723*
  atrophy of, *20*
    in Alzheimer's disease, *726*
    in Huntington's disease, 727
  cells of, 706
  concussion of, 719
  contrecoup lesions of, 719
  contusion of, 719
  copper deposition in, 557
  degenerative diseases of, 725–729
  demyelinating diseases of, 729–731
  edema of, 64, 707
    death due to, 64
  emboli in, 714
  ependymoma of, 724
  glioblastoma multiforme of, 722, *722*, *723*
  hemorrhage in, 64, *65*, 715–718
  herniation of, 707, *707*
  herpes simplex virus infection of, 711, *711*
  HIV infection of, *161*, 164–165, 711
    pathogenesis of, 162–163
  in galactosemia, 93
  in hydrocephalus, 707–708
  in lead poisoning, 230, *230*
  in shock, 713
  infarction of, 72, 713, 714, *715*
  infections of, 709–713
  ischemia of, 713
  laceration of, 719–720
  lacunae in, 714–715
  laminar necrosis of, 713
  Lewy bodies in, in parkinsonism, 729
  medulloblastoma of, 724
  metabolic disorders of, 732
  microaneurysms in, 715
  neurofibrillary tangles in, in Alzheimer's disease, *726*
  oligodendroglioma of, *723–724*
  parenchymal hemorrhage in, 715–717, *716*
    with subarachnoid hemorrhage, 718
  parenchymal injury to, 719–720
  plaques in, in Alzheimer's disease, 726–727, *727*
    in multiple sclerosis, 730
  thrombi in, 714
  trauma to, 718–720
  tumors of, 720–725, 721(t)
  vascular diseases of, 713–718
Brancher glycogenosis, 94
Branhamella catarrhalis infection, and pneumonia, 414
Breast(s), 631–641
  abscess of, 634
  cancer of, *178*, 636–641
  carcinoma in situ of, lobular, 639, *639*
  carcinoma of, 636–641
    clinical course of, 640–641
    colloid (mucinous), 638–639
    fibrocystic changes and, 634, *635*
    in male patients, 641
    infiltrating ductal, 638, *638*
    infiltrating lobular, 639
    intraductal, 637–638
    lobular, 639
    medullary, 638
    scirrhous, 638, *638*
    staging of, 640(t)
  comedocarcinoma of, 637–638

Breast(s) *(Continued)*
cysts of, 632, *632*
disease of, *631*, 631–641
ductal ectasia of, 634–635
enlargement of, in male patients, 641
fibroadenoma of, *178*, 635–636, *636*
fibrocystic changes in, 631–634
in gynecomastia, 641
inflammation of, 634–635
intraductal papilloma of, 636
Paget's disease of, 639
phyllodes tumor of, 636
sclerosing adenosis of, 633–634, *634*
traumatic fat necrosis of, 635
tumors of, 206, 635–641
Brenner tumor, 625
Brodie's abscess, 685
Bronchial carcinoid, 432
Bronchiectasis, 397–398, *398*
Bronchiolitis, chronic, 397
Bronchioloalveolar carcinoma, 429–430
Bronchitis, chronic, *396*, 396–397
Bronchogenic carcinoma, 428(t), 428–432, *430*, *431*
Bronchopneumonia, 411, 412, *412*, *413*. See also *Pneumonia*.
aspiration and, 414
Bronchopulmonary dysplasia, 388
Bronze diabetes, 554
Brown atrophy, 21
Brown tumors, of bone, 684
Bruton's disease, 154–155
Budd-Chiari syndrome, 530
Buerger's disease (thromboangiitis obliterans), 286(t), 293
Bulimia, 244
Bullous emphysema, *395*, 395–396
Burkitt's lymphoma (small noncleaved lymphoma), 359, *360*, 361(t)
chromosomal translocation and, 188–189, *189*
Epstein-Barr virus infection and, 202
Burn(s), 237–238
thermal, 237–238
Bursitis, 696

C
C3, activation of, 34, *35*, 36
in inflammation, 36
C3a, in inflammation, 36
C3b, in inflammation, 36
C5, in inflammation, 36
C5a, in inflammation, 28–29, 36
induction of leukocyte adhesion by, 28–29, *30*
Cachexia, cancer and, 206–207
Café-au-lait spots, in neurofibromatosis, 88
Caisson disease, 75
Calcific aortic stenosis, *23*, 318–319, *319*
Calcification, 22–23
dystrophic, 14, 22, 23, *23*
metastatic, 22, 23
Calcifying pancreatitis, 584
Calcium stones, in gallbladder, 562, 563, 563(t)
in kidney, 465–466
Calymmatobacterium granulomatis infection, 605
Campylobacter jejuni infection, 507
Cancer, 171–214. See also specific types, e.g., *Carcinoma*.
agents causing, 198–203
aging and, 182
AIDS-associated, 164
anaplasia in, 175, *175*, 176, *176*, 177
antibody-based therapy for, 206
cachexia associated with, 206–207
characteristics of, 174–181
chemicals causing, 199(t), 199–200
chromosomal alterations and, 193, 372(t)
clinical features of, 206–210
death rate from, 181, *182*
diagnosis of, 208–210, *209*

Cancer *(Continued)*
recombinant DNA technology in, 114–115
diet and, 259
differentiation in, 175–177, 180(t)
DNA viruses and, 202–203
effects of, on host, 206–208
environmental influences in, 182, 182(t)
epidemiology of, 181–184
epithelial. See *Carcinoma*.
etiology of, 198–203. See also *Carcinogenesis*.
extracellular matrix invasion by, *197*, 197–198
gene amplification and, 189, *189*, 193
geographic factors in, 181–182
grading of, 208
growth factor/growth factor receptors and, 186, 186(t), *188*
growth fraction in, 194, *194*
growth of, 178–179, 193–198, *194*, *195*
rate of, 177, 180(t)
hematogenous spread of, 180, *196*, 198
hereditary, 183(t), 183–184
heterogeneity in, 195, *195*
hormone secretion in, 206
host immune defenses against, 203–205, *204*
hyperplasia and, 22
immunodeficiency and, 205
immunotherapy for, 205–206
incidence of, 181, *181*
invasion by, local, 178–179, *197*, 197–198
latent period in, 194
lymphatic spread of, 180
mesenchymal. See *Sarcoma*.
metastasis of, 179–180, 180(t), *196*, 198
molecular basis of, 184–193, *185*. See also *Carcinogenesis*.
nomenclature applied to, 172–174, 174(t)
occupational, 182(t)
oncogenes and, 185–189, 186(t), *188*, 372(t)
oncogenic viruses and, 201–203
oncoproteins and, 185–187, 186(t)
paraneoplastic syndromes in, 207–208, 208(t)
pathogenesis of, *185*. See also *Carcinogenesis*.
pediatric cases of, 182–183
predisposing disorders in, 183, 183(t), 184
progression of, *195*, 195–196
radiation-induced, 200–201, 240–241
ras proteins and, 187, 188
rate of growth in, 177, 180(t)
RNA viruses and, 201
spread of, 180, *196*, *197*, 197–198
staging of, 208
sun exposure and, 201
suppressor genes and, 189–192
Trousseau's sign in, 72, 299
venous thrombosis in, 72, 299
vs. benign tumors, 174–179, 180(t)
Cancer cachexia, 206–207
Cancer suppressor genes, 189–192
Candidiasis, 423–424
esophageal, 423–424
oral, 423, 474
pulmonary, 424
vaginal, 423
Canker sores, 474
Cannabis sativa, effects of, 235–236
Capillary hemangioma, 301
Caplan's syndrome, 222
Caput medusae, 545
Carbohydrates, intracellular accumulation of, 18
Carbon dust, intracellular accumulation of, 19
Carbon monoxide, toxic effects of, 231–232
Carbon tetrachloride (CCl_4), liver injury due to, 9, *10*
Carbuncle, 44
Carcinoembryonic antigen, 210, 516–517
Carcinogen(s), chemical, 199(t), 199–200
occupational, 182, 182(t)
radiation, 200–201, 240–241
viral, 201–203

Carcinogenesis, 184–193, *185*
  chemical, 199(t), 199–200
  chromosomal alterations in, 193, 372(t)
  diet in, 259
  DNA viruses in, 202–203
  gene amplification in, 189, *189*, 193
  growth factors and growth factor receptors in, 186, 186(t), *188*
  loss of cancer suppressor genes in, 189–192
  molecular basis of, 192–193, *193*
  nuclear regulatory factors in, 186(t), 187
  oncogenes in, 185–189, 186(t), *188*, 372(t)
  oncogenic viruses in, 201–203
  oncoproteins in, 185–187, 186(t)
  radiation, 200–201, 240–241
  ras proteins in, 187, *188*
  RNA viruses in, 201
  signal-transducing proteins in, 186(t), 187, *188*
  sun exposure in, 201
Carcinoid, 517–519, *518*
  bronchial, 432
Carcinoid syndrome, 325, 519(t)
Carcinoma, 172–173, 174(t). See also *Cancer*; *Neoplasia*; *Soft tissue tumors*; *Tumor(s)*; and specific types.
  basal cell, of skin, 211–212, *212*
  bronchioloalveolar, 429–430
  bronchogenic, 428(t), 428–432, *430*, *431*
  embryonal, of testis, 592–593, *594*, 595(t)
  epidermoid. See *Carcinoma, squamous cell.*
  hepatocellular, 558–561, *560*
  large cell, of lung, 430
  of adrenal cortex, 674, *674*
  of ampulla of Vater, 566
  of biliary tract, 559, 560, 566
  of breast, 636–641
  of cervix, 612–615, *613–615*
  of colon, 514–517, *516*
  of colorectum, 514–517, *516*
  of endometrium, 619–620, *620*
  of esophagus, 482–483, *483*, 483(t)
  of extrahepatic biliary tract, 566
  of gallbladder, 565–566
  of kidney, 467–469, *468*
  of larynx, *435*, 435–436
  of liver, 558–561, *560*
  of lung, 428(t), 428–432, *430*, *431*
  of nasopharynx, 434–435
  of oral cavity, *177*, 475–476, *476*
  of pancreas, *585*, 585–586, *586*
  of parathyroid glands, 665
  of penis, 589
  of pituitary gland, 647
  of prostate, 597–599, *598*
  of rectum, 514–517
  of skin, 210–212, *211*, *212*
  of stomach, 490–493, 491(t), *492*
  of testis, 592, 593, *593*, 594, 595(t)
  of thyroid gland, 659–663
  of urinary bladder, 469–470, *470*
  of uterine cervix, 612–615, *613–615*
  of uterus, 619–620, *620*
  of vulva, 610
  renal cell, 467–469, *468*
  small cell, of lung, 430–431, *431*
  squamous cell, 173, 210
    of bladder, 470
    of cervix, 614
    of esophagus, 482, 483
    of larynx, 435, *435*
    of lung, 429, *430*
    of oral cavity, *177*, 475–476, *476*
    of penis, 589
    of skin, 210–211, *211*
    of vulva, 610
  transitional cell, of bladder, 469–470, *470*

Carcinoma in situ, 176, 179
  of breast, 639, *639*
  of cervix, *179*, 613, *614*
  of oral cavity, *476*
  of skin, 211
  of uterine cervix, *179*, 613, *614*
Carcinomatosis, meningeal, 725
Cardiac. See also *Heart.*
Cardiac amyloidosis, 167, 169, 170
Cardiac death, sudden, 313–314
Cardiac sclerosis, 530
Cardiogenic shock, 78, 78(t), 81
Cardiomyopathy, 327–329, *328*
  dilated (congestive), 327–328, *328*
  hypertrophic, *328*, 328–329, *329*
  ischemic, 313, *314*
  restrictive (obliterative), *328*, 329
Carotid artery, occlusion of, 714
Caseous necrosis, 13–14
Cat scratch disease, 42(t), 354
Cataracts, in galactosemia, 93
Cavernous hemangioma, 301, *301*
  of liver, *301*, 558
CCl₄ (carbon tetrachloride), liver injury due to, 9, *10*
CD4+ helper T cell(s), 118
CD8+ cytotoxic T cell(s), 118
Celiac sprue, 508–509
Cell(s), 3, 47–48
  accumulations in, 17–19
  acute injury to, 12–15
  adaptation by, 3, *4*, 20–23
  aging of, 10–11, *11*
  apoptosis of, 4, *14*, 14–15, *15*
  atrophy of, 20, 20–21. See also *Atrophy.*
  bacteria-induced injury to, 270–272
  calcification of, 14, 22–23, *23*
  death of, 3–4, *4*, 6, 12
  degeneration of, vacuolar, 12
  diphtheria toxin effects on, 271, *271*
  dysplasia of, 176, *176*. See also *Dysplasia.*
  dystrophic calcification of, 14, 22, 23, *23*
  fatty change in, 12, 17–18
  growth of, 47–52
    competence factors in, 48
    control of, 48–52
    cycle of, 47–48, *48*
      Rb protein in, 192, *192*
    cyclins in, 50
    G proteins in, 49–50
    growth factor receptor activation in, 48–49, *49*
    growth factors in, 48, 51–52
    growth-related genes in, 50
    guanosine triphosphatase (GTP) activating protein in, 49, 50
    inhibition of, 50–51
      transforming growth factor beta in, 51
    macrophages in, 51–52
    molecular events in, 48–50, *49*
    progression factors in, 48
    protooncogenes in, 50
    ras proteins in, 49, 50
    second messengers in, 49
    signal transduction in, *49*, 49–50
    transcription factors in, 50
    tyrosine kinase in, 49
  heterotopic rests of, 174
  hydropic change in, 12
  hyperplasia of, 21–22. See also *Hyperplasia.*
  hypertrophy of, 3, 21, *21*. See also *Hypertrophy.*
  injury to, 3–19, *4*
    aging and, 10–11
    apoptosis in, 4, *14*, 14–15, *15*
    bacteria-induced, 270–272
    causes of, 4–5
    diphtheria toxin in, 271, *271*
    free radical mediation of, 8, *8*, 9, *10*

Cell(s) *(Continued)*
  infection-induced, 268–272
  irreversible, 3
  mechanisms of, 5–12
  morphologic changes in, 12–15
  necrosis in, 3–4, 12–14, *13, 14*
  reversible, 3
    morphologic changes in, 12
  subcellular responses in, 15–17
  labile (continuously dividing), 47–48
  lysosomal storage in, 16, 95
  melanin accumulation in, 19
  metaplasia of, 22, *22.* See also *Metaplasia.*
  metastatic calcification of, 22, 23
  necrosis of. See *Necrosis.*
  permanent, 48
  quiescent (stable), 48
  rests of, heterotopic, 174
  swelling of, 12, *12*
  vacuolar degeneration of, 12
  virus-induced injury to, 268–270, *269*
Cell cycle, 47–48, *48*
  Rb protein in, 192, *192*
Cell membrane, injury to, 6–7, 7(t), 12. See also *Cell(s), injury to.*
  lipid peroxidation of, 9
Cellular immunity. See *T cell(s).*
Cellulitis, 44
Central hemorrhagic necrosis, of liver, 529–530
Central nervous system, 706–732. See also *Brain.*
Centrilobular (centriacinar) emphysema, 392, *392, 393*
Cerebellar hemorrhage, 716
Cerebral. See also *Brain.*
Cerebral abscess, 709–710
Cerebral amyloidosis, 167, 727
Cerebral aneurysm, 715, 717, *717*
Cerebral edema, 64, 707
Cerebral hemorrhage, 64, *65,* 715–718
Cerebral herniation, 707, *707*
Cerebral infarction, 72, 713, 714, *715*
Cerebral trauma, 718–720
Cervicitis, 611–612
  nongonococcal, 602
Cervix, 611–615. See also *Uterine cervix.*
Chagas' disease (trypanosomiasis), 326, 327, 479
Chancre, soft, 604–605
  syphilitic, *272,* 603
Chancroid, 604–605
Charcot-Bouchard aneurysm, 715
Chediak-Higashi syndrome, 17, 33
Chemical injury, 226–236
  nontherapeutic toxic agents in, 229–236, 230(t)
  therapeutic agents in, 227–229, 228(t)
Chemical mediators, of inflammation, 25, 33–39, *34,* 38(t)
  of type I (anaphylactic) hypersensitivity, 123, *124,* 125, 125(t)
Chemotaxis, in inflammation, *29,* 30, 36
  defective, 33
Chief cell hyperplasia, of parathyroid glands, 665, *665*
Child(ren). See also *Infant(s)* and *Newborn.*
  AIDS transmission to, 158
  cancer in, 182–183
  cretinism in, 649
  croup in, 434
  cystic fibrosis in, 91
  galactosemia in, 93
  liver disease in, 528–529
  malnutrition in, *243,* 243–244
  medulloblastoma in, 724
  neuroblastoma in, 676
  phenylketonuria in, 91
  polycystic kidney disease in, 465
  Reye's syndrome in, 529
  syphilis in, 604
  vaginitis in, 611(t)
Chlamydial infection, 262(t), 263
  genital, 602, 602(t), 605

Chlorpromazine, liver injury due to, 542
Chocolate cysts, 616, *617*
Chokes, 75
Cholangiocarcinoma, 559, 560, 566
Cholangiolitis, 561
Cholangitis, 561
  sclerosing, primary, *552,* 553, 554, 554(t)
Cholecystitis, 564–565
  acalculous, 564
  acute, 564, 565, *565*
  chronic, 564, 565
Cholelithiasis, 561–564, *563,* 563(t)
Cholera, 504, *505*
Cholestasis, 526
Cholesterol. See also *Lipoprotein(s).*
  metabolism of, 87
Cholesterol stones, 562, *563,* 563(t)
Chondroma, 172, 689
Chondrosarcoma, *692,* 692–693
Choriocarcinoma, in pregnancy, 630–631, *631*
  of ovary, 626
  of testis, 593–594, 595(t)
Choristoma, 174
Christmas disease, 383
Chromatin, sex (Barr body), 107
Chromosome(s), 105, *105*
  abnormalities of, 104–111
  alterations in, and cancer, 193, 372(t)
  deletion of, 106, *106*
  Philadelphia, in chronic myeloid leukemia, 189, *189,* 193, 369
  ring, 106, *106*
  sex, disorders of, 107, 109–111
  translocation of, 105–106, *106*
    and Burkitt's lymphoma, 188–189, *189*
    and cancer, 193, 372(t)
    and chronic myeloid leukemia, 189, *189,* 193, 369
    and Down's syndrome, 107, *109*
    and leukemia, 193, 372(t)
    and lymphoma, 193, 372(t)
    balanced reciprocal, 106, *106*
    Robertsonian (centric fusion type), 106, *106*
      and production of Down's syndrome, 107, *109*
Chronic granulomatous disease, 33
Chronic ischemic heart disease, 313, *314*
Chronic lymphocytic leukemia, 369–370
Chronic myeloid leukemia, 369, *369*
Chronic obstructive pulmonary disease (COPD), 391–398
Chrysotile, 224
Churg-Strauss syndrome, 286(t), 289–290
Chylocele, 590
Chylomicrons, 86–87, 279(t)
Chylothorax, 433–434
Chylous effusion, 330
Cigarette smoking, 219–220, *220,* 220(t)
  and atherosclerosis, 280
  and emphysema, 394
  and lung cancer, 428
Cirrhosis, 542, 542–558
  alcoholic, 545–547, *547,* 549, *550*
  α_1-antitrypsin deficiency and, 557, *558*
  biliary, *552,* 552–554, 554(t)
  classification of, 543
  extrahepatic obstruction and, 552, 553, 554
  fibrosis in, 542, 546, 547, *547,* 549, *551*
  hepatocellular carcinoma associated with, 559
  macronodular, 543, 546, 551, *551*
  micronodular, 543, 546, *547*
  pigment, 554–556, 555(t), *556*
  portal hypertension associated with, 544
  postnecrotic, 550–552, *551*
  Wilson's disease and, 557
Class I antigens, 120–121
Class II antigens, 121, 122
Class III proteins, 121
Clear cell adenocarcinoma, of vagina, 611

Clonal anergy, and self-tolerance, 137, *137*
Clonal deletion, and self-tolerance, 136–137, *137*
Clonality, of tumors, 184, *184*
Clostridial toxins, 271–272
Clostridium difficile infection, 506, *506*
Clotting system. See *Coagulation.*
Clubbing, of fingers, *688*, 688–689
Coagulation, 67–69, *68*, 378
    disorders of, 381–383
    endothelial cells and, 66, *66*
    in hemostasis, 67–69
    in inflammation, 36
    intravascular, disseminated, 73, 378–380
Coagulation cascade, *68*
Coagulative necrosis, 3–4, 13, *13*
Coagulative thrombi (red thrombi, stasis thrombi), 70
Coagulopathy, consumption, 73, 378
Coal macule, in lungs, 222
Coal nodule, in lungs, 222
Coal workers' pneumoconiosis, 19, 221(t), 221–223, *222*
Coarctation of aorta, 318
Cobalamin (vitamin B$_{12}$), 245(t)
    deficiency of, 245(t), 347–348, 731
Cocaine, effects of, *234*, 234–235
Coccidioidomycosis, 42(t), 423, *423*
Codman's triangle, 691
Cold antibody immunohemolytic anemia, 342–343
Colitis, amebic, 506–507
    Crohn's, 499
    pseudomembranous, *Clostridium difficile* infection and, 506, *506*
    ulcerative, 501–503, *502*
        vs. Crohn's disease, 501, 502(t), *503*
Collagen(s), 55
    abnormal, in Ehlers-Danlos syndromes, 104
    excess production of, in cirrhosis, 543, *543*
    in wound healing, 55
        degradation of, 56–57
        synthesis of, 53, 56
    platelet adhesion to, 67
Collagenase(s), in tumor invasion, 198
    in wound healing, 56–57
Colloid adenoma, of thyroid, 658
Colloid carcinoma (mucinous carcinoma), of breast, 638–639
Colloid goiter, 653
Colon, adenocarcinoma of, *175*, 516
    adenoma of, *510*, 510–514, *512*, *513*, 514(t)
        malignant transformation of, 192, *193*, 513, *514*
    amebiasis of, 506–507
    cancer of, 514–517
        adenoma-carcinoma sequence in, 192, *193*, 513, *514*
        diet and, 259, 515
        staging of, *517*, 517(t)
        ulcerative colitis and, 502
    Crohn's disease of, 499
    diverticular disease of, 495–497, *496*
    hemorrhoids in, 298, 498–499, 545
    hyperplastic polyp of, *510*, 511
    in familial adenomatous polyposis, 514, 514(t)
    in Gardner's syndrome, 514, 514(t)
    in Hirschsprung's disease (megacolon), 494–495, *495*
    inflammation of, 503–507
    juvenile polyp of, 511
    nonneoplastic polyps of, 511
    papilloma of, *173*
    polyp of, *510*, 510–514, *512*, *513*, 514(t)
        malignant transformation of, 192, *193*, 513, *514*
    pseudomembrane formation in, *Clostridium difficile* infection and, 506, *506*
    shigellosis of, 505
    sporadic adenomatous polyps of, 511–513
    tubular adenoma of, *510*, 512, *512*
    tumors of, 510–517
    ulcerative colitis, 501–503, *502*
    villous adenoma of, *510*, 512–513, *513*
Colorectal carcinoma, 514–517, *516*. See also *Colon, cancer of.*

Coma, hepatic, 527–528, 731–732
    hyperglycemic, 731
    nonketotic hyperosmolar, 574
Combined immunodeficiency, severe, 155–156
Comedocarcinoma, of breast, 637–638
Common variable immunodeficiency, 156
Compensatory emphysema, 395
Competence factors, in cell growth, 48
Complement system, 34
    activation of, 34, *35*, 36
    in inflammation, 34, 36
Compound nevus, 212, *213*
Compression atelectasis (passive atelectasis, relaxation atelectasis), 386, *386*
Concussion, 719
Condyloma, 603, 604
    cervical, 613
    vulvar, 609
Condyloma acuminatum, 604, 609
Condyloma latum, 603, 609
Congenital disease, definition of, 85
Congenital heart disease, 315(t), 315–318. See also individual types.
Congenital malformations, 103, 103(t)
Congenital megacolon (Hirschsprung's disease), 494–495, *495*
Congestion, 64
    hepatic, chronic passive, 306, *307*, 529
    pulmonary, left ventricular failure and, 64, 306
Congestive cardiomyopathy, 327–328, *328*
Congestive heart failure, 62, 63, *63*, 305–307
Congestive splenomegaly, 306
Congo red dye, in diagnosis of amyloidosis, 168
Conjugated hyperbilirubinemia, 525(t), 525–526, 527(t)
Connective tissue, disease of, 136
    repair by, 52–58. See also *Wound healing.*
    tumors of, 701–703
Conn's syndrome, 669
Constrictive pericarditis, 330
Consumption coagulopathy, 73, 378
Contraceptives, oral, adverse effects of, 72–73, 228–229
Contraction atelectasis (cicatrization atelectasis), 386, *386*
Contrecoup lesions, 719
Contusion, 236
    cerebral, 719
Coombs' test, 342
COPD (chronic obstructive pulmonary disease), 391–398
Copper, defective metabolism of, 557
Cor bovinum, 295
Cor pulmonale, 315, 315(t)
Cornea, copper deposition in (Kayser-Fleischer ring), 557
Coronary heart disease, 307–314, *308*. See also *Ischemic heart disease.*
Corrigan's pulse, 295
Corticotroph adenoma, 646–647
Corynebacterium diphtheriae infection, 271
    laryngeal, 434
Councilman bodies, 15, 537
Coup lesions, 719
Cranial arteritis (giant cell arteritis, temporal arteritis), 286(t), 290–291, *291*
Craniotabes, 250
Crescentic (rapidly progressive) glomerulonephritis, 450(t), 450–451, *451*
CREST syndrome (limited scleroderma), 151, 153
Cretinism, 649
Creutzfeldt-Jakob disease (subacute spongiform encephalopathy), 712–713
Crib death, 388(t), 388–389
Crigler-Najjar syndrome, 527(t)
Crohn's disease, 499–501, *500*
    vs. ulcerative colitis, 501, 502(t), *503*
Crooke's hyaline degeneration, of basophils, 668
Croup, 434
Cryoglobulinemia, 376
Cryptococcosis, 42(t), 424, 709
Cryptorchidism, 591

Cushing's disease, 646, 667
Cushing's syndrome, 666–669, *667, 668*
Cushing's ulcer, 486
Cutaneous T-cell lymphoma, 360
Cyanocobalamin (vitamin B$_{12}$), deficiency of, 245(t), 347–348
Cyclin(s), in cell growth, 50
Cyclooxygenase pathway, of arachidonic acid metabolism, 36, *37*
Cyclosporin, for transplant rejection, 135
Cyst(s), Bartholin's gland, 609
   breast, 632, *632*
   chocolate, 616, *617*
   dermoid, of ovary, 625, *625*
   follicle, 621
   Gartner's duct, 610
   luteal, 621
   nabothian, 612
   ovarian, 621–622
   renal, 464
   vulvar, 609
Cystadenocarcinoma, appendiceal, 521
   ovarian, 623, 624, *624*
Cystadenofibroma, ovarian, 625
Cystadenoma, 172
   appendiceal, 521
   ovarian, 623, *623*, 624
Cystic fibrosis, 89–91
Cystic medionecrosis, of aorta, 297, *297*
Cystic teratoma, of ovary, 625, *625*
Cystine stones, 466
Cystitis, 455
Cytogenetic disorders, 104–111
Cytokine(s), 38, 119–120
   fibrogenic, 51
   in fever, 45
   in granuloma formation, 131, *131*
   in hematopoiesis, 119–120
   in immunotherapy for cancer, 205–206
   in inflammation, 38, 45, 119
   in lymphocyte growth and differentiation, 119
   in natural immunity, 119
   in rheumatoid arthritis, 147
   in type I hypersensitivity, 125
   in type IV hypersensitivity, 131, *131*
Cytologic smears, in diagnosis of cancer, 209, *209*
Cytomegalovirus infection, 425–426, *426, 427*
Cytoskeleton, 16
   abnormalities in, 16–17
   and cell membrane injury, 7
Cytotoxic edema, 707
Cytotoxic T cell(s), 118
   in host defenses against cancer, 204
   in transplant rejection, 132, *133*
   in type IV hypersensitivity, 131–132
Cytotoxicity, antibody-dependent cell-mediated, in type II hypersensitivity, 126–127, *127*
   complement-mediated, in type II hypersensitivity, 126, *127*
Cytotrophoblast, 630

D

Dane particles, 533, *533*
Decompression sickness, 75
Defibrination syndrome, 73
Degenerative joint disease, 693–695, *694, 695*
Delayed type hypersensitivity, 123(t), *130*, 130–131
Delta agent hepatitis, 534
Dementia, in niacin deficiency, 254
   senile, 726
Demyelinating disease, 729–731
Dendritic cells, 119
Dense-deposit disease, 448

DeQuervain's thyroiditis, 657
Dermatomyositis, 153–154
Dermoid cyst, of ovary, 625, *625*
Desmoid(s), 58, 703
Desmoplasia, 175
Diabetes insipidus, 648
Diabetes mellitus, 569–580
   atherosclerosis in, 280, 575, 576, 577
   basement membrane thickening in, 575, 576
   bronze, 554
   clinical manifestations of, 579
   glomerular lesions in, 576–577, *577*
   glycogen deposition in, 18
   hyaline arteriosclerosis in, 576, *576*
   infections in, 579
   insulin-dependent, 569, 570(t)
   insulitis in, 571, 575
   islet cell lesions in, 575
   ketoacidosis in, 574
   Kimmelstiel-Wilson lesion in, 576
   metabolic derangements in, 574, *574*
   microangiopathy in, 575
   morphologic changes in, 574–579, *575–578*
   necrotizing papillitis in, 578
   nephropathy in, 576–578, *577, 578*
   neuropathy in, 578–579, 734
   non-insulin-dependent, 569, 570(t)
   nonketotic hyperosmolar coma in, 574
   ocular lesions in, 578
   pancreatic lesions in, 575, *575*
   pathogenesis of, 570–574, *571, 573*
   pyelonephritis in, 578
   renal lesions in, 576–578, *577, 578*
   retinopathy in, 578
   vascular lesions in, 575–576
Diarrhea, 504(t), 504–505
Differentiation-specific antigens, 204
Diffuse alveolar damage (DAD), 399(t), 399–401, *400*
DiGeorge's syndrome, 155
Dihydropteridine reductase, deficiency of, 92
Diphtheria, laryngitis in, 434
Diphtheria toxin, 271, *271*
Disaccharidase, deficiency of, 507
Discoid lupus erythematosus, 142
Dissecting aneurysm, 296, 296–298
Disseminated gonococcal infection, 601
Disseminated intravascular coagulation, 73, 378–380
Diverticulum (diverticula), colonic, 495–497, *496*
   esophageal, 479
   Meckel's, 494, *494*
   small intestinal, 494, *494*, 495
   Zenker's, 479
DNA oncogenic viruses, 202–203
Donovan bodies, 605
Down's syndrome (trisomy 21), 107
Drug abuse, 232(t), 232–236
Drug-induced hemolysis, 341, 342
Drug-induced injury, 227–229, 228(t)
Dubin-Johnson syndrome, 526, 527(t)
Duchenne's muscular dystrophy, 697–698
Ductus arteriosus, patent, 317
Duncan disease, 363
Duodenal ulcer, *45*, 487, 488, 489
Duret hemorrhage, 707, 720
Dysentery, bacillary, 505
Dysfunctional uterine bleeding, 616–617
Dysgerminoma, ovarian, 626
Dysplasia, 176, *176*
   bronchopulmonary, 388
   cervical, *176*
   fibrous, of bone, 688
Dysplastic nevi, 212–213
Dystrophic calcification, 14, 22, 23, *23*
Dystrophy, muscular, *697*, 697–698
   vulvar, 608

E
Eastern equine encephalitis, 711
EBV. See *Epstein-Barr virus.*
Ecchymosis, 64
Ectopic pregnancy, 628–629, *629*
Edema, 61–64
    causes of, 61–63, 62(t)
    cerebral, 64, 707
    heart failure and, 62, 63, *63*
    inflammatory, 27, 61
    liver diseases and, 62, 545
    lymphatic obstruction in, 62
    morphologic changes in, 63–64
    noninflammatory, 61
    pitting, 63
    pulmonary, 64, *64*, 306
    renal disease and, 62, 63
    sodium retention and, 61, 62, 63
    subcutaneous, 63, 64
Edwards' syndrome, *108*
Effusion, pericardial, 330
    pleural, 433
Ehlers-Danlos syndromes, 103–104
Electrical injury, 238
Elephantiasis, 62
Embolism, 73–75
    air, 75
    amniotic fluid, 75
    arterial, 74
    cerebral, 714
    fat, 74–75
    gas, 75
    paradoxical, 317
    pulmonary, 74, *74*, 406–408, *407*, *408*
    saddle, 74, 407, *407*
    septic, 77
    venous, 74
Embryonal adenoma, of thyroid, 658, *658*
Embryonal carcinoma, of testis, 592–593, *594*, 595(t)
Embryonal rhabdomyosarcoma, 702
Emphysema, 392–396
    bullous, *395*, 395–396
    centriacinar (centrilobular), 392, *392*, *393*
    compensatory, 395
    distal acinar (paraseptal), 393
    mediastinal (interstitial), 396
    panacinar (panlobular), *392*, 393, *393*
    pathogenesis of, 394, *394*
    senile, 395
Empty sella syndrome, 648, *648*
Empyema, of gallbladder, 565
Encephalitis, 709–712
    viral, *710*, 710–712, *711*
Encephalopathy, hepatic, 527–528, 731–732
    ischemic, 713
    metabolic, 731–732
    Reye's syndrome and, 528
    spongiform, 712–713
    Wernicke's, thiamine deficiency and, 253, 731
Enchondroma, 689
Endemic goiter, 653
Endocardial fibroelastosis, 329
Endocarditis, 323–325
    infective, 71, 323–324, *324*
    Libman-Sacks, 142–143, *143*, 325
    Loeffler's, 329
    marantic, 324
    nonbacterial thrombotic, 71, 324
    systemic lupus erythematosus and, 142–143, *143*, 325
    valvular vegetations in, 71, 323, 324, *324*
Endocrine pancreas, 569–581. See also *Pancreas.*
Endodermal sinus (yolk sac) tumor, of testis, 593
Endometrioid tumors, 624
Endometriosis, 616, *616*, *617*
Endometritis, 615

Endometrium, adenomyosis of, 615–616
    carcinoma of, 619–620, *620*
    estrogens and, 227–228
    hyperplasia of, 22, 617–618, *618*
    oral contraceptives and, 227–228
    polyps of, 618
    tumors of, 618–620
Endoplasmic reticulum, dilatation of, in cell injury, 12
Endothelial cells, adhesion molecules of, 29, 29(t)
    anticoagulant properties of, 66, *66*
    antiplatelet properties of, 65
    fibrinolytic properties of, 66
    in angiogenesis, 52, *53*
    in inflammation, 27, *28*
    injury to, in atherosclerosis, 280–281, *281*
        in disseminated intravascular coagulation, 378
        in hemostasis, 66
        in inflammation, 27, *28*
        in systemic sclerosis, 151
        in thrombogenesis, 69, *69*
    procoagulant properties of, 66, *66*
Endotoxemia, diffuse alveolar damage in, *400*
    shock in, 78, *79*
Endotoxins, bacterial, 271
Entamoeba histolytica infection, 266, 506–507
Enteritis, regional, 499
Enterocolitis, infectious, 503–507, 504(t)
    ischemic, 497
Enteropathogenic *Escherichia coli*, 505
Enteropathy, gluten-sensitive, 508
    hemorrhagic, acute, 497–498
        shock and, 80, *81*
Enterotoxin-induced diarrhea, 504–505
Environmental diseases, 217–259. See also individual pollutants.
Environmental pollution, 217–226, 218(t)
Enzymatic fat necrosis, of pancreas, 14, *14*, 581, 582, *582*
Eosinophil(s), in inflammation, 42
Eosinophilic granuloma, 377
Ependymal cells, 706
Ependymoma, 724
Epidermal growth factor, 51
    in wound healing, 56(t)
Epidermoid carcinoma. See *Squamous cell carcinoma.*
Epididymitis, 595
Epidural hematoma, 718, *719*
Epiglottitis, bacterial, 434
Epilepsy, post-traumatic, 720
Epispadias, 589
Epithelioid cells, in granuloma, 130, 131
Epstein-Barr virus infection, and Burkitt's lymphoma, 202
    and infectious mononucleosis, 351–353
    and nasopharyngeal carcinoma, 202, 434
Erosive gastritis, 484–485
Erythema chronicum migrans, in Lyme disease, 696
Erythema marginatum, in rheumatic fever, 322
Erythroblastosis fetalis, 343–344
Erythrocyte(s), disorders of, 334–350
Erythrocytosis, 350
Erythroleukoplakia, 475
Erythroplasia, 475
Esophagitis, 481–482
Esophagus, 478–483
    achalasia of, 478–479
    atresia of, 479
    Barrett's, 482
    cancer of, 482–483, *483*, 483(t)
    candidiasis of, 423–424
    diverticula of, 479
    hiatal hernia of, 480, *480*
    inflammation of, 481, 482
        reflux and, 481–482
    lacerations of, 480
    motor disorders of, 478–479
    rings of, 479
    stenosis of, 479

Esophagus *(Continued)*
 systemic sclerosis involving, 152
 varices of, 298, 480–481, *481*, 545
 webs of, 479
Essential hypertension, 459
 mechanisms of, *461*, 461–462
Estrogen(s), adverse effects of, 227–228
  and breast cancer, 637
  and gallstones, 563
  and vaginal carcinoma, 611
 deficiency of, and osteoporosis, 682
Ethanol. See *Alcohol* entries.
Ewing's sarcoma, 693
Exocrine pancreas, 581–586. See also *Pancreas.*
Exophthalmos, Graves' disease and, 652
Exostoses, 689
Exotoxins, bacterial, 271–272
Extracellular matrix, in spread of cancer, *197*, 197–198
 in wound healing, 55–56, *57*
Extrahepatic biliary tract, atresia of, 529
 obstruction of, and cirrhosis, 552, 553, 554
Extravascular hemolysis, 335
Extrinsic asthma, 389
Exudate, 27
Exudation, leukocyte, 28–30
Eye(s), destruction of, in vitamin A deficiency, 246, *247*
 dry, in Sjogren's syndrome, 149, 150
 lesions of, in diabetes mellitus, 578
 sarcoidosis involving, 404

F
FAB classification, of acute myeloblastic leukemia, 368(t)
Factor VIII deficiency, 382–383
Factor VIII–von Willebrand factor complex, 381–382, *382*
Factor VIII–von Willebrand factor deficiency, 381–382
Factor IX deficiency, 383
Fallopian tubes, 620–621
 implantation of fertilized ovum in, 628–629, *629*
 inflammation of, 620–621
Familial adenomatous polyposis, 514, 514(t)
Familial dysplastic nevus syndrome, 213
Familial hypercholesterolemia, 86–88
Familial Mediterranean fever, 167
Fasciitis, nodular (pseudosarcomatous), 700(t), 702–703
Fat, malabsorption of, cystic fibrosis and, 91
Fat embolism, 74–75
Fat necrosis, enzymatic, of pancreas, 14, *14*, 581, *582*
 traumatic, of breast, 635
Fat-soluble vitamins, 245(t)
 deficiency of, 245(t), 245–252
Fatty change, in cells, 12, 17–18
 in heart, 18
 in liver, 12, 17, *18*
  alcohol-induced, 17, 545, 546
  Reye's syndrome and, 529, *530*
 in myocardium, 18
Fatty streak, in atherosclerosis, *282*, 283, *283*
Felty's syndrome, 149
Female genital system, 607–631. See also specific parts.
Ferritin, in hemochromatosis, 556
 in iron metabolism, 345
Ferruginous bodies, 225
Fetal adenoma, of thyroid, 658
Fetor hepaticus, liver failure and, 527
Fever, blackwater, 345
 familial Mediterranean, 167
 in inflammation, 45
Fibril(s), amyloid, 165–166, *166*. See also *Amyloidosis.*
Fibrillin, defects in, in Marfan's syndrome, 86
Fibrinoid necrosis, of blood vessel walls, in hypersensitivity, 129, *130*
Fibrinolytic system, 68

Fibrinolytic system *(Continued)*
 in inflammation, 36
 promotion of activity of, endothelial cells in, 66
Fibrinous inflammation, 44, *44*
Fibroadenoma, of breast, *178*, 635–636, *636*
Fibroblast growth factor(s), 51
 basic, 52
 in wound healing, 56(t)
Fibroblastic meningioma, 725
Fibrocystic changes, in breast, 631–634
Fibrocystic disease, of pancreas, 90
Fibroelastoma, papillary, 331
Fibroelastosis, endocardial, 329
Fibrogenic cytokine(s), 51
Fibrolamellar carcinoma, of liver, 560
Fibroma(s), 172, 700(t), 701
 ovarian, 627, *627*
Fibromatosis, 700(t)
 aggressive, 58, 703
 deep, 700(t)
 superficial, 700(t)
Fibronectin, 55, *55*
 in wound healing, 55–56
Fibroplasia, in repair, 47
 pathologic, 58
Fibrosarcoma, 700(t), 701
Fibrosis, bone marrow, 373
 hepatic, cirrhosis and, 543, 549, *551*
  pipestem, *273*
  schistosomiasis and, *273*
 in inflammation, 42
 progressive massive, pulmonary, 222, *222*
 pulmonary, idiopathic, 401–403, *402, 403*
 systemic sclerosis and, 151
Fibrous atheroma, 284, *284*
Fibrous dysplasia, of bone, 688
Fibrous histiocytoma, 700(t), 701
 malignant, 700(t), 701–702, *702*
Fiedler's myocarditis, 327
Filariasis, 62
Fine-needle aspiration biopsy, 209
Fingers, clubbing of, *688*, 688–689
Fish oil–rich diet, beneficial effects of, 37
Flapping tremor, 527
Floppy valve syndrome, 86, 319
Foam cells, in atherosclerosis, *282*, *282*
Focal glomerulonephritis, 451
 in systemic lupus erythematosus, 143
Focal nodular hyperplasia, of liver, 558
Focal segmental glomerulosclerosis, *447*, 447–448
Folate, 245(t)
 deficiency of, 245(t), 347
Follicle cysts, of ovary, 621
Follicular adenoma, of thyroid gland, 658, *658*
Follicular carcinoma, of thyroid gland, 661, *661*
Follicular center cells, 356, *356*
Follicular hyperplasia, of lymph nodes, *353*, 353–354
Follicular lymphoma, *357*, 357–358, 361(t)
Folliculitis, 44
Foreign body granuloma, 43
Foreign body–type giant cells, 131
Fragile X syndrome, 111, *111*
Free radical(s), 8
 and inflammation, 10, 38
 and injury, to cell membranes, 7
  to cells, 8, *8*, 9, 10
French-American-British classification, of acute myeloblastic leukemia, 368(t)
Frontal bossing, 250
Full-thickness burns, 237
Fulminant hepatitis, 537–538
Fungal infection(s), 262(t), 263–264, 422–424. See also specific diseases.
 AIDS and, 164(t)
Furuncle, 44

G
Galactitol deposition, 92, 93
Galactokinase, deficiency of, 92
Galactose, metabolism of, *92*
Galactose-1-phosphate uridyl transferase, deficiency of, 92
Galactosemia, 92–93
Gallbladder. See also *Biliary tract.*
  calcium bilirubinate stones in, 562, 563, 563(t)
  carcinoma of, 565–566
  cholesterol stones in, 562, *563*, 563(t)
  empyema of, 565
  hydrops of, 565
  in cholelithiasis, 561–564, *563*, 563(t)
  inflammation of, 564–565, *565*
  mucocele of, 565
  pigment stones in, 562, 563, 563(t)
  porcelain, 565
  stones in, 561–564, *563*, 563(t)
Gallstones, 561–564, *563*, 563(t)
  pancreatitis associated with, 583
Gammopathy, monoclonal, 166–167, 375
Ganglioneuroma, 677
Gangliosidosis, 95(t), 97
Gangrene, of bowel, 497
  of lung, 425
Gardner's syndrome, 514, 514(t)
Gartner's duct cysts, 610
Gas embolism, 75
Gastric carcinoma, 490–493, 491(t), *492*
  advanced, 491(t), *492*
  early, 492
  ulcerative, 492, *492*
    vs. peptic ulcer, *493*
Gastric polyps, 490, 491(t)
Gastric ulcers, 486–490
Gastrinoma, 580–581
Gastritis, 484(t), 484–486
  acute (erosive, hemorrhagic), 484–485
  antral, hypersecretory, 485
  atrophic, 486
  chronic (nonerosive), 485–486
  fundal, 485
  Helicobacter, 485, *485*, 486, 488
  type A, 485
  type B, 485
Gastroenteritis, salmonellosis and, 505–506
Gastrointestinal tract, 473–521. See also specific organs.
  amyloidosis of, 169
  effects of shock on, 80, *81*
  helminthic infection of, 267
  radiation injury to, *241*, 242
  systemic sclerosis involving, 152
Gaucher cells, 95, *96*
Gaucher's disease, 95–96, *96*
Gene(s), amplification of, in carcinogenesis, 189, *189*, 193
  cancer suppressor, 189–192
  histocompatibility. See *HLA complex.*
Gene diagnosis, direct, 111–113, *112, 113*
Gene therapy, 84
Genetic diseases, 83–115. See also specific diseases.
  autosomal dominant, 85(t), 85–88
  autosomal recessive, 85(t), 88–98
    enzyme deficiency and, 89, *89*
  chromosomal, 104–111
    numerical, 104, 107, *108*
    structural, 104–106, *106*
  diagnosis of, 111
    allele-specific oligonucleotide probes in, 112, *113*
    direct detection of mutations in, 111–113, *112, 113*
    linkage analysis in, 113–114
    molecular, 83, 111–114
    recombinant DNA technology in, 83–84, 111–114
    restriction fragment length polymorphisms in, 113–114, *114*
  incidence of, 85
  mendelian, 85(t), 85–98

Genetic diseases *(Continued)*
  multifactorial, 98
  preneoplastic, 183, 183(t)
  sex-linked, 98
  variable modes of transmission of, 103–104
  X-linked, 85(t), 98
Genetic heterogeneity, 85
Genetics, 83
  classical, 83, *84*
  reverse, 83–84, *84*
Genital system, female, 607–631. See also specific parts.
  male, 589–606. See also specific parts.
Genome-based theories, of aging, 11, *11*
Germ cell tumor(s), of ovary, *622*, 625–626
  of testis, 591–595, 592(t), *592–594*, 595(t)
German measles (rubella), and congenital heart disease, 316
  and diabetes mellitus, 572
Gestational trophoblastic disease, 628–631
Ghon complex, 418, *419*
Giant cell(s), foreign body–type, 131
  HIV infection and, 159, *161*
  in granuloma, 43, *43*, 131
  in tumors, 175, *175*
  Langhans' type, 131
Giant cell arteritis (cranial arteritis, temporal arteritis), 286(t), 290–291, *291*
Giant cell myocarditis, 327
Giant cell tumor, of bone, *690*, 690–691
Giant fibroadenoma, of breast, 636
Giardiasis, 266, *266*, 504(t)
Gigantism, 645–646
Gilbert's syndrome, 526, 527(t)
Gingivostomatitis, herpetic, 474
Glial cells, 706
Glial nodules, 710
Glioblastoma multiforme, 722, *722, 723*
Glioma, brainstem, 723
Globoid cell leukodystrophy, 732
Glomangioma (glomus tumor), 302
Glomerulonephritis. See also *Nephritis.*
  acute proliferative (poststreptococcal, postinfectious), 449–450, *450*
  chronic, *452*, 452–453
  crescentic (rapidly progressive), 450(t), 450–451, *451*
  diffuse proliferative, 449–450, *450*
  focal (proliferative), 451
  immunologic mechanisms of, 440–443
  lupus erythematosus and, 143–144, *144, 145*
  membranoproliferative, *448*, 448–449
  membranous, 445–447, *446*
Glomerulosclerosis, *447*, 447–448
  diabetes mellitus and, 576–577, *577*
  focal segmental, *447*, 447–448
  nodular, 576
  reduction in renal mass and, 444, *444*
Glomerulus (glomeruli), 438, *439*, 440
  diseases of, 438–453, 440(t)
    pathogenesis of, 440–444
  injury to, *443*, 443–444
Glossitis, atrophic, in pernicious anemia, 348
  in riboflavin deficiency, 254, *254*
Glucocerebrosidase, deficiency of, 95
Glucose-6-phosphatase, deficiency of, 94(t)
Glucose-6-phosphate dehydrogenase, deficiency of, 341
Glucose transport units (GLUTs), 570
Gluten (gliadin), intolerance to, 508
Glycogen, intracellular accumulation of, 18, 93, 94(t)
  metabolism of, 93, *94*
Glycogen nephrosis, 578
Glycogen storage diseases, 18, 93–94, *94*, 94(t)
Glycosylation, nonenzymatic, in diabetes mellitus, 573
GM₂ gangliosidosis, 97, *97*
Goiter, 653–655
  colloid, 653
  diffuse, 653
  endemic, 653

Goiter *(Continued)*
  multinodular, 653–655, *654*
  nontoxic, 653–655
  plunging, 654
  simple, 653
  sporadic, 653
  toxic, 653–655
Goitrogens, 653
Goldblatt kidney, 461
Gonadotroph adenoma, 647
Gonococcal arthritis, 601
Gonorrhea, 600–601, *601*
Goodpasture's syndrome, 405–406
Gout, 99–103
  arthritis in, 99, 101, *101*, 102, 103
  classification of, 99, 99(t)
  clinical aspects of, 103
  in Lesch-Nyhan syndrome, 100
  inheritance of, 100–101
  morphologic features of, 101–103
  pathophysiology of, 100
  primary, 99, 99(t), 100
  renal lesions in, *102*, 103
  secondary, 99, 99(t), 100
  tophi in, 99, 102, *102*, 103
Grading, of cancer, 208
Graft(s), rejection of, 132–134, *134*
    prevention of, 135
Graft-versus-host disease, 135
Granular cell tumor, 700(t)
Granulation tissue, 52, *52*
  exuberant, 58
  in primary healing, 53
  in secondary healing, 54
Granuloma(s), 42–43, *43*, 130
  eosinophilic, 377
  epithelioid cells in, 130, 131
  foreign body, 43
  formation of, 130–131, *131*
    in tuberculosis, 418
  giant cells in, 43, *43*, 131
  immune, 43, 130–131, *131*
  noncaseating, in sarcoidosis, 403, *404*
  pyogenic, 300
Granuloma inguinale, 605
Granuloma pyogenicum, 300
Granulomatosis, Wegener's, 286(t), 289, *290*
Granulomatous arteritis, 290
Granulomatous colitis. See *Crohn's disease.*
Granulomatous disease, chronic, 33
Granulomatous inflammation, 42(t), 42–43, *43*, 130, 273. See also
    Granuloma(s).
Granulomatous thyroiditis, 657
Granulosa-theca cell tumors, 626–627, *627*
Graves' disease, 650–652, *651*
Ground-glass nuclei, in papillary thyroid carcinoma, 660
Growth factor(s), 48, 51–52
  cytokine, 51
  epidermal, 51
  fibroblast, 51
    basic, 52
  in carcinogenesis, 186, 186(t), *188*
  in wound healing, 56(t)
  platelet-derived, 51
  receptors for, activation of, 48–49, *49*
    in carcinogenesis, 186, 186(t), *188*
  transforming, 51
    in wound healing, 56(t)
Growth factor receptor(s), in carcinogenesis, 186, 186(t), *188*
  in normal cell growth, 48, 49, *49*
Growth hormone–secreting adenoma, 645–646
Growth-related gene(s), 50
  early, 50
  late, 50
Guanosine triphosphatase (GTPase) activating protein, in cell growth,
  49, 50

Guillain-Barré syndrome, 734
Gumma, 603
Gunshot wounds, 236
Guthrie screening test, 92
Gynecomastia, 641

H
Haemophilus ducreyi infection, 604–605
Haemophilus influenzae infection, and pneumonia, 413–414
Hageman factor, 34, *35*
Hairy cell leukemia, 370
Hairy leukoplakia, 474, 475
Halothane, liver injury due to, 542
Hamartoma, 174
Hamartomatous polyp, of colon, 514, 514(t)
Hand-Schuller-Christian disease, 377
Hashimoto's thyroiditis, 655–656, *656*
Healing, 53–58, *54*. See also *Repair.*
  by first intention, 53, *54*
  by second intention, 53–54, *54*
  cell-matrix interactions in, 55–56, *57*
  collagenases in, 56–57
  collagens in, 55
    degradation of, 56–57
    synthesis of, 53, 56
  extracellular matrix in, 55–56, *57*
  fibronectin in, 55–56
  growth factors in, 56(t)
  inflammation and, 25, 39
  laminin in, 56
  mechanisms of, 55–58
  metalloproteinases in, 56–57
  primary vs. secondary, 53–54
  proteoglycans in, 56
  wound strength in, 57
Heart, 305–331. See also *Cardiac* entries.
  amyloid deposition in, 167, 169, 170
  aortic valve of, calcific stenosis of, *23*, 318–319, *319*
    disease of, 319(t)
    infective endocarditis of, 324
  artificial valves of, complications of, 325, 344
  Aschoff bodies in, 320–321, *322*
  Barlow's disease of, 319
  beriberi affecting, 253
  carcinoid disease of, 325
  chronic ischemic disease of, 313, *314*
  congenital disease of, 315(t), 315–318
  congestive failure of, 62, 63, *63*, 305–307
  effects of shock on, 80
  endocardium of. See *Endocarditis.*
  failure of, congestive, 62, 63, *63*, 305–307
    edema in, 62, 63, *63*
    hepatic congestion in, 306, *307*, 529
    left-sided, 306
      pulmonary congestion in, 64, 306
    passive congestion in, 64
    pulmonary congestion in, 64, 306
    right-sided, 306–307
      edema in, 62, 63
      hepatic congestion in, 306, *307*, 529
  fatty change in, 18
  fibroelastoma of, 331
  glycogen deposition in, 94(t)
  hemochromatosis involving, 556
  hypertensive disease of, 314–315
  hyperthyroidism and, 650
  hypertrophy of, *21*, 314
  infarction of, 72, 308–313, *310*, 311(t)
  ischemic disease of, 307–314, *308*
    atherosclerosis and, 278
    chronic, 313, *314*
  lupus erythematosus involving, 142–143, *143*, 325
  malformations of, 315(t), 315–318

Heart *(Continued)*
  malpositions of, 318
  metastatic tumors of, 331
  mitral valve of, calcification of anulus of, 325
    disease of, 319(t)
      prolapse of, 319–320, *320*
  myocardium of. See *Myocardium.*
  myxedema, 649
  myxoma of, 331, *331*
  papillary fibroelastoma of, 331
  pericardial disease of, 329–330
  Pompe's disease and, 94(t)
  pulmonary disease and, 315, 315(t)
  rhabdomyoma of, 331
  rheumatic disease of, 320–323, *321, 322*
    arterial thrombi in, 73
  rheumatoid disease of, 330–331
  shock involving, 80
  systemic lupus erythematosus involving, 142–143, *143,* 325
  systemic sclerosis involving, 152
  thiamine deficiency affecting, 253
  thrombi in, 70, 71
  tumors of, 331
  valve(s) of, anomalies of, 318
    aortic, calcific stenosis of, *23,* 318–319, *319*
      disease of, 319(t)
      infective endocarditis of, *324*
    artificial, complications of, 325, 344
    disease of, 318–325, 319(t)
    floppy, 86, 319
    mitral, calcification of anulus of, 325
      disease of, 319(t)
        rheumatic, 322, *322*
      prolapse of, 319–320, *320*
      rheumatic disease of, 322, *322*
      vegetations on, 142–143, *143, 324*
    rheumatic disease of, 322
    thrombi on, 71
    vegetations on, 71
      infective endocarditis and, 323–324, *324*
      lupus erythematosus and, 142–143, *143,* 325
      nonbacterial thrombotic endocarditis and, 324
Heart failure cells, 306
Heavy-chain disease, 375, 376
Heberden's nodes, 693
Heinz body, 341
Helicobacter gastritis, 485, *485,* 486, 488
Helminths, 262(t), 264
  effects of, on hosts, 267
Helper T cell(s), 118
Hemangioendothelioma, 301
Hemangioma, 301
  capillary, 301
  cavernous, 301
  of liver, *301,* 558
Hemarthrosis, in hemophilia, 382
Hematocele, 590
Hematoma, 64. See also *Hemorrhage.*
  dissecting, *296,* 296–298
  epidural, 718, *719*
  retroperitoneal, 64
  subcutaneous, 64
  subdural, 718–719, *720*
Hematopoiesis, cytokines in, 119–120
Hematopoietic cells, transplantation of, 135
Hematopoietic/lymphoid systems, 333–383
  radiation injury to, 240
Hematoxylin body, 141
Hematuria, asymptomatic, 438
Hemochromatosis, 19, 554–556, 555(t), *556*
Hemoglobin A, nonenzymatic glycosylation of, 573
Hemoglobin S, 336
Hemoglobinuria, paroxysmal nocturnal, 342
Hemolysis, extravascular, 335
  intravascular, 334

Hemolytic anemia, 334–345. See also *Anemia, hemolytic.*
Hemolytic crisis, in hereditary spherocytosis, 336
Hemolytic disease of newborn, 126, 343–344
Hemolytic jaundice, 525
Hemopericardium, 330
Hemophilia, 382–383
Hemorrhage, 64–65
  anemia due to, 334
  cerebral, 64, *65,* 715–718
  colonic, mucosal, *81*
  Duret, 707, 720
  pulmonary, 405, 406, 407
    vs. pulmonary infarction, 77
  subarachnoid, 717–718
Hemorrhagic disorders, 64, 377–383
Hemorrhagic enteropathy, acute, 497–498
  shock and, 80, *81*
Hemorrhagic gastritis, 484–485
Hemorrhagic infarct (red infarct), 76, *76,* 77
  in brain, *715*
Hemorrhagic necrosis, of liver, 529–530
Hemorrhagic pancreatitis, 581, 582, *582*
Hemorrhoids, 298, 498–499, 545
Hemosiderosis, 19, 555–556
  pulmonary, 406
Hemostasis, 65–69
  coagulation in, 67–69
  endothelial cell injury in, 66
  platelets in, 66–67, *67*
Hemostatic plug, 67
Hemothorax, 433
Henoch-Schonlein purpura, 287–288
  glomerular disease in, 451
Hepar lobatum, 604
Heparan sulfate deposition, 97, 98
Heparin-like molecules, endothelial, 66
Hepatectomy, expression of protooncogenes following, 50, *50*
Hepatic. See also *Liver.*
Hepatic amyloidosis, 169
Hepatic encephalopathy, 527–528, 731–732
  in portal hypertension, 544, *544*
Hepatic failure, 526–528
  encephalopathy in, 527–528, 731–732
Hepatic nephropathy, 528
Hepatic vein thrombosis, 530
Hepatitis, 530–541
  acute, 536–537, *537*
  alcoholic, 545, 546, *546,* 549
  anicteric, 536
  autoimmune chronic, 541
  carrier state in, 538–539
  cholestatic, 536
  chronic, 539–541
  chronic active, *540,* 540–541
  chronic persistent, 539–540
  clinical manifestations of, 536–541
  delta agent, 534
  fulminant, 537–538
  icteric, 536
  infectious, 531
  long-incubation, 532
  lupoid (autoimmune), 541
  neonatal, 528–529
  non-A, non-B, 534
  serum, 532
  short-incubation, 531
  type A, 531(t), 531–532, *532*
  type B, 531(t), *532,* 532–534, *533*
    liver cancer associated with, 200, 202–203, 559
    mechanisms of liver injury in, 535
  type C, 531(t), 534–535
  type D, 531(t), 534
  type E, 531(t), 535
  viral, 530–541, 531(t)
Hepatocellular adenoma, 558

Hepatocellular carcinoma, 558–561, *560*
    aflatoxin and, 200, 559
    cirrhosis and, 559
    hepatitis B virus infection and, 200, 202–203, 559
Hepatocellular damage, drug-induced, 541–542, 542(t)
Hepatocyte. See *Liver.*
Hepatolenticular degeneration, 557
Hepatorenal syndrome, 528
Hepatotoxins, 541–542, 542(t)
Hereditary diseases, 83–115. See also *Genetic diseases.*
Hereditary hemorrhagic telangiectasia (Osler-Weber-Rendu disease), 300
Hereditary hyperbilirubinemia, 526, 527(t)
Hereditary malformations, 103, 103(t)
Hereditary nephritis, 451–452
Hereditary spherocytosis, 335–336
Heredofamilial amyloidosis, 167, 167(t), 168
Heredofamilial polyposis syndromes, 513–514, 514(t)
Hernia/herniation, cerebral, 707, *707*
    hiatal, 480, *480*
    inguinal, 590
    intestinal, 519
    subfalcine (cingulate), 707, *707*
    tonsillar, 707, *707*
    uncinate (uncal, transtentorial), 707, *707*
Heroin, effects of, 235
Herpes genitalis, 605–606
Herpes simplex inclusion body, *263*
Herpes simplex virus infection, cerebral, 711, *711*
    genital, 605–606
    oral, 474
Herpetic gingivostomatitis, 474
Heterolysis, 12
Heterophagy, 15, *15*
Heterotopic rests, 174
Hexosaminidase A, deficiency of, 97
Heymann nephritis, 442–443
Hiatal hernia, 480, *480*
Hirschsprung's disease (megacolon), 494–495, *495*
Histamine, 34
    in inflammation, 34
Histiocytes, sinus, 40
Histiocytoma, fibrous, 700(t), 701
    malignant, 700(t), 701–702, *702*
Histiocytosis, 376–377
    sinus, 354
Histocompatibility antigens. See *HLA complex.*
Histoplasmosis, 422
    chronic adrenocortical insufficiency in, 672
HIV (human immunodeficiency virus) infection, 157–165. See also *Human immunodeficiency virus (HIV) infection.*
HLA complex, *120*, 120–122
    diseases associated with, 122, 122(t)
    immune response to, 121–122
    in transplantation, 121, 132, *133*, 135
HLA matching, 135
Hodgkin's disease, 362–365
    Reed-Sternberg cell in, 362, *362*
    staging of, 362, 362(t)
    subtypes of, 363(t), 363–364, *364*, *365*
    vs. non-Hodgkin's lymphoma, 365(t)
Homans' sign, 72
HTLV-1 (human T-cell leukemia virus type 1), 201, *202*, 360
Human immunodeficiency virus (HIV) infection, 157–165
    central nervous system involvement in, 162–165, 711
    clinical features of, 164–165
    epidemiology of, 157–158
    etiology of, 158
    hairy leukoplakia in, 474, 475
    immunopathogenesis of, 158–162, *160*, 162(t)
    Kaposi's sarcoma in, 164, 302(t), 302–303, 474
    lymph nodes in, 165
    natural history of, 163–164
    non-Hodgkin's lymphoma in, 164, 165
    opportunistic infections associated with, 164, 164(t)

Human immunodeficiency virus (HIV) infection *(Continued)*
    oral lesions in, 474
    pathogenesis of, 158–163
    T cells in, 158–159, *160*, 161, 162, *162*, 162(t), 163
    thrombocytopenia in, 380
    transmission of, 157–158
    venereal disease and, 599–600
    virion structure in, 158, *158*
Human leukocyte antigens. See *HLA complex.*
Human papillomavirus, 202
    infection by, and cervical cancer, 613
        and condyloma, 604, 609, 613
        and penile cancer, 590
Human T-cell leukemia virus type 1 (HTLV-1), 201, *202*, 360
Humoral rejection, 134
Hunter's syndrome, 98
Huntington's disease, 727–728
Hurler's syndrome, 97–98
Hurthle cells, 656
Hyaline, alcoholic, 17, 546, *546*
Hyaline arteriolosclerosis, 462, *463*
    in diabetes mellitus, 576, *576*
Hyaline degeneration, of basophils, 668
Hyaline membrane(s), in adult respiratory distress syndrome, 400
Hyaline membrane disease, 387, *388*
Hydatidiform mole, 629(t), 629–630, *630*
Hydrocarbons, polycyclic, as carcinogens, 199
Hydrocele, 590
Hydrocephalus, 707–708
    communicating, 707
    noncommunicating, 707
Hydronephrosis, 466–467
Hydropericardium, 61. See also *Pericardial* entries.
Hydroperitoneum, 61
Hydropic change, in cells, 12
Hydrops, of gallbladder, 565
Hydrops fetalis, 343
Hydrostatic pressure, 61, *62*
    in edema, 61, 62, 62(t)
    in inflammation, *27*
Hydrothorax, 433
Hydroureter, 467
21-Hydroxylase deficiency, *670*
Hyperacute rejection, 132
Hyperadrenalism, 666–671
Hyperaldosteronism, 669
Hyperbilirubinemia, 524–526. See also *Jaundice (icterus).*
    conjugated, 525(t), 525–526, 527(t)
    hereditary, 526, 527(t)
    unconjugated, 525, 525(t), 527(t)
Hypercalcemia, 23
    causes of, 663(t)
    hyperparathyroidism and, 663
Hypercholesterolemia, 86–88
    and atherosclerosis, 279
    and endothelial injury, 281
    familial, 86–88
Hypercoagulability, 69–70
Hyperemia, 64. See also *Congestion.*
Hypergastrinemia, 580–581
Hyperglycemia. See also *Diabetes mellitus.*
    intracellular, 574
Hyperglycemic coma, 731
Hyperinsulinism, 580
Hyperlipidemia, and atherosclerosis, 279
    and endothelial injury, 281
Hyperosmolar coma, nonketotic, 574
Hyperparathyroidism, 663–666
    primary, 663–665
    secondary, 665–666
    skeletal disease in, 684
Hyperphenylalaninemia, 91, 92
Hyperpituitarism, 644–647
Hyperplasia, 21–22
    adrenocortical, congenital, 669–671

Hyperplasia *(Continued)*
  Cushing's syndrome and, 668, *668*
    diffuse, 668
    nodular, 668, *668*
  and cancer, 22
  breast, epithelial, 632–633, *633*
  chief cell, parathyroid, 665, *665*
  compensatory, 21–22
  congenital, adrenocortical, 669–671
  endometrial, 22, 617–618, *618*
  epithelial, breast, 632–633, *633*
  hepatic, 558
  parathyroid, 664–665, *665*
  pathologic, 22
  physiologic, 21–22
  prostatic, 596–597, *597*
  squamous, vulvar, 608
  thymic, 678
  thyroid, in Graves' disease, *652*
  vulvar, 608
Hypersecretory antral gastritis, 485
Hypersensitivity, 122–132
  type I (anaphylactic), 122–126, 123(t), *124*
    asthma as, 390–391
    clinical manifestations of, 125–126
    mast cells in, 123, *124*, 125, 125(t)
    mediators of, 125(t)
  type II (antibody-dependent), 123(t), 126–127, *127*
  type III (immune complex–mediated), 123(t), 127–130, *128*, *129*
    local (Arthus reaction), 129–130
    systemic, *128*, 128–129, *129*, *130*
  type IV (cell-mediated), 123(t), 130–132
    delayed, 123(t), *130*, 130–131
    granuloma formation in, 130–131, *131*
    T cell–mediated cytotoxicity in, 131–132
Hypersensitivity pneumonitis, 405, 405(t)
Hypersensitivity vasculitis (leukocytoclastic vasculitis) 286(t), 286–288, *287*
Hypersplenism, 383
Hypertension, 459–464, 462(t)
  atherosclerosis associated with, 280
  benign, 459
  essential, 459
  heart disease associated with, 314–315
  malignant, 459, 463, 464
  portal, 480–481, *544*, 544–545
  pulmonary, 408–409, 409(t)
    and heart disease, 315
  renal, 459, 461
  renovascular, 459
  secondary, 459
Hypertensive heart disease, 314–315
Hyperthermia, 238
Hyperthyroidism, 650
Hypertrophic cardiomyopathy, *328*, 328–329, *329*
Hypertrophic osteoarthropathy, *688*, 688–689
Hypertrophy, 21
  of left ventricle, *21*, 314
  of prostate, benign, 596–597, *597*
  of smooth endoplasmic reticulum of liver, barbiturate-induced, 16, *16*
  of striated muscle, 21
  of uterus, 21
Hyperuricemia, 99
Hyperuricemic asymptomatic gout, 103
Hyperviscosity syndrome, 376
Hypogonadism, male, 109–110
Hypoparathyroidism, 666
Hypopituitarism, 647–648
Hypoplasia, thymic, 155
Hypospadias, 589
Hypostatic pneumonia, pulmonary edema and, 64
Hypothermia, 238
Hypothyroidism, 649(t), 649–650

Hypovolemic shock, 78, 78(t), 81
  burns and, 237
Hypoxanthine guanine phosphoribosyl transferase, deficiency of, 100
Hypoxic-ischemic cell injury, 4, 77

I
IBD (inflammatory bowel disease), 499–503
  spondylitis associated with, 149(t)
Icterus (jaundice), 524–526, 525(t)
IDDM (insulin-dependent diabetes mellitus), 569, 570(t). See also
    Diabetes mellitus.
Idiopathic hypertrophic subaortic stenosis, 328
Idiopathic pulmonary fibrosis, 401–403, *402*, *403*
Idiopathic thrombocytopenic purpura, 380–381
Iduronidase (α-L-iduronidase), deficiency of, 97
IgA, deficiency of, 156
IgA nephropathy (Berger's disease), 451
IgE, in type I hypersensitivity, 123, *124*
Ileus, meconium, cystic fibrosis and, 90
Immotile cilia syndrome, 17
Immune complex deposition, in kidney, 129, 440–441, *442*
  in small blood vessels, 129, *130*
Immune complex–mediated hypersensitivity (type III hypersensitivity), 123(t), 127–128, *128*, *129*
  local, 129–130
  systemic, *128*, 128–129, *129*, *130*
Immune complex nephritis, 440–443, *441*, *442*
Immune complex vasculitis, 129, *130*, 286
Immune disorders, 117–160
Immune glomerulonephritis, cell-mediated, 443
Immune response, 121–122
  and cell injury, 4
  and host defenses against cancer, 203–205
  and inflammation, 40
  and rejection, 121, 132, *133*, 135
  and tissue injury, 122–132. See also *Hypersensitivity.*
Immune system, cells of, 117–119. See also *B cell(s)* and *T cell(s).*
  disorders of, 117–160
Immunity, cell-mediated, 117–118. See also *T cell(s).*
  humoral (antibody-mediated), 118
  natural, 119
  tumor, 203–206
Immunocyte dyscrasias, with amyloidosis, 166–167, 167(t), 376
Immunodeficiency, 154–165
  acquired, 157–165. See also *Human immunodeficiency virus (HIV) infection.*
  cancer associated with, 205
    HIV infection and, 164
  common variable, 156
  in Bruton's disease, 154–155
  in DiGeorge's syndrome, 155
  in thymic hypoplasia, 155
  in Wiskott-Aldrich syndrome, 156
  lymphocyte development in, *155*
  primary, 154–156
  secondary, 156–165
  severe combined (Swiss-type agammaglobulinemia), 155–156
  with thrombocytopenia and eczema, 156
  X-linked, 154–155
Immunoglobulin(s), 118
Immunoglobulin A, deficiency of, 156
  deposition of, in kidney, 451
Immunoglobulin E, in type I hypersensitivity, 123, *124*
Immunohemolytic anemia, 342(t), 342–343
Immunologic tolerance, 136–138
Immunoproliferative small intestinal disease, 493
Immunosurveillance, 205
Immunotherapy, for cancer, 205–206
Incised wound, 236
Inclusion bodies, viral, 252
Induction, of smooth endoplasmic reticulum of liver, barbiturate-induced, 16, *16*

Infant(s). See also *Child(ren)* and *Newborn*.
  AIDS transmission to, 158
  cystic fibrosis in, 91
  extrahepatic biliary atresia in, 529
  galactosemia in, 93
  phenylketonuria in, 91
  pyloric stenosis in, 484
  respiratory distress syndrome in, 387
  sudden death in, 388(t), 388–389
Infarct(s), 75–77. See also *Infarction*.
  bile, 553
  border-zone, 713
  red (hemorrhagic), 76, *76*, 77
    in brain, *715*
  subendocardial, 309–310, 312
  transmural, of intestine, 497, *497*, 498
    of myocardium, 308–312
  watershed, 713
  white (anemic), 76
Infarction, 65, 75–78. See also *Infarct(s)*.
  cerebral, 72, 713, 714, *715*
  clinical aspects of, 77–78
  development of, 77
  hepatic, 530
  intestinal, *497*, 497–498, *498*
  left ventricular, 310
  myocardial, 72, 308–313, *310*, 311(t)
    arterial thrombi in, 73
    diabetes mellitus and, 575
    ventricular thrombi in, 73, *73*
  pulmonary, 76, *76*, 407, *408*
    vs. pulmonary hemorrhage, 77
  right ventricular, 310, *310*
  splenic, *76*
Infection(s), host response to, 261–274
Infectious hepatitis, 531
Infectious mononucleosis, 351–353
Infective endocarditis, 71, 323–324, *324*
Inferior vena caval syndrome, 299
Inflammation, 25–45
  abscess formation following, 39, 44
  acute, 26–39
    cellular events in, 28–33
    chemical mediators of, 33–39, *34*, 38(t)
    definition of, 25
    outcomes of, 39
    resolution of, 39, *39*
    vascular changes in, 26–28, *27*, *28*
  arachidonic acid metabolites in, 36–37, *37*
  chemotaxis in, *29*, 30, 36
    defective, 33
  chronic, 39–45
    causes of, 39
    definition of, 25, 39
    fibrosis in, 42
    granulomatous, 42(t), 42–43, *43*
    macrophages in, 40–41, *41*, *42*
    progression to, from acute inflammation, 39
  clotting system in, 36
  complement system in, 34, 36
  connective tissue involvement in, 25, *26*
  cytokines in, 38, 45, 119
  endothelial injury in, 27, *28*
  eosinophils in, 42
  exudation in, 27
    leukocyte, 28–30
  fever in, 45
  fibrinolytic system in, 36
  fibrinous, 44, *44*
  free radicals in, 10, 38
  granulomatous, 42(t), 42–43, *43*, 130, 273. See also *Granuloma(s)*.
  increased vascular permeability in, 26, 27, 28, *28*, 36
  interleukins in, 38
  kinin system in, 34
Inflammation *(Continued)*
  leukemoid reaction in, 45
  leukotrienes in, 37, *37*
  local signs of, 26
  macrophages in, 40–41, *41*, *42*
  mononuclear, 272–273
  mononuclear phagocyte system in, 40, *41*
  morphologic patterns in, 44–45
  organization in, 44, 58
  outcomes of, 39
  oxygen-derived free radicals in, 10, 38
  phagocytosis in, 30–32, *32*, 36
    defective, 33
  plasma cells in, *40*, 42
  platelet-activating factor in, 37
  pseudomembranous, 434, 506
  purulent (suppurative), 44, 272
  resolution of, 39, *39*, 44, 58
  serous, 44
  suppurative (purulent), 44, 272
  systemic manifestations of, 45
  vascular changes in, 26–28, *27*, *28*, 36
  vascular leakage in, 27–28, *28*
  vasoactive amines in, 34
Inflammatory bowel disease, 499–503
  spondylitis associated with, 149(t)
Inguinal hernia, 590
Inhalant abuse, 236
Inhalation injury, 237
Inherited diseases, 83–115. See also *Genetic diseases*.
Inhibition, of cell growth, 50–51
  transforming growth factor beta in, 51
Insulin, metabolism of, 570
  resistance to, 573
Insulin-dependent diabetes mellitus, 569, 570(t). See also *Diabetes mellitus*.
  clinical manifestations of, 579
  pathogenesis of, 570–572, *571*
Insulin-secreting lesions, 580
Insulitis, 571, 575
Integrin receptors, 55
Interferon-alpha, in immunotherapy for cancer, 206
Interferon-gamma, in delayed hypersensitivity, 131
Interleukin(s). See also *Cytokine(s)*.
  in inflammation, 38
Interleukin-1, in inflammation, 38, *38*
  in wound healing, 56(t)
Interleukin-2, in delayed hypersensitivity, 131
  in immunotherapy for cancer, 205
Interleukin-8, in inflammation, 38
Interstitial emphysema (mediastinal emphysema), 396
Interstitial fluid, 61, *62*
Interstitial lung diseases, 389, 401–406
Interstitial nephritis, 453–457
Interstitial pneumonitis, 415
Intestine, 494–519
  angiodysplasia of, 498
  Crohn's disease of, 499–501, *500*
    vs. ulcerative colitis, 501, 502(t), *503*
  developmental anomalies of, 494
  herniation of, 519
  infarction in, *497*, 497–498, *498*
  infectious disease of, 503–507, 504(t)
  inflammatory diseases of, 499–503
  intussusception of, 519
  ischemic disease of, 497–498
  large. See *Colon*.
  obstruction of, 519, 519(t)
  small, adenocarcinoma of, 510
    argentaffinoma of, 517–519
    atresia of, 494
    cancer of, 510
    carcinoid of, 517–519
    Crohn's disease of, 499–501

Intestine *(Continued)*
    developmental anomalies of, 494
    duplication of, 494
    herniation of, 494
    immunoproliferative disease of, 493
    in celiac sprue, 508–509
    in disaccharidase deficiency, 507
    in regional enteritis, 499–501
    in tropical sprue, 509
    in Whipple's disease, 509
    infarction in, *497, 498*
    intussusception of, 519
    lymphoma of, 493
    malabsorption in, 507–509
    Meckel's diverticulum of, 494
    sarcoma of, 510
    stenosis of, 494
    tumors of, 509–510
   tuberculosis of, 421
   tumors of, 509–510. See also entries under *Colon.*
   vascular diseases of, 497–499
   volvulus of, 519
Intracanalicular fibroadenoma, of breast, 635
Intracellular accumulation(s), 17–19
Intracellular calcification, 23
Intracerebral hemorrhage, 64, *65,* 715–718
Intracranial hemorrhage, 715–718
Intracranial pressure, increased, 707
Intracranial tumors, 720–725, 721(t)
Intradermal nevus, 212
Intraductal carcinoma, of breast, 637–638
Intraductal papilloma, of breast, 636
Intraepithelial neoplasia, cervical (CIN), 612, 613
   vulvar, 610
Intrahepatic biliary tract, carcinoma of, 559, 560
Intravascular coagulation, disseminated, 73, 378–380
Intrinsic asthma, 389
Intrinsic factor, 348
Intussusception, 519
Inversion, chromosomal, 106, *106*
Ionizing radiation, injury due to, 239–241, *240, 241,* 242(t)
Iron deficiency anemia, 345–346
Iron overload, 554–556
Irradiation, injury due to, 239–241, *240, 241,* 242(t)
Irreversible injury, to cells, 3
    mechanisms of, 5–7, *6, 7*
Ischemia, cerebral, 713
   myocardial, 309(t), *312*
Ischemic acute tubular necrosis, 457, 458, *458*
Ischemic bowel disease, 497–498
Ischemic cardiomyopathy, 313, *314*
Ischemic encephalopathy, 713
Ischemic enterocolitis, 497
Ischemic heart disease, 307–314, *308*
   angina pectoris in, 307–308
   atherosclerosis and, 278
   chronic, 313, *314*
   coronary thrombosis in, 309
   myocardial infarction in, 308–313
   pathogenesis of, 308–310
   sudden cardiac death in, 313–314
Ischemic-hypoxic cell injury, 4
    mechanisms of, 5–7, *6*
Islet cell(s), 569
   adenoma of, *206,* 580, *580,* 581
   disorders of, 569–581
    diabetes mellitus due to, 569–580. See also *Diabetes mellitus.*
    neoplastic, 580–581
   tumors of, 580–581
Isochromosomes, 106, *106*
Ito cells, 543
   collagen production by, in cirrhosis, 543, *543*
ITP (idiopathic thrombocytopenic purpura), 380–381
Ixodes dammini, 696

J
Jakob-Creutzfeldt disease (subacute spongiform encephalopathy), 712–713
Jaundice (icterus), 524–526, 525(t)
   acute hepatitis and, 536
   hepatic failure and, 527
JC papovavirus, 712
Jejunum, giardiasis of, *266,* 504(t)
Joint(s), 693–696. See also *Arthritis.*
   bleeding into, in hemophilia, 382
   degenerative disease of, 693–695, *694, 695*
   hemosiderin deposition in, 556
   in Lyme disease, 696
   in rheumatic fever, 322
   in rheumatoid arthritis, 145, *695*
   in systemic lupus erythematosus, 144
   in systemic sclerosis, 152
   infection of, 696
   inflammation of. See *Arthritis.*
   monosodium urate crystal deposition in, 99, 101, 102
Junctional nevus, 212
Juvenile polyp, of colon, 511
Juvenile rheumatoid arthritis, 149

K
Kallikrein, 34
Kaposi's sarcoma, 302(t), 302–304, *303, 304*
   AIDS and, 164, 302(t), 302–303, 474
Kartagener's syndrome, 397
Karyolysis, 13
Karyorrhexis, 13
Karyotype, 104, *105.* See also *Chromosome(s).*
Kawasaki's disease (mucocutaneous lymph node syndrome), 286(t), 292–293
Kayser-Fleischer rings, 557
Keloid, 58
Keratitis, in riboflavin deficiency, 254
Keratoconjunctivitis sicca, in Sjogren's syndrome, 149, 150
Keratomalacia, vitamin A deficiency and, 246, *247*
Kernicterus, 343
Keshan disease, 257
Ketoacidosis, diabetic, 574
Kidney(s), 437–470. See also *Renal* entries.
   acute tubular necrosis of, 457–458, *458*
   amyloid deposition in, 169, *169,* 170
   arteriolosclerosis of, 462, *463*
    in diabetes mellitus, 577
   blood pressure regulation by, 460–461
   carcinoma of, 467–469, *468*
   cystic diseases of, 464–465
   diffuse cortical necrosis of, 458–459
   disease of, 437–470
    clinical manifestations of, 438
    edema in, 62, 63
    hyperparathyroidism associated with, 666
    osteodystrophy in, 684
   effects of shock on, 80, 457–458
   enlargement of, in glycogenosis, 94(t)
   epithelial cells of, swelling of, *12*
   failure of, 438
    acute, 438
    chronic, 438
    liver failure and, 528
    uric acid crystal deposition and, 103
   glomeruli of, 438, *439,* 440
    diseases of, 440(t), 440–453
    injury to, *443,* 443–444
   glycogen deposition in, 94(t)
   Goldblatt, 461
   gout involving, *102,* 103
   hyaline arteriolosclerosis of, 462, *463*
   immune complex deposition in, 129, 440–441, *442*

Kidney(s) *(Continued)*
  immunoglobulin A deposition in, 451
  in diabetes mellitus, 576–577, *577*
  in hydronephrosis, 466–467
  in hypertension, 459, 461
  in immune complex nephritis, 440–443
  in lipoid nephrosis, 445, *446*
  in nephritic syndrome, 449–453
  in nephrosclerosis, 462–464
  in nephrotic syndrome, 444–449
  in pyelonephritis, 453–456, 577–578
  in shock, 80, 457–458
  in systemic lupus erythematosus, 143–144, *144, 145*
  in systemic sclerosis, 152
  in urinary outflow obstruction, 465–467
  infection of, *453*
  interstitial diseases of, 453–459
  monosodium urate crystal deposition in, *102,* 103
  morphologic changes in, in diabetes mellitus, 576–578, *577, 578*
  multiple myeloma involving, 375–376
  papilla of, necrosis of, 454–455, 578, *578*
    in diabetes mellitus, 578
  polycystic disease of, 464–465, *465*
  reduction in mass of, effects of, 443–444, *444*
  stones in, 438, 465–466, 466(t)
  transplantation of, graft rejection in, 132–134, *134*
  tubules of, diseases of, 453–459
    lesions of, in diabetes mellitus, 578
    swelling of epithelial cells of, *12*
  tumors of, 467–470
  uric acid crystal deposition in, 103
  vascular disease of, 459–464
  vasodepressor substances produced by, 461
  Wilms' tumor of, 469
Kimmelstiel-Wilson lesion, 576
Kinin system, in inflammation, 34
Klebsiella pneumoniae infection, 272, 414
Klinefelter's syndrome, 109–110, 591, *591*
Knudson two-hit hypothesis, 190
Koilocytosis, 604, 609, *609*
Korsakoff's psychosis, thiamine deficiency and, 253, 731
Krabbe's disease, 732
Krukenberg tumor, 628
Kulchitsky cells, 432, 517
Kwashiorkor, 243, *243,* 244

L
Labile cells, 47–48
Laceration, 236
  cerebral, 719–720
  esophageal, 480
Lactase, deficiency of, 507
Lacunae, in brain, 714–715
Lacunar cell, in nodular sclerosis Hodgkin's disease, 363, *365*
Laminar necrosis, of brain, 713
Laminin, 56
  in wound healing, 56
  receptors for, on tumor cells, 198
Landry-Guillain-Barré syndrome, 734
Langerhans' cell(s), 119
Langerhans' cell histiocytosis, 377
Langhans' giant cells, 131
Lardaceous spleen, 169
Large intestine. See *Colon.*
Laryngitis, acute, 434
Laryngotracheobronchitis, 434
Larynx, carcinoma of, *435,* 435–436
  inflammation of, 434
  papilloma of, 435
  tumors of, 435–436
Lathyrism, 297

LE (lupus erythematosus), 139–145. See also *Systemic lupus erythematosus.*
Lead, toxic effects of, 229–231, *230, 231*
Leakage, vascular, in inflammation, 27–28, *28*
  in thermal burns, 28
Lecithin-sphingomyelin ratio, 388
Left-to-right cardiac shunts, 316–317
Left ventricle, failure of, 306
  pulmonary congestion in, 64, 306
  hypertrophy of, *21*
  infarction of, 310
  thrombi in, myocardial infarction and, 73, *73*
Legionella pneumophila infection, 414
Leiomyoma, 700(t), 702, *703*
  uterine, 177, 618, *619*
Leiomyosarcoma, 700(t), 702, *703*
  uterine, 619
Lens, galactitol deposition in, 93
  opacity of, in galactosemia, 93
  subluxation of, in Marfan's syndrome, 86
Leprosy, 42(t), *273*
Lesch-Nyhan syndrome, 100
Letterer-Siwe disease, 377
Leukemia, 365–372
  acute, 366–368
  acute lymphoblastic, 367, 367(t)
  acute myeloblastic, 367–368, *368,* 368(t)
  bone marrow infiltration in, 370, *370*
  central nervous system involvement in, 371
  chromosomal translocation and, 193, 372(t)
  chronic lymphocytic, 369–370
  chronic myeloid, 369, *369*
    chromosomal translocation and, 189, *189,* 193, 369
  etiology of, 371–372
  hairy cell, 370
  hepatomegaly in, 371
  lymphadenopathy in, 371, *371*
  lymphocytic (lymphoblastic), acute, 367, 367(t)
    chronic, 369–370
  morphologic changes in, *370,* 370–371, *371*
  myelocytic (myeloblastic, myeloid), acute, 367–368, *368,* 368(t)
    chronic, 369, *369*
      chromosomal translocation and, 189, *189,* 193, 369
  oncogenes in, 372(t)
  pathogenesis of, 371–372
  splenomegaly in, 370–371
Leukemia/lymphoma, T-cell, HTLV-1 in, 201, *202,* 360
Leukemoid reaction, in inflammation, 45
Leukocyte(s), disorders of, 350–377
  neoplastic, 354–377
  nonneoplastic, 350–354
  in inflammation, 33, 45
    activation of, *31,* 32
    adhesion of, 28–29, *29,* 29(t), *30*
    defects of, 33
    emigration of, 26, *29,* 29–30, *31*
    exudation of, 28–30
    margination of, 26, 28
    products of, 38
Leukocytoclastic vasculitis (hypersensitivity vasculitis), 286(t), 286–287, *287*
Leukocytosis, in infection, 45
  in inflammation, 45
  reactive, 351(t), 351–353
Leukodystrophies, 732
Leukoencephalopathy, progressive multifocal, 712
Leukopenia, 351
  in infection, 45
Leukoplakia, hairy, in AIDS, 474, 475
  oral, 474–475, *475*
  vulvar, 608
Leukotriene(s), 37
  in inflammation, 37, *37*
  in type I (anaphylactic) hypersensitivity, 125

Lewy bodies, 729
Libman-Sacks endocarditis, 142–143, *143*, 325
Lichen sclerosus, 608, *608*
Light-chain disease, 374
Limited scleroderma (CREST syndrome), 151, 153
  antinuclear antibodies in, 141(t), 151
Lines of Zahn, 70
Linkage analysis, 113–114
Lipid(s), intracellular accumulation of, 17–18
Lipid breakdown products, and cell membrane injury, 7
Lipid mediators, of type I (anaphylactic) hypersensitivity, 125
Lipid peroxidation, of cell membranes, 9
Lipofuscin, deposition of, in cells, 10
Lipogranuloma, formation of, in alcoholic liver disease, 546
Lipoid nephrosis (minimal change disease), 445, *446*
Lipoma, 700(t), 701
Lipoprotein(s), 279(t)
  high-density, 279, 279(t)
  in familial hypercholesterolemia, 86–88, *87*, *88*
  intermediate density, 87, 279(t)
  low-density, 279(t)
    metabolism of, 87, *87*
    oxidative modification of, and atherosclerosis, 282
    transport of, 87, *88*
  very low density, 87, 279(t)
Liposarcoma, 700(t), 701
Lipoxygenase pathway, of arachidonic acid metabolism, 36–37, *37*
Liquefactive necrosis, 13, *13*
Lisch nodules, in neurofibromatosis, 88
Liver, 523–561. See also *Hepatic* entries.
  abscess of, 561
  adenoma of, 558
  alcohol metabolism in, 232–233, 547–549, *549*
  alcoholic disease of, 545–550, *546–548*
  amyloid deposition in, 169
  angiosarcoma of, 558
  bilirubin metabolism in, 524. See also *Hyperbilirubinemia* and *Jaundice (icterus)*.
  cancer of, 558–561, *560*
    aflatoxin and, 200, 559
    cirrhosis and, 559
    hepatitis B and, 200, 202–203, 559
    hepatitis C and, 553, 559
    metastatic, *179*, 558
  cavernous hemangioma of, *301*, 558
  circulatory disorders of, 529–530
  cirrhosis of, *542*, 542–558. See also *Cirrhosis*.
  collagen deposition in, 543
  congestion of, chronic passive, 306, *307*, 529
  copper deposition in, 557
  disease of, in children, 528–529
  effects of shock on, 80
  endoplasmic reticulum of, effects of barbiturates on, 16, *16*
    effects of carbon tetrachloride on, 9, *10*
  enlargement of, in amyloidosis, 169
    in galactosemia, 93
    in glycogenosis, 94(t)
    in leukemia, 371
    in von Gierke's disease, 94(t)
  failure of, 526–528
    encephalopathy in, 527–528, 731–732
  fatty change in, 12, 17, *18*
    alcohol-induced, 17, 545, 546
    Reye's syndrome and, 529, *530*
  fibrosis of, cirrhosis and, 543, 549
    pipestem, *273*
    schistosomiasis and, *273*
  focal nodular hyperplasia of, 558
  galactitol deposition in, 93
  galactose-1-phosphate deposition in, 93
  glycogen deposition in, 94(t)
  hemangioma of, *301*, 558
  hemosiderin deposition in, 555–556, *556*
  in Budd-Chiari syndrome, 530
  in Crigler-Najjar syndrome, 527(t)

Liver *(Continued)*
  in hepatitis, 530–541. See also *Hepatitis*.
  in Reye's syndrome, 529, *530*
  in Rotor's syndrome, 527(t)
  in Wilson's disease, 557
  infarction of, 530
  infection of, viral, 530–541, 531(t). See also *Hepatitis*.
  injury to, alcohol-induced, 545–550
    carbon tetrachloride–induced, 9, *10*
    chlorpromazine-induced, 542
    drug-induced, 541–542, 542(t)
    halothane-induced, 542
    toxin-induced, 542(t)
  metastasis to, *179*, 558
  necrosis of, 550
    acute hepatitis and, 537
    alcoholic hepatitis and, 546, *546*
    bridging, 540, *540*
    chronic active hepatitis and, 540, *540*
    fulminant hepatitis and, 538, *538*
    hemorrhagic, 529–530
    massive, 527, 538, *538*
    piecemeal, 540, *540*
    submassive, 538
  nodularity of, cirrhosis and, 542–543
  nutmeg, 306, *307*
  regeneration of, 21–22
  sarcoidosis involving, 404
  schistosomiasis of, pipestem fibrosis in, *273*
  thrombosis in, 530
  transplantation of, 135
  tumors of, 558–561
  vascular disorders of, 529–530
  veno-occlusive disease of, 530
  viral infection of, 530–541, 531(t). See also *Hepatitis*.
Lobar pneumonia, 411, 412, *412*, *413*. See also *Pneumonia*.
Lobular carcinoma, of breast, 639
Loeffler's endocarditis, 329
Long-incubation hepatitis, 532
Lues. See *Syphilis*.
Lung(s), 385–433. See also *Pulmonary* entries.
  abscess of, 411(t), 424–425
  actinomycosis of, 416
  adenocarcinoma of, 429
  adult respiratory distress syndrome and, 399–401, *400*
  alveoli of, diffuse damage to, 399(t), 399–401, *400*
    emigration of inflammatory cells into, *31*
    immune-mediated inflammation of, 405
    wall of, *398*
  anthracosis of, 221–222
  asbestosis of, 221(t), 223–226, *225*
    and mesothelioma, 432
  atelectasis of, 386, *386*
  bacterial infection of, 411–414
  berylliosis of, 221(t), 226
  Branhamella catarrhalis infection of, 414
  bronchioloalveolar carcinoma of, 429–430
  brown induration of, 306
  candidiasis of, 424
  carcinoma of (bronchogenic carcinoma), 428(t), 428–432, *430*, *431*
  coal dust accumulation in, 19, 221(t), 221–223, *222*
  coccidioidomycosis of, 423, *423*
  congestion of, heart failure and, 64, 306
  cystic fibrosis involving, 90
  cytomegalovirus infection of, 426
  defense mechanisms of, 409–410, *410*
  diffuse alveolar damage in, 399–401, *400*
  edema of, 64, *64*
    alveolocapillary block associated with, 64
    hypostatic pneumonia associated with, 64
  embolism in, 74, *74*, 406–408, *407*, *408*
  fibrosis of, idiopathic, 401–403, *402*, *403*
    massive, progressive, 222, *222*
  fungal infection of, 422–424
  gangrene of, 425

Lung(s) *(Continued)*
  Haemophilus influenzae infection of, 413–414
  heart disease associated with, 315, 315(t)
  hemorrhage in, 405, 406, 407
    vs. pulmonary infarction, 77
  hemorrhagic infarction of, 76, *76*
  hemosiderosis of, 406
  histoplasmosis of, 422
  hyaline membrane disease and, 387, *388*
  hypersensitivity involving, 125, 390–391, 405
  idiopathic fibrosis of, 401–403, *402, 403*
  immune-mediated disease of, 405
  in asthma, 389–391
  in bronchiectasis, 397–398, *398*
  in bronchitis, 396–397
  in emphysema, 392–396
  in Goodpasture's syndrome, 405–406
  in systemic sclerosis, 152
  induration of, 306
  infarction of, 76, *76*, 407, *408*
    vs. pulmonary hemorrhage, 77
  infection of, 409–427, 411(t)
    cystic fibrosis and, 90
  injury to, air pollution and, 218(t), 219
  Klebsiella pneumoniae infection of, *272*, 414
  large cell carcinoma of, 430
  Legionella pneumophila infection of, 414
  mesothelioma of, 432–433
  mineral dust accumulation in, 220–226, *221*, 221(t)
  Mycobacterium tuberculosis infection of, 418, *419*, 420, *420, 421*
  mycoplasmal infection of, 415–416
  neonatal respiratory distress syndrome and, 386–388, *387, 388*
  nocardiosis of, 416
  obstructive disease of, 389–398
    chronic, 391–398
  pneumococcal infection of, 412–413
  Pneumocystis carinii infection of, 426–427, *427*
  pneumonias and, 411–416. See also specific infectious agents.
  progressive massive fibrosis of, 222, *222*
  Pseudomonas aeruginosa infection of, 414
  respiratory distress syndrome, adult, 399–401, *400*
    neonatal, 386–388, *387, 388*
  restrictive disease of, 389, 398–406
    acute, 399–401
    chronic, 401(t), 401–406
  sarcoidosis of, 404
  sclerosis of, vascular, 409
  shock, 80
  silicosis of, 221(t), 223, *224*
  small cell carcinoma of, 430–431, *431*
  squamous cell carcinoma of, 429, *430*
  Staphylococcus aureus infection of, 414
  Streptococcus pneumoniae infection of, 412–413
  toxic effects of oxygen on, 10, 399
  tuberculosis of, 418, *419*, 420, *420, 421*
  tumors of, 427–433
  type I (anaphylactic) hypersensitivity involving, 125, 390–391
  vascular disease of, 406–409
  vasculitis-associated hemorrhage in, 406
  viral infection of, *415*, 426
  Wegener's granulomatosis involving, 289, *290*
Lupus erythematosus, discoid, 142
  systemic, 139–145. See also *Systemic lupus erythematosus.*
Lupus erythematosus (LE) cell, 141
Lupus nephritis, 143, *144, 145*
Luteal cysts, 621
Lyme disease, 696
Lymph node(s), in AIDS, 165
  in inflammation, 43
  in sarcoidosis, 403
Lymphadenitis, reactive, 43, 353–354
Lymphadenopathy, in infectious mononucleosis, 352
  in inflammation, 44
  in leukemia, 371, *371*
Lymphangitis, 299

Lymphatic disorders, 299–300
Lymphatic spread, of cancer, 180
Lymphatics, 43
  in inflammation, 43
Lymphedema, 62, 299–300
Lymphoblastic lymphoma, 359, 361(t)
Lymphocyte(s). See also *B cell(s)* and *T cell(s).*
  atypical, in infectious mononucleosis, 352
  B. See *B cell(s).*
  development of, in immunodeficiency states, *155*
  differentiation of, cytokines in, 119
  growth of, cytokines in, 119
  in inflammation, 41–42, *42*
  T. See *T cell(s).*
Lymphocyte-depletion Hodgkin's disease, 363, *364*
Lymphocyte-predominance Hodgkin's disease, 363, *364*
Lymphocytic (lymphoblastic) leukemia, acute, 367, 367(t)
  chronic, 369–370
Lymphocytic meningitis, 709
Lymphoepithelioma, 435
Lymphogranuloma venereum, 605
Lymphoid/hematopoietic systems, 333–383
Lymphoid hyperplasia, paracortical, 354
Lymphoma, 354–365, 357(t), 361(t)
  AIDS and, 164, 165
  Burkitt's (small noncleaved lymphoma), 359, *360*, 361(t)
    chromosomal translocation and, 188–189, *189*
    Epstein-Barr virus infection and, 202
  chromosomal translocation and, 193, 372(t)
  diffuse large cell, *358*, 358–359, 361(t)
  diffuse non-Hodgkin's, 355, *356*
  etiology of, 371–372
  follicular (nodular), *357*, 357–358, 361(t)
  gastric, 493
  gastrointestinal, 493
  HIV infection and, 164, 165
  Hodgkin's, 362–365
    Reed-Sternberg cell in, 362, *362*
    staging of, 362, 362(t)
    subtypes of, 363(t), 363–364, *364, 365*
    vs. non-Hodgkin's lymphoma, 365(t)
  intestinal, 493
  lymphoblastic, 359, 361(t)
  malignant, 354–365
  morphologic changes associated with, 360–361
  nodular, 355, *356*
  non-Hodgkin's, 354–361, 357(t), 361(t)
    AIDS and, 164, 165
    diagnosis of, 361
    diffuse, 355, *356*
    diffuse large cell, *358*, 358–359, 361(t)
    follicular, *357*, 357–358, 361(t)
    gastric, 493
    gastrointestinal, 493
    HIV infection and, 164, 165
    intestinal, 493
    lymphoblastic, 359, 361(t)
    nodular, 355, *356*
    small lymphocytic, 357, 361(t)
    small noncleaved (Burkitt's lymphoma), 359, *360*, 361(t)
      chromosomal translocation and, 188–189, *189*
      Epstein-Barr virus infection and, 202
    staging of, 362(t)
    T-cell, cutaneous, 360
    vs. Hodgkin's disease, 365(t)
  oncogenes in, 372(t)
  pathogenesis of, 371–372
  small lymphocytic, 357, 361(t)
  small noncleaved (Burkitt's lymphoma), 359, *360*, 361(t)
    chromosomal translocation and, 188–189, *189*
    Epstein-Barr virus infection and, 202
  staging of, 362(t)
  T-cell, cutaneous, 360
Lymphotoxin, in delayed hypersensitivity, 131
Lyon hypothesis, 107, 111

Lysosomal acid maltase, deficiency of, 94(t)
Lysosomal storage diseases, 16, 94–97, *95*, 95(t)
Lysosome(s), 15–16

M
M protein, 374
Macroglobulinemia, Waldenstrom's, 374, 375, 376
Macronodular cirrhosis, 543, 546, 551, *551*
Macrophage(s), 40
  activation of, 40
  immune functions of, 118–119
  in cell growth, 51–52
  in HIV infection, *160*, 160–161
  in host defenses against cancer, 204–205
  in idiopathic pulmonary fibrosis, 402, *402*
  in inflammation, 40–41, *41*, *42*
  products released by, 40, *41*, 41(t), 51–52
Macrovesicular steatosis, in alcoholic liver disease, 546
Macule(s), coal, in lungs, 222
Major basic protein, 42
Major histocompatibility complex. See *HLA complex.*
Malabsorption syndromes, 507–509, 508(t). See also specific diseases.
Malaria, 344–345
Male(s), XYY, 110
Male breast, 641
Male genital system, 589–606
Malformation(s), arteriovenous, in brain, 718
  cardiac, 315(t), 315–318
  congenital, 103, 103(t)
  hereditary, 103, 103(t)
Malignant fibrous histiocytoma, 700(t), 701–702, *702*
Malignant hypertension, 459, 463, 464
Malignant lymphoma, 354–365
Malignant melanoma, 213–214
Malignant mesothelioma, 432–433
Malignant nephrosclerosis, *463*, 463–464
Malignant tumors. See *Cancer*; specific types (e.g., *Carcinoma*); and specific organs involved.
Mallory body, 17, 546, *546*
Mallory-Weiss syndrome, 480
Malnutrition, and cell injury, 4–5
  protein-energy, 242–244, *243*
Malpositions, of heart, 318
Malrotation, of large intestine, 494
Mammary duct ectasia, 634–635
Mammary gland. See *Breast(s).*
Mantoux test, 130, *130*, 131, 417
Marantic endocarditis, 324
Marasmus, 243, *243*, 244
Marfan's syndrome, 86
Marijuana, effects of, 235–236
Marrow. See *Bone marrow.*
Mast cells, in type I (anaphylactic) hypersensitivity, 123, *124*, 125, 125(t)
Mastitis, 634–635
Masugi nephritis, 441
Maternal age, and Down's syndrome, 107
McArdle's syndrome, 94(t)
McCune-Albright syndrome, 688
Mechanical injury, 236
  to red blood cells, and hemolytic anemia, 344
Meckel's diverticulum, 494, *494*
Meconium ileus, cystic fibrosis and, 90
Medial calcific sclerosis, 277–278
Mediastinal emphysema (interstitial emphysema), 396
Mediastinopericarditis, adhesive, 330
Mediator(s), cell-derived, of inflammation, 33, *34*
  chemical, of inflammation, 25, 33–39, *34*, 38(t)
    of type I (anaphylactic) hypersensitivity, 123, *124*, 125, 125(t)
  plasma-derived, of inflammation, 33, *34*
Medionecrosis, cystic, of aorta, 297, *297*
Mediterranean fever, familial, 167
Medullary carcinoma, of breast, 638
  of thyroid gland, *662*, 662–663

Medulloblastoma, 724
Megacolon, 494–495, *495*
  toxic, 503
Megaesophagus, 479
Megaloblastic anemia, 346–349
Meigs' syndrome, 627
Melanin, in albinism, 93
  intracellular accumulation of, 19
Melanocarcinoma, 213–214
Melanoma, 213–214
  nevi and, 213
  nodular, 214, *214*
  radial growth of, 213
  superficial spreading, 213–214
  vertical growth of, 213, 214
Membrane(s), basement. See *Basement membrane.*
  cell, injury to, 6–7, 7(t), 12. See also *Cell(s), injury to.*
    lipid peroxidation of, 9
    phospholipid loss in, 7
  hyaline, in adult respiratory distress syndrome, 400
    in neonatal respiratory distress syndrome, 387, *388*
  red blood cell, 335, *335*
Membranoproliferative glomerulonephritis, *448*, 448–449
Membranous glomerulonephritis (nephropathy), 445–447, *446*
  lupus erythematosus and, 144
MEN (multiple endocrine neoplasia), 675(t), 679(t), 679–680
Mendelian diseases, 85(t), 85–98
  autosomal dominant, 85(t), 85–88
  autosomal recessive, 85(t), 88–98
    enzyme deficiency and, 89, *89*
  X-linked, 85(t), 98
Meningeal carcinomatosis, 725
Meningioma, 724–725, *725*
Meningioma en plaque, 724
Meningitis, 708–709
  acute (purulent), *708*, 708–709
  acute lymphocytic (viral), 709
  chronic, 709
  cryptococcal, 424
  tuberculous, 709
Menorrhagia, 616
Mental retardation, in Down's syndrome, 107
  in fragile X syndrome, 111
  in galactosemia, 92
  in Klinefelter's syndrome, 110
  in phenylketonuria, 91
Mercuric chloride poisoning, 9
Mesangial lupus nephritis, 143
Mesenchymal tumors, benign, 174(t)
  malignant. See *Sarcoma.*
Mesenteric thrombosis, 497
Mesothelioma, 432–433
Metabolic diseases, of bone, 682–684
  of nervous system, 732
Metabolic encephalopathy, 731–732
Metachromatic leukodystrophy, 732
Metalloproteinases, in wound healing, 56–57
Metaplasia, 51
  apocrine, 632
  myeloid, with myelofibrosis, *373*, 373–374
  of columnar epithelial cells, *22*
Metastasis, 179–180, 180(t), *196*, 198
Metastatic calcification, 22, 23
Methyl alcohol, toxic effects of, 230(t)
Mice, transgenic, 84
Microaneurysm(s), cerebral, 715
  retinal, in diabetes mellitus, 578
Microangiopathic hemolytic anemia, 344
Microangiopathy, in diabetes mellitus, 575
Microcirculatory thrombosis, 73, 378
Microglia, 706
Micronodular cirrhosis, 543, 546, *547*
Microsomal ethanol-oxidizing system (MEOS), 548–549
Migratory thrombophlebitis, in cancer, 72, 299
Mikulicz syndrome, 404, 477

Miliary tuberculosis, 420, 421
Milk leg, 72
Milroy's disease, 300
Mineral dust pneumoconioses, 220–226, *221*, 221(t)
Minimal change disease (lipoid nephrosis), 445, *446*
Mitochondrial myopathies, 16
Mitochondrion (mitochondria), alterations in, 16
  damage to, in cell injury, 9, 12
Mitral valve, calcification of anulus of, 325
  disease of, 319(t)
  prolapse of, 319–320, *320*
  rheumatic disease of, 322, *322*
  vegetations on, infective endocarditis and, *324*
    lupus erythematosus and, 142–143, *143*
Mixed cellularity Hodgkin's disease, 363
Mixed tumor(s), 173, 174(t)
  of salivary glands, 173, *173*, 477, *478*
  of testis, 594, 595(t)
Mole, hydatidiform, 629(t), 629–630, *630*
  invasive, 630
Molecular diagnosis, of genetic diseases, 83, 111–114
Molecular events, in cell growth, 48–50, *49*
Monckeberg's medial calcific sclerosis, 277–278
Monoclonal gammopathy, 166–167, 375
Monoclonality, of tumors, assessment of, 184, *184*
Monocyte(s), 40
  in HIV infection, 161
Mononeuropathy, 733
Mononeuropathy multiplex, 733
Mononuclear inflammation, 272–273
Mononuclear phagocyte system. See also *Macrophage(s).*
  in inflammation, 40, *41*
Mononucleosis, infectious, 351–353
Monosodium urate crystal deposition, in joints, 99, 101, 102
  in kidney, *102*, 103
Monosomy, 104
Mosaic pattern, in Paget's disease of bone, 686–687, *687*
Mosaicism, 104
Motor neuron disease (amyotrophic lateral sclerosis complex), 729
Mouth, 473–477. See also *Oral cavity.*
  dry, in Sjogren's syndrome, 149, 150
Mucocele, of appendix, 521
  of gallbladder, 565
Mucocutaneous lymph node syndrome (Kawasaki's disease), 286(t), 292–293
Mucopolysaccharidoses, 95(t), 97–98
Mucormycosis, *264*, 424
Mucoviscidosis (cystic fibrosis), 89–91
Multifactorial inheritance (polygenic inheritance), 98, *98*
  disorders with, 98–103
Multifocal leukoencephalopathy, progressive, 712
Multinodular goiter, 653–655, *654*
Multiple endocrine neoplasia, 675(t), 679(t), 679–680
Multiple myeloma, 166, 374, 375, *375*, 376
Multiple sclerosis, 729–731, *730*
Mumps, 477
  orchitis in, 596
Mural thrombi, 70, *70*
Muscle, 696–700
  atrophy of, 697
  dystrophy of, *697*, 697–698
  glycogen deposition in, 94(t)
  hypertrophy of, 21
  in myasthenia gravis, *698*, 698–699
  in polymyositis-dermatomyositis, 153–154
  in trichinosis, *699*, 699–700
  inflammatory disease of, 697
    with cutaneous manifestations, 153–154
  systemic sclerosis involving, 152
  tumors of, 700(t), 702, *703*
Muscle phosphorylase, deficiency of, 94(t)
Muscular dystrophy, *697*, 697–698
Musculoskeletal system, 681–703
Myasthenia gravis, *698*, 698–699
  thymoma in, 679

Mycobacterium leprae infection, 42(t), *273*
Mycobacterium tuberculosis infection, 42(t), 416–422, *418*
  bone involvement in, 686
  chronic adrenocortical insufficiency in, 672
  intestinal, 421
  laryngitis in, 434
  meningitis in, 709
  miliary, 420, 421
  primary, 418–419, *419*
  pulmonary, 418, *419*, 420, *420*, *421*
  secondary (reactivation), 419–422, *420*
Mycoplasmal infection, 262(t), 263
  and pneumonia, 415–416
Mycoses, deep, 422–424
Mycosis fungoides, 360
Myelin figures, 5
Myelocytic (myeloblastic, myeloid) leukemia, acute, 367–368, *368*, 368(t)
  chronic, 369, *369*
    chromosomal translocation and, 189, *189*, 193, 369
Myelodysplastic syndromes, 368
Myelofibrosis, myeloid metaplasia with, *373*, 373–374
Myeloid metaplasia, with myelofibrosis, *373*, 373–374
Myeloma, multiple, 374, 375, *375*, 376
  amyloidosis in, 166
Myeloma nephrosis, 375–376
Myelopathy, vacuolar, in AIDS, 711–712
Myelophthisic anemia, 350
Myeloproliferative disorders, 372–374
Myocarditis, 326(t), 326–327, *327*
Myocardium, abscess of, *13*
  adaptation by, 3, *4*
  coagulative necrosis of, 13, *13*, *310*, 311–312
  death of, *4*
  disease of, 325–329
  fatty change in, 18
  hypertrophy of, 3
  infarction of, 72, 308–313, *310*, 311(t)
    arterial thrombi in, 73
    diabetes mellitus and, 575
    ventricular thrombi in, 73, *73*
  injury to, 3, *4*
  ischemia of, 309(t), *312*
  necrosis of, 13, *13*
    coagulative, 13, *13*, *310*, 311–312
    liquefactive, *13*
Myofibroblasts, in wound healing, 54
Myometrium, tumors of, 618–619
Myopathic glycogen storage disease, 94, *94*, 94(t)
Myopathy (myopathies), inflammatory, 697
  with cutaneous manifestations, 153–154
  mitochondrial, 16
Myositis, 697
  with cutaneous manifestations, 153–154
Myxedema, 649–650
  pretibial, 652
Myxoma, 331, *331*

N
Nabothian cysts, 612
Nasopharyngeal carcinoma, 434–435
  Epstein-Barr virus infection and, 202
Natural immunity, 119
  cytokines in, 119
Natural killer (NK) cells, 119, *119*
  in host defenses against cancer, 204–205
Necrosis, 12–14
  caseous, 13–14
  cerebral, laminar, 713
  coagulative, 3–4, 13, *13*
    of myocardium, 13, *13*, *310*, 311–312
  fat, enzymatic, of pancreas, 14, *14*, 581, 582, *582*
    traumatic, of breast, 635

Necrosis *(Continued)*
  fibrinoid, of blood vessel walls, in immune complex–mediated hypersensitivity, 129, *130*
  hemorrhagic, of liver, 529–530
  hepatic, acute hepatitis and, 537
    alcoholic hepatitis and, 546, *546*
    bridging, 540, *540*
    chronic active hepatitis and, 540, *540*
    fulminant hepatitis and, 538, *538*
    hemorrhagic, 529–530
    massive, 527, 538, *538*
    piecemeal, 540, *540*
    submassive, 538
  laminar, of brain, 713
  liquefactive, 13, *13*
  myocardial, 13, *13*, 310, 311–312
  pancreatic, 14, *14*, 581, 582, *582*
  pituitary, 647–648
  renal cortical, diffuse, 458–459
  renal papillary, 454–455, 578, *578*
    diabetes mellitus and, 578
  renal tubular, acute, 457–458, *458*
  vascular wall, fibrinoid, in immune complex–mediated hypersensitivity, 129, *130*
Necrotizing inflammation, 273
Necrotizing papillitis, 454–455, 578, *578*
  diabetes mellitus and, 578
Necrotizing vasculitis. See *Vasculitis.*
Negri body, 710
Neisseria gonorrhoeae infection, 600–601, *601*
Nelson's syndrome, 646
Neonate. See *Newborn* and see also *Child(ren)* and *Infant(s).*
Neoplasia, 171–214. See also *Cancer; Tumor(s)*; and specific types, e.g., *Carcinoma.*
  benign, 172, 174–179
    clinical features in, 206
    definition of, 172
    differentiation in, 175, 176, 180(t)
    effects of, on host, 206
    encapsulation in, 177, 178, *178*
    epithelial, 174(t)
    hormone secretion in, 206
    malignant change in, 184
    mesenchymal, 174(t)
    nomenclature applied to, 172, 174(t)
    vs. cancer, 174–179, 180(t)
  definition of, 172
  differentiation in, 175–177, 180(t)
  endocrine, multiple, 675(t), 679(t), 679–680
  epithelial, benign, 174(t)
    malignant. See *Carcinoma.*
  intraepithelial, cervical, 612, 613
    vulvar, 610
  malignant. See *Cancer* and specific types, e.g., *Carcinoma.*
  mesenchymal, benign, 174(t)
    malignant. See *Sarcoma.*
  mixed, 173, 174(t)
  nomenclature applied to, 172–174, 174(t)
  parenchyma in, 172
    differentiation of, 175
  rate of growth in, 177, 180(t)
  supporting stroma in, 172
  teratogenous, 173, 174(t)
Neovascularization (angiogenesis), 52, *53*
  in tumor growth, 194–195
Nephritic syndrome, 438, 449–453
Nephritis. See also *Glomerulonephritis.*
  analgesic usage and, 456–457
  anti–glomerular basement membrane, *441*, 441–442
  drug-induced, *456*, 456–457
  hereditary, 451–452
  Heymann, 442–443
  immune complex, 440–443, *441, 442*
  lupus, 143, *144, 145*
  Masugi, 441

Nephritis *(Continued)*
  tubulointerstitial, 453–457
Nephrolithiasis, 438, 465–466, 466(t)
Nephropathy, diabetic, 576–578, *577, 578*
  hepatic, 528
  IgA (Berger's disease), 451
  membranous, 445–447, *446*
  reflux, *455*, 455–456
  urate, 103
Nephrosclerosis, benign, 462, *463*
  malignant, *463*, 463–464
Nephrosis, glycogen, 578
  lipoid (minimal change disease), 445, *446*
  myeloma, 375–376
Nephrotic syndrome, 438, 444–449, 445(t)
  edema in, 62
Nephrotoxic acute tubular necrosis, 457, 458, *458*
Nervous system, 705–734
  AIDS involving, 162–165, 711–712
  central, 706–732. See also *Brain.*
  diabetes mellitus involving, 578–579, 734
  peripheral, 732–734
    AIDS involving, 712
  tumors of, 720–725, 721(t), 734
Neurilemmoma (schwannoma), 734
Neuroblastoma, 676–677, 677(t)
  amplification of N-*myc* gene in, *189*
  chromosomal alterations and, 677, *678*
Neurofibrillary tangles, in Alzheimer's disease, 17, 726
Neurofibroma, 88, 734
Neurofibromatosis, von Recklinghausen's, 88, 675(t), 734
Neurogenic shock, 78(t)
Neuroma, acoustic, 88
Neuronophagia, 710
Neuropathy, 733(t), 733–734
  demyelinating, 733(t), 734
  diabetic, 578–579, 734
  peripheral, 733(t), 733–734
  thiamine deficiency and, 252–253
Neuropeptides, in inflammation, 39
Neurotoxins, 731
Neutral proteases, in inflammation, 38
Neutropenia, 351
Nevus (nevi), 212–213
  acquired, 212
  compound, 212, *213*
  dysplastic, 212–213
  intradermal, 212
  junctional, 212
  pigmented, 212–213
  relationship of, to melanoma, 213
Newborn. See also *Child(ren)* and *Infant(s).*
  AIDS transmission to, 158
  cytomegalic inclusion disease in, 426, *426, 427*
  esophageal atresia in, 479
  gonococcal ophthalmia in, 601
  hemolytic disease in, 343–344
  hepatitis in, 528–529
  herpes in, 606
  jaundice in, 525
  mendelian disorders in, 85(t)
  respiratory distress in, 386–388, *388*
  vaginitis in, 611(t)
Niacin, 245(t), 254
  deficiency of, 245(t), 254, *254*
NIDDM (non–insulin-dependent diabetes mellitus), 569, 570(t). See also *Diabetes mellitus.*
Niemann-Pick disease, *96*, 96–97
Night blindness, 245(t), 246
Nitric oxide, 39
  effects of, on platelets, 65
Nitrosamines, as carcinogens, 200
N-*myc* gene, amplification of, in neuroblastoma, *189*
Nocardiosis, 416
Nocturnal hemoglobinuria, paroxysmal, 342
Nodular fasciitis (pseudosarcomatous fasciitis), 700(t), 702–703

Nodular glomerulosclerosis, in diabetes mellitus, 576–577, *577*
Nodular hyperplasia, of adrenal cortex, 668, *668*
  of prostate, 596–597, *597*
Nodular lymphoma, 355, *356*
Nodular melanoma, 214, *214*
Nodular sclerosis Hodgkin's disease, 363, *365*
Nodularity, hepatic, in cirrhosis, 542–543
Non-A, non-B hepatitis, 534
Nonbacterial thrombotic endocarditis, 71, 324
Nonenzymatic glycosylation, in diabetes mellitus, 573
Nongonococcal urethritis/cervicitis, 602
Non-Hodgkin's lymphoma, 354–361, 357(t), 361(t). See also *Lymphoma, non-Hodgkin's.*
  HIV infection and, 164, 165
Non–insulin-dependent diabetes mellitus, 569, 570(t). See also *Diabetes mellitus.*
Nonketotic hyperosmolar coma, 574
Nontoxic goiter, 653–655
Non-tropical sprue (celiac sprue), 508
Normal homeostasis, in cells, 3
Nuclear regulatory factors, in carcinogenesis, 186(t), 187
Nucleolar alterations, in cell injury, 12
Nucleolar pattern, on indirect immunofluorescence, 140
Nutmeg liver, 306, *307*
Nutritional diseases, 241–259
  and cell injury, 4–5
  and nervous system lesions, 252–253, 731

O
Oat cell carcinoma, of lung, 430
Obesity, 257–258, *258*
  and diabetes mellitus, 572–573
  and gallstones, 562
Obliterative cardiomyopathy, *328*, 329
Obliterative endarteritis, in syphilis, 603
Obstructive lung disease, 389–398
  chronic, 391–398
Occlusive thrombus. See *Thrombus (thrombi).*
Occupational tumors, 182(t)
Oligodendrocytes, 706
Oligodendroglioma, 723–724
Oligonucleotide probe, in diagnosis of α_1-antitrypsin deficiency, 112, *113*
Omphalocele, 494
Oncofetal antigens, 204
Oncogene(s), 185–189, 186(t), *188*
  activation of, 186(t), 187–189
  in leukemia, 372(t)
  in lymphoma, 372(t)
  protein products of, 185–187, 186(t)
Oncogenic viruses, 201–203
Oncoproteins, 185–187, 186(t)
Ophthalmia neonatorum, 601
Opportunistic infections, in AIDS, 164, 164(t)
Opsonins, 31, 262
Oral cavity, 473–477
  aphthous ulcers of, 474
  cancer of, 475–476, *476*, 476(t)
  candidiasis of, 423, 474
  carcinoma in situ of, *476*
  erythroplasia of, 475
  herpetic inflammation of, 474
  inflammatory lesions of, 473–474
  leukoplakia of, 474–475, *475*
    hairy, in AIDS, 474, 475
  squamous cell carcinoma of, *177*, 475–476, *476*
  ulcerative lesions of, 473–474
Oral contraceptives, adverse effects of, 72–73, 228–229
Orchitis, 595–596
Organization, in inflammation, 44, 58
  of thrombus, 71
Orthopnea, 306
Osler-Weber-Rendu disease, 300

Osmotic pressure, plasma, 61, *62*
  decreased, 61, 62, 62(t)
  in edema, 61, 62, 62(t)
  in inflammation, 27, *27*
Osteitis deformans (Paget's disease of bone), *686*, 686–688, *687*
Osteitis fibrosa cystica, 684
Osteoarthritis, 693–695, *694*, *695*
Osteoarthropathy, hypertrophic, *688*, 688–689
Osteochondroma, 689
Osteoclastoma (giant cell tumor of bone), *690*, 690–691
Osteodystrophy, renal, 684
Osteoid osteoma, 689
Osteoma, 689
Osteomalacia, 248, 250(t), 251, 684
Osteomyelitis, pyogenic, 684, *684*
  tuberculous, 685
Osteopenia (osteoporosis), 682(t), 682–684, *683*
Osteoporosis (osteopenia), 682(t), 682–684, *683*
Osteosarcoma, *691*, 691–692, *692*
Ostium primum, 316
Ostium secundum, 316
Ovary (ovaries), 621–628
  androblastoma of, 626
  Brenner tumor of, 625
  cancer of, 622–628, 623(t)
  chocolate cysts of, 616, *617*
  choriocarcinoma of, 626
  clear cell tumor of, 622(t), *622*
  cystadenocarcinoma of, 623, 624, *624*
  cystadenofibroma of, 625
  cystadenoma of, 623, *623*, 624
  cystic teratoma of, 625, *625*
  cysts of, 621–622
    chocolate, 616, *617*
    dermoid, 625, *625*
    follicle, 621
    luteal, 621
  dermoid cyst of, 625, *625*
  dysgerminoma of, 626
  endometrioid tumors of, 624
  fibroma of, 627, *627*
  follicle cysts of, 621
  germ cell tumors of, *622*, 625–626
  granulosa-theca cell tumors of, 626–627, *627*
  immature teratoma of, 625–626
  Krukenberg tumor of, 628
  luteal cysts of, 621
  mature teratoma of, 625, *625*
  metastasis of cancer to, 628
  monodermal teratoma of, 626
  mucinous tumors of, 624
  polycystic, 621–622
  serous tumors of, *623*, 623–624, *624*
  Sertoli-Leydig cell tumors of, 627
  sex cord–stromal tumors of, *622*, 626–627
  surface epithelial–stromal tumors of, *622*, 623–625
  teratoma of, *625*, 625–626
  thecoma of, 626
  tumors of, *622*, 622–628, 623(t)
    clinical manifestations of, 627–628
Oxygen. See also *Oxygen-derived free radical(s).*
  in injury, to cell membranes, 7
    to cells, 5, *5*, 8, *8*, 9, 10
    to lungs, 10
Oxygen-derived free radical(s), and inflammation, 10, 38
  and injury, to cell membranes, 7
    to cells, 8, *8*, 9, 10

P
PAF (platelet-activating factor), 37, 125, 125(t)
Paget's disease, of bone, *686*, 686–688, *687*
  of breast, 639
  of vulva, 609, *610*

Panacinar (panlobular) emphysema, *392*, 393, *393*
Pancoast's tumor, 431
Pancreas, 569–586
  carcinoma of, *585*, 585–586, *586*
  cystic fibrosis of, 90, *91*
  endocrine, 569–581
  enzymatic fat necrosis of, 14, *14*, 581, 582, *582*
  exocrine, 581–586
  fat necrosis of, 14, *14*, 581, 582, *582*
  fibrosis of, cystic, 90, *91*
  hemosiderin deposition in, 556
  inflammation of, 581–585
    acute, 581–584, *582*, *583*, 583(t)
    chronic, 584–585
  injury to, acute pancreatitis due to, 583
  islet cell disorders of, 569–581
    diabetes mellitus due to, 569–580. See also *Diabetes mellitus*.
    neoplastic, 580–581
  morphologic changes in, in diabetes mellitus, 575, *575*
  necrosis of, 14, *14*, 581, 582, *582*
  pseudocyst in, 582
  tumors of, 580–581, 585–586
    in multiple endocrine neoplasia syndrome I, 679–680
Pancreatic pseudocyst, 582
Pancreatitis, 581–585
  acute, 581–584, *582*, *583*, 583(t)
  alcoholic, 584
  calcifying, 584
  cholelithiasis and, 583
  chronic, 584–585
  edematous, 581
  hemorrhagic, 581, 582, *582*
Pancytopenia, in aplastic anemia, 349
  in myelodysplastic syndromes, 368
Panencephalitis, subacute sclerosing, 712
Panlobular (panacinar) emphysema, *392*, 393, *393*
Pannus, 146
Pantothenic acid, 245(t)
  deficiency of, 245(t)
Papanicolaou smears, in diagnosis of cancer, 209, *209*
Papillary carcinoma, of thyroid gland, *660*, 660–661
Papillary cystadenoma lymphomatosum (Warthin's tumor), 477–478
Papillary fibroelastoma, 331
Papillitis, necrotizing renal, 454–455, 578, *578*
  diabetes mellitus and, 578
Papilloma, 172, *173*
  bladder, 469
  breast, 636
  colonic, *173*
  genital, 604
  intraductal, of breast, 636
  laryngeal, 435
Papillomavirus, 202
  infection by, and cervical cancer, 613
    and condyloma, 604, 609, 613
    and penile cancer, 590
Paraesophageal hiatal hernia, 480, *480*
Paralysis agitans (idiopathic Parkinson's disease), 729
Paraneoplastic syndromes, 207–208, 208(t)
Paraphimosis, 589
Paraseptal emphysema (distal acinar emphysema), 393
Parathyroid glands, 663–666
  adenoma of, 664, *664*
  carcinoma of, 665
  hyperplasia of, 664–665, *665*
  hypersecretion of hormone by, 663–666
  inadequate hormone secretion by, 666
Parenchyma, of tumors, 172
  differentiation of, 175
Parkinsonism, 728–729
Parotid gland diseases. See *Salivary gland(s)*.
Paroxysmal nocturnal hemoglobinuria, 342
Partial hydatidiform mole, 629, 629(t), 630
Passive congestion, 64
  hepatic, in right ventricular failure, 306, *307*, 529
  pulmonary, in left ventricular failure, 64, 306

Patau's syndrome, *108*
Patent ductus arteriosus, 317
Paterson-Brown-Kelly syndrome, 479
Pathology, definition of, 3
Pavementing, of endothelium, in inflammation, 28
Peau d'orange, 300
Pediatric disease. See *Child(ren)*; *Infant(s)*; *Newborn*.
Peliosis hepatis, 530
Pellagra, 254, *254*
Pelvic inflammatory disease, 601, *621*
Penetrance, mendelian, 86
Penetrating wound, 236
Penis, 589–590
  balanoposthitis of, 589
  Bowen's disease of, 589
  carcinoma of, 589
  epispadias of, 589
  hypospadias of, 589
  phimosis of, 589
Peptic ulcer, 45, 487(t), 487–490, *488*, 488(t), *489*
  complications of, 490(t)
  duodenal, 45, 487, 488, 489
  gastric, 487–490, *489*
    vs. gastric carcinoma, *493*
Periarteritis nodosa (polyarteritis nodosa), 286(t), *288*, 288–289
Pericardial disease, 329–330
Pericardial effusion, 330
Pericarditis, 330
  in systemic lupus erythematosus, 142
Periorbital edema, 63
Peripheral nervous system, 732–734
  AIDS involving, 712
  axonal degeneration in, 732
  disorders of, 733(t), 733–734
  in diabetes mellitus, 578–579, 733(t), 734
  regeneration in, 732
  segmental demyelination in, 732–733, *733*
  tumors of, 734
  wallerian degeneration in, 732
Perivascular cuffing, in syphilis, 603
Permanent cells, 48
Permeability, vascular, increased, in inflammation, 26, 27, 28, *28*, 36
Pernicious anemia, 347–349, *349*
  chronic gastritis and, 485
  neurologic changes in, 731
Peroxidation, of cell membranes, 9
Petechiae, 64
Peutz-Jeghers syndrome, 514, 514(t)
PG. See *Prostaglandin* entries.
Phagocytes. See also *Phagocytosis* and *Macrophage(s)*.
  in inflammation, 40, *41*
Phagocytosis, 15
  in inflammation, 30–32, *32*, 36
    defective, 33
Pharyngitis, acute, 434
Phenobarbital, effects of, on smooth endoplasmic reticulum of liver, *16*
Phenylalanine hydroxylase, deficiency of, 91–92
Phenylketonuria, 91–92
Pheochromocytoma, 675(t), 675–676, *676*
Philadelphia chromosome, in chronic myeloid leukemia, 189, *189*, 193, 369
Phimosis, 589
Phlebothrombosis, 70, 71, 72, 299
Phlegmasia alba dolens, 72
Phospholipids, antibodies against, in lupus erythematosus, 140
  in thrombogenesis, 70
  loss of, in cell membrane, 7
Phosphorylase, muscle, deficiency of, 94(t)
Phyllodes tumor, 636
Physical agent–related injury, 236–241
  to cells, 4
Pick's disease, 726
Pigeon breast deformity, 250
Pigment(s), intracellular accumulation of, 18–19
Pigment cirrhosis, 554–556, 555(t), *556*

Pigment stones, 562, 563, 563(t)
Pigmented nevi, 212–213
Pili, gonococcal, 600
Pilocytic astrocytoma, 723
"Pink puffers," 395
Pinocytosis, 15
Pipestem fibrosis, of liver, *273*
Pitting edema, 63
Pituitary apoplexy, 645
Pituitary gland, 643–648
  ACTH-secreting adenoma of, 646, 667
  adenoma of, 644(t), *644–646*, 644–647
    Cushing's disease due to, 646, 667
  atrophy of, 648, *648*
  carcinoma of, 647
  cells of, 643–644, 644(t)
  corticotroph adenoma of, 646–647
  empty sella syndrome and, 648
  excess hormone secretion by, 644–647
  gonadotroph adenoma of, 647
  growth hormone–secreting adenoma of, 645–646
  hormone-secreting adenoma of, *645*, 645–647, *646*
  hypofunction of, 647–648
  necrosis of, 647–648
  nonsecretory (null cell, chromophobe) adenoma of, 647
  posterior, 648
  prolactinoma of, 646, *646*
  Sheehan's necrosis of, 647
  somatotroph adenoma of, *645*, 645–646
  tumors of, 644–647
PKU (phenylketonuria), 91–92
Placenta, infection and inflammation of, 628
  tumors of, 629–630
Plaque(s), athcromatous, *284*, 284–285, *285*
  cerebral, in Alzheimer's disease, 726–727, *727*
    in multiple sclerosis, 730
  pleural, in asbestosis, *225*, 225–226
  senile, in Alzheimer's disease, 726–727, *727*
Plasma, colloid osmotic pressure of, 61, *62*
    decreased, 61, 62, 62(t)
    in edema, 61, 62, 62(t)
    in inflammation, 27, *27*
Plasma cell(s), in inflammation, *40*, 42
Plasma cell dyscrasias, 374–376
  with amyloidosis, 166–167, 167(t)
Plasma membrane. See *Cell membrane.*
Plasmacytoma, 374
Plasmids, 262
Plasmin, in inflammation, 36
Plasminogen activator(s), 68–69
Plasminogen-plasmin system, 68–69
Plasmodium species, infection by, 344–345
Platelet(s), 66
  activation of, 67
  adhesion of, to collagen, 67
    to endothelial cells, inhibition of, 65
  ADP release by, 67
  aggregation of, 67
  alpha granules in, 66
  deficiency of, 380–381
  electron-dense bodies in, 66
  in hemostasis, 66–67, *67*
  release reaction by, 67
  secretion by, 67
Platelet-activating factor, 37
  in inflammation, 37
  in type I (anaphylactic) hypersensitivity, 125
Platelet-derived growth factor, 51
  in wound healing, 56(t)
Platelet factor 3, 67
Pleiotropy, genetic, 85
Pleomorphic adenoma, 173, *173*, 477, *478*
Pleura, inflammation of, *44*, 433
  mesothelioma of, 432–433
  plaques on, in asbestosis, *225*, 225–226
Pleural effusion, 433

Pleural space, air in, 433
  blood in, 433
  chyle in, 433–434
  effusion in, 433
  fluid in, 433
Pleuritis, 433
Plummer-Vinson syndrome, 346
Plunging goiter, 654
Pneumococcal pneumonia, 412–413
Pneumoconiosis (pneumoconioses), 220–226, *221*, 221(t)
  asbestos exposure and, 221(t), 223–226, *225*
  beryllium exposure and, 221(t), 226
  coal workers', 19, 221(t), 221–223, *222*
  mineral dust, 220–226, *221*, 221(t)
  silica inhalation and, 221(t), 223, *224*
Pneumocystis carinii infection, 426–427, *427*
Pneumonia, 411(t), 411–416
  acute bacterial, 411(t), 411–414, *412*, *413*
  atypical, 411(t), 415–416
  Branhamella catarrhalis infection and, 414
  bronchial, 411, 412, *412*, *413*
    aspiration and, 414
  chronic, 411, 411(t)
  emigration of inflammatory cells in, *31*
  Haemophilus influenzae infection and, 413–414
  hypostatic, pulmonary edema and, 64
  interstitial, desquamative, 402
  Klebsiella pneumoniae infection and, *272*, 414
  Legionella pneumophila infection and, 414
  lobar, 411, 412, *412*, *413*
  mycoplasmal, 415–416
  pneumococcal, 412–413
  Pneumocystis carinii infection and, 426–427, *427*
  Pseudomonas aeruginosa infection and, 414
  Staphylococcus aureus infection and, 414
  Streptococcus pneumoniae infection and, 412–413
  tuberculous, 420
  viral, *415*
Pneumonitis, 411
  hypersensitivity, 405, 405(t)
  interstitial, 401
Pneumothorax, 433
Poisoning, 4, 226. See also specific agents.
Poliomyelitis, 710
Pollutant, definition of, 218
Pollution, 217–226
  air, 218(t), 218–219, 219(t)
  environmental, 217–226, 218(t)
  pneumoconioses due to, 220–226, *221*, 221(t)
  smoking and, 219–220, *220*, 220(t)
Polyarteritis nodosa, 286(t), *288*, 288–289
Polycyclic hydrocarbons, as carcinogens, 199
Polycystic kidney disease, adult, 464–465, *465*
  childhood, 465
Polycystic ovaries, 621–622
Polycythemia, 350, 350(t)
Polycythemia vera, 372–373
Polygenic inheritance (multifactorial inheritance), 98, *98*
  disorders with, 98–103
Polymyalgia rheumatica syndrome, 290
Polymyositis-dermatomyositis, 153–154
  antinuclear antibodies in, 141(t)
  morphologic changes in, 153–154, *154*
Polyneuropathy, 733
  acute idiopathic, 734
  thiamine deficiency and, 252–253
Polyp(s), 172
  adenomatous, of colon, *510*, 510–514, *512*, *513*, 514(t)
    of stomach, 490, 491(t)
  cervical, 612
  colonic, *510*, 510–514, *512*, *513*, 514(t)
    malignant transformation of, 192, *193*, 513, *514*
  endometrial, 618
  gastric, 490, 491(t)
  hamartomatous, of colon, 514, 514(t)
  hyperplastic, of colon, *510*, 511

Polyp(s) *(Continued)*
 of stomach, 490, 491(t)
 juvenile, of colon, 511
 nonneoplastic, of colon, 511
 uterine, 618
 uterine cervical, 612
 vocal cord, 435
Polyploidy, 104
Polyposis, heredofamilial, 513–514, 514(t)
Pompe's disease, 94, 94(t)
Porcelain gallbladder, 565
Port-wine stain, 301
Portal hypertension, *544,* 544–545
 intrahepatic, 544, *544*
 posthepatic, 544, *544*
 prehepatic, 544, *544*
Portal vein thrombosis, 530
Portosystemic shunts, 545
Posterior pituitary syndromes, 648
Postgonococcal urethritis, 602
Postinfectious (acute proliferative, poststreptococcal) glomerulone-
 phritis, 449–450, *450*
Postinfectious (tropical) sprue, 509
Postmortem clots, vs. venous thromboses, 70
Postnecrotic cirrhosis, 550–552, *551*
Postrenal azotemia, 438
Poststreptococcal (acute proliferative, postinfectious) glomerulonephritis, 449–450, *450*
Potato node, 403
Pott's disease, 686
Pregnancy, amniotic fluid embolism in, 75
 choriocarcinoma in, 630–631, *631*
 diseases of, 628–631
 ectopic, 628–629, *629*
 granuloma pyogenicum occurring in, 300
 hydatidiform mole in, 629(t), 629–630, *630*
 invasive mole in, 630
 placental inflammations and infections in, 628
 trophoblastic disease in, 628–631
 tubal, 628, *629*
 tumor (granuloma pyogenicum) occurring in, 300
 venous thrombosis in, 72
Pregnancy tumor, 300
Preneoplastic disorders, 183, 183(t), 184
Prerenal azotemia, 438
Pretibial myxedema, 652
Primary healing, 53
Prinzmetal's angina, 307
Progression, tumor, *195,* 195–196
Progression factors, in cell growth, 48
Progressive massive fibrosis, of lungs, 222, *222*
Progressive multifocal leukoencephalopathy, 712
Prolactinoma, 646, *646*
Prolapse, mitral valve, 319–320, *320*
Proliferative glomerulonephritis, diffuse, 449
 focal, 451
 in systemic lupus erythematosus, 143–144
Proliferative retinopathy, in diabetes mellitus, 578
Prostaglandin(s), 36
 in inflammation, 36, 37, *37*
Prostaglandin D_2, in type I (anaphylactic) hypersensitivity,
 125
Prostaglandin I_2 (prostacyclin), effects of, 36
 on platelets, 65
 vs. effects of thromboxane, 67
 in inflammation, 36, *37*
Prostate, 596–599
 bacterial infection of, 596
 benign hypertrophy of, 596–597, *597*
 carcinoma of, 597–599, *598*
 inflammation of, 596
 nodular hyperplasia of, 596–597, *597*
Prostatitis, 596
Prosthetic heart valves, complications of, 325, 344
Protein C, 68

Protein-energy malnutrition, 242–244, *243*
Protein S, 68
Proteinuria, 438, 444
Proteoglycan(s), 56
 in wound healing, 56
Protooncogene(s), 185. See also *Oncogene(s).*
 expression of, after partial hepatectomy, 50, *50*
 in cell growth, 50
Protozoal infection(s), 262(t), 264
 AIDS and, 164(t)
 diarrhea due to, 504(t)
 gastrointestinal, 266–267
Proud flesh, 58
Psammoma bodies, in meningioma, 725
Pseudocyst, pancreatic, 582
Pseudolymphoma, 150
Pseudomembranous colitis, *Clostridium difficile* infection and, 506,
 506
Pseudomonas aeruginosa infection, and pneumonia, 414
 in cystic fibrosis, 90
Pseudomyxoma peritonei, 521, 624
Pseudopolyp, 502, *502*
Pseudosarcomatous fasciitis (nodular fasciitis), 700(t), 702–703
Psoriatic arthropathy, 149(t)
Psychosis, Korsakoff's, thiamine deficiency and, 253, 731
Pulmonary. See also *Lung(s).*
Pulmonary abscess, 411(t), 424–425
Pulmonary alveolus (alveoli), diffuse damage to, 399(t), 399–401, *400*
 emigration of inflammatory cells into, *31*
 immune-mediated inflammation of, 405
 wall of, *398*
Pulmonary anthracosis, 221–222
Pulmonary congestion, left ventricular failure and, 64, 306
Pulmonary edema, 64, *64*
 alveolocapillary block associated with, 64
 drug addiction and, 235
 hypostatic pneumonia associated with, 64
Pulmonary embolism, 74, *74,* 406–408, *407, 408*
Pulmonary fibrosis, idiopathic, 401–403, *402, 403*
Pulmonary hemorrhage, 405, 406, 407
 vs. pulmonary infarction, 77
Pulmonary hemorrhagic infarction, 76, *76*
Pulmonary hemosiderosis, 406
Pulmonary hypertension, 408–409, 409(t)
 and heart disease, 315
Pulmonary infarction, 76, *76,* 407, *408*
 vs. pulmonary hemorrhage, 77
Pulmonary infection, 409–427, 411(t)
 cystic fibrosis and, 90
 edema and, 64
Pulmonary stenosis, 318
Pulmonary vascular sclerosis, 409
Pulseless disease (Takayasu's arteritis), 291–292
Puncture wound, 236
Purine, synthesis of, 99, *100*
Purpura, 64
 Henoch-Schonlein, 287–288
 idiopathic thrombocytopenic, 380–381
 palpable, 287
 thrombotic thrombocytopenic, 381
Purulent (suppurative) inflammation, 44, 272
Purulent meningitis, *708,* 708–709
Pyelonephritis, 453
 acute, 453–455, *454*
 chronic, 455
 vesicoureteral reflux–associated, *455,* 455–456
 diabetes mellitus and, 577–578
Pyknosis, 13
Pyloric stenosis, 484
Pyogenic granuloma, 300
Pyogenic infection(s), 44, 272
Pyogenic osteomyelitis, 684, *684*
Pyosalpinx, 601
Pyridoxine (vitamin B_6), 245(t)
 deficiency of, 245(t), 255

Q
Quiescent cells, 48

R
Radiation injury, 239–241, *240*, *241*, 242(t)
 and carcinogenesis, 200–201
 to cells, 10, 240
Radical(s), free, 8
 and inflammation, 10, 38
 and injury, to cell membranes, 7
  to cells, 8, *8*, 9, 10
Radon, 241
Rapidly progressive (crescentic) glomerulonephritis, 450(t), 450–451, *451*
ras proteins, 187, *187*
 in carcinogenesis, 187, 188
 in cell growth, 49, 50
 mutant, 188
Raynaud's disease, 293–294
Raynaud's phenomenon, 293
 in systemic sclerosis, 153
Rb protein, in cell cycle, 192, *192*
Reactivation tuberculosis (secondary tuberculosis), 419–422, *420*
Reactive arthropathy, 149(t)
Recanalization, of thrombus, *71*, 71–72
Receptor(s), acetylcholine, antibodies to, 698
 binding of ligands to, in cell growth, 48
 growth factor, activation of, 48–49, *49*
  in carcinogenesis, 186, 186(t), *188*
 integrin, 55
 laminin, in cancer cells, 198
 T-cell, 117–118, *118*
Recessive genetic diseases, autosomal, 85(t), 88–98
 enzyme deficiency and, 89, *89*
 X-linked, 98
Recombinant DNA technology, 83–84
 and allele-specific oligonucleotide probing, 112, *113*
 and detection of identity, 115
 and diagnosis, 84
  of cancer, 114–115
  of genetic diseases, 83–84, 111–114
  of infectious diseases, 114
  of tumors, 114–115
 and direct gene diagnosis, 111–113, *112, 113*
 and gene therapy, 84
 and linkage analysis, 113–114
 and restriction fragment length polymorphism analysis, 113 114, *114*
Rectum, carcinoma of. See *Colon, cancer of.*
Red blood cell(s), disorders of, 334–350
Red thrombi (coagulative thrombi, stasis thrombi), 70
Reed-Sternberg cell, 362, *362*
Reflux, vesicoureteral, 454
 chronic pyelonephritis associated with, *455*, 455–456
Reflux esophagitis, 481–482
Regeneration, 47–52
 axonal, 732
 cell cycle in, 47–48
 cell types in, 47–48
 control of cell growth in, 48–52
 endothelial, and leakage, in inflammation, 28, *28*
 hepatic, 21–22
Regional enteritis, 499–501
Reid index, 396
Reiter's syndrome, 149(t)
Rejection (immunologic rejection), 132–134, *134*
 HLA antigens in, 121, 132, *133*, 135
 prevention of, 135
 T cell–mediated, 132, *133*
 vasculitis in, 134, *134*
Release reaction, by platelets, 67
Renal. See also *Kidney(s).*
Renal ablation glomerulopathy, 443–444, *444*

Renal cell carcinoma, 467–469, *468*
Renal cortical necrosis, 458
Renal failure, 438
 acute, 438
 chronic, 438
 gout and, 103
 liver failure and, 528
Renal hypertension, 459, 461
Renal osteodystrophy, 684
Renal stones, 438, 465–466, 466(t)
Renal transplantation, graft rejection in, 132–134, *134*
 prevention of, 135
Renal tubule(s), diseases of, 453–459
 lesions of, in diabetes mellitus, 578
Renal vasodepressor substances, 461
Rendu-Osler-Weber disease, 300
Renin-angiotensin system, in blood pressure regulation, 460, *460*
Renomegaly, in glycogenosis, 94(t)
Renovascular hypertension, 459
Repair, 47–59
 connective tissue in, 47, 52–58
  wound healing and, 53–58, *54*. See also *Wound healing.*
 inflammation and, 25, 39, 58–59, *59*
 pathologic aspects of, 58
 regeneration in, 47–52
  cell cycle and, 47–48
  cell types and, 47–48
  control of cell growth and, 48–52
Resolution, of inflammation, 39, *39*, 44, 58
Respiratory distress syndrome, in adults, 399(t), 399–401, *400*
 in newborn, 386–388, *388*
Respiratory system, 385–436. See also *Lung(s)* and *Pulmonary* entries.
 infection of, 266, 409–427, 434
 upper, lesions of, 434–436
Rest(s), heterotopic, 174
Restriction fragment length polymorphisms, 113
 in diagnosis of genetic diseases, 113–114, *114*
Restrictive cardiomyopathy, *328*, 329
Restrictive lung disease, 389, 398–406
 acute, 399–401
 chronic, 401(t), 401–406
Retina, morphologic changes in, in diabetes mellitus, 578
Retinoblastoma, 183
 pathogenesis of, 189–190, *191*
Retinoic acid, 245
Retinoids, 245, *245*
Retinol, 245
Retinopathy, diabetic, 578
 hypertensive, 459
Retroperitoneal hematoma, 64
Reverse genetics, 83, *84*
Reversible injury, to cells, 3
 mechanisms of, 5, *6, 7*
 morphologic changes in, 12
Reye's syndrome, 529, *530*
Rh incompatibility, 343
 complement-mediated cytotoxicity in, 126
Rhabdomyoma, 700(t), 702
 of heart, 331
Rhabdomyosarcoma, 700(t), 702
 anaplastic, *175*
Rheumatic fever, 320, *321*
Rheumatic heart disease, 320–323, *321, 322*
 arterial thrombi in, 73
Rheumatoid arthritis, 145–149, *146, 148*
 heart disease associated with, 330–331
 juvenile, 149
 vs. degenerative arthritis, *695*
Rheumatoid heart disease, 330–331
Rheumatoid subcutaneous nodules, 146–147
Riboflavin (vitamin B$_2$), 245(t), 253
 deficiency of, 245(t), 253–254, *254*
Rickets, 248, 250, *250*, 250(t), 684
Rickettsial infection, 262(t), 263

Riedel's thyroiditis, 655
Right ventricle, enlargement of, 315
 failure of, 306–307
  edema in, 62, 63
  hepatic congestion in, 306, *307*, 529
 infarction of, 310, *310*
Ring(s), esophageal, 479
Ring chromosome, 106, *106*
RNA oncogenic viruses, 201
Robertsonian translocation (centric fusion type translocation), 106, *106*
 and production of Down's syndrome, 107, *109*
Rocky Mountain spotted fever, 263
Rolling hiatal hernia, 480, *480*
Rotor's syndrome, 526, 527(t)
Rubella (German measles), and congenital heart disease, 316
 and diabetes mellitus, 572
Rupture, of aorta, 64, *237*
 in Marfan's syndrome, 86
 of blood vessels, 64
Russell bodies, 18

S
Saber shins, 604
Sacroiliitis, in spondyloarthropathies, 149(t)
Saddle deformity, of nasal septum, 604
Saddle embolus, 74, 407, *407*
Sago spleen, 169
Salicylism, 229
Salivary gland(s), diseases of, 476–478
 inflammation of, 477
 sarcoidosis of, 404, 405
 tumors of, 477–478
  mixed, 173, *173*, 477, *478*
  Warthin's, 477–478
Salmonellosis, 505–506
Salpingitis, 620–621
Salpingo-oophoritis, 601
Sarcoidosis, 42(t), 403–405, *404*
Sarcoma, 172, 174(t)
 Ewing's, 693
 Kaposi's, 302(t), 302–304, *303, 304*
  AIDS and, 164, 302(t), 302–303, 474
 osteogenic, *691*, 691–692, *692*
 small intestinal, 510
 synovial, 700(t), 702
Sarcoma botryoides, 611, 702
Scarring, 53, 58–59, *59*. See also *Wound healing* and *Repair*.
 abnormal, 58
 infection and, 273
 inflammation and, 25, 39
Schatzki's rings, 479
Schaumann bodies, in sarcoidosis, 403
Schistosomiasis, 42(t)
 pipestem fibrosis of liver in, *273*
Schwannoma (neurilemmoma), 734
Scleroderma (systemic sclerosis), 150–153
 antinuclear antibodies in, 141(t), 151
Sclerosing adenosis, of breast, 633–634, *634*
Sclerosing cholangitis, primary, *552*, 553, 554, 554(t)
Sclerosing panencephalitis, subacute, 712
Sclerosis, amyotrophic lateral, 729
 arterial, 277–285. See also *Atherosclerosis*.
 cardiac, 530
 medial calcific, 277–278
 multiple, 729–731, *730*
 pulmonary vascular, 409
 systemic, 150–153
Scrotum, disorders of, 590
Scurvy, 255
Segmental demyelination, 732–733, *733*
Selenium deficiency, 257

Self-tolerance, 136–137, *137*
 loss of, 138, *138*
Seminiferous tubules, alterations in, in Klinefelter's syndrome, 109–110, *591*
Seminoma, 592, *593*, 595(t)
Senile amyloidosis, 167, 169
Senile dementia, 726
Senile emphysema, 395
Senile hyperinflation, 395
Senile plaques, in Alzheimer's disease, 726–727, *727*
Septic embolus, 77
Septic shock, 78, 78(t), 81
 and diffuse alveolar damage, 399
Serositis, lupus erythematosus and, 142
Serotonin, 34
Serous cystadenocarcinoma, of ovary, 623, *624*
Serous cystadenoma, of ovary, 623, *623*
Serous effusion, pericardial, 330
Serous inflammation, 44
Serous tumors, of ovary, *623*, 623–624, *624*
Serpentine chrysotile, 224
Sertoli-Leydig cell tumors, 627
Serum hepatitis, 532
Serum sickness, acute, 128
Severe combined immunodeficiency, 155–156
Sex chromatin (Barr body), 107
Sex chromosome(s), disorders of, 107, 109–111
Sex cord–stromal tumors, of ovary, *622*, 626–627
Sex-linked diseases, 98
Sexually transmitted diseases (venereal diseases), 599–606, 600(t). See also specific diseases.
Sézary's syndrome, 360
Sheehan's syndrome, 647
Shigellosis, 505
Shock, 78–81
 burns and, 237
 cardiogenic, 78, 78(t), 81
 classification of, 78(t)
 clinical course of, 81
 disseminated intravascular coagulation in, 80, 378
 effects of, 78, 80
  on adrenal cortex, 80
  on gastrointestinal tract, 80, *81*
  on heart, 80
  on kidneys, 80
  on liver, 80
  on lungs, 80, 399
 endotoxic, 78, *79*
 hypovolemic, 78, 78(t), 81
  burns and, 237
 irreversible stage of, 80
 morphologic changes in, 80–81
 neurogenic, 78(t)
 pathogenesis of, *79*
 septic, 78, 78(t), 81
  and diffuse alveolar damage, 399
 stages of, 78, *79*, 80
Shock lung, 80, 399
Short-incubation hepatitis, 531
Shunt(s), cardiac, left-to-right, 316–317
  right-to-left, 317–318
 portosystemic, 545
Sialadenitis, 477
Sicca syndrome, 149
Sickle cell anemia, *336*, 336–337, *337*
Sickle cell disease, diagnosis of, direct gene, 112, *112*
Sidestream smoke, effects of, 220. See also *Smoking*.
SIDS (sudden infant death syndrome), 388(t), 388–389
Sigmoid colon, diverticula of, 496
Signal transduction, in cell growth, *49*, 49–50
Silicosis, 40, 221(t), 223, *224*
Singer's nodes, 435
Sinus histiocytes, 40
Sinus histiocytosis, 354
Sipple's syndrome, 679(t), 680

Sjogren's syndrome, 149–150, *150*, 477
  antinuclear antibodies in, 141(t)
Skeletal muscle, 696–700. See also *Muscle*.
  glycogen deposition in, 94(t)
Skeletal system, 681–693. See also *Bone*.
  abnormalities of, in Marfan's syndrome, 86
Skin, as barrier to infection, 265
  basal cell carcinoma of, 211–212, *212*
  cancer of, 210–214
  carcinoma in situ of, 211
  hemosiderin deposition in, 556
  infection of, 265
  melanoma of, 213–214
  nevi of, 212–213
  polymyositis involving, 153–154
  sarcoidosis involving, 404
  squamous cell carcinoma of, 210–211, *211*
  systemic lupus erythematosus involving, 142, *143*
  systemic sclerosis involving, 152, *152*
  tumors of, 210–214
Skip lesions, in Crohn's disease, 500
Skip metastases, 180
Skull, Paget's disease of, 687, *687*
SLE (systemic lupus erythematosus), 139–145. See also *Systemic lupus erythematosus*.
Sliding hiatal hernia, 480, *480*
Slow viruses, 201
  cerebral infection by, 712
Small intestine, disorders of, 494–510. See also *Intestine, small*.
Smog, 218
Smoking, 219–220, *220*, 220(t)
  and atherosclerosis, 280
  and emphysema, 394
  and lung cancer, 428
Smooth endoplasmic reticulum of liver, barbiturate-induced hypertrophy of, 16, *16*
  carbon tetrachloride–induced swelling of, 9, *10*
Smooth muscle tumors, 702
Sodium homeostasis, in blood pressure regulation, 460–461
Sodium retention, and edema, 61, 62, 63
Soft chancre, 604–605
Soft tissue tumors, 700(t), 700–703
Solar keratosis, 211
Somatotroph adenoma, *645*, 645–646
Sorbitol, 574
Southern blot analysis, in diagnosis of sickle cell disease, 112, *112*
Spherocytosis, hereditary, 335–336
Sphingolipidoses, 95(t)
Sphingomyelin deposition, 95, *96*
Sphingomyelinase, deficiency of, 96
Spider angioma, 528
Spider cells, 331
Spider telangiectasia, 300, 528
Spleen, amyloid deposition in, 169
  congestive enlargement of, 306
  disorders affecting, 383
  enlargement of. See *Splenomegaly*.
  Gaucher cells in, 95, *96*
  infarction of, *76*
  lardaceous, 169
  Niemann-Pick disease involving, *96*
  sago, 169
  sarcoidosis involving, 404
  sphingomyelin deposition in, *96*
  systemic lupus erythematosus involving, 144–145
Splenomegaly, 383
  congestive, 306
  in amyloidosis, 169
  in Gaucher's disease, 96
  in hairy cell leukemia, 370
  in hereditary spherocytosis, 336
  in infectious mononucleosis, 352
  in leukemia, 370–371
  in myeloid metaplasia, 373

Splenomegaly *(Continued)*
  in portal hypertension, 545
  in sickle cell anemia, 337
Spondylitis, ankylosing, 149(t)
  HLA-B27 and, 122, 139
  inflammatory bowel disease and, 149(t)
Spondyloarthropathies, 149, 149(t)
Spongiform encephalopathy, 712–713
Sporadic goiter, 653
Sprue, celiac, 508–509
  postinfectious (tropical), 509
Squamous cell carcinoma, 173, 210
  of bladder, 470
  of cervix, 614
  of esophagus, 482, 483
  of larynx, 435, *435*
  of lung, 429, *430*
  of oral cavity, 475–476, *476*
  of penis, 589
  of skin, 210–211, *211*
  of vulva, 610
Squamous hyperplasia, of vulva, 608
Stable cells, 48
Staging, of cancer, 208. See also specific cancer types.
Staphylococcus aureus infection, and pneumonia, 414
Stasis, in blood flow, and thrombogenesis, 69
  in inflammation, 26
Stasis thrombi (coagulative thrombi, red thrombi), 70
Status asthmaticus, 391
Steatosis, macrovesicular, in alcoholic liver disease, 546
Stein-Leventhal syndrome, 621–622
Stenosis, aortic, *23*, 318–319, *319*
  esophageal, 479
  pulmonary, 318
  pyloric, 484
  small intestinal, 494
Stiff lung syndrome, in systemic sclerosis, 153
Still's disease, 149
Stomach, 484–493
  carcinoma of, 490–493, 491(t), *492*
    advanced, 491(t), *492*
    diffuse type of, 491, 491(t), *492*
    early, 492
    intestinal type of, 491, 491(t), *492*
    ulcerative, *492*, *492*
      vs. peptic ulcer, *493*
  in pernicious anemia, 348, 486
  inflammation of, 484(t), 484–486. See also *Gastritis*.
  lymphoma of, 493
  peptic ulcer of, 487–490, *489*
    vs. gastric carcinoma, *493*
  polyps of, 490, 491(t)
  pylorus of, stenosis of, 484
  tumors of, 490–493
  ulcers of, 486–490
    benign vs. malignant, *493*
    peptic, 487–490, *489*
      vs. gastric carcinoma, *493*
    stress, *486*, 486–487
Stomatitis, aphthous, 474
  herpetic, 474
Storage diseases, 17
  glycogen, 18, 93–94, *94*, 94(t)
  lysosomal, 16, 94–97, *95*, 95(t)
Streptococcal infection, and glomerulonephritis, 449
  and pneumonia, 412–413
  and rheumatic fever, 320
Streptococcus pneumoniae infection, 412–413
Stress ulcers, *486*, 486–487
Stroke, 714
Stroma, supporting, of tumors, 172
Struma lymphomatosa (Hashimoto's thyroiditis), 655–656, *656*
Struma ovarii, 626
Sturge-Weber syndrome, 675(t)

Subacute sclerosing panencephalitis, 712
Subacute spongiform encephalopathy (Creutzfeldt-Jakob disease), 712–713
Subacute thyroiditis, 657
Subarachnoid hemorrhage, 717–718
Subcellular responses, to injury, 15–17
Subcutaneous edema, 63, 64
Subcutaneous hematoma, 64
Subcutaneous nodule(s), rheumatoid, 146–147
Subdural hematoma, 718–719, *720*
Subendocardial infarct, 309–310, 312
Subfalcine (cingulate) herniation, 707, *707*
Subluxation, of lens, in Marfan's syndrome, 86
Subperiosteal abscess, 685
Sudden cardiac death, 313–314
Sudden infant death syndrome (SIDS), 388(t), 388–389
Sun exposure, and cancer, 201
Superficial spreading melanoma, 213–214
Superficial venous thrombosis, 72
Superior vena caval syndrome, 299
Superoxide. See also *Oxygen-derived free radical(s).*
    and cell injury, 8, *8*, 9
Suppressor T cell(s), in self-tolerance, 137, 138
Suppurative arthritis, 696
Suppurative inflammation (purulent inflammation), 44, 272
Surfactant, 387
Swelling, of cells, 12, *12*
    of endoplasmic reticulum of liver, carbon tetrachloride–induced, 9, *10*
    of renal tubular epithelial cells, *12*
Swiss-type agammaglobulinemia, 155–156
Syncytial meningioma, 725
Syncytiotrophoblast, 630, 631
Syndecan, 56
Synovial sarcoma, 700(t), 702
Syphilis, 42(t), 602–604
    aortitis and aortic aneurysm in, *295*, 295–296
    chancre in, *272*, 603
Systemic immune complex–mediated hypersensitivity, 128, 128–129, *129*, *130*
Systemic lupus erythematosus, 139–145
    antinuclear antibodies in, 141(t)
    cardiac involvement in, 142–143, *143*, 325
    clinical manifestations of, 145
    diagnostic criteria for, 140(t)
    distribution of lesions in, 142(t)
    endocarditis in, 142–143, *143*, 325
    etiology of, 139–141
    genetic factors in, 140
    glomerulonephritis in, 143–144, *144*, *145*
    immunologic factors in, 141
    joint involvement in, 144
    nephritis in, 143, *144*, *145*
    nongenetic factors in, 140–141
    pathogenesis of, 139–141
    pericarditis in, 142
    renal involvement in, 143–144, *144*, *145*
    serositis in, 142
    skin lesions in, 142, *143*
    splenic onion-skin lesions in, 145
    tissue injury in, 141
    valvular vegetations in, 142–143, *143*, 325
    vasculitis in, 142, *142*
Systemic sclerosis, 150–153
    antinuclear antibodies in, 141(t), 151
    cardiac lesions in, 152
    clinical course of, 152–153
    esophageal involvement in, 152
    etiology of, 151, *151*
    fibrosis in, 151
    gastrointestinal lesions in, 152
    immunologic abnormalities in, 151
    joint lesions in, 152
    muscular lesions in, 152
    pathogenesis of, 151, *151*

Systemic sclerosis *(Continued)*
    pulmonary lesions in, 152, 153
    Raynaud's phenomenon in, 153
    renal lesions in, 152
    skin lesions in, 152, *152*
    stiff lung syndrome in, 153
    vascular injury in, 151

T
T cell(s), 117–118
    as antitumor effector mechanism, 204
    differentiation of, *355*
    in AIDS, 158–159, *160*, 161, 162, *162*, 162(t), 163
    in antigen recognition, 121, *121*, 122
        and transplant rejection, 132, *133*
    in cell-mediated hypersensitivity, 131–132
    in HIV infection, 158–159, *160*, 161, 162, *162*, 162(t), 163
    in host defenses against cancer, 204
    in HTLV-1 infection, 201
    in rheumatoid arthritis, 147
    in self-tolerance, 137, 138
    in transplant rejection, 132, *133*
    in type IV hypersensitivity, 131–132
T cell–mediated cytotoxicity. See also *Cytotoxic T cell(s).*
    in type IV hypersensitivity, 131–132
T cell–mediated rejection, 132, *133*
T-cell leukemia/lymphoma, 360
    HTLV-1 in, 201, *202*
T-cell lymphoma, cutaneous, 360
T-cell receptor, 117–118, *118*
T-cell tolerance, 137
    helper, 137
        bypass of, 138, *138*
Takayasu's arteritis (pulseless disease), 291–292
Tangles, neurofibrillary, in Alzheimer's disease, 17, 726
Tay-Sachs disease, 97, *97*
Telangiectasia, hereditary hemorrhagic, 300
    spider, 300, 528
Temporal arteritis (cranial arteritis, giant cell arteritis), 286(t), 290–291, *291*
Tensile strength, of wounds, 57
Teratoma, 173, 174(t)
    ovarian, *625*, 625–626
    testicular, 594, *594*, 595(t)
Testis (testes), 591–596
    atrophy of, in cryptorchidism, 591
        in Klinefelter's syndrome, 109, 591, *591*
    cancer of, 591–595
    choriocarcinoma of, 593–594, 595(t)
    embryonal carcinoma of, 592–593, *594*, 595(t)
    germ cell tumors of, 591–595, 592(t), *592–594*, 595(t)
    inflammation of, 595–596
    mixed tumors of, 594, 595(t)
    seminoma of, 592, *593*, 595(t)
    teratoma of, 594, *594*, 595(t)
    torsion of, 590
    tumors of, 591–595, 592(t), *592–594*, 595(t)
    undescended, 591
    yolk sac tumor of, 593, 595(t)
Tetrahydrocannabinol, 235
Tetralogy of Fallot, *317*, 317–318
Thalassemia, 338–339, *340*, 340(t), 341
    point mutations in β-globin gene and, 339, *339*
Thecoma, 626
Therapeutic agents, injury by, 227–229, 228(t)
Thermal injury, 237–238
    vascular leakage in, 28
Thiamine (vitamin B₁), 245(t), 252
    deficiency of, 245(t), 252–253, *253*, 731
Thrombin, pro- and anticoagulant roles of, 66
Thromboangiitis obliterans (Buerger's disease), 286(t), 293
Thrombocytopenia, 380–381
    with immunodeficiency and eczema, 156

Thrombocytopenic purpura, idiopathic, 380–381
  thrombotic, 381
Thromboembolism, 65, 73
  pulmonary, 406–408, *407, 408*
Thrombogenesis, 69–70. See also *Thrombosis; Thrombus (thrombi).*
  antiphospholipid antibodies and, 70
  endothelial cell injury and, 69, *69*
  hypercoagulability and, 69–70
  stasis and, 69
  turbulence and, 69
Thrombomodulin, 66
Thrombophlebitis, 72, 299
  migratory, in cancer, 72, 299
Thrombosis, 65–73. See also *Thrombogenesis; Thrombus (thrombi).*
  arterial, 70, 71
    embolization of, 71, 74
    florid atherosclerosis and, 73
    myocardial infarction and, 73
    obstruction by, 72, 73
    rheumatic heart disease and, 73
  clinical aspects of, 72–73
  coronary, *308,* 309
  hepatic vein, 530
  mesenteric, 497
  microcirculatory, 73, 378
  pathogenesis of, 65–70
  portal vein, 530
  venous, 70, 71, 299
    cancer and, 72, 299
    contraceptive use and, 72–73
    deep, 72
    embolization of, 71, 72, 74
    lower extremities as site of, 70, 72
    postoperative, 72
    pregnancy and, 72
    superficial, 72
    vs. postmortem clot, 70
Thrombotic endocarditis, nonbacterial, 71, 324
Thrombotic thrombocytopenic purpura, 381
Thromboxane, effects of, 36
  vs. effects of prostacyclin, 67
  in inflammation, 36, *37*
Thrombus (thrombi), 65. See also *Thrombogenesis; Thrombosis.*
  aortic, *70*
  arterial, 70–74
  cardiac, 70, 71
  cardiac valve, 71
  cerebral, 714
  coagulative (red, stasis), 70
  left ventricular, myocardial infarction and, 73, *73*
  microcirculatory, 73, 378
  morphology of, 70–72
  mural, 70, *70*
  occlusive, 70
  organization of, 71
  recanalization of, *71,* 71–72
  red (coagulative, stasis), 70
  stasis (coagulative, red), 70
  venous, 70–74, 299
Thrush, 423, 474
Thymoma, 678–679
Thymus, 678–679
  hyperplasia of, 678
  hypoplasia of, 155
  in myasthenia gravis, 698
  in self-tolerance, 137
  tumors of, 678–679
Thyroid gland, 649–663
  adenoma of, *658,* 658–659
  autoantibodies against, 651, 655
  carcinoma of, 659(t), 659–663
    anaplastic, 661
    follicular, 661, *661*
    medullary, *662,* 662–663
    papillary, *660,* 660–661

Thyroid gland *(Continued)*
  enlargement of (goiter), 653–655
  excess hormone release by (hyperthyroidism), 650
  Graves' disease of, 650–652, *651*
  hyperplasia of, in Graves' disease, *652*
  inadequate hormone production by (hypothyroidism), 649
  inflammation of, 655–657
  metastasis of cancer to, 663
  nodules of, 657
  tumors of, 657–663
Thyroiditis, 655–657
  chronic (silent), 657
  Hashimoto's, 655–656, *656*
  Riedel's, 655
  subacute (DeQuervain's, granulomatous), 657
Thyrotoxicosis, 650
Tissue thromboplastic substances, 378
Tobacco smoking, 219–220, *220,* 220(t)
  and atherosclerosis, 280
  and emphysema, 394
  and lung cancer, 428
Tolerance, B-cell, 137
  self, 136–137, *137*
    loss of, 138, *138*
  T-cell, 137
    helper, 137
      bypass of, 138, *138*
Tongue, atrophic, in pernicious anemia, 348
  in riboflavin deficiency, 254, *254*
  cancer of, 475–476
Tonsillar herniation, 707, *707*
Tophi, in gout, 99, 102, *102,* 103
Torsion, of testis, 590
Total body irradiation, 241, 242(t)
Toxic goiter, 653–655
Toxic oxygen radicals. See *Oxygen-derived free radical(s).*
Toxic shock syndrome, 611, 611(t)
Trace elements, 256, 257(t)
  deficiency of, 256–257, 257(t)
Transforming growth factor alpha, 51
  in wound healing, 56(t)
Transforming growth factor beta, 51
  in inhibition of cell growth, 51
  in wound healing, 56(t)
Transfusion reaction, complement-mediated cytotoxicity in, 126
Transgenic mice, 84
Transient ischemic attacks, 714
Translocation. See *Chromosome(s), translocation of.*
Transmural infarct, of intestine, 497, *497,* 498
  of myocardium, 308–312
Transplantation, bone marrow, 135
  graft-versus-host disease following, 135
  kidney, graft rejection in, 132–134, *134*
    prevention of, 135
  liver, 135
  rejection in, 132–134, *134*
    HLA antigens and, 121, 132, *133,* 135
    prevention of, 135
    T cell–mediated, 132, *133*
    vasculitis associated with, 134, *134*
Transplantation antigens, tumor-specific, *203,* 203–204
Transtentorial (uncal, uncinate) herniation, 707, *707*
Transthyretin, 166
Transudation, 27
Traumatic fat necrosis, of breast, 635
Traveler's diarrhea, 499, 504(t)
Treponema pallidum infection, 42(t), 602–604
  aortitis and aortic aneurysm in, *295,* 295–296
  chancre in, *272,* 603
Trichinosis, 264, *265,* 699, 699–700
Trisomy (trisomies), 104, 107, *108*
Trisomy 21 (Down's syndrome), 107
Trophoblastic disease, gestational, 628–631
Tropical sprue (postinfectious sprue), 509
Trousseau's sign, 72, 299

Trypanosomiasis (Chagas' disease), 326, 327, 479
Tubal pregnancy, 628, *629*
Tuberculin test, 130, *130*, 131, 417
Tuberculosis, 42(t), 416–422, *418*
  arthritis and, 686
  bone involvement in, 686
  chronic adrenocortical insufficiency in, 672
  intestinal, 421
  laryngitis in, 434
  meningeal, 709
  miliary, 420, 421
  primary, 418–419, *419*
  pulmonary, 418, *419*, 420, *420*, *421*
  secondary (reactivation), 419–422, *420*
  testicular, 595
Tubular adenoma, of colon, *510*, 512, *512*
Tubular necrosis, acute, 457–458, *458*
Tubule(s), renal, diseases of, 453–459
    lesions of, in diabetes mellitus, 578
    swelling of epithelial cells of, *12*
  seminiferous, alterations in, in Klinefelter's syndrome, 109–110, *591*
Tubulointerstitial nephritis, 453–457
Tumor(s), 171–214. See also *Cancer* and specific types, e.g., *Carcinoma.*
  AIDS-associated, 164
  angiogenesis of, 194
  benign, 172, 174–179
    clinical features of, 206
    definition of, 172
    differentiation of, 175, 176, 180(t)
    effects of, on host, 206
    encapsulation of, 177, 178, *178*
    epithelial, 174(t)
    hormone-secreting, 206
    malignant change in, 184
    mesenchymal, 174(t)
    nomenclature applied to, 172, 174(t)
    vs. cancer, 174–179, 180(t)
  clonality of, assessment of, 184, *184*
  definition of, 172
  desmoid, 58, 703
  diagnosis of, recombinant DNA technology in, 114–115
  differentiation of, 175–177, 180(t)
  epithelial, benign, 174(t)
    malignant. See *Carcinoma.*
  hormone-secreting, 206
  malignant. See *Cancer* and specfic types, e.g., *Carcinoma.*
  mesenchymal, benign, 174(t)
    malignant. See *Sarcoma.*
  mixed, 173, 174(t)
  monoclonality of, assessment of, 184, *184*
  nomenclature applied to, 172–174, 174(t)
  parenchyma of, 172
    differentiation of, 175
  rate of growth of, 177, 180(t)
  supporting stroma of, 172
  teratogenous, 173, 174(t)
Tumor angiogenesis factor, 194
Tumor-associated antigens, 204
Tumor markers, 210
Tumor necrosis factor, in inflammation, 38, *38*
  in wound healing, 56(t)
Tumor necrosis factor alpha, in delayed hypersensitivity, 131
  in endotoxic shock, 78
Tumor-specific antigens, 203
Tumor-specific transplantation antigens, *203*, 203–204
Turcot's syndrome, 514(t)
Turner's syndrome, *110*, 110–111
Type I hypersensitivity (anaphylactic type hypersensitivity), 122–126, 123(t), *124*
  clinical manifestations of, 125–126
  mast cells in, 123, *124*, 125, 125(t)
  mediators of, 125(t)
    primary, 123, *124*, 125
    secondary, *124*, 125

Type II hypersensitivity (antibody-dependent hypersensitivity), 123(t), 126–127, *127*
Type III hypersensitivity (immune complex–mediated hypersensitivity), 123(t), 127–130, *128*, *129*
  local (Arthus reaction), 129–130
  systemic, *128*, 128–129, *129*, *130*
Type IV hypersensitivity (cell-mediated hypersensitivity), 123(t), 130–132
  delayed, 123(t), *130*, 130–131
  granuloma formation in, 130–131, *131*
  T cell–mediated cytotoxicity in, 131–132
Typhoid fever, 505
Typhus fever, 263
Tyrosinase, deficiency of, 93
Tyrosine kinase, activation of, 48, *49*
  in cell growth, 49

U
Ulcer(s), 44–45
  aphthous, 474
  Cushing's, 486
  duodenal, peptic, *45*, 487, 488, 489
  gastric, 486–490
    benign vs. malignant, *493*
    peptic, 487–490, *489*
      vs. gastric carcinoma, *493*
    stress, *486*, 486–487
  oral, 474
  peptic, *45*, 487(t), 487–490, *488*, 488(t), *489*
    complications of, 490(t)
    duodenal, *45*, 487, 488, 489
    gastric, 487–490, *489*
      vs. gastric carcinoma, *493*
    stress, *486*, 486–487
Ulcerative colitis, 501–503, *502*
  vs. Crohn's disease, 501, 502(t), *503*
Uncinate (uncal, transtentorial) herniation, 707, *707*
Unconjugated hyperbilirubinemia, 525, 525(t), 527(t)
Unconventional agent encephalopathy, 712–713
Undescended testis, 591
Upper respiratory tract, lesions of, 434–436
Urate nephropathy, 103
Uremia, 438
Urethritis, gonococcal, 601
  nongonococcal, 602
  postgonococcal, 602
Uric acid, elevated serum levels of, 99
Uric acid crystal deposition, in kidney, 103
Uric acid stones, 103, 466
Urinary bladder, carcinoma of, 469–470, *470*
  infection/inflammation of (cystitis), 455
  papilloma of, 469
  stones in, 466
  tumors of, *469*, 469–470
Urinary collecting system, tumors of, 469–470
Urinary outflow obstruction, 465–467
Urinary tract infection, 438, *453*, 453–456
Urokinase-like plasminogen activator, 68–69
Urolithiasis, 465–466, 466(t)
Uterine cervix, 611–615
  carcinoma in situ of, *179*, 613, *614*
  carcinoma of, 612–615, *613–615*
    Papanicolaou smear in, *209*
  condyloma of, 613
  dysplasia of, *176*, 613–614
  infections of, 602, 612
  inflammation of, 611–612
  polyps of, 612
  tumors of, 612–615
Uterus, body of, 615–620. See also *Uterine cervix.*
  adenomyosis of, 615–616
  bleeding from, dysfunctional, 616–617
  carcinoma of, 619–620, *620*
  endometrial hyperplasia of, 22, 617–618, *618*
  endometrial tumors of, 618–620

Uterus, body of *(Continued)*
    endometriosis of, 616, *616, 617*
    endometritis of, 615
    hypertrophy of, 21
    leiomyoma of, 177, 618, *619*
    leiomyosarcoma of, 619
    myometrial tumors of, 618–619
    polyps of, 618
    tumors of, 618–620

V
Vacuolar degeneration, 12
Vacuolar myelopathy, in AIDS, 711–712
Vagina, 610–611
    candidiasis of, 423
    congenital anomalies of, 610
    inflammation of, 610–611, 611(t)
    sarcoma botryoides of, 611, 702
    tumors of, 611
Vaginitis, 610–611, 611(t)
Valvular heart disease, 318–325, 319(t). See also *Heart, valve(s) of.*
Varicella-zoster virus, 710
Varices, esophageal, 298, 480–481, *481*, 545
Varicose veins, 298
Vascular diseases, 277–304. See also *Artery (arteries)*; *Vein(s).*
    cerebral, 713–718
    diabetes mellitus and, 575–576
    hepatic, 529–530
    intestinal, 497–499
    pulmonary, 406–409
    renal, 459–464
Vascular tumors, 300–304
Vascularization (angiogenesis), 52, *53*
    in tumor growth, 194–195
Vasculitis, 286(t), 286–293
    acute rejection of kidney and, 134, *134*
    immune complex, 129, *130*, 286
    polymyositis-dermatomyositis and, 153
    systemic lupus erythematosus and, 142, *142*
Vaso-occlusive crisis, in sickle cell anemia, 338
Vasoactive amines, in inflammation, 34
Vasodepressor substances, renal, 461
Vasodilatation, in inflammation, 26
Vasogenic edema, of brain, 707
Vegetation(s), on heart valves, 71
    in infective endocarditis, 323–324, *324*
    in nonbacterial thrombotic endocarditis, 324
    in rheumatic heart disease, *321*, 322
    in systemic lupus erythematosus, 142–143, *143*, 325
Vehicular accidents, 236
Vein(s), blood flow in, stasis in, 69
    carcinoma invading, 180
    disorders of, 298–299
    emboli in, 74
    thrombi in. See *Venous thrombosis.*
Vena cava, inferior, obstruction of, 299
    superior, obstruction of, 299
Venereal diseases (sexually transmitted diseases), 599–606, 600(t).
    See also specific diseases.
Veno-occlusive disease, of liver, 530
Venous blood flow, stasis in, 69
Venous disorders, 298–299
Venous embolism, 74
Venous thrombosis, 70, 71, 299
    cancer and, 72, 299
    contraceptive use and, 72–73
    deep, 72
    embolization of, 71, 72, 74
    lower extremities as site of, 70, 72
    postoperative, 72
    pregnancy and, 72
    superficial, 72
    vs. postmortem clot, 70
Ventricular septal defect, 316

Verocay bodies, 734
Very low density lipoproteins, 87, 279(t)
Vesicoureteral reflux, 454
    chronic pyelonephritis associated with, *455*, 455–456
Vibrio cholerae infection, 504, *505*
Villous adenoma, of colon, *510*, 512–513, *513*
Viral encephalitis, *710*, 710–712, *711*
Viral hepatitis, 530–541, 531(t). See also *Hepatitis.*
Viral infection(s), 262, 262(t). See also specific diseases and organs.
    AIDS and, 164(t)
    cell injury in, 268–270, *269*
    diarrhea due to, 504(t)
    gastrointestinal, 266
Viral meningitis, 709
Viral myocarditis, 326, *327*
Viral pneumonia, *415*
Virilism, adrenal, 669
Virus(es), oncogenic, 201–203
Vitamin(s), 245(t)
    deficiency of, 244–256, 245(t)
Vitamin A, *245*, 245–246
    deficiency of, 245(t), 246, *247*
    toxicity of, 247
Vitamin B_1 (thiamine), 245(t), 252
    deficiency of, 245(t), 252–253, *253*, 731
Vitamin B_2 (riboflavin), 245(t), 253
    deficiency of, 245(t), 253–254, *254*
Vitamin B_6 (pyridoxine), 245(t)
    deficiency of, 245(t), 255
Vitamin B_{12} (cobalamin), 245(t)
    deficiency of, 245(t), 347–348, 731
Vitamin C (ascorbic acid), 245(t)
    deficiency of, 245(t), 255–256, *256*
Vitamin D, 245(t), 247, 248
    deficiency of, 245(t), 248, *249, 250*, 250(t), 250–251
    metabolism of, 247–248, *249*
Vitamin E, 245(t), 251
    deficiency of, 245(t), 251
Vitamin K, 245(t), 252, *252*
    deficiency of, 245(t), 252
Vocal cord nodules, 435
Volvulus, 519
von Gierke's disease, 93–94, 94(t)
von Hippel–Lindau disease, 675(t)
von Recklinghausen's disease, 88, 675(t)
    of bone, 684
von Willebrand's disease, 67, 382
von Willebrand's factor, 67, 381
Vulva, 608–610
    carcinoma of, 610
    condyloma of, 609
    cysts of, 609
    dystrophy of, 608
    inflammation of, 608
    intraepithelial neoplasia of, 610
    leukoplakia of, 608
    lichen sclerosus of, 608, *608*
    non-neoplastic epithelial disorders of, 608
    Paget's disease of, 609, *610*
    squamous hyperplasia of, 608
    tumors of, 609–610
Vulvitis, 608

W
Waldenstrom's macroglobulinemia, 374, 375, 376
Wallerian degeneration, 732
Warm antibody immunohemolytic anemia, 342
Warthin's tumor (papillary cystadenoma lymphomatosum), 477–478
Waterhouse-Friderichsen syndrome, 673, *673*
Watershed infarct, 713
Water-soluble vitamins, 245(t)
    deficiency of, 245(t), 252–256
Web(s), esophageal, 479
Wegener's granulomatosis, 286(t), 289, *290*

Wermer's syndrome, 679(t), 679–680
Wernicke's encephalopathy, thiamine deficiency and, 253, 751
Whipple's disease, 509, *509*
White blood cell(s), disorders of, 350–377. See also *Leukocyte(s).*
White infarct (anemic infarct), 76
Wilms' tumor, 469
Wilson's disease, 557
Wiskott-Aldrich syndrome, 156
Wound(s). See also *Wound healing* and *Repair.*
  contraction of, 54
  gunshot, 236
  healing of. See *Wound healing* and see also *Repair.*
  incised, 236
  penetrating, 236
  perforating, 236
  puncture, 236
Wound healing, 53–58, *54.* See also *Repair.*
  adhesive glycoproteins in, 55
  by first intention, 53, *54*
  by second intention, 53–54, *54*
  cell-matrix interactions in, 56–56, *57*
  collagenases in, 56–57
  collagens in, 55
    degradation of, 56–57
    synthesis of, 53, 56
  extracellular matrix in, 56–56, *57*
  fibronectin in, 55–56
  growth factors in, 56(t)
  laminin in, 56
  mechanisms of, 55–58
  metalloproteinases in, 56–57
  modifying factors in, 58
  primary vs. secondary, 53–54

Wound healing *(Continued)*
  proteoglycans in, 56
  tensile strength achieved in, 57

X
X chromatin (sex chromatin), 107
X chromosome, 107
  fragile, 111, *111*
45,X karyotype, 110
Xanthoma, in diabetes mellitus, 579
  in familial hypercholesterolemia, 87
Xeroderma pigmentosum, 183, 201
Xerophthalmia, 245(t), 246
Xerostomia, in Sjogren's syndrome, 149, 150
X-linked agammaglobulinemia, 154–155
X-linked diseases, 85(t), 98
47,XXY karyotype, 109
XYY karyotype, 110

Y
Y body, 109
Y chromosome, 109
Yersinia enterocolitica infection, 507
Yolk sac tumor, of testis, 593, 595(t)

Z
Zenker's diverticulum, 479
Zinc deficiency, 256–257
Zollinger-Ellison syndrome, 580–581

Portions of this book, including text and illustrations, have appeared previously in *Robbins Pathologic Basis of Disease,* fourth edition, by Ramzi S. Cotran, Vinay Kumar, and Stanley L. Robbins, published by W.B. Saunders Company in 1989. The following figures and tables appeared in *Robbins Pathologic Basis of Disease:*
Figures:
1–1, 1–2, 1–3, 1–4, 1–5 (modified), 1–17, 1–18, 1–20, 2–8, 2–10, 2–11, 2–14, 2–18, 2–19, 2–21, 4–3, 4–12, 5–1, 5–7, 5–8, 5–9, 5–10, 5–12, 5–21, 5–27, 6–2, 6–3, 6–7, 6–9, 6–11, 6–18, 6–22, 6–27, 6–28, 7–5, 7–8, 7–9, 7–15, 7–16, 7–21, 7–25, 7–26, 7–35, 8–1, 8–3, 8–4, 8–5, 8–7, 8–14, 8–15, 8–20, 8–21, 8–22, 8–23, 8–24, 8–25, 8–26, 8–29, 9–1, 9–2, 9–3, 9–4, 9–5, 9–7, 9–10, 9–11, 9–12, 9–13, 10–10, 10–17, 11–2, 11–8, 12–3, 12–4, 12–6, 12–7, 12–8, 12–9, 12–13, 12–14, 12–15, 12–17, 12–22, 12–23, 12–26, 13–3, 13–5, 13–7, 13–9, 13–11, 13–14, 13–16, 13–17, 13–19, 13–26, 13–28, 13–32, 14–6, 14–8, 14–9, 14–13, 14–16, 14–20, 15–1, 15–3, 15–7, 15–19, 15–26, 18–1, 19–1, 19–7, 19–8, 19–16, 19–19, 19–20, 19–21, 19–26, 19–30, 19–32
Tables:
2–4, 5–2, 5–3, 5–4, 6–2, 6–3, 6–4, 6–9, 6–11, 6–12, 7–2, 9–2, 12–1, 12–3, 12–4, 12–10, 12–14, 13–1, 19–2, 19–3, 22–2